CLINICAL INTEGRATION

Population Health and Accountable Care

Third Edition

EDITORS

Ken Yale | Thomas A. Raskauskas
Joanne Bohn | Colin Konschak

FOREWORD BY
David B. Nash

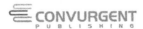
CONVURGENT
PUBLISHING

ISBN-13:   9780991234547
ISBN-10:   0991234545

Convurgent Publishing, LLC
4445 Corporation Lane, Suite #227
Virginia Beach, VA 23462
Phone: (877) 254-9794, Fax: (757) 213-6801
Web Site: www.convurgent.com
E-mail: info@convurgent.com

Special Orders.

Bulk Quantity Sales.
Special discounts are available on quantity purchases. Please contact sales@convurgent.com.

Library of Congress Control Number: 2014956283

Bibliographic data:

Clinical Integration. Population Health and Accountable Care, Third Edition / Ken Yale, Thomas A. Raskauskas, Joanne Bohn, Colin Konschak

p. cm.

1. Clinical integration. 2. Clinically integrated networks. 3. Healthcare reform. 4. Health information technology. 5. Clinical quality. 6. Care coordination. 7. Behavioral health. 8. Population health. 9. Operational standards.

ISBN: 9780991234547

Credits
Corresponding Editor: Joanne Bohn (jb@km4i.com)

THE EDITORIAL TEAM

Ken Yale, DDS, JD, is Vice President of Clinical Solutions at ActiveHealth Management, a research-based, advanced clinical decision support and care management company. Previously he founded and built innovative health companies in medical management, health data analytics, and patient engagement. Before building businesses, he held senior government posts in the White House, United States Senate, and as a commissioned officer in the U.S. Public Health Service. He currently holds a teaching appointment in predictive analytics in healthcare with the University of California.

Thomas A. Raskauskas, MD, is CEO of President of St. Vincent's Health Partners, Inc. (SVHP), a physician hospital organization in southwestern Connecticut. He graduated from Georgetown University School of Medicine in Washington, D.C. in 1985, and is a Board Certified Obstetrician Gynecologist. He started his career in private practice in Salem, Massachusetts, and has held teaching appointments through the Medical Schools at Harvard University, Brown University, Michigan State University and Quinnipiac University. Dr. Raskauskas has been a medical director overseeing a multispecialty multi-site clinic, and a Chief Medical Officer for a multi-state Medicaid managed care plan in the Midwest. He served in the United States Navy as a Medical Officer.

Joanne Bohn, MBA, is a published author, book designer, and corresponding editor on contemporary healthcare topics, and principal for KMI Communications, LLC. Bohn is a PhD candidate in Public Health Sciences with a specialization in Health Management at the University of Louisville School of Public Health and Information Sciences.

Colin Konschak, MBA, FACHE, FHIMSS, is the managing partner and CEO of the Virginia Beach, Va.-based management consulting firm, Divurgent. Divurgent provides services related to Clinical and Revenue Cycle Transformation, as well as Strategic Planning services to providers, payers, and healthcare focused vendors.

ACKNOWLEDGEMENTS

We want to thank our families, co-workers, and leadership at our respective organizations, for all their support and understanding as we developed the third edition, and previous editions, of this book.

In particular, Dr. Ken Yale wishes to extend special thanks to his family, especially his wife, Minna Yale, and children. Without their support, patience, and putting up with him, this laborious effort never would have been attempted. In addition, Dr. Yale is grateful for industry mentors, colleagues and friends, especially at ActiveHealth Management, NeoCare, Healthagen, and Aetna, whose humor and dedication have been a constant source of inspiration.

Joanne Bohn would like to thank mentors and faculty at the University of Louisville for their help in expanding a foundation of theoretical knowledge of health systems, public health and sociology topics over the past two years which contributed to the content development of this book.

To the hardworking staff of St. Vincent's Health Partner's Inc, their efforts in becoming the nation's first URAC accredited clinically integrated network is greatly appreciated along with their contributions to the development of this book.

And, without the original vision and insight of Dr. Bruce Flareau, who started us down this path in the first and second edition, this third edition would not have been possible. We are grateful for his original contributions that helped initiate and enable our efforts in the design and compilation of this latest collaborative work.

Finally, we wish to thank all the authors of the individual chapters for their knowledge, insight, content, and patience. We have worked with all of them, some for years, yet the endeavor of a book with multiple revisions can wear thin even the best of friendships. To the authors we owe a huge debt of gratitude, for without them this book would not be the excellent work it has become. All brilliance is theirs as authors, and all mistakes ours as editors.

Again, thank you!

PREFACE

Third Edition

Clinical Integration. Population Health and Accountable Care, Third Edition provides a fresh set of insights and new information on the evolution of Clinically Integrated Networks (CINs), Accountable Care Organizations (ACOs), Patient-Centered Medical Homes (PCMHs) and other new models of provider collaboration across the United States (U.S.) healthcare system. Since the second edition was released in November 2011, the industry has seen significant growth in the formation of these new clinical and business models as large integrated delivery networks such as Banner Health Systems, Vanderbilt University Medical Center (VUMC), St. Vincent's Health Partners, BayCare Physician Partners, Emory Clinically Integrated Network, the University of California, Los Angeles Health System, and many others have made transformational efforts to establish new, sustainable models of care finance and delivery.

The second edition noted that these organizations "are legitimate collaborations of otherwise competing providers (hospitals and/or physicians) organized in a way that improves efficiencies in care delivery (including quality improvement and cost reduction)." These innovative models are rapidly growing as disruptive innovations in the market for care delivery. The need to focus on population health and care management is at the forefront of priorities for C-suite executives, including chief executive officers (CEO), chief financial officers (CFO), chief technology officers (CTO), chief data officers (CDO), chief information officers (CIO), chief medical information officers (CMIO), chief medical officers (CMOs), and others. This book draws on the expertise of these C-suite executives implementing these new models in the field, and is written especially for a leadership audience interested in their experiences.

These provider-based organizations and their leaders recognize the need for a renewed emphasis on care coordination, integrated health information technology, consumer and patient engagement, risk and financial management, and provider network development. To meet these new challenges, leaders are establishing a culture of collaboration focused on continuously improving quality, while enhancing clinical and operational efficiency and effectiveness to improve affordability. Leaders of these new provider models are dealing with accelerated change fomented by health reform that is helping implement new ways healthcare services will be financed and delivered.

The transformation of the U.S. healthcare system is underway, and is driven by the needs of payers, patients, and providers for new and improved population health management services, and evolving to better serve individual consumers as new technologies such as predictive analytics enable a retail approach. Paradoxically, this new retail, individual consumer approach encourages distributed technologies and social media that can enable improvements in health and care for the population as a whole.

Structure of This Book

The third edition transitions from the second edition collaborative work of its four original authors to a 14-chapter anthology, each chapter authored by industry experts and edited by the second edition authors. This new edition provides a refresh on the issues covered in the second edition, along with introducing a number of new topics. Patient engagement, care coordination, behavioral health, and industry standards are new areas of importance for provider-sponsored organizations that are discussed for the first time in this edition.

In addition, new laws and regulations that impact the evolution of PCMH, ACO, and CIN are also covered. These include new requirements for Meaningful Use of Electronic Health Records (EHRs), Medicare Shared Savings Program-Accountable Care Organization (MSSP), the Patient Protection and Affordable Care Act's insurance mandate, and the most recent final rules of the Health Insurance Portability and Accountability Act (HIPAA), among other regulatory matters promulgated since the last edition of this book was released. Each chapter concludes with chapter highlights along with a set of study questions to stimulate critical thinking about the material covered.

Audience for This Book

The audience for this collaborative anthology is multi-faceted. The content covered is expanded to meet the needs of several industry stakeholders including:

- *Physician Leaders and Practitioners* - Hospitals, health systems, and physician practices continue to look for insights into best practices and lessons learned in advancing the development of their organizations.

- *Payers* – Health insurance plans, self-insured employers, union and association sponsored plans, and other plan sponsors face constant and continued pressure as health insurance reforms continue to impact and alter the way health and care is financed and delivered. Both intended and unintended consequences of health reform will be felt for years to come.

- *Healthcare Policy Makers* – Policy makers continue to monitor the impact of a changing healthcare ecosystem, and ponder both the practical impact of reforms in place, as well as ways to improve the system. With the ripple effect of health reform still being felt, an updated, industry-leading reference manual, with key insights and practical applications, will support research and health policy development.

- *Healthcare Law* - Health law practices are critical for any health organization, and provide legal and strategic support needed by physican practices, health systems, and hospital organizations in navigating the legal and regulatory issues central to establishment, growth and governance of new provider-led organizations.

- *Academic and Research* - Medical school, public health, and healthcare administrations, as well as other programs interested in an advanced understanding of new care delivery models with a focus on provider organizations.

- *Consumers* – Consumers are increasingly called upon to understand and function within a rapidly changing healthcare system. The advent of health insurance exchanges, with their myriad of different products, require a sophisticated understanding of insurance not previously needed in the days before the Affordable Care Act. This book is designed to make the changes more understandable and accessible as consumers increasingly must manage their own health, care, and insurance.

In closing, this latest edition is a significant addition to the print and digital reference collection of healthcare leaders. Many new developments have occurred since release of the second edition, which this new anthology helps address. We believe this book will provide a roadmap through the many complex issues that must be considered in the rapidly changing healthcare environment.

TABLE OF CONTENTS

Chapter 11. Non-Traditional Mental Health and Substance Use Disorder Services as a Core Part of Health in CINs and ACOs.......380

Chapter 12. Improving Future Care Through Comparative Effectiveness Research..426

Contributors

CHAPTER 1

Ken Yale, DDS, JD,
VP, ActiveHealth Management

Thomas A. Raskauskas, MD, CEO,
St. Vincents Health Partners, Inc.

Joanne Bohn, Principal,
KMI Communications, LLC

Colin Konschak, MBA, FACHE,
CEO, Divurgent

CHAPTER 2

Robert Steiner, MD, PhD,
Professor, Health Management and
Systems Sciences, University of
Louisville School of Public Health
and Information Sciences

John Morse, MBA
Chief Development Officer
Department of Family and Geriatric
Medicine
University of Louisville School of
Medicine

Isaac J. Myers II, MD
Chief Health Integration Officer
Baptist Health
President
Baptist Health Medical Group

CHAPTER 3

Thomas A. Raskauskas, MD, CEO,
St. Vincents Health Partners

Joanne Bohn, Principal,
KMI Communications, LLC

CHAPTER 4

Thomas A. Raskauskas, MD, CEO,
St. Vincents Health Partners, Inc.

CHAPTER 5

Brian Nichols, JD, MBA
Partner
Robinson & Cole, LLP

CHAPTER 6

Deborah S. Smith, MN, RN-BC,
Product Development Principal
URAC

CHAPTER 7

Thomas A. Raskauskas, MD, CEO,
St. Vincents Health Partners, Inc.

Joanne Bohn, Principal,
KMI Communications, LLC

CHAPTER 8

Michael G. Hunt, DO, CMO/CMIO,
St. Vincents Health Partners, Inc.

Colleen Swedberg MSN, RN, CNL,
Director for Care Coordination and
Integration
St. Vincents Health Partners, Inc.

CHAPTER 9
Kylanne Green, CEO
URAC

CHAPTER 10

Holton Walker, Head of Health IT
Solutions
ActiveHealth Management
President, Langdon Moore

Ken Yale, DDS, JD,
VP, ActiveHealth Management

CHAPTER 11

Roger Kathol, MD,
President, Catesian Solutions, Inc.
Professor, Internal Medicine and
Psychiatry, University of Minnesota

Steve Melek,
Principal & Consulting Actuary
Milliman

Susan Sargent,
President, Sargent Healthcare
Management Advisors, LLC

Lee Sacks, MD
EVP and CMO Advocate Healthcare
and CEO Advocate Physician
Partners

Kavita K. Patel, MD, MS, Fellow and
Managing Director,
Engelberg Center for Healthcare
Reform, Brookings Institution

CHAPTER 12

Ken Yale, DDS, JD,
VP, ActiveHealth Management

CHAPTER 13

Ewa Matuszewski,
CEO, Medical Network One

Thomas A. Raskauskas, MD CEO,
St. Vincents Health Partners, Inc.
Ken Yale, DDS, JD,
VP, ActiveHealth Management

CHAPTER 14

Ken Yale, DDS, JD,
VP, ActiveHealth Management

Thomas A. Raskauskas, MD, CEO,
St. Vincents Health Partners, Inc.

Joanne Bohn, Principal,
KMI Communications, LLC

Colin Konschak, MBA, FACHE,
CEO, Divurgent

Foreword

Clinical Integration: Population Health and Accountable Care
Third Edition

Editors: Ken Yale, et al.

Clinical Integration, Population Health, and Accountable Care are all enormously important concepts as the healthcare industry transforms itself now five years post-passage of the Affordable Care Act. Can a disparate group of authors give sufficient attention to each of these broad topics in a way that makes good sense? The answer to this question for Ken Yale and his colleagues is a resounding "yes"!

As the Founding Dean of the nation's only School of Population Health, I have the privilege of interacting with amazing faculty and students, both on our campus and across the nation, (for our asynchronous online courses). Rarely have I come across a "one stop shopping" textbook, that so neatly packages the critical issues facing the nation and our healthcare system.

Kudos to Ken Yale, Tom Raskauskas, Joanne Bohn, and Colin Konschak. Somehow they managed to assemble a team of experts to tackle all of the front page stories characterizing our current system, including such topics as reframing primary care and patient-centered medical homes, the future of leadership, network evolution, the quality challenge, and many others. I particularly enjoyed chapter 3, the future of leadership and chapter 6, the quality challenge—two topics that have been of continuous interest to me in the last 30 years in academic medicine.

The chapter on the future of leadership does a nice job in summarizing current research in this ever evolving field, and it makes nice connections with work exclusively in the clinical realm. Chapter 6, on the connection between quality accountability and continuous improvement, is similarly well designed and structured. From neophytes to experts, there is something for everyone in nearly every chapter. The references provide an opportunity for a deeper dive for those who are so inclined.

Yale and his colleagues are well suited for such a herculean undertaking. With extensive expertise in both the clinical and managerial realm, the editors exercise good judgment in not only selecting authors, but in the hard work of binding the manuscript together--tying the threads, connecting the dots, and making it all read seamlessly. This is a heavy lift indeed.

Another feature of this "one stop shopping guide" are the concluding discussion questions and chapter highlights that follow each section. Not everyone will be drawn to every chapter. The discussion questions and summary highlights provide an efficient approach for those readers simply shopping for specific sections. In a book that literally covers the waterfront, one reader is unlikely to examine every ship and every dock on the horizon.

As a Dean, I would like to assign this book to every faculty member and every student too! If we all utilize this book as our core curriculum, we would be making lots of progress in deepening our understanding of this complex system in which we all study and work. The building blocks are all here and Yale and his colleagues have built the sturdy foundation for any reader to pursue.

Kudos to Yale and the team for delivering such clarity on a subject whose very enormity would have simply overwhelmed and discouraged most others who ventured into it. I am only hoping that all the stakeholders will take the time to thoughtfully go through this book and garner the take home messages. With so much at stake for the very future of our country, I'm keeping my fingers crossed.

David B. Nash, MD, MBA
Dean, Jefferson School of Population Health

Chapter 1. Continuing the Momentum

Ken Yale | Thomas A. Raskauskas

Joanne Bohn | Colin Konschak

Tipping Points are a reaffirmation of the potential for change and the power of intelligent action. (Gladwell, 2000)

Malcolm Gladwell
American Author

CHAPTER 1 LEARNING OBJECTIVES

✓ Understand the paradigm-shift taking place across the healthcare industry.

✓ Discuss four key areas of change driving the Care Revolution Era.

✓ Recognize the significance and impact of the social determinants of health on the provider's efforts to drive improvement in care delivery.

✓ Understand the basic regulatory issues for the formation and structure of CINs and ACOs.

Background

In this chapter we provide an overview of key topics to be addressed in depth throughout this book. This edition transitions from the collaborative work of its four original authors to a 14-chapter anthology authored by a wide variety of subject matter experts from across the industry. This refresh on the original issues covered in the second edition, also introduces a number of new topics. Patient engagement, care coordination, and behavioral health are a few of the new topics covered in detail in new chapters of this edition.

Introduction

Across the United States (U.S.) over the past several years, physician practices, hospitals, and payer organizations have engaged in new and evolvingg ways of delivering patient care in their communities. A continuous transformation has been underway, linked to several factors driving change throughout the industry. Perhaps the 'tipping point' was reached in the second half of the past decade when the Medicare Modernization Act of 2003 started the transition to new models of care. This transition, chronicled in government legislation and demonstration projects, was spawned by the realization of massive future costs and care burdens of the aging Baby Boomer population, the need to shift from a volume-driven to a value-driven model of care, medical technology innovation, health information technology adoption, and increased awareness of the impact of social determinants on health of a population. Figure 1-1 illustrates the factors in this shift, which may be called the "Care Revolution Era."

Figure 1-1. Industry Paradigm Shift

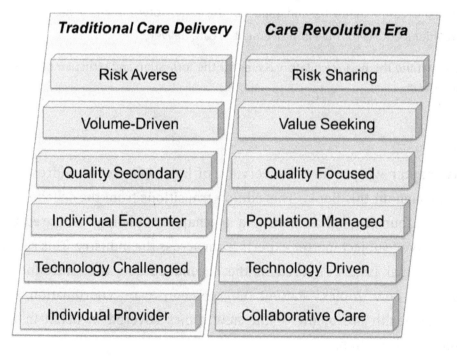

Today, in the Care Revolution Era, we are entering a new time where the relationship dynamics between patient and physician, physician and facility, and all three of these groups are making a paradigm shift in their relationships with each other and with payers. New laws, regulations, technologies, policies, organizational models, and evidence-based practices are changing the landscape for future care delivery teams and the knowledge workers that support them. Paul Starr, a well known health policy pundit, wrote in his 1981 book, *The Social Transformation of American Medicine*, on factors in transformations (e.g., "epic of progress") that occur over time in healthcare:

> The history of medicine has been written as an epic of progress, but it is also a tale of social and economic conflict over the emergence of new hierarchies of power and authority, new markets, and new conditions of belief and experience. (Starr, 1982)

All of these factors, and many others to be discussed throughout this book, contribute to the need for re-examination of the healthcare system and revolutionary change in the quality of care, delivery, and payment for patient services. The ACA was a catalyst for this change, with its policy focus on improving population health as part of the Three Part Aim. (Centers for Medicare and Medicaid Services, April 7, 2011)

In light of this new policy focus, in 2013 the Institute of Medicine (IOM) established the Roundtable for Population Health Improvement and issued their initial report, entitled *Population Health Implications of the Affordable Care Act: A Workshop Summary*. Efforts such as this, and many others, highlight the national shift to addressing care at the population level.

To help make this shift happen, the problems with health care quality, affordability, and accessibility are being addressed throughout the healthcare system. New and innovative models of care have been introduced in reaction to the new emphasis on population health and requirements of the ACA. The new models of care include Clinically Integrated Networks (CINs) and Accountable Care Organizations (ACOs).

These major changes and new models of care were predicted during the 2008 Presidential campaign. During the campaign, Presidential candidate Barack Obama, noted,

> Simply put, in the absence of a radical shift toward prevention and public health, we will not be successful in containing medical costs or improving the health of the American people. (Fielding, Tilson, & Richland, December 2008)

One of the key challenges the health care industry has been working to address is the reimbursement system. Under the current fee-for-service payment system, each procedure is paid, regardless of outcome. This "pay for procedure" approach has contributed to inefficiency, over-utilization, and waste.

In 2006, the IOM released a report that brought attention to many of the problems with the fee-for-service system. The IOM stated this system "reward(s) excessive use of services; high-cost, complex procedures; and lower-quality care."(Institute of Medicine & Committee on Redesigning Health Insurance Performance Measures, 2006) This reimbursement model has resulted in a volume-driven system that contributes to suboptimal quality of care and concurrent increases in the cost of healthcare. The policy reforms and innovations in care delivery facilitated by the ACA are meant to address these perverse incentives in the healthcare system.

At the time of the second edition of this book, healthcare expenditures in the United States had risen at an annual rate of 2.4% faster than the rate of growth in gross domestic product (GDP) and national healthcare expenditures had grown to 17.6% of total GDP. (Kaiser Family Foundation, March 2009) Also, national health expenditures as a share of GDP were projected to increase to 19.3% by 2019. (Center for Medicare and Medicaid Services, 2009) However, fast forward two and half years and the complex effects of new policy, technology, unsteady demand for services, the economic recession, and population demographics have all contributed to a slow down in healthcare spending. In a December 2013 *New England*

Journal of Medicine article, Blumenthal and colleagues provided an assessment of this slow down in spending. and noted that while there is debate as to what caused this decrease in spending, a few of the dynamics included: a slowing trend in diffusion of some medical technologies, greater cost sharing that has put more burden on consumers, the focus on efforts to reduce certain hospital costs (such as unnecessary readmissions), and a moderating of healthcare service prices. (Blumenthal, Stremikis, & Cutler, 2013)

With this as a backdrop, what is the current state of affairs for providers, including hospitals, health systems, and medical group practices today, and what is the historical and regulatory basis for the emerging CINs and ACOs? And what are some of the contemporary factors influencing the growth and operation of these new models of care and reimbursement? The authors of this third edition explore these questions, and share their experiences, to shed light on the current state and future directions of the industry.

The CIN: State of Affairs

Trends and lessons learned from the managed care era and more recent demonstration projects have fostered a number of innovations in care delivery, quality improvement, and payment reform. One such innovation— the focus of this book series and its third edition—is the continued growth and expansion of new business models such as CINs and ACOs. The ACO concept originated from work done by researchers at the Dartmouth-Brookings Institute, and piloted in the Medicare Physician Group Practice Demonstration Project. The demonstration and Congressional testimony provided sufficient interest for the U.S. federal government to support advancement of the ACO model in the ACA, and spawned development of private payer ACO initiatives. Additional details on the final results of the Physician Group Practice demonstration can be found in the September 2012 final report on the demonstration. (Centers for Medicare and Medicaid Services, September 2012)

CINs, as defined by the U.S. Federal Trade Commission (FTC), are legitimate collaborations of otherwise competing providers (hospitals and/or physicians, for example) organized in a way that improves efficiencies in care delivery (including quality improvement and cost reduction) for the benefit of consumers that outweigh any potential anticompetitive effects (such as fixing prices among competitors). If providers meet specific criteria for clinical integration, the federal government will not be prevent them from collaborating and even negotiating prices with payers, without running afoul of antitrust laws that prohibit competitors from illegal price setting.

CINs have become an integral part of the Care Revolution Era and provide many of the tools required for operating a Medicare or private payer ACO. In addition, the FTC and Department of Justice (DOJ) Antitrust Division issued their final *Statement of Antitrust Enforcement Policy Regarding ACOs Participating in the Medicare Shared Savings Program* to clarify how providers may legitimately collaborate in these ACA-created entities. In that document, these two federal government agencies (who jointly enforce the federal antitrust laws) proposed a new policy to treat Medicare ACOs similar to CINs and apply existing guidance they use to determine whether collective activities by otherwise competing providers (such as negotiating or setting prices) are per se illegal, fall under more lenient "rule of reason" analysis, or certain "safety zones" where the providers' collective actions will not be challenged, absent extraordinary circumstances. (Department of Justice, 2011) New developments in their statement included:

a) application to all types of collaborations between independent providers and provider groups participating in a Medicare ACO program; and

b) removal of requirements for mandatory antitrust review.

To fall within the "safety zones", providers need to share substantial financial risk and meet certain requirements for how much of the market for their services they control. Substantial risk sharing, the antitrust agencies believe, shows that providers have a financial incentive to be efficient, control costs and improve quality, ultimately benefiting the consumer – which is the primary goal of the antitrust agencies. Medicare ACOs are designed to be responsible for the cost and quality of care, and therefore should fall within the safety zones, if properly established.

If a joint venture among providers does not qualify for a safety zone, for example it does not share substantial financial risk, it may still qualify for more lenient "rule of reason" scrutiny if it meets other requirements. The antitrust agencies generally require providers to establish an active and ongoing program to identify, evaluate and modify practice patterns by the physicians participating in the organization that also creates a high degree of interdependence and cooperation among the physicians to control costs and ensure quality. (Department of Justice & Federal Trade Commission, 1996b) If one considers the medical home as an effort to transform a physician practice, the CIN is a medical home multiplied by many, otherwise independent primary and specialty care physicians who collaborate to create a new service that benefits consumers through higher quality and lower costs, rather than trying to merely negotiate to increase prices.

According to the antitrust agencies, a legitimate clinically integrated network collaboration may include:

(1) establishing mechanisms to monitor and control utilization of health care services that are designed to control costs and assure quality of care; (2) selectively choosing network physicians who are likely to further these efficiency objectives; and (3) the significant investment of capital, both monetary and human, in the necessary infrastructure and capability to realize the claimed efficiencies. (Department of Justice & Federal Trade Commission, 1996b)

The goal is to design a service that benefits consumers with lower costs and improved care, expanding consumer choice with increased competition, and therefore is "procompetitive."(Department of Justice & Federal Trade Commission, 1996a) Collective negotiation of prices with payers must be "reasonably necessary and ancillary" to these core goals.

Experience with clinical integration and meeting FTC/DOJ criteria leads to a number of areas of emphasis for an effective and efficient provider operation that meets the requirements for CINs:

- Physicians: Physicians lead the development of quality, cost, and access initiatives, and are responsible for creating a new service that improves care and costs for consumers;

- Interdependence: collaboration, information sharing, and building physician affinity;

- Care coordination: primary and specialty care participation in coordinating care;

- Clinical protocols: used for a wide range of diseases and conditions;

- Clinician responsibility: to ensure compliance with clinical protocols;

- Infrastructure: appropriate systems and processes to meet the goals and objectives, and training available for everyone involved;

- IT integration: use of appropriate information technology and clinical decision support;

- Performance: monitoring and improvement of physician performance, including feedback and specific action taken;

- Outcomes: measurable outcomes that demonstrate improved quality and affordability; and

- Results: ability to report results, provide feedback, and improve poor performance.

(Yale, Jenrette. 2010)

Once an entity is legitimately clinically integrated, with appropriate infrastructure and processes to improve quality and lower costs, it can collectively negotiate prices with payers for the new services developed.

This provides an overview of the legal issues for CIN formation. These organizations have grown in number recently, and are continuing to be adopted and implemented at an accelerated pace. It's an innovative and evolving business model helping forge a path of innovation for hospitals, physicians, care provider teams, and payers in the Care Revolution Era.

Current Environmental Factors

The renaissance age for the healthcare industry currently unfolding includes the transformation of business models, health outcomes, interventions, and industry direction. In Gareth Morgan's 1986 work, *Images of Organization*, one of the topics discussed was the evolutionary process in which organizations dynamically adapt (or don't) to their constantly changing environment. In his "ecological philosophy," he noted,

> As organizations assert their identities they can initiate major transformations in the social ecology to which they belong. They can set the basis for their own destruction. Or they can create the conditions that will allow them to evolve along with the environment. (Morgan, 1986)

The healthcare industry has experienced major changes in the last four decades that confirm the truth of this ecological philosophy.

Paul Starr wrote of the demise of the cottage industry structure for physicians and the rise of the managed care industry in the 70s and 80s. Today, in the midst of the Care Revolution Era, we see a continuation of that evolution in the new focus on population health and continued emphasis on improved quality, accessibility and affordability of care. But, as Morgan noted, it is critical for organizations to adapt to their changing environment in order to survive. For physicians, other provider organizations, and payers that have dealt with major market and environmental changes, this is even more true today.

The IOM, in their 2001 report, *Crossing the Quality Chasm: A New Health System for the 21st Century*, identified four causes of inadequate care. Changes underway in these areas help illustrate the changing environment.

(Institute of Medicine & Committee on Quality of Health Care in America, 2001) Figure 1-2 identifies these four areas.

Figure 1-2. Areas of Change Fueling the Care Revolution Era

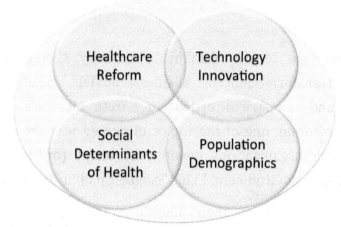

These four areas have fueled the need to adopt a new way of delivering healthcare, such as clinically integrated organizations, as a business model for healthcare delivery. A few thoughts on each of these areas of change:

Healthcare Reform

Major federal government healthcare reforms have included the 2003 Medicare Modernization Act, 2009 American Recovery and Reinvestment Act, 2010 Patient Protection and Affordable Care Act, and in 2013 the final privacy and security rules from the Health Information Portability and Accountability Act. These laws helped usher in an infusion of innovation with greater focus on electronic health records (EHRs) and health information exchange (HIE), start-up of Medicare ACOs, greater support for the transition to value-based contracting, and a continued refinement of the industry's efforts to ensure consumer protection of health information.

Technology Innovation

Innovation in healthcare has accelerated, in the form of new business models such as CINs, requiring new technologies such as predictive analyticis, mobile health, and telehealth,; and new processes for people to work together. Key to successful health reform is figuring how to make innovations sustainable. In his 2008 keynote address to the World Economic Forum in Davos, Switzerland, Victor J. Dzau, MD, new President of the Institute of Medicine and former Chancellor of Health Affairs at Duke University, noted the importance of "ideas, people and integrity" combined with "development, ownership and diffusion" for growth of sustainable innovations in healthcare. (Dzau, 2008)

In the course of finding innovations, the industry encounters both incremental and disruptive innovations, as described by Clayton M. Christensen and colleagues in their book *The Innovator's Prescription: A Disruptive Solution for Health Care.* Here the "disruptive value network" was described as a dynamic and "complicated system" that would invoke new business models, capabilities and ways of working together to provide better care for patients. (Christensen, Grossman, & Hwang, 2009) The CIN is well positioned to serve as the nucleus of this new medical care model— embracing the new challenges that lie ahead.

Population Demographics

The population can be segmented based on many characteristics, including age, race, gender, ethnicity, and geographic region. Each demographic segment faces different epidemiologic burdens, barriers to care, quality issues, and cost conundrums. Today patients are more informed by information available on the Internet that has fueled the growth of consumer and crowd wisdom as well as potential for patient engagement.

For CINs, understanding population demographics is an important element of the business model. The makeup of the patient population and network capabilities are important considerations in contractual relationships with payer organizations. Figure 1-3 provides one example of the wide variation in age of the United States population, as represented in a pyramid. (US Census Bureau, 2013)

Figure 1-3. Population Pyramid: U.S. Age Distribution

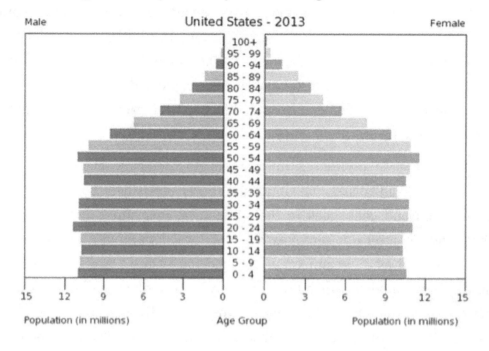

Given the impact of the Baby Boomer segment in the United States, one can envision the shift to prevention and chronic care needed by CINs. Figure 1-3 illustrates the buldge of this population segment and the ripple effects that will occur in future decades.

Social Determinants of Health

One of the major challenges, increasingly recognized by the healthcare establishment, is the integral relationship between medical care and the social determinants of health. Social determinants of health include factors such as housing, income, access to healthy foods, social support networks, education level, behavioral risk factors, stigma, and discrimination. These factors are issues that can impact all individuals and segments of the population. (Dean, Williams, & Fenton, 2013) In the World Health Organization's 2008 report, *Closing the Gap in a Generation, Health Equity through Action on the Social Determinants of Health*, a key element to improving population health was the need to address social and economic policies in communities. (Word Health Organization & Commission on Social Determinants of Health, 2008)

For the CIN, understanding the influence of these factors on the health of the population served is essential. Clinical leadership needs to engage with community partners to drive medical care and preventive services for each population segment in a community. (Terrell & Bohn, 2012) Striving to identify and deliver the most effective treatment plans for patients based on the spectrum of their needs, taking into account social determinants, has been a historical challenge but one that CINs, ACOs and other care provider organizations can work toward improving. In 2013, the nation saw the initiation of accountable care communities with the first such program in Akron, OH as described in the IOM's 2013 report, *Population Health Implications of the Affordable Care Act: A Workshop Summary.* (Institute of Medicine & Board on Population Health and Public Health Practice, 2013) In these communities, there is a collaborative, multidisciplinary effort among health care delivery organizations, community partners, faith-based organizations, and public health service providers. These comprehensive projects hold the promise of addressing the challenges posed by social determinants.

Forthcoming Chapters

This book is focused on new and evolving healthcare business models -- specifically CINs, ACOs, and the collaborative ventures they foster. This third edition contains chapters prepared by a collection of authors that cover a spectrum of interests, from hospitals, health systems, health plans, medical group practices, affiliated providers, healthcare organizational leaders, practicing physicians, accreditation organizations, academic researchers, and medical educators.

New chapters have been developed for this edition on care coordination, new accreditation standards for CINs, the importance of behavioral health service integration for CINs and ACOs, and patient engagement.

Future Direction

The cottage industry that once symbolized the healthcare industry continues to disappear with the formation of value-based, interconnected networks such as CIN and ACO. The future for CINs and ACOs is bright, serving a role in helping improve healthcare. The influence of the ACA and its many underlying policies and programs will be touched on throughout this book. To achieve sustainable growth of new business models, it will be essential to recognize the importance of new technologies, policies, and management practices, as a collective set of tools to enable care providers to establish new processes that allow achievement of the Triple Aim. The Care Revolution Era is unfolding before us. It's our responsibility to recognize the significance of this new Era, and how it can improve health and wellness for current and future generations.

CHAPTER 1 DISCUSSION QUESTIONS

Discussion questions are provided for team building or class exercises. Answers for all questions are provided in Appendix C.

Question Number	Question
1	What was a central focus of the ACA noted in the chapter?
2	What are the six elements of the Care Revolution Era?
3	What is one industry shift that results from the Baby Boomer demographic segment's influence on health services?
4	What are some of the factors included in the social determinants of health and what is one strategy that CINs may take to address their effect on community and population health?
5	What is one novel approach noted in the chapter being piloted in some communities as a way to improve collaboration and population health?
6	What are the four areas that help illustrate the changing environment in the Care Revolution Era?

CHAPTER 1 HIGHLIGHTS

✓ Introduces the concept of the Care Revolution Era - a phenomenon where relationship dynamics between patients, phsyicians, and payers are undergoing a paradigm shift.

✓ Emphasized work of the IOM describing the industry shift to focus on population health management.

✓ Discussed challenges of restructuring the payment and delivery systems.

✓ Highlighted the slowdown in healthcare spending that had been reported in 2013, and various reasons for the moderation in spending.

✓ Defined CINs and described their place as an integral part of the Care Revolution Era.

✓ Provided an overview of the FTC/DOJ requirements underpinning CINs.

✓ Described four areas that illustrate the changing environment that seem to be fueling the Care Revolution Era: a) healthcare reform, b) technology innovation, c) social determinants of health, and d) population demographics.

CHAPTER 1 REFERENCES

Blumenthal, D., Stremikis, K., & Cutler, D. (2013). Health care spending--a giant slain or sleeping? *New England Journal of Medicine*, 369(26), 2551-2557. doi: 10.1056/NEJMhpr1310415

Center for Medicare and Medicaid Services. (2009). National health expenditure projections 2009-2019. Retrieved from http://www.cms.gov/NationalHealthExpendData/25_NHE_Fact_Sheet.asp - TopOfPage

Overview and Intent of the Medicare Shared Savings Program., Vol. 76, No. 67, *Federal Register*, 19533 (April 7, 2011).

Centers for Medicare and Medicaid Services. (2012, September). Evaluation of the Medicare Physician Group Practice Demonstration Project. Final Report. Retrieved from http://www.cms.gov/Medicare/Demonstration-Projects/DemoProjectsEvalRpts/Downloads/PhysicianGroupPracticeFinalReport.pdf

Christensen, C. M., Grossman, J. H., & Hwang, J. (2009). Introduction. In *The Innovator's Prescription: A Disruptive Solution for Health Care* (pp. xxviii-xxx). New York, NY: McGraw-Hill.

Dean, H. D., Williams, K. M., & Fenton, K. A. (2013). From Theory to Action: Applying Social Determinants of Health to Public Health Practice. *Public Health Reports*, 128(Supplement 3), 1-4.

Statement of Antitrust Enforcement Policy Regarding Accountable Care Organizations Participating in the Medicare Shared Savings Program (2011).

Department of Justice, & Federal Trade Commission. (1996a). Statements of Antitrust Enforcement Policy on Healthcare. Statement 3. Hospital Joint Ventures Involving Specialized Clinical Or Other Expensive Health Care Services. Department of Justice: Retrieved from http://www.justice.gov/atr/public/guidelines/1791.pdf

Department of Justice, & Federal Trade Commission. (1996b). Statements of Antitrust Enforcement Policy on Healthcare. Statement 8. Physician Network Joint Ventures. Department of Justice: Retrieved from http://www.justice.gov/atr/public/guidelines/1791.pdf

Dzau, V. J. (2008). Innovation in Healthcare in Emerging Economies. Paper presented at the World Economic Forum Davos, Switzerland.

Fielding, J. E., Tilson, H. H., & Richland, J. H. (2008, December). Medical Care Reform Requires Public Health Reform: Expanded Role for Public Health Agencies. In *Improving Health. A Prevention Policy Paper Commissioned by Partnership for Prevention: Partnership for Prevention*.

Gladwell, M. (2000). Conclusion. Focus, Test and Believe. *The Tipping Point. How Little Things Can Make A Big Difference* (pp. 259). New York, NY: Back Bay Books.

Institute of Medcine, & Board on Population Health and Public Health Practice. (2013). Chapter 3. Current Models for Integrating a Population Health Approach into Implementation of the Affordable Care Act. In *Population health implications of the Affordable Care Act, Workshop Summary* (pp. 7-10). Washington, DC: The National Academies Press.

Institute of Medicine, & Committee on Quality of Health Care in America. (2001). Underlying Reasons for Inadequate Quality of Care. In *Crossing the Quality Chasm: A New Health System for the 21st Century* (pp. 25-33). Washington, DC: National Academies Press.

Institute of Medicine, & Committee on Redesigning Health Insurance Performance Measures, P., and Performance Improvement Programs. (2006). Summary. In *Rewarding Provider Performance: Aligning Incentives in Medicare* (pp. 4). Washington, DC: National Academies Press.

Kaiser Family Foundation. (2009, March). Trends in health care costs and spending.

Morgan, G. (1986). Chapter 8. Unfolding Logics of Change. Organization as Flux and Transformation (Toward a New View of Organizational Evolution and Change). In *Images of Organization* (pp. 245). Newbury Park, CA: Sage Publications, Inc.

Starr, P. (1982). The Social Origins of Professional Sovereignty. In *The Social Transformation of American Medicine* (pp. 4). New York, NY: Harper Collins.

Terrell, G. E., & Bohn, J. M. (2012). Figure 4. Collaborative Clinical Leadership Model. In *MD 2.0: Physician Leadership for the Information Age, From Hero to Duyukdv* (pp. 42). Tampa, FL: American Academy of Physician Executives.

US Census Bureau. (2013). Population pyramid of the U.S. population distribution by age for 2013. Retrieved from http://www.census.gov/population/international/data/idb/region.php?N= Results &T=12&A=separate&RT=0&Y=2013&R=-1&C=US

World Health Organization, & Commission on Social Determinants of Health. (2008). *Closing the Gap in a Generation, Health Equity through Action on the Social Determinants of Health*. Geneva, Switzerland: World Health Organization.

Yale, K., Jenrette, J. (2010, November). *ACO Technologies: Performance and Reporting Tools*. Presentation to World Congress Leadership Summit on Accountable Care Organizations West. San Diego, CA,

Chapter 2. Re-Framing Primary Care and Patient-Centered Medical Homes in the Lens of Complexity, Culture and Relationship-Centered Care

Robert Steiner | John Morse

Isaac J. Myers II

Evidence of the benefits of a health system with a strong primary care base is abundant and consistent.

Barbara Starfield, Shi, & Macinko, 2005

CHAPTER 2 LEARNING OBJECTIVES

✓ Describe the characteristics of primary care as a foundation for an effective healthcare system.

✓ Discuss the importance of primary care for assuring population health.

✓ Discuss how the major epidemiologic transitions of health care in the U.S. apply to the development of the Patient-Centered Medical Home (PCMH) model.

✓ Describe the roles of the chronic care model and healthcare financing reform in the development of PCMH.

✓ Describe the roles that complexity perspectives in management might play in the clinical transformation process of PCMH.

✓ Define "relationship-centered care" and "culture of caring" as applicable to the evolution of the PCMH.

Introduction

The landscape for medical care, and especially primary care, is changing in the United States (U.S.), in part due to the Patient Protection and Affordable Care Act (ACA). The ACA began implementation in 2010 as a national, legislative means for health insurance reform. Prior to the ACA and the Health Information Technology for Economic and Clinical Health Act (HITECH), the United States did not have a comprehensive, national government policy for enhancing primary care. The changes associated with implementation of the ACA are broad and multi-factorial. (Kaiser Foundation, 2013)

Healthcare in the United States is the most expensive among all nations in the world, yet we fail to achieve better health outcomes than the other developed countries. In such comparative rankings, the United States ranks in last or near-last place on dimensions of access, efficiency, and equity. (Davis, Squires, Schoen, 2014)

The United States consistently ranks lower in measures of health status among developed countries, and yet it ranks highest among national expenditures for health. (Avendano & Kawachi, 2014) Health care spending in the United States increased from $148 per person per year in 1960, to $1,834 in 1985 and $8,233 in 2010. (OCED, 2012) Similarly, over the same 50 years, life expectancy in the United States increased from 69.8 years in 1960, to 78.7 years in 2010. (OECD, 2012) Many consider the expense of medical care to be worth the costs, although the magnitude of the causal associations with improved longevity and quality of life are small, from a societal perspective. Others cite the unsustainability of rising health care costs as a matter of national and global concern.

How did we as a nation reach such a status? What are the solutions? How does primary care and the Patient-Centered Medical Home (PCMH) fit within the new and evolving health reform context? How can the status of primary care be improved? These are key questions this chapter shall address, using perspectives from complexity sciences, within the context of culture, as applied to the dynamic relationships that evolve between people, technology and social health policies. (Esterhay, 2014) The concepts of emergence and self-organization provide new avenues for thinking about policies and issues of healthcare reform, especially in primary care arenas. (McDaniel Jr, Jordan, & Fleeman, 2003; McDaniel & Driebe, 2001; Plsek, 2001) These topics will be our focus for proposed innovations that favor development of primary care, PCMH, CIN and ACO.

Finally, we propose the PCMH as the organizing construct around which CINs and Accountable Care Organizations (ACOs) can succeed. We review the historical background of PCMH, and the current healthcare reform context that makes PCMH appealing, and even necessary, to improve population health.

Health Care Reform and the ACA

The central aim of the ACA is to increase health insurance coverage in order to make healthcare more affordable and accessible for U.S. citizens. (Ormond, 2011) By providing opportunities for more people to enroll in private health insurance, Medicaid, and federally qualified health plans (FQHP), more people will have access to public and private insurance for healthcare services. Thus, demand for primary care services will likely increase as a result of implementing the ACA. HITECH serves as an impetus for the development of health information technologies (HIT), electronic medical records (EMR) and patient administrative systems that enhance primary care by integrating and coordinating clinical information between multiple providers of healthcare services. These new technologies are not limited to medical practices alone, as pharmancies, clinical laboratories, vision and dental services, speciality care, and providers of other clinical services also contribute information.

Developing HIT and EMR capabilities represents a national, politically-sanctioned, attempt to make mainstream clinical information networks linking various providers in medical care. Previously, most efforts to develop HIT focused on health information for billing. As a result, a vast array of claims data has been created and is held by public and private payers. In addition, means to link the clinical contents of EMRs and other non-financial information is less well developed. Linking clinical content and allowing inter-operability would be useful to develop evidence supporting new quality improvement strategies, and improve a variety of care processes, such as facilitating transitions between and within healthcare settings. Inter-operability of EMR and HIT can also provide new means for health services research to study and improve population health.

Although some attention has been given to developing access to clinical, pharmacy, disease registry and other data within healthcare systems, these efforts are usually provider focused, and there is insufficient attention to person-centered data about the social and behavioral determinants of health. The social and behavioral determinants of health, according to the Institute of Medicine (IOM), are key components of individual "functional status, and the onset and progression of disease". (IOM, 2014) Understanding and acting upon these determinants could assist physician offices, hospitals, and health systems to apply more effective treatments and procedures, based on evidence provided by Big Data and other sources of information.

The premises of the ACA are consistent with the broad principles embodied in the World Health Organization (WHO) Alma-Ata Declaration, including the notion that "...health ... is a fundamental human right", and "...the attainment of the highest possible level of health is a most important world-wide social goal...." (WHO, 1978) Furthermore, the Alma-Ata Declaration cited the development of primary care as the key means to the attainment of this goal and for the WHO program entitled "Health for All".

From these perspectives, primary care:

> ...forms an integral part both of the country's health system, of which it is the central function and main focus, and of the overall social and economic development of the community. It is the first level of contact of individuals, the family, and community with the national health system bringing health care as close as possible to where people live and work,

and constitutes the first elements of a continuing health care process. (Mahler, 1981)

Success in healthcare reform and transformation is often discussed in terms of the Triple Aim. (Berwick, Nolan, & Whittington, 2008) The Triple Aim is a concept developed by Dr. Donald Berwick to describe the elements of a well functioning health system, including quality of care, costs and outcomes. The Triple Aim is: improving population health, enhancing the patients' experiences of care and reducing costs per capita. (Stiefel M. 2012) The union of primary care with Clinically Integrated Networks (CINs) represents one possible way to concurrently attain Triple Aim success. The Triple Aim is now the framework for the U.S. National Quality Strategy of the U.S. Department of Health and Human Services, Centers for Medicare and Medicaid Services, and many other organizations. (Stiefel, Perla, & Zell, 2010)

Relationship-Centered Care

We posit that all people participating in medical care are in complex adaptive relationships, and that the experiences of "health" and "culture" are emergent, self-organizing properties of complex adaptive human systems. Improving health is then synonymous with interactive and interdependent processes, whereby exchanges with diverse people (e.g., patients with physicians and other clinicians in the context of family and community) provide novel avenues for therapeutic change and for generating insights to facilitate approaches to health and wellness. Hence, the context of relationship-centered care (RCC) is a key concept for this chapter.

RCC advances a humanistic approach toward patient care, especially for primary care. (Suchman, 2006) RCC includes concepts from patient-centered care (McWhinney, 1972) and rests upon the foundation of the bio-psycho-social model of healthcare for individals in a social context (G. L. Engel, 1977, 1979), and a socio-cultural-ecologic model for the collective, or societal aspects, of population health. (Steiner, 2014) RCC places a priority on humanism in healthcare and community development; it offers technology as a tool for people to use to facilitate better health, rather than using selected tools as a touted sole solution. As such, RCC is a means to bridge the diverse cultures of complementary approaches between the medical, techhological, and social aspects of population health.

Philosophic Views of Primary Care

Primary care represents a generalist's approach to health concerns of patients and populations. Primary care is a component of healthcare systems that can effectively address the majority of medical needs for common conditions among people of all ages. There is ample evidence to support the role of primary care as a means to improve and sustain the health status of societies and nations. (Barbara Starfield, 1991, 1998; Barbara Starfield et al., 2005)

Notions of primary care can evoke iconic images about what primary care is, including vestiges of its historic roots and concepts of what it might become. Characters from popular culture, like Marcus Welby, MD or James Kildare, MD, conveyed their passion for the profession of medicine, and their altruistic concerns for patients in need, often extending beyond the confines of traditional medical care establishments, like hospitals and clinics, into homes and social settings. The physician was often portrayed as a humanistic caregiver, typically depicted either as a kind "hero" or compassionate "heroine," whereby each would willingly go to extremes to visit the sick and render care to those in need (see Figure 2-1 below). This characterization is part of the history and culture of the United States, and fits within the context and history of evolving cultural traditions of healthcare systems, including Western scientific biomedicine.

A more common notion now is that primary care providers (PCPs) include "ordinary" physician generalists and other trained clinicians. Far from ordinary, primary care physicians do have special training and skills. Primary care clinicians are trained to make diagnoses from undifferentiated health conditions, interwoven patterns of the signs of disease and symptoms of illness, within the context of unique arrays of embedded social health concerns and resources. These patterns are then integrated into disease entities with specific approaches to treatment within the allopathic, biomedical model. Yet, the components of wellness and comprehensive care for individuals also lie within the context of families and society. To address this context, PCPs can offer comprehensive healthcare services for patients and their families, in their social and community environment, over the entire course of their lifespans – from cradle to grave. PCPs also facilitate the judicious mobilization of personal, family, and community resources to alleviate the signs and symptoms of disease, while attempting to buffer the impact of suffering through the judicious use of psychosocial and community resources.

Figure 2-1. Examples of Primary Care Providers Depicted through History[*]

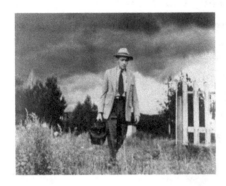 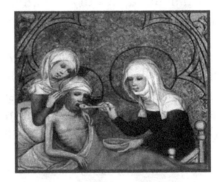

Humanism in the clinical practice of medicine and nusing has been characterized by altruism and compassion throughout the ages and across cultures.

The late Dr. Barbara Starfield, a leading authority on primary care and former professor of Health Policy and Management at the Johns Hopkins Bloomberg School of Public Health, defined primary care as:

---

[*] Black and white portrait is of Dr. Ernest Ceriani makes a house call on foot, Kremmling, Colorado, 1948. Accessed November 25, 2014 at http://life.time.com/history/life-classic-eugene-smiths-country-doctor/#1. The color drawing shows *St. Catherine Attends the Sick*, accessed at on Dec 9, 2014 at
http://www.ldysinger.com/ThM_580_Bioethics/webcourse/x-nurs-sist.jpg

> ...that aspect of a health services system that assures person-focused care over time to a defined population, accessibility to facilitate receipt of care when it is first needed, comprehensiveness of care in the sense that only rare or unusual manifestations of ill health are referred elsewhere, and coordination of care such that all facets of care (wherever received) are integrated. (Barbara Starfield, 2001a)

In her work, Dr. Starfield described four pillars of primary care practice: first-contact for care; continuity of care over time; comprehensiveness of care, including concern for the whole person rather than one disease or one physiologic system; and coordination of care with other parts of the health care system. (Barbara Starfield, 1998) These four pillars are not only the foundation for PCMH, but could also be for CIN and ACO.

Adequate primary medical care services are seen as a necessary foundation for a healthy community. The IOM report on Primary Care (1996) recommended the adoption of a new definition for primary care:

> ...as the provision of integrated, accessible health care services by clinicians who are accountable for addressing a large majority of personal health care needs, developing a sustained partnership with patients, and practicing in the context of family and community. (Donaldson, Yordy, Lohr, & Vanselow, 1996)

Primary care is designed to be one of the most cost-effective forms of health care, and it is associated with better and more equitable distribution of measures for population health, when compared to similar results for specialty care, in comparable international settings. (Barbara Starfield et al., 2005) For example, developed countries with strong primary care services have lower overall expenditures for healthcare, and the populations show better measures for health status indicators. (Fleming, 1993; Barbara Starfield, 2001b)

None of the developed societies in these studies, however, used the ACO model to develop their primary care services. Whether the transformation of healthcare systems in the United States will be successful within the dynamic context of the ACA and the evolving forms for PCMH and ACOs, as measured by the Triple Aim, is a question to be evaluated over the next several decades. Here we will review select evidence available to date, focusing on primary care - with an emphasis on conclusions from systematic reviews and meta-analyses, where available.

Historic Context, Epidemiologic Transitions and the Development of PCMH

PCMH may be considered a historic extension of the bio-psycho-social model, in contrast to the biomedical model. The biomedical model is based upon a positivist approach, in which medical therapeutics are applied to the "body-machine" -- a model that supports using technology fixes to counter the signs and symptoms of disease and illness. Yet, there are other approaches to medical care. For example, Engel first proposed a bio-psycho-social model in 1977 (G. L. Engel, 1977, 1979), and this model was taken up as a standard for training a more humanistic approach to medical care. Within the discipline of Family Medicine, the unit for awareness, influence and treatments included both the patient and family, with continuity expressed as continuous care from cradle-to-grave. (Borrell-Carrió, Suchman, & Epstein, 2004; G. Engel, 1990) The emphasis of Family Medicine changed the perspectives from care of individuals, viewed as independent from their social context, toward active, feeling, motivated patients as people in the psycho-social context of family and community.

The U.S. healthcare system and its primary care delivery have evolved through several historic movements, based upon the advent of new technologies, training models, available resources and evolving modes of finance and organizational structure for healthcare delivery. Long-term, adaptive changes in healthcare have emerged from processes within the socio-cultural ecology of developing societies. (Steiner, 2014) For example, Omran described the progression, stages of development, and changes in healthcare over more than a century, and called these stages "epidemiological transitions." Each transition has profoundly influenced aspects and approaches to population health in the U.S.. (Omran, 1971, 2005)

The focus on an early epidemiological transition, beginning more than a century ago, was on the control of communicable diseases. This issue remained prominent as other epdiemiological transitions emerged. Next, during the 1970s, a new transition shifted the focus in the United States toward addressing the impact of chronic diseases, and the impact on the growing numbers of people identified with these illnesses and conditions. Most of the emphasis was associated with preventing mortality, through risk reduction programs, first in medical settings but then expanding to community based, health education campaigns. The emphasis remained on preventing disease, without addressing the social context of health and illness.

New approaches are needed to address societal health concerns from the perspective of the community. The WHO has defined the "social determinants of health" as the circumstances in which people are born, live, work and play. These circumstances are in turn, shaped by a wider set of economics, social policies, and political forces. They all have an impact on health and medical care. There is evidence of a new conceptual model for promoting wellness in health policies and private-sector health plans. (Diener, 2009) This new model looks at issues beyond disease management and includes the social fabric of where we work, play, and learn. This may represent a new epidemiological transition that includes socially-enmeshed health concerns.

These three major epidemiological transitions correspond to the historic development of different frameworks for medical care. The first epidemiologic transition was associated with a disease-oriented model, the second transition favors a patient-centered model, and the third model invokes population health. Medical technologies tend to follow the focus of each new epidemiologiocal transition. For example, the disease-oriented model included use and development of antibiotics and vaccines, which were accompanied by better sanitation methods to assure the safety of food and clean water to reduce the disease burden of the population. These efforts provided both treatments and prevention from many communicable diseases.

From the perspective of the epidemiological transitions and historic patterns of technology adoption and development of health systems, PCMHs are designed to better address the needs of patients with chronic illnesses. To align with the newest epidemiological transition, the PCMH also needs to address population health aspects, such as the adequacy and accessibility of the community resource-base for disease prevention, assuring health protection, and fostering well-being. In short, PCMHs need to pay particular attention to the social determinants of health. And attention to population health has become part of the evolution of PCMH.

PCMH is now best described as a model or philosophy of primary care that is patient-centered, comprehensive, team-based, coordinated, accessible, and focused on quality and safety. (PCPCC, 2014) This newly proposed PCMH model is evolving away from a "disease-centered model", and toward a "person-centered model."

PCMH is both an established and continuously evolving construct. The American Academy of Pediatrics (AAP) first mentioned medical homes in 1967, followed by the American Academy of Family Physicians (AAFP) in 2004. (Green et al., 2004) The Joint Principles of the Patient-Centered Medical Home, collaboratively sponsored by professional societies representing members from the generalist traditions in medical care, including AAP, AAFP, American College of Physicians (ACP), and the American Osteopathic Association (AOA), describe the characteristics of the PCMH. (Patient-Centered Primary Care Collaborative, 2007) Major milestones for primary care and the medical home, from 1967–2013, are highlighted in the Patient-Centered Primary Care Collaborative (PCPCC) website (www.pcpcc.org).

Figure 2-2. Family Medicine is the Foundation for the PCMH[*]

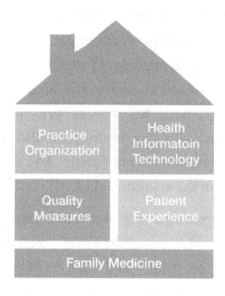

The PCMH is an approach to improve primary care by requiring that primary care practices deliver care differently than traditions and styles of care that evolved in the fee-for-service (FFS) model. Although individual definitions of PCMH may vary, all major stakeholders agree that the PCMH encompasses five major principles (Moreno L, Peikes DN, Krilla A. 2010):

1. **A patient-centered orientation toward the whole person,** requiring understanding the patient's and the family's structures, needs and preferences, their neighborhood and social context, and providing the patient's entire range of care needs.

2. **Comprehensive, team-based care**, which relies on a team of providers that might include physicians, nurses, pharmacists, nutritionists, social workers, information technology specialists, and practice managers, to meet the patient's care needs.

3. **Care coordination and/or integrated care** across all aspects of the health care system, including medical providers, mental health

---

[*] Source: Maine Health Management Coalition. Payment Reform. Accessed online November 26, 2014 at http://www.mehmc.org/about-us/what-we-do/payment-reform/.

specialists and behavioral health care, as provided by specialists, hospitals, and skilled nursing facilities, via home health workers and/or community services and support personnel, and other providers who see the patient.

4. **Continuous access to care** with shorter waits to get appointments, enhanced hours for clinical services, and alternative methods of communication, including e-mail and telephone.

5. **A systems-based approach to quality and safety**, including: (a) using evidence-based medicine and clinical decision-support tools to guide decision-making, as evidenced by attainment of quality indicators, (b) the practice and the indicators include patients and families participation in performance measurement and improvement, (c) patient satisfaction that is measured and then acted upon, and (d) the practice actively participates in population health management. (Esterhay, 2014)

Assessments of the impact of PCMH are only recently becoming available. For example, practices that attained PCMH recognition status had lower costs for Medicare patients than practices that did not attain recognition. (van Hasselt M, McCall N, Keyes V, Wensky SG, Smith KW. 2014; Fogarty, 2014) Reports from PCPCC show consistency between industry and academic reports for cost savings associated with implementing PCPCC. (PCPCC, 2012) But these results are early, and comprehensive examinations of the overall impact of the PCMH model, rather than a comparison of component outcomes, do not yet exist.

PCMH and the Chronic Care Model

The focus of PCMH includes a clinical orientation to the whole person, providing care for patients over their entire life span, with expertise and attention to acute care, chronic care, preventive services, and end of life care. Care is coordinated and/or integrated across all elements of the complex health care system (e.g., subspecialty care, hospitals, home health agencies, nursing homes) and within the patient's community (e.g., family, public and private community-based services). Clinical care is facilitated by disease registries, health information technology and information exchange, and other means to assure that patients get the indicated care when and where they need and want it, in a culturally and linguistically appropriate manner. Effective, high quality care and patient safety are three hallmarks of the medical home.

The ACP issued a policy monograph about the Advanced Medical Home (AMH). (ACP, 2005) One of the key attributes of the AMH was an emphasis on the Chronic Care Model (CCM), as originally designed and implemented by Dr. Ed Wagner and associates. (Rothman & Wagner, 2003; Wagner, Austin, & Von Korff, 1996) This recommendation is important as treatment of chronic illness is a major stress on the current healthcare system and a factor in rising financial expenditures within the United States. (Vogeli et al., 2007)

The components of the CCM are consistent and compatible with those of the PCMH. Common elements and activities include: enhancing capacities to link clinical services with community resources and policies; delivery system re-design, with emphasis on team care to support engaging and activating patients with skills in self-management; clinical information systems, including EMRs, as an aid for care, including case management and disease management; and the availability of on-site decision support tools for clinicians and staff. Concurrently transforming a practice to PCMH, while building the infrastructure of the CCM, seems like a reasonable and efficient strategy to meet the challenges of a reformed health system by improving patient-centered outcomes.

Patient-Centered Medical Homes and Reforming the Health Care Reimbursement Model

Payment reforms for primary care physicians are necessary to assure success of PCMH. The Group Health feasibility study of PCMH (Reid et al., 2010), and other reports about incorporating behavioral health into PCMH (Brandon, Bair, & Kathol, 2011), conclude that providing additional time with patients with multiple comorbidities (one of the principles of the

PCMH model) may require downsizing patient panels for practices and/or providers, with the concurrent risk of incurring additional financial losses as a result of such actions. There is evidence that inadequate time for person-centered consultations may be a stimulus for some physicians to use testing or referrals to specialists as a means to solve clinical questions. (González-González et al., 2007) PCMH and team-based care can include the provision "in house" of specialty care services for select, highly prevalent conditions. This is discussed later, in the innovations section.

Collaborative care models, such as PCMH, CIN, and ACO, typically employ case managers to ensure proper diagnosis, treatment and follow-up of patients. (Compton, 2012) Adding nurse case managers to physician practices creates new costs, especially in practices not used to these services, and as a result many PCMH do not add these new resources. Without assistance from case managers, some experts suggest that the size of primary care physician panels might need to be reduced by a third, in order to accommodate the extra time needed for implementing evidence-based guidelines. (Brandon et al., 2011) Naturally, reimbursements for such a large reduction in panel size must compensate clinicians for the extra time and resources used to integrate services, or new methods will be needed to address financial concerns. One paradoxical finding in the current, FFS payment scheme that pays specialists more for equivalent services is that the complexity and breadth of care provided by PCP, measured by the numbers of diagnostic codes accounting for 50% of codes used by physicians, is far higher when compared to the number of codes used by specialists. (Freeman, Patterson, Bazemore, 2014) In other words, PCPs generally treat patients with more complex arrays of medical conditions, yet they are paid less than specialists.

Health care reimbursement is complex, making it difficult for any proposed changes in physician reimbursement for services. In 1992, after years of discussion, debate, and legislation, the Health Care Financing Administration (HCFA, now called the Centers for Medicare & Medicaid Services, or CMS) implemented the Resource-Based Relative Value Scale

(RBRVS), a system that consolidated and standardized physician payment by assigning relative value units (RVUs) for all professional services. The RBRVS had two main goals: to contain the total cost of all physician services, and to correct the imbalance between payments for purely cognitive clinical encounters, which are the main services provided by primary care physicians (e.g., office visits, consultations, preventive medicine visits, collectively known as evaluation and management, or E&M services) and procedural services mainly delivered by specialists (e.g., surgery, interpretation of diagnostic tests).

However, neither of these original goals has been achieved. Compensation to primary care physicians is woefully behind physicians who perform procedures. The RBRVS has been cited as having a number of flaws, including: the full range of office-based E&M activities are not captured by the Current Procedural Terminology (CPT) code set; RBRVS places relatively high values on procedural services; and there are no measures of intensity for complex outpatient E&M care. (Kumetz & Goodson, 2013) It is interesting to note that the Relative Value Scale Update Committee (RUC) that makes relative value recommendations to CMS, is composed mostly of specialty physicians, so changes favoring primary care alone will likely be politically difficult. (AMA, 2014)

For example, PCPs who provide services to complex patients with multiple co-morbidities do not have adequate coding mechanisms to reflect the value of their decision-making and care coordination services, especially in comparison to procedure-based providers. This has led to a severe payment disparity between providers of non-invasive types of care and those who perform procedure-centered clinical work. For example, the total income gap, or relative shortfall, for primary-care physicians compared to specialists has increased from an average 61% in 1995 to 89% in 2008. In other words, on average, procedurally-oriented specialists are now compensated at rates that are nearly twice that for primary care physicians. (Moses et al., 2013)

Escalating costs and the growing imbalance between primary and specialty care have increased the urgency of calls for fundamental reform of the health care payment system. (Rosenthal M.B., 2008b) The dominant FFS model of financial reimbursement offers more rewards to providers who perform high volume and high intensity services, rather than rewarding value of care delivered. One approach to diminish the differences between specialty care services and primary care services is to bolster incentives for high quality outcomes for all providers involved in PCMH. As this book goes to press, CMS will reimburse for care coordination for beneficiaries with two or more chronic conditions. It will be interesting to see how these will be used and how they will be accepted by beneficiaries, as the services are provided at a cost to the beneficiary.

The forms of reimbursement a PCP receives for clinical services can influence the future of primary care workforce development. Each type of payment system may result in different quantities and patterns of care. (Gosden et al., 2000) For example, under both salary and capitation payment systems, the PCPs know in advance the amount of payment they will receive before any care is provided. Some PCPs are paid an annual salary to work a set number of hours per week per year. Salaried payments to PCPs are usually not associated with any encouragement or discouragement for any level of patient care. Capitation systems pay PCPs a set amount per patient registered with them or currently in their care. Capitation systems include prospective payment, which may encourage PCPs to contain costs, potentially underutilizing necessary care.

FFS payment systems reimburse the PCP for each item of service provided (the fee usually depends on the type of service) and payment occurs after care has been provided. Overall, evidence from a review of only four studies suggests that PCPs paid by FFS provide a higher quantity of primary care services, when compared with PCPs under capitation and PCPs receiving salaries. However, the evidence for impact of payment systems is not sufficiently robust to be used and/or applied in every policy context. (Gosden et al., 2000) Therefore, depending on the level of the fee, there may be an incentive to deliver more care, in order to attain threshold values and so inflate the clinician's personal income. An alternative option is for the clinicians to provide less care during each patient encounter, in order to attain a higher volume of patients and services, or as a means to see other patients whose payer may provide better financial incentives.

There are also regional variations in healthcare spending, quality and outcomes. This is demonstrated by the well-known Dartmouth Healthcare Atlas, which has published variations in utilization of health resources for over 20 years in the United States. According to the Atlas, Medicare enrollees in higher-spending regions receive more care than those in lower-spending regions, but they do not have better health outcomes or satisfaction with care. (Fisher E.S., et al., 2003b) Fisher demonstrated that quality of care and clinical outcomes do not necessarily improve as the regional costs of care increase. The increased costs of care were mostly attributed to increases in activities associated with supply-sensitive specialist physicians. (Fisher et al., 2003a, 2003b; Fisher, & Wennberg, 2003c)

Fisher and associates suggest that preference-based care and supply-sensitive care are two forms of healthcare services most associated with escalating costs in the United States. (Fisher & Wennberg, 2003d)

Atul Gawande, MD, MPH, a surgeon, author, and Harvard University professor, published a 2009 article in the *New Yorker* magazine that made similar findings about costs and regional variations between two towns in Texas, each associated with different cultures of medical care. (Gawande, 2009) Physicians in the town of McAllen, Texas were reported to be most interested in receiving high reimbursement rates. Accordingly, they allegedly "gamed" the healthcare system by ordering excessive numbers of tests, performing many procedures with low likelihood of yielding clinically useful results, and requesting many consultations with their specialty peers, all as a means to attain their payment goals. The comparison physician groups in El Paso, Texas described themselves as more altruistic, with interests in good patient outcomes. They made their best efforts toward benefiting patients, and they also managed to keep overall costs lower.

Despite much higher costs and the provision of more clinical services by physicians, McAllen patients were not healthier in comparison to those in El Paso. Gawande reported that physician behaviors can escalate the costs of healthcare without improving the health status of patients. Potential solutions to the cost-quality conundrum identified by Fisher and Gawande include greater use of clinically-based medical decision-making to better align costs, effectiveness and desired clinical outcomes. (Sox, Higgins, & Owens, 2013)

PCMH, Complexity and the Clinical Transformation Process

Transformation of primary care, including changes to clinical and business processes, and continuous improvement, are major features of PCMH adoption for the individual practice. However, published findings are mixed as to both the effectiveness and results of these changes. In June 2006, the American Academy of Family Physicians launched the first National Demonstration Project (NDP) to test a model of the PCMH in a diverse national sample of 36 family practices. (Nutting et al., 2009) NDP was designed to evaluate whether facilitated change toward adoption of PCMH among select Family Medicine clinics was more effective than self-directed change processes. After slightly more than two years, both groups showed only small improvements in condition-specific quality of care measures, but there were no changes in measures of patient experience of care. (Jaén et al., 2010) For example, EHR adoption (one of the major tenets of PCMH) was recognized as a new technology that demanded time, service learning and adaptation among all personnel, rather than being a "plug-and-play" type of tool. In short, all clinical and staff personnel needed to adapt to new techniques and technologies, and adaptation is a slow process. Replicate studies over time may show larger changes in quality outcomes after the practices adapt to organizational changes.

Crabtree and associates 15-years of research on program development highlighted the limitations of viewing primary care practices in mechanistic terms, as per the current and traditional approaches to quality improvement. (Crabtree et al., 2011) They propose a theoretical perspective that views primary care practices as dynamic complex adaptive systems (CAS), with "agents" (e.g., people serving in different roles, including clinicians, staff, technicians, patients and families, etc.) who each have capacities to learn, and the freedom to act in unpredictable ways. (Miller, Crabtree, Nutting, Stange, & Jaén, 2010)

There are advantages to viewing healthcare interventions as processes within CAS. A major finding from follow-up studies of the NDP is that,

> ...although it is feasible to transform independent practices into the NDP conceptualization of a PCMH, this transformation requires tremendous effort and motivation, and benefits from external support. Most practices will need additional resources for this magnitude of transformation. (Crabtree et al., 2010)

Clinical transformation to PCMH was recognized as a feasible but difficult task as it involved changes in all aspects of work flow and work routines. (Solberg et al., 2014) A survey of items correlated with systems changes within PCMH were nearly all from categories of patients, organizational change and culture. (Solberg, et al., 2014) It appears that no single mechanistic change in clinic operations will result in improvements. Rather, multi-faceted strategies will likely be required, and each practice may need to find its own approach to fit its own unique situation, personnel and qualities of relationship. As Solberg and associates report, "There may not be any silver bullets that work for all or even most clinics."(Solberg, et al., 2014, p. 456) Thus, effectively transforming PCP into PCMH is a task that will take a long time to accomplish, with a lot of effort from all members of the clinical team.

The notions of generalizability of strategies to implement a PCMH and the necessity for specific leadership skills within complex, prototypic organizations are questioned in the NDP framework. Rather, the authors emphasize the individual agents and the qualities of their interactions and relationships. It is from this complex array of diverse, interactive qualities among agents that the transformation of the PCMH organization can emerge. Transformation is seen as a phenomenon that depends upon the qualities of the interactive, dynamic whole, rather than the properties of any one or group of individuals. As such, what works in one practice may not work in another. Stated from a more positive perspective, there are many different approaches to achieving good outcomes. (Crabtree et al., 2005)

Crabtree states that the CAS approach provides a better theoretical framework for grounding quality improvement strategies. Accordingly, CAS approaches are more likely to achieve success than the use of more conventional prescriptive, top-down methods. (Crabtree et al., 2011) The CAS framework strongly emphasizes that quality improvement interventions should not only use the perspectives of complex systems, but continual reflection and attendance to the qualities of relationships within the present situation ("mindful awareness") is also needed by the participating agents. Mindful awareness is thus a key element in the transformation process to PCMH.

According to the CAS, the human element of people in relationships as caring "agents" is the starting point for effectively treating patients with diseases and medical needs, helping to reduce individual patient health risks within the PCMH, improving the collective health status of community-based populations, and evaluating the success of each aspect of health and medical care. Attention to the dynamics and qualities of interactive processes between agents is essential for progress within the CAS framework, more so than prioritizing conventional strategies that focus upon distant outcomes. The latter tend to be imposed externally by conventional leaders within (or upon) a top-down hierarchy. The CAS framework is well-suited for bottom-up methods, interpersonal relating, and consensus development. This is often a missing piece in more conventional, strategic, top-down approaches to organizational transformation.

It is likely that both bottom-up and top-down methods are necessary for effective change within organizations, including practice sites attempting to be PCMH, as well as communities and societies interested in adopting this model. (Grol, Wensing, Eccles, & Davis, 2013) Shared leadership, rather than a single dominant physician leader within PCMH, may be one means to success, especially when attempting to overcome divisions within a clinical practice involving administrative support staff. (Crabtree et al., 2008) Contributing to the sustainability of networks of leaders, providers, patients and care-givers may be one variety of CAS- approach to organizational management that is at least as important as traditional care models for individuals.

Success will likely depend upon the presence of adaptive reserves, and the capacities of healthcare leaders to improve the practice of medicine, from primarily technically-oriented sciences to a more relationship-centered model of care. (Klein, Laugesen, & Liu, 2013; Thygeson, Morrissey, & Ulstad, 2010) In addition, most practices will need additional support and resources to make a meaningful transformation. (Crabtree et al., 2010) The costly habit of substituting technical interventions for situations that require adaptive work is a prevalent problem in modern medicine – one that represents a failure of adaptive leadership. (Thygeson et al., 2010; p. 1014)

Transformation to PCMH in a CAS context requires that clinicians develop fresh perspectives on clinical, organization and systems issues, so they can engage with patients with the awareness that all parties are facing social, technical and/or adaptive challenges. These changes represent a paradigm shift in health services in many societies. As such, transforming to a PCMH by focusing on qualities of relationships within clinical service sites represents a change in culture. Consistent with RCC, we might call this a transformation to a "culture of caring".

Addressing Primary Care Workforce Issues

Physician supply and demand in the United States is a complex phenomenon, especially because of federal government laws that subsidize physician training and changes brought about by implementation of the ACA. (Kirch, Henderson, & Dill, 2012) Physician supply issues include the aging of current practicing physicians, static growth in the number of graduate medical education (GME) residency training positions supported by the federal government, and the apparent preferences of younger physicians to work fewer hours. Physician demand issues include increased utilization by an enlarging and aging population, economic growth, and increased demand caused by expanded health insurance coverage from the ACA.

Access to affordable care is another physician supply and demand issue, and an important aspect of success in delivery of primary care. Although access cannot be denied to hospital-based emergency care, by federal law, that point of entry to the healthcare system is not efficient. Despite massive expenditures, disparities exist in access to healthcare, as exemplified by 20% of the population that were residing in federally designated health professions shortage areas (HPSA) in 2007. (Kirch & Vernon, 2008)

Demand for primary care services is projected to increase through 2020, due largely to aging and population growth and, to a lesser extent, expanded health insurance coverage under the ACA. In addition, there are many projections and opinions about physician shortages, especially within the context of the ACA. In 2020, the U.S. may face shortages of 45,400 primary care physicians and 46,100 medical specialists—a total of 91,500 too few doctors. (Kirch et al., 2012) These authors project a shortage of 64,100 physicians, even if the ACA were not implemented.

Population growth will be the greatest driver of expected increases in primary care demand, according to some authors, while aging and insurance coverage expansion will also contribute to utilization, but to a smaller extent. These authors cite population growth as the most important issue driving the need for more physicians, accounting for 33,000 additional physicians, while 10,000 additional physicians will be needed to accommodate the aging population. Next, insurance coverage expansion will require more than 8,000 additional physicians, a 3% increase in the current workforce. The total number of office visits to primary care physicians is projected to increase from 462 million in 2008 to 565 million in 2025, driven mostly by population growth and aging. After incorporating insurance expansion, the United States will require nearly 52,000 additional primary care physicians by 2025. (Petterson et al., 2012)

The United States needs sufficient family physicians and other primary care providers to form the foundation of a health care system that meets the Triple Aim. At the present time, 32% of practicing physicians in the United States are primary care providers, with 12.7% being family physicians, 10.9% general internists, 6.8% general pediatricians, and 1.6% general practitioners. (COGME, 2010) Only 16 - 18% of medical students who obtained positions through the National Resident Matching Program in 2010 are likely to select and practice primary care. (Iglehart, 2010) Among those who elect to pursue Internal Medicine specialties, only about 20% remain in primary care. (Schwartz, 2012) A Council on Graduate Medical Education (Council) report called for an increase in the percentage of U.S. primary care physicians to at least 40% of the total U.S. physician workforce. Currently, this goal is not being met. (COGME, 2010)

Most internists are lured away from primary care by the higher incomes of sub-specialties in internal medicine, such as cardiology or gastroenterology. Specialists have higher mean salaries compared to primary care, often by a factor of 2-3x or more. The Council also called for a narrowing of the payment gap between primary care and specialty care physicians. (COGME, 2010) For example, Family Medicine physicians had the lowest mean annual salaries ($185,740), as well as the lowest fill rate in residency positions with programs that provided care for elderly patients (42.1%). (Ebell, 2008) The remaining primary care residency positions are often filled with international medical graduates.

The trends in numbers of graduates from U.S. medical schools who chose primary care residencies are not favorable. (AHRQ, 2012) Also, increasing enrollment in U.S. medical schools does not necessarily translate into an increase in the percentage of U.S. physicians entering Family Medicine. Decreased matriculation of primary care physicians from graduate medical education is a reflection of the choices made by young physicians. Only one in six medical students now state intention to enter into primary care. Changes in values among younger physicians make the shortage worse, due to their expressed desire for control of their time, more so than the long hours being on-call to attend to patients' needs. (Arnetz, 1997)

Most solutions for the projected workforce shortage of primary care providers, especially for primary care physicians, have long lead times for attaining educational and professional certification goals. Traditional training of medical doctors includes 3-4 years for an undergraduate degree, four years for medical school training, and 3-5 years for residency training and fellowships. New models for medical school reduce training to three years. (Emanuel & Fuchs, 2012) There are calls for discussions about the financial, educational, and policy ramifications of national initiatives to promote primary care. (Mullan, 2003)

On the other hand, some disagree with fast-tracking graduate medical education or using non-physician "surrogates" as physician-extenders. For example, given the increasing complexity of medical care systems, there are calls for physicians to attain additional advanced degrees, including MPH, MBA, MMM, MHA, or other degrees. (Linney, 1998) A new four year dual-degree program (M.D., Sc.M.) in Primary Care and Population Health at the Warren Alpert Medical School at Brown University provides training in leadership skills, public health policy and the impact of the social determinants of health, as well as relevant medical knowledge and clinical management skills. (AAMC, 2013) Medical schools in Louisville, Kentucky, New York, Kansas, Indiana, Texas, North Carolina and many others have rural medicine rotations for students and residents that will likely promote selection and completion of primary care residencies.

CMS Innovation projects are supporting transformation of primary care. CMS has funded and implemented multi-payer reform initiatives that are currently being conducted by states to make advanced primary care practices more broadly available. The demonstrations will evaluate whether advanced primary care practice will reduce unjustified utilization and expenditures, improve the safety, effectiveness, timeliness, and efficiency of health care, increase appropriate patient decision-making, and increase the availability and delivery of care in underserved areas. For example, the Michigan Primary Care Transformation Project (MiPCT) is a three-year multi-payer project aimed at improving health in the state, making care more affordable, and strengthening the patient-care team relationship. MiPCT is state-wide in scope and is one of the largest PCMH projects in the nation, with approximately 400 primary care practices and 1900 primary care physicians and mid-level providers. (CMS, 2014a)

There are new approaches to more fully develop medical students' interests in primary care and the attractiveness of PCMHs at multiple universities. (AAMC, 2013) For example, the University of California, San Francisco (UCSF) administers the Program in Medical Education for the Urban Underserved (PRIME-US) to provide clinical experiences with populations at the lower spectrum of the social gradient of health. However, the current freeze on Medicare support to teaching hospitals for graduate medical education at 1996 levels by Congress limits the feasibility for expanding the supply pipeline for the physician workforce at most academic medical centers. Nevertheless, Title VII funding and new Health Resources and Services Administration (HRSA, an agency in the U.S. Department of Health and Human Services) initiatives for the Teaching Health Center program provide new opportunities for increasing the numbers and proportions of primary care physicians through collaboration between academic health centers and community health centers. (Rieselbach RE, et.al. 2013)

Other new programs have been announced and implemented by CMS. One initiative offers $840 million in funding to provider networks, professional associations, and other organizations providing education and training in the transition to value-based health care. The "Transforming Clinical Practice Initiative" is a 4-year project designed to support 150,000 clinicians in sharing, adapting and further developing comprehensive quality improvement strategies, which are expected to lead to greater improvements in patient health and reduction in health care costs. Funding is awarded in two general areas: "practice transformation networks" that involve peer-to-peer learning and "support and alignment networks" that involve learning opportunities created by professional associations, societies, and other organizations. (CMS, 2014c)

Finally, non-physician extenders in primary care include advanced registered nurse practitioners (ARNP) and physicians' assistants (PA). They are also part of the care team in PCMH, CIN, ACO, and other models of care and they are a new resource group to help alleviate the primary care physician shortage. Cochrane reviews of the outcomes of nurse practitioners demonstrate that:

> ...appropriately trained nurses can produce as high quality care as primary care doctors and achieve as good health outcomes for patients. However, this conclusion should be viewed with caution given that only one study in the review was statistically powered to assess equivalence of care. Many studies in the review had methodological limitations, and patient follow-up was generally 12 months or less. (Laurant, et. al., 2004)

Many ARNPs are electing to serve with and as specialists, rather than with PCPs. The combination of a fragmented health care system, high debt levels among medical students, the quicker timeline for graduation of ARPNs, and the continuing disparity in earnings between specialists and PCP may serve to further devalue primary care physicians in the eyes of patients and potential new medical school recruits. More time will be needed to see how the potential for competition or collaboration between physician and non-physician clinicians will play out.

Innovations in Primary Care and PCMH

Transformation within PCMH, CIN and ACO allows different forms of innovation to be tried and tested. Alternatively, some innovations may become the rationale for transforming existing practices into PCMH, CIN or ACO. We suggest five areas often addressed by PCMH, CIN and ACO that may be considered innovations within primary care:

1. Integrating Behavioral and Mental Health with Primary Care

2. Making Effective Linkages with Public Health to Address Social Determinants of Health

3. Employing Lay Community Health Workers to Address Cultural Health Issues

4. Aligning New Metrics with Financial Incentives

5. Adopting a Complexity Paradigm for Transformational Change

Each topic is briefly addressed here.

1. Integrating Behavioral and Mental Health with Primary Care

Models for integrating behavioral and mental health practices into primary care have been proposed. (Manderscheid & Kathol, 2014; Baird M, Blount A, Brungardt S, Dickinson P, Dietrich A, Epperly T, et al., 2014; See also Chapter 11.) These authors compare three different models: the classic referral model, the bi-directional model, and the integrated model, whereby mental and behavioral health specialists provide relevant clinical and support services for the PCMH. The authors also review current models for providing medical and mental health services to patients, describe an alternative model for integrating behavioral health into primary care settings, and cite evidence that clinical improvements and cost savings are possible for patients with depression or anxiety, using integrated models. Tierney and associates (2014) report on two successful models for ACO that integrate behavioral health services with primary care. The characteristics of the models differ, but the PCP retains the role as primary coordinator of care and services in each realm.

Kathol and associates reported that the biggest barrier to integrating behavioral health care in primary care settings is financial. (Kathol, Butler, McAlpine, & Kane, 2010) Physical health and mental health are interactive, with estimates that about a third of patients with a medical condition will also have a mental health diagnosis, and about two-thirds of mental health patients will have a co-existing medical condition. However, current reimbursement methods for mental and behavioral categories are segregated from those for primary care. (Menachemi, Matthews, Ford, &

Brooks, 2007) Kathol and associates suggest a model for co-locating primary care and mental health services. They cite means to achieve success, based on interviews with key informants from integrated models, and suggest that models that integrate services for mental health and primary care will likely best utilize a transformational approach, rather than an "add-on" approach. Paths to success include a culture shift in both the clinical and administrative domains, and a clear vision that favors population health. (Kathol, Butler, McAlpine, & Kane, 2010) Chapter 11 has a detailed discussion from Dr. Kathol and his colleagues.

Collaborative care for the management of depressive disorders was recommended as a proven and effective strategy by the Community Guide for Preventive Services in June 2010. It was the topic of an extensive systematic review and meta-analyses. (Thota et al., 2012) Thota and her associates provided robust evidence for the effectiveness of collaborative care in improving depression symptoms, adherence to treatment, response to treatment, remission and recovery from symptoms, improvements in measures of quality of life and functional status, and satisfaction with care for patients diagnosed with depression. She also noted that collaborative care interventions provide a supportive network of professionals and peers for patients with depression, especially at the primary care level. Similarly, in 2012, the Community Guide for Preventive Services recommended support for legislation for parity and coverage of mental health benefits.

2. Making Effective Linkages with Public Health to Address the Social Determinants of Health

Linking activities in Public Health with PCMH may be one means to address the social determinants of health. As previously mentioned, social determinants of health are the circumstances in which people are born, live, work, and play. They are shaped by a wide set of economic, social policy, and political forces that are external to the traditional realm of healthcare. Sir Michael Marmot has generalized findings from many research studies, including the Whitehall II Studies, into a concept known as the "social gradient of health."(Marmot, MG 2013; Marmot MG, 2006; Marmot MG, et al., 1991)

Marmot observed that the poorest of the poor, around the world, tend to have the worst health status. Within countries, evidence shows that people with lower socioeconomic position tend to have the worst health status, as compared to their peers and neighbors with more resources. There are decrements in health status that run in a social gradient of good health, for those with the highest social status, to the poorest health status for those at the bottom of the socio-economic spectrum. (Adler NE, et al., 1994; Marmot, MG, 2006)

Both the social determinants of health and other disease-oriented measures follow a social gradient of health. A social gradient was identified for the presence or absence of diseases, risk factors, and community resources -- such as adequacy of housing and education. (M. Marmot, 2013) The poor tend to have a greater prevalence and incidence of diseases, risk factors, and less access to community resources, such as adequate housing and education. The social gradient of health is ubiquitous. It is present for those with only slightly lesser status in comparison to a more affluent or higher ranking person or group, such that even Vice Presidents in an organization, for example, are more likely to show relative decrements in health status when compared to measures among Presidents or CEOs. (Marmot, 2013)

Galea and associates showed that the magnitude of cause-specific death rates attributable to the social determinants of health are comparable to those from diseases. (Galea, Tracy, Hoggatt, DiMaggio, & Karpati, 2011) Steiner argues for an approach to manage the resource-base of the social determinants of population health as a complement to the disease-oriented approach of medical care for individuals. Risk in such a socio-cultural-ecologic approach to population health is defined as the lack of access to common social resources, such as adequate food and housing, and educational attainment. The resource base for social health can be measured through wellness indicators that are independent but interactive with measures of disease and illness. (Steiner, 2014)

The current epidemiological transition, with a focus on socially-enmeshed health concerns, is complex -- with no simple treatment or cure from any external noxious agent or problematic situation. Rather, the solutions to socially-enmeshed health concerns may lie within the fabric of society itself. When considering socially-enmeshed health concerns, Kartman eloquently stated, "...the ecology of human disease must start with the social fabric.... The starting point is not disease or the prevalence of infection, and it is not epidemiology -- it is the social unit."(Kartman, 1967; p. 745)

In essence, a change in culture may be a possible solution for socially-enmeshed health concerns.

Therefore, making effective linkages between PCMH and public health is a means for enabling the tripartite cycle for public health: to assess, improve and assure better population health through the design and implementation of effective health policies. (Institute of Medicine, 1988) This three part cycle for public health seems a reasonable contextual arena for developing innovations in PCMH. Health policy is one way of making new social norms.

To understand the importance of public health in the PCMH context, we must look beyond the costs to the healthcare system, and account for societal losses, such as losses to employers from diminished productivity or increased absenteeism, or even inability of some people to find or keep a job due to declines in social role performance, sometimes associated with mental health issues. For example, evidence indicates that collaborative care for management of depressive disorders provides good economic value, including results from multiple cost-benefit and cost-utility studies. (Jacob et al., 2012) However, Jacob points out that a selection bias is present in the review, in that all studies examined consistently used the perspective of the healthcare system, rather than a societal perspective to assess the true impact on public health. In addition, the studies reviewed only included patients who were already enrolled within existing sites and/or programs. They did not address people who were lost to follow-up or marginalized from society as a result of their disease, nor did the studies include those who were fired from their jobs or who performed poorly while at their jobs, resulting in lost wages and lost productivity, respectively. These and other public and social health perspectives will likely enlarge the scope and magnitude of financial considerations at risk. Yet, public health policy solutions are often much less expensive to implement, compared to biomedical solutions.

The meaning of population health is a problem within research designs about the effectiveness and impact of PCMH, CIN and ACO, as most studies are typically limited to population sectors, such as "covered lives", rather than attending to all residents within a geo-political area, which is the traditional purview of public health. As such, systematic reviews more often represent measures of efficacy, rather than effectiveness, in that they include only patients who accessed the medical care system. This selection and information bias limits the generalizability of the results to the societal or public health perspectives, rather than the more narrow population health construct, as typically defined and implemented in CIN and ACO.

3. Employing Lay Community Health Workers to Address Cultural Health Issues

Historically, lay community health workers (LCHW) helped to create conditions in which people can be healthier within a community or neighborhood. LCHW include members of the community who are not healthcare professionals that assist with outreach to vulnerable, low-income, and underserved populations, and federal government defined "navigators:" trained workers who assist new and prospective enrollees to access ACA-established Health Insurance Exchanges, including expanded Medicaid services and access to FQHPs.

As trusted community members who also understand the health and social service systems, LCHWs are uniquely positioned to work within communities to address the social determinants of health. (Rosenthal, Wiggins, Ingram, Mayfield-Johnson, & De Sapiens, 2011) Researchers should be careful to differentiate between LCHW facilitating medical treatment interventions from those who influence social support for their patients and contacts although these services are often integrated in practice

There is a rich literature and history associated with cultural traditions of LCHW. One example includes *promotores de salud* (Spanish: promoters of [good] health), who assist with management of diabetes, asthma and other chronic conditions, especially among Latino neighborhoods or groups. *Promotores* are active in the west and southwest United States (Ferrer et al., 2013). Another version of LCHW include *doulas* (Greek: female servant; also known as "labor coaches" or "birth attendants"), who typically assist women with child-bearing and related family issues. (Hartmann et al., 2012) The CDC, Department of Health and Human Services, and most public health agencies support these roles for *doulas*. (CDC, 2011)

LCHW are categorically promoted within the ACA, to serve as liaison for community residents who are not accessing the medical care system in effective ways. Multiple systematic reviews of the research literature are available, and the results are cohesive and supportive of LCHW. One Cochrane report, however, states:

> Overall, lay health worker programs appear to be effective for some kinds of healthcare, but there is not yet enough evidence to say that this is true for all or most kinds of healthcare. Compared to usual care, lay health worker programs to increase immunization (vaccination) in children and adults and programs to improve health in people with lung infections and malaria may be effective. These programs may also be effective in increasing breastfeeding, and in decreasing death in the elderly through providing home aide services.... It is also not known how best lay health workers should provide services and how much training they need to be effective. (Lewin et al., 2005)

Social support from LCHW is a well-known factor in the etiology, progression and recovery from disease, at both the individual and collective levels. (Cohen & Wills, 1985; Broadhead, Kaplan, James, et. al., 1983) Social support is also a family and community resource that can be cultivated to aid those with the most need and fewest resources. Common cultural backgrounds between LCHW and community members may serve to overcome embedded socio-cultural barriers to favor improved health. (N. Adler et al., 2007)

Peer-specialists are people, including former patients, who have a "lived experience" with mental illness or with successful recovery. They are another form of LCHW, and can serve as allied mental health workers. Peer-specialists may interact with patients to enhance outcomes (M. Salzer, Schwenk, & Brusilovskiy, 2010; M. S. Salzer, 2010), although Thota found a smaller effect for this group, when compared to the outcomes for case managers, such as nurses and social workers. (Thota et al., 2012) Skill levels for peer-specialists and case managers should be reported in future studies, and perhaps periodically assessed in clinical practices, to better substantiate the evidence and the benefits.

Rather than being seen as a lesser trained health worker, LCHWs represent a different, and sometimes preferred, type of health worker for some groups of patients and community residents. (Glenton et al., 2013) Indeed, the close relationships between LCHWs and recipients of medical care are an asset that can be cultivated to improve outreach programs and care, especially when health extends beyond the domain of medical care services, and into social determinants of health. Likewise, using LCHW as resources for people involved in the criminal justice system may be an innovative approach to reduce recidivism. (Csete & Cohen, 2010; Sauber & Vetter, 2013)

4. Aligning New Metrics with Financial Incentives

Metrics focus attention on what is perceived to be important. (Stange et al., 2014) New business and clinical models with new dimensions of healthcare, such as PCMH, CIN and ACO, require new metrics.

Measures for continuity of care, for example, are not commonly used to evaluate success within PCMH. Yet the continuity and qualities of relationships between patients and providers are potent influences for developing meaningful, satisfactory and successful medical encounters and outcomes. (B. Starfield & Horder, 2007; Wagner et al., 2012) Lower financial reimbursements for PCP tend to support efforts to increase patient volume. This may lead to more referrals to specialists, rather than spending extra time with patients and families to manage the complicated constellations of signs, symptoms and treatment options that may be present. Yet this pattern of healthcare delivery is expensive and detracts from continuity of care. (Berenson et al., 2008) Metrics for continuity of care are a topic of international research efforts. (Uijen et al., 2012) Some questionnaires, such as the Primary Care Assessment Tool (PCAT), show psychometric properties as evidence for validity of the measurement scale in association with patients' reported satisfaction ratings with their clinical experiences in primary care. (Rocha et al., 2012)

We propose a new method for reimbursement of primary care providers, based upon metrics for continuity of care. In keeping with names for past incentives, this new incentive might be called "pay for continuity of care." There is evidence that measuring longitudinal continuity of care with instruments such as the General Practice Assessment Questionnaires (GPAQ and GPAQ-R) are useful for measuring and evaluating continuity of care (Roland, Roberts, Rhenius, & Campbell, 2013). Likewise, others have suggested incentivizing payments for continuity of care in the United Kingdom. (Freeman & Hughes, 2010) Family Medicine researchers from the United States have suggested that first applying metrics and building infrastructures to support highly leveraged activities in primary care, including care for patients with depressive symptoms and common mental health issues, will best serve continuity of care and positive encounters for patients and providers. (Eidus, Pace, & Staton, 2012)

There are other means to increase payments to primary care providers, including regulatory means at the state level directed at insurers. The Insurance Commissioner for Rhode Island initiated a regulatory agenda to increase the percentage of total annual medical spending within the state for primary care services from 6% to 11%, for a small group of fully-insured individuals. The increases in reimbursed payments to primary care providers were to be implemented over time, increasing by one percent each year for five years. (Koller CF, Brennan TA, Bailit MH, 2010) The increase in primary care spending is mandated, and is to be in the form of pay-for-performance compensation, rather than increasing the standard fees for medical services. The specification of the minimum goal of increased spending for primary care at 11% of total medical spending came from comparisons to the spending levels for primary care among high performing, integrated medical care delivery systems, such as Geisinger in Pennsylvania, Group Health Cooperative of Puget Sound and others. This is a project that will be followed closely, with evaluation reports to follow.

5. Adopting a Complexity Paradigm for Transformational Change in Evolving PCMH

Complexity approaches within health care are prominent in popular and professional literature. (McDaniel Jr & Driebe, 2001; McDaniel, Driebe, & Lanham, 2013) All people participating in medical care (and, indeed, any human activity!) are involved in complex adaptive relationships. Schneider & Somers highlight a tendency for many people to reify the idea of complexity, despite its nature as an abstraction or a means to explain applications in the context of organizational dynamics. (Schneider & Somers, 2006) Paley and Eva succinctly state, "Complexity systems mimic design; they are not examples of it."(Paley & Eva, 2011, p. 273.)

They argue that there is no conceptual link between order and design in complexity; indeed that link with human intentionality is severed, by the very definitions of "emergence" and "self-organization". Within a self-organizing system, "...there is no blueprint and no plan... such that individuals act unilaterally without reference to the possible structures or global order that they (might) create."(Paley & Eva, 2011, p. 273)

One implication of the complexity model is that culture itself may be viewed as an emergent phenomenon of a collective aspect of a population. Culture is a shared, interactive relational resource created by the interactions and shared values among people living together in society. Some have suggested that RCC be the more appropriate terminology for

PCMH, as it goes beyond our implicit cultural notions of individualism, to include complexity notions, such as relationships with practitioners and providers, as well as with family, neighbors, community, and society. (Nolan, Keady, & Aveyard, 2001)

The name "relationship-centered care" (RCC) really implies that the patient is a co-learner and a team member who attends and participates in a primary care practice site. (W.L. Miller et al., 2010) This aspect of RCC implicates the notion of transformational change. The depth of change required by RCC for traditional clinical settings to become a PCMH involves a difficult and transformational process, and is better viewed as an ongoing journey rather than a goal. (Stange, 2014; Stange et al., 2014)

Transformational change also requires transformational leadership. There are differences between traditional leaders and transformational leaders. Traditional leaders and managers apply known solutions to known problems. Traditional leadership describes a role, rather than a set of behaviors; it places power within the position rather than within the context and presence of relationships. (Plowman & Duchon, 2008) The traditional leadership model assumes that the world is knowable and that strategic planning and exercising control can bring about desired outcomes. Three problems limit the utility of traditional leadership: linear thinking, lack of awareness of organizational culture, and lack of preparedness for innovation or disruption. (Weberg, 2012) On the other hand, transformational leadership attempts to empower employees to participate in changing the conversations that will lead to organizational change.

For transformation to occur, organizational change must emerge through collaboration and input of stakeholders at all levels. The congruence and diversity of values in communities, between organizational leaders, stakeholders, and community members, is a key determinant of success. (Hoffman, Bynum, Piccolo, & Sutton, 2011) Changing the deep assumptions of the organization that drive unconscious thinking, reacting and behaviors requires new ways of acting and interacting with the informal culture. Relating to goals, principles and people in organizations in this manner is not a static process. Thus, the local resources and qualities of interactive relationships among team members within a given site are determining factors for the culture that will serve as an invisible foundation for the transformation of any practice into a PCMH.

Conclusions and Forward Looking Thoughts

Primary care is the backbone for CIN and ACO, helping transform healthcare and achieve success in the Triple Aim. Primary care reforms in the ACA include fostering innovation in the delivery of care, with an emphasis on PCMH and ACO care models that are intended to lead to better clinical outcomes and patient care experiences. Medicare and Medicaid payments to primary care providers are temporarily increased by the ACA, and are accompanied by proposed investments for the continuing development of the primary care workforce. Push-back on these initiatives seems inevitable, as part of the political processes at the federal and state government levels that includes many professional healthcare groups competing for the same resources.

The path to PCMH may be slow and arduous for many PCPs, staff and organizations. However, to achieve the Triple Aim, patterns of entrenched, inefficient daily operations within routine primary care clinical practices need to change. These changes can be accomplished by transforming primary care services toward the PCMH model. The transition to PCMH practice means panel sizes may decrease, new personnel may need to be hired, adaptation to new and expensive technologies will occur, and may not be welcome. But transforming clinical practices requires disrupting existing processes to begin to make changes. (Hwang J, Christensen CM. 2008) All stakeholders involved with developing each local PCMH must adapt. This is no easy task, nor can it be accomplished in a short timeframe. Similarly, the foundations of scientific reasoning are changing (Kuhn, 1976), accompanied by changes in the basic sciences of organizational management. (Anderson, 2013; McDaniel et al., 2013) All these developments can assist with the transition from traditional primary care to PCMH.

PCMH acts as a focal point for primary care in an integrated delivery system that better serves population health. As such, the PCMH is a gateway to the larger health system, including hospital, special medical care and other stakeholders. (Shaljian & Nielsen, 2013) Delivery system redesign can improve health of populations, improve patient experiences with the delivery of healthcare services, and reduce per capita costs for such services. (Clark, 2014; Pollack, Raney, & Vanderlip, 2012) There is evidence that incentives work, both for clinical improvements and from costs perspectives. (Ratzliff, Christensen, & Unützer, 2014; Unützer et al., 2012)

However, to achieve the goals of the Triple Aim, medical specialties and tertiary care medicine can no longer continue to dominate the design, finances and power relationships within the healthcare system. Rather, there must be a transition to develop more effective and attractive primary care services. This includes evidence-based clinical preventive services, facilitation of community engagement and health promotion, and addressing wellness and the social gradient of health at a societal level.

The top-down notion of tertiary care referral hospitals and specialists as the drivers of healthcare must give way to an added importance for the evolving roles of primary care and PCMH. This shift could serve as a marker for successful implementation of health reform. The RCC model, presented here, adds a social dimension to the issues that influence health and care, including normal everyday social functioning of people - at school and work, home with family and at leisure activities with friends. Normal social role functioning is also an indicator and predictor of good health and well-being. (Talley, Kocum, Schlegel, Molix, & Bettencourt, 2012) New metrics may be useful for such social dimensions, including routine measures for generic quality of life. (Stange et al., 2014)

Society might also look to health-related quality of life (HRQL) as an indicator of social health and well-being. The content and metrics for various forms of HRQL questionnaires are diverse. There are no clear cut guidelines for the proper use of generic and disease-specific measures of HRQL in research and evaluations. Similarly, there are no consensus-based guidelines for assessing subjective rating and/or objective assessment of the different dimension present in our life experiences.

Using global HRQL measures can indicate the presence of un-diagnosed disease and functional limitations that may be hidden from the medical care system. For example, depressive symptoms, whether they are diagnosed or not, typically have high impact upon measures of quality of life. However, the separation between medical and behavioral health treatment and reimbursement for these categories of illness may mask the clinical appraisal of depression among cases treated within the biomedical context. Routine measures for HRQL could complement the focused perspective of the disease-oriented biomedical model and assist with a paradigm shift to favor resource-based, wellness-oriented health strategies and policy development at a societal level. (Diener, 2009; Steiner, 2014)

Focusing on health and well-being as an asset needs to be a higher priority, on par with reducing risks associated with disease. (Frieden, 2010; Healthy People 2020) Health and well-being could include ensuring children who attend school are not hungry, sleepy or afraid, in order to learn and develop well. Likewise, workers with minor recurring aliments, like headaches, back pain or undiagnosed affective disorders, which cannot perform well at their jobs, may benefit from medical attention more so than punishment for lack of productivity and presenteeism. (Aronsson, Gustafsson, & Dallner, 2000; Kessler et al., 2006) Social and ecologic models for health address situations like these, and may be more effective at achieving the goals of the Triple Aim, rather than relying solely on access to the biomedical model of care.

Complexity science is a new framework for studying organizations. Complexity offers a new view of science and the world of phenomena, based upon interactions and interdependence. Because interdependence is a major requirement of CIN, delivery systems attempting to make the change to accountable care could learn much from complexity science and how complex systems can adapt to change. Foundational concepts for complexity emerged from systems thinking, theoretical biology, non-linear dynamics, network sciences, complex adaptive systems, and others. Each of these basic sciences included aspects of interaction, inter-dependence, and attention to social and environmental contexts. Complexity-informed leadership may be key to development of PCMH, CIN, and ACO. This form of leadership requires adaptive capacity, interactions within internal and external environments, including social, business, financial, and political networks, where groups readily encounter unpredictable issues and deal with them as learning opportunities.

The role of the complexity leader is to remove barriers within the organization, so that innovations can emerge from the interactive relationships involving the stakeholders. This involves developing productive, collaborative relationships among multiple stakeholders and partners. Each relationship is based upon trust between individuals and organizations. In short, success in the new health ecosystem, and within and between PCMH, CIN and ACO, requires a foundation of trust between stakeholders. Social capital must be engendered among stakeholders for new organizations to succeed. (Putnam, 1995)

This is not just a philosophic discussion about science, harmony and humanism. There are practical implications to be considered when moving from a traditional, reductionist framework of science, based solely on comparative measurements of objective phenomena, to an ecologic perspective, including socio-cultural approaches, where context is important, and indeed may be viewed as a determining factor for most outcomes. (Bayliss et al., 2014)

Contextual perspectives are useful as they permit a vantage point for discernment of new patterns that might emerge from older traditional perspectives – those that involve the same agents, in the same clinics, with the same patients, but are each viewed from new perspectives and performing with fresh enthusiasm for caring. Seeing the fresh perspectives and patterns among the myriads of interactions that are possible among people, technologies and organizations in clinical practice is part of the delight that is possible in transforming from traditional practice to a sustained PCMH model for primary care, based upon a socio-cultural-ecologic view of population health, and perhaps even a notion about possibilities for creating an Enlightened Society! (Mipham 2013)

"...no health care system can be complete without primary care."

(Donaldson et al., 1996, p.3)

CHAPTER 2 DISCUSSION QUESTIONS

Discussion questions are provided for team building or class exercises. Answers for all questions are provided in Appendix C.

Question Number	Question
1	Name and discuss at least four characteristics of primary care.
2	How are the concepts of chronic care model, insurance reform and healthcare financing reform related to the development of PCMH?
3	Why are HIT and EMR important for the development of PCMH, ACO and CIN?
4	What is the Triple Aim? How is it related to PCMH?
5	How do the topics of complexity in management and relationship-centered care relate to PCMH?

CHAPTER 2 HIGHLIGHTS

✓ The landscape for medical care, and especially for primary care, is changing in the United States, in part from implementing the Patient Protection and Affordable Care Act (ACA). The central aim of the ACA is to increase health insurance coverage in order to make healthcare more affordable and accessible for U.S. citizens. Demand for primary care medical services will likely increase as a result of ACA implementation.

✓ The Triple Aim (quality, costs and outcomes) is now the framework for the US National Quality Strategy for the US Department of Health and Human Services, Centers for Medicare and Medicaid Services, and many other organizations.

✓ Relationship-centered care (RCC) advances a humanistic approach toward patient care, especially for primary care. RCC places a priority on humanism in healthcare and community development; it offers technology as a tool for people to use to facilitate better health, rather than as a touted sole solution. RCC includes concepts from patient-centered care, and rests upon the foundation of the bio-psycho-social model of healthcare and emerging models for the socio-cultural-ecologic aspects of population health.

✓ Patient-Centered Medical Homes (PCMH) are now best described as a model or philosophy of primary care that is patient-centered, comprehensive, team-based, coordinated, accessible, and focused on quality and safety. The newly proposed PCMH model is evolving away from a "disease-centered model" and toward a "person-centered model" of population health.

✓ Payment reforms for primary care physicians are necessary to assure success of PCMH.

✓ Clinical transformation to PCMH is recognized as a feasible, but difficult, task, as it involves a changes in all aspects of work flow and work routines. A survey of items that were correlated with systems changes within PCMH were nearly all from categories of patients, organizational change and culture.

✓ The means to transform PCHM by engendering qualities of relationship as desired within the clinical service sites for patients and families represents a change in culture. Consistent with RCC, we might call this a transformation of the "culture of caring."

CHAPTER 2 REFERENCES

AAMC American Association of Medical Colleges, (2013, April 23) Successful Primary Care Programs: Creating the Workforce We Need: Hearing before the Committee on Health, Education, Labor, and Pensions (HELP), Subcommittee on Primary Health and Aging, United States Senate. Retrieved from https://www.aamc.org/download/334538/data/aamcstatementforsenatehelpsubcommitt eehearingonprimarycareworkf.pdf

ACP, American College of Physicians. (2005). *The Advanced Medical Home: A Patient-Centered, Physician-Guided Model of Health Care.* Philadelphia: American College of Physicians.

Adler, N., Stewart, J., Cohen, S., Cullen, M., Roux, A., Dow, W., & Evans, G. (2007). Reaching for a healthier life: Facts on socioeconomic status and health in the US. The John D. and Catherine T. MacArthur Foundation Research Network on Socioeconomic Status and Health.

Adler, N. E., Boyce, T., Chesney, M. A., Cohen, S., Folkman, S., Kahn, R. L., & Syme, S. L. (1994). Socioeconomic status and health: the challenge of the gradient. *American Psychologist*, 49(1), 15.

AHRQ, Agency for Healthcare Research and Quality. (2012, January). *Primary Care Workforce Facts and Stats: Overview.* Retrieved from http://www.ahrq.gov/research/findings/factsheets/primary/pcworkforce/index.html

AMA Amecian Medical Association website, The RSV Update Committee. Retrieved from http://www.ama-assn.org/ama/pub/physician-resources/solutions-managing-your-practice/coding-billing-insurance/medicare/the-resource-based-relative-value-scale/the-rvs-update-committee.page

Anderson, R. A. (2013). Commentary on "Health care organizations as complex systems: new perspectives on design and management" by Reuben R. McDaniel, Dean J. Driebe, and Holly Jordan Lanham. *Advances in Health Care Management*, 15, 27-36.

Arnetz, B. B. (1997). Physicians' view of their work environment and organization. *Psychotherapy and Psychosomatics*, 66(3):155-62.

Aronsson, G., Gustafsson, K., & Dallner, M. (2000). Sick but yet at work. An empirical study of sickness presenteeism. *Journal of Epidemiology and Community Health*, 54(7), 502-509.

Avendano, M., & Kawachi, I. (2014). Why do Americans have shorter life expectancy and worse health than do people in other high-income countries? *Annual Review of Public Health*, 35, 307-325. doi: 10.1146/annurev-publhealth-032013-182411

Baird M, Blount A, Brungardt S, Dickinson P, Dietrich A, Epperly T, et al. (2014). Joint Principles: Integrating Behavioral Health Care into the Patient-Centered Medical Home. *Annals of Family Medicine*, 12(2):183-5. doi: 10.1370/afm.1633

Bayliss, E. A., Bonds, D. E., Boyd, C. M., Davis, M. M., Finke, B., Fox, M. H., . . . Lachenmayr, S. (2014). Understanding the context of health for persons with multiple chronic conditions: moving from what is the matter to what matters. *Annals of Family Medicine*, 12(3), 260-269. doi: 10.1370/afm.1643

Berenson, R. A., Hammons, T., Gans, D. N., Zuckerman, S., Merrell, K., Underwood, W. S., & Williams, A. F. (2008). A house is not a home: keeping patients at the center of practice redesign. *Health Affairs*, 27(5), 1219-1230. doi: 10.1377/hlthaff.27.5.1219

Berwick, D. M. (2011). Launching accountable care organizations—the proposed rule for the Medicare Shared Savings Program. *New England Journal of Medicine*, 364(16). doi: 10.1056/NEJMp1103602

Berwick, D. M., Nolan, T. W., & Whittington, J. (2008). The triple aim: care, health, and cost. *Health Affairs*, 27(3), 759-769. doi: 10.1377/hlthaff.27.3.759

Bitton, A., Martin, C., & Landon, B. E. (2010). A nationwide survey of patient centered medical home demonstration projects. *Journal of General Internal Medicine*, 25(6), 584-592. doi: 10.1007/s11606-010-1262-8

Black, A. D., Car, J., Pagliari, C., Anandan, C., Cresswell, K., Bokun, T., . . . Sheikh, A. (2011). The impact of eHealth on the quality and safety of health care: a systematic overview. *PLoS Medicine*, 8(1), e1000387. doi:10.1371/journal.pmed.1000387

Borrell-Carrió, F., Suchman, A. L., & Epstein, R. M. (2004). The biopsychosocial model 25 years later: principles, practice, and scientific inquiry. *Annals of Family Medicine*, 2(6), 576-582.

Brandon, S. T., Bair, B., & Kathol, R. (2011). Commentary: Understanding the Importance of Time in Delivering Evidence-based Major Depression Treatment to Geriatric Patients in the Primary Care Setting. *Clinical Geriatrics*, 19(1), 40-43.

Broadhead W. E., Kaplan B. H., James S. A., Wagner E. H., Schoenbach V. J., Grimson R, Heyden S, Tibblin G, Gehlbach S. H. (1983, May). The epidemiologic evidence for a relationship between social support and health. *American Journal of Epidemiology*, 117(5):521-37.

CDC, Centers for Disease Control Prevention. (2011). CDC's Division of Diabetes Translation Community Health Workers/Promotores de Salud: Critical Connections in Communities. Retrieved from http://www.cdc.gov/diabetes/projects/pdfs/comm.pdf

Chaudhry, B., Wang, J., Wu, S., Maglione, M., Mojica, W., Roth, E., Shekelle, P. G. (2006). Systematic Review: Impact of Health Information Technology on Quality, Efficiency, and Costs of Medical Care. *Annals of Internal Medicine*, 144(10), 742-752.

Clark, J. and Wrightson, S. (2014). Behavioral Health and PCMH. *Journal Kentucky Academy Family Physicians*, 80(Spring 2014), 8-10.

CMS Centers for Medicare and Medicaid Services, Press Center. (2014a). *Medicare's delivery system reform initiatives achieve significant savings and quality improvements - off to a strong start.* Retrieved from http://www.cms.gov/Newsroom/MediaReleaseDatabase/Press-Releases/2014-Press-releases-items/2014-01-30.html

CMS Centers for Medicare and Medicaid Services. (2014b). *Innovation Center Home, Innovation Models, Multi-Payer Advanced Primary Care Practice.* Retrieved from http://innovation.cms.gov/initiatives/Multi-Payer-Advanced-Primary-Care-Practice/

CMS Centers for Medicare and Medicaid Services. (2014c). *Innovation Center Home, Transforming Clinical Practice Initiative.* Retrieved from http://www.cms.gov/Newsroom/MediaReleaseDatabase/Fact-sheets/2014-Fact-sheets-items/2014-10-23.html

COGME, Council on Graduate Medical Education. (2010). *Advancing Primary Care - Twentieth Report.* Retrieved from http://www.hrsa.gov/advisorycommittees/bhpradvisory/cogme/reports/twentiethreport.pdf

Cohen, S., & Wills, T. A. (1985). Stress, social support, and the buffering hypothesis. *Psycholological Bulletin*, 98(2), 310.

Compton, M.T. (2012). Systemic organizational change for the collaborative care approach to managing depressive disorders. *American Journal of Preventive Medicine*, 42(5), 553-555. doi: 10.1016/j.amepre.2012.01.016

Crabtree, B. F., McDaniel, R. R., Nutting, P. A., Lanham, H. J., Looney, A., & Miller, W. L. (2008). Closing the physician-staff divide: a step toward creating the medical home. *Family Practice Management*, 15(4), 20.

Crabtree, B. F., Miller, W. L., Tallia, A. F., Cohen, D. J., DiCicco-Bloom, B., McIlvain, H. E., Stange, K. C. (2005). Delivery of clinical preventive services in family medicine offices. *The Annals of Family Medicine*, 3(5), 430-435.

Crabtree, B. F., Nutting, P. A., Miller, W. L., McDaniel, R. R., Stange, K. C., Jaén, C. R., & Stewart, E. (2011). Primary care practice transformation is hard work: insights from a 15-year developmental program of research. *Medical Care*, 49(Suppl), S28. doi: 10.1097/MLR.0b013e3181cad65c

Crabtree, B. F., Nutting, P. A., Miller, W. L., Stange, K. C., Stewart, E. E., & Jaén, C. R. (2010). Summary of the National Demonstration Project and recommendations for the patient-centered medical home. *The Annals of Family Medicine*, 8(Suppl 1), S80-S90. doi: 10.1370/afm.1107

Csete, J., & Cohen, J. (2010). Health benefits of legal services for criminalized populations: the case of people who use drugs, sex workers and sexual and gender minorities. *The Journal of Law, Medicine & Ethics*, 38(4), 816-831. doi: 10.1111/j.1748-720X.2010.00535.x

Davis, K. S., Squires D., and Schoen C. (2014, June). *Mirror, Mirror on the Wall, 2014 Update: How the Performance of the U.S. Health Care System Compares Internationally*. Retrieved from http://www.commonwealthfund.org/publications/fund-reports/2014/jun/mirror-mirror

Diener, E. (2009). *Well-being for public policy*. New York, NY: Oxford University Press.

Donaldson, M. S., Yordy, K. D., Lohr, K. N., & Vanselow, N. A. (1996). *Primary care: America's health in a new era*. Washington, DC: National Academies Press.

Ebell, M. H. (2008). Future salary and US residency fill rate revisited. *The Journal of the American Medical Association*, 300(10), 1131-1132. doi:10.1001/jama.300.10.1131

Eidus, R., Pace, W. D., & Staton, E. W. (2012). Managing patient populations in primary care: points of leverage. *The Journal of the American Board of Family Medicine*, 25(2), 238-244. doi: 10.3122/jabfm.2012.02.100224

Emanuel, E. J., & Fuchs, V. R. (2012). Shortening medical training by 30%. *The Journal of the American Medical Association*, 307(11), 1143-1144. doi: 10.1001/jama.2012.292

Engel, G. (1990). The essence of the biopsychosocial model: from 17th to 20th century science. *A new medical model: a challenge for biomedicine*, 86-107.

Engel, G. L. (1977). The need for a new medical model: a challenge for biomedicine. *Science*, 196(4286), 129-136. doi: 10.1126/science.847460

Engel, G. L. (1979). The biopsychosocial model and the education of health professionals. *General Hospital Psychiatry*, 1(2), 156-165.

Esterhay, R. J., Nesbitt, L. S., Taylor, J. H., Bohn, H. J. (2014). *Population Health: Management, Policy, and Technology*. Virginia Beach, VA: Convurgent Publishing, LLC.

Federal Trade Commission, U.S. Department of Justice and Federal Trade Commission. (1996). Statements of Antitrust Enforcement Policy in Health Care.: Retrieved from http://www.justice.gov/atr/public/guidelines/0000.htm

Ferrer, R. L., Schlenker, C. G., Romero, R. L., Poursani, R., Bazaldua, O., Davidson, D., . . . Corona, B. A. (2013). Advanced primary care in San Antonio: linking practice and community strategies to improve health. *The Journal of the American Board of Family Medicine*, 26(3), 288-298. doi: 10.3122/jabfm.2013.03.120238

Fisher, E. S., Wennberg, D. E., Stukel, T. A., Gottlieb, D. J., Lucas, F. L., & Pinder, E. L. (2003a). The implications of regional variations in Medicare spending. Part 1: the content, quality, and accessibility of care. *Annals of Internal Medicine*, 138(4), 273-287.

Fisher, E. S., Wennberg, D. E., Stukel, T. A., Gottlieb, D. J., Lucas, F. L., & Pinder, E. L. (2003b). The implications of regional variations in Medicare spending. Part 2: health outcomes and satisfaction with care. *Annals of Internal Medicine*, 138(4), 288-298.

Fisher, E. S., & Wennberg, J. E. (2003c). Health care quality, geographic variations, and the challenge of supply-sensitive care. *Perspectives in Biology & Medicine*, 46(1), 69-79.

Fisher, E. S., Wennberg, J. E., Fisher, E. S., & Wennberg, J. E. (2003d). Health care quality, geographic variations, and the challenge of supply-sensitive care. *Perspectives in Biology & Medicine*, 46(1), 69-79.

Fleming, D.M. (1993). The European study referrals from primary to secondary care.

Fogarty C. T., Mauksch L. (2014). Commentary by the American College of Physicians on the "Joint Principles: Integrating Behavioral Health Care into the Patient-Centered Medical Home". *Annals of Family Medicine*, 12(2), 186-7. doi: 10.1037/fsh0000038

Freeman, G., & Hughes, J. (2010). Continuity of care and the patient experience. London: The King's Fund.

Freeman J., Pettereson S., Bazemore A. (2014). Accounting for Complexity: Aligning Current Payment Models with Breadth of Care by Different Specialities. *American Family Physician*. Dec 1;90(11):790.

Frieden, T. R. (2010). A framework for public health action: the health impact pyramid. *American Journal of Public Health*, 100(4), 590-595. doi: 10.2105/AJPH.2009.185652

Galea, S., Tracy, M., Hoggatt, K. J., DiMaggio, C., & Karpati, A. (2011). Estimated deaths attributable to social factors in the United States. *Ameridan Journal of Public Health*, 101(8), 1456-1465. doi: 10.2105/AJPH.2010.300086

Gawande, A. (2009). The cost conundrum. *The New Yorker*, 1, 36-44.

Glenton, C., Colvin, C. J., Carlsen, B., Swartz, A., Lewin, S., Noyes, J., & Rashidian, A. (2013). Barriers and facilitators to the implementation of lay health worker programmes to improve access to maternal and child health: qualitative evidence synthesis. *Cochrane Database of Systematic Reviews*, 10. doi: 10.1002/14651858.CD010414

González-González, A. I., Dawes, M., Sánchez-Mateos, J., Riesgo-Fuertes, R., Escortell-Mayor, E., Sanz-Cuesta, T., & Hernández-Fernández, T. (2007). Information needs and information-seeking behavior of primary care physicians. *Annals of Family Medicine*, 5(4), 345-352.

Gosden, T., Forland, F., Kristiansen, I., Sutton, M., Leese, B., Giuffrida, A., Pedersen, L. (2000). Capitation, salary, fee-for-service and mixed systems of payment: effects on the behaviour of primary care physicians. *Cochrane Database of Systematic Reviews*, 3(3).

Green, L. A., Graham, R., Bagley, B., Kilo, C. M., Spann, S. J., Bogdewic, S. P., & Swanson, J. (2004). Task Force 1. Report of the task force on patient expectations, core values, reintegration, and the new model of family medicine. *Annals of Family Medicine*, 2(suppl 1), S33-S50.

Grol, R., Wensing, M., Eccles, M., & Davis, D. (Eds.). (2013). *Improving patient care: the implementation of change in health care*. Hoboken, NJ: John Wiley & Sons.

Hartmann, K. E., Andrews, J. C., Jerome, R. N., Lewis, R. M., Likis, F. E., McKoy, J. N., . . . Walker, S. H. (2012). *Strategies to reduce cesarean birth in low-risk women*.

Health Care Cost Institute. (2012). *2011 Health Care Cost and Utilization Report*. Retrieved from http://www.healthcostinstitute.org/2011report

Hoffman, B. J., Bynum, B. H., Piccolo, R. F., & Sutton, A. W. (2011). Person-organization value congruence: How transformational leaders influence work group effectiveness. *Academy of Management Journal*, 54(4), 779-796. doi: 10.5465/AMJ.2011.64870139

Hwang J, Christensen C. M. (2008). Disruptive innovation in health care delivery: a framework for business-model innovation. *Health Affairs*, 27(5), 1329-35. doi: 10.1377/hlthaff.27.5.1329

Iglehart, J. (2010). Health Reform, Primary Care, and Graduate Medical Education. *New England Journal of Medicine*, 363(6), 584-590. doi: doi:10.1056/NEJMhpr1006115

Iglehart, J. K. (2011). Assessing an ACO prototype—Medicare's physician group practice demonstration. *New England Journal of Medicine*, 364(3), 198-200. DOI: 10.1056/NEJMp1013896

Committee for the Study of the Future of Public Health, Institute of Medicine. (1988). The future of public health. Washington, DC: National Academy Press. Retrieved from http://iom.edu/Reports/1988/The-Future-of-Public-Health.aspx

Committee on the Recommended Social and Behavioral Domains and Measures for Electronic Health Records, Board on Population Health and Public Health Practice, Institute of Medicine. (2014). *Capturing Social and Behavioral Domains in Electronic Health Records: Phase 1*. Washington, DC: The National Academies Press.

Jackson, G. L., Powers, B. J., Chatterjee, R., Prvu Bettger, J., Kemper, A. R., Hasselblad, V., . . . Williams, J. J. W. (2013). The Patient-Centered Medical HomeA Systematic Review. *Annals of Internal Medicine*, 158(3), 169-178. doi: 10.7326/0003-4819-158-3-201302050-00579

Jacob, V., Chattopadhyay, S. K., Sipe, T. A., Thota, A. B., Byard, G. J., & Chapman, D. P. (2012). Economics of collaborative care for management of depressive disorders: a community guide systematic review. *American Journal of Preventive Medicine*, 42(5), 539-549. doi: 10.1016/j.amepre.2012.01.011

Jaén, C. R., Ferrer, R. L., Miller, W. L., Palmer, R. F., Wood, R., Davila, M., . . . Stange, K. C. (2010). Patient Outcomes at 26 Months in the Patient-Centered Medical Home National

Demonstration Project. *Annals of Family Medicine*, 8(Suppl 1), S57-S67. doi: 10.1370/afm.1121

Kaiser Foundation. (2013). Summary of the Affodable Care Act (#8061-02) Focus on Health Reform: Kaiser Family Foundation. Accessed online November 26, 2014 at http://kff.org/health-reform/fact-sheet/summary-of-the-affordable-care-act/

Kartman, L. (1967). Human ecology and public health. *American Journal of Public Health and the Nations Health*, 57(5), 737-750.

Kathol, R. G., Butler, M., McAlpine, D. D., & Kane, R. L. (2010). Barriers to physical and mental condition integrated service delivery. *Psychosomatic Medicine*, 72(6), 511-518. doi: 10.1097/PSY.0b013e3181e2c4a0

Keleher, H., Parker, R., Abdulwadud, O., & Francis, K. (2009). Systematic review of the effectiveness of primary care nursing. *International Journal of Nursing Practice*, 15(1), 16-24. doi: 10.1111/j.1440-172X.2008.01726.x

Kern, L. M., Edwards, A., & Kaushal, R. (2014). The Patient-Centered Medical Home, Electronic Health Records, and Quality of Care. *Annals of Internal Medicine*, 160(11), 741-749. doi: 10.7326/M13-1798

Kessler, R., Akiskal, H., Ames, M., Birnbaum, H., Greenberg, P., Jin, R., Wang, P. (2006). Prevalence and effects of mood disorders on work performance in a nationally representative sample of US workers. *American Journal of Psychiatry*, 163(9), 1561-1568.

Kirch, D. G., Henderson, M. K., & Dill, M. J. (2012). Physician workforce projections in an era of health care reform. *Annual Review of Medicine*, 63, 435-445. doi: 10.1146/annurev-med-050310-134634

Kirch, D. G., & Vernon, D. J. (2008). Confronting the complexity of the physician workforce equation. *The Journal of the American Medical Association*, 299(22), 2680-2682. doi: 10.1001/jama.299.22.2680

Klein, D. B., Laugesen, M. J., & Liu, N. (2013). The Patient-Centered Medical Home: A Future Standard for American Health Care? *Public Administration Review*, 73(s1), S82-S92. DOI: 10.1111/puar.12082

Koller C. F., Brennan T. A., Bailit M. H. (2010). Rhode Island's Novel Experiment to Rebuild Primary Care from the Insurance Side. *Health Affairs*, 29(5):941-7. doi: 10.1377/hlthaff.2010.0136

Kuhn, T. S. (1976). The Structure of Scientific Revolutions (Chicago, 1962). *KuhnThe Structure of Scientific Revolutions 1962*.

Kumetz, E. A., & Goodson, J. D. (2013). The Undervaluation of Evaluation and Management Professional ServicesCurrent Procedural Terminology Deficiency ImpactThe Lasting Impact of Current Procedural Terminology Code Deficiencies on Physician Payment. *CHEST Journal*, 144(3), 740-745. doi:10.1378/chest.13-0381

Laurant, M., Reeves, D., Hermens, R., Braspenning, J., Grol, R., & Sibbald, B. (2004). Substitution of doctors by nurses in primary care. *Cochrane Database System Review*, 4.

Lewin, S., Dick, J., Pond, P., Zwarenstein, M., Aja, G., Van Wyk, B., Patrick, M. (2005). Lay health workers in primary and community health care. *Cochrane Databas System Review*, 1.

Linney, B. (1998). Why become a certified physician executive? *Physician Executive*, 24:50-52.

Mahler, H. (1981). *The Meaning of" health for All by the Year 2000*. World Health Organization.

Manderscheid, R., & Kathol, R. (2014). Fostering sustainable, integrated medical and behavioral health services in medical settings. *Annals of Internal Medicine*, 160(1), 61-65-65. doi: 10.7326/M13-1693

Marmot, M. (2013). Fair Society, Healthy Lives. *Inequalities in Health: Concepts, Measures, and Ethics*, 282. doi: 10.1016/j.puhe.2012.05.014

Marmot, M. G. (2006). Status syndrome: a challenge to medicine.[see comment]. *The Journal of the American Medical Association*, 295(11), 1304-1307.

Marmot, M. G., Smith, G. D., Stansfeld, S., Patel, C., North, F., Head, J., Feeney, A. (1991). Health inequalities among British civil servants: the Whitehall II study.[see comment]. *Lancet*, 337(8754), 1387-1393.

McDaniel Jr, R. R., Jordan, M. E., & Fleeman, B. F. (2003). Surprise, surprise, surprise! A complexity science view of the unexpected. *Health Care Management Review*, 28(3), 266-278.

McDaniel, R. R., & Driebe, D. J. (2001). Complexity science and health care management. In (ed.) *Advances in Health Care Management*, 2, 11-36.

McDaniel, R. R., Driebe, D. J., & Lanham, H. J. (2013). Health Care Organizations as Complex Systems: New Perspectives on Design and Management. *Advances in Health Care Management*, 15, 3-26.

McWhinney, I. R. (1972). Beyond diagnosis: an approach to the integration of behavioral science and clinical medicine. *New England Journal of Medicine*, 287(8), 384-7.

Menachemi, N., Matthews, M. C., Ford, E. W., & Brooks, R. G. (2007). The influence of payer mix on electronic health record adoption by physicians. *Health Care Management Review*, 32(2), 111-118.

Miller, R. H., & Sim, I. (2004). Physicians' use of electronic medical records: barriers and solutions. *Health Affairs*, 23(2), 116-126.

Miller, W. L., Crabtree, B. F., Nutting, P. A., Stange, K. C., & Jaén, C. R. (2010). Primary care practice development: a relationship-centered approach. *Annals of Family Medicine*, 8(Suppl 1), S68-S79. doi: 10.1370/afm.1089

Mipham S. (2013). The Shambhala Principle: Discovering Humanity's Hidden Treasure. New York, NY: Random House, LLC.

Moreno, L., Peikes, D. N., Krilla, A. (2010). Necessary But Not Sufficient: The HITECH Act and health information technology's potential to build medical homes: Agency for Healthcare Research and Quality, US Department of Health and Human Services.

Moses, H., Matheson, D. H., Dorsey, E. R., George, B. P., Sadoff, D., & Yoshimura, S. (2013). The anatomy of health care in the United States. *The Journal of the American Medical Association*, 310(18), 1947-1964. doi:10.1001/jama.2013.281425

Mullan, F. (2003). The future of medical education: A call for action. *Health Affairs*, 22(4), 88-90.

Nielsen M., Langner B., Zema C., Hacker T., Grundy P. (2012) Benefits of Implementing the Primary Care Patient-Centered Medical Home. Washington: Patient-Centered Primary Care Collaborative.

Newhouse, R. P., Stanik-Hutt, J., White, K. M., Johantgen, M., Bass, E. B., Zangaro, G., Heindel, L. (2011). Advanced practice nurse outcomes 1990-2008: a systematic review. *Nursing Economics*, 29(5), 1-21.

Nolan, M., Keady, J., & Aveyard, B. (2001). Relationship-centred care is the next logical step. *British Journal of Nursing*, 10(12), 757.

Nutting, P. A., Crabtree, B. F., Miller, W. L., Stange, K. C., Stewart, E., & Jaén, C. (2011). Transforming physician practices to patient-centered medical homes: lessons from the national demonstration project. *Health Affairs*, 30(3), 439-445. doi: 10.1377/hlthaff.2010.0159

Nutting, P. A., Miller, W. L., Crabtree, B. F., Jaen, C. R., Stewart, E. E., & Stange, K. C. (2009). Initial lessons from the first national demonstration project on practice transformation to a patient-centered medical home. *Annals of Family Medicine*, 7(3), 254-260. doi: 10.1370/afm.1002

Omran, A. R. (1971). The Epidemiologic Transition: A Theory of the Epidemiology of Population Change. *Milbank Quarterly*, 49(4), 509-538. doi: 10.2307/3349375

Omran, A. R. (2005). The Epidemiologic Transition: A Theory of the Epidemiology of Population Change. *Milbank Quarterly*, 83(4), 731-757. doi: 10.1111/j.1468-0009.2005.00398.x

Ormond, B. A. (2011). Assuring Access to Care Under Health Reform: The Key Role of Workforce Policy.

Paley, J., & Eva, G. (2011). Complexity theory as an approach to explanation in healthcare: a critical discussion. *International Journal of Nursing Studies*, 48(2), 269-279. doi: 10.1016/j.ijnurstu.2010.09.012

PCPCC, Patient-Centered Primary Care Collaborative, P. (2007). Joint principles of the patient centered medical home. Retrieved from http://www.pcpcc.net

PCPCC, Patient-Centered Primary Care Collaborative. (2014). Joint Principles of the Patient Centered Medical Home. Retrieved from http://www.pcpcc.net

PCPCC. Patient-Centered Primary Care Collaborative (2012). Benefits of Implementing the Primary Care Patient-Centered Medical Home: A Review of Cost and Quality Results. Retrieved from http://www.pcpcc.net

Petterson, S. M., Liaw, W. R., Phillips, R. L., Rabin, D. L., Meyers, D. S., & Bazemore, A. W. (2012). Projecting US primary care physician workforce needs: 2010-2025. *Annals of Family Medicine*, 10(6), 503-509. doi: 10.1370/afm.1431

Plowman, D. A., & Duchon, D. (2008). Dispelling the myths about leadership. Complexity leadership: Part I: Conceptual foundations, 129-153.

Institute of Medicine, Committee on Quality of Health Care in America, & Plsek, P. (2001). Redesigning health care with insights from the science of complex adaptive systems. In *Crossing the quality chasm: A new health system for the 21st century.* (pp. 309-322). Washington, DC: National Academies Press.

Pollack, D., Raney, L., & Vanderlip, E. (2012). Integrated Care and Psychiatrists. In H. L. McQuistion, W. E. Sowers, J. M. Ranz & J. M. Feldman (Eds.), *Handbook of Community Psychiatry* (pp. 163-175). New York, NY: Springer.

Putnam, R. D. (1995). Bowling alone: America's declining social capital. *Journal of Democracy*, 6, 68.

Ratzliff, A. H., Christensen, C., & Unützer, J. (2014). Building Value-Added Teams to Care for Behavioral Health Needs in Primary Care. In P. Summergrad & R. G. Kathol (Eds.), *Integrated Care in Psychiatry* (pp. 103-126). New York, NY: Springer.

Reid, R. J., Coleman, K., Johnson, E. A., Fishman, P. A., Hsu, C., Soman, M. P., . . . Larson, E. B. (2010). The group health medical home at year two: cost savings, higher patient satisfaction, and less burnout for providers. *Health Affairs*, 29(5), 835-843. doi: 10.1377/hlthaff.2010.0158

Rieselbach, R.E., Crouse B.J., Neuhausen K, Nasca T.J., Frohna J.G.. (2013). Academic medicine: A key partner in strengthening the primary care infrastructure via teaching health centers. *Academic Medicine.* 88(12):1835-43. doi: 10.1097/ACM.0000000000000035

Rittenhouse, D. R., Shortell, S. M., & Fisher, E. S. (2009). Primary care and accountable care—two essential elements of delivery-system reform. *New England Journal of Medicine*, 361(24), 2301-2303. doi: 10.1056/NEJMp0909327

Rocha, K. B., Rodríguez-Sanz, M., Pasarín, M. I., Berra, S., Gotsens, M., & Borrell, C. (2012). Assessment of primary care in health surveys: a population perspective. *European Journal of Public Health*, 22(1), 14-19. doi: 10.1093/eurpub/ckr014

Roland, M., Roberts, M., Rhenius, V., & Campbell, J. (2013). GPAQ-R: development and psychometric properties of a version of the General Practice Assessment Questionnaire for use for revalidation by general practitioners in the UK. *BMC Family Practice*, 14(1), 160. doi: 10.1186/1471-2296-14-160

Rosenthal, E. L., Wiggins, N., Ingram, M., Mayfield-Johnson, S., & De Zapien, J. G. (2011). Community health workers then and now: an overview of national studies aimed at defining the field. *Journal of Ambulatory Care Management*, 34(3), 247-259. doi: 10.1097/JAC.0b013e31821c64d7

Rosenthal, M. B. (2008a). Beyond pay for performance—emerging models of provider-payment reform. *New England Journal of Medicine*, 359(12), 1197-1200. doi: 10.1056/NEJMp0804658

Rosenthal, M. B. (2008b). Beyond Pay for Performance — Emerging Models of Provider-Payment Reform. *New England Journal of Medicine*, 359(12), 1197-1200. doi:10.1056/NEJMp0804658

Rothman, A. A., & Wagner, E. H. (2003). Chronic illness management: what is the role of primary care? *Annals of Internal Medicine*, 138(3), 256-261.

Salzer, M., Schwenk, E., & Brusilovskiy, E. (2010). Certified peer specialist roles and activities: Results from a national survey. *Psychiatric Services*, 61(5), 520-523. doi: 10.1176/appi.ps.61.5.520

Salzer, M. S. (2010). *Certified peer specialists in the United States behavioral health system: an emerging workforce Mental Health Self-Help* (pp. 169-191). New York, NY: Springer.

Sauber, S. R., & Vetter, S. R. S. H. J. (2013). *The Human services delivery system: Mental health, criminal justice, social welfare, education, health services*. New York, NY: Columbia University Press.

Schneider, M., & Somers, M. (2006). Organizations as complex adaptive systems: Implications of complexity theory for leadership research. *Leadership Quarterly*, 17(4), 351-365.

Schwartz, M. D. (2012). The US primary care workforce and graduate medical education policy. *The Journal of the American Medical Association*, 308(21), 2252-2253. doi: 10.1001/jama.2012.77034

Scott, A., Sivey, P., Ait Ouakrim, D., Willenberg, L., Naccarella, L., Furler, J., & Young, D. (2011). The effect of financial incentives on the quality of health care provided by primary care physicians. *Cochrane Database of Systematic Reviews*, 9(9). doi: 10.1002/14651858.CD008451

Shaljian, M., & Nielsen, M. M. (2013). Managing Populations, Maximizing Technology.

Solberg, L. I., Asche, S. E., Fontaine, P., Flottemesch, T. J., & Anderson, L. H. (2011). Trends in quality during medical home transformation. *Annals of Family Medicine*, 9(6), 515-521. doi: 10.1370/afm.1296

Solberg, L. I., Crain, A. L., Tillema, J. O., Fontaine, P. L., Whitebird, R. R., Flottemesch, T. J., . . . Crabtree, B. F. (2014). Challenges of medical home transformation reported by 118 patient-centered medical home (PCMH) leaders. *Journal of the American Board of Family Medicine*, 27(4), 449-457. doi: 10.3122/jabfm.2014.04.130303

Sox, H. C., Higgins, M. C., & Owens, D. K. (2013). *Medical decision making*. Hoboken, NJ: John Wiley & Sons.

Stange, K. C. (2014). On-the-Ground Wisdom About Care Integration. *Annals of Family Medicine*, 12(4), 375-377. doi: 10.1370/afm.1682

Stange, K. C., Etz, R. S., Gullett, H., Sweeney, S. A., Miller, W. L., Jaén, C. R., Glasgow, R. E. (2014). Metrics for Assessing Improvements in Primary Health Care. *Annual Review of Public Health*, 35, 423-442. doi: 10.1146/annurev-publhealth-032013-182438

Stange, K. C., Zyzanski, S. J., Jaén, C. R., Callahan, E. J., Kelly, R. B., Gillanders, W. R., . . . Miller, W. L. (1998). Illuminating the'black box'. A description of 4454 patient visits to 138 family physicians. *Journal of Family Practice*, 46(5), 377.

Stanton M. W., Rutherford M. K. (2005). The high concentration of U.S. health care expenditures. *Research in Action*, Issue 19. AHRQ Pub. No. 06-0060.

Starfield, B. (1991). Primary care and health: a cross-national comparison. *The Journal of the American Medical Association*. 266(16), 2268-2271.

Starfield, B. (1998). Primary care: balancing health needs, services, and technology. New York, NY: Oxford University Press.

Starfield, B. (2001a). Basic concepts in population health and health care. *Journal of Epidemiology and Community Health*, 55(7), 452-454.

Starfield, B. (2001b). New paradigms for quality in primary care. *British Journal General Practice*, 51(465), 303.

Starfield, B., & Horder, J. (2007). Interpersonal continuity: old and new perspectives. *British Journal General Practice*, 57(540), 527-529.

Starfield, B., Shi, L., & Macinko, J. (2005). Contribution of primary care to health systems and health. *Milbank Quarterly*, 83(3), 457-502.

Steiner R. W., Wainscott B. (2014). Envisioning an Expanded Model for Population Health: Toward a Socio-Cultural-Ecologic Model, Based on Resources and Relationships. In R. Esterhay, et.al. (Ed.), *Population Health. Management, Policy, and Technology, First Edition* (pp. 112 - 161). Virginia Beach, VA: Convurgent Publishing.

Stiefel M, N. K. A. (2012). *Guide to Measuring the Triple Aim: Population Health, Experience of Care, and Per Capita Cost.* IHI Innovation Series white paper.

Stiefel, M. C., Perla, R. J., & Zell, B. L. (2010). A healthy bottom line: healthy life expectancy as an outcome measure for health improvement efforts. *Milbank Quarterly*, 88(1), 30-53.

Suchman, A. L. (2006). A new theoretical foundation for relationship-centered care. Complex responsive processes of relating. *Journal General Internal Medicine*, 21 Suppl 1, S40-44.

Talley, A. E., Kocum, L., Schlegel, R. J., Molix, L., & Bettencourt, B. A. (2012). Social roles, basic need satisfaction, and psychological health the central role of competence. *Personality and Social Psychology Bulletin*, 38(2), 155-173. doi: 10.1177/0146167211432762

Thota, A. B., Sipe, T. A., Byard, G. J., Zometa, C. S., Hahn, R. A., McKnight-Eily, L. R., Anderson, C. W. (2012). Collaborative care to improve the management of depressive disorders: a community guide systematic review and meta-analysis. *American Journal of Preventive Medicine*, 42(5), 525-538. doi: 10.1016/j.amepre.2012.01.019

Thygeson, M., Morrissey, L., & Ulstad, V. (2010). Adaptive leadership and the practice of medicine: a complexity-based approach to reframing the doctor–patient relationship. *Journal of Evaluation in Clinical Practice*, 16(5), 1009-1015. doi: 10.1111/j.1365-2753.2010.01533.x

Tierney K., Saunders A., Lewis V., Creating Connections: An Early Look at the Integration ofBehavioral Health and Primary Care in Accountable Care Organizations, The Commonwealth Fund, December 2014.

Toussaint, J., Milstein, A., & Shortell, S. (2013). How the Pioneer ACO Model Needs to Change: Lessons From Its Best-Performing ACO. *The Journal of the American Medical Association*, 310(13), 1341-1342. doi: 10.1001/jama.2013.279149

Uijen, A. A., Heinst, C. W., Schellevis, F. G., van den Bosch, W. J., van de Laar, F. A., Terwee, C. B., & Schers, H. J. (2012). Measurement properties of questionnaires measuring continuity of care: a systematic review. *PLoS ONE* [Electronic Resource], 7(7), e42256. doi: 10.1371/journal.pone.0042256

Unützer, J., Chan, Y.-F., Hafer, E., Knaster, J., Shields, A., Powers, D., & Veith, R. C. (2012). Quality improvement with pay-for-performance incentives in integrated behavioral health care. *American Journal of Public Health*, 102(6), e41-e45. doi: 10.2105/AJPH.2011.300555

van Hasselt M, McCall N., Keyes V., Wensky S. G., Smith K. W. (2014). Total Cost of Care Lower among Medicare Fee-for-Service Beneficiaries Receiving Care from Patient-Centered Medical Homes. *Health Services Research*. doi: 10.1111/1475-6773.12217

Vogeli, C., Shields, A. E., Lee, T. A., Gibson, T. B., Marder, W. D., Weiss, K. B., & Blumenthal, D. (2007). Multiple chronic conditions: prevalence, health consequences, and implications for quality, care management, and costs. *Journal of General Internal Medicine*, 22(3), 391-395.

Wagner, E. H., Austin, B. T., & Von Korff, M. (1996). Organizing care for patients with chronic illness. *Milbank Quarterly*, 74(4), 511-544.

Wagner, E. H., Coleman, K., Reid, R. J., Phillips, K., Abrams, M. K., & Sugarman, J. R. (2012). The changes involved in patient-centered medical home transformation. *Primary Care: Clinics in Office Practice*, 39(2), 241-259. doi: 10.1016/j.pop.2012.03.002

Weberg, D. (2012). Complexity leadership: A healthcare imperative. Paper presented at the Nursing forum.

Welch, W. P., Miller, M. E., Welch, H. G., Fisher, E. S., & Wennberg, J. E. (1993). Geographic variation in expenditures for physicians' services in the United States. *New England Journal of Medicine*, 328(9), 621-627.

WHO, World Health Organziation. (1978). Declaration of Alma Ata: Report of the international conference on primary health care. Alma Atta, USSR.

WHO, World Health Organziation. (2014). Health 2020. A European policy framework and strategy for the 21st century. Prevalence.

Chapter 3. The Future of Leadership

Thomas A. Raskauskas

Joanne Bohn

A true leader has the confidence to stand alone, the courage to make tough decisions, and the compassion to listen to the needs of others. He does not set out to be a leader, but becomes one by the equality of his actions and the integrity of his intent. (Kruse, October 16, 2012)

General Douglas MacArthur
U.S. Army 5-Star General
(1880-1964)

Chapter 3 Learning Objectives

✓ What are some of the building blocks for CIN or ACO leader success?

✓ Define 3 styles of leadership that can be applied and adopted by leaders of CINs and or ACOs.

✓ Understand the importance of governance to the CIN or ACO and the level at which governance boards engage and provide direction.

✓ Recognize some of the current challenges facing leaders of CINs and ACOs in today's dynamic healthcare environment.

✓ Understand the importance of "Network and Alliance Engagement" and 'Relational Connectors' for the CIN or ACO leader.

✓ Be able to define the new concept: "Accountable Care Network" (ACN).

Introduction

Traditional leadership roles in medicine have been hierarchical, based on longevity in the organization, and unrelated to the skill set of the individual. As health care changes intervene, including enacted reforms, novel delivery models, innovations in reimbursement, antitrust requirements, and managing populations rather than encountering individuals, today's healthcare leaders need multiple skills that have not been required in the past. Engaging the right persons in governance and leadership of Clinically Integrated Networks (CINs) and Accountable Care Organizations (ACOs) is critical to success. This chapter will cover key conceptual building blocks for successful leaders, styles of leadership, and the importance of governance in the strategy and oversight of CINs and ACOs.

Leaders of healthcare organizations have confronted challenges in the past. The present transformation of healthcare resulting from health reforms and the search for value compounds the challenges. Some of the past and current challenges include:

◆ A highly professional workforce concentrated in silos;

◆ Traditional physician training that tends to inhibit collaboration;

◆ Lengthy and demanding training to develop clinical skills and knowledge that may delay the development of leadership skills;

◆ An industry in transition from a fee-for-service model to a quality and performance driven model;

◆ Exponential increase in quality measure reporting for clinical performance;

◆ A large and growing body of laws and regulations that attempt to ensure proper healthcare, but also stifle innovation; and

◆ An increasingly complex external environment (e.g., payer reimbursement changes, state licensing requirements, and antitrust laws) requiring a high level of business acumen to function.

(Berwick 1996, Stoller 2009)

The transformation to CINs and ACOs requires new leadership styles. Because each community and its complement of healthcare providers are unique, the leadership required to achieve the goals of CINs and ACOs has never been greater. In addition to dealing with the challenges described throughout Chapter 2, the CIN and ACO also need skills and knowledge in managing change. Large-scale organizational transformations require leaders who also understand the emotional turmoil their personnel may undergo, and the complex disruptions and interdependencies that develop among participants as innovations are introduced.

A 1996 quote from Dr. Donald Berwick may serve as a theme for this section: "Effective leaders challenge the status quo both by insisting that the current system cannot remain and by offering clear ideas about superior alternatives." (Berwick 1996) Along with implementing change and addressing challenges, leaders of CINs and ACOs must welcome innovations that challenge the status quo. There are several essential building blocks for leaders of CIN/ACO and a variety of leadership styles that leaders can adopt in their efforts to further develop these new delivery models.

Building Blocks for CIN/ACO Leaders

In order for providers to continue to evolve, physician engagement at the leadership level is essential. In fact, it has been noted that, "...involving physicians in the governance of provider organizations improves communication and builds trust..." (Colla, Lewis et al. 2014) Strong communications and trust are essential to achieve greater integration of clinical and staff resources, adoption of innovations, and improvement of access, quality and cost. CIN and ACO leaders need foundational skills to support evolution and growth. Figure 3-1 illustrates a set of building blocks to develop and refine new organizational models. This conceptual model is based on two core leadership pillars — Shared Purpose and Shared Culture. Following Figure 3-1 is a description of each of these building blocks.

Figure 3-1. Building Blocks for CIN and ACO Leaders

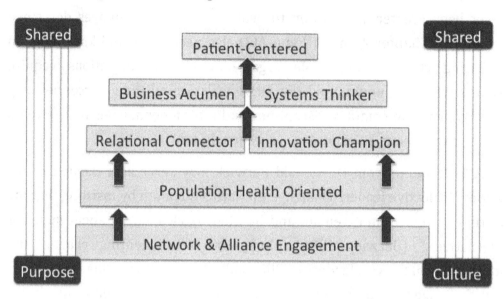

Shared Purpose - it is important for a leader to establish a common bond and positive motivating force, as noted by Lee and Cosgrove in their 2014 article, *Engaging Doctors in the Health Care Revolution*. (Lee and Cosgrove 2014) Underlying this shared purpose is professional will and personal humility, as noted in the best seller, *Good to Great*. (Colins 2001) Physician-leaders need this trait to help their organizations achieve goals and engage and drive collaborative multidisciplinary teams. This is not only a good management principle, but also a matter of regulatory compliance, as CINs are required by federal antitrust laws to have every physician share and understand common goals to improve care and lower costs for the benefit of consumers, and demonstrate interdependence in practice – all elements of a shared purpose.

Shared Culture - Three key elements compose Shared Culture — mission, values, and engagement. First, the leader of any CIN or ACO must be able to communicate the mission and vision for the organization to internal and external groups. Second, each CIN or ACO has a set of values that serve as their business ethics tenets. The values support strategic direction and help guide decisions large and small that impact the organization and its patients, community, and other stakeholders. Third, any CIN or ACO leader must possess the ability to drive engagement of clinical and administrative staff in the culture of the organization, and serve as an agent of change when necessary. Whether it is an existing culture they choose to embrace or a shift in culture, they need to have everyone on board. This element is magnified in a CIN, where engagement of physicians is critical to demonstrating compliance with regulations and achieving goals of cost reduction and quality improvement.

Network and Alliance Engagement - The formation of physician networks is a basic requirement of CINs and ACOs and carries regulatory compliance implications. To develop the necessary networks and alliances, the organization needs to amass clinical talent, maintain needed affiliations with community providers, and operate within the regulatory framework. A key ingredient for healthcare leaders is to "embrace connectivity and openness." This was highlighted in a 2012-2013 IBM survey of CEOs from multiple industries across 64 countries. (Randall, Brian Leavy et al. 2014) Facilitating greater connectivity, enabled by the Internet and social media, can create new incentives, new collaborations, and increase opportunities for new networks and alliances that allow further growth.

Population Health Oriented- Modern medicine in the United States is shifting toward an emphasis on population health. The focus of the Medicare Shared Savings Program was to improve the health of the assigned population. (Centers for Medicare and Medicaid Services April 7, 2011) The meaning of population health varies depending on one's perspective, but one definition is in a 2013 *American Journal of Public Health* article:

> ...the health outcomes of a group of individuals, including the distribution of such outcomes within the group...population health also includes patterns of health determinants, policies and interventions that connect the two. (Kindig and Stoddart 2003)

As defined in this book, "accountable care" generally means providers being accountable for the cost and quality of care for a defined population. If providers are fully accountable for both the clinical and financial outcomes, a function health insurance plans and managed care organizations have performed for years, then population health may be generally defined as medical and financial risk management to ensure clinical quality and financial solvency. Providers are adopting medical and financial management services and processes from health plans and managed care organziations, which focus on needs of the populations served, and increasingly social determinants of health. CIN and ACO leaders need to maintain awareness of the needs of the population they serve and the changing social determinants that impact the health of their communities.

Relational Connectors- Leaders of CINs and ACOs need to operate as connectors for their organizations and in their communities. Two related points from the literature on the importance of this building block are conveners and explorers In the book, *Finding Allies, Building Alliances: 8 Elements That Bring and Keep People Together*, Mike Leavitt and Rich McKeown describe the connector role as "convener of stature". (Leavitt and McKeown 2013) This role applied to a CIN or ACO leader means an influential leader with the ability to bring together key parties to drive collaboration. In *The Tipping Point: How Little Things Make a Big Difference*, Malcom Gladwell discusses the concept of Connectors, noting that,

> ...in the case of Connectors, their ability to span many different worlds is a function of something intrinsic to their personality, some combination of curiosity, self-confidence, sociability, and energy. (Gladwell 2001)

What Gladwell emphasizes when applied to the CIN or ACO, is the importance of exploring all the nodes in the community ecosystem that, when leveraged and connected properly, can benefit the ultimate goal of the CIN or ACO. Serving as a 'Relational Connector' builds new relationships and strengthens existing ones. Leaders who exercise this skill become increasingly valuable to their organizations and the greater communities.

Innovation Champion- Driving and embracing innovation is essential for healthcare leaders. Incorporating innovation into the fabric of a new CIN or ACO is not easy. As Hill and colleagues noted in *Collective Genius*,

> The rhetoric of innovation is often about fun and creativity, but the reality is that innovation is hard work and can be a very taxing, uncomfortable process, both emotionally and intellectually. (Hill, Brandeau et al. 2014)

Championing innovation for the CIN or ACO means aligning resources and setting priorities so the organization remains agile, open and flexible — while operating within legal and regulatory requirements. It also means finding ways to accelerate evaluation and adoption of new technologies, services, business operating models, and payment mechanisms and processes. In the book, The *6 Ps of Physician Leadership. A Primer for Emerging and Developing Leaders*, Flareau noted,

> The field of innovation is critical to follow and monitor for every physician leader as the technology revolution we are all impacted by infiltrates the intricacies of every element of how we practice, pay for, and care for the patients in our community. (Flareau and Bohn 2013)

What Flareau noted as important for physician leaders is applicable to all healthcare leaders. Without a focus on new innovations healthcare organization could find themselves obsolete at one of the most critical times in the history of healthcare.

Systems Thinkers- Originating in the field of engineering, systems thinking means understanding interrelationships of complex entities and the ways that individual components affect the function of the whole. Systems thinking is part of the foundation of the "learning organization" which can support progress of the CIN and ACO. (Senge 1990, Pisapia, Reyes-Guerra et al. 2005) Novel systems will emerge as new CINs and ACOs are formed. (Leavitt and McKeown 2013) Invoking a systems approach to problem solving, oriented to people, processes, and technologies is a powerful tool for physician, nursing, and all healthcare leaders.

Business Acumen- Leaders of CINs and ACOs need core skills in management, communications, finance, and social sciences to strengthen their abilities to lead their organizations in new directions. Physicians and nurses are getting more formal advanced business education to support new leadership roles. With greater business acumen these leaders will have the ability to better lead their organizations in a financially stable and solvent way, and communicate to physician peers, clinical teams, administrative staff, payers, and competing providers a vision and path based on solid financial and operational considerations.

Patient-Centered- The last of the building blocks we present for consideration, and perhaps most important for new provider business models, is a patient-centered focus. The ultimate goal for every CIN, ACO or any other healthcare delivery model is delivery of safe, effective, efficient, quality, affordable, and coordinated care that supports achieving or surpassing desired and targeted health outcomes for the individual and population. This is a tradition, and very provider focused approach, which needs infusion of a patient perspective. In *Core Communication Competencies in Patient-Centered Care*, Boykins noted,

> Patient centered care is care based on a partnership between the patient, their families, and the health care provider that is focused on the patient's values, preferences, and needs. (Davis-Boykins 2014)

This is a typical definition of patient-centeredness, and takes a different perspective than the traditional provider-focused approach. Note the lack of "targeted health outcomes," as these might be irrelevant to the patient – for example they might not care whether the HbA1C "Control is <7% for a Selected Population." (NCQA, 2014) The emphasis, instead, is on a "partnership of equals," where both parties contribute to the relationship. This partnership requires trust among the parties, a trait lacking in some patient-provider relationships. Significant changes in perspective and approach is needed to achieve the trust required for a partnership of equals. (Stanford University, 2014) Patient engagement is a key factor in this new approach.

Patient-centered care and patient engagement are critical to achieving provider goals. In, *Early Lessons From Four 'Aligning Forces For Quality' Communities Bolster The Case For Patient-Centered Care*, Roseman and colleageus notes it plays an important role in the quality of care received, thus impacting provider metrics such as quality improvement efforts and patient experience:

> ...engaging patients in quality improvement efforts prompts changes that can include increasing engagement in their own care and improving their experiences with the health care system. (Roseman, Osborne-Stafsnes et al. 2013)

The building blocks reviewed here serve as a set of management tools for healthcare leaders in their efforts to guide CIN or ACO. These new care delivery models are evolving and these building blocks equipped leaders with skills and tools to operate in the new healthcare environment.

Leadership Styles

Leaders typically subscribe to a particular style based on their personal traits, strengths, experiences, and the situation faced in their organization. Given the current challenges in healthcare, several leadership styles may be considered by healthcare leaders. The styles described here include situational, transformational, and servant (see Table 3-1). (Schwartz and Tumblin 2002, Xirasagar, Samuels et al. 2006, Chaudry, Jain et al. 2008) Each is applicable to healthcare organizations — especially those forming CINs and ACOs. Leaders of these new models must bring management expertise an unwavering commitment to quality and excellence, and agility that allow them to conform their style to the current challenges. While each organization and community has particular features, requirements, goals, and objectives, they can reach a higher level of performance with the help of a leader who understands how to apply different leadership styles as they are needed.

Table 3-1. Leadership Styles and Successful ACO/CIN Implementation

Style	Description
Situational (Chaudry, Jain et al. 2008)	• Adaptable to specific situations. • Leader assumes one of four roles: coaching, supporting, delegating, or leading. • Understands need for workers' empowerment and recognition. • Leader knows his or her strengths but adjusts when needed. • Recognizes the need for change.
Transformational (Xirasagar, Samuels et al. 2006)	• Influences subordinates to move toward "ethically inspired goals transcending self-interest". • Four central components: "idealized influence, inspirational motivation, intellectual stimulation, and individualized consideration". • Facilitates team growth through individualized mentoring or coaching relationships.
Servant (Schwartz and Tumblin 2002)	• Engages in active listening. • Demonstrates empathy for workers and peers. • Strong communicator of concepts. • Possesses strong persuasive abilities. • "Exerts a healing influence on individuals and institutions". • Establishes a community in the workplace.

Each leadership style is beneficial in the development of a CIN or ACO. The transformational style of leadership, for example, may be the best approach where the organization faces severe challenges, such as revenue losses and imminent closure, and dramatic change is needed to ensure survival. In this example, physicians and other staff must see beyond their traditional roles and operations to achieve a new level of effort that changes the way they do business.

Understanding the skills necessary for the different types of situations will enable leaders to successfully implement CIN and ACO.

Who Drives the Bus?

Securing the right leader for each CIN or ACO is critical. One of the most important steps is selection of physician leaders. Medicare ACOs require physician leadership. The American Medical Association (AMA), Institute for Healthcare Improvement, NCQA, Medicare Payment Advisory Commission, and other organizations have all endorsed this requirement. Ensuring physicians are the source of medical decisions and leadership, and they are both clinically and financially committed to the new ways of doing business, is critical to ensuring that goals are met across the organization. The insistence on physician leadership is related in part to past experience with HMOs in the 1990s, and the recent experience with Medicare demonstration projects in the 2000s.

In contrast to the Health Maintenance Organization (HMO) model, in which payers primarily used various methods of physician oversight (such as utilization management) to control costs, the physician-led CIN or ACO model is intended for physicians to focus on patient care and clinical outcomes, help patients achieve or maintain health, and thereby indirectly lower the total cost of care while improving quality. An associated change is the shift from the utilization review metrics of the past to the quality outcome-driven measures of the present and future. Although experience is beginning to show that quality metrics focusing on appropriate care do not necessarily reduce costs and many provider led organizations find they need to adopt utilization review measures as well (more about that in later chapters).

As the U.S. healthcare system evolves, different networks and partnerships will emerge with changing industry dynamics. To navigate these new situations, physician leadership will be essential. One national survey indicated that,

> Fifty-one percent of the respondent ACOs identified themselves as physician led, and another 33 percent reported that they were jointly led by hospitals and physicians. (Colla, Lewis et al. 2014)

The question of "who drives the bus?" is clearly answered by physicians, engaged at leadership levels to address the challenges in transitioning to a value-based model of care.

CIN and ACO are intended to achieve economies of scale in care delivery, enable joint contracting with insurers, and increase quality and coordination of care while reducing costs. Clinical integration helps accomplish these initiatives, and is a necessary building block of an ACO. A formal clinically integrated network is necessary where the majority of physicians are not employed by the ACO entity. It is an especially attractive model in any situation where independent physicians wish to retain their autonomy while engaging with a larger organization collectively focused on quality, integration, collective negotiation, cost reduction, and health care value for the consumer. Figure 3-2 provides an illustration of a path to move from a CIN to formation of an ACO and the potential for growth of an Accountable Care Network (ACN).

Figure 3-2. Network Progression[*]

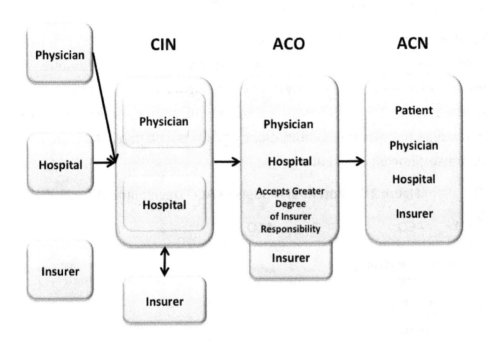

Reinhart and Esterhay conceptually advanced Figure 3-2, originally illustrated in the second edition of this book, in their final chapter of *Accountable Care: Bridging the Health Information Technology Divi*de. They also defined the Accountable Care Network:

> Just as a CIN is a necessary building block of an ACO, an ACO is a necessary building block for an ACN. An ACN would be comprised of three or more separate business entities such as a physician group, hospital, and insurer with a formal shared vision, mission, network strategy, and network governance structure. (Reinhart and Esterhay 2012)

The other critical element of an ACN is a more direct patient engagement strategy that may involve innovative use of mobile health information

---

[*]Original illustration developed based on BDC Advisors presentation to VHA on Clinical Integration (slide 2). Accessed online June 29, 2011, at http://bdcadvisors.com/presentations.asp

technologies and social media for communication and collaborative use of patient records by providers and patients.

As physicians and hospitals integrate their activities through various arrangements, new opportunities will emerge to improve value and economies of scale through shared services. Figure 3-3, expanded from its illustration in the 2nd edition with a sixth model, shows some of these new arrangements in potential combinations of ACO participants. (Devers 2009, Rittenhouse, Shortell et al. 2009)

Figure 3-3. Potential Models of ACO Development

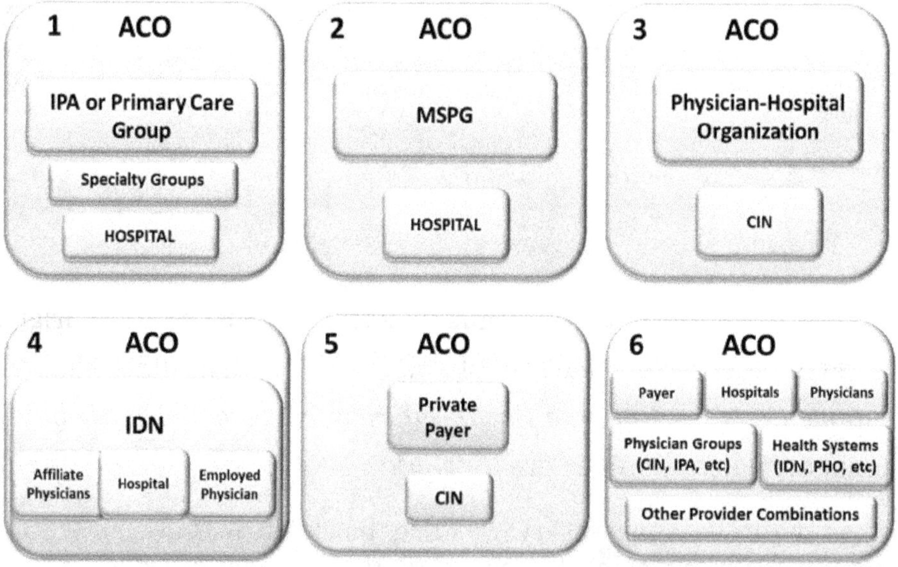

Additional configurations are possible, including academic medical centers as integrated delivery networks, and virtual models (Blue Shield of California April 22, 2009) that combine health systems, physician groups, and payer organizations for collaborative care coordination. The models referenced in Figure 3.3 are intended as representative examples rather than an exhaustive list of all arrangements that will shape the future. Following are more detailed descriptions of these models.

1: IPA-directed ACO - This model positions the independent practice association (IPA) or primary care physician group in the lead role of the ACO, with specialty groups and hospitals in a subordinate position. This model also brings the medical home to the forefront in the new entity and allows physicians (both primary care and specialists) flexibility in creating exclusive or nonexclusive contracts. An alternative approach is to have primary care physicians under exclusive contracts, but allow specialists to work across multiple ACOs within the community.

2: MSPG-directed ACO - In this model the multispecialty physician group (MSPG, such as Mayo and Cleveland Clinics) directs the ACO with the hospital subordinated to the MSPG. Here physicians (primary care and specialists) work in an ACO with nonexclusive contracting rights, and the ACO partners with hospitals and ancillary service providers (laboratories, skilled nursing facilities, rehabilitation clinics, and the like) to support clinical integration.

3: PHO-directed ACO - This model places the physician-hospital organization at the center of the ACO. The physician hospital organization (PHO) creates partnerships with physician practices, and the entire collaboration serves as a collective risk-bearing organization. The PHO also negotiates contracts for the physician practices (primary or specialty care) as part of clinical and financial integration. Sutter Health and Scripps Health in California, and Advocate Health in Chicago are examples of this model. (Boland, Polakoff et al. 2010, Shortell, Casalino et al. 2010)

4: IDN-directed ACO - The fourth model places the integrated delivery network (IDN) at the forefront of the ACO. An IDN is usually a formal integrated network of hospitals and physicians, who combine to contract and deliver a set of services. The IDN has the option of exclusive or nonexclusive contracting with primary care practices and specialty care groups regardless of whether they are affiliated or unaffiliated with the IDN. In addition, the IDN has control over hospital medical staff organizations, which could be under exclusive contracts with the IDN to support the required level of services needed for beneficiary care under the ACO. Examples of these arrangements are Kaiser Permanente, Intermountain Healthcare in Utah and southeastern Idaho, and the Henry Ford Health System in Michigan.

5: Private payer-directed ACO - This model is based on a private payer forming a direct partnership with physicians, creating a physician-only CIN that subcontracts for hospital or other services. This ACO could also be formed with IPAs or MSPGs, as it intends the private payer to serve as the partner to provide needed financial support for infrastructure development such as health information technology, population data aggregation, and training. As the purpose of the ACO is to improve population health for the populations it serves, it would contract separately with hospitals and ancillary service providers for inpatient care, tests, rehabilitation, and other services when needed. Contracting with physicians may be more rigid; that is, the ACO may require more exclusive relationships. This is particularly important for Medicare ACOs that designate a specific number of beneficiaries for the ACO. Even though the payer serves as a principal partner under this model, accountability for patient care could still reside at the local level with a governance board headed by physician leaders.

6: Private payer partnership ACO – This model is a hybrid, intended to combine the best of all organizations. Physicians and hospitals in many cases have not much experience with managing risk and medical services to financial and clinical targets. In addition, few payers outside of traditional, vertically integrated IDNs (e.g., Kaiser, Intermountain Health) have the knowledge of the local market to know how best to reduce waste and control costs. Recognizing the strengths of each organization, the partnership ACO draws on the best practices of each organization to improve both, and create an ACO that is truly accountable for both financial costs and clinical quality. Building on the medical and financial/risk management, actuarial, and health information technologies of the insurance company, the hospital and physician can more confidently focus on clinical practice. Relying on the clinical expertise of physicians and hospitals, the insurance company can focus on what it does best, using predictive analytics and risk management capabilities to ensure organization solvency and financial sustainability. This kind of partnership is built on trust, and exhibits qualities rarely found in traditional healthcare stakeholder relationships. Successful examples of this partnership include Aetna and Banner Health Network, a model explored in later chapters.

Governance

"Good governance requires letting management run the show." (Bass and Cammarano 2014) As Bass and Cammarona note, it is imperative for governing boards to allow hospital management to run the operations. Establishing and maintaining trust between board members and senior management helps facilitate communication, oversight, and key decisions that drive success. The AMA released a set of 13 principles to guide ACO establishment, one of which is a governance principle.[*] The ACO governance principle identifies four elements necessary for effective governance:

- Medical decisions should be made by physicians;

- Governance should be by a board of directors elected by the ACO's professionals;

- Physician leadership should be licensed in the state in which the ACO operates and licensed for the active practice of medicine in the ACO's service area; and

- The ACO's governing board should be separate from and independent of the hospital's board of directors (when a hospital is part of the ACO entity).

---

[*] Interim meeting of the American Medical Association House of Delegates. Accountable care organization (ACO) principles; November 2010; San Diego, CA. Accessed online July 20, 2011 at http://op.bna.com/hl.nsf/id/bbrk-8b5szv/$File/ACOandAMA.pdf

Instituting effective governance in CINs and ACOs requires a long-term focus and understanding of broader economic and community issues impacting the organization. Morrisette summarized that it,

> ...includes decisions which might fundamentally change the nature and scope of the firm, especially to hospitals which are predominantly nonprofit institutions with volunteer boards of directors. (Morrissette 2012)

Effective governance is a critical element of leadership. Board members are trustees of the organization who provide strategic oversight and advisement to senior management teams — often operating as volunteers. They help steer the organization toward achievement of its mission and vision.

Future Direction

Ultimately the principal focus of each CIN or ACO leader should be achieving the goals for which the organization was developed, with a patient-centered focus — hence the importance of physician executive experience with patient care. With a both patient-facing clinical experience, and business expertise, the physician executive can lead the organization in a multi-disciplinary fashion, understanding all aspects of the new organization. In *MD 2.0: Physician Leadership for the Information Age*, Grace Terrell, said it best,

> In the complex environment of contemporary health care, physicians find themselves at a critical juncture in history that beacons a call for leadership across the profession. (Terrell and Bohn 2012)

Meeting this call to leadership requires mastery of essential skills as presented in this chapter. In addition, leaders in healthcare organizations have an added ethical duty to focus on the physician-patient relationship and the health of their communities given the constant challenges they will face in the future. (Souba 2011)

CHAPTER 3 DISCUSSION QUESTIONS

Discussion questions are provided for team building or class exercises. Answers for all questions are provided in Appendix C.

Question Number	Question
1	What are the six types of ACO models listed in the chapter?
2	What are three styles of leadership discussed in the chapter?
3	What are 'Relational Connectors' and how does Malcolm Gladwell's "The Tipping Point" fit in to the concept?
4	What are the four elements necessary for effective ACO governance according to the AMA?
5	What is the Accountable Care Network (ACN) concept? Where was it first cited?
6	What are the two pillars of the Building Blocks for CIN and ACO Leaders (found in Figure 3-1)?

CHAPTER 3 HIGHLIGHTS

✓ Provided a new conceptual model of the Building Blocks for a CIN or ACO Leader. These building blocks include shared purpose, shared culture, network & alliance engagement, population health oriented, relational connector, innovation champion, business acumen, systems thinking, and patient-centered.

✓ Covered six types of potential ACOs as built on those in the 2nd edition.

✓ Reviewed three styles of leadership: situational, transformational and servant.

✓ Emphasized the importance of physician leadership for strategic steering of CINs and ACOs.

✓ Listed the AMA's principles for effective governance.

✓ Discussed the importance of organizational governance, as a critical element of leadership.

✓ Identified key challenges facing healthcare leaders.

✓ Covered the concept of an Accountable Care Network (ACN) as an extension of the health care organizations and their integration with key stakeholders.

CHAPTER 3 REFERENCES

Bass, K. H. and Cammarano, T. W. (2014). A matter of perspective. The best boards respect the line between governing and managing. *Trustee*, 67(3), 27-29, 21.

Berwick, D. M. (1996). A primer on leading the improvement of systems. *BMJ*, 312(7031), 619-622.

Blue Shield of California (2009, April 22). Blue Shield of California, Catholic Healthcare West and Hill Physicians Medical Group to Pilot Innovative New Care. *Reuters.*

Boland, P., et al. (2010). Accountable care organizations hold promise, but will they achieve cost and quality targets? *Managed Care,* 19(10), 12-16, 19.

Centers for Medicare and Medicaid Services (2011, April 7). Overview and intent of the Medicare Shared Savings Program., Vol. 76, No. 67, Federal Register: 19533.

Chaudry, J., et al. (2008). Physician leadership: the competencies of change. *Journal of Surgical Education,* 65(3), 213-220. doi: 10.1016/j.jsurg.2007.11.014

Colins, J. (2001). Level 5 leadership. In *Good to Great: Why Some Companies Make the Leap and Others Don't* (pp. 17-40). New York, NY, Harper Business.

Colla, C. H., et al. (2014). First national survey of ACOs finds that physicians are playing strong leadership and ownership roles. *Health Affairs,* 33(6), 964-71. doi: 10.1016/j.juro.2014.10.083

Davis-Boykins, A. (2014). Core communication competencies in patient-centered care. *ABNF Journal,* 25(2), 40-45.

Devers, K. J. (2009). Can accountable care organizations improve the value of health care by solving the cost and quality quandaries?

Flareau, B. and Bohn, J.M. (2013). Principles of business. In *6 Ps of Physician Leadership. A Primer for Emerging and Developing Leaders* (p. 69). St. Petersburg, FL, Kumu Press.

Gladwell, M. (2001). The law of the few. Connectors, mavens, and salesmen. In *The Tipping Point. How Little Things Can Make a Big Difference* (p. 49). New York, NY, Back Bay Books.

Hill, L. A., et al. (2014). Collective genius. *Harvard Business Review,* 92(6), 94-102.

Kindig, D. and Stoddart, G. (2003). What is population health? *American Journal of Public Health,* 93(3), 380-383.

Kruse, K. (2012, October 16). 100 Best quotes on leadership. *Forbes.* Retrieved from http://www.forbes.com/sites/kevinkruse/2012/10/16/quotes-on-leadership/

Leavitt, M. and McKeown, R. (2013). Committed leadership. In *Finding Allies, Building Alliances: 8 Elements That Bring and Keep People Together* (pp. 68-69). Hoboken, NJ: Jossey-Bass.

Leavitt, M. and McKeown, R. (2013). *Finding Allies, Building Alliances: 8 Elements That Bring and Keep People Together.* Hoboken, NJ: Jossey-Bass.

Lee, T. H. and Cosgrove, T. (2014). Engaging doctors in the health care revolution. *Harvard Business Review,* 92(6), 104-111.

Morrissette, S. G. (2012). Governance issues in the transition to accountable care: A case study ofsSilver cross hospital. *Hospital Topics*, 90(4), 104-112. doi: 10.1080/00185868.2012.737755

National Committee on Quality Assurance. (2015) HEDIS® Volume 2: Technical Specifications for Health Plans.

Pisapia, J., et al. (2005). Developing the leader's strategic mindset: Establishing the measures. *Leadership Review*, 5(1), 41-68.

Randall, et al. (2014). Leading in the connected era. *Strategy & Leadership,* 42(1), 37-46.

Reinhart, J. and Esterhay, R. (2012). Chapter 11. The new horizon—A network transition to individual and population health. In *Accountable Care: Bridging the Health Information Technology Divide, First Edition* (pp. 395-396). B. Spooner, B. Reese and C. Konschak. Virginia Beach, VA, Convurgent Publishing.

Rittenhouse, D. R., et al. (2009). Primary care and accountable care—two essential elements of delivery-system reform. *New England Journal of Medicine*, 361(24), 2301-2303. doi: 10.1056/NEJMp0909327

Roseman, D., et al. (2013). Early lessons from four 'aligning forces for quality'communities bolster the case for patient-centered care. *Health Affairs*, 32(2), 232-241. doi: 10.1377/hlthaff.2012.1085

Schwartz, R. W. and Tumblin, T. F. (2002). The power of servant leadership to transform health care organizations for the 21st century economy. *Archives of Surgery*, 137(12), 1419-1427.

Senge, P. (1990). *The Fifth Discipline: The Art and Practice of the Learning Organization.* New York, NY, Knopf Doubleday Publishing Group.

Shortell, S. M., et al. (2010). How the Center for Medicare and Medicaid Innovation should test accountable care organizations. *Health Affairs*, 29(7), 1293-1298. doi: 10.1377/hlthaff.2010.0453

Souba, W. W. (2011). The being of leadership. *Philosophy, Ethics, and Humanities in Medicine*, 6(5), 1-11. Retrieved from http://www.peh-med.com/content/6/1/5

Stanford University. (2014). What is an ePatient. MedicineX 2014 Conference. Retrieved from http://medicinex.stanford.edu/what-is-an-epatient-2/

Stoller, J. K. (2009). Developing physician-leaders: a call to action. *Journal of General Internal Medicine*, 24(7), 876-878.

Terrell, G. E. and Bohn, J. M. (2012). Chapter 8: The next generation. *MD 2.0: Physician Leadership for the Information Age. From Hero to Duyukdv* (p. 134). Tampa, FL, American College of Physician Executives.

Xirasagar, S., et al. (2006). Management training of physician executives, their leadership style, and care management performance: an empirical study. *American Journal of Managed Care*, 12(2), 101-108.

Chapter 4. Network Evolution

Thomas A. Raskauskas

In the realm of ideas, everything depends on enthusiasm; in the real world, all rests on perseverance.

Johann Wolfgang von Goethe
German Writer and Statesman
1749-1832

CHAPTER 4 LEARNING OBJECTIVES

✓ Understand the elements necessary to establish a CIN/ACO.

✓ Understand the importance of timelines for development of a CIN/ACO.

✓ Understand the importance of strategic planning and budget development for CINs/ACOs.

✓ Increase awareness of federal agencies (e.g., Federal Trade Commission and Internal Revenue Service) on formation of a CIN/ACO.

Overview

Primary care physician practices provide the underpinnings of patient-centered care that become the foundation for Accountable Care Organizations (ACOs) and Clinically Integrated Networks (CINs), as discussed in Chapter 2. In the contemporary health system these organizations, their physicians and care teams are increasingly called upon to improve effectiveness and efficiency, facilitate coordination of care, and manage care, including care transitions. From a global view, these efforts can be seen as part of a broader societal transition, or "network effect." As described in *Heading Toward a Society of Networks: Empirical Developments and Theoretical Challenges,*

> Western societies are moving towards a society of networks, i.e., a society, in which the formal, vertically integrated organization that has dominated the 20th century is replaced or at least complemented by

consciously created and goal-directed networks. (Raab & Kennis, 2009)

Getting a CIN or ACO initiated requires coordination with a network of providers and technology vendors, collaboration with payers, partnering with patient groups, oversight of government agencies, and involvement of other organizations across a spectrum of stakeholders. All these stakeholders, when properly combined, create a network effect of new collaborations and services that improve quality and affordability for the consumer, and effect change and align participants with the vision of the new organization.

The term "providers," in this context, includes care delivered by those working with patients both within, and beyond, the primary care office. This includes all providers of care in the continuum that result in the total care and total cost of care of the patient. As networks are developing, each transition needs to be identified to understand what potential providers must be included. These may be hospitals and hospital systems, physician specialists, skilled nursing facilities, home health care, durable medical equipment agencies, pharmacies, nurse care managers, community health workers, family caregivers, public health agencies, social service agencies, and any other provider of care, including the patient. In developing the network, it is important to understand that each provider plays a role in care and cost, and how much care improvement and cost control the network wants to provide will determine the extent to which providers are included in the network beyond the primary care office.

When the CIN or ACO advances to a multi-payer model, the complexity of the care processes typically increase as providers care for multiple patient populations with new ways of delivering, evaluating, and receiving compensation for care. In this chapter we discuss a number of tactical issues to consider in establishing the CIN/ACO network.

CIN/ACO: The Tactical Framework

Creation of a CIN or ACO requires a new operational infrastructure. As the Medicare ACO model has taken shape under the 2010 Patient Protection and Affordable Care Act (ACA), and private payer initiatives continue to flourish, a number of common infrastructure elements have been identified.

To begin, the Federal Trade Commission's (FTC) guidelines for a CIN provide a broad framework for establishing the elements of a provider network. The guidelines include:

1. Establishing mechanisms to monitor and control utilization of health care services that are designed to control costs and assure quality of care;
2. Selectively choosing network physicians (and other providers of care) who are likely to further these efficiency objectives; and
3. The significant investment of capital, both monetary and human, in the necessary infrastructure and capability to realize the claimed efficiencies. (Department of Justice and Federal Trade Commission, 1996)

And although the FTC guidelines have been updated and revised over the years, including advisory opinions and a joint FTC/Department of Justice (DOJ) guidance document to provide additional clarity for Medicare ACO, the core principles set forth in 1996 are still relevant.

Elements of a Network Operation

Establishing a CIN or ACO is essentially the creation of a new business entity comprised of multiple organizations brought together to create a new service designed to improve quality and affordability for the benefit of consumers. This new entity requires each organization to participate in the administration, management, and delivery of health and wellness services, usually in a specific geographic region. There are many descriptions of essential elements of CINs, but here the discussion will focus on the elements in Figure 4-1, especially elements the FTC reinforced in its Norman PHO Advisory Opinion. (Federal Trade Commission, 2013)

Figure 4-1. Elements of the Network Operation

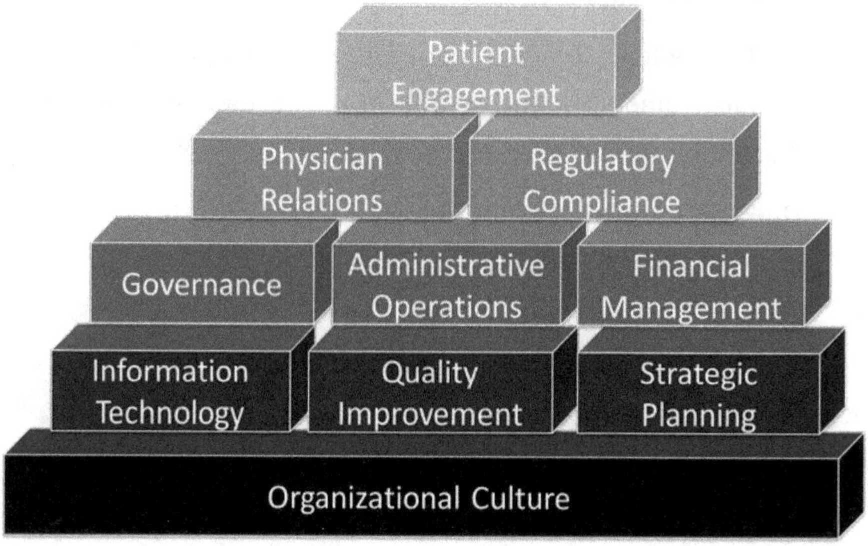
Patient Engagement
Physician Relations
Regulatory Compliance
Governance
Administrative Operations
Financial Management
Information Technology
Quality Improvement
Strategic Planning
Organizational Culture

Patient Engagement

One of the important drivers in the Care Revolution Era is the need for patient engagement to empower patients as participants in their own care, and improve each patient's experience with care providers and healthcare systems. Different interventions can improve health by changing the patients' "social environment" and their abilities to handle and solve problems on their own through better self-management. (Hibbard & Greene, 2013) Every CIN, ACO, Patient-Centered Medical Home (PCMH), and care team has goals of improving the health of the patient population and experience with the care delivery system, improving quality, and lowering costs of care— all parts of the Triple Aim. Patient-centered care has also been identified as one of the six IOM goals to improve the U.S. health system.

To drive patient-centered care the CIN or ACO must continually evaluate the quality of care patients receive, including their experience with the care system. A 2013 New England Journal of Medicine article, entitled *The Patient Experience and Health Outcomes,* identified three areas to consider in measuring patient experience: a) specific events, b) "patient-provider interactions", and c) timely assessment of the patient's experience of the care they receive. (Manary, Boulding, Staelin, & Glickman, 2013)

To foster a more patient-centric perspective, each CIN and ACO must incorporate into its operations policies, procedures, rules and guidelines a patient-centered perspective, from the bedside to the boardroom. Successful patient engagement efforts can include improved outreach to patients through patient experience surveys, engagement of patients in quality improvement initiatives, and most importantly focused efforts on patient-provider partnering to improve communications, decision making, health literacy, and ultimately achieve better health outcomes. (Ishikawa, Hashimoto, & Kiuchi, 2013; Roseman, Osborne-Stafsnes, Amy, Boslaugh, & Slate-Miller, 2013) This "360–degree" approach ensures that executives, physicians, nurses, and other key stakeholders have an opportunity to hear directly from the patients and gain unfiltered insight to the value their organization is delivering.

Information Technology

The technology infrastructure of any CIN or ACO must have certain essential elements. Health information technology is the driver of connectivity. These topics will be discussed in more detail in Chapter 10, but a number of operational issues are introduced here.

Health information technology is rapidly becoming the backbone of healthcare services, due to government mandates requiring its use and efficiencies required by new provider-based models of care. Although electronic medical record implementations are in full swing, electronic medical records (EMRs) by themselves are insufficient to manage an ACO or CIN. In fact, successful population health management has been done with little to no EMR technology at all. Instead, early adopters have relied on paper-based registry systems in which relevant patient care information is entered into a common repository for quality reporting and proactive care management. As EMRs become more prevalent and functional, manual entry will become less necessary and larger amounts of information will be available for refined, direct patient care and population health management.

CINs and ACOs also need to acquire the ability to analyze data and report on physician performance, which is usually a legal requirement for these organizations as well. The ability to collect and use appropriate data that measures physician performance and patient outcomes, such as clinical, claims, laboratory, and pharmacy data, are important for programs to succeed. Claims data can be collected directly from each physician or hospital management system, but billed charges are not always as useful as adjudicated claims. Adjudicated claims may be obtained from payers, or more commonly, from regional clearinghouses, but it is sometimes difficult to connect the claims data to the right patient and provider. Many providers, therefore, rely on EMR clinical data to fulfill their data requirements. Laboratory data should include all relevant laboratory providers within the market, including hospital and physician office-based laboratories. This brings its own challenges. And finally, pharmacy data can come from e-prescribing directly or more commonly from pharmacy benefit managers. Electronic medical record clinical data is becoming more useful as EMR vendors recognize the importance of performance metrics for their provider clients. Finally, "exogenous" data that adds both patient reported, and consumer derived data give an additional amount of information key to understanding lifestyle and consumer behavior outside the healthcare environment.

Claims data are perhaps most important, as payers use them to analyze total population health, cost of care, stratify risk, identify individual patients for interventions, identify quality and related performance metrics on which to base CIN/ACO reimbursement, and attribution for enhanced physicians payment. Because of their long history and detailed nature, claims data may be the only way to obtain historical patient treatment information, providing the basis for ACO benchmarking and shared savings analysis.

As systems mature clinical information is being aggregated directly from medical records and combined with claims data. Start-up operations, however, may have to to focus on near term high-value investments, such as billed charges that can be mined with readily available software applications. Many vendors are emerging in this space with data aggregation, analytic, and reporting capabilities. In addition to aggregate repositories, population-based care management is largely dependent on ways to identify, intervene, and co-manage patients using this data. Cross-system cohort management and patient identification capabilities, building links between clinical and claims databases as well as between disparate clinical medical records, are essential to helping ACOs effectively manage populations.

Helping physicians implement EMRs is a consideration for start-up and ongoing operations of a CIN or ACO because of the need to access and manage patient information from multiple points of care, provide care management support and coordination, and measure performance. In addition, it is important to have a portal allowing patients to access their information, contribute relevant patient-reported data, and for clinical teams and self-management tools increasingly critical in a patient-centered and value-based system.

In the age of the Internet and with the social media and mobile communications revolution, health information for patients is now more important than ever. CINs and ACOs must introduce processes that strengthen patient engagement and self-management by ensuring access to information and tools so that patient-centeredness criteria are met. (Federal Register Volume 76 Number 67, April 7, 2011a) Success in patient self-management requires the use of such enabling technologies as EMRs, mobile platforms, predictive analytics, personal health records, electronic communications, and remote monitoring. To support implementing these tools, CMS initiated the Meaningful Use of Electronic Health Records Program in 2009, including reimbursement opportunities for eligible professionals to defray the cost of implementation. Some of the goals of the Meaningful Use program include setting up a structure and evaluation criteria to improve the interoperability of systems, strengthen quality, and improve safety. These programs can be leveraged to benefit the establishment of ACOs.

Over the last decade the patient population has been enabled in this technology driven era with iPads™, smart phones, laptops, and "apps" that support these various platforms. The asymmetries of information that once existed between health professional and patient have changed in light of universal access to information via the Internet. CINs, ACOs and their participants can use these technologies to support patients, increase trust, and improve care delivered and health outcomes.

Governance

Launching a CIN or ACO requires a strong, agile, and multidisciplinary group of stakeholders engaged to ensure the success and sustainability of the new organization. A passion for clinical and administrative transformation, and a cultural transition from fee-for-service operations to a value-oriented way of delivering care, is essential. Depending on the configuration and path chosen, the leadership structure of the organization will vary. A common characteristic is having a physician-led system with the necessary operational processes and infrastructure in place to work effectively toward improving patients' experience and clinical outcomes, and lowering cost while improving quality and value.

Forming the board involves detailed discussions about voting rights, initial and ongoing criteria for membership, incentive compensation formulas, care management programs, and most importantly the quality of care and other indicators used to measure performance. Sub-committees of the board commonly include credentialing, quality or clinical performance, nominations, and contracting. Committees vary in scope, type, and number, depending on the CIN and or ACO configuration, but they must address these fundamental issues and involve physicians so they understand their roles and responsibilities to meet performance metrics and enhance the value of care delivered. An industry leader in CIN establishment is Advocate Physician Partners in Illinois. Their 2013 Value Report summarized the governance model employed in the nineth year of their clinical integration program.

Advocate Physician Partners - Clinical Integration Program Governance

"At any given time, over 100 Advocate Physician Partners member physicians hold governance positions on various boards and committees that guide the measure development process and monitor results. Advocate Physician Partners requires all board and committee members to participate in a comprehensive governance orientation program, an annual conference and business conduct programs to ensure they fully understand their duties and obligations. In addition, new leaders participate in a mentoring program in collaboration with an existing physician leader. Real physician representation in governance has facilitated a strong sense of group identity, enabled rapid expansion of the Program and fostered acceptance of ever more challenging performance goals and measures by the general physician membership." (Advocate Physician Partners, 2013)

Advocate Physician Partners includes more than 3,800 physicians. Over the years it has established programs that have achieved significant improvement in population health along with a positive economic impact. The excerpt above demonstrates the deep commitment and level of involvement from physicians in the strategic guidance of the program. Moreover, it shows the need to involve physicians in the development of performance goals against which they will be measured, and the importance of their acceptance of changes needed to move from a procedure-based to a performance-based system

Additionally, Shields and colleagues noted, "This arrangement creates a structure that enables physicians and hospitals to work together to improve care with common quality and cost effectiveness goals." (Shields, Patel, Manning, & Sacks, 2011) The article further noted the importance of collaboration to drive improvements in quality. As one of the nation's leading examples of CIN operation, Advocate's 2014 Value Report illustrated an innovative array of interventions diffused across care settings that led to an increased level of care coordination and cost control in 2013.

(Advocate Physician Partners, 2014)

Physician involvement and governance is even more critical for organizations of otherwise independent physicians interested in becoming a CIN, but not a full-risk ACO. This is because the antitrust enforcing agencies require physician involvement and collaboration from the beginning, to ensure every physician is committed to the goals of cost containment and quality improvement, and collective price negotiations are reasonably necessary and ancillary to achieve that goal. Moreover, without the financial risk of an ACO, the CIN will draw greater scrutiny from the federal government to ensure anti-competitive collusion does not occur.

Physician / Provider Relations

Selective identification, recruitment and retention of a panel of physicians and other providers capable of meeting all needs of the patient population is essential for every CIN and ACO. Physician relations is a dynamic field as the roles and responsibilities of physicians in today's healthcare environment and society are changing. Decades ago the physician's role involved autonomy, control, and prestige in both professional responsibilities and community status. Healthcare reforms and other changes over the last two decades have resulted in a shift from provider-centric to patient-centric care, and this change is affecting the entire medical profession. Autonomy and control are giving way to an emphasis on collaboration, empowerment of others, and performance evaluation based on data-driven analysis and evidence. The "cottage industry" solo, private practice environment continues to shrink amid declining reimbursements and greater physician employment by hospitals, integrated health systems and other provider organizations. In light of these issues, managing CIN/ACO physician relations is increasingly vital. Clinical integration is growing across the industry, and will certainly intensify the need for stronger relations to retain the base of providers to meet organization commitments.

Important components of physician relations include a physician champion, strong physician network manager or director, and a physician relationship team. The network manager should be hired early in the formation of the organization. The physician network team puts many demands on physicians, necessitating much planning in the physician relations department. As physicians are increasingly being asked to serve as leaders in addition to their patient care responsibilities, it is often helpful for physicians to partner with healthcare administrators who can focus on overseeing the strategic and day-to-day operations of provider organizations. Beyond the leadership team, every physician in the CIN or ACO needs a relationship that best promotes collaboration and attainment of the goals created and agreed upon by the organization. Having dedicated physician relationship team members that put a face and a name on the CIN or ACO is a way to bring to life the organization on a personal level. Certainly physician-to-physician relations are key to success, but they should be supplemented by a relationship team that facilities bidirectional communication.

Regardless of how the relational functions are staffed or managed, ensuring maintenance of physician engagement, at all levels, is paramount to success of the new organization.

While physician recruitment does not take place officially until after the legal entity is formed and a physician participation agreement created, the recruitment process begins from the moment the first steering committee is convened. As CIN or ACO processes develop, a comprehensive communication and marketing plan is essential to recruit physicians. Value to physicians and setting expectations for network participants should be central to a communication plan.

A key component of the recruitment process is finding the so-called "right docs" for your organization. Generally, high-volume, high-quality, and low-cost providers are sought. How to identify and access the information necessary to identify these characteristics, particularly in markets in which the creating entity does not have insurance data to rely upon for intelligence, is not simple. Health systems that employ physicians can look in their own data or third-party administrator information, and others may extrapolate from hospital-based data. In most cases insurers have the richest data source through claims, and most have already identified physicians with the best outcomes. CINs and ACOs should consider partnering with insurers willing to share information and interested in partnerships (see Aetna-BHN example in Chapter 14). Another mechanism is to have a third party survey physicians targeted as potential members of the provider practice network. Regardless of the process, efforts should be undertaken early to assess this aspect of network formation.

In addition to "who gets on the bus", network recruitment must look at service coverage, in order to have adequate health services to meet the goals and objectives of the organization. Of course, this and other activities should always keep in mind antitrust rules, and the right approach helps to ensure laws, regulations, or guidelines are not violated. The approach must focus on ensuring improved quality and lower costs for the benefit of the consumer, and making sure the physician fully understands not only their role and the benefits, but also their responsibilities and how they are held accountable. The legal aspects of this step are discussed further in Chapter 5, and must be considered in the recruitment process.

ACOs and CINs need to consider other resources needed by the newly developing network in addition to traditional provider relation roles. An important part of any arrangement that looks to drive efficiencies and value is finding and using resources already available in the community. The challenges of increasing costs, shrinking budgets and price compression have created resource and socioeconomic challenges. To help improve efficiency and cost-effectiveness CIN and ACO leaders should seek out community and social service resources already available and build them into their operational plans. This can be accomplished by establishing a community engagement plan that builds strong ties with all services available, including those of managed care payers and social service providers. (Jarousse, 2010) Other organizations already providing services that could be part of the plan include area employers, school systems and clinics, economic development agencies, social service agencies, and safety net providers. Identifying the spectrum of stakeholders and nurturing their collective resources to optimize performance is another network effect that will not only benefit the new organization but also the entire community.

The United States is at a turning point in how we deliver care. The CIN and ACO focus on value rather than volume implies a greater focus on the community and improving total population health. Building on the network effect by using existing community and social services helps fulfill the CIN and ACO goals of operational soundness while improving the health of the community and creating an agile organization able to adjust course when needed based on community needs and future changes that inevitably occur as healthcare reform evolves.

Quality Improvement

The ability to measure physician and network clinical quality and outcomes performance is at the heart of all CIN and ACO activities. Not only is this critical to the efficiencies expected of CINs and ACOs, but it is also a requirement of federal government agencies (i.e., FTC, CMS, etc.), and necessary to determine proper compensation plans for participating physicians. Paraphrasing Lord Kelvin, "...you can't manage what you can't measure," (Stellman, 1998) and measuring physician performance is required for CIN and ACO management and enhanced reimbursement. The concept that, "Each physician must make his or her practice data and medical records available for the network's review and analysis" was emphasized by the FTC in the Norman PHO decision. (Federal Trade Commission, 2013)

Finding methods to provide accurate intelligence on clinical quality and outcomes to share with physicians and clinical teams is critical. Quality and performance initiatives include clinical quality improvement, administrative process improvement, organizational change management, educational programming for clinicians and physicians, and executive scorecard reporting on programs throughout the organization. Claims analysis and clinical decision support tools can be used to analyze data, develop goals, and monitor progress.

Choosing and focusing on the most important clinical and administrative programs is an early task for the quality and compensation committees. For organizations deciding to clinically integrate with independent physicians, the relationship must focus on improved clinical outcomes and bringing enhanced value to the consumer. Moreover, if an integrated network wishes to function as a single contracting entity, antitrust laws require the network to prove that it can both monitor and deliver greater value to the consumer in the form of improved outcomes, or risk FTC legal challenges.

Clinicians are best suited to judge the available data and take the most appropriate courses of action to improve quality and reduce costs for an individual patient. It takes expert systems, predictive analytics, and clinical decision support tools, however, to understand the entire breadth and depth of evidence-based guidelines, the latest medical findings, up-to-date evidence-based medicine, and individual patient environmental factors. Whether looking at specific conditions such as diabetes, asthma, or looking at avoidable events like all-cause hospital readmission, the network needs to develop quality and performance improvement programs informed by clinical decision support technologies that set care management and quality goals, identify care opportunities, notify clinicians, and measurably improve outcomes.

Development of goals and benchmarks to measure quality and outcomes improvement is a critical step for the CIN or ACO. Several factors should be considered in the selection of these goals. Looking at disease prevalence, population health characteristics, greatest opportunities for improvement, local expertise, and readiness to implement change are only a few of the considerations to be taken into account.

Once the quality goals have been selected, the care management initiatives around those goals must be developed, widely communicated, and put into place. This process may include a team of management staff, such as registered nurses or midlevel providers who assist physicians in caring for patients across practice types and locations. Here one begins to see the need for more advanced technologies for identification, stratification, intervention, and communication. In addition to monitoring patients and the care provided in physician offices and hospitals, efforts need to be coordinated among all providers, including home care, post-acute care, hospital facilities and other remote settings.

Patient communication, including education, follow-up reminders, and other interventions, is important for patient self-management and improving the quality and health of the managed population. Proactive engagement of patients, including persons without visible signs and symptoms who are at risk for serious illness, is challenging for some physicians and their office staff. Having effective clinical decision support systems, an office communication strategy, and close relationships with patients has proven to be invaluable. Often the office staff members of the referral team and other clinician participants are best positioned to interact with patients and form the network that coordinates the patient experience.

Scorecards measuring physician performance at the individual patient and total population levels should guide the physicians so they can see progress and their relative status within the organization. Transparency of reporting, once agreed to by the clinician participants, is a powerful motivator in helping move the CIN or ACO to a higher level of performance, and is necessary to identify progress toward goals and enhanced reimbursement.

Financial Management

A simplified view of the financial starting point for a CIN or ACO is to look at how dollars flow into and out of the organization. The two issues considered here are: capital to fund the organization and its ongoing operations, and distribution of funds to providers in some kind of enhanced payment, such as shared savings, quality bonuses, or other contractual payments paid to providers for meeting performance goals.

The budget and finance issues must first be addressed at the board level within the governance structure. Top-level executives will need accurate information regarding the status of clinical operations performance, and visibility to health outcomes in order to have an informed perspective on performance against benchmarks and other quality measures. Once performance goals are determined and communicated, the CIN or ACO can evaluate the effectiveness of its service delivery, make appropriate payment to providers for improved performance, and change course as needed to move toward greater quality and performance.

Initial funding sources of network revenue are determined by the corporate structure. For a physician hospital organization (PHO), as an example, membership fees including initial and ongoing subscription fees matched by the hospital provide an initial revenue stream to fund the PHO. Other legal structures may include funding from third-party payers, self-insurance products, physicians, health systems and private investors. Joint ventures can involve second and third capital calls depending on the status of the network. In other arenas, health systems have been the exclusive source of startup capital to make such ventures operational. The Internal Revenue Service (IRS) has posted a special bulletin (Internal Revenue Service, 2011) to provide guidance for tax-exempt organizations participating in these ventures so as not to jeopardize their tax status.

A common funding approach is for the proposed entity to approach third-party payers requesting creation of a shared risk pool, based on mutually agreed-upon goals. Ideally the network will select goals that will bring value to the patients, providers, and payers. One benefit of this approach is that a single set of goals is easier to implement than negotiating different goals with each payer.

With negotiated contracts in hand, and funding of a shared risk pool in place, we now turn to the distribution of funds.

Financing compensation of physicians, care provider teams, and other ACO participants is a complex challenge that involves managing the revenue cycle, setting benchmarks and quality goals, regulatory/stakeholder reporting, ensuring accuracy of medical coding and provider attribution, and overseeing audit and risk management functions. Administering these functions under the Medicare ACO program is made more complicated by regulations and requirements, such as one-sided and two-sided risk models. Each risk model has a complex set of rules and calculations with benchmarks, quality metrics, other factors regarding the ACO's beneficiary population, and their linkage to determining the share of financial incentives or losses by the ACO participants, based on outcomes achieved. (Mulvany, 2011)

How does a network manage a shared risk pool and distribute the funds equitably to physicians and other participants and ancillary providers based on documented performance? No single model will fit all situations; however, a few principles can be outlined. First, the distribution model should have criteria for both individual and group performance. This feature offers physicians an incentive to collaborate on improving the overall performance of the CIN or ACO, and also encourages the "interdependence" required by federal regulation and guidelines. Second, there are usually financial incentives that individual physicians are eligible to earn. Depending on physician affiliation and attribution, there may be a desire to weigh payments based on fully delegated or only partially delegated membership or affiliation. Another consideration for bonus eligibility might be patient volume, such that a physician who manages a large volume of patients within a network receives greater weight than one who manages a smaller number. For example, highly productive physicians might have greater eligibility than less productive physicians. This approach must be carefully designed, however, so as to avoid overutilization rather than rewarding only higher quality and participation. Again, no one size fits all in analyzing these complex issues, and the compensation plan usually changes over time with changing population characteristics and physician performance. The best way to begin is to look at what others have done and engage the leadership in creating a model that works in the specific situation currently at hand.

Distribution of funds to providers must have a quality and appropriate utilization of services component to be in compliance with the FTC guidelines to avoid antitrust action. An example of distribution of funds is illustrated in Figure 4-2.

Figure 4-2. CIN Distribution of Funds Example[*]

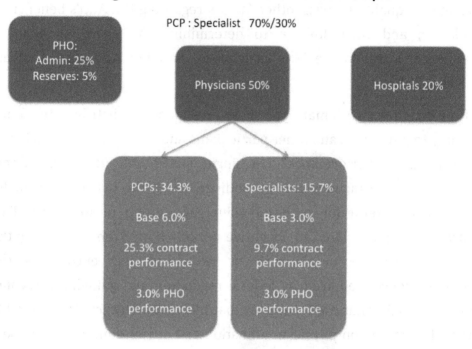

In this model, shared savings are distributed to the PHO along with reserves, to the hospital, and to the physicians. The physicians' shared savings are distributed based upon three components: base amount, contract performance and PHO performance. The base amount is distributed regardless to the number of patients or quality performance, as it reflects the reimbursement for infrastructure changes within the practice to participate in the organization and meet performance standards. The contract performance is distributed based upon success at meeting quality metrics. Finally, the PHO performance components are for the so-called "good citizenship" metrics of the PHO, such as patient satisfaction surveys, participating in learning activities, involvement in committees, meeting

---

[*] CIN funds distribution model developed by St. Vincent's Health Partners, Inc. Bridgeport, CT.

meaningful use requirements, in network referrals, and other such activities.

Payer Relations

CINs/ACOs are tasked with improving the quality of care for a targeted population while reducing costs, and participating in the resulting savings. Various healthcare stakeholders, both public and private, have similar goals. In terms of public payers CINs/ACOs need to consider Medicare, Medicaid and Children's Health Insurance Programs (CHIPs). Medicare is the primary payer for those over 65 years of age and certain disabled persons, while state Medicaid programs cover low-income, disabled, maternal, and pediatric subpopulations. CHIPs, some of which are also administered by Medicaid, serve low-income children not covered by Medicaid due to income ceilings. Private payer organizations, such as self-insured employers and health insurance plans, provide coverage for the largest segment of our nation's population, including individual coverage from health insurance exchanges. Each of these payer organizations has different goals and objectives, is affected by health insurance reforms, and all must be taken into consideration in setting up a CIN or ACO.

Other forces at work make it imperative to interact with payers. The changing structure of regional markets is a major concern to payers as they see continued consolidation of health systems and physician groups (including primary and specialty care) that can shift the balance of power in contract negotiations. (Carroll, 2011) The potential for hospitals and physician groups to concentrate market power and illegally leverage such power in negotiating prices for health services is one of the reasons for increased antitrust review by the FTC (Federal Register Volume 76 Number 67, April 7, 2011b). CINs and ACOs must carefully consider both how they establish their integration and the potential impact on the local market.

An important operational consideration for a new CIN or ACO as they start to organize is engaging third-party payers and gauging their willingness to collaborate. Collaboration may take several forms, including funding of shared risk pools, participating in network contracting, or other payment incentives to move from episodes of care to population- and value-based payment methodologies. This variation means opening discussions early with each payer and finding mutual opportunities to develop relationships. Payers may not initially be able or willing to collaborate for a number of reasons. Increasingly, however, some payers are innovating and looking to enhance hospital and physician ability to provide the type and quality of care they do best while contributing the actuarial, underwriting, risk management, data mining, and clinical decision support services that payers do best. (see Aetna/Banner Health Network (BHN) example in Chapter 14)[*]

Administrative Operations

Administrative issues within a CIN or ACO are similar to that of any business, and include management, finance, human resources, budget, performance measurement, continuous quality improvement, internal communication and coordination, development schedules, and resource allocation. These issues also include managing inherent business risks and developing mitigation strategies. Finally they require developing and improving the processes, policies, procedures, and workforce necessary to make the network successful.

A challenge of starting up a CIN or ACO is establishing operations prior to establishing a network, and setting priorities for organization development. For this reason, a proper budget and strategic plan must be in place. One of the biggest issues facing new CINs and ACOs is underestimating the resources required for successful operations. Under resourcing will most certainly predetermine the new organization's demise. To make the kinds of sustainable change needed for a successful CIN or ACO means adequate resources and a culture of change that touches every

---

[*] One example of an innovative approach to collaboration is the Aetna Accountable Care Solution services. Accessed online August 14, 2011, at http://www.aetnaacs.com/accountable-care-solutions.html

aspect of the organization in such a way that real change can occur and be maintained. A composite of good management skills, disciplined project management, and transparent dashboard reporting are required for adequate administration. In any case, managing operations takes adequate resources, a clear roadmap, and well-defined milestones.

A National Association of ACOs (NAACO) survey, conducted to determine sary startup costs of an ACO, reported startup costs of at least $4 million in capital. (National Association of ACOs, 2014) The report also cited CMS estimates for startup to be $1.8 million. The American Hospital Organization, however, estimates startup costs from $11.6-$26.5 million.

One of the first functional areas to be addressed in setting up operations is health information technology. The U.S. and global healthcare communities are in the midst of a technological revolution on many levels as technology solutions affect the processes, clinicians, and patients in every aspect of healthcare finance, administration, and delivery. In light of the cost of implementation, health information technology must be addressed early in the planning stages of an ACO or CIN.

Payer relations are perhaps the second most important operational issue for a new CIN or ACO to address. Establishment of a clinical integration program requires joint contracting with payers. As an organization moves toward the ACO model, providers and hospitals may assume more risk in the new organization as they accept more responsibility for quality and outcomes traditionally assumed by the payer. Transference and sharing of risk is an ongoing process that needs to be carefully administered as new care delivery models are put in place.

A third critical operational area involves ensuring legal compliance to meet requirements of federal and state government antitrust and insurance agencies, and IRS regulations on taxation of shared savings and distributions.

A fourth important area in setting up operations is quality and outcomes measurement and performance reporting. Monitoring, analyzing, and reporting to executives and team members on quality and outcomes allows transparency, course correction, and continuous improvements in clinical services – all critical operational elements of a CIN or ACO. With new health information technologies, performance can be continuously monitored, corrective actions can be taken, and rewards given where positive economic and clinical impacts are demonstrated and verified.

Strategic Planning

Healthcare executives increasingly find they must maintain a keen sense of awareness of the changing environment in which they operate. This includes continually developing and refining strategies that look to the future for new opportunities, and mitigation of political, economic, and technological threats to the operations of the organizations they lead. In *Redefining Health Care: Creating Value-based Competition on Results*, Porter and Teisberg noted, "Health care delivery cries out for strategy, given the stakes, the scale, and the sheer complexity of the task." (Porter & Teisberg, 2006c)

The magnitude of change facing the U.S. healthcare system is enormous. The pace of technological change, impact of federal reforms such as the ACA, continuous tinkering and manipulation of laws and regulations by the U.S. Congress and Executive branches of government, seemingly annual renegotiation of vendor and payer contracts, and increasing need for greater patient engagement, all contribute to the volume of change and complexity of the system. But ultimately, Porter and Teisberg believe the one key priority for every healthcare organization in dealing with change should be "superior patient value."(Porter & Teisberg, 2006a)

In light of the need for strategy that ultimately leads to superior value for the patient, every CIN or ACO should have multi-disciplinary teams that focus on short-term and long-term strategic planning, with the patient in mind. Often these efforts start at the board level (a traditional top-down approach). In order to effectively drive strategic planning and strategy development, an understanding is also needed of the complexity characteristics of every provider, payer, and hospital relationship, and the patient population – more of a bottom-up approach.

The strategy development team should also look at government issues and community partnerships. Strategy team members help increase broad awareness of changes in the community environment in which the organization operates, and help ensure legal compliance and reporting requirements are met, as well as changing requirements of private and public payers. Organizations can use many different processes in developing the strategic plan; however, some basic questions should be answered at the inception of a planning process, including:

- What is our mission and vision for the future of our organization?

- What is the demographic composition of the patient population we serve?

- What is the composition of the physicians who could be part of a network we develop, and what is the political dynamics among the different provider groups?

- What services do our patients need today and in the future?

- What resources (e.g. staff, technology, financial capital) are needed?

- What payers currently exist in the community, how is the payer mix changing, and what do we anticipate future payers will look like?

- What goals and objectives related to the organization's clinical operating efficiency, financial performance, quality, and safety will enhance our delivery of healthcare services for the population served?

The answers to these questions will vary depending on the provider organization's environment, resources, and capabilities. Five key initiatives are suggested in Table 4-1 as a framework for any CIN or ACO's start-up strategic planning efforts.

Table 4-1. CIN / ACO Start-up Planning Framework

Category	Description
Establish Mission and Vision	The mission and vision of a CIN or ACO should be developed, communicated, and embraced throughout the organization. Each organization should focus on its mission — e.g., to deliver excellence in health care services to improve population health and consumer value.
Situational Awareness	Understanding the environment in which the CIN or ACO and its stakeholders are operating is critical to success. Healthcare leaders involved in the governance of CINs and ACOs need to assess the political, economic, societal, and industry issues that affect their organization. Some issues may include: • Market innovations in care delivery, • The impact of regulatory changes, • Public or private payer funding and contracting, • Best practice and their potential adoption, • Competitive market assessments, • Multi-sectoral alliances and similar collaborations among stakeholders, and the legal structures of such collaborations, • Market perception of patient population, partners, vendors, and other stakeholders. Improving the situational awareness of physicians, healthcare executives, and care teams helps ensure decisions will improve their future prospects, and their ability to improve care of their patient population.
Weaknesses and Threats	Weaknesses and threats exist at the individual and organizational level. Only through self-awareness and an ability to recognize and admit weaknesses can they be identified, discussed, and plans made to mitigate. Threats to any CIN or ACO can be both external and internal. External threats may come in the form of contract renegotiations, competing health service providers, and new government legislation, regulation or health policies. Internal threats may include low morale, problems with

Category	Description
	staff retention, and technology adoption challenges.
Intelligence Network	As a complex adaptive system, the U.S. healthcare system exhibits two important characteristics: agents and interactions. McDaniel and Driebe noted "The one characteristic that … agents all share is that they can process information and can react to changes in that information." Second, 'interactions' of these agents form patterns of relationships that drive and influence business processes, alliances, contracts, patient engagement, and ultimately improved care, lower costs, and satisfaction with care delivery. (McDaniel & Driebe, 2001) Each CIN or ACO should develop their intelligence network in the "macro" sense: that feeds off the existence of these agents and interactions among individuals and organizations. The macro forces, including state and federal government activities, need to be monitored so the organization may proactively respond and adapt.
Systemic Innovation	To thrive in the ever-changing environment, healthcare organizations must welcome and embrace innovation. Industry-leading healthcare organizations participate in initiatives that expanded their operational boundaries and created new and improved services through sustaining and disruptive innovations. (Christensen, Grossman, & Hwang, 2009) Over the years many innovations have been tested and adopted by CMS for diffusion throughout the U.S. healthcare system. In an address to the World Economic Forum, Duke University's Chancellor for Health Affairs, Victor J. Dzau, noted an important framework for "determinants of innovation." (Dzau, 2008) These determinants are development, ownership, and diffusion. The realization of each determinant requires ideas, people and integrity. According to Dr. Dzau (who assumed the role of president of the Institute of Medicine in July 2014 (Husten, 2014)) these determinants strengthen innovations that enable the growth of CIN and ACO.

Regulatory Compliance

Contracts, regulatory compliance, and managing the unending flow of changing federal and state healthcare laws are significant issues faced by all healthcare providers. They take on added significance in a CIN or ACO context due to additional Federal and State laws and regulations that apply to these new business models. Contracts with payer organizations will continue to be important for CIN and ACO revenue. Federal and state antitrust law has always governed relationships among providers and with payers. But in a CIN or ACO situation they take on added significance because of the close relationship between the parties that could be construed as improper collusion, if not carefully constructed.

The FTC is most concerned with the local market economic impact of organizations controlling the supply of services, especially if they focus on profit maximization for the benefit of their own organization, instead of improving the value of care delivered to the consumer. Ensuring fair trade and preventing the development of monopolies is a major concern.

Negotiation and contracting activities require the services of legal professionals as intermediaries and counsel to CIN, ACO, and managed care executives, especially given potential changes in antitrust regulations and waivers. Preventing market dominance while allowing for the growth of clinical integration programs that produce procompetitive benefits is a goal of the FTC, and crucial to the success of CINs and ACOs. These issues are discussed in more detail in Chapter 5.

Managing compliance involves a host of regulatory issues and is part of managing any contemporary healthcare organization. There are a myriad of issues, ranging from patient safety, privacy and confidentiality, financial stewardship, and managing the legal medical record, especially when you engage in continuity of care across care settings and among traditionally disparate care providers. To ensure these issues are covered appropriately, an internal compliance program that includes a designated compliance officer is crucial to provide objective oversight and reporting. The Final Rule issued in November 2011 called for five elements of a compliance plan to be in place for all Medicare ACOs:

1. Assign a specific compliance official/officer who reports directly to the

ACO's governing board.

2. Put in place mechanisms that "identify and address compliance problems directly related to the ACO."

3. Establish a method/system for employees or contractors of ACO participants to report compliance issues regarding the ACO's operations.

4. Provide a compliance training program for all employees and contractors of the ACO.

5. Have a requirement for employees and contractors of the ACO to report any "suspected violations of the law to appropriate law enforcement agencies."

(Federal Register Volume 76 Number 212, November 2, 2011)

Culture

The last element presented here is one of the most important. It is the underlying culture of the organization. While an entire chapter, or even a book, could be dedicated to the importance of culture in the Care Revolution Era, two points noted here are: how culture is created, and the importance of consistent mindful or "heedful" actions.

The general culture and values within every U.S. provider organization have evolved over the last century as the healthcare industry has matured. Throughout this maturation process, the culture of physician practices, hospital organizations and most recently payers has been through "norm formation around critical incidents." (Schein, 1990) Incidents as defined by Schein, a quarter century ago, can be thought of as medical errors, which healthcare organizations are still grappling with today. They can also be defined as disruptions, such as the beginning of Medicare and Medicaid in 1965, or the landmark reforms created by the ACA, which is transforming the way healthcare services are delivered, paid for, and accessed. This is one way that culture has evolved, as a reaction to external incidents that come along occasionally.

For the FTC, and especially in the context of a CIN, culture must be established proactively, and instilled from the beginning. To start, the governing board of the CIN must set the tone for the organization, showing that its goals and objectives are consistent with improving quality and lowering costs, to benefit the consumer with a better service. Second, the infrastructure and organization established must have a culture of compliance with laws and regulations and continuous improvement in services and delivery that drives quality and lowers costs. Finally, the culture must be acknowledged and practiced all the way to the front line physicians and other members of the care team, who must demonstrate their understanding and execution of the culture of improved quality and efficiency. Not only is it important for these cultural imperatives to be established and implemented, but federal government regulators will test to see if the culture has been proactively infused within the organization, and if it permeates and is understood by all clinicians, staff, and actions of the organization.

A second part of healthcare organization culture is a mindful focus on mission-critical systems, and constant striving to improve patient safety. As noted in the article, *Collective Mind in Organizations: Heedful Interrelating on Flight Decks*, Weik and Roberts state there is "...a pattern of heedful interrelations of actions in a social system" (Weick & Roberts, 1993) that when done well can decrease error rates, lead to improved standardization of operations, and improve the reliability of systems (organizational and technological).

The culture of each provider organization has always focused on patient care. As CINs and ACOs evolve as networks of interlocking entities, their culture must evolve to focus on the additional parameters of quality improvement and cost reduction. This is done through greater collaboration and interdependency, skills not normally taught in medical school nor fostered in a pay-for-procedure environment. As the cottage industry continues to dissolve, a different and unifying culture focused on value-driven systems and organizations will continue to mature.

Building a CIN: Work Plan

As part of the development of a CIN or ACO, a work plan should be developed and revisited periodically to record progress, and change and update as the situation warrants. An example of a set of work plans is provided below in Figures 4-2 through 4-5 from St. Vincent's Physician Partners in Bridgeport, CT. St. Vincent's Health Partners, as part of its business plan, developed timelines for key strategic components of organizational functions: financial management, operations, quality and utilization, and information technology.

Figure 4-2. Financial Management Timeline

	Start	Finish	June	July	Aug	Sept	Oct	Nov	Dec
Budget Development	6/4/2012	12/31/2012							
Identify initial network providers	6/4/2012	12/31/2012							
Estimate patient population	6/4/2012	8/31/2012							
Identify IT capital needs	9/1/2012	10/31/2012							
Develop dashboard reports	9/1/2012	12/31/2012							
Develop initial disbursement plan	6/4/2012	8/31/2012							
Contract with payers	6/4/2012	12/31/2012							

Figure 4-3. Operations Development Timeline

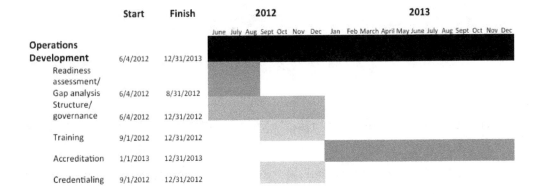

	Start	Finish	2012							2013												
			June	July	Aug	Sept	Oct	Nov	Dec	Jan	Feb	March	April	May	June	July	Aug	Sept	Oct	Nov	Dec
Operations Development	6/4/2012	12/31/2013																			
Readiness assessment/ Gap analysis	6/4/2012	8/31/2012																			
Structure/ governance	6/4/2012	12/31/2012																			
Training	9/1/2012	12/31/2012																			
Accreditation	1/1/2013	12/31/2013																			
Credentialing	9/1/2012	12/31/2012																			

Figure 4-4. Quality and Utilization Review Development Timeline

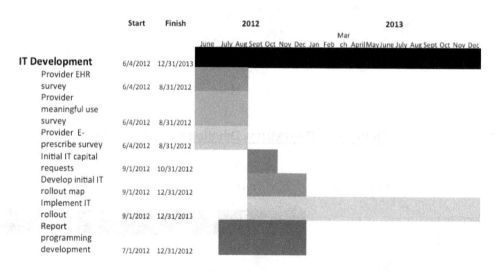

	Start	Finish	2012	2013
			June July Aug Sept Oct Nov Dec Jan Feb March April May	June July Aug Sept Oct Nov Dec
Quality and Utilization Review Development	6/4/2012	12/31/2013		
Establish quality metrics	7/1/2012	12/31/2012		
Develop dashboard quality reporting	7/1/2012	12/31/2012		
Develop provider quality compliance program	7/1/2012	12/31/2012		
Develop patient satisfaction survey	7/1/2012	12/31/2012		
Develop patient satisfaction dashboard	7/1/2012	12/31/2012		
Develop utilization metrics	7/1/2012	12/31/2012		
Develop dashboard utilization reporting	7/1/2012	12/31/2012		
Survey PCPs for PCMH readiness	6/4/2012	12/31/2012		
PCMH accreditation for PCPs	9/1/2012	12/31/2013		

Figure 4-5. Information Technology Development Timeline

	Start	Finish	2012	2013
			June July Aug Sept Oct Nov Dec Jan Feb March April	May June July Aug Sept Oct Nov Dec
IT Development	6/4/2012	12/31/2013		
Provider EHR survey	6/4/2012	8/31/2012		
Provider meaningful use survey	6/4/2012	8/31/2012		
Provider E-prescribe survey	6/4/2012	8/31/2012		
Initial IT capital requests	9/1/2012	10/31/2012		
Develop initial IT rollout map	9/1/2012	12/31/2012		
Implement IT rollout	9/1/2012	12/31/2013		
Report programming development	7/1/2012	12/31/2012		

These timelines kept the organization on task, and were also used as a roadmap for its strategy to become accredited as a clinically integrated network. By frequently visiting the timelines, St. Vincent's Health Partners was successful in obtaining both value based contracts and Clinical

Integration accreditation by the URAC industry standards and accreditation organization.

Future Direction

Regardless of the model and path chosen by healthcare leaders and teams implementing a CIN or ACO, each of the elements described in this chapter should be addressed. Ultimately the question must be asked, to whom are the operations of the CIN or ACO accountable? Our answer is to the patients, the communities in which they live, the populations to whom they are accountable, and to the taxpayers and consumers who pay for the health system and its services. The physician-patient relationship is sacred and serves as a unifying focus for all activities in the healthcare industry. And without the patient there is no need for the technology, the facilities, or the staff to care for and support them.

So in this Care Revolution Era, we are confronted with establishing new healthcare organizations — innovative and agile care delivery networks that leverage medical care, wellness, social services, and new technologies to help improve comprehensive population health. Networks of historically competing organizations are coming together to form ACOs and CINs for care delivery extending beyond historical and traditional geographic boundaries. We are reinventing a system that has evolved over the last hundred years, a system that has been fragmented and broken, with a lack of market competition and overregulation of the structure that has evolved. (Porter & Teisberg, 2006b) The industry made significant changes through the managed care era but now we enter the period of accountable care and new "network effects." Operations may be physician led, but significant know-how must be obtained from other stakeholders, including patients, who have additional experience to fuel the pipelines of innovation and continuously improve quality and affordability.

The current system complexity must be managed better to reduce fragmentation, and make better use of technologies for patients' benefit. New value alliances (Leavitt & McKeown, 2013) and stronger partnerships are being formed among historically competing players throughout the industry in order to help CINs and ACOs work more effectively, embrace innovation, and focus on the Triple Aim for the good of the health of the nation's population.

CHAPTER 4 DISCUSSION QUESTIONS

Discussion questions are provided for team building or class exercises. Answers for all questions are provided in Appendix C.

Question Number	Question
1	What are two essential elements of culture for a CIN or ACO as discussed in the chapter?
2	What is a "takeaway" from the St. Vincent's Health Partners CIN Development Workplan case example in the four figures illustrated in the chapter?
3	What are the five key initiatives in the CIN/ACO Start-up Planning Framework? How might you apply these initiatives to your own organization?
4	Regarding physician/provider relations, what is the key transition that has taken place with the shift from a provider centric focus in the industry to a patient-centric focus (as noted in the chapter)?
5	Patient engagement was noted as one of the essential elements and building blocks in the evolution of any network. What are some key considerations for patient engagement (and patient experience as a part of patient engagement) as discussed in the chapter?

CHAPTER 4 HIGHLIGHTS

✓ Ten elements to address in building a clinically integrated network were identified in Figure 4-1 of the chapter. These elements were: patient engagement, strategic planning, quality improvement, administrative operations, regulatory compliance, financial management, information technology, physician relations, governance, and organizational culture.

✓ Five elements for a CIN/ACO Planning Framework were discussed as: establishing a mission and vision, situational awareness, recognize weaknesses and threats, develop a strategic view of the intelligence network for the CN or ACO, and continuously look for work to enstill systemic innovations.

✓ The Advocate Physician Partners program was noted as one of the leadng CINs in the nation. Collaboration was noted as important to drive improvement in quality and their innovative array of interventions diffused across care settings, led to an increased level of focus on care coordination and cost control in 2013.

✓ Culture in healthcare organizations is a foundational and essential underpinning element for every successful CIN or ACO venture. There are many important elements of how values are instilled but two points addressed in the chapter were the ways that culture is created andthe importance of consistent (e.g. heedful) actions.

✓ The chapter noted that new innovative and agile care delivery networks are being established to help improve comprehensive population health and that new value alliances are needed to help CINs and ACOs embrace innovation for the good of the health of the nation's population.

CHAPTER 4 REFERENCES

Advocate Physician Partners. (2013). 2013 Value Report. Retrieved from http://www.advocatehealth.com/documents/app/2013ValueReport-Complete.pdf; 2014 Value Report. Retrieved from http://www.advocatehealth.com/documents/app/FINAL2014ValueReport.pdf

Carroll, J. (2011). FTC antitrust rules offer hope of limiting ACO market power. *Managed care (Langhorne, Pa.)*, 20(5), 5-7.

Christensen, C. M., Grossman, J. H., & Hwang, J. (2009). The Role of Disruptive Technology and Business Model Innovation in Making Products and Services Affordable and Accessible. In *The Innovator's Prescription. A Disruptive Solution for Health Care* (pp. 3-8). New York, NY: McGraw Hill.

Department of Justice and Federal Trade Commission. (1996). Statement on Policy Enforcement on Physician Network Joint Ventures. Statement 8(B)1. Retrieved from http://www.ftc.gov/sites/default/files/attachments/competition-policy-guidance/statements_of_antitrust_enforcement_policy_in_health_care_august_1996.pdf

Dzau, V. J. (2008). Innovation in Healthcare in Emerging Economies. Retrieved from http://www.dukemedicine.org/Leadership/Chancellor/transforming_medicine/lectures_and_writings/3%20d.%20Innovation%20Healthcare%20Davos%20Remarks%201-24-2008.pdf

Federal Register Volume 76 Number 67. (2011, April 7a). II(B)(9)(b). Processes to Promote Patient Engagement and II(B)(10). Patient Centeredness Criteria. pp. 19547–19548.

Federal Register Volume 76 Number 67. (2011, April 7b). II(I)(4)(c). Competition, Price, and Access to Care. pp. 19630–31.

Federal Register Volume 76 Number 212. (2011, November 2). II(H)(4)(a). Compliance plans. pp. 67952. Retrieved from http://www.gpo.gov/fdsys/pkg/FR-2011-11-02/pdf/2011-27461.pdf

Federal Trade Commission. (2013). Norman PHO Advisory Opinion. Washington, DC: Federal Trade Commission Retrieved from http://www.ftc.gov/sites/default/files/documents/advisory-opinions/norman-physician-hospital-organization/130213normanphoadvltr_0.pdf

Hibbard, J. H., & Greene, J. (2013). What the evidence shows about patient activation: better health outcomes and care experiences; fewer data on costs. *Health Affairs*, 32(2), 207-214. doi: 10.1377/hlthaff.2012.1061

Husten, L. (2014, February 19). Victor Dzau Leaving Duke to Head the Institute of Medicine. *Forbes*. Retrieved from http://www.forbes.com/sites/larryhusten/2014/02/19/victor-dzau-leaving-duke-to-head-the-institute-of-medicine/

Notice Regarding Participation in the MSSP through an ACO, Notice 2011-20 C.F.R. (2011).

Ishikawa, H., Hashimoto, H., & Kiuchi, T. (2013). The evolving concept of patient-centeredness in patient-physician communication research. *Social Science and Medicine*, 96, 147-153. doi: 10.1016/j.socscimed.2013.07.026

Jarousse, L. A. (2010). Leadership in the era of reform. *Hospitals & Health Networks*, 84(11), 5p following 33, 31.

Leavitt, M., & McKeown, R. (2013). *Finding Allies, Building Alliances: 8 Elements That Bring - and Keep - People Together.* San Francisco, CA: Jossey-Bass Publishers.

Manary, M. P., Boulding, W., Staelin, R., & Glickman, S. W. (2013). The patient experience and health outcomes. *New England Journal of Medicine*, 368(3), 201-203. doi: 10.1056/NEJMp1211775

McDaniel, R. R., & Driebe, D. J. (2001). Complexity science and health care management. *Advances in Health Care Management*, 2, 11-36.

Mulvany, C. (2011). Medicare ACOs no longer mythical creatures. *Healthcare Financial Management: Journal of the Healthcare Financial Management Association*, 65(6), 96-104.

National Association of ACOs. (2014). National ACO Survey Conducted November 2013. Retrieved from https://www.naacos.com/pdf/ACOSurveyFinal012114.pdf

Porter, M. E., & Teisberg, E. O. (2006a). Defining the right goal: Superior patient value. In *Redefining Health Care: Creating Value-based Competition on Results* (pp. 155). Boston, MA: Harvard Business School Publishing.

Porter, M. E., & Teisberg, E. O. (2006b). Introduction In *Redefining Health Care: Creating Value-based Competition on Results* (pp. 3). Boston, MA: Harvard Business School Publishing.

Porter, M. E., & Teisberg, E. O. (2006c). Strategic implications for health care providers. In *Redefining Health Care: Creating Value-based Competition on Results* (pp. 151). Boston, MA: Harvard Business School Publishing.

Raab, J., & Kennis, P. (2009). Heading toward a society of networks empirical developments and theoretical challenges. *Journal of Managed Inquiry*, 18(3), 198-210. doi: 10.1177/1056492609337493

Roseman, D., Osborne-Stafsnes, J., Amy, C. H., Boslaugh, S., & Slate-Miller, K. (2013). Early lessons from four 'Aligning Forces For Quality' communities bolster the case for patient-centered care. *Health Affairs*, 32(2), 232-241. doi: 10.1377/hlthaff.2012.1085

Schein, E. H. (1990). Organizational culture. *American Psychologist*, 45(2), 109-119.

Shields, M. C., Patel, P. H., Manning, M., & Sacks, L. (2011). A model for integrating independent physicians into accountable care organizations. *Health Affairs*, 30(1), 161-172. doi: 10.1377/hlthaff.2010.0824

Stellman, J. M. (1998). Lord Kelvin, May 3, 1883 Lecture: Electrical units of measurement encyclopaedia of occupational health and safety (Vol. 1, pp. 73): International Labour Organization.

Weick, K. E., & Roberts, K. H. (1993). Collective mind in organizations: Heedful interrelating on flight decks. *Administrative Science Quarterly*, 38, 357-381.

Chapter 5. Regulatory Matters and Antitrust Issues

Brian Nichols

Bona fide clinical integration by health care providers with the potential for significant cost savings and quality improvements may be demonstrated by the network of health care providers implementing an active and ongoing program to evaluate and modify practice patterns by the network's physician participants and create a high degree of interdependence and cooperation among the physicians to control costs and ensure quality.

> *Richard A. Feinstein, Former Director of the Bureau of Competition at the FTC Statement of the FTC Before the Subcommittee on Consumer Protection, Product Safety, and Insurance Committee on Commerce, Science & Transportation, United States Senate, July 16, 2009*

CHAPTER 5 LEARNING OBJECTIVES

✓ Understand the basic antitrust issues of concern for CINs and ACOs.

✓ What are the waivers for tax-exempt organization participation in ACOs?

✓ What are five types of conduct to be avoided by CINs and ACOs in order to reduce the likelihood of antitrust investigations?

✓ How does the Stark Law apply to CINs and ACOs?

✓ Know the three landmark laws that form the framework for antitrust law enforcement.

Background

Regulatory issues for hospitals, health systems, physicians and other providers are extensive and complex. A wide range of regulations already cover many aspects of hospital and physician office clinical activities and administrative operations, including coding and reimbursement, anti-kickback laws, self-referral prohibitions, fraud prevention and detection, antitrust laws, and others. In many cases, these rules and regulations seek to limit or prohibit certain activities that can be viewed as fundamental to

Accountable Care Organization (ACO) and Clinically Integrated Network (CIN) business models, such as joint agreements to negotiate prices, payment of financial incentives, and financial risk bearing.

Here we focus on some exceptions to these rules and regulations, and related guidance issued by federal regulators that have been promulgated to meet the needs of CINs and ACOs and to further public and private interest in the development of integrated care networks. These exceptions involve antitrust, anti-kickback, and tax laws and regulations.

This chapter is designed to be an overview for providers as they implement CINs and ACOs. Because the following material is an overview and not meant to give legal advice, the reader is strongly encouraged to seek competent legal representation.

Medicare Shared Savings Program (MSSP) ACO

A number of federal agencies have released guidance regarding payment reform and accountable care arrangements between independent health care providers. The guidance has been issued due to creation of the MSSP and the increasing popularity of similar arrangements involving private payers.

This chapter deals mainly with these laws, waivers and other important laws and regulations that affect the creation and operation of ACOs and CINs.

Antitrust Issues and Laws

Antitrust issues are discussed first because of the large and growing body of law in this field, and because integration among and between hospitals and physicians, a fundamental activity of CIN and ACO, raises major antitrust issues. Over the last couple decades antitrust laws and regulations applied to health care settings have evolved, especially in areas such as price fixing, market concentration in specific geographic areas, and non-price competition. (Jacobs and Rapoport 2004)

The basic antitrust rule is that any activities between competitors, such as physicians who practice as separate and independent business entities in the same market, that involve setting or "fixing" prices restrain trade are in violation of antitrust laws and are by definition ("per se") illegal. (1982) There are, however, instances in which joint arrangements between otherwise competing physicians can improve efficiencies, bring economies of scale, and increase competition. In fact, the Health Maintenance Organization Act of 1973 recognized this potential and encouraged collective activity by physicians, causing a conflict with the fundamental antitrust prohibition against collective actions by otherwise competing sellers of services. As a result, the federal government has worked to define situations in which joint activities do improve competition and will not be deemed per se illegal. Here we look at some of the ways the federal government has defined allowable joint activities.

Collective activity by physicians and hospitals that might otherwise be per se illegal will be allowed if procompetitive results of the activity can be found, such as improvement in quality or lowered costs that outweigh the potential anticompetitive impact. A balancing test called the "rule of reason" analysis, which compares the procompetitive effects of the activities against their anticompetitive effects, is generally used by the Federal Trade Commission (FTC) to determine whether an activity is illegal. Both case law and statements by the federal government indicate the FTC will scrutinize the joint activities in balancing the procompetitive results against the anticompetitive effects. Activities reviewed by the FTC have included whether providers create a product or service new and different from what existed previously; whether the persons participating in the venture share substantial financial risk; and whether care delivery has been integrated in such a way that procompetitive results justify joint price negotiation. (U.S. Department of Justice and Federal Trade Commission 1996) Fundamental to rule of reason analysis is a review of the facts behind the joint venture pricing arrangements. To avoid per se treatment, agreements to set and negotiate prices must be "reasonably necessary" or "ancillary" to achieve procompetitive efficiencies.

Although the American Medical Association and others have argued that antitrust laws should not apply to the "learned professions," such as physicians, engineers, and lawyers, the Supreme Court overturned the learned professions exception to the Sherman Act in the 1975 decision *Goldfarb v. Virginia State Bar.* (1975) Since that decision, FTC scrutiny of physicians and hospital collaborations began in earnest and has continued to this day. A 2007 article in a Journal of Health Law noted:

> . . . as early as 1976, the FTC was challenging physician attempts to thwart competition by denying reimbursement to physicians providing services to HMOs, penalizing physicians who accepted salaries or payment on other than a fee-for-service basis or limiting price competition by other means. (Greaney 2007)

Antitrust Laws

Antitrust laws are enforced by the Antitrust Division of the Department of Justice (DOJ), FTC, state attorneys general, and private suits brought by plaintiffs. In the healthcare industry the FTC ensures fair pricing of health services and products within and across geographic markets and enforces laws that prohibit any activity that restrains trade. Congress has passed a body of antitrust laws the DOJ and FTC use to enforce fair trade in the Unites States and global marketplace. Three laws form the framework for antitrust enforcement: the Sherman Act of 1890, the Federal Trade Commission Act of 1914, and the Clayton Act of 1914. The Sherman Act, the first United States antitrust law, prohibits unreasonable restraint of trade, including "every contract, combination, or conspiracy in restraint of trade and any monopolization, attempted monopolization, or conspiracy or combination to monopolize."

The Federal Trade Commission Act created the FTC; it bans "unfair methods of competition and unfair or deceptive acts or practices." The Clayton Act "prohibits mergers and acquisitions where the effect may be substantially to lessen competition, or to tend to create a monopoly." The

Clayton Act has been amended over the years, notably by the Robinson-Patman Act of 1936 banning "discriminatory pricing and allowances in dealings between merchants;" and the Hart-Scott-Rodino Act of 1976 requiring advance notice of large planned mergers to the FTC. (U.S. Department of Justice and Federal Trade Commission 1996)

Antitrust Issues Facing CINs and ACOs

CINs and ACOs require collaboration among and between hospitals and physicians to obtain the economies of scale necessary to reduce cost and improve quality. One way to collaborate for greater efficiency is through a joint venture or agreement whereby providers band together to achieve greater efficiency and collectively negotiate their fees with payers. Such collective negotiation with single signature authority for hospital and physician contracting is generally considered anticompetitive and hence problematic. Competitive pressures and government reform efforts, however, are resulting in unprecedented mergers, acquisitions, and the formation of new alliances. Many of the new structures have economies of scale that are procompetitive and bring down the cost of care while increasing quality and accessibility. Because these efficiencies are sought by all stakeholders, exceptions to the antitrust rules have been created for certain kinds of organizations and the government is looking at new waivers for other categories of joint arrangements. The antitrust laws, regulations, and exceptions are important for any hospital or physician collaboration.

In 1996 the FTC and DOJ issued their Statements of Antitrust Enforcement Policy in Health Care in 1996 (hereinafter referred to as the Joint Statements). The Joint Statements provide basic guidance to the healthcare industry on collaborative arrangements that comply with antitrust laws, introduced the clinical integration concept and create "safety zones." Since the Joint Statements were released the FTC has set forth numerous rulings and pursued many lawsuits against physician and hospital organizations for collective activity, many of which have been pronounced illegal as they have not found significant, procompetitive improvements in quality of care and reductions in costs necessary to outweigh potentially anticompetitive effects.

The Joint Statements and Case Studies

The FTC and DOJ Joint Statements form the current framework for guidance on collaborative arrangements between and among hospitals and physicians. (U.S. Department of Justice and Federal Trade Commission 1996) Of particular importance to ACOs and CINs are Statements #8 (enforcement policy on physician network joint ventures) and #9 (enforcement policy on multiprovider networks). These two statements provide a framework of rules applied by the FTC in its rule of reason analysis to determine whether joint ventures are legitimate networks producing procompetitive efficiencies that outweigh their anticompetitive effects.

If competitors are economically integrated and share substantial financial risk, arrangements that set prices and are ancillary to the procompetitive benefits achieved either fall under a safety zone, or may be reviewed under rule of reason analysis. When providers agree to share financial risk of overutilization of resources, they have an incentive to reduce costs and it becomes necessary for them to agree on the prices charged for services to manage the financial risk. The Joint Statements describe several financial risk sharing arrangements, including capitation, percent of premium, withholds, shared savings, global fee, and all-inclusive case rates. ACOs, by definition are a risk sharing or bearing entity; still need to document how financial risk is shared.

For CINs that don't share substantial financial risk or meet safety zone requirements, but wish to collaborate to negotiate prices, the analysis is more detailed and depends on the facts of the situation. Statement #8 defines a clinically integrated network as:

> ...implementing an active and ongoing program to evaluate and modify practice patterns by the network's physician participants and create a high degree of interdependence and cooperation among the physicians to control costs and ensure quality. This program may include:

(1) Establishing mechanisms to monitor and control utilization of health care services that are designed to control costs and assure quality of care;

(2) Selectively choosing network physicians who are likely to further these efficiency objectives; and

(3) The significant investment of capital, both monetary and human, in the necessary infrastructure and capability to realize the claimed efficiencies.

(U.S. Department of Justice and Federal Trade Commission 1996)

A joint arrangement between or among hospitals or physicians must meet the requirements discussed above to avoid being labeled per se illegal, and instead be reviewed by the FTC under the rule of reason analysis. Rule of reason analysis will determine whether economic actions collectively taken by the participants are highly likely to create procompetitive benefits for consumers and whether any pricing or market allocation arrangements are reasonably necessary to achieve the procompetitive efficiencies.

To assist with legitimate healthcare integration, the DOJ and FTC jointly issued a healthcare industry report in 2004 that identified four primary indicia of clinical integration, as outlined below in Figure 5-1. (U.S. Department of Justice and Federal Trade Commission 1996, Department of Justice and Federal Trade Commission July 2004)

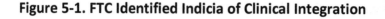

Figure 5-1. FTC Identified Indicia of Clinical Integration

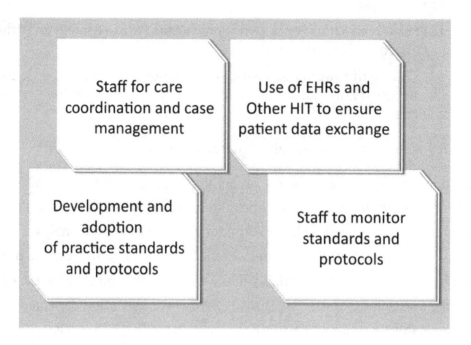

Implementation of these elements of clinical integration requires proper planning and the right people, processes and technology. To begin, recruiting and retaining the clinical and administrative staff necessary to meet all the indicators of clinical integration is critical. Administration and management personnel are needed to help develop, measure, and maintain practice standards and protocols. Appropriate staff members are needed to monitor standards and protocols, enabling implementation of an "ongoing program to evaluate and modify practice patterns." This process requires development of benchmarks and report cards so that everyone knows how they are doing and that clinical quality improvements are being achieved. Staffing for care coordination, including physicians and other clinicians as nursing care managers and other ancillary personnel is are usually needed to ensure appropriate care continues between office visits. Care coordination requires both primary and specialty care participation, and appropriate transitions between physicians, which may be facilitated by clinicians or non-clinicians. Health information technology staff and management are also needed to meet these requirements.

Processes, and policies and procedures to implement them, are necessary to meet the legal requirements of clinical integration and accountable care. Practice standards and protocols should focus on creation of clinical protocols from evidence-based guidelines and other medical and scientific findings to create agreed upon benchmarks against which clinicians may be measured and practice patterns modified for clinical improvement. Measurable outcomes are critical for the program to succeed.

Many medical organizations develop and adopt clinical practice standards and protocols through committees including physicians and other clinicians. It is important for the physicians to be involved in both development and adoption of the protocols, as they will be called upon to follow them and regulators will scrutinize whether the physicians demonstrate a commitment to the goals of improved quality and cost reduction. The protocols may also use clinical, safety, and other quality metrics developed by external regulatory agencies and such industry-developed guidelines as the National Quality Forum, Joint Commission standards, CMS Hospital Quality Initiative metrics, and Agency for Healthcare Research and Quality guidelines. Moreover, clinical and business process redesign is crucial to ensuring an "active and ongoing program" is implemented and adopted by physicians and clinicians.

Case Studies: GRIPA

Four FTC opinions are provided here as examples of clinical integration; three of these opinions pre-date implementation of the ACA. First is the ruling by the FTC in 2007 regarding the Greater Rochester Independent Practice Association (GRIPA) in their evaluation of that entity's clinically integrated program. A 2010 Robert Wood Johnson Foundation policy paper summarized the FTC's opinion:

> GRIPA offers an example of a clinically integrated physician arrangement that successfully met the FTC's standard as set forth in the revised 1996 Statements. GRIPA positioned its venture as one offering a

new health care product that would combine clinical practice with an integrated clinical improvement program designed to improve the quality of care and create efficiencies in the practice of medicine. GRIPA claimed that this new product would be "intertwined" with its proposed joint contracting practices with payers (health insurance companies) on behalf of its 500 independent and hospital-affiliated primary care physicians and specialists in practice across 40 separate areas. The FTC agreed that collective bargaining was reasonably necessary to achieve the program's likely efficiencies. (Burke and Rosenbaum 2010)

In the FTC's GRIPA opinion the agency provided in-depth analysis of each element of clinical integration and validated that GRIPA's proposed clinical improvement services program showed evidence that the program was likely to produce substantial cooperation among participating physicians. (Federal Trade Commission September 17, 2007) On the subject of physician collaboration, the FTC's opinion indicated that GRIPA presented appropriate clinician responsibility and interdependence in a number of collaborative initiatives with its physicians that planned to implement or build "from its risk-sharing program as evidencing the physicians' clinical integration through the proposed program."

The FTC's plan also included expanding the scope of diseases that GRIPA covered in its disease management services; ensured nonexclusivity options for contracting; and established a clinical integration committee comprising 12 physicians. (Federal Trade Commission September 17, 2007) The FTC recommended in its conclusion that the Commission not challenge GRIPA's clinical integration program as its joint negotiation of contracts was "reasonably related to" GRIPA's ability to achieve potential efficiencies and in view of the "pro-competitive potential of GRIPA's proposed program."(Federal Trade Commission September 17, 2007)

Case Studies: TriState Health Partners

A second opinion rendered by the FTC was the TriState Health Partners, Inc. (TriState) in April 2009. (Federal Trade Commission April 13, 2009) TriState was a physician-hospital organization (PHO) located in Maryland with over 200 physicians engaged in a multiprovider network joint venture.

In this case TriState proposed a clinical integration program that would require a joining fee of $2,500 per physician with no additional investment required (which met the financial risk requirement). TriState also proposed joint contracting among all member physicians to maximize the number of patients in the program and the engagement of physicians to maximize the integration of care services within the network. TriState met a similar but slightly more extensive set of clinical integration requirements than GRIPA. Its collaborative physician activities are aligned with the four primary indicators noted above.

TriState went further in demonstrating clinical integration program through their physician engagement, governance, and peer review. These elements indicate deeper commitment by physicians in the network to ensure an emphasis on quality improvement in patient care and controlling costs.

Case Studies: Advocate Physician Partners

A third opinion to note is that of Advocate Physician Partners (Advocate) and its clinical integration program. Advocate's Chief Executive Officer, Lee B. Sacks M.D., indicated in a May 2008 presentation that the goal of its program is,

> ...to drive targeted improvements in health care quality and efficiency through our relationship with every major insurance plan offered in the Chicago metropolitan area, thus uniting payer, employer, patients, and physicians in a single program to improve outcomes. (Sacks May 29, 2008)

The Advocate Clinical Integration Program (CIP) was launched on January 1, 2004. It was initially controversial as some stakeholders thought that collective activities by independent physicians to jointly negotiate contracts with fee-for-service health plans were illegal. The activities of Advocate drew FTC scrutiny and a lawsuit by a major national health plan. After years of investigation, the FTC issued a consent decree in 2006 specifically allowing Advocate's CIP to proceed, including the contracting practices. The consent decree was the first time the FTC granted such permission, but the commission also commented that it would continue to monitor the CIP. (Federal Trade Commission December 29, 2006, Federal Trade Commission December 29, 2006) We can see from the Advocate Physician Partners' 2011 Value Report on Clinical Integration that a number of benefits were derived from the program.

Advocate's efforts demonstrate the economic impact on its community and improvements in population health in the market it serves. Proving measurable benefits to the community, consumers, and patients is crucial to a successful clinical integration program and compliance with existing FTC rulings and regulations.

Case Studies: Norman PHO

In the most recent FTC advisory opinion and the first in over four years as well as the first opinion post implementation of the 2010 Patient Protection and Affordable Care Act (ACA), the FTC reviewed the CIN activities of Norman PHO. (Federal Trade Commission February 13, 2013) The Norman PHO was founded in 1994 by a physicians' association and a health system. Its approximately 280 physician members were primary care physicians and specialists on the medical staff of the health system's hospitals. Norman PHO proposed to develop a non-exclusive CIN for members to establish and enforce adherence to clinical practice guidelines and increase transparency and visibility of practice. Norman PHO planned to develop clinical guidelines for 50 disease-specific conditions and developed an electronic platform with a clinical decisions support system, and e-prescribing and electronic medical records capability. All participating providers in the CIN were required to adhere to the clinical guidelines, participate on a Norman PHO committee, pay a membership fee and annual dues and were subject to a withhold on reimbursements from payers to support the CIN's infrastructure. In addition, participating providers were required to maintain equipment and licenses necessary to access Norman PHO's electronic platform. (Federal Trade Commission February 13, 2013)

The FTC applied the rule of reason analysis to Norman PHO's CIN activities because it determined that such activities were designed to create efficiencies in care that benefit patients and payers and the pricing arrangements were reasonable and necessary to integration. Under the rule of reason analysis, the FTC determined that Norman PHO's pro-competitive benefits were likely to outweigh any anti-competitive effects. The FTC noted that Norman PHO's payment arrangements were structured in such a way that competitive activity was not limited. Specifically, payers were not required to contract with all of the health system's hospitals and the arrangements did not contain any provisions requiring payers to direct or otherwise steer patients to providers within Norman PHO's CIN. (Federal Trade Commission February 13, 2013)

The foregoing cases are examples of FTC approval of clinical integration programs; however, there are other cases in which the commission did not approve joint activities by physicians and hospitals. Cases of interest include *Arizona v. Maricopa County Medical Society*;(1982) Evanston Northwestern Health System;(Federal Trade Commission August 6, 2007) and North Texas Specialty Physicians. (2008, Federal Trade Commission September 12, 2008) Each case or administrative opinion has its unique circumstances, but ultimately each comes down to the rule of reason balancing of anticompetitive actions versus procompetitive effects, including improvements in quality and reductions in cost of healthcare services in each geographic market.

Federal District Court Decision: FTC; State of Idaho v. St. Luke's Health System, Ltd.

On January 24, 2014, a district court in Idaho found that the acquisition of the assets of the Saltzer Medical Group by St. Luke's Health System (St. Luke) violated federal and state antitrust laws. (U.S. District Court of Idaho January 24, 2014) The Court permanently enjoined the acquisition and ordered St. Luke's to fully divest itself of the physicians and assets obtained from the Group. St. Luke's, a not-for-profit health system composed of six hospitals, an emergency room facility, a children's hospital, a cancer referral center, and more than 100 clinics, acquired the assets of the Medical Group, the largest independent primary physician practice in Idaho, with 44 physician employees. Although the Medical Group's physicians were not employed by St. Luke's following the acquisition, the physicians entered into a five-year professional services agreement with St. Luke's and provided St. Luke's with the right to manage the Medical Group's daily operations, to negotiate payer contracts, and to establish rates and charges for services provided by the Medical Group's physicians. As a result, St. Luke's controlled 80 percent of the primary care physicians in the service area.

The FTC and other local health care providers, including two hospital competitors, filed suit against St. Luke's, claiming the acquisition violated antitrust laws. In its complaint, the FTC alleged that St. Luke's acquisition of independent physician groups in the geographic area had created a "single dominant provider" of adult primary care services, which resulted in increased bargaining leverage and the ability to negotiate higher rates with payers, thereby increasing overall health care costs to the consumer. The FTC also alleged that any claim of promoting efficiency and quality of care following the acquisition did not negate the potential for anticompetitive harm.

Although the Court commended St. Luke's effort to improve patient outcomes, an accomplishment it noted that St. Luke's would likely have achieved, the Court determined that the anticompetitive effects of the acquisition outweighed these benefits and, therefore, violated both federal and state antitrust laws. Specifically, the Court stated that the acquisition would give St. Luke's the power to (1) negotiate higher reimbursement rates and (2) raise rates for ancillary services provided by St. Luke's and physicians affiliated with St. Luke's, thereby raising the cost of health care. The Court's ruling illustrates how antitrust laws apply to physician buyouts by hospitals looking to create an integrated health care delivery system.

As health systems strengthen their relationships with physician practices and develop both ACOs and CINs, one compelling truth appears: the primary reason for these participants to come together must be improving quality and value in healthcare services. Discussions and negotiations must focus on both economic incentives (such as joint contracting) and improvements in quality and value of services. Otherwise the initiative will violate legal, regulatory, and antitrust requirements from the outset. Table 5-1 provides examples of activities and conduct that has historically been viewed positively by the FTC while Table 5-2 (Federal Register 2011) provides examples of conduct to avoid to reduce likelihood of antitrust investigations.

Table 5-1. Conduct Historically Viewed Favorably by the FTC

Favorable Conduct
Setting pro-competitive goals, for example, improving quality of care and lowering health care costs.
Development and implementation of, and enforcement of compliance with, universal clinical protocols.
Physician investment in the CIP.
Collection and sharing of clinical outcomes across the CIP.

Table 5-2. Conduct to Avoid to Reduce Likelihood of Antitrust Investigation

Type of Conduct to Avoid
Taking actions to keep commercial payers from directing or incentivizing patients to choose certain providers.
Implicit or explicit linkage of sales (through pricing policy) of ACO services to commercial payers' purchase of other services from providers outside the ACO including providers affiliated with an ACO participant.
Except for primary care physicians, "contracting with other ACO physician specialists, hospitals, ambulatory service centers, or other providers on an exclusive basis, thus preventing or discouraging them from contracting outside the ACO, either individually or through other ACOs or provider networks."
"Restricting a commercial payer's ability to make available to its health plan enrollees cost, quality, efficiency, and performance information to aid enrollees in evaluating and selecting providers in the health plan…"
"Sharing among the ACO's provider participants competitively sensitive pricing or other data that they could use to set prices or other terms for services they provide outside the ACO."

Antitrust Safety Zones

One of the most important steps taken by the DOJ and FTC in allowing the development of CINs is the creation of antitrust safety zones for ACOs participating in the MSSP based on participant's percentage share of common services within their designated primary service areas. The guidance is also instructive with respect to the development of commercial ACOs and their integration activities outside of the MSSP. (Federal Register 2011)

If an ACO falls within the safety zone, it is considered unlikely to raise anti-competitive concerns and the DOJ and FTC will not challenge the ACO, except in cases of improper conduct. An ACO outside of the safety zone may still be legal, provided it does not interfere with competition in relevant markets. Qualification for the safety zone does not protect an ACO from private causes of action, but it may be harder to maintain a private cause of action against an ACO in a safety zone.

To be classified within the safety zone, an ACO whose participants provide the same service (a common service) must have a combined market share of 30 percent or less for each such common service in each participant's primary service area (PSA). A PSA is the least number of zip codes from which the ACO participant obtains at least 75 percent of its patients.

For purposes of evaluation of the safety zone only, a "service" is defined as: (1) physician specialties; (2) major diagnostic categories for inpatient facilities; and (3) outpatient categories (as defined by CMS) for outpatient facilities. The DOJ and FTC consider each physician, practice group, and inpatient facility to have its own PSA. Inpatient facilities are analyzed separately, even if they are part of the same hospital system.

To calculate PSA shares for a common service, the ACO must (1) identify each common service, (2) identify the PSA for each participant who provides the common service, and (3) calculate the ACO's share in the PSA of each such participant. A newly formed ACO may need to estimate expected participation.

The safety zone's availability depends in part on whether an ACO participant is an exclusive- or non-exclusive participant in the ACO. To be eligible for the safety zone, the ACO must allow non-exclusive participants to contract with commercial payers independent of the ACO. It is important to note that hospitals and ambulatory surgery centers must participate in ACOs on a non-exclusive basis, regardless of the hospital's or ambulatory surgery center's market share.

Under the safety zone's "dominant provider limitation," if the ACO includes a participant that has a greater than 50 percent share of any service in its PSA that no other ACO participant provides to patients in that PSA, then (1) such participant must be non-exclusive to the ACO and (2) the ACO cannot require commercial payers to contract with it on an exclusive basis, or otherwise restrict any commercial payer's ability to contract with other ACOs or provider networks. In addition, under the safety zone's "rural exception", an ACO may include one physician per specialty from each rural county, as well as rural hospitals (as defined in the DOJ/FTC Statement), both on a non-exclusive basis and still qualify for the safety zone, even if the inclusion of these physicians causes the ACO's share of any common service to exceed 30 percent in any ACO's PSA for that service.

The safety zone is available for the duration of an ACO's participation agreement with CMS, provided the ACO continues to meet the safety zone's requirements.

Additional Guidance for ACOs Outside the Safety Zone

Failure to fall within the safety zone does not necessarily mean that an ACO is unlawful. An ACO will not raise competitive concerns if it does not interfere with competition. The FTC and the DOJ have advised ACOs with high PSA shares or other indicia of market power to avoid the following types of conduct that may raise anti-competitive concerns:

- Discouraging or restricting commercial payers from incentivizing or otherwise directing patients to certain providers within or outside of the ACO;

- Tying sales of ACO services to services outside of the ACO, whether implicitly or explicitly;

- Entering into exclusive contracts with ACO physicians, hospitals or other providers, which prevent or discourage them from contracting outside of the ACO; and

- Restricting the ability of commercial payers to provide data on cost, quality, efficiency and performance to health plan enrollees, if such data is similar to information used in the Shared Savings Program.

Expedited Antitrust Review

Newly formed ACOs that have not yet signed contracts, or negotiated, with commercial payers and have not participated in the Shared Savings Program that need additional antitrust guidance may request a voluntary, expedited 90-day review of their formation and planned operation. An ACO comprised of providers who previously negotiated contracts with commercial payers is not considered "newly-formed."

To obtain an expedited review, an ACO should submit a completed cover sheet (available on the DOJ's and FTC's websites) along with a request for review, to both the DOJ and FTC *prior* to entering into the Shared Savings Program. The DOJ and FTC will determine which agency will conduct the review. The reviewing agency will examine the potential anti-competitive effects of the proposed ACO and, to the extent possible, will utilize the rule of reason analysis in its review.

Upon receiving notice of which agency will conduct the review, the ACO must submit comprehensive documentation to the reviewing agency, including its ACO application, documents discussing its business strategies and the type and level of competition among the ACO's participants and information regarding the common services provided by the ACO's participants to patients from the same PSA. Within 90 days of receiving all information requested, the reviewing agency will inform the ACO whether it likely, potentially, or does not likely raise competitive concerns. If it appears that the ACO may raise competitive concerns, then the agency may further investigate the ACO and take any enforcement action that it deems appropriate, whether before or during such ACO's participation in the Shared Savings Program. Both the ACO's request for review, and the reviewing Agency's response, will be made public. This review process replaces the FTC's traditional investigation procedures, such as those utilized by the FTC in the Advocate decision discussed above.

Application of Certain Fraud and Abuse Rules to ACOs and CINs

Stark Law

The Stark Law (Section 1877 of the Social Security Act 42 U.S.C. 1395(nn)) is also known as the physician self-referral law. The Stark law is a civil statute that prohibits physicians from making referrals for "designated health services" reimbursable by Medicare or Medicaid, including hospital services, to entities with which they or their immediate family members have a financial relationship, unless a specific exception to the referral prohibition applies. (Title 42 Public Health and Welfare) The Stark Law also prohibits an entity from presenting a claim for payment for any designated health services provided under a prohibited referral. For the purposes of the Stark Law, a financial relationship is defined as a direct or indirect (1) ownership or investment interest of a referring physician their immediate family members in an entity that provides a designated health service or (2) compensation arrangement between the referring physician and an entity that provides a designated health service. (Title 42 Public Health and Welfare)

Designated health services that include the following:

- Clinical laboratory services;
- Physical therapy, occupational therapy, and speech-language pathology services;
- Radiology and certain other imaging services;

- Radiation therapy services and supplies;

- Durable medical equipment and supplies;

- Parenteral and enteral nutrients, equipment, and supplies;

- Prosthetics, orthotics, and prosthetic devices and supplies;

- Home health services;

- Outpatient prescription drugs; and

- Inpatient and outpatient hospital services.

(Health Care Financing Administration January 4, 2001)

Penalties for violation of the Stark Law include denial of reimbursement for services provided in violation, repayment of amounts paid in violation, exclusion from federal healthcare programs, and civil monetary penalties (up to $15,000 per improper claim presented, up to $100,000 per arrangement or scheme intended to circumvent the statute, and/or up to $10,000 per day for failure to adhere to the law's reporting requirements). Violators of the Stark Law may also be subject to fines of up to three times the amount paid in violation, as well as other penalties, under the federal False Claims Act.

In practice, all business relationships entered into by physicians that involve the referral of services implicate the Stark Law, including, but not limited to employment arrangements, the provision of administrative or other services to a hospital or health care entity, space and equipment leases, physician investments and physician recruitment arrangements. As noted above, there are a number of statutory and regulatory exceptions to the Stark Law that protect certain narrowly-defined business arrangements, provided that the arrangement meets all of the applicable exception's requirements.

Below are a few examples of commonly used Stark Law exceptions and some of the requirements associated with the exceptions:

- *Physician Recruitment*: hospitals can provide remuneration to assist a physician group that refers patients to the hospital in recruiting a new physician only in limited circumstances, and only if certain requirements are met.

- *Rental of Office Space*: a hospital can lease space to a physician group that refers patients to the hospital only if the lease arrangements satisfies a number of conditions, such as, all rent to be paid for the entire term of the lease is set in advance and the rent is set at fair market value, the lease agreement is set out in writing and has a term of at least one year.

- *Personal Service Arrangements*: a physician can refer patients to an entity for designated health services if the nature of the compensation relationship between the physician and the entity is a "personal service arrangement" for certain services, such as medical director services. In order to fall within the exception, the compensation paid cannot be dependent on referral of patients from the physician and must be set at fair market value.

- *Electronic Health Records Arrangement*: this exception protects items and services provided by a hospital to a physician that are used to develop an electronic health record system, provided that certain conditions are met, including that the physician pays 15% of the cost of such items and services before receipt of the items and/or services.

Federal Anti-Kickback Statute and Safe Harbors

The Anti-Kickback Statute (42 U.S.C. § 1320a-7b) makes it a criminal offense to provide remuneration in order to induce a party to (1) refer an individual for goods or services payable by a federal health care program or (2) purchase, lease, order, arrange for or recommend the purchase, lease, or order of goods or services payable by a federal health care program. (Social Security Act) For purposes of the Anti-Kickback Statute, "remuneration" includes the transfer of anything of value, directly or indirectly, covertly or overtly, in cash or in-kind. In order for an arrangement to violate the Anti-Kickback Statute, the federal government must prove that remuneration was provided "knowingly and willfully" to induce referrals or the purchasing, leasing or ordering of good or services covered by Medicare or Medicaid or the arranging or recommending of the purchase, lease or order of goods or services covered by Medicare or Medicaid. An Anti-Kickback Statute violation can be established if even one purpose of the arrangement is to induce referrals, purchases, leases or orders of goods or services covered by Medicare or Medicaid. (1985)

Any person or entity that violates the Anti-kickback Statute could face criminal penalties up to $25,000 and/or be imprisoned for not more than five years. Additionally, the Secretary of the Department of Health and Human Services has the authority to exclude providers, including individuals or entities who have committed any of the prohibited acts, from participation in the Medicare or Medicaid programs.

Regulatory Safe Harbors provide immunity from violations of the Anti-Kickback Statute for narrowly defined arrangements. Below are a few examples of commonly used Anti-Kickback Statute Safe Harbors and some of the requirements associated with the Safe Harbors:

- *Discount Safe Harbor:* this Safe Harbor protects discount offered by vendors of goods and services provided that certain conditions regarding reimbursement for the discounted goods or services and discount is accurately reported.

- *Personal Services and Management Contracts Safe Harbor*: Civil Monetary Penalties Law.

The federal Civil Monetary Penalties Law (42 U.S.C. § 1320a-7a) provides for the imposition of civil monetary penalties against:

- any person (including an organization, agency, or other entity) who offers or transfers remuneration to a beneficiary of a federal or state healthcare program that the person knows or should know is likely to influence the beneficiary's selection of a particular provider, practitioner, or supplier of any item or service for which payment may be made, in whole or in part, by a federal or state healthcare program; or

- any hospital who offers or makes payments to a physician to reduce or limit services to Medicare or Medicaid beneficiaries under that physician's direct care.

(Social Security Act)

Violation of the Civil Monetary Penalties Law can subject a person to fines of $50,000 for each such act, in addition to liability for three times the total amount of remuneration paid or received in each act and exclusion from the Medicare and Medicaid programs. (Social Security Act)

Examples of conduct that may be prohibited by the Civil Monetary Penalties Law includes:

- Offering patients grocery store gift cards to encourage preventative health screenings;

- Offering physicians financial incentives for discharging a patient early following surgery or otherwise limiting necessary care;

- Offering patients preventative health services at no charge to the patient; and

- Conducting home safety checks for patients who are about to discharged from a hospital.

Each of the Stark Law, the Anti-Kickback Law and the Civil Monetary Penalties Law limit the ability of physicians, physician groups and other health care entities from entering into certain business arrangements that are commonplace outside of the healthcare industry. For example, other industries commonly offer discounts or other financial incentives in order to generate business and to draw in customers. As outlined above, such activities are heavily regulated and may be prohibited conduct.

In October 2011, the Centers for Medicare & Medicaid Services ("CMS") and the Department of Health & Human Services' Office of the Inspector General (OIG) issued certain fraud and abuse waivers (the Waivers) to encourage the development of Accountable Care Organizations (ACOs) participating in the MSSP. (Federal Register 2011) The Waivers are specific to the MSSP, and do not apply to other integrated models for health care delivery, including the Pioneer ACO Model and other models developed in conjunction with private payers for health care services.

The Waivers

1. The Pre-Participation Waiver

The Stark law, the AKS and the Gainsharing CMP do not apply to start-up arrangements that pre-date an ACO's participation agreement with CMS, provided that certain conditions, as outlined below, are met (the Pre-Participation Waiver). For the purposes of the Pre-Participation Waiver, a start-up arrangement refers to medical or non-medical items, services, facilities or goods that are used to create or develop an ACO if such items, services, facilities or goods are provided by the ACO, ACO participants, ACO providers and suppliers or providers or supplies that are outside of the ACO. Examples of a start-up arrangement include, but are not limited to, infrastructure creation, hiring of new staff, developing care coordination processes, providing incentives to attract primary care physicians to join the ACO and capital investments in the ACO.

The Pre-Participation Waiver will apply to a start-up arrangement if the following conditions have been met.

- The start-up arrangement must be entered into by parties with a good-faith intention to (i) develop an ACO that will participate in the Shared Savings Program in a "target year" and (ii) submit a completed application to participate in the Shared Savings Program in such target year. Participants in the start-up arrangement must include the ACO or an ACO participant that is eligible to form an ACO. The Pre-Participation Waiver will not apply if the parties to a start-up arrangement include drug and device manufacturers, distributors, durable medical equipment suppliers, or home health suppliers.

- The parties to a start-up arrangement must take diligent steps develop and ACO that would participate in the Shared Savings Program in the target year and satisfy requirements regarding governance, leadership and management of the ACO.

- The ACO's governing body must make and duly authorize a bona fide determination that the start-up arrangement is reasonably related to the purposes of the Shared Savings Program.

- The documentation of the arrangement must be contemporaneous with the establishment of the arrangement, the documentation of the authorization of must be contemporaneous with the authorization, and the documentation of the diligent steps must be contemporaneous with the diligent steps. All documentation must be maintained for ten years and include: (i) a description of the start-up arrangement, the parties involved in the start-up arrangement, the date of the arrangement, the purpose(s) of the arrangement; the items, services, facilities and/or goods covered by the arrangement and the financial terms of the start-up arrangement; (ii) the date and manner of the authorization of the start-up arrangement by the ACO's governing body, including the basis for the determination by the ACO's governing body that the arrangement is reasonably related to the purposes of the Shared Savings Program; and (iii) a description of the diligent steps taken to form an ACO, including the actions undertaken and the manner in which the actions relate to the development of an ACO that would be eligible for a participation agreement.

- Public disclosure of the start-up arrangement.

If an ACO fails to submit an application for participation in the MSSP by the last available application due date for the target year, such ACO must submit a statement on or before the last applicable application due date for the target year in a form and manner to be determined by the Secretary outlining the reasons for such failure.

The application of the Pre-Participation Waiver and will end on (i) the start date of the ACO's participation agreement, (ii) the denial date if an ACO's application is denied, except with respect to any arrangement that qualified for the waiver before the date of the denial notice, in which case the waiver period would end on the date that is six months after the date of the denial notice, (iii) the earlier of the MSSP application due date or the date that the ACO submits a statement regarding its failure to submit such an application. If an ACO failed to submit an application but plans to do so, it may apply for an extension of the Pre-Participation Waiver. An ACO may use the Pre-Participation Waiver, including any extensions, only one time.

Examples of arrangements that could qualify for protection by the Pre-Participation Waiver:

- Providing hardware and software to primary care physicians and/or physician groups who become ACO participants.

- Offering recruitment assistance to physician groups who recruit new primary care providers to the geographic area served by the ACO.

2.   The ACO Participation Waiver

The Stark Law, the AKS and the Gainsharing CMP are waived with respect to arrangements of an ACO, for one or more of its participants or its ACO providers or suppliers if each of the following conditions are met (the Participation Waiver):

- The ACO has entered into a participation agreement with CMS and remains in good standing;

- The ACO satisfies requirements regarding governance, leadership and management of the ACO;

- The ACO's governing body must make and duly authorize a bona fide determination that the arrangement is reasonably related to the purposes of the MSSP;

- The documentation of the arrangement must be contemporaneous with the establishment of the arrangement, the authorization, and with the diligent steps. All documentation must be maintained for ten years and include: (i) a description of the arrangement, the parties involved in the arrangement, the date of the arrangement, the purpose(s) of the arrangement; the items, services, facilities and/or goods covered by the arrangement and the financial terms of the arrangement; and (ii) the date and manner of the authorization of the arrangement by the ACO's governing body, including the basis for the determination by the ACO's governing body that the arrangement is reasonably related to the purposes of the MSSP.

- Public disclosure of the arrangement.

Examples of arrangements that could qualify for protection by the Participation Waiver:

- Lease of space to ACO participants at below fair market value if such lease facilitates continuity of care services.

- Offering incentives to attributed patients to participate in preventative care and/or post-acute care services.

If the arrangement meets the aforementioned conditions, the application of the Participation Waiver will begin on the start date of the ACO's participation in the MSSP and end six months after the earlier of (i) the expiration of the ACO's participation agreement with CMS or any renewal period, or (ii) the date on which the ACO voluntarily terminates the participation agreement. If an ACO's participation in the Shared Savings Program is terminated by CMS, application of the waiver will end on such termination date.

3. Medicare Shared Savings Distribution Waiver

The application of the Stark law, the AKS and the Gainsharing CMP are waived with respect to distributions of shared savings earned by an ACO during its participation in the Shared Savings Program (i) to or among ACO participants, ACO providers or suppliers, and individuals and entities that were ACO participants or ACO providers or suppliers during the year in which the shared savings were earned by the ACO, or (ii) for activities that are reasonably related to an ACO's participation in and operations under the

MSSP (the Shared Savings Distribution Waiver). The waiver of the application of the Gainsharing CMP to distributions of shared savings is limited to payments made directly or indirectly by a hospital to a physician that are not made knowingly to induce the physician to reduce or limit medically necessary items or services to Medicare or Medicaid patients. CMS and the OIG will interpret medically necessary in accordance with existing Medicare rules and standards of practice. The Shared Savings Distribution Waiver applies only to ACOs that have entered into a participation agreement with CMS and are in good standing under such participation agreement.

4. Compliance with the Stark Law

CMS and the OIG have waived the application of the AKS and the Gainsharing CMP to any financial relationship between or among the ACO, ACO participants and ACO providers or suppliers that is (i) reasonably related to the purposes of the MSSP, and (ii) provided such financial relationship implicates the Stark law and fully complies with an exception to the Stark law. If a financial relationship meets these conditions, and the ACO has a participation agreement with CMS and remains in good standing under such participation agreement, application of the waiver of the AKS and the Gainsharing CMP will begin on the start date of the ACO's participation agreement and will end on the earlier of (i) the expiration of the participation agreement or (ii) the date of which the ACO's participation agreement has been terminated. CMS and the OIG are soliciting comments on whether this Waiver should continue to apply for a period of time after the ACO's participation agreement expires or terminates.

5. Waiver for Patient Incentives

Application of the Beneficiary Inducement CMP and the AKS are waived with respect to items or services provided to Medicare or Medicaid beneficiaries by an ACO participating in the MSSP, the ACO's participants or providers or suppliers for free or at below fair market value if: (i) the ACO has a participation agreement with CMS and is in good standing under such participation agreement; (ii) there is a reasonable connection between the items or services provided and the beneficiary's medical care; (iii) the items or services are in-kind (i.e. not patient copayments or deductibles); and (iv) the items and services are preventive in nature or advance a certain clinical goal, including, adherence to a treatment or drug regime or management of a chronic disease or condition (the Waiver for Patient Incentives). If an arrangement meets these conditions, the Waiver for Patient Incentives will apply beginning on the start date of the participation agreement and will end on the earlier of the expiration of the participation agreement or the termination of the participation agreement.

Internal Revenue Service Implications

Two federal tax issues of concern to ACOs are nonprofit status and taxability of unrelated business income. These issues affect physicians, hospitals, integrated delivery networks, and CINs as new business relationships are created in forming ACOs. It is important to understand whether clinical and financial integration initiatives affect tax status and whether nonprofit organizations are an asset to a newly formed ACO.

The IRS has issued guidance regarding involvement of tax-exempt hospitals or other healthcare organizations (i.e. § 501(c)(3) organizations) in the MSSP. (Internal Revenue Service 2011, Internal Revenue Service October 20, 2011) This guidance confirms that participation in an ACO through the MSSP in accordance with the rules and regulations relating to the proper creation and maintenance of such MSSP or ACO will not, in and of itself, affect the tax consequences for a tax-exempt participant.

The charitable exemption under Section 501(c)(3) of the Internal Revenue Code (the Code) exempts qualified entities from federal taxation on their income. Qualified companies include those which are organized and operated exclusively for charitable, scientific, or educational purposes, provided no part of the organization's net earnings inures to the benefit of any private shareholder or individual. The IRS has long recognized the promotion of health as a charitable purpose, however, a health institution will not qualify as having a charitable purpose if it is privately owned and is run for the profit of the owners. Notwithstanding an entity's status as tax exempt, unrelated business taxable income (that is the gross income derived from any unrelated trade or business regularly carried on by the company) is not exempt from taxation.

Tax-exempt entities participate in ACOs as partners, shareholders, or otherwise, along with other private non-tax exempt entities. Tax-exempt organizations that take part in ACOs and the MSSP have expressed concern that payments received under the MSSP may be viewed as inuring to the benefit of an insider or provide an impermissible private benefit that would jeopardize their tax-exempt status. The IRS recognizes that participation in ACOs and Shared Savings Programs is expected to reduce health costs and lessen the government's burden and IRS does not want to discourage participation in these programs. As such, the IRS has determined it will not automatically treat tax-exempt entities that receive shared savings as having received prohibited benefits provided they comply with the Code and the IRS Guidance.

Organizations will have different levels of involvement in a Medicare ACO based on contractual arrangements and their specific role in the new organization. Understanding the flow of funds, capital contributions, and economic benefits to all parties are key to managing these new care delivery models, and help ensure tax laws are followed.

The IRS has stated that a tax-exempt organization can participate in the MSSP through an ACO provided the participation does not result in (a) any net earnings inuring to the benefit of its board members, officers, key management employees or other insiders or (b) the ACO being operated for the benefit of private parties participating in the ACO. The IRS will determine whether either of these conditions exists by reviewing the facts and circumstances of the arrangement in accordance with the charitable exemption provisions of the Code.

There are no specific federal income tax rules related to a tax-exempt entity's participation in the MSSP through an ACO. All tax-exempt entities are required to comply with the Code to ensure their tax-exempt status is not negatively affected. To provide guidance to the tax-exempt entities participating in an ACO and the MSSP, the IRS established a five-factor test to determine whether participation results in inurement or impermissible benefit:

- The terms of the tax-exempt organization's participation in the MSSP through the ACO (including its share of shared savings or losses and expenses) are set forth in advance in an arm's length written agreement.

- CMS has accepted the ACO into, and has not terminated the ACO from, the MSSP. Termination of an ACO from the MSSP does not automatically jeopardize the tax-exempt status of a participant. The IRS will review all relevant facts and circumstances, including whether the ACO acts to further charitable purposes even after its termination from the MSSP.

- The tax-exempt organization's share of economic benefits derived from the ACO (including its share of MSSP payments) is proportional to the benefits or contributions it provides to the ACO. The IRS takes into account all contributions that the tax-exempt organization makes to the ACO, in whatever form, including property, cash and services, in determining whether the economic benefits received are proportional to the tax-exempt organizations contributions. If the tax-exempt organization receives an ownership interest in the ACO, the ownership interest received is proportional and equal in value to its capital contributions to the ACO and all ACO returns of capital, allocations and distributions are made in proportion to ownership interests. If the economic benefits are not proportional, the IRS may view such disparity as impermissible excess benefit to an ACO participant.

- The tax-exempt organization's share of the ACO's losses (including its share of shared losses) does not exceed the share of ACO economic benefits to which it is entitled; and

- All contracts and transactions entered into by the tax-exempt organization with the ACO and the ACO participants, and by the ACO with the ACO's participants and any other parties, are at fair market value.

The satisfaction of any one of the foregoing factors will not necessarily be determinative of whether participation in the ACO will result in inurement to insiders or impermissible benefit. The IRS will have discretion in making such a determination based on all of the relevant facts and circumstances of the ACO.

It is also important to note that even if certain aspects of an organization's conduct does not further a charitable purpose or results in unrelated business income, such conduct will not automatically impact the organization's tax-exempt status. The IRS will analyze all of the facts and circumstances of such situations under the general tax rules and regulations applicable to tax-exempt organizations.

State Laws and Regulations

State governments have antitrust and other laws that impact healthcare organization activities. State authorities have responsibilities for regulating health insurance payers, administering state Medicaid programs, and even health reform initiatives within their state boundaries. Responsibility for maintaining fair and open competition in each state's geographic market is shared by federal and state authorities. (Hellinger 1998)

State Medicaid agencies are responsible for administration of state Medicaid programs. Medicaid Fraud and Abuse offices monitor and enforce laws preventing fraudulent activities. Enforcement of federal civil monetary and criminal penalties is an important component of state antifraud and abuse activities. As Medicaid-focused ACOs develop, state Medicaid offices will be engaged at some level to ensure that new healthcare organizations meet legal requirements.

Future Legislative Impact

As this chapter illustrates, federal and state laws have a significant impact on the planning and formation of new healthcare organizations. The impact of ACOs (public and private) and CINs will change the landscape of how healthcare services are financed and delivered. As the Medicare Shared Saving Program evolves, lessons will be learned and regulations be revised to respond to needs of ACOs. New CINs and ACOs should ensure that government affairs regulatory activities closely cover state government agencies as they have the ability to issue new rules and regulations that affect the operations of these new care delivery organizations. Ensuring resources are in place to monitor government policies and rule-making processes at both federal and state levels will allow CIN and ACO leaders to mitigate risk, deal with changes, and adjust operating or financial plans accordingly.

Innovations that emerge throughout the industry will result in new modes of operation for healthcare providers as changes in the delivery system bring about closer integration to achieve greater efficiencies that improve quality and reduce costs, benefiting patients and their communities. Continuing the roadmap series illustrated by Flareau, Yale, Bohn, and Konschak in the second edition, four initiative areas they identified are still of merit for CINs and ACOs to address throughout their efforts to launch and manage their new organizations.

1. *Formation and ongoing management of the joint venture.* Oversight from the CIN's or ACO's executive governance board, with physician leadership and involvement of all key participants, is required to ensure compliance and manage change.

2. *Regulatory monitoring, especially in the formative stages of these organizations.* A complete understanding of complex regulations is important to be compliant with the most current rules of federal, state and local government agencies.

3. *Clinical and financial integration.* Elements of clinical integration include 1) staff for care coordination and case management; 2) adoption of practice standards and protocols; 3) use of EHR to ensure patient data exchange; and 4) having staff in place to monitor standards and protocols.

4. *Compliance with FTC, DOJ, DHHS, CMS, IRS, and other government regulatory bodies.* This is an ongoing initiative that ensures continued compliance over time.

Planning for these areas should involve the CEO, senior executives, legal counsel, government affairs experts, and other staff from across the CIN/ACO. Typically this planning requires board involvement and establishment of a regulatory compliance committee coordinated by a government affairs expert and a compliance officer.

> **DISCLAIMER:** The intent of this chapter is not to provide legal guidance but to raise awareness of many issues, many of which are related to the fields of antitrust and other regulatory laws. It is recommended that readers engage competent legal counsel for themselves and/or their organizations on any specific application of laws and regulations. It is also recommended to retain counsel for necessary communication with government agencies regarding opinions needed on potential CIN or ACO models.

Future Direction

Changes to federal and state laws and regulations will continue to have a significant impact on the evolution of CINs and ACOs. To be successful, organizations must build and maintain clinical integration programs that have both positive economic impacts and improve the quality of healthcare. As joint ventures are proposed among competitors (horizontal) and partners throughout the healthcare supply chain (vertical) in the development of CINs and ACOs, federal and state agencies will monitor markets for anticompetitive behavior to ensure procompetitive effects of improved quality and lower costs mitigate any potential economic harm to consumers. (Besanko, Dranove et al. 2004)

As these market changes tale place, federal and state regulators should evaluate the implications of allowing the "effects of monopoly extraction" (reducing competition in some regions to stimulate innovation for the benefit of all) over against ensuring the "effects of monopoly extension."(Raskovich and Miller September 2010)

Clinical integration programs are essential to the structure of ACOs, and will continue to evolve. Those who are involved in developing new relationships among physician practices, hospital organizations, and other suppliers of services and products should ensure that key staff members are in place to deal with the challenges and risks that will continue to emerge with future changes in federal and state laws and regulations.

CHAPTER 5 DISCUSSION QUESTIONS

Discussion questions are provided for team building or class exercises. Answers for all questions are provided in Appendix C.

Question Number	Question
1	How can an ACO take advantage of the pre-participation waiver?
2	Can an ACO member provide electronic health records software to physician participants in the ACO?
3	Do the MSSP Waivers apply to ACOs participating in private payer arrangements?
4	What are four innovation areas identified in the second edition that still hold merit for CINs and ACOs to develop closer integration within the construct of antitrust regulations?
5	What guidance did the IRS issue in 2011 regarding involvement of tax-exempt hospitals or other healthcare organizations in the Medicare Shared Savings Program?
6	What conditions must be met for the Stark Law, to be waived with respect to arrangements of an ACO?
7	What are the three landmark laws that form the framework for antitrust law enforcement?
8	What types of conduct should be avoided by CINs and ACOs to reduce the likelihood of antitrust investigation?

CHAPTER 5 HIGHLIGHTS

✓ There are three landmark laws that form the framework of antitrust regulations that include: Sherman Act of 1890, the Federal Trade Commission Act of 1914, and the Clayton Act of 1914.

✓ The FTC identified four indicia of clinical integration that include: a) staff for care coordination and case management, b) use of EHRs and other HIT to ensure patient data exchange, c) development and adoption of practice standards and protocols, and d) staff to monitor standards and protocols.

✓ Two federal tax issues of concern to ACOs are nonprofit status and taxability of unrelated business income.

✓ Four innovation initiative areas identified in the second edition and carried over here to the third edition for CINs and ACOs to continue to develop tighter integration include:

  o *Formation and ongoing management of the joint venture,*

  o *Regulatory monitoring, especially in the formative stages of these organizations,*

  o *Clinical and financial integration,*

  o *Compliance with FTC, DOJ, DHHS, CMS, IRS, and other government regulatory bodies.*

✓ In light of the need for compliance with the Stark Law, CMS and the OIG have waived the application of the AKS and the Gainsharing CMP to any financial relationship between or among an ACO, ACO participants, and ACO providers or suppliers that is (i) reasonably related to the purposes of the MSSP, and (ii) provided such financial relationship implicates the Stark law and fully complies with an exception to the Stark law.

CHAPTER 5 REFERENCES

(1975). Goldfarb vs. Virginia State Bar, 421 U.S. 773

(1982). Arizona v Maricopa County Medical Society, 457 U.S. 332.

(1985). U.S. v. Greber, 760 F.2d 68, 69 (3rd Cir. 1985), cert. denied, 474 U.S. 988.

(2008). North Texas Specialty Physicians v. FTC, 528 F.3d 346

Besanko, D., et al. (2004). Competitors and competition. In *Economics of Strategy*. (pp. 218-223). Hoboken, NJ, John Wiley and Sons, Inc.

Burke, T. and S. Rosenbaum, J., (2010). Accountable care organizations: Implications for antitrust policy. *BNA's Health Law Reporter*, 19.

Department of Justice and Federal Trade Commission (2004, July). Improving health care: a dose of competition. Retrieved from http://www.justice.gov/atr/public/health_care/204694/chapter2.htm - 4b3

Federal Register (2011). Statement of Antitrust Enforcement Policy Regarding Accountable Care Organizations Participating in the Medicare Shared Savings Program. 76(209): 67026-67032.

Federal Register (2011). Statement of Antitrust Enforcement Policy Regarding Accountable Care Organizations Participating in the Medicare Shared Savings Program. IV.B. ACOs Outside the Safety Zone. 76(209): 67029.

Federal Register (2011). Statement of Antitrust Enforcement Policy Regarding Accountable CareOrganizations Participating in the Medicare Shared Savings Program. IV.B(1) Conduct to Avoid. 76(209): 67029.

Federal Trade Commission (2009, April 13). Tristate Health Partners Advisory Opinion. Retrieved October 8, 2014, from http://www.ftc.gov/policy/advisory-opinions/tristate-health-partners-inc.

Federal Trade Commission (2007, August 6). Commission Rules that Evanston Northwestern Healthcare Corp.s Acquisition of Highland Park Hospital Was Anticompetitive.

Federal Trade Commission (2006, December 29). Analysis of agreement containing consent order to aid public comment in the matter of Advocate Health Partners, et al., file No. 031 0021. Retrieved from http://www.ftc.gov/os/caselist/0310021/061229ana0310021.pdf

Federal Trade Commission (2006, December 29). FTC charges Chicago-area doctor groups with price fixing.

Federal Trade Commission (2013, February 13). Norman PHO Advisory Opinion. Retrieved from http://www.ftc.gov/policy/advisory-opinions/norman-physician-hospital-organization

Federal Trade Commission (2008, September 12). FTC issues final order on remand in case of North Texas Specialty Physicians.

Federal Trade Commission (2007, September 17). GRIPA advisory opinion (Detailed analysis of FTC review of GRIPA evidence for meeting the indicia of clinical integration). Retrieved from http://www.ftc.gov/sites/default/files/documents/advisory-opinions/greater-rochester-independent-practice-association-inc./gripa.pdf

Greaney, T. L. (2007). Thirty years of solicitude: Antitrust law and physician cartels. *Houston Journal of Health Law and Policy*, 7, 189-226.

Health Care Financing Administration (2001, January 4). 42 CFR Parts 411 and 424. Federal Register. Physician self-referral, final rule (Stark I- Phase I), Vol. 66, No. 3. 856–904.

Hellinger, F. J. (1998). Antitrust enforcement in the healthcare industry: the expanding scope of state activity. *Health Services Research*, 33(5 Pt 2), 1477.

Internal Revenue Service (2011). IRS Notice 2011-20, 2011-16 I.R.B 652. Retrieved from http://www.irs.gov/pub/irs-drop/n-11-20.pdf

Internal Revenue Service (2011, October 20). IRS Fact Sheet: Tax-Exempt Organizations Participating in the Medicare Shared Savings Program through Accountable Care Organizations FS-2011-11. Retrieved from http://www.irs.gov/pub/irs-news/fs-2011-11.pdf

Jacobs, P. and J. Rapoport (2004). Regulation and antitrust policy in health care. In *The Economics of Health and Medical Care*. Sudburry, MA, Jones and Bartlett Publishers.

Raskovich, A. & Miller, N. H. (2010, September). Cumulative innovation and competition policy. Department of Justice Economic Analysis Group Discussion paper. Retrieved from http://www.justice.gov/atr/public/eag/262643.pdf

Sacks, L. B. (2008, May 29). Presentation at Federal Trade Commission Clinical Integration Workshop.

Social Security Act Sec. 1128B. [42 U.S.C. 1320a–7a(a)5. Criminal Penalties for Acts Involving Federal Healthcare Programs.

Social Security Act Sec. 1128B. [42 U.S.C. 1320a–7a(a). Criminal Penalties for Acts Involving Federal Healthcare Programs.

Social Security Act Sec. 1128B. [42 U.S.C. 1320a–7b. Criminal Penalties for Acts Involving Federal Healthcare Programs.

Title 42 Public Health and Welfare. 42 U.S.C. § 1395nn. Limitation on certain physician referrals. Retrieved from http://www.gpo.gov/fdsys/pkg/USCODE-2010-title42/pdf/USCODE-2010-title42-chap7-subchapXVIII-partE-sec1395nn.pdf

Title 42 Public Health and Welfare. 42 U.S.C. § 1395nn.a(2) Limitation on certain physician referrals. In Office Ancillary Services. Retrieved from http://www.gpo.gov/fdsys/pkg/USCODE-2010-title42/pdf/USCODE-2010-title42-chap7-subchapXVIII-partE-sec1395nn.pdf

U.S. Department of Justice and Federal Trade Commission (1996). Statements of Antitrust Enforcement Policy in Health Care. Retrieved from http://www.ftc.gov/sites/default/files/documents/reports/revised-federal-trade-commission-justice-department-policy-statements-health-care-antritrust/hlth3s.pdf

U.S. Department of Justice and Federal Trade Commission (1996). Statements of Antitrust Enforcement Policy in Health Care. Statement 8.4(a). Retrieved from http://www.ftc.gov/sites/default/files/documents/reports/revised-federal-trade-commission-justice-department-policy-statements-health-care-antritrust/hlth3s.pdf

U.S. Department of Justice and Federal Trade Commission (1996). Statements of Antitrust Enforcement Policy in Health Care. Statement 8.B(1). Determining When Agreements Among Physicians in a Physician Network Joint Venture Are Analyzed Under the Rule of

Reason. Retrieved from
http://www.ftc.gov/sites/default/files/documents/reports/revised-federal-trade-
commission-justice-department-policy-statements-health-care-antritrust/hlth3s.pdf

U.S. Department of Justice and Federal Trade Commission (1996). Statements of Antitrust
Enforcement Policy in Health Care. Statement 8.C(1). Examples of Physician Network Joint
Ventures. Retrieved from
http://www.ftc.gov/sites/default/files/documents/reports/revised-federal-trade-
commission-justice-department-policy-statements-health-care-antritrust/hlth3s.pdf

US. District Court of Idaho (2014, January 24). Saint Alphonsus Meducal Center- NAMPA,
Inc, Treasure Valley Hospital Limited Partnership, Saint Alphonsus Health System, Inc., and
Saint Alphonsus Regional Medical Center v. St. Lukes Health System, Ltd. (Case No. 1:12-CV-
00560-BLW (Lead Case)) And Federal Trade Commission v. St. Lukes Health System, Ltd
(Case No. 1:13-CV-00116-BLW). Memorandum Decision and Order.

Chapter 6. The Quality Challenge- Accountability for Continuous Improvement

Deborah S. Smith

Many of these incremental changes that we have seen...
have been really focused on cost control,
and really the question is:
has any of that added any value to our patients?

José R. Sánchez, LMSW, LCSW
President and CEO,
Norwegian American Hospital
Chicago, IL
November 15, 2013

CHAPTER 6 LEARNING OBJECTIVES

✓ Describe the context for provider accountability for measurement and reporting of quality data in healthcare delivery.

✓ Iterate a current understanding of "quality healthcare" based on how it has been defined by recognized leaders.

✓ Review trends in healthcare performance measurement.

✓ See how accountability for quality depends on performance measurement and reporting.

✓ Explore in a case study how practice transformation can come through performance transparency.

✓ Discuss data needs for population health management accountability by Medical Homes, CINs, and ACOs.

A Landscape of Issues

The challenges faced by providers in demonstrating delivery of quality healthcare today are entwined with performance measurement and reporting. Establishing the framework and infrastructure for performance monitoring, measurement, and reporting on population health management indicators is a critical success factor for value-based healthcare organizations. This is true for Medical Home, Clinical Integration and Accountable Care ventures of all types, including the state and federal government sponsored Accountable Care Organization (ACO) programs and commercial private payer ACOs.

In an era of care delivery transformation mandates, measurement and reporting accountability is important not only for performance reporting to purchasers but also is imperative for internal understanding of the achievement and improvement record as practices and networks evolve. Performance feedback to participating providers is an essential building block for these ventures, and possibly the only way to reward performance, incentivize real improvement, and allow these new models to be financially viable. Providers are also anxious to know how they are doing when compared to peers. James L. Holly, MD, CEO of the South East Texas Medical Associates (SETMA) said in a presentation "Metrics are like a healthcare 'Global Positioning System': it tells you where you are, where you want to be, and how to get from here to there."(Holly March 30, 2012)

But before exploring facets of accountability in today's quality challenges, let us very briefly look back at some sentinel milestones in the development of measurement importance since one of the first, large scale quality initiatives: the nineteenth century collection of mortality data and infection rates practiced by Florence Nightingale. While there is evidence that patient outcome data were being collected at the hospital of the University of Pennsylvania as early as the middle of the eighteenth century, the first end-results hypothesis was proposed by Dr. E.A. Codman at Massachusetts General in the early twentieth century, thus beginning the movement toward performance measurement as an index of quality in healthcare. (Loeb 2004) Twenty-first century measurement and reporting has taken leaps forward from where we were prior to 2000. Avedis Donabedian was the first to focus the discipline of healthcare quality measurement on the outcomes research model of "structure, process and outcomes" evaluation that served as the prevailing paradigm since the 1960s. Since that era, many healthcare leaders focused on quality delivery approaches, such as the balanced scorecard. (Curtright, Stolp-Smith et al. 2000, Voelker, Rakich et al. 2001, Grigoroudis, Orfanoudaki et al. 2012) The scorecard sometimes is called a "dashboard." (Curtright, Stolp-Smith et al. 2000)

A balanced scorecard is a performance management tool that links organization goals to individual actions, and allows leadership to track and monitor individual performance. It has been found useful to integrate clinical organizations because it incorporates the perspective of various stakeholder-critical success factors, such as quality, operational, and financial goals. As Voelker described it, the balanced scorecard has been favored by healthcare executives because it is a "methodology that converts an organization's vision and strategy into a comprehensive set of linked performance and action measures that provide the basis for sound strategic measurement and management." (Curtright, Stolp-Smith et al. 2000)

To achieve quality outcomes through a systematic, value-based approach to quality management and performance measurement, some healthcare providers follow best practices as outlined by the Malcom Baldrige Criteria. (National Institute of Standards and Technology, Baldrige Performance Excellence Program, 2014) The Baldrige Criteria for Healthcare are published by the National Institute of Standards and Technology (NIST), an agency of the U.S. Department of Commerce. The Baldrige Criteria promote an integrated performance management framework adapted to healthcare specifically from its roots in nonprofit business. The NIST offers self-assessment tools to assist in development of an organizational profile via examination of organizational strengths and weaknesses in relationship to market challenges. Self-assessment leads to alignment of resources and identification of opportunities to improve communication, productivity, and effectiveness. As depicted in Figure 6-1, the Baldrige self-assessment examines seven aspects of organizational management and performance: Leadership; Strategic planning; Customer focus; Measurement, analysis, and knowledge management; Workforce focus; Operations focus; and Results. (National Institute of Standards and Technology, Baldrige Performance Excellence Program, 2014)

Figure 6-1. The Baldrige multidimensional value-based process for development of an organizational profile through self-assessment

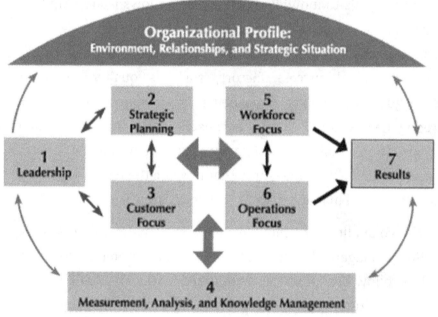

Organization engagement in the Baldrige process centers on the core concept of organizational learning which "moves an organization from reacting to problems to preventing them" and taking steps toward more mature processes. This is also a balanced, multi-dimensional process encompassing infrastructure, process and quality outcomes. Measurement and analysis of data are the tools for continuous performance improvement. The result is said to be delivery of "ever-improving value to patients, customers, and stakeholders, which contributes to organizational sustainability". (National Institute of Standards and Technology, Baldrige Performance Excellence Program, 2014)

For a contemporary clinical practice organization, value-based improvements in quality and accountability have been shown to come from five strategies: integration of providers in practice; transformative patient-centered processes; patient safety through coordination of care; progression to an increasingly sophisticated digital infrastructure; and reliance at the point of service on nationally-recognized, locally adopted care guidelines. The SETMA model, developed by a group of practitioners and highlighted later in this chapter, adds to these characteristics their assumptions about the usefulness of public reporting of performance data they believe give an indication of whether the patient's care is going in the right direction. Their metrics address the range of essential quality characteristics embraced by the SETMA practitioners, which include: access, outcome, patient experience, process, structure and costs of care. (Holly March 30, 2012)

In 2001 the Institute of Medicine (IOM) acknowledged a need to build support for health systems' delivery design change. (Committee on Quality of Healthcare in America, Institute of Medicine, 2001) Recognizing the difficulties faced by providers, the report says:

> Between front line clinical care teams and the healthcare environment lies an array of healthcare organizations, including hospital, managed care organizations, medical groups, multispecialty clinics, integrated delivery systems, and others. Leaders of today's healthcare organizations face a daunting challenge in redesigning the organization and delivery of care to meet the aims set forth in this report. They face pressures from employees and medical staff, as well as from the local community, including residents, business and service organizations, regulators, and other agencies. It is difficult enough to balance the needs of those many constituencies under ordinary circumstances. It is especially difficult when one is trying to change routine processes and procedures to alter how people conduct their everyday work, individually and collectively. (Committee on Quality of Healthcare in America, Institute of Medicine, 2001)

The industry has responded to the 2000 and 2001 IOM Reports with numerous healthcare quality management initiatives focused on improving processes, cost and outcomes. However, as recently written by this author,

> America continues to search for answers to ongoing healthcare challenges: costs remain unsustainably high, care processes are fragmented, and care outcomes reflect the disappointing conclusion that the U.S. health system is expensive and not very effective. There still are too many preventable errors. (Smith 2014)

Understanding Quality

So how is quality healthcare defined and understood? Three expert organizations emerge in the literature: The IOM, the Commonwealth Fund, and the Institute for Healthcare Improvement (IHI).

First, the IOM 2001 *Crossing the Quality Chasm* report identified six aims for healthcare improvement, saying that healthcare should be characterized as outlined in Table 6-1. (Committee on Quality of Healthcare in America, Institute of Medicine 2001)

Table 6-1. Six Dimensions of Quality from the IOM Crossing the Quality Chasm Report

Dimension	Description
Safe	Avoiding injuries to patients from the care that is intended to help them.
Effective	Providing services based on scientific knowledge to all who could benefit and refraining from providing services to those not likely to benefit (avoiding underuse and overuse).
Patient Centered	Providing care that is respectful of and responsive to individual patient preferences, needs, and values and ensuring that patient values guide all clinical decisions.
Timely	Reducing waiting times and harmful delays for both those who receive and those who give care.
Efficient	Avoiding waste, in particular waste of equipment, supplies, ideas,

Dimension	Description
	and energy.
Equitable	Providing care that does not vary in quality because of personal characteristics such as gender, ethnicity, geographic location, and socioeconomic status.

Then, in 2008, the Commonwealth Fund Commission on a High Performance Health System expanded understanding of quality when it identified six attributes of an ideal healthcare delivery system:

1. Patients' clinically relevant information is available to all providers at the point of care and to patients through electronic health record systems.

2. Patient care is coordinated among multiple providers, and transitions across care settings are actively managed.

3. Providers (including nurses and other members of care teams) both within and across settings have accountability to each other, review each other's work, and collaborate to reliably deliver high-quality, high-value care.

4. Patients have easy access to appropriate care and information, including after hours; there are multiple points of entry to the system; and providers are culturally competent and responsive to patients' needs.

5. There is clear accountability for the total care of patients.

6. The system is continuously innovating and learning in order to improve the quality, value, and patients' experiences of healthcare delivery.

(Shih 2008)

And after the U.S. healthcare system received a 66% scorecard rating from the Commonwealth Fund Commission (cited above) and the CMS pay-for-performance (P4P) Premier demonstration project and other P4P efforts showed slow progress on all six of the IOM quality dimensions. Don Berwick from the Institute for Healthcare Improvement (IHI) outlined a framework for quality care. (Berwick, Nolan et al. 2008) He introduced the linked goals of the now well-recognized, driving principle behind the formation of ACOs: the Triple Aim. According to the Triple Aim,

> Improving the U.S. healthcare system requires simultaneous pursuit of three aims: improving the experience of care, improving the health of populations, and reducing per capita costs of healthcare. Preconditions for this include the enrollment of an identified population, a commitment to universality for its members, and the existence of an organization (an "integrator") that accepts responsibility for all three aims for that population. The integrator's role includes at least five components: partnership with individuals and families, redesign of primary care, population health management, financial management, and macro system integration. (Berwick, Nolan et al. 2008)

Figure 6-2. IHI Triple Aim Diagram
(Institute for Healthcare Improvement 2014)

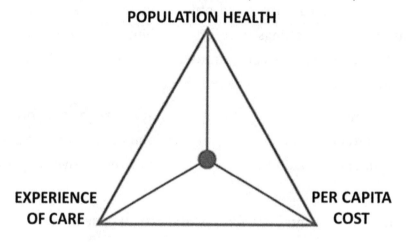

In the provider sector, the incentives for quality improvements in care delivery, cost and outcomes generally arise from continued emphasis on government and commercial pay-for-performance models. Such models may shift both risk and accountability to the provider. By following the Triple Aim precepts, provider organizations not only improve care, but attain performance metrics resulting in reimbursement increases. Thus, demonstrable improvements in the three quality dimensions defined by the Triple Aim are key to provider sustainability for the future.

Trends in Healthcare Performance Measurement

URAC Vice President for Research and Measures, Marybeth Farquhar, PhD, in an internal document wrote about 2010 Patient Protection and Affordable Care Act (ACA)-era trends in healthcare performance measurement. She said:

"There are implications for the use of performance measures as payment reform models become more prevalent. The emerging trends are:

- Optimal approaches to measuring performance and assessing care quality are still experimental,

- There continues to be a large body of measures (structure and process, some outcome measures) available for measuring performance.

- Measures should focus on the continuum of care rather than on discrete clinical services. Health outcomes are emphasized, specifically changes in functional status, morbidity and quality of life,

- Complex measurement strategies may be beneficial for complex organizations or systems such as the use of multiple data sources for quality information,

- Standardized but flexible measures and measure sets may address the needs of the integrated payment reform models.

- Composite measures or measure sets will be important in reporting on quality,

- Efficiency and resource use measures may be useful in assessing quality, although they should not be the sole indicator used.

- As payment models blend together, complex measurement strategies may be required to assess quality, and

- Structure of care measures may be relevant in the near term.
(URAC internal memorandum, 2013)

A 2011 RAND report identified areas for further measure development and refinement that emerge across various payment reform models, including:

- Health outcome measures that can be used to assess care for populations:
  - Health status measures (functional status and quality of life)
  - Safety outcomes (preventable harms attributable to healthcare)
- Care coordination measures (including measures that assess care transitions);
- Measures of patient and caregiver engagement (measures that assess the participation of patients and caregivers in their care);
- Measures of structure (particularly management measures and health information technology utilization measures that address new organizational types);
- Composite measures that combine outcome, process, structure, patient experience, cost, and other measure types;
- Efficiency measures that combine quality and resource use measures;
- Clinical and socio-demographic risk profiles of providers' patient populations; and
- Measures of access to care and measures to detect provider avoidance of high-risk patients.
(Schneider, Hussey et al. 2011)

The IOM has identified several existing gaps in the current measure sets, and suggests four approaches to measure development.

1. *Comprehensive measurement:* 'A performance measurement system should advance the core purpose of the health care system and foster

improvements in all six aims identified in the *Quality Chasm* report: safety, effectiveness, patient centeredness, timeliness, efficiency, and equity.' (Committee on Quality of Healthcare in America, Institute of Medicine, 2001)

2. *Longitudinal measurement:* "Standardized performance measures should characterize health and healthcare both within and across settings and over time."

3. *Individual patient-level, population-based, and systems-level measurement:* "Measurement and measures should assess the health and healthcare of both individuals and populations and the many systems within which care is provided."

4. *Shared accountability:* "Measurement should not be constrained by the absence of a current, identifiable, single responsible agent." (e.g., accountability should rest with the team of care givers, not one specified individual or entity)."

(Committee on Redesigning Health Insurance Performance Measures, Payment, IOM 2006)

Accountability in CMS Measurement and Reporting Programs

The Center for Medicare and Medicaid Innovation (CMMI) was established, in part, to create alternative government payment models - including ACOs - based on the goal of achieving the Triple Aim. The CMMI established the Pioneer ACO demonstration program to test how well ACOs and other cost-containment programs integrate and coordinate care, improve quality and contain costs. (Boyarsky and Parke 2012) The initial Pioneer ACOs were 32 integrated health delivery systems with longstanding experience in managing care. Pioneer ACOs were not only to share in savings generated, but face a financial risk if they didn't meet certain financial and quality performance thresholds. The Medicare Shared Savings Program (MSSP) is a permanent program enacted as part of the ACA. The ACA built upon the

Medicare Physician Group Practice (PGP) demonstration project and the Premier Hospital Quality Incentive Demonstration (HQID) to design the MSSP-ACO, a Medicare-only ACO. Under the MSSP, physicians and other providers voluntarily form ACOs for a Medicare population defined by CMS, and share in savings generated beyond a minimum threshold if they maintain their performance on CMS mandatory quality metrics.

The CMS measures align with the first arm of the 2001 IHI Triple Aim shown in Figure 6-1. CMS identified four quality domains and also aligned closely with the Physician Quality Reporting System (PQRS; a pay-for-reporting program in Medicare) for eligible professionals within an ACO.

Figure 6-3. Four Quality Domains of CMS MSSP ACOs

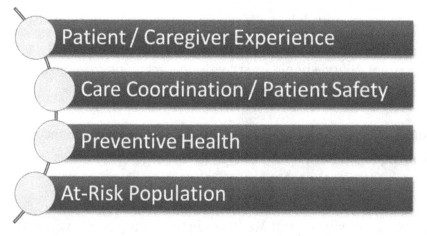

CMS settled on 33 required quality measures for the MSSP and Pioneer ACO provider participants after initially proposing 65. The 33 measures focus predominantly on ambulatory care, given the primary care focus of the MSSP and the method of Medicare beneficiary attribution to each provider. Nationally-recognized measures were selected based on the belief that the measures would have high-impact on the quality of care delivered, and ensure appropriate care would not be withheld (underutilization) as a way to force savings and "game" the system to achieve higher savings to share. These measures, derived from the four quality domains, are summarized in Table 6-2. (RTI International August 15, 2014)

Table 6-2. Measures for use in 2014 for establishing quality performance standards that ACOs must meet for CMS shared savings

Domain	Measure	Number	Source(s)
Patient/caregiver Experience	CAHPS Scores	7 measures	AHRQ, CMS
Care coordination/patient safety		6 measures	AHRQ, CMS, AMA-PCPI/NCQA
Preventive Care		8 measures	AHRQ, CMS, AMA-PCPI/NCQA & QIP
At-risk population		5 measures & 2 composites	
	Diabetes	1 measure & 1 composite consisting of 5 measures	NCQA, MCM
	Hypertension	1 measure	NCQA
	Ischemic Vascular Disease	2 measures	NCQA
	Heart Failure	1 measure	AMA/PCPI/ACC/AHA/AMA
	Coronary Artery Disease	1 composite consisting of 2 measures	AMA/PCPI/ACC/AHA/AMA

The impact of the four composite measures is that 33 measures are actually scored as 23.

ACOs are responsible for selecting and paying for a CMS-approved vendor to administer the CAHPS for ACOs experience of care survey. The CAHPS for ACOs is based on the Clinician and Group (CG) CAHPS. For claims-based measures, ACOs do not need to collect or submit data. Provider participants are required to attest to Meaningful Use of EHRs; data are collected and calculated for the practices.

Claims based measures include:

- Risk standardized all condition readmissions;
- Ambulatory sensitive admissions for COPD or Asthma in older adults;
- Ambulatory sensitive admissions for heart failure; and
- Percent of primary care physicians who qualify for EHR program incentive payment.

2014 and 2015 benchmark scores were established using 2012 fee-for-service claims data. 2013 CAHPS data from fee-for-service Medicare beneficiaries were used to set benchmarks for patient experience. The ACO-7 CAHPS: Health status/functional status measure has no benchmark and is considered a pay-for-reporting indicator. Benchmarks are stratified by percentile from 30th to 90th. For 2015, it is expected that the number of required measures will rise to 37, though some measures will be retired and replaced. Proposed new measures are based on claims data, so the burden of reporting could be reduced by one metric. (Gordon 2014)

Currently proposed changes are intended to bring reporting requirements in line with changes to clinical practice and streamline the reporting demand.

> The new measures include whether patients say providers educated them about the cost of medications; the rate of patients who are admitted to a skilled-nursing facility within 30 days of leaving the hospital; and all-cause unplanned readmissions for patients with diabetes, heart failure or multiple chronic conditions. CMS also proposed a replacement measure for medication management and a modification to its requirement for electronic health-record adoption and suggested removing some measures related to the treatment of diabetes, ischemic vascular disease and coronary artery disease. (Evans 2014)

Preliminary Results from Pioneer and MSSP ACO programs

Both the Pioneer and MSSP ACO programs are supposed to improve quality, decrease costs, and allow both payer and provider to share in savings while transforming how care is delivered and patients experience the delivery system – all elements of the Triple Aim. Actual experience, however, based on preliminary results has been somewhat disappointing.

Measures adopted by CMS are quality-only, and do not focus explicitly on resource use or reducing costs. It has been reported that,

> CMS believes that specific measures addressing utilization or high-cost services are unnecessary to incentivize ACOs to address costs, and that the incentives offered by shared savings will be sufficient to engender lower cost. (Integrated Healthcare Association October 2011)

However, the rate of Pioneer and MSSP participant withdrawal may actually indicate otherwise.

One disappointment is that both government ACO programs are hazarding attrition as the consequences of risk assumption begin to take hold. Before negative reimbursement consequences could be applied, one third of the Pioneer ACOs dropped out of the program. Some of them opted to join the portion of the MSSP program that only rewarded their savings. Now CMS is contemplating requiring all ACOs to face some financial risk based on their performance in the second round of applications. As a result, nearly one third of the existing participating groups in the regular MSSP program have said they don't anticipate seeking to continue in the MSSP program. And in fact, at the end of November, 2014, CMS announced changes in the savings thresholds so that participants could continue in the program with less risk.

Year one results from both the Pioneer and the MSSP programs were released in January 2014. The January release extends the available Pioneer program results initially reported in July 2013, and includes the first two rounds from April and July 2012 MSSP start dates. Published analyses concur that modest gains in delivery of higher quality of care were damped by the finding that overall reductions in spending were not significant enough to qualify the participants for shared savings distributions under the CMS rules. (Petersen and Muhlestein 2014, Kocot, Mostashari et al. February 7, 2014)

Petersen and Muhlestein, in their Health Affairs blog "ACO Results – What we know so far," report that all Pioneer and all but five MSSP ACOs successfully reported quality metrics to CMS. Pioneer programs showed improvement where comparable data was available. (Petersen, Muhlstein et al. 2013) The 2013 Pioneer data showed "notable success" with quality scores higher than industry benchmarks. Reporting was the only requirement for the MSSP programs at the first stage of participation.

Kocot, et. al. conclude that the results "suggest great potential for ACOs to bend the overall cost growth curve" and "it is unreasonable to expect a majority of ACOs to be able to satisfy both criteria for shared savings – reducing costs and improving quality" – in their early years of transformation. The authors cite as barriers the considerable challenge faced by ACO providers in effective data collection and reporting supported by adequate HIT systems, and the need for reinforcement of changes in behavior necessary for transformation through incentives to providers and patients. They speculate, however, that there is enough substance in the cost savings from the CMS perspective for financial sustainability of these ACO programs. (Kocot, Mostashari et al. February 7, 2014) Though not all agree with the authors' conclusion, CMS appears to be moving toward new regulations in 2015 or 2016 and CMMI is gathering reactions to population-based payments that will encourage greater care coordination and financial accountability.

Data analysis on ACO metrics by the Leavitt Partners Center for Accountable Care Intelligence included state Medicaid and commercial ACOs as well as the Pioneer and MSSP participants. Oregon is the leading example of a state program with published results. The Oregon Health Authority showed a decrease in cost of care for 19 of 21 financial indicators, but posted only a marginal overall savings. February 2014 quality measures reported a 13% decline in ER visits and an 8% reduction in all-cause re-hospitalizations and one third less chronic condition related hospitalizations. But it is noted that "it remains to be seen if shared savings will offset investment costs."(Petersen, Muhlstein et al. 2013)

Some data have been published on commercial ACO performance, but Leavitt Partners found comparisons difficult. Not only is there a high degree of variability in organization among commercial ACOs, but lack of uniformity in measurement and reporting is a barrier. And few commercial ACOs have publicly reported results.

A Model of Practice Transformation through Performance Transparency

Practice transformation depends on the commitment of practitioners and willingness to work in the context of the Triple Aim and national aims and priorities. One compilation of national aims and priorities is The National Healthcare Quality Improvement Strategy (NHQIS).

The NHQIS was first published in March 2011, as required by the ACA. It is led by the Agency for Healthcare Research and Quality (AHRQ) on behalf of the U.S. Department of Health and Human Services. National aims were articulated in a Report to Congress. (Agency for Healthcare Quality and Research March 2011) These national aims "guide and assess local, state and national efforts to improve healthcare quality."(Farquhar 2011)

Table 6-3. Aims of the National Quality Strategy articulated by AHRQ

National Aims for Quality Improvement
Better Care: Improve overall quality by making healthcare more patient-centered, reliable, accessible, and safe.
Healthy People/Healthy Communities: Improve the health of the U.S. population by supporting proven interventions to address behavioral, social and environmental determinants of health in addition to delivering higher-quality care.
Affordable Care: Reduce the cost of quality healthcare for individuals, families, employers, and government.

From these aims, and under the leadership of AHRQ, six priorities have emerged based upon research, input from a broad range of stakeholders, and examples from around the country. These priorities have the potential for rapidly improving health outcomes and increasing the effectiveness of care for all populations. (Farquhar 2011)

Table 6-4. Initial Priorities for Achieving Quality U.S. Healthcare

National Quality Priorities
1. Making healthcare safer by reducing harm caused in the delivery of care.
2. Ensuring that each person and family is engaged as partners in their care.
3. Promoting effective communication and coordination of care.
4. Promoting the most effective prevention and treatment practices for the leading causes of mortality, starting with cardiovascular disease.
5. Working with communities to promote the wide use of best practices to enable healthy living.
6. Making quality care more affordable for individuals, families, employers, and governments by developing and spreading new healthcare delivery models

The IHI Triple Aim concept for redesign of healthcare delivery is to create a system around its three dimensions of healthcare: the experience of the individual; the health of a defined population; per capita cost for the population. The system imagined by the IHI Innovations Team include: focus on individuals and families; redesign of primary care services and structures; population health management; cost control platform; and system integration and execution. (Institute for Healthcare Improvement 2014) In such a system it is envisioned that quality is defined from the perspective of an individual member of a population as shown in Figure 6-4. (Institute for Healthcare Improvement 2014)

Figure 6-4. IHI Triple Aim Enterprise Design: A Paradigm for Healthcare Redesign and System Development

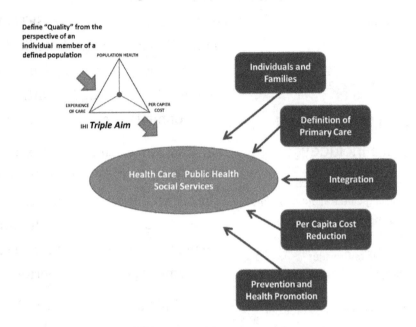

The following case study demonstrates how a multispecialty medical group centered in Beaumont, Texas, has used its commitment to the Triple Aim to realize success for its physician partners, its patients, and the communities it serves. It also makes the point that data collected and analyzed at the point of care is the most powerful motivator for practice transformation leading to improvements in population health.

Case Study: Southeast Texas Medical Associates

Southeast Texas Medical Associates, LLP (SETMA) was founded in 1995 by James L. Holly, M.D. and four others to create a medical group which would integrate all of the various components of a family's health needs in a multi-specialty setting. SETMA adopted the Triple Aim and translated it into the *SETMA Way* and *The SETMA Model of Care* as "improved processes of healthcare delivery, improved outcomes of healthcare, with both existing in a sustainable systems approach." (Southeast Texas Medical Associates 2014) From the practices of four physicians with 21 employees, SETMA has grown successfully into a mid-size multi-specialty group with 40 providers and over 250 employees with its own charitable foundation providing patient financial assistance for needed care. And, uniquely, SETMA now holds Patient Centered Medical Home recognition from all four issuing bodies: AAAHC, NCQA, URAC, and The Joint Commission.

The key to this model is the real-time ability of providers to measure their own performance at the point-of-care. This is done with multiple displays of quality metric sets, and real-time aggregation of performance.

SETMA's seven clinical locations are integrated electronically through a single EMR platform. Through it, SETMA providers have access to patient records at all area hospitals, emergency departments, nursing homes, as well as from all SETMA providers' homes and clinics. Enabled by the EMR, SETMA began using its website in 2009 for public reporting of provider performance by individual provider name on over 300 quality metrics. Dr. Holly said in a 2012 presentation "a single or a few quality metrics does not change outcomes, but fulfilling 'clusters' and 'galaxies' of metrics at the point-of-care can and will change outcomes."(Holly March 30, 2012) The concepts of multiple metrics on a single condition and tracking of multiple health issues at the point of service are illustrated in the following two figures. SETMA believes that,

> ...the power of quality metrics, like the benefit of the GPS, is enhanced if the healthcare provider and the patient are able to know the coordinates

SETMA's Model of Care includes:

- Personal Performance Tracking One Patient at a Time
- Auditing of Performance by Panel or Population
- Analysis of Provider Performance Statistical Analysis
- Public Reporting By provider Name at www.setma.com
- Quality Assessment and Performance Improvement"

– their performance on the metrics -- while care is being received. (Holly March 30, 2012)

Figure 6-5. A "*cluster*" is seven or more quality metrics for a single condition, i.e., diabetes, hypertension, etc.

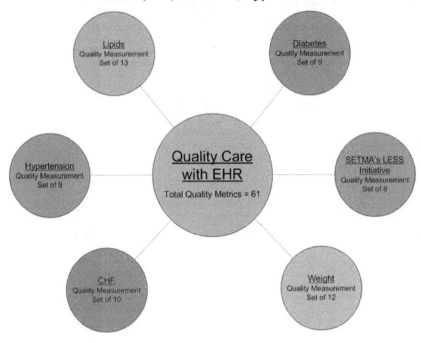

Figure 6-6. A "*galaxy*" is multiple clusters for the same patient, i.e., diabetes, hypertension, lipids, CHF, etc.

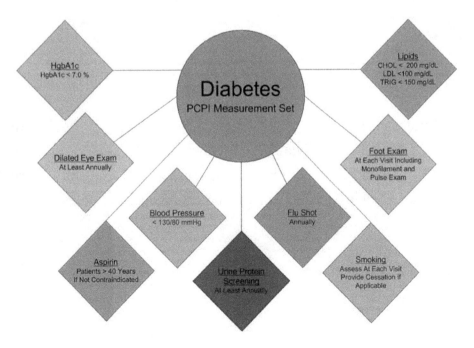

A Clinical Case Example

In 2009, SETMA launched a Business Intelligence software solution for real-time analytics. Trending revealed that from October-December, 2009, many patients were losing HbA1C control. Further analysis showed that these patients were being seen and tested less often in this [holiday] period than those who maintained control.

A 2010 Quality Improvement Initiative included writing all patients with diabetes encouraging them to make appointments and get tested in the last quarter of the year. A provider - patient contract was made, which encouraged celebration of holidays while maintaining dietary discretion, exercise and testing. In 2011, trend analysis of the data showed that the holiday-induced loss of control had been eliminated. (Holly March 30, 2012)

Chart 6-1. Trends of HbA1C show relative stability during the 2011 holiday period. (Holly March 30, 2012)

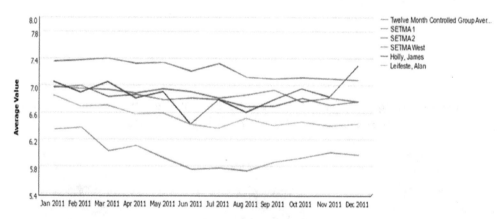

Statistical analysis by SETMA shows the impact on the health of populations as well as individuals. SETMA is able to analyze patterns to explain why one population or one patient is not to goal while others are. As shown in the example below, the analysis includes such variables as:

- Frequency of visits;
- Frequency of testing;
- Number of medications;

- Change in treatment if not to goal;
- Attended Education or not;
- Ethnic disparities of care; and
- Age and Gender variations, etc.

Chart 6-2. A 2012 analysis illustrates the usefulness of data to show patterns amenable to intervention that will change outcomes. (Holly March 30, 2012)

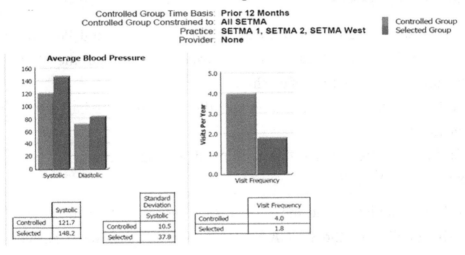

Chart 6-3. Comprehensive Diabetes measures are reported by physician for 2011. (Holly March 30, 2012)

Location	Provider	\<120	120-129	130-139	140-149	150-159	160-169	170-179	≥180	Not Present	\<75	75-79	80-89	90-99	100-109	≥100	Not Present
						YELLOW ZONE		RED ZONE						YELLOW ZONE		RED ZONE	
SETMA 1	Aziz	26.6%	31.8%	19.2%	13.6%	5.0%	2.9%	0.3%	0.7%	0.0%	55.0%	13.1%	25.6%	5.5%	0.3%	0.3%	0.1%
	Duncan	35.1%	35.3%	18.4%	8.0%	1.1%	0.8%	0.0%	0.0%	1.3%	50.1%	9.7%	35.1%	3.8%	0.0%	0.0%	1.3%
	Henderson	36.3%	33.1%	18.1%	7.8%	2.9%	1.0%	0.3%	0.3%	0.2%	55.4%	11.8%	28.1%	4.0%	0.2%	0.3%	0.2%
	Murphy	30.5%	29.4%	23.0%	9.5%	3.6%	2.2%	0.8%	0.8%	0.2%	48.5%	8.1%	33.9%	7.2%	1.7%	0.4%	0.2%
	Palang	10.5%	33.2%	29.4%	26.2%	6.5%	2.0%	0.5%	0.0%	1.7%	54.4%	5.0%	32.4%	5.7%	0.7%	0.0%	1.7%
	Thomas	14.0%	41.2%	21.1%	14.9%	6.1%	1.8%	0.9%	0.0%	0.0%	28.1%	14.9%	50.0%	6.1%	0.0%	0.0%	0.9%

By looking more closely at trending results, trends can be extrapolated into the future and begin to predict what will happen. By analyzing past trends of patients who have been readmitted to the hospital, they have been able to predict the factors they believe are likely to reduce a patient's risk of unnecessary readmission to the hospital. They found three actions that played a significant role in keeping patients from coming back to the hospital unnecessarily:

1. The patient received their Hospital Care Summary and Post Hospital Plan of Care and Treatment Plan (previously called the Discharge Summary) and the time of discharge.
2. A 12-30 minute care coaching call the day after discharge from the hospital.
3. Seeing the patient in the clinic within 5 days after discharge."

(Holly March 30, 2012)

Other examples of the more than 30 categories of performance data available publicly on the SETMA website are locally developed, such as the Transitions of Care audit and the SETMA Physician's Role in Hypertension Management. Other performance metrics include NQF, PQRS and HEDIS measures.

> *Once you "open your books on performance" to public scrutiny; the only place you have in which to hide is excellence!*
> Larry Holly, MD
> SETMA Founder

The SETMA experience validates what many believe to be the most powerful change agent: the internal commitment of physician champions to transformation of healthcare service delivery for their own satisfaction and betterment of patient health status. The SETMA growth and financial success story shows us one path to sustainability in a value-based market environment, built on performance measurement and transparency, using the EMR as its database.

Data Needs of the Medical Home, CIN and ACO

The preponderance of quality reporting historically was performed with a dependence on claims-based billing system information. Claims data has often been considered inaccurate, in part because of coding errors but also due to lack of granularity, and thus contested by many providers when used for purposes other than procedure-based payment. Billing data often is not specific enough for satisfactory analysis to support practice transformation or the goals of population health management. For example, claims or billing data can tell you whether a blood test was billed, but may not provide the results of the test or its relevance to patient care. So dependence on claims data supports reliance on process measures and is a barrier to examination of health status outcomes, both for individuals and populations.

Early clinical-based quality reporting systems - far less mature than billing counterparts - were not able to effectively or efficiently support analysis of information from disparate systems and locations. Newer clinical reporting systems obtain test results, clinical interventions, and sometimes relevant outcomes accessible via structured data. Most clinical systems are challenged, however, by the needs of multi-site medical homes, joint ventures, and networks because of the multiplicity of changing performance metrics and lack of uniformity among legacy systems in practice settings. The emergence of data warehouse repositories and their ability to integrate disparate data has moved forward the ability of joint ventures and networks to aggregate, analyze and compare practice performance data.

The patient registry has also emerged as an important and powerful tool, paving the way for more robust outcomes measurement in a larger number of settings. The registry is a list of persons and their conditions or variance from acceptable care or metrics, drawn from claims or clinical data. The registry is a low-cost tool afforded by many practices in early stages of transformation and those in safety net settings. However, as in the

SETMA story, the gold standard remains the uniform platform and ease of interoperability between practice settings.

Data reporting from remote monitoring, quantified-self, and telemedicine devices is the next frontier. This data may help to enrich clinical and claims data, with remote devices measuring, recording, and reporting a wide variety of real-time personal information such as blood pressure, heart rate, glucose levels, and weight, etc.

URAC standards for Clinical Integration and Accountable Care require participating providers to engage in "performance measurement and reporting procedures." Measurements/metrics are defined by the integrated network, including criteria for inclusion and exclusion, calculation methods, and performance thresholds. Selected measures may be created by the accredited organization or adopted from external sources, such as payer/purchaser contracts, public reporting requirements, or government (e.g., CMS) metrics. Measures and metrics are linked to the value-driven, consumer-oriented goals of these ventures. Because of the close alignment with FTC anti-trust guidelines, joint ventures such as Clinically Integrated Networks (CINs) must have measures in place to evaluate and modify practice patterns.

Accreditation standards include the need for performance monitoring to confirm that established goals related to improved health, enhanced efficiency, and controlled healthcare costs in the population served are being met, and transparent reporting. Performance measurement and reporting is integral to the type of care management and coordination central to integrated care models. Providers are encouraged to implement and measure both processes and outcomes derived from nationally accepted, locally adopted guidelines for clinical care of acute and chronic conditions. Chronic conditions and patients with multiple co-morbidities are the principal focus to achieve population health status gains and thus cost efficiencies. Consistent with the Triple Aim, consumer experience also is a required measure. Performance measurement and reporting is supported in the accredited organization by health information systems. The URAC Accountable Care standards require sophisticated electronic systems, while CINs are acknowledged to be in various stages of development along the pathway to accountability.

Whatever the organization's digital capabilities, URAC expects no less than annual performance monitoring, analysis and reporting of individual practitioners, groups, locations, as well as organization-wide. In accredited organizations, data are put to use to make improvements in quality, efficiency, and value. Accountable care standards include additional expectations for tracking of gaps in care triggering in-reach and outreach activities. In-reach activities are actions taken to close gaps in care when the patient is in contact with the practice. Organizations are encouraged to strive toward data liquidity and interoperability of clinical information across care settings to enable good communication and appropriate action when patients contact any part of the organization. Electronic clinical decision support tools are mandatory to support the accountable network's quality and utilization performance improvement metrics tracking and reporting.

Importance to Providers of the ICD – 10 Challenges

The International Statistical Classification of Diseases and Related Health Problems (ICD) is a classification system used to record signs and symptoms of disease and conditions, and related procedures. The system is useful for coding diagnoses and procedures for billing purposes and epidemiology studies. The ICD-9 system, used since the 1970s in the United States, is scheduled to be replaced by the ICD version 10 (ICD-10) in October 2015, which is more accurate and has more granular information on conditions and procedures.

Claims remain an important source of data on a national or payer-specific scale, but coding of the clinical record is also an important strategy for the future of population health management. Inefficiencies are inherent in some clinician-produced point-and-click, structured clinical documentation. Such systems as SNOMED[1] use exhaustive libraries to codify what they can recognize from within the clinical record and are far more specific to clinical conditions than the more traditional claims-based billing system codes. ICD-10 coding is a movement to close that gap, with greater amounts of more detailed and reliable data.

It will be very important for Medical Homes, CINs and ACOs to work to assure that an effective and hopefully seamless transition takes place with the conversion from ICD-9 to ICD-10. There are many positive benefits to be gained once ICD-10 is in place. First, the level of detail and specificity in patient health data will increase exponentially as a result of this transition. ICD-10-coded health records will provide new levels of information to help identify gaps and disparities in care, track effectiveness of treatment plans and measure health outcomes, thus supporting accountability and promoting the ability to receive related financial rewards. Second, as CIN/ACO operations increasingly focus on improving performance measurement and reporting, these new code sets will increase the quality of health data and awareness of clinical root causes, diagnoses, and plans of care, yielding greater actionable detail valuable to providers, patients engaged in self-management, and payers.

While the U.S. healthcare system waits for full ICD-10 implementation, increasingly smart technology such as Natural Language Processing (NLP) software is beginning to automate the recognition of free text entries and voice-to-text conversions, allowing codification of the medical record without the workflow intrusion of point-and-click documentation. The

---

[1] SNOMED CT (Systematized Nomenclature of Medicine--Clinical Terms) is a comprehensive clinical terminology, originally created by the College of American Pathologists (CAP) and, as of April 2007, owned, maintained, and distributed by the International Health Terminology Standards Development Organization (IHTSDO), a not-for-profit association in Denmark. SNOMED CT is one of a suite of designated standards for use in U.S. Federal Government systems for the electronic exchange of clinical health information and is also a required standard in interoperability specifications of the U.S. Healthcare Information Technology Standards Panel.

entire U.S. system will be challenged with the transition to ICD-10 coded data, required by October 1, 2015 under the new HIPAA rules.

The new ICD-10 diagnostic codes increase item specificity in many ways as outlined in tables 6-5 and 6-6. (American Medical Association 2010)

Table 6-5. Differences between ICD-9 and ICD-10 Diagnostic Codes

ICD-9	ICD-10
3-5 characters	3-7 characters
Approximately 13,000 codes	Approximately 68,000 codes
Space limitation to increase codes	Flexible system able to increase number of codes
Lacks specificity	Increased level of specificity
Lacks laterality	Codes include laterality (right vs. left)

In addition to new diagnostic codes, the ICD-10 transition introduces new procedure code sets. These code sets are used to report services and procedures in ambulatory care and physician office settings.

Table 6-6. Differences between ICD-9 and ICD-10 Procedure Code Sets

ICD-9	ICD-10
3–5 characters	7 characters
Approximately 3,000 codes	87,000 codes with availability to expand
Lacks specificity	Increased level of specificity
Lacks laterality	Codes include laterality (right vs. left)
Based on outdated technology	Reflects current medical and device-related terminology
Uses generic terminology for body part references	Has more specific terminology for body part references
Lacks descriptions of methodology and approaches for procedures	Will have expanded descriptions of methodologies and approaches to procedures
Inadequate definition of procedures	Precisely defines procedures with detail regarding body part, approach, any device used, and other qualifying information

The basic ICD-10 codes are endorsed through the World Health Organization's World Health Assembly and have been in use in 25 other countries since 1994. This shift to a new code set clearly places an administrative burden on the industry – and hence repeated delays have been allowed. But ICD-10 is necessary in order to clarify our understanding of population health data originating from both inpatient and ambulatory care settings and thereby enabling greater improvements in quality of care across the country.

Organizations Engaged in Measure Development

While uniformity of quality measures and methods for reporting remains a goal and some parties do collaborate, a variety of organizations and agencies set the requirements for provider reporting and accountability. With payers and regulators being powerful forces, providers seeking favorable payment strategies often negotiate different arrangements with different payers, and as a result are required to meet multiple expectations with varied metrics. Accreditors and professional societies also play an important role in establishing benchmarks for excellence. Some of the government and private nonprofit organizations engaged in setting quality measures include:

Agency for Healthcare Research and Quality (AHRQ): AHRQ is an agency within DHHS providing a clearinghouse for quality measures, coordination of evidence-based guidelines, and annual reporting of clinical quality measures at the national level. It also manages the Consumer Assessment of Healthcare Providers and Systems (CAHPS) patient satisfaction surveys.

American Medical Association (AMA): A national association for physicians, the AMA convened the Physician Consortium for Performance Improvement® (PCPI) in 2000. Since that time, the PCPI has grown to include participants from over 170 organizations and has identified a PCPI portfolio that includes measures in more than 46 clinical areas with over 280 measures across 46 measure sets. The mission of the PCPI is to align patient centered care, performance measurement and quality improvement. The PCPI develops evidence-based performance measures that are clinically meaningful and are used in national accountability and quality improvement programs.

Centers for Medicare and Medicaid Services (CMS): CMS requires mandatory reporting of quality measures by hospitals, physicians, and other providers of products and services. CMS' Measures Management System provides a standardized process for ensuring "that CMS will have a coherent, transparent system for measuring quality of care delivered to its beneficiaries. (Centers for Medicare and Medicaid Services 2014) This system has been developed in coordination with the public, including other organizations mentioned in this section. CMS collaborates with such private nonprofit organizations as The Joint Commission and the American Medical Association to develop quality measures required for regulatory compliance, including the Hospital Outpatient Quality Data Reporting Program, the Physician Quality Reporting System, and Hospital Compare.

National Committee for Quality Assurance (NCQA): The NCQA is a certification and accreditation organization for patient centered medical home initiatives, health plan accreditations, disease and case management, and other healthcare provider certification and recognition programs. The NCQA provides and governs the development of the Healthcare Effectiveness Data and Information Set (HEDIS) ambulatory care measures. HEDIS reporting has been selected as the sole measurement accepted by CMS for health plans participating in the marketplaces created by the ACA.

National Quality Forum (NQF): The NQF focuses on building consensus on national healthcare priorities and goals for quality measurement and performance improvement. It endorses consensus standards for performance measurement. As new quality measures are developed and tested for ACOs the NQF may play a vital role in validating these measures prior to their official use and application.

The Joint Commission (TJC): Hospitals and health systems maintain TJC accreditation regarding their clinical care processes, ability and performance on specific quality measures, and standards of care as one way of achieving deemed status with CMS Conditions of Participation. TJC has been involved in performance measurement since the mid-1980s and launched its ORYX® initiative in 1999 integrating outcomes and other performance measure data into the accreditation process. "Over time, the ORYX® measures have evolved into standardized sets of valid, reliable, and evidence-based quality measures."(Joint Commission 2012) In June 2010 The Joint Commission categorized its process core performance measures into accountability and non-accountability measures, placing an emphasis on accountability measures. In 2012, The Joint Commission introduced the Top Performers on Key Quality Measures™ program. This initiative recognizes accredited hospitals that attain excellence on accountability measure performance. TJC has had a number of collaborative efforts with CMS and other industry stakeholders throughout its history of measurement development.

URAC: URAC promotes healthcare quality through its accreditation, education, and measurement programs. URAC offers over 30 accreditation and certification programs for health plans, provider organizations, pharmacies and physician practices and networks. These accreditation programs include health plans and networks, healthcare utilization management, case management, Patient-Centered Medical Homes (PCMHs), pharmacy benefits management, and disease management. As of this writing, URAC offers the only recognition for Clinical Integration and has recently launched a comprehensive Accountable Care accreditation program that addresses requirements for success by the CMS ACOs as well as those in the private/commercial sector and state and local governments. URAC's approach to measurement is to align its performance measures with the national quality endeavors of the federal, state, and local governments to address key health issues of population groups. Furthermore, the clinical quality requirements are flexible and adaptable, allowing organizations to adopt quality measures that fit their local markets and individual requirements, rather than a one-size-fits-all quality approach.

Efforts toward establishment of standardized, uniform quality measures have been led by NQF, NCQA, AMA, TJC, and CMS collectively but thus far the industry has not obtained consensus on standards for evaluating the quality of healthcare. The lack of consensus is partly due to the changing nature of medicine, shifts in population disease burden, demographics, and development of new quality metrics. Uniformity is also difficult because of the different definitions of quality followed by different payer organizations and the resulting need for performance measures that fit local markets. Moreover, recent emphasis has been on cost of care more than on health status outcomes. That will change as the United States moves toward a more broadly defined population health management scheme as a widespread care management and payment strategy.

Future Direction

Recent published research and policy reports take the position that the measures of the past are not necessarily the measures of the future. What has been shown to date is not sufficiently focused on demonstrating the outcomes of a value-based proposition. A June 2014 "Report to the Congress: Medicare and the Healthcare Delivery System", by the Medicare Payment Advisory Commission (MedPac) says:

> A fundamental problem with Medicare's current quality measurement programs, particularly in fee-for-service (FFS) Medicare, is that they rely primarily on clinical process measures for assessing the quality of care provided by hospitals, physicians, and other types of providers—measures that may exacerbate the incentives in FFS to overprovide and overuse services and contribute to uncoordinated and fragmented care. In addition, some of these process measures are often not well correlated to better health outcomes, there are too many measures overall, and reporting the data needed for the measures places a heavy burden on providers. (Medicare Payment Advisory 2013)

Providers have criticized existing reporting requirements repeatedly for inconsistency of demand and wide variation in methodology. The burden placed on providers by various sources has been seen as onerous because of the lack of a universal agreement on approach and methodology for data collection, analysis and reporting. In addition, many practitioners have not had the digital infrastructure required to readily support electronic data capture for efficient data gathering, quality reporting, and resulting payment adjustments. And where the demand has been greatest, in state and federal government programs, many providers are the least able to access needed capital to purchase empowering hardware and software.

As Jerod Loeb in 2004 wrote on behalf of the The Joint Commission, the perspective of public policy makers and large purchasers is that "performance measurement should be an integral part of the everyday business of healthcare."(Loeb 2004) And thus we find ourselves now in an era embarking on increased accountability for both processes and outcomes related to cost and quality even though methodological problems identified by Loeb, including measurement standardization, data quality and integrity, risk adjustment, validity of analysis and reporting, remain today. (Loeb 2004)

CHAPTER 6 DISCUSSION QUESTIONS

Discussion questions are provided for team building or class exercises. Answers for all questions are provided in Appendix C.

Question Number	Question
1	What are the six dimensions of quality and how do you think they might be measured?
2	What metrics would you choose to evaluate achievement of the three aspects of the Triple Aim using process measures?
3	What metrics would you choose to evaluate achievement of the three aspects of the Triple Aim using outcome measures?
4	Why is transparency of data the gold standard?
5	Why is measurement and reporting accountability important to practice transformation?

CHAPTER 6 HIGHLIGHTS

✓ Establishing the framework and infrastructure for performance monitoring, measurement and reporting on population health management indicators is a critical success factor for value-based healthcare organizations.

✓ Quality in healthcare is understood definitively by:

   o The IOM in the 2001 Crossing the Quality Chasm report six aims for healthcare improvement: safe, effective, patient-centered, timely, efficient and equitable;

   o In 2008, the Commonwealth Fund Commission on a High Performance Health System "six attributes of an ideal healthcare delivery system; and

   o IHI's Triple Aim of improving patient experience of care and the health of populations, and reducing per capita cost of care.

✓ Emerging payment models demand accountability through measurement and reporting for pay for performance and other contractual financial incentives and penalties.

✓ Well-developed organizations demonstrate the ability to be accountable and transparent when health information technology capability is robust.

✓ It is beneficial to look beyond the CMS experience in accountability to the several other organizations engaged in measures development for the future.

✓ Measurement, reporting, transparency and accountability in healthcare is likely here to stay as policy makers and purchasers retain their interest in cost control and quality improvement.

CHAPTER 6 REFERENCES

Agency for Healthcare Quality and Research (2011, March). Report to Congress: National Strategy for Quality Improvement in Health Care. Retrieved from http://www.ahrq.gov/workingforquality/nqs/nqs2011annlrpt.pdf

American Medical Association (2010). Fact Sheet 2: The Difference Between ICD-9 and ICD-10. Retrieved from http://www.nationalfamilyplanning.org/document.doc?id=775

Berwick, D. M., et al. (2008). The triple aim: care, health, and cost. *Health Affairs,* **27**(3): 759-769.

Boyarsky, V. and R. Parke (2012). The Medicare Shared Savings Program and the Pioneer Accountable Care Organizations. *Milliman Healthcare Reform Briefing Paper.*

Centers for Medicare and Medicaid Services (2014). *Measures Management System.* Retrieved from https://www.cms.gov/Medicare/Quality-Initiatives-Patient-Assessment-Instruments/MMS/MeasuresManagementSystemBlueprint.html

Committee on Quality of Healthcare in America and Institute of Medicine (2001). Chapter 2. Improving the 21st Century Health Care System. In *Crossing the Quality Chasm. A New Health System for the 21st Century* (pp.44-53). Washington, DC: National Academies Press.

Committee on Quality of Healthcare in America and Institute of Medicine (2001). Chapter 5. Building Organizational Supports for Change. In *Crossing the Quality Chasm. A New Health System for the 21st Century* (pp. 111-144). Washington, DC: National Academies Press.

Committee on Redesigning Health Insurance Performance Measures, et al. (2006). Chapter 4. Moving Forward: What Should Be Measured? In *Performance Measurement. Accelerating Improvement*(p. 85). Washington, DC, National Academies Press.

Curtright, J. W., et al. (2000). Strategic performance management: development of a performance measurement system at the Mayo Clinic. *Journal of Healthcare Management,* 45: 58-68.

Evans, M. (2014). Physician fee schedule would modify Medicare ACO measures. *Modern Healthcare.* Retrieved from http://www.modernhealthcare.com/article/20140703/NEWS/307039940.

Farquhar, M. (2011). "URAC Measures Strategy." 2.

Farquhar, M. (2011). "URAC Measures Strategy." 3.

Gordon, D. (2014). *CMS to Increase Quality Measures for MSSP ACOs: 4 Things to Know.* Retrieved from http://www.beckershospitalreview.com/accountable-care-organizations/cms-to-increase-quality-measures-for-mssp-acos-4-things-to-know.html

Grigoroudis, E., et al. (2012). Strategic performance measurement in a healthcare organisation: A multiple criteria approach based on balanced scorecard. *Omega,* 40(1): 104-119. doi: 10.1016/j.omega.2011.04.001

Holly, J. L. (2012, March 30). *The Importance of Data Analytics in Physician Practice.* Massachusetts Medical Society.

Institute for Healthcare Improvement (2014). The IHI Triple Aim. Retrieved from http://www.ihi.org/Engage/Initiatives/TripleAim/pages/default.aspx

Institute for Healthcare Improvement (2014). Institute for Healthcare Improvement Website. Retrieved from www.ihi.org

Integrated Healthcare Association (2011, October). *Explanation of Performance Measurement and Payment. Framework for the Medicare Shared Savings Program*. Retrieved from http://www.iha.org/pdfs_documents/Memo_ACOPMFramework_102711_FINAL.pdf

Joint Commission (2012). *Specifications Manual for Joint Commission National Quality Core Measures*. Retrieved from https://manual.jointcommission.org/releases/TJC2013A/

Kocot, L., S,, et al. (2014, February 7). *Year One Results from Medicare Shared Savings Program: What it Means Going Forward*. Retrieved from http://www.brookings.edu/blogs/up-front/posts/2014/02/07-results-medicare-shared-savings-program-kocot-mostashari

Loeb, J. M. (2004). The current state of performance measurement in health care. *International Journal for Quality in Health Care*, 16(suppl 1), i5-i9.

Medicare Payment Advisory, C. (2013). *Report to the Congress: Medicare and the health care delivery system*, MedPAC.

National Institute of Technology and Ba ldrige Performance Excellence Program (2014). *2013–2014 Health Care Criteria for Performance Excellence*. Retrieved from http://www.nist.gov/baldrige/publications/hc_criteria.cfm

Petersen, M. & Muhlestein, D. (2014). *ACO Results: What We Know So Far*. Retrieved from http://healthaffairs.org/blog/2014/05/30/aco-results-what-we-know-so-far/

Petersen, M., et al. (2013). *Growth and dispersion of accountable care organizations: August 2013 update*. Washington, DC: Leavitt Partners.

RTI International (August 15, 2014). *Accountable Care Organization 2014 Program Analysis Quality Performance Standards Narrative Measure Specifications*. Retrieved from http://www.cms.gov/Medicare/Medicare-Fee-for-Service-Payment/sharedsavingsprogram/Downloads/ACO-NarrativeMeasures-Specs.pdf

Schneider, E. C., et al. (2011). *Payment reform: analysis of models and performance measurement implications*, Rand Corporation.

Shih, A. (2008). Organizing the US health care delivery system for high performance. *Commonwealth Fund*.

Smith, D. (2014). Leading Delivery Models Emphasize Care Coordination for Chronic Conditions. *CASE IN POINT: Advanced Care Coordination*.

Southeast Texas Medical Associates (2014). "About SETMA." Retrieved from http://www.setma.com/about-setma/

Voelker, K. E., et al. (2001). The balanced scorecard in healthcare organizations: a performance measurement and strategic planning methodology. *Hospital Topics*, 79(3), 13-24.

Chapter 7. Financial Implications: The Physician's View

Thomas A. Raskauskas

Joanne Bohn

We see healthcare shifting from a procedure reimbursement, where in this country doctors are reimbursed for how many procedures they conduct, to a world where people will be reimbursed for the outcomes - did the patient actually get better, and what was the total cost of the cycle of care.

John Sculley
Former CEO of Apple
1939-Present

CHAPTER 7 LEARNING OBJECTIVES

✓ Understand the transition taking place moving the industry away from traditional fee-for-service models and toward value-based reimbursement models.

✓ Be able to describe the four types of bundled payment care models.

✓ Recognize the importance of risk in reimbursement models.

✓ Be able to articulate some of the financial management related challenges that have emerged for CINs due to enacted federal healthcare laws.

✓ Know the elements of new reimbursement models advocated by the American Medical Association's Innovator's Committee.

✓ Be able to describe the types of models within the Medicare Shared Savings Program.

✓ Know three elements of the 'financial roadmap' to help ensure CIN financial success.

Introduction

The cost of health care services in the United States (U.S.) is still extremely high for the value delivered. In response, the Society of General Internal Medicine established the National Commission on Physician Payment Reform in 2012. This commission released a report in 2013 that offered 12 key recommendations for improving the U.S. cost of care and payment system. In it they noted, "The United States health care system is plagued by the twin ills of high cost and uneven quality. Health care spending in the United States represents 18 percent of gross domestic product or $8,000 per person annually." (Commission on Physician Payment Reform, March 2013)

The commission's report centered on a key recommendation: to end fee-for-service physician payments within 5-years. While this recommendation also mirrors the new financial reform focus of the Centers for Medicare and Medicaid Services (CMS), a subsequent article by Selker, Kravitz and Gallagher noted, "An increased focus on payment mechanisms that reward value and efficiency could inadvertently diminish the patient-centered focus that characterizes high-quality healthcare."(Selker, Kravitz, & Gallagher, 2014)

In essence, this tension symbolizes the complexity and inherent challenge in reforming the finances of the U.S. healthcare system. We all wish to lower cost, improve quality and shift to a "value-based" system, but what are trade-offs and hidden consequences?

For Clinically Integrated Networks (CINs) and Accountable Care Organizations (ACOs), organizations that are predominantly led by physician executives, managing the continued fee-for-service (FFS) reimbursements, while making the shift to pay-for-performance systems, while at the same time making strategic programmatic changes in operations to capture provider and systems level financial incentives tied to quality measures, pose immense challenges. Managing these changes is all part of the physician executive's focus on profit/loss and revenue cycle management for the organizations for which they maintain executive custodianship. They are joined in this endeavor by board-level governance groups. These critical players, and how they help evolve the healthcare financial ecosystem, will be key to building sustainable and financially strong CINs, ACOs, and their Patient-Centered Medical Homes (PCMHs) infrastructures.

The strategic redesign of the nation's healthcare system involves changing contractual relationships of stakeholders and shifting the balance of financial risk that has historically been shared by physicians, hospitals, payers (both public and private) and patients. While the passage of the 2010 Patient Protection and Affordable Care Act (ACA) was a step toward universal coverage and mandated health insurance for all U.S. citizens, there still exists a complicated network for consumers, patients and stakeholders to understand about access to health care services and who pays for those services. Ultimately a larger percentage of the total bill is shifting to consumers and patients as the nation struggles to reduce the ever increasing costs that are covered by health plan payers, hospitals, government agencies, and safety net organizations.

This chapter provides an overview from the physician executive and Chief Financial Officer (CFO) perspective on some of the challenges encountered as they move toward a more value-centric and quality driven approach that delivers results—improved quality for consumer and patient populations at lower total costs. In addition, this chapter is intended to build upon and expand some of the original material from *Chapter 9 Financial Perspectives*, of the second edition of this book.

Challenges Affecting Finances of CINs and ACOs

Health care delivery organizations face a number of challenges that affect their financial health. Many of these challenges are related to recent healthcare reforms, contained in laws and regulations such as the 2009 American Recovery and Reinvestment Act (ARRA), ACA, 2011 final rule on the Medicare Shared Savings Program, and the 2013 final HIPAA rule. These landmark federal health reforms, and others, have resulted in payment pilot projects, novel risk sharing arrangements, new pay-for-performance models, among other financially related system-level initiatives. Some of the most pressing payment reform challenges resulting from all these changes include:

- Payment pressures from government-funded programs and unresolved sustainable growth rate adjustments in Medicare payments to physicians and their practices; (Centers for Medicare and Medicaid Services, 2014b)*

- CMS Meaningful Use penalties starting in 2014 for providers who have not achieved compliance. The payment adjustment is 1% per year and is cumulative for every year that an eligible professional is not a meaningful user. (Centers for Medicare and Medicaid Services, 2014a) The maximum cumulative payment adjustment can reach as high as 5% by 2018. (Centers for Medicare and Medicaid Services, March 2014)

- New penalties from CMS in the Physician Quality Reporting System (PQRS) - eligible professionals who do not satisfactorily report data on quality measures for covered professional services will be subject to a payment adjustment under PQRS beginning in 2015 which will be 1.5% less than the Medicare Physician Fee Schedule (MPFS) amount for that service. For 2016 and subsequent years, the payment adjustment is 2.0%. (Federal Register Volume 78 Number 237, December 10, 2013)

- Expansion of the CMS recovery audit contractor (RAC) program to all institutional providers and adoption of the RAC program concept by private payers. (Centers for Medicare and Medicaid Services, 2014c)

- Delay in implementation of the 10th revision of the International Statistical Classification of Disease (ICD-10). (Centers for Medicare and Medicaid Services, 2014b)

- Funding transformation of health services with novel reimbursement models. Rapidly changing reimbursement methodologies, including new value-based purchasing, risk-adjusted diagnosis related groups (DRGs),

---

* 1 year extension signed April 1, 2014.

medical homes, and other initiatives not completely integrated in all practices, nor are they consistent across payers.

- Increase in aging physician population, over 60, near retirement, or opting for early retirement. (Young, Chaudhry, Rhyne, & Dugan, 2011)

- Increase in employment of physicians by hospital systems or large groups with the resulting decrease in solo and small practices. (The Physicians Foundation, September 2012)

Financial reform in healthcare is not new. Several industry-level payment reform policies have been enacted over the last 30 years. The timeline in Figure 7-1 depicts several key reforms, some of which made significant changes in the financial operations of the U.S. healthcare system. The piloting, testing and implementing of many of these programs contributed to the emergence of CINs, ACOs, PCMHs and other innovative models.

Figure 7-1. 30 Years of Health Services Payment Reform Models & Programs

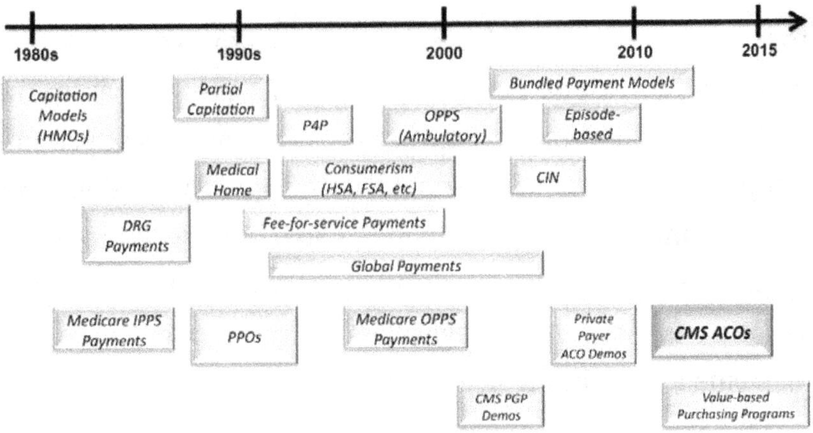

Note: Boxes only indicate an approximate market entry point for each program or model

The capitation models of the 1980s brought about significant changes with the advent of the managed care era. In succession came such transformative new programs as diagnosis-related group payments, other new Medicare payment models, the consumer movement with health savings and flexible savings accounts, and other reimbursement reform models such as bundled and global payments. As new models of reimbursement are introduced, concerns from consumer groups need to be considered, such as the potential for underutilization of needed services.

A FFS system lowers the risk of underutilization. However, because providers are rewarded for the volume of services prescribed (pay-for-procedure), overutilization becomes another issue. For Medicare ACOs, the U.S. Department of Health and Human Services (DHHS) monitors risk sharing to ensure that ACOs do not underutilize care for at-risk patients. If any participant in a Medicare ACO program is found to avoid delivering services to certain "at-risk beneficiaries," that ACO participant will not only be placed under sanctions (including being put on probation or termination from the Medicare Shared Savings Program [MSSP]), but he or she may also forfeit their mandatory 25% withholding of shared savings. (Federal Register Volume 76 Number 67, April 7, 2011c)

New and Transitional Payment Models

With the rapidly changing landscape of healthcare reimbursement, a number of different reimbursement models are currently being co-developed in the public and private sector. These models affect not only the physician practice, but reimbursement to hospitals and other providers of care. Common in all the models is movement from volume-based care to value based care, and moving from individual care transactions to payment for population management. Regardless of the model, there are several common elements, as outline by the American Medical Association (AMA):

- *The new models encourage clinical integration*: move toward effective team-based care by improved care coordination and efficient transitions of care resulting in decreased readmissions and unnecessary services.

- *Efficiently allocate limited resources*: Utilize newer technologies at care transitions, avoiding face-to-face encounters but utilizing IT and telecommunications infrastructure (telehealth and telemedicine).

- *Rebalance the healthcare workforce*: rebalancing the workforce away from specialty care to primary care to improve population health.

- *Encourage competition between providers*: reward care demonstrating improved quality at a lower cost in the free market setting.

- *Foster provider accountability*: Providers become accountable for outcomes both clinically and financial in the population, providing interdependent care.

(AMA Innovators Committee, 2012)

Every CIN and ACO must contend with multiple issues in financial risk-sharing and strategy. Issues that are coming to the forefront as these care delivery models mature, include financial risk for the CIN/ACO, risk adjustment of the patient, and understanding the total cost of care.

Financial Risk

We start with the assumption that a certain degree of financial risk is unavoidable for hospitals and physician practice organizations in a CIN or ACO. One of the qualification criteria for Medicare ACOs includes the ability to take on greater degrees of risk based on capabilities and infrastructure in place that allow management of complexity and risk among ACO participants and patient populations. The agreements among ACO participants link higher levels of risk assumed to higher potential incentives. The incentives may be achieved by improving quality of care and population health for the entire panel of patients or certain disease conditions targeted for improvement under the ACO. Unless the practice or hospital has been optimized already to meet quality measures and productivity, the infrastructure needed to achieve the quality goals and incentives and reduce risk is through clinical integration.

Patient Risk Adjustment

In terms of patient risk adjustment, "risk scores" are assigned to patients based upon algorithms that take into account the intensity of services and cost of care related to beneficiaries based on their demographics, diagnosed conditions, past cost experience, and future potential costs. The ACO's ability to effectively manage clinical risk associated with individual patients while simultaneously focusing on total population health management may be directly correlated with its incentive payments received. Two factors that affect risk scores and incentive payments are accurate assessment of beneficiary health status and the intensity of medical coding (i.e. the completeness of diagnostic codes assigned to beneficiaries). If an ACO increases coding intensity there is the potential for a favorable increase in the risk score associated with the beneficiary. In light of this possibility, CMS proposed they would retain the option of auditing ACOs in this area for appropriate coding practices and risk adjustment methodologies. (Federal Register Volume 76 Number 67, April 7, 2011b) This is an issue that ACO leaders must understand to safeguard against perceptions of inappropriate changes in risk scores (e.g. "upcoding") or triggering CMS audits. Medical management and health information technology staff can help monitor this issue, which may also involve changes in the primary care and specialist provider mix.

Total Cost of Care

As new models of reimbursement develop, a better understanding of total cost of care is needed. Cost of care is defined differently, based on the perspective of whom is paying or receiving payments, from the insurer or employer. (Painter & Cernew, March 2012) As stated in the Robert Wood Johnson (RWJ) publication,

> Consumers, businesses, oversight bodies, and other stakeholders encounter these same issues in every industry. And in every industry, the costs, prices, and total spending are often easily understandable. But not in health care. Why? (Painter & Cernew, March 2012)

From a patient viewpoint, cost of care is defined by out-of-pocket expenditures that include co-pays and deductibles. From a provider viewpoint, cost is defined by the amount an insurer or employer reimburses for the service. This does not necessarily correspond to the actual costs to the provider for the care delivered — overhead, equipment, time, etc. that goes into rate setting. From the insurer and employer viewpoint, total cost of care is the amount paid for each employee for all the medical costs in a fiscal year. This cost varies from provider to provider, and region to region. It is because of this variation of cost that CMS created new innovation models for reimbursement, some of which are mandated by statute, while others are in development through the new Center for Medicare and Medicaid Innovation (CMMI). The CMMI was established by section 1115A of the Social Security Act (as added by section 3021 of the ACA). Congress created CMMI for the purpose of testing "innovative payment and service delivery models to reduce program expenditures ...while preserving or enhancing the quality of care for those individuals who receive Medicare, Medicaid, or Children's Health Insurance Program (CHIP) benefits." (Centers for Medicare and Medicaid Services) The CMMI has focused on the following priorities:

- Testing new payment and service delivery models;

- Evaluating results and advancing best practices; and

- Engaging a broad range of stakeholders to develop additional models for testing.

Private payers have followed with the development of models requiring providers to take financial risk and be accountable for outcomes. The balance of this chapter will review various payment models under development by both public and private payers. Payment models that are at the level of the practice and only between provider and patient, such as various cash-only and concierge models will not be discussed.

CMS Reimbursement Models under the Affordable Care Act (ACA)

Through the CMMI, there have been many new payment design pilots throughout the country. The models range from the formation of ACOs (as in the MSSP and Pioneer ACO programs), State Innovation Model Designs, care for pregnant women, care at federally qualified health centers, and many more listed on the CMMI website. (Centers for Medicare and Medicaid

<u>Services)</u> The discussion below will concentrate on the Medicare and/or Medicaid reimbursement models most widely adopted by physicians in ACOs or in concert with hospital and post-acute systems of care.

1. *Medicare Shared Savings Program (MSSP-ACO)*

As described by CMS, the Medicare Shared Savings Program-Accountable Care Organization (MSSP-ACO) was established "to facilitate coordination and cooperation among providers to improve the quality of care for Medicare Fee-For-Service (FFS) beneficiaries and reduce unnecessary costs. Eligible providers, hospitals, and suppliers may participate in the Shared Savings Program by creating or participating in an ACO." (Centers for Medicare and Medicaid Services) The MSSP was designed to: promote accountability for care; coordinate care; invest in infrastructure and redesign care process.

CMS introduced two risk options for Medicare ACOs in the ACA. The first option is a one-sided risk model and the second is a two-sided risk model. The CMS Medicare ACO compensation model starts with the normal FFS Parts A and B payments to individual providers for claims submitted to CMS. The second part of the model is the ACO shared savings program process, involving the two risk-bearing models. Currently, there have been four rounds of MSSP participants, which, coupled with the Pioneer ACOs, brings the number of Medicare ACOs to 366.

The **one-sided model** is intended for organizations that are less mature in the infrastructure, systems, physician relations, and processes needed to run an ACO, and includes the majority of MSSP participants. The implication is that the one-sided model gives ACO participants a lower level of risk in the first and second-year performance periods. In exchange for not being responsible for losses, ACO participants also accept a lower percentage of shared savings (up to 50%) based on their quality performance scores plus a lower potential increase in their shared savings rate (up to 2.5%) for the inclusion of rural health clinics or federally qualified health centers in their network.

The **two-sided risk model** is intended for more mature organizations that have strong infrastructure, advanced health information technologies, Department of Justice (DOJ) / Federal Trade Commission (FTC)-approved clinical integration programs, strong physician relations, and advanced quality improvement programs and processes in place to positively impact patient care. This model is the one adopted by the Pioneer MSSP programs. ACO participants adopting this model start off the first performance period accepting a greater degree of risk that includes responsibility for sharing in losses. But with this greater degree of risk comes greater potential for rewards, with a higher percentage of earned shared savings (up to 60%) based on quality performance scoring plus a higher potential shared savings rate (up to 5.0%), based on the inclusion of rural health clinic or federally qualified health centers in their network. Figure 7-2 (originally illustrated in the 2nd Edition) provides an overview of MSSP-ACOs.

Figure 7-2. CMS MSSP-ACO Compensation Model Overview[*]

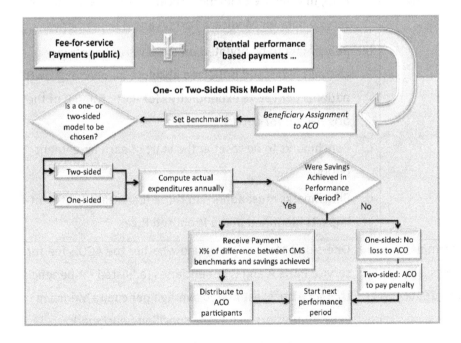

---

[*] Figure 7-2 was originally created in the 2nd edition book, *Clinical Integration. A Roadmap to Accountable Care.* (2011). Authors acknowledge this model is subject to change pending future changes by CMS to the MSSP-ACO program.

If participating in an MSSP, providers need to understand the financial elements, beneficiary assignment, financial benchmarks, and determination of the shared savings along with potential payouts. Table 7-1 provides a summary of these elements. This description is not intended to cover every element and issue, but provides some of the highlights.

Table 7-1. Financial Element Highlights of CMS ACO Shared Savings Program

Element	Key Points
CMS ACO agreement period	a. Minimum 3-year agreement between ACO and DHHS. Each ACO is evaluated in each year of the agreement period.
Beneficiary assignment	a. Beneficiaries are assigned to ACOs in which they are receiving a plurality of primary care physician services but they are not limited to seeing only those primary care physicians who participate in the ACO.
Setting financial benchmarks (HR 3590, 2010c)	a. Estimate a benchmark for every agreement period for each ACO, making use of its most recent three years of fee-for-service data for Medicare Parts A and B beneficiaries. b. Benchmark to be updated on the basis of beneficiary characteristics and projected absolute amount of growth in national per capita expenditures for Parts A and B of the original fee-for-service program. c. Benchmarks to be reset at the start of each agreement period. d. Benchmarks must adhere to three technical adjustment impacts identified in the Proposed Rule.
1) Determine savings (HR 3590, 2010b)	a. **One-sided Model:** Determine whether the ACO's fee-for-service Parts A and B beneficiaries (adjusted for beneficiary characteristics) estimated average per capita Medicare expenditures are below the specified benchmark. 1. **Shared Savings:** Must be below the minimum savings rate (sliding scale) based on number of beneficiaries and minimum quality performance requirements.

Element	Key Points

	2. Passes the net savings threshold and is eligible for net 2% of benchmark in shared savings or may be eligible for **up to 7.5%** shared savings. Will receive a shared savings payment **up to 50%** based on quality performance.
	
	 b. **Two-sided model**: Determine whether the ACO's fee-for-service Parts A and B beneficiaries (adjusted for beneficiary characteristics) estimated average per capita Medicare expenditures are below the specified benchmark.
	
	    1. **Shared Savings:** Must be below the minimum savings rate of 2% based on number of beneficiaries and minimum quality performance requirements.
	
	    2. Passes the net savings threshold and is eligible for net 2% of benchmark in shared savings or may be eligible for **up to 10%** shared savings. Will receive a shared savings payment **up to 60%** based on quality performance.
	
	    3. **Shared Loss Rate**: based on the inverse of the ACO's final sharing rate.
	
	    4. **Loss Recoupment Limits**: 5% in performance period 1, 7.5 % in performance period 2, 10% in performance period 3. *One-sided ACOs* in performance period 3 their loss recoupment limit is 5%.

Payments of shared savings to ACO (HR 3590, 2010d)	a. When ACO meets requirements, a percentage (determined by DHHS) of the difference bet*ween the bench*mark and the "estimated average per capita Medicare expenditures adjusted for beneficiary characteristics" for the agreement period will be paid to the ACO and remainder goes to CMS. b. DHHS will set a limit on the total shared savings that can be paid to any ACO.

Organizations should monitor federal rule making for new developments that emerge as the program continues to evolve.

After the first year experience with the MSSP-ACO program, CMS reported that,

> Savings from both the Medicare ACOs and Pioneer ACOs exceed $380 million...While ACOs are designed to achieve savings over several years, not always on an annual basis, the interim financial results released for the Medicare Shared Savings Program ACOs show that, in their first 12 months, nearly half (54 out of 114) of the ACOs that started program operations in 2012 already had lower expenditures than projected. Of the 54 ACOs that exceeded their benchmarks in the first 12 months, 29 generated shared savings totaling more than $126 million – a strong start this early in the program. In addition, these ACOs generated a total of $128 million in net savings for the Medicare Trust Funds. ACOs share with Medicare any savings generated from lowering the growth in health care costs while meeting standards for high quality care. Final performance year-one results will be released later this year. (Department of Health and Human Services, January 30, 2014)

2. *Value-based Purchasing Programs*

Value-based purchasing is considered by many as another phrase for pay-for-performance. According to CMS,

> Value-based purchasing is a concept that links payment directly to the quality of care provided and is a strategy that can help transform the current payment system by rewarding providers for delivering high quality, efficient clinical care. (Federal Register Volume 76 Number 67, April 7, 2011a)

As such, value-based purchasing can include the MSSP-ACO.

Section 3001 of the ACA creates a hospital value-based purchasing program. This is the latest of a number of similar programs. In 2005 Congress passed the Deficit Reduction Act (DRA). Section 5001(b) of the DRA called for DHHS to develop a plan for a hospital value-based purchasing program. (Centers for Medicare and Medicaid Services, January 17, 2007; U.S. Senate, 2005) That law as well as other efforts helped development of a broader set of value-based purchasing programs. In 2009 CMS released "Roadmap for Implementing Value Driven Healthcare." (Centers for Medicare and Medicaid Services, January 2009b) That report presented the CMS roadmap as a three- to five-year plan for multiple value-based purchasing program initiatives that would work in concert with ACOs and other incentive-oriented programs.

The ACA Section 3001 defines hospital value-based payments as incentives to hospitals that meet performance standards based on quality measures for a minimum number of cases for specific conditions and procedures within a given fiscal year. In addition to the hospital value-based purchasing program, the CMS roadmap provides plans for starting value-based purchasing programs for nursing homes,(Centers for Medicare and Medicaid Services, January 2009a) home health care, and physician services related to the PQRS program.

The ACA also contains Section 3007: Value-Based Payment Modifier under the Physician Fee Schedule. (HR 3590, 2010a) This section requires the establishment of a value-based payment modifier that physicians or groups of physicians will be eligible for during specific performance periods. These payments will be based on performance measured against specific quality standards to be released by January 1, 2012. The rule making will take place in 2013 and reporting will begin in 2015.

3. *Bundled Payments for Care Improvement (BPCI) Initiative*

In January 2013, CMS announced its bundled payment demonstration, involving four different model designs. Recognizing that payment for episodic care that is uncoordinated, not based upon quality or outcomes, CMS devised four different bundled payment models to incentivize providers to provide more coordinated, quality outcome based care, resulting in cost savings. Table 7-2 below provides a description of the models. (Centers for Medicare and Medicaid Services, January 2013)

Table 7-2. Bundled Payment Models

Category	Description
Model 1:	Under Model 1, the episode of care is defined as the inpatient stay

Category	Description
Retrospective Acute Care Hospital Stay Only	in the acute care hospital. Medicare will pay the hospital a discounted amount based on the payment rates established under the Inpatient Prospective Payment System used in the original Medicare program. Medicare will continue to pay physicians separately for their services under the Medicare Physician Fee Schedule. Under certain circumstances, hospitals and physicians will be permitted to share gains arising from the providers' care redesign efforts. Participation will begin as early as April, 2013 and no later than January, 2014 and will include most Medicare fee-for-service discharges for the participating hospitals.
Model 2: Retrospective Acute Care Hospital Stay plus Post-Acute	In Model 2, the episode of care will include the inpatient stay in the acute care hospital and all related services during the episode. The episode will end either 30, 60, or 90 days after hospital discharge. Participants can select up to 48 different clinical condition episodes.
Model 3: Retrospective Post-Acute Care Only	For Model 3, the episode of care will be triggered by an acute care hospital stay and will begin at initiation of post-acute care services with a participating skilled nursing facility, inpatient rehabilitation facility, long-term care hospital or home health agency. The post-acute care services included in the episode must begin within 30 days of discharge from the inpatient stay and will end either a minimum of 30, 60, or 90 days after the initiation of the episode. Participants can select up to 48 different clinical condition episodes.
Model 4: Acute Care Hospital Stay Only	Under Model 4, CMS will make a single, prospectively determined bundled payment to the hospital that would encompass all services furnished during the inpatient stay by the hospital, physicians, and other practitioners. Physicians and other practitioners will submit "no-pay" claims to Medicare and will be paid by the hospital out of the bundled payment. Related readmissions for 30 days after hospital discharge will be included in the bundled payment amount. Participants can select up to 48 different clinical condition episodes.

Private Payer Reimbursement and Compensation Reform

Private payers have been experimenting with various payment reforms for many years (also known as pay-for-performance, alternative quality contracts, and collaborative care payments), as noted earlier in this chapter.

What is common with many of the models currently underway is that FFS reimbursement at the point of care is the base reimbursement, with various other payment methodologies added to the FFS payment. Many insurers hope to transform care by gradually increasing the amounts at risk in the form of quality and outcomes based payments, as well as shared savings, and decreasing the proportion of provider income derived from FFS. The following discussion provides an overview of some of the payment models added to the FFS structure. As CMS MSSPs are growing, commercial insurers are benefiting from practice transformation, and are changing their reimbursement to more closely align with the MSSP-ACO reimbursement models.

Shared Savings

A recent publication found that many payers use ACO shared savings payments. (Premier Inc, 2013) Additionally, many were upside risk only. There has been criticism that commercial payers are benefiting from CMS' efforts in transforming practices, but not providing the depth and amount of shared savings payments as CMS. National payers such as Aetna, Cigna, Blue Cross Blue Shield and United have various forms of shared savings. Risk corridors vary in these models, as do amount of savings paid to the ACO. Additionally, each insurer has other reimbursement components than shared savings in their respective ACO contracting.

Bundled Payments

One of the frequently discussed methods of payment reform is bundled payment. In one form of bundled payments, the payer provides a set amount for a particular episode of care, starting from the point of hospital admission for a specified procedure through discharge and possibly post-acute care requirements, based on the terms set for the payment bundle (including an adjustment factor for severity of the case). This type of payment bundle may be negotiated by the physician and provider organization (such as hospital organizations), agreeing to a package of services for treating specific conditions that yields a single payment received and allotted on the basis of the agreement. (Evans, 2010) A number of organizations have tested and used payment bundling.

When bundled payments are adopted, managing episodes of care and total population health become more important. The movement toward managing inter-episodes of care (also known as care coordination or transitional care) is an outgrowth of the need to better manage patients' overall health, and is associated with medical management and the evolution of CIN and ACO programs. Geisinger Health System's ProvenCare® program has demonstrated the value of improving "episode-based coordination of care," in which physicians and other stakeholders effectively collaborate to improve the clinical processes along the entire care continuum to "minimize avoidable complications" in coronary artery bypass graft surgeries. (Goldsmith, 2010)

The Prometheus Payment Model may be the most well-known of bundled payment designs. It was developed and funded by the Robert Wood Johnson Foundation in 2006. (de Brantes, Rosenthal, & Painter, 2009) The Prometheus model was set up to compensate provider organizations in two ways. First, the model calculated an evidence-informed case rate (ECR®)—that is, a patient-specific budget adjusted for the severity and complexity of the case. The ECR® was translated into a bundled budget for all necessary interventions, accounting for the entire episode of care and services provided by the physicians, hospitals, laboratories, pharmacies, and post-acute care facilities and services. The Prometheus model also provides an allowance in addition to the ECR® to compensate for typically known potentially avoidable costs (PACs).

When care provider teams manage a full episode of care in an efficient and high-quality manner and avoid the occurrence of PACs they are rewarded by keeping a portion of the PAC allowance unused in the patient's episode. This bundled budget concept differs from bundled payments in that providers are still reimbursed on the basis of FFS claims from payers; however, the budgets for the bundled services for specific types of episodes of care are compared to actual costs on a quarterly basis that includes a review of PACs that were avoided. When savings are achieved they result in bonuses for the provider teams and organizations involved. Four organizations are involved in piloting the Prometheus Model; including:

- Health Partners of Minneapolis, MN
- Crozer-Keystone Health System, Philadelphia, PA
- Employers Coalition on Health, Rockford, IL
- Spectrum Health, Grand Rapids, MI

(Robert Wood Johnson Foundation & Health Care Incentives Improvement Institute, July 2010)

A recent example of projects involving bundled payment comes from Arkansas Medicaid. With Medicaid budgetary shortfalls looming, in 2010 the Arkansas Department of Human Services designed the Payment Improvement Initiative to change the state's Medicaid payment structure to support and reward providers who consistently deliver high-quality, coordinated, and cost-effective care. (Thompson, J., November 2012) Episodes of care, or bundles, were developed initially for five episodes, as demonstrated in Figure 7-3 below. Since then, episodes have been expanded to include other episodes, and have also been adopted by commercial payers in Arkansas.

Figure 7-3. Bundled Payment Models from Arkansas Payment Improvement Initiative[*]

2012: Episode-based payment launched for 5 episodes

	Wave 1 episodes	Principle Accountable Provider
Hip/knee replacements	• Surgical procedure plus all related claims from 30 days prior to procedure to 90 days after	• Orthopedic surgeon • Hospital
Perinatal (non NICU)	• Pregnancy-related claims for mother from 40 weeks before to 60 days after delivery • Excludes neonatal care	• Delivering provider • If separate providers perform prenatal care and delivery, both providers are PAPs (shared accountability)
Ambulatory URI	• 21-day window beginning with initial consultation • Excludes inpatient costs and surgical procedures	• Provider for the first in-person URI consultation
Acute/post-acute CHF	• Hospital admission • Care within 30 days of discharge	• Hospital
ADHD	• 12-month episode • Includes all ADHD services + pharmacy costs (with exception of initial assessment)	• Could be the PCP, mental health professional, and/or the RSPMI provider organization, depending on the pathway of care
Developmental disabilities	• Assessment or annual review plus 12 months of DD services	• Primary DD provider

Global Payments

The global payment model provides a physician or provider organization a single payment to cover all the costs of care for a person's treatment requirements during a specific period of time regardless of the number of inpatient episodes they experience. (Miller, June 2010) Global payments are intended to contain costs and reduce the use of unnecessary services, encourage efficiency, integration, and coordination of services. They are already being widely used by many organizations, including integrated delivery networks, independent practice associations, and multispecialty physician groups. Global payment models are similar to the bundled

[*] Figure 7-3 illustration from the November 2012 National Governors Assocation Annual Conference presentation by Joseph Thompson, MD, MPH titled, *Arkansas Payment Improvement Initiative. Improving Quality, Containing Cost.* Retrieved from http://www.nga.org/files/live/sites/NGA/files/pdf/2013/1305SIMThompson.pdf

payment model. The primary difference between global payments and bundled payments is that a bundled payment is set for a specific episode of care, while global payments are not dictated by episodes treated by a physician or provider organization.

Global payment models vary based on the amount of risk assumed by the provider organization and the methods used to limit risks. Risks can be limited based on services included in the global payment and what, if any, adjustments are considered when evaluating provider performance.

Each payer–provider global payment arrangement considers multiple methodological variations. Typically, no two arrangements are the same for providers contracting with multiple plans and for payers contracting with multiple providers. Plans and providers report variations in global payment arrangements including:

- Which patients are included (e.g., Medicare, Medicaid, commercial);
- Which products are included (e.g., fully insured, self-insured, HMO, PPO);
- How to determine which patients are under the provider's care (e.g., patients specify and lock in provider, patients are attributed to providers based on de facto provider use);
- Which covered services are included (e.g., all covered services, all services except pharmacy, all services except mental health, professional services only, primary care services only, etc.);
- Methodology and technology used for risk adjustment;
- Methodology used for adjustment for catastrophic claims;
- How risk is limited based on performance levels around a target, (e.g., in some types of arrangements providers can be at risk for +/– 10% of what their fee-for-service payments would have been, with the payer retaining the balance of the risk);
- How providers outside the globally paid organization are contracted and paid;

- Level of fee-for-service payments or withholds made prior to reconciliation; and
- Timing and data sharing for reconciliation payments.

The most widely used current example of global payment is for obstetrical care. For years, Obstetricians have been paid a single global fee for care provided for a pregnancy, including the prenatal care, delivery and postpartum care. Below is an example of an insurer's global payment structure for obstetrical care:

The following services are included in the global OB package (CPT codes 59400, 59510, 59610, 59618).

- All routine prenatal visits until delivery (approximately 13 for uncomplicated cases);
- Initial and subsequent history and physical exams;
- Recording of weight, blood pressures and fetal heart tones;
- Routine chemical urinalysis (CPT codes 81000 and 81002);
- Admission to the hospital including history and physical;
- Inpatient Evaluation and Management (E/M) service provided within 24 hours of delivery;
- Management of uncomplicated labor;
- Vaginal or cesarean section delivery (limited to single gestation; for further information see Multiple Gestation section);
- Delivery of placenta (CPT code 59414);
- Administration/induction of intravenous oxytocin (CPT codes 96365 - 96367);
- Insertion of cervical dilator on same date as delivery (CPT code 59200);
- Repair of first or second degree lacerations;
- Simple removal of cerclage (not under anesthesia);
- Uncomplicated inpatient visits following delivery;
- Routine outpatient E/M services provided within six weeks of delivery;

and

- Postpartum care only (CPT code 59430).

(United Healthcare, effective September 1, 2013)

More recently, insurers are looking to provide prospective payment to providers for global care for chronic disease management to incent better care coordination and quality of care. In particular, looking at the cost of diabetes and congestive heart failure (CHF), it is recognized that the care has been episodic, poorly coordinated, with high hospital readmissions and poor overall quality of care. Insurers are looking to control the cost of care by providing global fees for the total cost of care for disease treatments such as diabetes and CHF.

Organizations using variations of global payment models include Kaiser Permanente, MassHealth, (Massachusetts Medicaid Program), the Veterans Health Administration, and Blue Cross/Blue Shield of Massachusetts (BCBSMA). (Heit & Dorsey, 2009) Another organization, Northeast Health Systems Physician Hospital Organization, established a five-year alternative quality contract (AQC) program in 2010 with a global payment model as the basis of its reimbursement strategy. (Becker's Hospital Review, May 26, 2010)

Care Coordination Fees

Many insurers are moving to provide payment for care management in the form of care coordination fees. These fees are a response to providers requesting reimbursement for services that have been traditionally provided, yet not reimbursed. The payments are usually paid in a set per-member per-month structure, ranging from $2-$5 per member per-month by an insurer. These are paid directly to primary care providers, or the CIN/ACO for members attributed either prospectively or retrospectively depending on the insurers' methodology. (Lewis, McClurg, Smith, Fisher, & Bynum, 2013)

Prospective attribution can be assigned by two different methodologies. In the "gate keeper" model, monthly eligibility listings are provided in which beneficiaries are required to select a primary care physician (PCP) and the PCP or CIN/ACO knows ahead of time their patient population. The other method assigns members based upon historical use of services in a prior timeframe, usually 1-3 years. The advantage of prospective payment is the CIN/ACO knows ahead of time whom its members are, and how to allocate resources to provide necessary preventive care and chronic disease management. The down side is that providers are responsible for members that may not utilize resources within the CIN/ACO, yet the CIN/ACO is financially responsible. Retrospective attribution is performed at the end of the actual performance year based upon utilization of resources by the member. The disadvantage of this method is that CINs/ACOs may provide care and services to members that will not ultimately be assigned to them, thus wasting resources on non-members of the CIN/ACO. The advantaged of retrospective attribution is that providers will only be responsible for those who utilize the CIN/ACO services.

Traditional Pay for Performance

Various forms of pay for performance have been used in healthcare for decades. The model is most often added to the fee for service payments, based upon achieving certain threshold or benchmarks for certain standards of care for services delivered, such as immunizations or breast and cervical cancer screening. These methods have not achieved the results for which they have been designed, mainly because the amounts provided for achieving the benchmarks have been too low, and efficiency of care is not taken into account. (AMA Innovators Committee, 2012) For pay for performance to be effective, it must provide sufficient reimbursement to achieve the care desired, and allow for development of the necessary infrastructure. This is thought to be more of a transitional method to help with practice transformation rather than a final reimbursement model for value based care.

Risk Shifting

Payment reform is having an impact on provider organizations, physicians, and payers, potentially redesigning the health finance and delivery systems in fundamental ways. From the physician's perspective, payment reform requires an understanding of the risks and rewards, as well as knowing who bears the burden of risk between the stakeholders, including physicians, hospitals, and payers (including employer, government, and commercial plans). Figure 7-4 illustrates a progression of payment models on the basis of financial risk.

Figure 7-4. Payment Model Reforms and Risk[*]

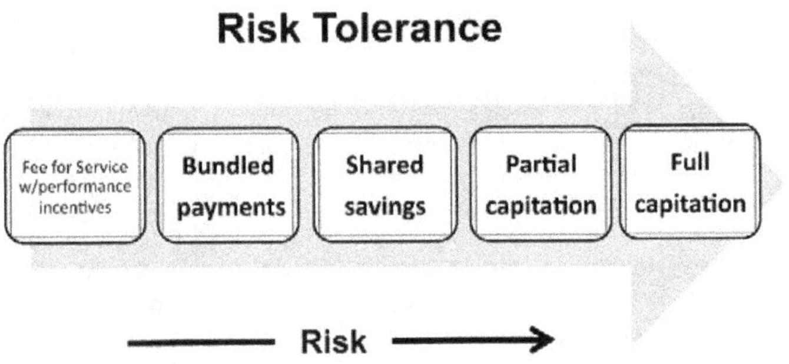

Risk Tolerance

| Fee for Service w/performance incentives | Bundled payments | Shared savings | Partial capitation | Full capitation |

——— Risk ———➔

In this illustration, the shared savings programs (public and private) fall between other models in the risk tolerance continuum. At one end of the continuum is the FFS system, which government and industry are moving away from in preference for some kind of value-based or pay-for-performance reimbursement. At the other end is full capitation, in which physicians bear a greater burden of risk with these contracts, but which usually presents a commensurate potential for increased financial reward. (Welch & Welch, 1995)

Table 7-3 describes a three-level payment model with a central focus on increasing the level of risk and reward accepted by the healthcare provider

---

[*] Illustration provided from BDC Advisors presentation slide in January 2011 for second edition of this book.

and greater need to manage total population health in moving from Level 1 to Level 3. (McClellan, McKethan, Lewis, Roski, & Fisher, 2010)

Table 7-3. ACO Payment Models

Level I Asymmetric shared savings	Level 2 Symmetric Model	Level 3 Partial Capitation Model
• Continue operating under current insurance contracts / coverage models (e.g. FFS)	• Payments can still be tied to current payment system, although ACO could receive revenue from payers and distribute funds to members (depending on ACO contracts)	• ACO receives mix of FFS and prospective fixed payment
• No risk of losses if spending exceeds targets	• At risk for losses if spending exceeds targets	• If successful at meeting budget and performance targets, greater financial benefits
• Most incremental approach with least barriers for entry	• Increased incentive for providers to decrease costs due to risk of losses	• If ACO exceeds budget, more risk means greater financial downside
• Attractive to new entities, risk-adverse providers, or entities with limited organizational capacity, range of covered services, or experience working with other providers	• Attractive to providers with some infrastructure or care coordination capability and demonstrated track record	• Only appropriate for providers with robust infrastructure, demonstrated track record in finances and quality and providing relatively full range of services

Levels of risk may be an important consideration for ACO readiness assessment. Level 1 aligns with an ACO at a lower level of readiness to accept risk, which could mean it also lacks the infrastructure to manage clinical or financial risk. Level 2, the symmetric model, gives ACO physicians greater opportunities for shared savings. Organizations interested in this level of risk/reward should have a stronger infrastructure and capabilities in place to accept greater accountability for care of the patient population in question. Level 3 represents a greater assumption of risk and reward, and could be an ACO at a higher level of capabilities, with more advanced systems, greater financial backing, and perhaps a clinically integrated network infrastructure.

While the FTC has specific requirements for CINs, clinical integration may be implemented differently for ACOs because they have different objectives. The objectives of a CIN are to collectively negotiate physician payment rates with payers, while the ACO typically becomes like a payer, negotiating global premium and shared savings rates with patients, or with groups of patients owned by a payer (government, employer, health plan, etc.). The benefits and infrastructure of a clinical integration program have been studied and validated, and it should be seriously considered by any organizations participating in the Medicare ACO program. Whether or not an organization has an immediate goal of becoming an ACO, establishing a strong CIN program helps set the foundation for future participation in shared savings and similar programs, and builds the healthcare provider organization's capacity to understand quality and cost, improve margins, and accept and manage higher levels of risk necessary under newer reimbursement models and scenarios progressing from Level 1 to Level 3.

Each ACO will ultimately determine its level of acceptable risk, based on its ability to tolerate risk as influenced by the strength of its infrastructure, financial strength, and other capabilities. As the industry continues to advance the various pay-for-performance models, physicians will continue to see decreasing FFS payments but have increasing opportunities to earn additional compensation by demonstrating positive patient outcomes, meeting quality standards, and demonstrating improvement in performance.

Health care reform has spawned the development and testing of new payment models; as a result the financial environment for physicians, hospitals, and other providers will continue to evolve. Academic medical centers and physician training programs will help prepare current and future physicians for the new compensation models they will confront. (Griner, 2010)

Future of Payment Reforms

The next generation of payment and reimbursement models is crystallizing through the efforts of countless physicians, hospitals, health insurance plans, government agencies, researchers, policy analysts, and healthcare executives.

The concept of a learning organization is applicable to the healthcare industry. In the area of payment reform an abundance of new payment models and incentive programs have been piloted and demonstrated for years, with results providing feedback to leaders and policy makers. Given the complexity of the financial issues and time required to design, test, implement, collect data, and analyze incentive programs, the learning system concept provides a philosophy as well as a model to convey the evolution of the healthcare industry and point the best path forward. This concept is similar to continuous quality improvement, and is designed to strengthen performance. The learning system model illustrated in Figure 7-5 is a possible path—which could have many variations—for the continued evolution of a CIN/ACO in its financial reimbursement model maturation.

Figure 7-5. The Learning System: Payment Reform Progression

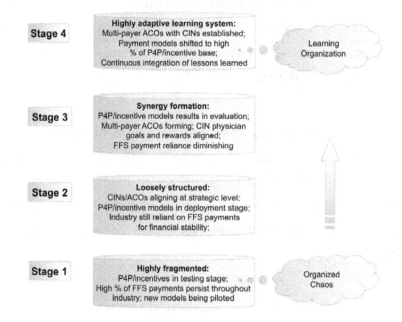

The four-stage model is based on the "Stages of Evolution of the Design of Health Organizations" provided by the Institute of Medicine. (Institute of Medicine, 2001) This application of the model focuses on the transition away from FFS payments toward an increasingly higher percentage of incentive and pay-for-performance payments for physician and provider compensation. It also features the evolution of the system toward better-organized and clinically integrated multi-payer models. The IOM, CMMI, and others are collectively leading progress along this path. In addition, private sector stakeholders, such as trade associations and commercial health insurance plans, are collaborating with physicians and hospitals to introduce new reimbursement models that are proving effective. As results of CIN/ACO implementations and new payment approaches translate into lessons learned, and best practices emerge, the industry will continue to advance toward Stage 4 as a highly adaptive learning system.

The Financial Roadmap

CIN/ACO initiatives require strong governance, financial, and administrative models. Physician leaders should partner with senior financial leaders, including Chief Financial Officers (CFOs), practice administrators and others, on the financial stewardship of their organizations. This partnering is important to set the strategic agenda for reimbursement and physician compensation policies and processes, as well as financial and contracting relationships. Understanding the risk tolerance of the organization is a critical function requiring the engagement of physician executives and administrators early in planning and decision-making. An organization at an early point in its establishment may be more inclined to focus efforts on creating a CIN as a precursor to pursuing an ACO. A greater tolerance of risk, and commensurate greater rewards, can be anticipated as ACOs mature and deal more effectively with the complexities associated with delivering higher value healthcare services while retaining accountability and responsibility for the results.

The CIN/ACO needs to evaluate several elements to ensure financial success and sustainability. First is *risk tolerance assessment*, which can be viewed as a continuous monitoring activity, or as a functional evaluation at the point of critical executive decision-making.

Second, and key to the longevity of every healthcare organization, is the need to *proactively engage in revenue cycle management*. The CIN/ACO will have increasing responsibility for risk management as it evolves, and must have a strong financial team to manage the flow of reimbursements, physician/staff compensations, and expenses associated with day-to-day operations. This will also require visibility into quality and performance objectives; an understanding of whether or not objectives are being met; and the ability to respond and change course when necessary. Physician leaders and others from across multi-disciplinary areas will need to see monthly, and sometimes weekly or daily, updates to ensure funds are flowing properly through the organization's financial system.

Third, *physician compensation* is a critical element of the financial roadmap. Physicians are the lifeblood of these entities because they are responsible for directing patients/beneficiaries to hospital facilities and outpatient centers for inpatient or outpatient services. Compensation models are changing along with reimbursement models and physicians who are better equipped to understand data about their practices, how they are performing, and whether they are meeting quality metrics and continuous improvement goals, will be better prepared to assume greater financial risk and rewards. They will also be better positioned to engage more actively in new models of care finance and delivery. As the industry shifts away from FFS reimbursement, the physician workforce is adjusting its financial compensation plans to better align with pay-for-performance realities adopted throughout the industry.

The fourth element to address in the financial management of healthcare organizations is *auditing*. Audits are a frequently occurring activity needed to ensure the integrity of organizations. Both internal compliance staff and external parties, including CMS, public accounting firms, state health departments, the Internal Revenue Service and others, conduct periodic audits. In a CIN and ACO this function takes on added importance. In the case of an MSSP-ACO the financial facts can make a big difference as to whether an organization succeeds or fails. And if history is any indication, rarely do the financial results recorded by CMS match the results recorded by the entity participating in the program. One of the editors of this book has personal experience with this issue. When CMS evaluated the program he and his team were running, they found the savings goals had not been met – meaning that CMS would not pay any additional amount – but worse, the organization where the editor was working at the time would have to refund a large advance payment that had already been made by CMS. Working diligently, the editor and his financial officer found errors made by the third-party, contracted actuaries used by CMS. This all came to a denouement with a potentially confrontational conference call with the CMS program manager, his boss, her boss, 12 other CMS listeners, the outside actuarial firm, the editor and his CEO, CFO, General Counsel, Chief Technology Officer (CTO), Chief Operating Officer (COO), and Chief Medical Officer (CMO). After explaining the error to this large group, there was a pregnant silence, after which the outside actuarial firm retained by CMS said "yes, I think you're right, let's take this back and see what happened here." And, after realizing their mistake, the editor's organization was able to keep the fees, obtain additional payments, and did not have to pay anything back. If it were not for careful and painstaking audit activities, established all along the way, the outcome might have been different.

The last critical element is financial *capital management.* New resources, and the capital to finance them, are necessary to establish new care delivery models. While capital management is listed on the map, it is not least in importance. Without appropriate management of this function a CIN or ACO will not have the ability to secure and maintain needed resources and infrastructure. Many healthcare provider organizations have had to realign major initiatives in light of economic challenges stemming from the financial downturn, landmark federal health and social policy reforms, and major technology implementation and adoption requirements. As healthcare organizations work their way back to financial health, if they wish to participate in new health finance and delivery models, they will need to secure and allocate funds necessary to start and sustain new operational capabilities.

Future Directions

A number of financial challenges and risks need to be navigated in establishing and operating CINs and ACOs. Many can be mitigated by engagement of stakeholders and careful planning. Healthcare provider organizations have the challenge of evaluating and determining the reimbursement models to adopt, including risks and rewards associated with different configurations. As the industry continues to move toward a pay-for-performance and value-driven culture, FFS reimbursements will continue to decline, resulting in a shift in payment methods as organizations work toward the design and implementation of new financial management and care delivery models. Much will depend on actions taken by physicians, hospitals, and other health system stakeholders; whether CMS, commercial insurers and employers see evidence they are getting value for funds spent; and whether additional funding should go towards the healthcare system or diverted to other pressing government or private programs.

Another challenge presented by the ACA is the new health insurance exchanges. As insurance exchanges opened in 2013 and the nation's insured population increases, there may be an influx of new patients across all demographic groups coming into primary care practices and hospital organizations. (Clemans-Cope, Kenney, Buettgens, Carroll, & Blavin, 2012; Schoen, Doty, Robertson, & Collins, 2011) There are substantial workforce challenges in managing the increased workload. The operational burden of higher demand for services, including the new focus on quality and value that is becoming a central theme, will prove to be equally challenging. The formation of CINs and ACOs, with their repositioning of accountability and risk while increasing the potential reward, will serve as one way to deal with the new environment and help mitigate such challenges. (Epstein et al., 2014)

Establishing meaningful and realistic financial objectives that account for the transition in risk will be essential for physicians and hospitals to improve the quality of care and get paid appropriately. Organizations that embrace a collaborative governance approach will be better positioned to report performance to leadership and take corrective actions that improve population-based care and benefit from financial reforms.

CHAPTER 7 DISCUSSION QUESTIONS

Discussion questions are provided for team building or class exercises. Answers for all questions are provided in Appendix C.

Question Number	Question
1	What are some points to consider in developing a plan for managing increasing risk for the CIN/ACO while working in a largely fee-for-service oriented market?
2	What are the five elements of a financial roadmap for CINs and ACOs discussed in the chapter?
3	How is the four-stage learning system model (from the IOM's 2001 *Crossing the Quality Chasm* report) applied to payment model evolution?
4	What are global payments for CINs and ACOs and what is one of the most important benefits from their use and adoption?
5	What are the four categories of bundled payment models from CMS's bundled payment demonstration?

CHAPTER 7 HIGHLIGHTS

✓ The current fee for service reimbursement model has led to rewarding providers for volume of care rather than quality of care.

✓ As the health care system is evolving to value-based reimbursement models, organizations will need to transition from the fee for service to multiple, new quality based reimbursement models, while simultaneously evolving the capabilities to provide better coordination of care throughout the care continuum.

✓ Careful financial planning and mapping strategies as organizations move away from the fee for service model is necessary to remain financially sound.

✓ Physicians need to develop new skills to better understand and deal with risk adjustment, financial risk, and the total cost of care. These skills will be required to aid in the evolution of networks toward true clinical integration and accountability for the quality and cost of care.

✓ Understanding and adapting to new reimbursement models will be critical to the success of health care organizations.

✓ Three important elements of the CIN 'financial roadmap' discussed in the chapter were physician compensation, proactive engagement in revenue cycle management, and risk tolerance assessment.

CHAPTER 7 REFERENCES

AMA Innovators Committee. (2012). Physician Payment Reform Early Innovators Share What They Have Learned: American Medical Assocation.

Becker's Hospital Review. (2010, May 26). BCBS of Massachusetts, Northeast Health Systems sign 5-year global payment deal [Press release]. Retrieved from http://www.beckershospitalreview.com/hospital-financial-and-business-news/bcbs-of-massachusetts-northeast-health-systems-sign-5-year-global-payment-deal.html

Centers for Medicare and Medicaid Services. About the CMS Innovation Center. Retrieved from http://innovation.cms.gov/about/index.html

Centers for Medicare and Medicaid Services. Innovation Models. Retrieved from http://innovation.cms.gov/initiatives/index.html#views=models

Centers for Medicare and Medicaid Services. Medicare Shared Savings Program. Retrieved from http://www.cms.gov/Medicare/Medicare-Fee-for-Service-Payment/sharedsavingsprogram/index.html?redirect=/sharedsavingsprogram/

Centers for Medicare and Medicaid Services. (2014a). Meaningful Use Program Overview. Retrieved from http://www.cms.gov/Regulations-and-Guidance/Legislation/EHRIncentivePrograms/Meaningful_Use.html

Protecting Access to Medicare Act of 2014 (2014b).

Centers for Medicare and Medicaid Services. (2014c). Recovery Audit Program- Recent Updates (May 2014). Retrieved from http://www.cms.gov/Research-Statistics-Data-and-Systems/Monitoring-Programs/Medicare-FFS-Compliance-Programs/Recovery-Audit-Program/Recent_Updates.html

Centers for Medicare and Medicaid Services. (2007, January 17). Issues Paper: DHHS Medicare hospital value-based purchasing plan development. Retrieved May 19, 2014, from http://www.cms.gov/Medicare/Medicare-Fee-for-Service-Payment/AcuteInpatientPPS/Downloads/Hospital_VBP_Plan_Issues_Paper.pdf

Centers for Medicare and Medicaid Services. (2009a, January). Medicare demonstrations. Nursing home value-based purchasing program. Retrieved from http://www.cms.gov/DemoProjectsEvalRpts/MD/itemdetail.asp?filterType=none&filterByDID=-99&sortByDID=3&sortOrder=descending&itemID=CMS1198946&intNumPerPage=10

Centers for Medicare and Medicaid Services. (2009b, January). Roadmap for implementing value driven healthcare in the traditional Medicare fee-for-service program. Retrieved from https://www.cms.gov/QualityInitiativesGenInfo/downloads/VBPRoadmap_OEA_1-16_508.pdf

Centers for Medicare and Medicaid Services. (2013, January). Bundled Payments for Care Improvement (BPCI) Initiative: General Information. Retrieved from http://innovation.cms.gov/initiatives/Bundled-Payments/index.html

Centers for Medicare and Medicaid Services. (2014, March). Payment Adjustments & Hardship Exceptions Tipsheet for Eligible Professionals. Retrieved from http://www.cms.gov/Regulations-and-Guidance/Legislation/EHRIncentivePrograms/Downloads/PaymentAdj_HardshipExcepTipSheetforEP.pdf

Clemans-Cope, L., Kenney, G. M., Buettgens, M., Carroll, C., & Blavin, F. (2012). The Affordable Care Act's coverage expansions will reduce differences in uninsurance rates by race and ethnicity. *Health Affairs*, 31(5), 920-930. doi: 10.1377/hlthaff.2011.1086

Commission on Physician Payment Reform. (2013, March). Report of the National Commission on Physician Payment Reform. Retrieved from http://physicianpaymentcommission.org/wp-content/uploads/2013/03/physician_payment_report.pdf

de Brantes, F., Rosenthal, M. B., & Painter, M. (2009). Building a bridge from fragmentation to accountability—the Prometheus payment model. *New England Journal of Medicine*, 361(11), 1033-1036. doi: 10.1056/NEJMp0906121

Department of Health and Human Services. (2014, January 30). Press Release- Medicare's delivery system reform initiatives achieve significant savings and quality improvements - off to a strong start. Retrieved from http://www.hhs.gov/news/press/2014pres/01/20140130a.html

Epstein, A. M., Jha, A. K., Orav, E. J., Liebman, D. L., Audet, A.-M. J., Zezza, M. A., & Guterman, S. (2014). Analysis Of Early Accountable Care Organizations Defines Patient, Structural, Cost, And Quality-Of-Care Characteristics. *Health Affairs*, 33(1), 95-102. doi: 10.1377/hlthaff.2013.1063

Evans, J. (2010). The Current state of bundled payments. *American Health and Drug Benefits*, 3(4).

Federal Register Volume 76 Number 67. (2011a, April 7). I(A). Introduction and Overview of Value-Based Purchasing. p. 19530.

Federal Register Volume 76 Number 67. (2011b, April 7). II(F)(4). Establishing an Expenditure Benchmark. pp. 19604-19606.

Federal Register Volume 76 Number 67. (2011c, April 7). II. (H) Monitoring; Actions prior to termination; Termination, suspension, and repayment of Shared Savings. pp. 19648-19650.

Federal Register Volume 78 Number 237. (2013, December 10). Medicare and Medicaid Programs: Hospital Outpatient Prospective Payment and Ambulatory Surgical Center Payment Systems and Quality Reporting Programs; Hospital Value-Based Purchasing Program; Organ Procurement Organizations; Quality Improvement Organizations; Electronic Health Records (EHR) Incentive Program; Provider Reimbursement Determinations and Appeals; Final Rule. pp. 74825-75200. Retrieved from http://www.gpo.gov/fdsys/pkg/FR-2013-12-10/html/2013-28737.htm

Goldsmith, J. (2010). Analyzing shifts in economic risks to providers in proposed payment and delivery system reforms. *Health Affairs*, 29(7), 1299-1304. doi: 10.1377/hlthaff.2010.0423

Griner, P. F. (2010). Payment reform and the mission of academic medical centers. *New England Journal of Medicine*, 363(19), 1784-1786. doi: 10.1056/NEJMp1005413

Heit, M., & Dorsey, K. P. S. (2009). Global Payments to Improve Quality and Efficiency in Medicaid: Concepts and Considerations. Prepared for the Massachusetts Medicaid Policy Institute. Boston, MA: Massachusetts Medicaid Policy Institute.

HR 3590. (2010a). Patient Protection and Affordable Care Act, §3007. Value-based payment modifier under the physician fee schedule (2010).

HR 3590. (2010b). Patient Protection and Affordable Care Act, §3022(d)(1)(B)(i). Determining savings (2010).

HR 3590. (2010c). Patient Protection and Affordable Care Act, §3022(d)(1)(B)(ii). Determining benchmarks (2010).

HR 3590. (2010d). Patient Protection and Affordable Care Act, §3022(d)(2). Payments for shared savings (2010).

Institute of Medicine, & Committee on Quality of Health Care in America. (2001). Building Organizational Supports for Change. In *Crossing the Quality Chasm. A New Health System for the 21st Century* (pp. 111-117). Washington, DC: National Academies Press.

Lewis, V. A., McClurg, A. B., Smith, J., Fisher, E. S., & Bynum, J. P. W. (2013). Attributing patients to accountable care organizations: performance year approach aligns stakeholders' interests. *Health Affairs*, 32(3), 587-595. doi: 10.1377/hlthaff.2012.0489

McClellan, M., McKethan, A. N., Lewis, J. L., Roski, J., & Fisher, E. S. (2010). A national strategy to put accountable care into practice. *Health Affairs*, 29(5), 982-990. doi: 10.1377/hlthaff.2010.0194

Miller, H. (2010, June). Comprehensive care payment Pathways for physician success under healthcare payment and delivery reforms (p. 26): American Medical Association.

Painter, M. W., & Cernew, M. E. (2012, March). Counting change measuring health care prices, costs and spending: Robert Wood Johnson Foundation. Retrieved from http://www.rwjf.org/content/dam/web-assets/2012/03/counting-change

Premier Inc. (2013). Payor Partnerships Insights form Premier's PACT Population Health Collaborative. Retrieved from https://www.premierinc.com/wps/wcm/connect/6b9aad65-3d93-4bf4-8041-b3091a335d2f/Payor-Partnership-White-Paper-6+3.pdf?MOD=AJPERES

Robert Wood Johnson Foundation, & Health Care Incentives Improvement Institute. (2010, July). Prometheus payment: On the frontlines of health care payment reform.

Schoen, C., Doty, M. M., Robertson, R. H., & Collins, S. R. (2011). Affordable Care Act reforms could reduce the number of underinsured US adults by 70 percent. *Health Affairs*, 30(9), 1762-1771. doi: 10.1377/hlthaff.2011.0335

Selker, H. P., Kravitz, R. L., & Gallagher, T. H. (2014). The National Physician Payment Commission recommendation to eliminate fee-for-service payment: balancing risk, benefit, and efficiency in bundling payment for care. *Journal of General Internal Medicine*, 29(5), 698-699. doi: 10.1007/s11606-014-2787-z

The Physicians Foundation. (2012, September). A survey of America's physicians: practice patterns and perspective. Retrieved from http://www.physiciansfoundation.org/uploads/default/Physicians_Foundation_2012_Biennial_Survey.pdf

Thompson, J., (November 2012). Joseph Thompson, MD, MPH titled, *Arkansas Payment Improvement Initiative. Improving Quality, Containing Cost.* Retrieved from http://www.nga.org/files/live/sites/NGA/files/pdf/2013/1305SIMThompson.pdf

United Healthcare. (effective 2013, September 1). Oxford Health Plan Policy Administrative 200.9 T0 Obstetrical Policy: Reimbursement Policy United Healthcare.

Deficit Reduction Act (DRA) (2005).

Welch, W. P., & Welch, H. G. (1995). Fee-for-data: a strategy to open the HMO black box. *Health Affairs*, 14(4), 104-116.

Young, A., Chaudhry, H. J., Rhyne, J., & Dugan, M. (2011). A census of actively licensed physicians in the United States, 2010. *Journal of Medical Regulation*, 96(4), 10-20.

Chapter 8. Coordinating Care—Transforming the Delivery Process

Michael G. Hunt

Colleen Swedberg

Alone we can do so little; together we can do so much. (Keller, 2013)

Helen Keller
American Author
1880-1968

CHAPTER 8 LEARNING OBJECTIVES

✓ Exposure to new Care Coordination models resulting from healthcare reform.

✓ Understand how Care Coordination facilitates organizational achievement of the "Triple Aim".

✓ Exposure to a systematic approach to identifying care coordination challenges.

✓ Understand the symbiosis of Clinical Integration and Care Coordination.

✓ Understand how Care Coordination is a component of medical management and its effect on population health management

Overview

The purpose of care coordination is to improve the health of each member of a population, assist a provider network's delivery of care to reflect quality and appropriate access that help determine the patient's experience, and collaborate with provider network participants to decrease and control the costs of healthcare for consumers and patients served by the network. This purpose reflects the goals of the "Triple Aim." (Beasley, 2009)

Care coordination should be the driving force to help manage the member population while engaging local healthcare resources to "manage" patient care. Care coordination is the foundation of medical management that oversees the entire population, or a specific population subset attributed to an organization. This function within each Clinically Integrated Network (CIN) and Accountable Care Organization (ACO) focuses attention on standardization of processes to assure efficient patient care transitions among providers and sites of care and meeting the medical care requirements for both chronic and preventative care. Care coordination serves a central role in monitoring the population at-large and empowering local facilities, especially the primary care provider, in case managing the patient locally. The successful maturation of care coordination is critical when organization take on full risk with payer contracts.

Both care coordination and case management are mutually exclusive professional roles while being interdependent. Case management should occur directly with the patient while medical services are rendered (ED, inpatient, ambulatory service center). Case management functions best when local team members bring into play the relationship between the physician (provider) and the patient. Localized case management is positioned to activate a complete treatment plan using the most current medically relevant information.

INSIGHT: The model differentiates care coordination at the enterprise level and case management at the most local level. Case management exploits the patient provider relationship fully, where care coordination manages the population at-large and is reliant on effective case management locally.

As a function of clinically integrated services, case management may include education, treatment, referral, and other clinical services (coordination and scheduling of services, facilitation and confirmation of medical information transfer (portability), and resolves actual and perceived patient barriers to continuous care). The case manager directly interacts with the patient. Care coordination may include coordination of medical activities, medical information portability, and resolution of patient/facility barriers when case management needs additional resources. Care Coordination (at the enterprise level) institutionalizes and enculturates standardized processes for patient care and collaboration, monitors the population at large, facilitates individual care, and supplements case management activities when necessary from the enterprise level. Care coordination is the macro healthcare controller, while case management manages healthcare issues at the individual patient level. Care coordination requires continuous communication with case managers and medical professionals, access to "real-time" medical information that is portable, and guides local facilities to optimize workflow and patient out-reach.

Access to highly developed diagnostic tests and interventions, delivered in state-of-the-art institutions that are not connected, contributes to duplication of effort and an expensive health care system in the United States. (National Quality Forum, 2010) There is a perception that more sophisticated or a greater number of interventions equates to better health care. Public education about the need to understand outcomes and cost has lagged behind promotion of advances in science and technology. As a result, healthcare in the United States is intricate, highly specialized, over utilized, and expensive.

Yet while care may be delivered in a technically correct fashion within various specialties, the intricacies and specialization have led to fragmentation, in which one clinical provider often does not know what another is doing with the same patient. (National Quality Forum, 2013) Further, the complexity of care today is such that patients frequently do not understand how to care for themselves after they leave the clinical setting, even following a simple primary care visit. This situation creates a dangerous, unnecessarily complicated, and bewildering environment for patients—putting at risk of harm the very people the system seeks to serve, with sometimes disastrous consequences. (National Quality Forum, 2010)

In fact, fragmentation is a characteristic of the U.S. health care system. The system is designed to provide care and services to individuals and help them survive an episodic acute illness event. (Robinson, 2010) Multiple, specialized providers care for people with chronic illnesses. Chronic care for a single illness is often provided without knowledge of medications and care given by other specialty providers. (Reuben, 2007) Ball et. al. describes the context as systems, structures and processes that have evolved over time and have been cobbled together with unaligned assumptions in each silo. (Ball, Merry, & Verlaan-Cole L, 2013) Patients move from silo to silo within the system. A lack of coordination gives rise to 'misuse, over use, [and] underuse' of resources. (Chassin & Galvin, 1998)

Ideally, the health care system should be designed to interface with people so as to make it possible for them to have the care they need and want, can understand that care, and can assume communication occurs between providers. Various models, approaches, processes and interventions have emerged over time to address the gaps in communication and coor dination inherent in the current system. These efforts are mostly band aids trying to patch a broken system rather than designs that have developed systematically and organically and can be validated and replicated, to improve value and quality outcomes with the appropriate use of data.

More than a decade ago the Institute of Medicine (IOM) published a landmark study, *Crossing the Quality Chasm –a New Healthcare System for the 21st Century* which served as a trumpet call for revamping the U.S. health care system. (Committee on Quality of Healthcare in America & Institute of Medicine, 2001) It is frequently referenced in the medical literature, programming, and academia. The study calls for improvements in six dimensions of health care performance: safety, effectiveness, patient-centeredness, timeliness, efficiency, and equity; and it asserts that those improvements cannot be achieved within the constraints of the existing system of care. It provides a rationale and a framework for the redesign of the U.S. health care system at four levels: patients' experiences; the "microsystems" that actually give care; the organizations that house and support microsystems; and the environment of laws, rules, payment, accreditation, and professional training that shape organizational action. (Berwick, 2002) These microsystems and the organizations that house them are fertile ground for care coordination.

Response to the IOM mandate to redesign the health care system is emerging, with coordination of care at the center. For example, the American Hospital Association in a 2011 presentation to its membership addressed the health care landscape, suggesting a shift is required from the volume based 'first curve' economics with stand-alone acute inpatient hospitals, to a value-based 'second curve' economics system, including realigned incentives, partnerships with shared risk, IT utilization for population management and increased coordination. (American Hospital Association, 2011)

Health reform laws, mainly the 2010 Patient Protection and Affordable Care Act (ACA) is a defining moment in addressing the deficiencies outlined in the Quality Chasm report. The ACA targets realigning providers' financial incentives, encouraging more efficient organization and delivery of health care, and investing in preventive and population health – all elements of care coordination. Provisions in the ACA extend health insurance coverage to 32 million uninsured Americans, potentially improving access to care and equity but making care coordination even more important as the ranks of insured seeking care swell. (Davis, June 23, 2010) The legislation encourages new delivery models, such as ACOs, CINs, medical homes, health homes, and transitional care interventions, which offer incentives to providers for coordinating and improving care for chronically ill populations. (Volland, Schraeder, Shelton, & Hess, 2012) The American Recovery and Reinvestment Act included approximately $19 billion to expand the use of health information technology – another key element in coordination of care.

Defining Care Coordination

Health care coordination, in its simplest form, involves providers, patients, and other caregivers working together to deliver health care services. In context of the ACA and new government regulations, it is also designed to meet the "Triple Aim" of improved quality, lowered costs and better patient satisfaction.

The healthcare industry and health professionals have not solidified a concept or single definition for care coordination. Many have incorrectly equated collaboration with coordination. Stille et al distinguish between care coordination and collaboration, noting that care coordination is not synonymous with collaborative care, which is simply the act of working together. (Stille, Jerant, Bell, Meltzer, & Elmore, 2005) By contrast, coordination according to Stille involves the regulation of participants to produce higher-order functioning and involves the integration of inputs from multiple entities towards a common goal. Care coordination is sometimes thought of as case management, but there are differences here too. Understanding these differences can help further define care coordination.

Not surprisingly, given the complexity and fragmentation of the healthcare system, coordination of care is the 'subject du jour' in health care redesign discussions. 'Coordination' is generally defined as the process of organizing people, groups or things in order to make them work together effectively. (Macmillan Dictionary, 2013)

Various nationally recognized health quality organizations have defined 'care coordination'. For example, the National Quality Forum (NQF) defines care coordination as "a function that helps ensure that the patient's needs and preferences for health services and information sharing across people, functions, and sites are met over time."(National Quality Forum, 2006) This definition is purposely patient-centric, does not even specify providers or organizations, and adds a time element. NQF elaborates on this definition by emphasizing information-rich, patient and patient-centered characteristics and the purposeful intention to deliver the right care to the right patient at the right time. NQF refers to care coordination as a function that allows communication across settings and between episodes of care to limit medical errors, reduce costs, and limit the pain a patient bears from care plans not integrated to meet the patient's unique needs. Further, arising from the work of the NQF and the National Priorities Partnership, care coordination is described as ensuring that patients' needs and preferences for healthcare services are understood and that they are shared as patients move from one healthcare setting to another or to home, as care is transferred from one healthcare organization to another or is shared among primary care professional and specialists. (National Priorities Partnership, 2008)

The federal government Agency for Healthcare Research and Quality (AHRQ) defines care coordination as,

> ...the deliberate organization of patient care activities between two or more participants (including the patient) involved in a patient's care to facilitate the appropriate delivery of health care services. Organizing care involves the marshalling of personnel and other resources needed to carry out all required patient care activities and is often managed by the exchange of information among participants responsible for different aspects of care. (Agency for Healthcare Research and Quality, 2011)

Care coordination here is a brokering of services for patients to ensure that needs are met and services are not duplicated by professionals participating in the same patient care. This definition does specify health professionals and others involved, including the patient, and references "other resources," which alludes to community and social services, reflecting the close relationship of this agency to government Public Health Services. AHRQ further elaborates its concept of care coordination through supporting information sharing across providers, patients, and types and levels of service, sites and time frames.

Care coordination and case management have also been used interchangeably within healthcare. For example, the Case Management Society of America defines case management as a collaborative process of assessment, planning, facilitation, care coordination, evaluation, and advocacy for options and services to meet an individual's and family's comprehensive health needs through communication and available resources to promote quality, cost-effective outcomes. (Case Management Society of America, 2013) The National Coalition on Care Coordination defines care coordination as,

> ...a client-centered, assessment-based interdisciplinary approach to integrating health care and social support services in which an individual's needs and preferences are assessed, a comprehensive care plan is developed, and services are managed and monitored by an identified care coordinator following evidence-based standards of care. (National Coalition on Care Coordination, 2013)

In this definition the two roles do not appear to be distinct.

Table 8-1 compares and contrasts the proposed care coordination concept and literature-defined case management roles. SVHP Transition Leadership Team Presentation June 5, 2014, St. Vincent's Medical Center.

Table 8-1. Comparison between Care Coordination and Case Management

Category	Care Coordination	Case Management
Targeted Population	Organizational attributed patients	Individual patient
Education and outreach (inform and motivate	Primary: Organizational Providers Secondary: Patient	Patient
Disease Management	Oversees organizational care delivery success	Provides care for the patient
Communication	Organizational and	Individual patient and

Category	Care Coordination	Case Management
	individual members	care team
Goals	Network directed	Patient/Payer/facility directed
Care Delivery	Population management	Medical service and individual care management
Processes	System standardization	Process and implementation focused
Relationship	Primary – Local healthcare team Secondary - Patient	Primary - Patient Secondary – Local healthcare team
Network Resource	Utilize network	Utilize individual clinician
Use of Health Information Technology	Primary – Network and population management Secondary – Patient/Practice/Panel	Primary - Patient/Practice/Panel Secondary – Network and population management
Measure of Success	Population outcomes	Patient outcomes

These roles and the professionals that occupy them have significant impact on the delivery of population health management services and each organization's ability to operationalize them to effect patient care. These roles are distinctly unique, although in practice there is overlap, and have different foundational processes in the delivery of healthcare services for the population served. Notice the categories and how each role is differentiated. This chapter elaborates on these categories and what they mean for the effective delivery of health care services for CINs and ACOs.

Case management identifies appropriate providers and facilities throughout the continuum of care, ensuring that available resources are used timely and cost-effectively. Case management functions better when the environment allows direct communication between the case manager, client, and healthcare provider. The Commission for Case Manager Certification's premise is that "...everyone benefits when clients reach their optimum level of wellness, self-management, and functional capability."(Commission for Case Management Certification, 2013) Case management facilitates wellness and autonomy through advocacy, assessment, planning, communication, education, resource management, and service facilitation. All intervention is based on the needs and values of the client.

The Library of Medicine defines case management as a traditional term for the activities that a physician or other health care professional normally performs to ensure the coordination of the medical services required by a patient. (Slee, Slee, & Schmidt, 2008) The definition of case management includes the activities of evaluating the patient, planning treatment, referral, and follow-up so that care is continuous and comprehensive and payment for the care is obtained.

Improving Chronic Illness Care's website describes care coordination as a "deliberate organization of patient care activities between two or more participants involved to facilitate the delivery of health care services". (Improving Chronic Care (ICC), 2013) Consequently, the providers managing a patient's care share clinical information and have clear, shared expectations about the patient's needs and their role in providing care. By supporting and managing the transition between participants, the patient's receipt of medical care is enhanced. Care coordination engages families during care plan development and "manages" care expectations.

Improving Chronic Illness Care website delineates the principles of care coordination to include: accessibility, individualization, family alignment, promotion of solutions to systemic problems, and attention to outcome. (Improving Chronic Care (ICC), 2013) It describes effective care coordination to be activities which promote:

- Continuous evaluation of community and environmental resources (community programs, community agencies, resource guide, relationship building with program/agency staff, develop coalitions),

- Utilization of screening tools reflective of different conditions,

- Performing needs assessment (interview family for needs, strengths, and resources),

- Development of individual family support plans (review patient needs with the family), and

- Implementing and monitoring patient care plans, and revise the plan as needed. (Improving Chronic Care (ICC), 2013)

The Commission for Case Manager Certification (CCMC) states that care coordination falls within the domain of a case manager. When looking at healthcare organization operationalization of care coordination, many institutions define care coordination as a function performed by a case manager and not as a unique professional role. (Commission for Case Management Certification, 2013) This cacophony of definitions and perspectives highlights the fragmentation of the industry and how each professional group defines care coordination to their benefit.

Models of Care Coordination versus Case Management

In 2011, the Institute for Healthcare Improvement published a white paper detailing potential care coordination models. (Institute for Healthcare Improvement, 2011) The first model was led by a nurse with support from a case manager, behaviorist, elder worker, and others to coordinate care between direct care providers; assure appropriate and timely access to services, pharmaceuticals, and durable medical equipment; teach, coach, and develop self-management strategies for chronic and acute illness, and mental health problems; and promote optimal primary care home management. The intensity of patient contact was tiered. The care coordination activities were stratified into three levels. The third level is development of a comprehensive treatment plan incorporating family dynamics, understanding long-term diverse resource requirements to facilitate continuous patient care, and facilitating continual communication between providers to effectively manage the patient's ongoing medical needs. Attention to quality metrics and organizational outcome metrics is required to justify the intensity of intervention and level of resource utilization.

In another model, Tufts Health Plan attempts to change behaviors and align economic incentives by coordinating care and focus on cost and quality care through promotion of effective settings that use care management to engage plan members and providers. The National Institutes of Health has also published data detailing case management outcomes, concluding that the most effective programs focused on engaging patients during inpatient services and connecting the patient to increased utilization of community-based services. The programs seem more effective for patients of medical disease versus mental health issues.

Care coordination models are also included as components of Medical Home models. Care coordination is described in that context as providing patient care oversight and support by aligning community agencies, hospitals/emergency facilities, and medical specialist through communication and information connectivity to ensure accountable patient care. Through the Medical Home model, care coordination can follow the patient through each care transition. This means that information must accompany the patient care event and precede and send information timely to record and transmit proper patient care information.

Antonelli et al. described how a busy pediatric practice used care coordination to serve children with special care needs within a practice setting. (Balanced Budget Act, 1997) These patients were complex and totaled 11% of the empanelled patients while consuming 25% of the total encounters during the measurement period. They required staff time four times longer than typical pediatric patients. Coordination of care included processing referrals, consulting with schools or educational programs, and oversight for psychosocial issues. (Antonelli, McAllister, Popp, & Fund, 2009)

A significant aspect of healthcare reform is transforming the delivery of care from a volume-based, per-visit (fee-for-service) model to a value-based model. In this new, value-based world, health care providers take a significant role to "manage" a population and all services rendered to their patients, regardless of multiple organizations participating in their care, with the goal of ensuring quality, cost-effective care is experienced by all their patients.

> *INSIGHT:* Value based care is blind to the number of patients requiring medical intervention. The expectation is that each patient receive quality cost-effective treatment plans. Successful treatment of patients is dependent upon providers managing populations respecting that the patient may receive out-of-network intervention. Managing the patient in all transitions is critical to evaluate and manage the total cost-of-care. Quality care must be measured in all transitions. As organizational networks solidify, providers must work together and minimize any negative effect of out-of-network visits.

As ACOs become effective, they will oversee and become more responsible for the total care of their population, and each individual member. The member may receive care from more than one healthcare organization, yet the ACO is charged to "coordinate" the care, reduce overall cost of care, and preserve the quality rendered. Because of the focus on value, resulting "challenges" of quality and assumption of the risk of the cost of care, an integrated network that decides to become a risk-bearing ACO will logically strive to use medical professionals within its own organization to manage these challenges and overcome barriers to refer within the group.

Review of the Literature

Published studies show mixed impacts on health outcomes and costs from care coordination, and there is little agreement on the design of care coordination interventions. When managing patients and populations, interventions that studies have shown to be effective include: transitions of care (care when transferring between healthcare facilities/professionals), medication management, patient engagement and self-management, education (community based programs), patient direct outreach, intermediary between patient and provider, and social support. A common theme running through the studies is that careful attention to detail is required to cost-effectively manage each patient and the overall population.

The available literature on care coordination is characterized by an array of models, processes and activities focusing on differing populations with varying complexity, all being defined as care coordination. A common element of these models is the intent to arrange disparate aspects of the care of a patient or groups of patients in an organized fashion. The entire continuum of care is represented in the literature on care coordination including variations in age, condition, health concern, population, provider and setting. The unit of care may be static or spread out over time it may refer to the organizing of activities during a single episode of care and setting or between settings such as in transitional care, or it may refer to a set of activities over sequential and differing episodes of care. The coordination may be during acute care or it may refer to care of those with chronic disease in ambulatory, home, or other settings.

In an attempt to study whether care coordination improves the quality of care and how it affects cost, the Balanced Budget Act of 1997 mandated the Secretary of Health and Human Services conduct and evaluate care coordination programs and their effect on cost in the Medicare fee-for-service settings. (U.S. Congress, 1997) Eligible fee-for-service Medicare patients (primarily with congestive heart failure, coronary artery disease, and diabetes) who volunteered to participate between April 2002 and June 2005 in 15 care coordination programs were randomly assigned to treatment or control (usual care) groups. Hospitalizations, costs, and some quality-of-care outcomes were measured with claims data for 18,309 patients enrolled through June 2006. A patient survey 7 to 12 months after enrollment provided additional quality-of-care measures.

Peikes et al. summarized the outcomes of the Balanced Budget Act of 1997 study of care coordination. (Peikes, Chen, Schore, & Brown, 2009) Only two programs (Mercy Medical Center and Georgetown) had favorable statistically significant treatment-control differences in hospitalizations and sizable differences (−9.3% and −14.0%, respectively) in Medicare expenditures and one of those was not viable for the long term. Many of the other programs showed improvements in quality of care or cost containment but not both, or the improvements were either not statistically significant or applied only to a segment of the population and not the entire study group. The authors suggest that the most effective intervention for care coordination may be a combination of an ongoing model with five components they found to be most effective, combined with a proven transitional care model to prevent hospital readmissions.

Comparing the two programs with the most positive results, with the 10 unsuccessful programs, Piekes et al. note five differences worth noting. First, both of the successful programs averaged nearly one in-person contact per month per patient. Second, these two programs had favorable effects on populations with average monthly Medicare expenditures in a middle range of approximately $900 and $1,200 (most of the other programs had populations with much higher costs and terminal stages of illness, e.g., class 4 CHF), whereas only 1 of the 10 unsuccessful programs enrolled a mix of beneficiaries with average Medicare expenditures in this range. This finding suggests that programs may need to target patients who are neither at too low a risk of acute illness and hospitalizations for the program to have effects, nor so seriously ill that it is too late for interventions to have an effect. Third, in both programs, treatment group members were significantly more likely than control group members to report being taught how to take their medications. Fourth, care coordinators worked closely with local hospitals, and in fact the successful programs were hospital-based, which provided the programs with timely information on patient hospitalizations and enhanced their potential to manage transitions and reduce short-term readmissions. Finally, care coordinators in both programs had frequent opportunities to interact informally with physicians.

Volland et al. presents a detailed overview of the emerging research evidence on two approaches to primary care for the chronically ill, and the patient populations that benefit from their different perspectives and approaches to care: transitional care and comprehensive care coordination. (Volland et al., 2012) They concluded that both approaches have yet to demonstrate success in reducing total health care costs, although certain components of the models are potentially cost-effective when included in comprehensive efforts to manage the healthcare needs of adults with multiple chronic conditions. Targeting the appropriate level of interventions for individuals based on their health profile, educational background, and knowledge of the healthcare system and other resources are key in the effectiveness of these approaches when it comes to health outcomes and cost.

The two models of transitional care that Volland et al. review the Transitional Care Model developed by Mary Naylor and the Care Transitions Intervention developed by Eric Coleman, have shown reduced re-admissions and costs. Although the two models differ in approach, both engage patients with chronic illnesses while hospitalized; follow patients intensively post-discharge (for four to twelve weeks); engage in medication reconciliation; use a transitional coach or team to manage clinical, psychosocial, rehabilitative, nutritional, and pharmacy needs; teach or coach patients about medications, self-care, and symptom recognition and management; and, remind and encourage patients to keep follow up appointments.

An example of a comprehensive care coordination program is ValueOptions, a national company that provides employee assistance, health and life coaching, healthy connections engagement centers, reporting, Medicaid management programs, work/life solutions, and telepsychiatry. (Maryland Department of Health and Mental Hygiene, 2013) This comprehensive care coordination program utilizes a health information system to automate the reporting and tracking of patient care. They employ predictive modeling and risk stratification to "manage" high-risk comorbid populations and develop a locally-based, multi-disciplinary team to assist with transitions of care for the individual patient. The individual (along with person-specific barriers) is the focal point of their program. Their patient outreach is tailored to the individual. Additionally, they engage providers to meet the individual requirements of each patient. This model exemplifies a common strategy for managing healthcare at the patient level.

A growing evidence base suggests services that address social factors with an impact on health, such as transportation and caregiver support, can make these new models of care more effective. Examining early evidence from seven innovative care models, each with strong social support service components, Sheir et al. note that the evidence suggests coordinated efforts to identify and meet social needs of patients can lead to lower health care use and costs, and better outcomes for patients. (Shier, Ginsburg, Howell, Volland, & Golden, 2013)

Similarly, Claiborne defines three care coordination models that incorporate social services: centralized team model, regionalized, and provider-based. (Claiborne, 2006) The goal of these models is to integrate bio-psychosocial interventions for specific at-risk patients. The activity occurs primarily by phone and can offer enhanced services such as transportation, and housing assistance. Care coordinators screen and assess for quality of life and health status, educate patients, organize referrals, screen for psychosocial issues, assist and problem solve service need, advocate patient entitlements through public and private services, crisis intervene for mental health, coach self-care practices and adherence to treatment plans, and monitor patient progress and care.

Gittell et al. studied coordination within health systems using established scientific work around organization theory, especially as it relates to organizational social capital. (Gittell, Seidner, & Wimbush, 2010) Organizational social capital has been shown to improve performance by enabling employees to access resources that are embedded within a given network and by facilitating the transfer and sharing of knowledge. The related topic of relational coordination identifies dimensions of relationships integral to the coordination of work that is highly interdependent, uncertain and time-constrained – all characteristic of health care. Their study of nine hospitals revealed that relational coordination leads to high performance work practices and improved outcomes. There are seven dimensions validated in their fieldwork that have since been validated in subsequent studies, including: frequent, timely, accurate, problem-solving communication, and relationships of shared goals, shared knowledge and mutual respect. (Gittell, 2011)

Mapping the Challenges of Care Coordination

The pace of change caused by economic pressures and health reforms require the ability to move nimbly to incorporate best practices in care delivery. Yet information about rapidly evolving system threatens to overwhelm, and the availability of information through the Internet, social media, and other avenues challenges the capacity of organizations to consistently remain abreast of new findings, new models, and innovations in health care delivery, and maintain a robust vetting process to decide which changes to adopt.

In a rapidly changing healthcare environment, many organizations recognize the need for a disciplined, theoretical framework. Having the framework ensures maintaining perspective in the face of a growing breadth and depth of innovations, novel care models, and other care coordination challenges, without compromising the need to remain flexible, take risks, and learn through successes and failures. Regularly returning to evaluate care coordination work and its challenges against a framework permits rapid cycles of change without losing sight of known components. This is particularly true where there is no agreed upon set of competencies or measures for care coordination. It also maintains a process, independent of the changing whims or biases of individuals.

Therefore, we believe it is not only beneficial, but necessary to connect the process of mapping the challenges of care coordination to a framework that provides the theoretical foundation and logic to the mapping. To that end, the work of Houdt et al. is particularly pertinent. Houdt et al. provided an overview of the current theoretical frameworks for care coordination and performed an in-depth analysis of all identified theoretical frameworks to clarify key concepts related to care coordination. (Van Houdt, Heyrman, Vanhaecht, Sermeus, & De Lepeleire, 2013)

In that study, the 2007 Agency for Healthcare Research and Quality (AHRQ) review of five care coordination frameworks is used as the benchmark for the identification of theoretical frameworks around care coordination and to show how theoretical thinking can enrich the study of care coordination. Houdt et al. then searched through the PubMed/Cochrane database and found seven other frameworks that had emerged between 2007 and 2010. Together with the five frameworks in the AHRQ study, an in-depth analysis was performed of all of the frameworks (n=12).

Houdt et al. identified 14 care coordination concepts in the analysis of the frameworks: external factors, structure, tasks characteristics, cultural factors, knowledge and technology, need for coordination, administrative operational processes, exchange of information, goals and roles, quality of relationships, patient outcomes, team outcome, and organizational or inter-organizational outcome. These key concepts are put forward by the authors as a means to facilitate the selection of a useful theoretical framework for developing, studying and evaluating care coordination strategies. Two of the twelve frameworks emerged as being the most comprehensive because they incorporate more of the key concepts when compared with the other frameworks: the Relational Coordination Theory for exploring care coordination within an organization and the Multi-level Framework which can be used to study care coordination between organizations.

The Multi-level Framework is relevant to a CIN because it proposes that organizational design shapes networks. Gittell et al. argue effectively that the same formal practices that give rise to effective coordination at one level can also be used proactively to generate effective coordination at other levels. By using the same organizational mechanisms within and between organizations, CINs are strengthened resulting in greater quality and efficiency. (Gittell & Weiss, 2004)

The organization design practices described in the Multi-Level Framework are: cross-functional routines or protocols, information systems, functional boundary spanners and cross-functional meetings. Integration is also achieved through the use of control mechanisms including shared incentives, shared performance measures and supervision. In examining the organization design literature, Gittell notes that traditional organization perspective underestimates the autonomy of departments within an organization, while overestimating the autonomy of organizations from each other. However, the problems of achieving effective coordination both within and across organizations are comparable in that both require deliberate design interventions to creative effective networks for coordination.

The 14 key concepts identified in the theoretical frameworks analysis are mapped to care coordination challenges in the fishbone diagram (see Figure 8-1). This type of diagram was chosen because of its ability to illustrate the complexity of the topic and give clarity to the major themes involved. The fishbone is a scientific tool used to identify and clarify causes of an effect of interest. (Nelson E.C., Batalden, & Godfrey, 2007) This mapping facilitates the systematic exploration of the key concepts to consider while retaining the confidence of the foundation of the research process from which they emerged, the goal of such an analysis is to improving work in the organization. As the experience of care coordination grows, modifications to this model may emerge.

Figure 8-1. Care Coordination Fishbone Diagram

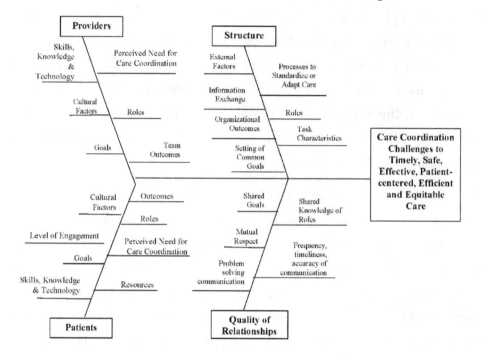

Care Coordination Challenges Fishbone Diagram

The fishbone diagram is comprised of the 14 key care coordination concepts grouped into four major categories (the big bones attaching to the spine), allowing them to be mapped to the care coordination challenges. Within each major category are multiple concepts which can be explored further for their contribution as specific causes of challenges to care coordination. In addition to serving as a mapping tool, the fish bone is an assessment tool and a model to launch improvement work. The exploration and potential improvement will depend on the characteristics and priorities of the organization interested in improving its care coordination. This mapping process is important as it provides a strategy with which to approach existing and future care coordination challenges.

As previously noted, the major care coordination concepts comprise the big bones and the various key concepts are listed on the smaller bones. Some of the key concepts recur in each of the major categories because the challenge is expressed differently within the category and merits a unique response. The major categories are: (1) structure, (2) patients, (3) providers, and (4) quality of relationships. Although the authors did not set out to do so, the categories resonate strongly with the four levels of the IOM redesign in the IOM's 2001 *Crossing the Quality Chasm* report described by Berwick: the organizations that house and support microsystems and the environment of laws, rules, payment, accreditation, and professional training that shape organizational action (these two levels correspond to the 'structure' category); patients' experiences ('patients' category) and the "microsystems" that actually give care ('providers' category).

Structure

Under the concept of 'Structure' the following elements are clustered: external factors, processes to standardize or adapt care, information exchange, task characteristics, roles, goals, and outcomes. Aspects of structure considered when discussing care coordination challenges include the physical and organizational characteristics that support and direct care delivery. They also include the number of participating providers and provider organizations, their specializations and how they are grouped, the amount of information required to manage the care of the patient or patient group, and existing linkages between the entities. As noted previously, a major challenge that patients often unwittingly face in accessing health care is a formal system of care characterized by 'silos' because of poor linkages and accountability between and within entities. The Structure category is designed to address these challenges.

The 'External factors' linked with structure include national and state health policy, economic factors, dependency on regulations, and existing resources. Political leaders in health care must wisely steward revenue, develop appropriate policies and should remain connected to and learning from disciplines outside of healthcare. Historically, business acumen, policy and leadership theory, and organizational design have not been a part of medical, nursing or allied health curriculums. These cross-cutting dimensions should be infused through undergrad and graduate medical education to help address these challenges ingrained in healthcare. There should be recognition of the value of involving complementing expertise from outside healthcare, at both a macro and a micro level.

An example of an external factor is coding of patient care by physicians. How does a practitioner ensure that documentation and coding for reimbursement sufficiently and appropriately reflect the care being provided? An analysis of the fishbone for coding practices at the organization level may reveal a significant difference between national benchmarks and local utilization by providers. This may lead to creation of a 'cheat sheet' for major diagnoses coding, letting physicians understand the significance of diagnosis specificity, and appreciate the targeted and timely information at point of care. With the added reimbursement from proper coding of previously hidden procedures, it's possible that other activities physicians wish to do around patient care, but have been unable to afford, such as care coordination, may be within reach. Additionally, breaking the silos between hospital coders and provider is underappreciated, and ambulatory practices should consider embedding coders to improve diagnostic accuracy.

Evidence-based practice, another external factor, extends to the ability to monitor advances in other industries which may have relevance to healthcare. An example from the last decade in the published work of Provonost and Gawande is the recognition by open minded health care workers of safety principles which have been successfully developed and applied to improve processes in the aviation industry and can be applied in health care. The safety practices honed in aviation are now being modified, applied and scaled up in health care with compelling impact on patient outcomes. (Gawande, 2009; Provonost, September 3, 2013)

'Administrative operational processes' to standardize or adapt care are a part of the overall structure category. Impersonal methods involving standardized arrangements and minimal feedback, such as the rote application of guidelines, create an inflexible structure that may result in standardized care but not care that is adaptive or improving. Personal methods that communicate between individuals and teams with considerable feedback, and group methods with joint planning and decision making with maximum feedback, are methods which standardize or adapt care and improve processes. (Gittell & Weiss, 2004)

The 'Exchange of information' garners much attention in the literature. Different expectations about the information needed, lack of accountability, failure to provide timely and consistent information between providers and settings, lack of standardization based on best practice, and role clarification all are challenges involved in 'the exchange of information'. The relationship to outcomes is well documented, for example in the area of exchange of information about the patient's medication list between providers and settings, an area fraught with frustration and known lapses. Medication reconciliation is quickly becoming a standard best practice, shown to result in better quality care and reduced costs and errors.

The benefits of health information exchange and electronic record communication are assumed for the purposes of this chapter and can be read about in detail elsewhere. However, clinicians and administrative staff complain about the limitations and frustrations associated with electronic communication. Care coordination is affected by the capacity of practice staff to access and respond to information, and access should improve when it is sent electronically, but this is a capacity which varies considerably amongst practitioners. Different electronic record systems mean that 'work-a-rounds' have to be created for exchange of information, which is cumbersome and takes time. Maximizing existing EMR capabilities to overcome perceived difficulties requires more time and resources than many primary care practices can afford. (O'Malley, Grossman, Cohen,

Kemper, & Pham, 2010) Overflow of information and "alert fatigue" has become common - just because a fax is sent or a record available does not necessarily help if there are multiple pages to read, or as one cardiac nurse said:

> 'We're glad to get the referral but to have to wade through all that paper when we are pressed for time – never mind find the medication list – is just too much.'

The concept 'Characteristic of the care coordination task' is placed within the structure of care coordination. Much could be written from an anecdotal perspective about the tasks associated with coordinating care at the point of service. As previously noted, a major challenge is the lack of standardization of the process of coordinating patient care, especially during transitions and across settings. The variability in skills needed and the lack of certainty in outcomes contributes to the lack of standardization. (Van Houdt et al., 2013)

Some tasks may seem simple but require maturity and/or knowledge on the part of the clinician for optimal results. For example, in the case of delegation of a follow up phone call to a patient following transition out of the hospital, if the information needed can be determined by a question as straightforward as: 'What transportation have you arranged for your appointment tomorrow?' one may have reasonable confidence in the information gleaned. Considerable experience is required, however, on the part of the clinician to gain rapport with the patient quickly through such a 'cold call', to know how to ask the question and be able to identify less obvious issues that may need to be addressed. The patient may have every intention of going to the appointment, but lacks the resources necessary to get there and feels ashamed to disclose the problem. A checklist of possible phrases to use may be helpful in bringing to light issues that may be more obvious in a face-to-face encounter.

Another task is the timely and pertinent documentation of care management and care coordination. Because it is a longitudinal activity, spanning multiple settings and involving multiple practitioners, the work and value of documentation is a challenge. How much detail is needed for providers? What level of information needs to pass from one entity to another? Does software incorporate 'tickler' systems or just-in-time workflow tasks?

Coordination of care activities take time. The time is difficult to quantify, the results difficult to connect to outcomes and therefore difficult to justify for reimbursement. Making phone calls to different agencies, closing loops between service providers such as referral sources or when making referrals, analyzing data to target interventions all take time, which is not embedded in a fee-for-service models of payment. With the advent of value-based purchasing and accountable care, the value of care coordination activities may increase as providers assume more risk for the outcomes.

Patients

The second care coordination concept category is 'patients.' Embedded in this category are the cultural factors pertaining to patients, the perceived need for care coordination, patient resources, level of engagement, patient knowledge of and use of technology, roles, goals, and outcomes.

To state the obvious: patients vary greatly in their health status, health literacy, available resources, engagement with the health care system and their (or their caregiver's) ability to manage care. With the degree of specialization in healthcare, clinical information about patients can be highly complex and involve multiple disease processes. Cultural factors that may be critical to patient choice and healing, such as attitudes, beliefs, preferences, family situation and values factor into their participation in the health care system. Gittell and Wiess note that clinical, social and administrative information is not easily codified for transmission amongst providers. (Gittell & Weiss, 2004) Care coordination as part of population management is challenged by the need to use limited resources wisely with as many patients as possible without losing the specificity that may be necessary to engage individual patients and build their capacity to self-manage health care.

The patient and family caregiver are typically the only common thread in all settings and by default have to coordinate their care. (E.A. Coleman, 2003 Apr; Eric A. Coleman & Berenson, 2004) A challenge is that they often lack the skills, knowledge, confidence or connection with the kind of health coaching that effectively does that coordination. As mentioned previously, many patients live with multiple chronic conditions, complex health care needs and functional limitations that require comprehensive care coordination. Challenges exist in effectively engaging them in their own care, leveraging resources, and incorporating best practices using technology. In care coordination, patient centeredness is a constant challenge and requires intentional, sustained patient feedback.

Patients may not even perceive the need for coordination. Even if they do understand the need for coordination and have the capacity to coordinate their own care, they may not be willing to take responsibility for coordination. As the administrator of one emergency department said,

> 'We the health workers have created this in the health care system: because we have done everything for them and kept them in a passive role we have fostered a generation of patients who do not expect to participate in their care; they expect to just be recipients of care.'[*]

This speaks to the validity of role clarification and goal setting, not just among providers or healthcare organizations, but also between patients, their caregivers, and systems of care.

Providers

The key concepts clustered around the category of Providers overlap somewhat with the Patient category but are expressed differently: skills and knowledge, proficiency with technology, perceived need for care

---

[*] Per business meeting discussion with administrator of the Emergency Department at the October 1, 2013 Care Coordination Subcommittee meeting in Bridgeport, CT.

coordination, and roles, goals and outcomes. The coordination dimension to health care is sometimes recognized by providers as common sense, but may be perceived as near impossible to execute due to a system entrenched in episodic and setting-specific payment silos. The status quo and absence of precedence in doing anything different also contributes to a lack of expectation. A physician may express anger over a delayed hospital lab report while ignoring a lack of timely communication of results from other clinicians.

There is a lack of education and skill about the relevance of data, benchmarking and population management. Physicians also struggle with the challenges of running practices without formal business or leadership education. In one review of the literature, Stille et al. note that in order to effectively accomplish the tasks of coordination, physicians need training in building teams whose education and skills respond to the physicians' panel of patients and whose roles are clearly defined, especially for the sake of the patient's understanding. (Stille et al., 2005)

Providers have 'new initiative fatigue' and are rightly skeptical about the difference promised by the next change. On the other hand, there is a deep seated desire to be part of excellent work, and hope their efforts are not wasted in the pursuit of better health for patients.

Expectations or lack of expectations is an unfortunate phenomenon that erodes the edges of care coordination efforts. Providers do not expect to take responsibility for the patient in transition. Coordination mechanisms are well intentioned but generally are ad=hoc and seem to collapse when those involved in the process leave the system. Providers do not expect patients will be able to take responsibility for their personal health information or medication list nor do they expect communication from providers in other specialties and settings. Providers do not experience nor expect accurate and timely communication from others in the system, despite evidence related to improved outcomes with robust two-way communication. Clinicians work in parallel rather than collaboratively, which leaves patients at risk for disjointed, ineffective care. (Stille et al., 2005) Opportunities to standardize the referral process abound but without common goals and role clarification it is unlikely to happen.

One specialist noted,

'I have worked for 20 years in this system and what we are talking about is a culture change. Physicians have been historically very competitive and worked hard to hold on to their piece of the action and are very suspicious of each other. We have to change that culture so that we are on the same team for the sake of the patient. It will take a change in the culture.'*

Clinicians in urgent care centers feel that community physicians do not respect them and feel they are treated disrespectfully, particularly by specialists. When ambulatory or ED settings reach out to primary care physicians they find it difficult to get past the gate keepers to speak with the physicians for effective hand offs and become discouraged in doing so. Clinicians in the community are ignored by the hospitalists who do not know them and are not incentivized to keep the loop closed.

It takes time, effort and persistence to disseminate evidence-based practice effectively. When clinicians have read the literature, return to school or participate in work groups, there is more awareness of best practices and of the need to work toward models that demonstrate better outcomes. The adage 'it takes seven times for an adult to hear something' was never truer than with the area of sustainable change in a health care system, working with providers. Providers are constantly pushed for time, balancing multiple agendas, and stressed about risk management. Consistent messaging over time as well as using principles of adult learning are just as important for the providers as it is for patients. Indeed, it is important to demonstrate with the providers what they are being challenged to do with patients.

---

* Per business meeting discussion with a specialist at the October 10, 2013 Quality & Utilization Review Committee meeting in Bridgeport, CT.

Relationships

Quality of relationships is another major challenge for care coordination. Perceived status differences among caregivers, and between caregivers and patients, undermine and challenge effective communication needed in coordinating patient care. Status differences between organizations in the continuum of care, such as the traditionally higher status a hospital has over other providers in the community, has also posed an obstacle to care coordination across the continuum. (Gittell & Weiss, 2004)

Addressing high-performance work practices that foster relational coordination is an opportunity for improved organizational performance. (Gittell et al., 2010) This includes selection of employees that have not only the technical skills but also team building skills, mutual respect, cross functional conflict resolution abilities, participation in shared rewards, who can appreciate cross functional face-to-face meetings, and respect the role of boundary spanners.

Our experience has shown how fragmented the relationships may be, and includes limited collaboration that crosses organizational boundaries and was initiated because of specific shared goals, such as reduction of re-hospitalization rates. These experiences involved Medicare intermediaries or forward thinking hospital systems managing heart failure patients. A local collaborative between hospitals and nursing homes, for example, generated important work around the use of personal health records and patient responsibility for medication lists. However, it stalled at the execution phase because of lack of shared resources and the time and leadership required on the part of all the stakeholders to persist in development of a sustainable model.

Factors contributing to quality of relationships on the fishbone chart include roles and goals. The patient centered medical home, for example, focuses on roles and relationships between roles in primary care practice, leveraging relationships to improve outcomes. Improved organizational performance is influenced by shared goals, appreciation for the overall work process, understanding by network participants of their own tasks, the tasks of others, and how they relate to overall work processes. Having respect for the work of others encourages members to value those contributions and consider the impact of their actions, further reinforcing the inclination to act with regard for the overall work process. This web of relationships reinforces the frequency, timeliness, accuracy and problem-solving nature of communication, enabling participants to effectively coordinate the work processes in which they are engaged. (Gittell, 2011)

Disrespect is one of the potential sources of division among those who play different roles in a given work process. Occupational identity serves as a source of pride, as well as a source of invidious comparison. Gittell describes how members of distinct occupational communities often have different status and may bolster their own status by actively cultivating disrespect for the work performed by others. When members of these distinct occupational communities are engaged in a common work process, the potential for these divisive relationships to undermine coordination is apparent. By contrast, respect for the competence of others creates a powerful bond, and is integral to the effective coordination of highly interdependent work.

Sample questions in each of the key dimensions posed by Gittell contribute to the mapping of challenges in the area of quality of relationships and suggest directions for improvement. For example, if the work process being examined is the caliber of handoff communication that occurs as patients move between provider settings, the following questions can be posed to providers in the different settings:

- *Frequent Communication*: How frequently do people in each of the groups communicate with you about the patient population in transition between your facilities?

- *Timely Communication*: Do people in the groups communicate with you in a timely way about the patients in transition?

- *Accurate Communication*: Do people in the groups communicate with you accurately about the patients in transition?

- *Problem Solving Communication*: When a problem occurs with patients in transition, do the people in the groups blame others or work with you to solve the problem?

- *Shared Goals*: Do people in the groups share your goals regarding patients in transition?

- *Shared Knowledge*: Do people in each of the groups know about the work you do with patients in transition?

- *Mutual Respect*: Do people in the groups respect the work you do with patients in transition?(Gittell, 2011)

Making these questions open ended and the use of 'why?' may glean helpful information on which to base improvements.

The fishbone tool allows an organization to map the challenges facing successful operationalization of care coordination and explore their causes. The four major groupings: structure, patients, providers and quality of relationships reflect the major issues facing healthcare organizations in implementing care coordination.

The Recommended Care Coordination Model

Care coordination has a vital role within a clinically integrated healthcare organization. It is distinct from case management. Nevertheless, case management has a broad and varied role within an organization. The case manager in an inpatient department or ambulatory clinic works directly with the patient and physician (Primary Care Provider [PCP]) or specialist). The manager directly engages the patient with their care and services, educates the patient about disease management, facilitates solutions, and overcomes barriers that inhibit effective care. Many hospitals utilize case managers to assist with transfer to sub-acute facilities and follow-up after discharge. Larger organizations may use case managers to follow patient populations for specific disease prevention programs, to limit readmissions, etc. Many organizations incorporate case managers in their electronic home monitoring (telemedicine) to follow patients within a specific population to minimize disease complications and readmissions. For example, congestive heart failure patients can be transitioned home with scales and blood pressure monitors that are used to automatically send biometric values to case managers who monitor these patients' chronic disease and maximize ambulatory treatment efficacy. Case managers assist with discharge follow-up, and tailor medical service referrals to reflect the individual's needs. A common operational issue that distinguishes case management from care coordination is that once a patient is discharged the case manager no longer works with the individual, or continued contact is narrowly focused to the exclusion of other chronic diseases or healthcare issues.

Care coordinators, on the other hand, reinforce the culture of the integrated network and the inherent linkages they instill among physicians, hospitals, and skilled nursing facilities. Care coordinators, based at the corporate/enterprise level, do not necessarily have direct patient contact. Instead, they utilize patient-specific and population medical data to constantly oversee the attributed patients of the organization. Attribution is a function of a payer/employer identifying the PCP responsible for the patient. The PCP member of a clinically integrated network organization is interdependent with the other physicians, and therefore the collective patient population of all PCPs determines the population of the organization.

With the corporate/enterprise level care coordinator, information technology is utilized to effectively organize attributed patients based upon risk, care gap alerts, and transition status (for example between home, hospital, ED, urgent care), to focus resources of the enterprise, reduce barriers to care, and enable/encourage the local network provider to effectively manage the individual patient. When the local facility is unable to effectively assist an individual the care coordinator may assist directly. Care coordination facilitates enculturation of process standardization to more effectively serve patients within the population. Care coordinators reinforce, encourage, and monitor patient care using information technology to monitor attributed patient care processes (standardized playbook adherence) through constant vigilance of reporting dashboards for patient care.

Care coordination has greater potential to be effective when clinical integration is fully implemented. Clinical integration uses evidence-based science to guide care of an individual patient and the greater population. Clinical integration allows all members of the healthcare team to utilize evidence-based guidelines, care transition requirements, healthcare metrics, and patient engagement requirements to effectively manage patients. Standardization throughout the organization allows for patient and population reporting to monitor and manage short and long-term medical issues/challenges facing patients.

The metrics used to follow quality, cost, and efficiency can be reported to organizational members with actionable data to guide patient level efforts. A "Playbook" that lists all payer required quality metrics, evidence-based preventative and chronic disease management, and minimal requirements for effective transition of patients between healthcare providers/facilities allows patients' data to be presented to care coordinators to guide institutional patient care with actionable communication with providers. The "Playbook" serves as the reference from which each practice can develop protocols and internal processes to allow all team members to function at their highest skill level, provide focused attention to high risk patients, and manage the population of patients with diverse care challenges. Effective local case management utilizing institutional evidence-based guidelines will allow increasingly more individuals to achieve improved health and system-wide care coordination monitoring processes and consequently will improve the health of the population.

Communication within the healthcare organization happens continuously to meet patient specific medical challenges. Population data is delivered monthly to allow the practice/facility level staff to focus local resources to make the most impact on patient health. For example, best practice dictates that if a patient is discharged from a hospital or emergency department, the patient needs follow-up by a physician within 7-14 days.

The following case study provides an example of how care coordination serves as an integral part of improving service delivery in the primary care setting.

Case Study: Primary Care Physician's Practice

This thriving independent primary care practice has multiple offices in a geographic span of 20 miles. This physician group leads the network's vision to transform healthcare to achieve the "Triple Aim". Recently as part of the CIN, this practice has been in the process of making an application to NCQA for Patient Centered Medical Home (PCMH) status. The Practice Manager has no prior experience in a PCMH model or precepts and was charged by the physician owner to lead the application process which she has done. Patient satisfaction surveys in the waiting rooms and the hiring of an APRN are two recent practice enhancements made to complete the application.

The PHO has monthly patient care meetings with each practice. The agenda includes: (1) response to previously identified issues, (2) identify new challenges, (3) review of the patient and practice population, (4) review of the active care plans of high risk patients, (5) review of the Playbook, and (6) evaluate the PCMH application progress. The meeting identified existing patients with high prospective risk, readmission risk, patients who had utilized the emergency department (ED) in the prior 12 months and the patients past due for prevention tests.

Two patients were brought to the attention of the practice physicians: one was a female patient who used the ED frequently (five times in the prior year due to ambulatory sensitive conditions). The Practice Manager made a note in the electronic medical record in anticipation of an already scheduled visit that month. At the next month's care coordination meeting she was able to report that the physician discussed the ED visits with the patient and developed a more appropriate emergency plan with her. Relevant to that plan, as part of its PCMH application, the practice had recently adjusted its after-hours telephone messaging system to

Case Study: Primary Care Physician's Practice

encompass safe access options communicated for the patients. Care Coordination staff will continue to support the local practice's monitoring of this and other patient's appropriate utilization but the patient is now aware of her physician's recommendations for her evidenced based care which is an effective predictor of behavioral change.

The Care Coordinator also reviewed a 57 year old male listed on the inpatient report and identified to have a high prospective risk. He has a severe complex cardiac disease with significant loss of ejection fraction (5% to 10%). During the past year, he had been an in-patient three times (total of 19 days), in observation twice, elective inpatient admission twice for procedures, and to the ED. In the month prior the PCP said that the patient had been non-compliant in the past with all aspects of care and recommendations related to medications, dietary restrictions and follow up and had not cooperated with the PCP. The PCP was extremely frustrated with the patient and considered that the patient might consider another physician.

The Care Coordinator had collaborated with the network's heart failure (HF) clinic to follow the patient after the current hospitalization as part of the care plan facilitating the patient to connect to the network. The care coordinator learned from the HF clinic that he had refused to use the facility in the past. During the hospitalization, the attending cardiologist requested that an HF clinic nurse see the patient and try to convince him to go to the clinic. One of the HF clinic nurses did go visit the patient making a personal connection and advised him of the benefits of the clinic and how it worked. The patient reluctantly agreed to go to the clinic and an appointment was set for five days after discharge. The Care Coordinator recommended specifying incremental goals with which the patient could be successful.

Despite skepticism of the staff and physicians, the patient kept his appointment. The HF clinic's goal was to prevent a 30 day readmission and successfully educate the patient about better dietary choices, medication compliance, and self-monitoring techniques to decrease his symptoms and improve the quality of his life while living with heart failure. He was also instructed about the importance of carrying a current medication list with him at all times and showing the list at each health care appointment. This was accomplished because the patient kept his follow-up visits to the heart failure clinic over a period of four months. His wife and physicians receive frequent updates allowing the family to participate and reinforce the patient to participate with the care plan. At times, he has been impatient and stated he wasn't coming back but he has returned for each visit so far, has successfully decreased weight and has not been readmitted in four months. For this patient, the appropriate setting for care was the HF clinic. The PCP and HF clinic are now working as a team leading to successful patient engagement.

Clinical integration improves the ability for the healthcare team to share data between members of the organization to effectively follow the patient. This case study illustrated how care mangers organize and arrange for the follow-up of each patient, while care coordinators validate organizational success to meet the follow-up requirements. When the system is challenged, care coordination quickly identifies the barriers and begins to effect organizational adaptation to assure patient and population care.

Care coordinators are presented population data detailing those who are at risk of disease complications. They communicate with PCPs and specialists to aggressively manage patients thereby reducing their overall risk. Additionally, care coordinators share with each practice location patients who have not met disease or preventative care measures and summarizes for the practice where their focus will be most successful. Ideally, communication with each practice location is continuous to manage individual patients and periodically to manage patient-centered groups. An example is the bundle of tests recommended at regular intervals for the organization's diabetic patients: LDL, urine, hemoglobin A1C, foot and eye exams. Using information systems and health data (e.g., electronic medical records, claims data, etc.) the practices can tailor their patient outreach to anticipate test needs and to close gaps.

When the patient requires medical service not offered within the network, or the patient utilizes non-network services, care coordination is vital to evaluate and monitor the quality and cost of that care to develop strategic organizational growth and manage the cost-of-care to affect organizational shared saving programs. Given the intra and inter-organizational healthcare opportunities described, one can begin to appreciate how complicated the Multi-Level Framework becomes.

Medical management is differentiated from services. Medical services are the face-to-face patient-directed healthcare events. These include the physician-patient visit/event, and other health care encounters such as radiologic study and counseling by a nutritionist. Medical services are rendered to each individual patient. Case management is a component of services offered directly to the patient. This is done locally as close to the patient as possible to insure that socioeconomic barriers are considered and factored into the individual care plan. The care plan may be developed by various numbers of healthcare professionals, but the plan respects the patient's desire for care. Case management coordinates resources and opportunities to uphold the care plan and assure the patient of its success. The plan updates with each healthcare contact and change in patient status.

Care of patients with chronic disease continues to demonstrate disparities with care provision. Less than 50% of diabetic patients have timely eye exams. Many diabetics fail to have an HbA1C evaluated at least two times per year. Actual follow-up after hospitalization or emergency room evaluation within recommended time frames frequently are not completed and these realities continue to increase the cost-of-care. Using a "Playbook" construct reinforces expectation and allows for identification of care delivery concerns. Even though case management programs have been institutionalized for many years, readmission rates, patient-care follow-up, and disease management measures still remain national challenges.

Clinical integration can minimize failure to facilitate patient data portability, improves intra organizational communication, minimizes the cost-of-care by reducing redundant services, and facilitates the right care at the right time with the right resource. Table 8-2 is a sample from an organizational "Playbook" detailing the minimum recommendation for diabetic care. The sample illustrates the measured metrics to be reported, the evidence-based recommendations to care for a diabetic patient, and allows providers and their support staff to anticipate patient needs to demonstrate quality care.

Table 8-2. Playbook Recommendations for Diabetic Care

WHO?	WHAT?	WHEN?
Adults ages 18-75 years with	➤ Check at least once annually: ○ LDL-C level (target measure is	During measurement

WHO?	WHAT?	WHEN?
diabetes mellitus	<100 mg/dL) o Urine micro albumin or macro albumin or treatment of nephropathy o Neuropathy screen or evidence of medical attention to existing neuropathy o Blood pressure (Target measure is <140/90) o Tobacco use status (Target measure is # non-users) o Comprehensive foot examination o Dilated eye exam by ophthalmologist/optometrist o Serum creatinine & calculated GFR o BMI	year During measurement year
	➢ Check HbA1C at least 2 times annually; target measure is <8% for most patients (2-4 times based on goal)	In previous 2 years
	➢ Prescribe at least 2 generic diabetic medications with at least 80% days covered since first Rx	In the previous 12 months
		Every visit
	➢ Two or more face-to-face visits for diabetes	
	➢ CCD printed; includes action plan	
Adults ages 18-75 years with diabetes mellitus and ischemic	Documented daily aspirin or antiplatelet medication use	During the measurement year

WHO?	WHAT?	WHEN?
vascular disease	(ACCEPTED CONTRAINDICATIONS: Anticoagulant use, Lovenox (enoxaparin) or Coumadin (warfarin) Any history of gastrointestinal (GI)* or intracranial bleed (ICB) Allergy to aspirin (ASA) *Gastroesophogeal reflux disease (GERD) is not automatically considered a contraindication but may be included if specifically documented as a contraindication by the physician. The following may be exclusions if specifically documented by the physician: Use of non-steroidal anti-inflammatory agents Documented risk for drug interaction Uncontrolled hypertension defined as 180 systolic, 110 diastolic Other provider documented reason for not being on ASA therapy)	

Future

"Flooding the Triple Aim zone"

Healthcare organizations have institutionalized various models of care coordination and case management. Few detailed descriptions have appeared in medical literature. Clinical integration is more than a proposed vision or philosophy; it should be an organizational mission that adapts to the perturbations of healthcare reform. Growing evidence, Einthoven et al., suggests that greater organizational integration is associated with higher quality and efficiency (such as reduced mortality secondary to myocardial infarction). (Enthoven & Tollen, 2005)

The American Hospital Association defines clinical integration as needing to facilitate the coordination of patient care across conditions, providers, settings, and time in order to achieve care that is safe, timely, effective, efficient, equitable, and patient-focused. (American Hospital Association, February 2010) To achieve clinical integration we need to promote changes in provider culture, redesign payment methods and incentives, and modernize federal laws. Care coordination is the adhesive within a healthcare network that promotes recognition for evidence-based medicine and utilization of standardized medical delivery accentuating patient/provider communication and compliance to individual care plans.

Larger organizations are more likely to use organized care management processes compared to smaller organizations. Additionally, independent physician associations (IPA) are twice as likely to use effective care management processes as small groups without IPA affiliation. Medical Services are the patient care events occurring in each member's facilities. The services are face-to-face and include office visits, consultations, inpatient admissions, emergency department visits, special nursing facility admission, etc. Medical management is a total approach to managing attributed population while facilitating and focusing efforts to achieve preventative health maintenance while addressing existing chronic disease issues of each patient. Several authors (Ahgren, Axelsson, and others) have described horizontal clinical integration as the services within a facility and vertical clinical integration as services provided at the organizational level to "manage" the population while empowering each patient care location to successfully manage their empaneled patients. (Ahgren & Axelsson, 2007)

The following case study illustrates how taking advantage of system-wide information systems, care coordinators monitor all patients attributed to the PHO and facilitate internal data analysis distribution to each practice and physician. The data specifically articulates the patients attributed, and provides actionable guidance for each practice to focus local efforts to manage those patients with high risk or significant risk change, over utilizers of emergent services, those recently admitted, and the list of patients needing preventative care. Additionally enterprise care coordinators assist the local case managers with direct patient outreach for highly complicated patients requiring additional personalization to achieve disease management.

Case Study: Primary Care Physician and Urgent Care

A 44 year old Type 2 Diabetic was identified in monthly data review of the PCP's attributed patients. The care coordinator flagged the patient as requiring closer attention because the Emergency Department (ED) was used six times within a year. The primary and secondary diagnoses for the ED visits were all ambulatory sensitive conditions. The Care Coordinator contacted the PCP who was unaware of the patient's history of ED visits, having not been consulted or given feedback by the ED. The last scheduled appointment for this patient was three months prior and he had been a 'no show'. He had last come for an appointment eight months before and then had been a 'no show' a month later. The patient had not responded to phone call reminders from PCP's office.

After reviewing the risk data, system utilization data, and overdue care alerts, the care coordinator purposefully contacted the PCP to review the patient's medical challenges. The PCP verbalized frustration because the patient seemed unengaged. The PCP reviewed patient data (from various sources including insurance claims). After discussion with the PCP, a care plan was developed.

The care coordinator attempted to engage the patient telephonically (voicemail), and after several attempts, direct patient contact was made (Friday afternoon). The care coordinator briefly described the care coordination program, the medical neighborhood concept, the need to maintain a relationship with a PCP, timely prevention testing, medication management, glucose management, less copays, and limited ED visits. The Patient was initially suspicious of the intervention, but willing to talk.

The patient said he was unable to go to the PCP during day because of his current work jobsite restrictions. He stated 'It's funny that you should call me - I ran out of

Case Study: Primary Care Physician and Urgent Care

my Metformin a few days ago. Twice I called my CVS and they got refills, first 10 pills and then 6 but I ran out a few days ago.' When the CVS Care Coordinator asked him about checking his blood sugar he responded: 'Well I left my glucometer at the place that I moved from so no - I haven't been checking that for a while.' He stated that he has continued to take his insulin. He had never been to an Urgent Care and denied knowledge that it is an appropriate alternative to the ED.

Through discussions with the PCP, the Urgent Care manager and the patient, he was redirected to the Urgent Care within blocks of his home and instructed to follow up with an appointment at the PCP within a week. The Urgent Care manager prepared the staff to receive the patient, and he was able to be assessed after work, received a prescription for his diabetic medication which he obtained at the pharmacy that night.

To reinforce the best practice transition protocol (described in the Playbook), the Urgent Care staff was reminded to communicate to the PCP about the visit. The patient was asked to make a follow-up appointment with the PCP. Finally, after one unavoidable cancellation and 2 phone calls from the PCP's practice and the Care Coordinator, he was seen by the PCP. Because he needed a glucometer, one was provided (supplied by a local vendor) during his follow-up visit.

Subsequently, new patient care alerts indicated additional testing was past due (past due 25 months: LDL-C, HbA1C). When the Care Coordinator requested to the HbA1C and LDL results, the PCP noted to his surprise that he did not have them and was going to have the patient come to get the script and go to the lab. The Care Coordinator recommended electronic orders to Quest Lab and a call was made to the patient to get the lab tests done. The patient was happy to go directly to the lab and avoid an extra copay. The next day he did go to the lab. The labs, which were abnormal, were available during the next follow-up PCP appointment for review.

In summary care coordination will:

1. Utilize patient and population data analysis to effectively promote preventive care.

2. Utilize data to manage chronic disease.

3. Utilize data to achieve payer quality and utilization requirements.

    a. Readmission

    b. ED utilization

     c. Ambulatory sensitive conditions

4. Coordinate system-wide patient management with payers.

     a. Coordinate care coordination activities to maximize patient outreach

         i. Collaborate with disease management activities provided by insurers

5. Strategically communicate with members of the clinically integrated network to maximize location specific activities to achieve practice-level success.

Figure 8-2 illustrates how clinical integration focuses on clinical outcomes, patient experience and engagement, and utilization of services. In the proposed model, a clinically integrated network must consider each of these components as distinct entities that continuously interact and are not "managed" in silo. Current case management models focus on patient engagement with limited attention to outcome and cost. The reason that case management is well accepted is that healthcare organizations strengths predominate by provider directed care to a patient/customer. The case manager will filter outreach according to facility immediate disease/service strategies. In a functioning clinically integrated organization, the focus is not facility-based championed by local stakeholders, but population-based for the attributed patients to the whole organization. Care coordinators work with each member of the organization to enculturate standardized patient care initiatives with respect to preventative and disease management, transition of care observance, and agnostic payer quality initiatives.

Care coordination actions significantly contributes to a clinically integrated network's success to achieve the "Triple Aim". CMS and other leading organizations repeatedly report that five to seven percent of the population consumes a large proportion of healthcare resources. These actions allow the network to operationalize population management to reduce the risk of the most complicated patients while addressing the needs of each patient within the population.

Health information technology is a vital component to arm care coordinators with the data necessary to achieve the stated goals. Additionally, the health information technology pulls data from disparate systems into meaningful reports necessary to effectively manage a population served by a clinically integrated network. Clinical outcomes and transparency will determine which organizations successfully adapt to healthcare reform. Successful organizations are able to use technology to evaluate quality care, manage chronic disease, and anticipate care gaps. Healthcare organizations will increasingly need to meet patient expectation and provide professional quality care. Ultimately, public reporting of organizational success achieving competitive levels of quality will reinforce patient engagement and assure that organizational patient attribution is preserved.

When considering a multi-level framework, an organization must be continuously aware of challenges external to the organization (public policy, national and state legislation, local competition). Structure within the organization is vital to withstand uncontrollable external perturbations. Healthcare organizations that achieve national recognition for achieving clinical integration excellence have the structure to manage a network that meets the "Triple Aim" goals. A network of medical providers exists in various levels of accomplishment and care coordination engenders the organizational culture of transformation. Change is not dictatorial but developed through relationships. Care coordination becomes the organizational glue that binds each member of the network to reach patient care goals that encompass the patient but affects the population at-large.

Authors such as Hernandez and Burns have differentiated the delivery of integrated healthcare through horizontal and vertical integration. (Burns & Pauly, 2002; Hernandez, 1999) Horizontal integration occurs when healthcare organizations consolidate and utilize economies of scale to benefit from purchasing, shared physical plant, shared capital, and spreading fixed costs over a larger base of operation. Additionally, a large organization could benefit from a wider patient base to make multiple service lines profitable. These organizations typically utilized the size to steer patients to a central "hub" facility. Unfortunately, realization of scaled savings has not been well demonstrated. Vertical integration attempts to provide patient care using multiple organizations seamlessly. The goal is to utilize providers and facilities that demonstrate cost-effective high quality care. Case management typically reinforces the horizontal approach to healthcare delivery, while care coordination's strength is to provide vertical care to the patient and population.

Vertical integration focuses on the care of a patient population. Successful vertical integration requires collaboration between aligned organizations and providers. Historically, horizontal care of the patient has not met with reduced healthcare cost. Consequently, public policy is driving alternative models. Intuitively organizations such as ACOs and PHOs that are responsible for populations of patients should be able to contain costs between economically competing entities to provide overall comprehensive patient care. These models of care, focused on population health and care coordination, should result in reductions in healthcare costs. Vertical care tested in small projects has demonstrated success.

Comparisons of facility charges are abundant in the literature. The cost of a hospital charge per day versus special nursing facility is dramatic. Greater attention is focusing on how to utilize the right setting to effectively provide patient care services. Unfortunately, barriers to using cost-effective settings are challenged by healthcare policy, and unfamiliarity with individual setting capabilities. Additionally, strong leadership is necessary to develop a clinically integrated network that offers significant options of patient care settings to advantageously provide quality cost-effective patient directed care.

Figure 8-2. Clinical Integration: A Vertically Integrated System

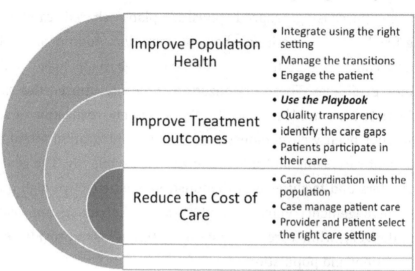

Improve Population Health	• Integrate using the right setting • Manage the transitions • Engage the patient
Improve Treatment outcomes	• *Use the Playbook* • Quality transparency • identify the care gaps • Patients participate in their care
Reduce the Cost of Care	• Care Coordination with the population • Case manage patient care • Provider and Patient select the right care setting

Clinical integration in a mature healthcare system facilitates a patient to receive medical services in the right setting such as a patient's home, nursing facility, physician office, urgent care, or hospital. Clinical integration is the glue that combines medical services (direct patient care) and medical management (population health management) working in tandem to serve the individual without losing focus on the medical issues challenging the population. Clearly defining the roles of case management and care coordination as offered in the model provides a healthcare organization the vision to direct patient care to achieve the right care, at the right time, in the right setting, with the whole healthcare team participating in the care centered on the patient, respecting the patient, and affecting improved health of the population, one patient at a time and serving the whole population at large.

CHAPTER 8 DISCUSSION QUESTIONS

Discussion questions are provided for team building or class exercises. Answers for all questions are provided in Appendix C.

Question Number	Question
1	The fishbone diagram demonstrates the most common challenges facing an organization. How do you use the fishbone to meet the ever-changing organizational stressors that prevent high quality patient care?
2	What are the actionable features of the proposed care coordination model? How does it answer the Triple Aim?
3	Describe how the proposed care coordination model contributes to the goals of clinical integration.
4	Describe the difference between case management and care coordination.

CHAPTER 8 HIGHLIGHTS

✓ The purpose of care coordination is to meet the Triple Aim.

✓ Care Coordination is a unique role and distinctly different than case management.

✓ Care Coordination is most effective within a clinically integrated network.

✓ The fishbone diagram mapping care coordination challenges facilitates analysis by organizations of the challenges and their causes for solution development.

CHAPTER 8 REFERENCES

Agency for Healthcare Research and Quality. (2011). Chapter 2. What is care coordination?: Care coordination measures atlas. Retrieved from http://www.ahrq.gov/professionals/systems/long-term-care/resources/coordination/atlas/chapter2.html

Ahgren, B., & Axelsson, R. (2007). Determinants of integrated health care development: chains of care in Sweden. *The International Journal of Health Planning and Management*, 22(2), 145-157.

American Hospital Association. (2011). Hospitals and care systems of the future. AHA Committee on Performance Improvement Report. Retrieved from http://www.aha.org/content/11/hospitals-care-systems-of-future.pptx

American Hospital Association. (2010, February). Clinical integration – The key to real reform. Retrieved from http://www.aha.org/research/reports/tw/10feb-clinicinteg.pdf

Antonelli, R. C., McAllister, J. W., Popp, J., & Fund, C. (2009). Making care coordination a critical component of the pediatric health system: a multidisciplinary framework.

Balanced Budget Act of 1997. Pub L No. 105-33.

Ball, T., Merry, M., & Verlaan-Cole L. (2013). Designing & Creating "Second Curve" Healthcare Systems. Retrieved from http://www.cicatelli.org/tpp/files/Designing%20%20Creating%20Second%20Curve%20Healthcare%20Systems1.pdf

Beasley, C. (2009). The triple aim: Optimizing health, care, and cost. *Healthcare Executive*, 24, 64-66.

Berwick, D. M. (2002). A user's manual for the IOM's 'Quality Chasm'report. *Health Affairs*, 21(3), 80-90.

Burns, L. R., & Pauly, M. V. (2002). Integrated delivery networks: a detour on the road to integrated health care? *Health Affairs*, 21(4), 128-143.

Case Management Society of America. (2013). What is a case manager? Retrieved from http://www.cmsa.org/Home/CMSA/WhatisaCaseManager/tabid/224/Default.aspx

Chassin, M., R., & Galvin, R., W. (1998). The urgent need to improve health care quality: Institute of Medicine National Roundtable on Health Care Quality. *The Journal of the American Medical Association*, 280(11), 1000-1005.

Claiborne, N. (2006). Effectiveness of a care coordination model for stroke survivors: a randomized study. *Health & Social Work*, 31(2), 87-96.

Coleman, E. A. (2003, Apr). Falling through the cracks: Challenges and opportunities for improving transitional care for persons with continuous complex care needs. *American Geriatric Society*, 51(4), 549-555.

Coleman, E. A., & Berenson, R. A. (2004). Lost in transition: challenges and opportunities for improving the quality of transitional care. *Annals of Internal Medicine*, 141(7), 533-536.

Commission for Case Management Certification. (2013). FAQs about Case Management. Retrieved from http://ccmcertification.org/health-care-organizations/faqs-about-case-management

Committee on Quality of Healthcare in America, & Institute of Medicine. (2001) *Crossing the Quality Chasm. A New Health System for the 21st Century*. Washington, DC: National Academies Press.

Davis, K. (2010, June 23). U.S. ranks last among seven countries on healthcare performance. *Healthcare IT News*. Retrieved from http://www.healthcareitnews.com/news/us-ranks-last-among-seven-countries-healthcare-performance

Enthoven, A. C., & Tollen, L. A. (2005). Competition in health care: it takes systems to pursue quality and efficiency. *Health Affairs*, 24(5), 1383.

Gawande, A. (2009). *The Checklist Manifesto: How to get Things Right*. New York, New York: Metropolitan Books.

Gittell, J. H. (2011). Relational Coordination: Guidelines for Theory, Measurement and Analysis Retrieved from http://rcrc.brandeis.edu/downloads/Relational_Coordination_Guidelines_8-25-11.pdf

Gittell, J. H., Seidner, R., & Wimbush, J. (2010). A relational model of how high-performance work systems work. *Organization Science*, 21(2), 490-506. doi: org/10.1287/orsc.1090.0446

Gittell, J. H., & Weiss, L. (2004). Coordination networks within and across organizations: A Multi-level Framework*. *Journal of Management Studies*, 41(1), 127-153.

Hernandez, S. R. (1999). Horizontal and vertical healthcare integration: lessons learned from the United States. *HealthcarePapers*, 1(2), 59-66.

Improving Chronic Care (ICC). (2013). Care coordination. Retrieved from http://www.improvingchroniccare.org/index.php?p=Care_Coordination&s=326

Institute for Healthcare Improvement. (2011). Care coordination model: Better care at lower cost for people with multiple health and social needs. Retrieved from http://www.ihi.org/knowledge/Pages/IHIWhitePapers/IHICareCoordinationModelWhitePaper.aspx

Keller, H. (2013). Helen Keller Quotes. Retrieved from http://www.successories.com/iquote/author/830/helen-keller-quotes/1

Macmillan Dictionary. (2013). Definition of Coordination. Retrieved from http://www.macmillandictionary.com/us/dictionary/american/coordination

Maryland Department of Health and Mental Hygiene. (2013). Comprehensive Care Management Program. Retrieved from http://dhmh.maryland.gov/bhd/Documents/ValueOptionsComprehensiveCareManagementProgram.pdf

National Coalition on Care Coordination. (2013). What is Care Coordination? . Retrieved from http://www.nyam.org/social-work-leadership-institute-v2/care-coordination/

National Priorities Partnership. (2008). National Priorities and Goals: Aligning Our Efforts to Transform America's Healthcare. Washington, DC: National Quality Forum.

National Quality Forum. (2006).NQF-Endorsed® Definitions and Framework for Measuring Care .

Coordination. from http://www.qualityforum.org/Home.aspx

National Quality Forum. (2010). Quality Connections: Care Coordination. Retrieved from www.qualityforum.org

National Quality Forum. (2013). Effective Communication and Care Coordination. Retrieved from http://www.qualityforum.org/Topics/Effective_Communication_and_Care_Coordination.aspx

Nelson E.C., Batalden, P. B., & Godfrey, M. M. (2007). *Quality by Design*. San Francisco, CA: Jossey-Bass.

O'Malley, A., S., Grossman, J., M., Cohen, G., R., Kemper, N., M., & Pham, H. H. (2010). Are electronic medical records helpful for care coordination? Experiences of physician practices. *Journal of General Internal Medicine*, 25(3), 177-185. doi: 10.1007/s11606-009-1195-2

Peikes, D., Chen, A., Schore, J., & Brown, R. (2009). Effects of care coordination on hospitalization, quality of care, and health care expenditures among Medicare beneficiaries: 15 randomized trials. *The Journal of the American Medical Association*, 301(6), 603-618. doi: 10.1001/jama.2009.126

Provonost, P. (2013, September 3). A Powerful idea from the nuclear industry. Retrieved from http://thehealthcareblog.com/blog/tag/peter-pronovost/

Reuben, D., B. (2007). Better care for older people with chronic diseases: an emerging vision. *The Journal of the American Medical Association*, 298(22), 2673-2674.

Robinson, K., M. (2010). Care coordination: A priority for health reform. *Policy, Politics, & Nursing Practice*, 11(4), 266-274. doi: 10.1177/1527154410396572

Shier, G., Ginsburg, M., Howell, J., Volland, P., & Golden, R. (2013). Strong social support services, such as transportation and help for caregivers, can lead to lower health care use and costs. *Health Affairs*, 32(3), 544-551. doi: 10.1377/hlthaff.2012.0170

Slee, D. A., Slee, V. N., & Schmidt, H. J. (2008). *Slee's Health Care Terms* (Fifth ed.). Sudbury, MA: Jones and Bartlett's Publishers.

Stille, C. J., Jerant, A., Bell, D., Meltzer, D., & Elmore, J. G. (2005). Coordinating care across diseases, settings, and clinicians: a key role for the generalist in practice. *Annals of Internal Medicine*, 142(8), 700-708.

U.S. Congress. Balanced Budget Act of 1997 (1997).

Van Houdt, S., Heyrman, J., Vanhaecht, K., Sermeus, W., & De Lepeleire, J. (2013). An in-depth analysis of theoretical frameworks for the study of care coordination. *International Journal of Integrated Care*, 13.

Volland, P. J., Schraeder, C., Shelton, P., & Hess, I. (2012). The transitional care and comprehensive care coordination debate. *Generations*, 36(4), 13-19.

Chapter 9. Standards for the CIN

Kylanne Green

It takes a lot of courage to release the familiar and seemingly secure, to embrace the new. But there is no real security in what is no longer meaningful. There is more security in the adventurous and exciting, for in movement there is life, and in change there is power.

Alan Cohen
1954 - Present
American Entrepreneur

CHAPTER 9 LEARNING OBJECTIVES

✓ Understand the importance of national performance standards and accreditation across the healthcare industry.

✓ Explore how clinical integration fits into the continuum of care from patient centered medical homes to total population management.

✓ Examine how accreditation advances excellence in clinical integration.

✓ Understand how accreditation process readies networks for optimum development and then verifies that objectives have been met.

Introduction

In today's markets, healthcare leaders seek to establish optimum arrangements that will enable care providers to avail themselves of innovative payer opportunities while meeting demands for improved care of patient populations. New ventures spawned by these innovative opportunities, such as Accountable Care Organizations (ACOs) and Clinically Integrated Networks (CINs), are designed to use the strengths of available medical professionals, address recognized gaps in care and promote performance transparency. This chapter explores how to envision, organize and execute these new undertakings, assisted by the tools of accreditation and performance standards.

The enabling and validating pathways for integration and accountability are found in the URAC accreditation process for CINs and ACOs. CINs are a means to organize health care delivery that can ready provider groups to become sustainable through market responsiveness and accountability. URAC is a not-for-profit healthcare accreditation organization committed to strategies that foster consumer empowerment and protection and health care management, innovation, and improvement. URAC accreditation standards show the way to integration and accountability and provide validation of successful progression and achievement.

An accredited CIN is a provider collaboration that may be horizontally or vertically structured. A CIN may take many forms and may include one or more hospitals or a health system, aligned or employed physicians, independent practices and other service providers. The network coordinates care and is collectively responsible for cost and quality of care for a group of patients for whom they have contracted to provide services. Evolving beyond traditional hospital or primary care environments, a group of providers forming a CIN transforms itself into broader networks of providers and services operating in a well-coordinated, cohesive manner across the healthcare neighborhood. The resulting entity is established to develop, govern and administer an active, ongoing program of clinical initiatives to improve care delivery patterns and thus the quality of health care services. Successful practice transformation can be demonstrated through measurement and reporting of greater effectiveness, and efficiency-resulting cost savings.

Following the URAC standards roadmap while transitioning to an entity with these objectives supports systematic achievement of the IHI Triple Aim of optimizing healthcare performance. Providers take the lead in these ventures to pursue the three essential healthcare system dimensions articulated by IHI: improving the patient experience of care (including quality and satisfaction); improving the health of populations; and reducing the per capita cost of care. (Institute for Healthcare Improvement, 2014)

CINs occupy a vital place in the health care system and URAC's provider accreditation continuum. As the healthcare industry transitions to a more value-based, prevention-minded, population-management model, URAC has promulgated performance standards that emphasize patient centeredness, adoption of health information systems, care coordination, population health, and transparency in performance measurement and reporting. As Figure 9-1 shows, clinical integration resides in a space between Patient-Centered Medical Homes (PCMH) and the full risk bearing ACOs. While the CIN may accept risk, the ACO is a more sophisticated, technologically buoyed and advanced population management entity. The ACO may evolve from the integrated CIN foundation and ultimately may take many commercial and government-sponsored forms, as recently reported by Leavitt Partners. (Peterson & et. al., June 2014) Certainly this kind of innovation will continue in this era of population oriented accountability, and yet unseen arrangements will emerge. Figure 9-1 also provides a high level illustration of the building blocks of higher order networks that are the foundation of URAC accreditation programs.

Figure 9-1. URAC Accreditation Building Blocks

Accreditation Building Blocks

Fee for Service | Health Care Delivery | PCMH | Clinical Integration | Accountable Care | Health Care Financing and Management | Pay for Performance

Medical Home / Primary Care Practitioners | Provider Network / Specialty Providers | Clinically Integrated Networks / Systems | Accountable Care Organizations

Evolution of the Delivery System

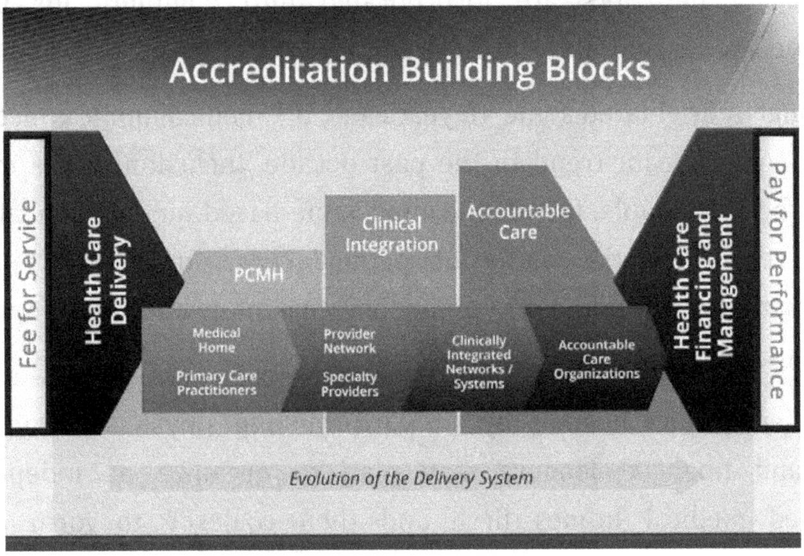

The building blocks for population health management move a health care organization progressively from the current "fee-for-service" state of payment for volume of services to payment for the demonstrated value of those services as evidenced by improved patient outcomes and efficient health care delivery. URAC's programs expedite this progression as primary-care providers work to achieve the aims of a medical home, develop integrative relationships among themselves and with specialty providers, and operate with greater efficiency and performance improvement purpose within a network of various types and levels of healthcare providers and groups. These networks bring together otherwise independent provider practices to form a vibrant interactive health care neighborhood in the markets they serve.

URAC Provider Care Integration and Coordination Model

The URAC accreditation model for assisting organizations with their journey to a higher level of quality and affordability is dynamic, scalable and not prescriptive. And while it appears the relationship of the three programs (i.e., PCMH, CIN, ACO) should be linear, networks and neighborhoods can grow in varied ways depending on the construct and needs of the local market. URAC provider recognition programs also embrace small as well as large organizations. With primary care as the base in PCMH, specialty and multispecialty networks are incorporated into eligibility for Clinical Integration and Accountable Care accreditations.

Although it originated some 40 years ago, the medical home concept has become a mainstream trend in the past decade. Inclusion of the medical home in the sustainable, forward leaning value-based models of healthcare delivery recognizes the value of patient centeredness and practice transformation as a foundation for collaborative integration and population health management.

Provider groups headed by forward-thinking physicians and other clinical and financial leaders may plan to organize as independent unaffiliated medical homes first, and then coalesce to form a CIN.

Alternatively, a CIN forms and becomes a driver for development and incorporation of medical homes in its network. An Accountable Care entity also may be the catalyst.

As provider-driven ventures, all of these self-governing organizations can create alignment of incentives and develop the infrastructure necessary to embrace a successful, financially viable and sustainable future. Medical home formation contributes consistency in point of service philosophy and approach to patient centered care, improved processes and better outcomes. The PCMH has contributed more than one important philosophical building block of clinical integration, including the roots of population health management. Most importantly, patient centeredness is the heart of both of these models. Patient centered organizations provide enhanced access to services provided by multidisciplinary teams and integrate patient engagement strategies. The medical home may provide the springboard for care coordination across the continuum of care, necessary for a CIN to operate legally and effectively.

The nucleus of care coordination embodied in the defined medical neighborhood enables these types of organizations to improve patterns of care delivery. Such improvements promote the opportunity to move into clinical integration and to accountable care.

The URAC advisory group that developed the clinical integration accreditation standards established baseline capabilities by alignment with the published FTC guidance, first published in 1996. (Department of Justice and Federal Trade Commission, 1996) The capabilities outlined in the original FTC guidelines also serve as the foundation for Accountable Care. Thus, in the progression of URAC recognition, integrated network organizations are expected to achieve CIN accreditation as a pre-requisite to Accountable Care.

URAC's model of provider accreditations permits network development and practice transformation along many different clinical service lines. After all, these organizations are intended to be market-driven and clinician led, and every market has their unique needs for clinical services. URAC recognizes that when it comes to point of care, all healthcare is local. So, networks essentially are medical neighborhoods for providers and patients.

URAC's model is flexible. For example, an organization can be an accredited CIN without necessarily having the primary-care focus inherent in medical homes. Some specialty networks have been among the first to embrace the URAC CIN accreditation process. The standards do require linkages – either in or out of network – between primary care practitioners and specialists, including those in behavioral health, believed to be essential for care coordination and population health management.

An appreciation of the clinician leadership, strong governance, and objectives of clinical coordination must pervade the formative organization. But how does a would-be CIN proceed? How does it know what the critical success factors are, and whether all parts of the integrating organization are pulling the same way? Creation of noteworthy integration efforts requires planning and implementation of a complex combination of both broad arrangements and the myriad of details necessary to draw disparate health care providers together and maintain allegiance to a network-wide set of goals. The URAC standards emphasize the processes and structures known to promote success: leadership, governance and management; information systems; care coordination; and measurement and reporting. Thomas Raskauskas, MD, President/CEO St. Vincent's Health Partners, in Bridgeport, CT, has said that he advises following URAC CIN standards as a roadmap to successful formation of a CIN and ACO.

In a highly strategic manner, successful leaders will discern the best arrangements to fit the geography and demography of its market and attributed populations, and fully leverage provider strengths. Top of license practice has been recommended for optimal care coordination. (National Transitions of Care Coalition, May 2008) Physician leadership is responsible for creating an inclusive, collaborative culture. The hallmark of these organizations is that they embrace point of care improvements such as effective exchange of clinical information necessary to coordinate care, and foster safe transitions from one setting or one provider to the next. The successful CIN is both clinically and financially integrated.

Ever present throughout the formation and operation of these initiatives is the obligation to justify the intense financial inter-dependencies and collaborations of otherwise competing providers. Improvements and efficiencies in care delivery, and resulting benefits to consumers, must outweigh potentially anticompetitive effects of such activities, as payer contract negotiations can demonstrate. Satisfying the Federal Trade Commission (FTC) and Department of Justice (DOJ) requires being continually aware that failure to convincingly operate as a clinically integrated network with an attendant beneficial consumer-oriented impact on care has been known to invite antitrust scrutiny. The FTC has articulated the requisite areas of demonstrated focus, and successful ways of serving the interests of consumers as: improvements in quality in terms of consumer outcomes; utilization conservation; and cost efficiencies. (Department of Justice and Federal Trade Commission, 1996) Adherence to URAC accreditation standards and demonstration of measured results from alterations in practice patterns will stand as evidence of the resolve to be financially sustainable, consumer focused, and population health oriented at the same time.

Roles of Accreditation

Accreditation programs are the health care industry's mechanisms to advance the adoption of systems, processes and performance requirements according to predetermined criteria and consistent, agreed-upon national standards. The accreditor develops an evaluative, rigorous, transparent and comprehensive process to examine whether an applicant organization meets predetermined criteria.

URAC, the only accreditor to offer Clinical Integration accreditation, launched its program in 2013 to address the needs of practices and providers as they develop and operate CINs, and evolve their organizations towards accountable care. Clinical Integration accreditation is one of three provider-oriented URAC accreditation initiatives and complementary to the URAC Patient Centered Medical Home and Accountable Care accreditations. Each is designed to build capabilities to create and operate a financially viable patient-centered organization using management strategies and tools for clinical and business information systems, population health, and care coordination. Care coordination has been said to be central to the achievement of FTC requirements.

URAC believes that accreditation standards and their interpretations must be comprehensive and thorough, but not rigid. There is much work involved in bringing providers together to clinically integrate and provide coordinated services. What happens in a CIN is heavily dependent on local providers and locally distinct populations, and therefore each developing CIN must have flexibility to sort out priorities and approaches without adhering to one-size-fits-all structures.

URAC's Clinical Integration standards are applicable to any kind of structure as long as the organization meets the definition of a clinically integrated network. Because the standards are broadly carved, the elements of accreditation are reasonably applied to vertically integrated networks involving inpatient facilities coupled with ambulatory care as well as to horizontal networks organized along the same level of care.

Accreditation standards can be applied to the configuration and progression of CINs at every stage of development. The standards have been used as a guide to the initial formation of a CI structure and operation, as noted above, or they can be a validation and refinement of a CIN already in place. Advanced, highly integrated organizations in the course of their ongoing development likely will have followed many of the precepts upon which the URAC CIN accreditation standards are based. However, many applicant organizations do find they have gaps in organization or execution of CI characteristics that the rigor from the accreditation process assists them to identify and address.

The URAC accreditation process is interactive and educational for the applicant organization. The first of two steps in the process consists of an online review of documents and materials uploaded into a secure extranet. A knowledgeable and experienced accreditation reviewer is then assigned to each application. The reviewer works with the applicant organizations to ensure that documents demonstrate consistency with the expectations in the standards. Once that state is achieved, then an onsite visit is scheduled wherein the URAC reviewer evaluates and verifies actual performance consistency with the documentation submitted. Some on-sites are face-to-face, while others may be conducted remotely and online. This is done through a dialogue with the organization to allow better understanding of the organization's application of its interpretation of the standards. Results of the survey are forwarded to URAC's Accreditation Committee at the end of the onsite review for determination of accreditation status.

Accreditation processes for integrated organizations are built on a foundation common to all integrated and accountable networks, comprised of four pillars of clinical integration: leadership and governance, organizational alignment, coordinated care, and evolving technology for an integrated infrastructure. Together these four pillars mark the characteristics of a successful integrated venture that fulfills the responsibilities for producing results beneficial to consumers. In these practice models, leadership and governance is provider dominated and driven by provider interests. Alignment of business interests with integrated clinical practice leads to opportunities for rewarding provider network participation, improvements in practice patterns, and medical neighborhood formation. Planning for technology acquisition is critical in this age of measurement and accountability and the standards support planned transition from paper to digital integration. These pillars (Figure 9-2) in the URAC accreditation standards are examined in following sections.

Figure 9-2. Foundations for Clinical Integration Found in URAC Standards

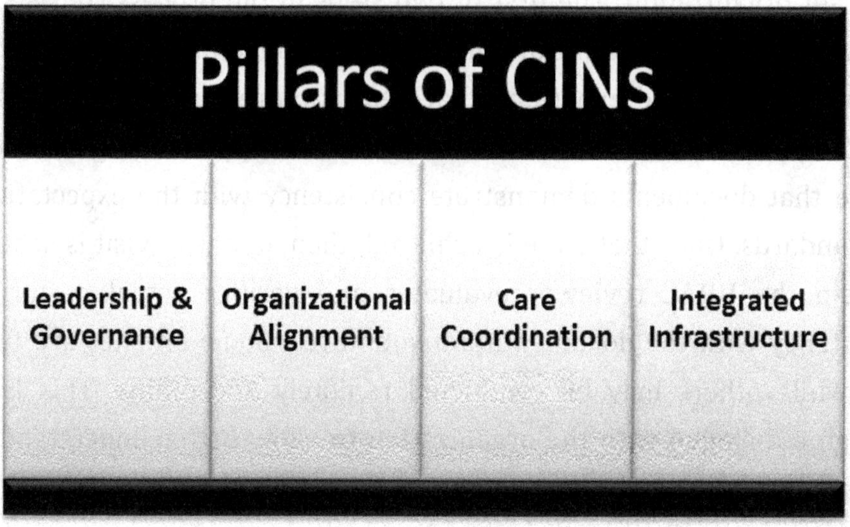

Pillars of CINs

| Leadership & Governance | Organizational Alignment | Care Coordination | Integrated Infrastructure |

Governance: Leading, Protecting

URAC standards capture sound business practices for whatever type of venture is seeking accreditation. The URAC CIN standards begin by recognizing the the importance of structural and contractual foundations for a successful network. Oversight by clinical leaders is critical for the governing body.

For example, a governing body must provide oversight of systems to assure provider acceptance of performance goals, compliance with all applicable federal and state laws and regulations, and promotion of clinical practices consistent with goals of the CIN and grounded in evidence-based medicine.

From the outset, URAC standards validate the twin goals of financial sustainability and clinical transformation. Everything that follows flows from objectives for improved clinical quality, health outcomes, and cost efficiency. At its core, the CIN is market driven. The driving business model is wedded to local consumer interests. The standards reflect the philosophy that CIN leadership must be provider driven. Participating providers are contracted to adhere to the CIN's goals and the methods of their attainment.

Provider contracts cover requirements, rewards and provider protections – establishing the seriousness of the effort to transform practice patterns. Because of the inherent challenges in local market responsiveness and the demand for successful clinical outcomes, URAC requires that clinical practitioners lead the self-governing integrated organization.

Consistent with its market-oriented goals, the governing body determines the clinical program approach within the network business model. Clinicians and business management professionals come together to make sure all participants are assigned the right roles and responsibilities to facilitate the agreed-upon clinical and financial approaches. Provider led governance also is responsible for determining how clinicians will use scientific evidence and acknowledged best practices to reduce variation and thus make coordination viable and clinical outcome goals achievable.

Viewed as part of the total accreditation, governance is not the major thrust, but it is foundational because it establishes how disparate providers work together. Good governance and structure promote the soundness perceived to be required for assurance of consumer protection in the long run. The same principles apply to the ACO.

Provider interests are articulated not only in the elements that speak to provider dominance in leadership, but also in those addressing remediation processes when performance falls short and an opportunity is given to resolve identified performance deficiencies. Through the standards, providers are afforded explicit description of the requirements for provider participation in CIN activities, including investment of time, finances, and other resources. A provider dispute resolution process is also required of all accredited CINs.

Another initial issue essential to moving ahead is satisfying federal, and often state, government requirements that the accumulation of otherwise competing providers around contractual arrangements for health care is offset by observable benefits. Standards in place for CINs have been devised to be consistent with the DOJ and the FTC rulings and requirements.

Accreditation is not tantamount to attaining a safe harbor, but it provides reasonable guidance toward that end.

Alignment

Organizational alignment begins at the top. It doesn't end until it reaches into the farthest extensions of the integrating network, all the way to the treatment of individual patients. Here is where thoughtful and thoroughly executed business agreements take on importance. Business agreements contain and reinforce the organization's standard operating procedures: the structure of the organization, the scope of the business arrangement, and how that arrangement will affect consumers in terms of improving clinical quality, healthcare outcomes and cost efficiency - in other words achievement of the Triple Aim.

Alignment also means philosophical cohesion among providers collaborating for both clinical and financial integration. The parties must agree on clinical parameters, such as patient-centeredness. Clinically, evidence-based guidelines must be identified for targeted conditions and adherence agreed upon to meet the needs of the population. Guidelines form the basis of focused priorities for practice pattern improvement and measurement of quality outcomes. A challenge for every CIN is the timely exchange of pertinent clinical information so care is improved and costs reduced; and each party must recognize and do its part to move in this direction. Financial integration speaks to the success of the network as a whole and to alignment of financial incentives and rewards among all network providers and at all levels of the network.

In addition to requiring contracts and agreements defining the organized venture and leadership structures, URAC standards elucidate other important infrastructure elements and characteristics of a successful network. These include:

- Management responsibilities;

- Staff and provider training requirements for effective participation in an integrated network;
- Consumer safety; and
- Financial integration and fiduciary responsibility.

Thus, there are protections for the interests of consumers as well as those of providers.

Standards provide clarity to principles required to function as a clinically integrated entity. Where a CIN falls short of expectations, or is unable to achieve successful implementation, the accreditation process assists the organization to identify the gaps and categorizes them according to priority and impact.

Clinical Management and Coordination

While an organization's leadership, governance, regulatory status, and organizational alignment provide the enabling framework for formation of a CIN, its ultimate success rests on the redesign of the clinical environment. Clinical integration demands the capability of rendering superior, high-quality, coordinated care services to its designated population. Coordination of care and sharing of clinical data is expected throughout the medical neighborhood between all appropriate providers. There is an interdependence required in the formation of the provider team. The goals of coordination are streamlined care, improving cost and affordability, facilitated by effective communication. Care coordination is the job of every member of the expanded healthcare team. One outcome of good care coordination is error reduction. Coordination and collaboration are anticipated in network operations and demonstrated through performance measurement and reporting.

In addition to care coordination, effective clinical management in an accredited CIN includes:

- Selection, appropriate use, and implementation of clinical practice protocols;

- A focus on relevant chronic care and co-morbidities;

- Support for patient-centeredness, consumer self-management and safe transitions of care; and

- Patient care integration through linkages and referrals between primary care and specialists, including mental health and substance use disorder providers and other service agencies.

Population health receives significant attention in the CIN as well as the Accountable Care accreditations because success requires the organization to effectively and efficiently serve the designated population. The successful organization analyzes and stratifies its target population, identifying those at risk, and prioritizing strategies aimed at improving specific outcomes related to the needs of the population and goals of the organization. The standards envision that CINs will target patients with higher risk for chronic illness, or those with multiple chronic morbidities.

Successful CIN leaders, management, and provider participants understand that the ability of a CIN to achieve cost-reduction and quality-improvement objectives is dependent on the daily execution of integrated collaborative activity. Often that means taking an extra step to ensure the optimum use of professionals to facilitate objectives such as population health management or medication adherence.

Clinical leaders select the areas of focus based on their population: It might include diabetes for all age strata, congestive heart failure for the Medicare-age population, perhaps obstetrics if they have a younger population. An organization's leadership must provide the necessary oversight to ensure providers are following guidelines, and the organization has to produce results and evaluate outcomes demonstrating the impact on achievement of the CIN's clinical and financial goals.

URAC publishes a Clinical Integration Accreditation self-assessment tool to help organizations identify key areas of concentration as they consider the steps they must take to demonstrate core aspects of clinical integration, and ready their organization for accreditation. For example, in the area of care coordination, an accreditation-ready organization is developing or already possesses:

- Documents that clinically integrated providers participate in required training.

- Written agreements that address the rights of clinically integrated providers to resolve performance issues.

- Signed agreements with clinically integrated providers that address expectations regarding such essential components as clinical practice and/or evidence-based guidelines, quality standards, performance measurement and reporting, provider rights to resolve performance deficiencies, and mechanisms to resolve disputes.

- Written policies and documented procedures for clinical management that address such matters as provider consensus for adopting performance metrics, measuring actual performance as compared with established benchmarks, coordinating referrals for network patients, and establishing criteria for when patients need case management.

In addition the organization must ensure that its population management program has criteria for individual assessments and care plans, provision of health education information, and prevention and wellness communications.

Physicians and other practitioners must be at the forefront of activity related to setting clinical priorities and enforcing them. It is not enough to assert that the doctors were involved in selecting clinical practice protocols, and that they weighed in on the goals for improving clinical practices, etc. Each physician must contractually agree to the clinical priorities, how they are enforced, and demonstrate understanding of the new ways of doing clinical practice designed to transform the delivery and efficiency of care.

Some organizations do better than others in documenting all that is required to receive and maintain clinical integration accreditation. There needs to be documentation of activities showing how the organization helped motivate physicians to participate in the discussions and keep good records. Leadership can leverage the standards with physician practices to emphasize that documentation standards are important to follow to demonstrate their agreement and determination to execute organization goals allowing government antitrust scrutiny to be withheld and the organization to operate legally.

Integration Infrastructure

Demonstrating and documenting quality in a CIN are among the critical capabilities vested in the construction and intelligent implementation of information systems and infrastructure. For governance to ably create, communicate and align incentives, and for clinicians to play their roles in a coordinated system, there has to be a unifying and accessible information network readily available. Technology and infrastructure, when sophisticated and ubiquitous, supports decision-making, record-keeping, population management, and performance assessment. However, URAC recognizes that one of the largest challenges for CINs is the existence of a multiplicity of legacy information systems in provider networks.

The information systems standards require four clinical functions to be in place:

1. Support for clinically integrated practice;

2. Exchange of clinical information among members of the healthcare team;

3. Capability to produce comparative reports; and

4. Identification and stratification of at-risk members of the attributed population.

URAC standards also address the need for business systems to support network operations and reporting requirements.

The accreditation process acknowledges the essential role of technology in the success of a CIN by emphasizing core standards that encourage planning for technology acquisition over time. Reporting requirement standards are more easily met in organizations having some level of automation. It may not be an EHR, especially for components not covered by the HITECH Act, but some type of web-based registry or warehouse is needed.

The Clinical Integration Accreditation self-assessment tool highlights the importance of health information systems, showing applicants that in order to be successful in the accreditation process their information systems must be able to support the essential components of clinical integration. Examples from the self-assessment tool include provider communication, care collaboration and management, evaluation of system usage by network providers, comparative reporting for individual and group practice performance, and adoption and dissemination of performance metrics.

The URAC approach acknowledges the complexity of building a strong and sustainable IT infrastructure. The accreditation process gives ample allowance to phase in higher levels of automation that power system wide communication, care coordination, and well-documented and defined results. The prevailing perspective is that organizations cannot do all of this at once. The preferred route is assessing the status quo, planning for improved capabilities and acquisition over time, setting timelines based on planned capital assets and practitioner acceptance, and working on objectives until completed or making adjustments as conditions change.

Whatever is built must support the providers in their specific network objectives, and not just in their own internal environment. The systems must have the ability to handle the operational needs of the network. These integration-minded accreditation standards for CINs are intended to guide the network's planners and implementers to include essential functions at the beginning stages of upgrading or adding IT systems.

URAC recognizes that networks may be at any given point on the continuum of health information technology implementation. The expectation is that the organization has a plan to implement and is working toward that implementation. This plan demonstrates to URAC, FTC, payers and others that performance management oversight is ongoing.

Flexible Approaches

As part of the Clinical Integration Standards development process, an advisory committee consisting of 40 subject matter experts recruited from throughout the healthcare industry helped to draft the standards. The draft standards were then published for public comment. Information received during the public comment period was reviewed by the expert panel and the standards were then revised as needed. The draft standards were further validated through the beta testing process. Eight physician led organizations participated, provided further comment on the standards, and made recommendations for improvement. This multi-step process produced a clinical integration standard set that provides a solid foundation for the industry, and based on the reality that a flexible approach is needed to accommodate ongoing changes underway in the healthcare ecosystem.

When any organization applies for accreditation, URAC provides educational training to help that organization identify the intent of the standards, understand how the organization may demonstrate compliance, and what will be required during the online "desk top" and onsite evaluation. Included is information on the mandatory standards. Any organization must meet the intent of applicable mandatory standards in order to attain accreditation.

URAC recommends that the organization identify a team to work on the accreditation application and that leaders select a project chief. The successful accreditation process begins with network leadership allocating budgetary and staff resources to the initiative. The project team then conducts a gap analysis to determine what processes, documentation, and reporting requirements are in place and which must be developed.

Successful applicants have identified this as a step that helps to determine the scope of the work needed and to set reasonable goals for the submission of the application.

The next step is being in alignment with the afore-mentioned DOJ/FTC antitrust guidelines for healthcare. Networks must be organized to improve quality and constrain costs through coordinated care, not to increase prices. This may necessitate a cultural change. When organizing to the extent that relationships with unaffiliated providers are built into the care network, the FTC Guidance requires that there has to be economic benefit to the consumer. The FTC Guidance (as updated through the Norman PHO decision) is clear that the purpose of organizing is not only to command greater reimbursement but to provide better care and contain costs. (Federal Trade Commission, February 13, 2013) Advances in population health along with reduction in the costs of care are what policymakers and purchasers are after.

A Case of Urgency for Accreditation

Current market environments and previous attempts to aggregate providers in a region can skew the odds for or against the approval and acceptance of CINs. In Connecticut, for example, the formation of a physician/hospital organization (PHO) comprising 98 percent of the physicians in and around the city of Danbury resulted in a federal investigation and action to disband the PHO in 1995 on antitrust grounds. (Marx, 1995) Twenty years later, that event still caused a lack of confidence and trust between physicians and entities wanting to integrate.

With that failed attempt in the background, a PHO in Bridgeport, Conn., called St. Vincent's Health Partners decided it had to seek independent assurances that the clinically integrated network it was forming met legal guidelines, it would be organized and operated according to requirements all participants understood, and they would agree to a cohesive structure for coordinating clinical and financial services. "All participants, including St. Vincent's Medical Center, 100 physicians in practices owned by the hospital, and 100 more independent physicians, helped create and then live by a "playbook" that spelled everything out," said Colleen Swedberg, MSN, RN, CNL, Director for Care Coordination and Integration at St. Vincent's Health Partners.[*]

The URAC accreditation application process helped shape policies and procedures necessary to establish a network that improved the level of quality service and clinical efficiency, as required by federal regulators and the patient population. The leadership started with a plan to implement the organization, but also decided to pursue accreditation during the formative stages. The accreditation process both validated some aspects and guided change in others. The very organizational design was being informed along the way by URAC standards, Swedberg explained.

Follow-through was continuously on the minds of St. Vincent's Health Partners leaders as physicians signed up and began to fold operations into the network. An essential aspect was cooperation among providers on behalf of a single patient, a marker for the attention to clinical quality and efficiency that leads to good outcomes, and a step necessary to satisfy regulators. The playbook, for example, has a section on executing patient transitions. More than 100 transitions were identified, taken from best practices outlined by recognized authorities, including information that needs to accompany the patient and what each face-to-face interaction needs to embody.

St. Vincent's Health Partners was mindful that the reasons the Danbury network fell afoul of the federal law in 1995 was not only due to a failure of leadership, but also a less-than-complete understanding of legal realities by the participating practices, said Michael G. Hunt, DO, Chief Medical Officer/Chief Medical Information Officer of St. Vincent's Health Partners. Because of the misperceptions, and because physicians are not naturally

---

[*] Comment by Colleen Swedberg on January 14, 2014 at URAC Review meeting at St. Vincent Health Partners in Bridgeport, CT.

knowledgeable about rules pertaining to antitrust and collusion, Dr. Hunt noted that St. Vincent's network wanted to be guided and validated as openly and clearly as possible from the very beginning by URAC.[*]

The logic of accreditation, and its grasp by top leadership, enabled the network-building to proceed without wasting time at the onset, especially as to how it should be set up, and communicate clear expectations among the membership. With this information, St. Vincent's Health Partners got a head start, and became the first accredited clinically integrated network on March 1, 2014.

Future Directions

The first clinical-integration accreditation reviews supplied the foothold and learning experiences for the program. Clinical integration in healthcare will continue as new approaches to payment, based on the value of services, drive organizational approaches that mesh with incentives to produce greater value through efficiency and care coordination. Within developing CINs, relationships with PCMHs require definition, and the presence or absence of goals to attain ACO risk-based status should be clear, to allow smooth integration. The way forward for URAC includes development of additional tools and strategies to guide the field through new operational challenges brought on by the evolution of value-based payment approaches.

Besides scrutinizing the actual structure of integration, accreditation can advance the sustainability and acceptance of CINs by using the process to solve new challenges around payment when they arise. The close alignment of the URAC standards with published guidance from the DOJ and FTC gives accredited organizations some sense of ease and safety in the evolving market as providers continue to innovate. And as it nurtures clinical integration, URAC is refining and strengthening the relationship between its clinical integration accreditation program and the complementary

---

[*] Comment by Dr. Michael Hunt on January 14, 2014 at URAC Review meeting at St. Vincent Health Partners in Bridgeport, CT.

accreditation objectives of PCMH and ACO. As it applies and refines clinical integration standards, URAC will continue to have in mind that a CIN can take an increasing number of forms. As of this writing, successful CIN accreditation applicants include both multidisciplinary and specialty networks. For the subset of healthcare systems around the country that has engaged in a substantial amount of clinical integration, applying URAC's accreditation approach would supply objective verification of success in meeting nationally-based standards.

The ways in which health care is practiced, paid for, and deployed are clearly changing. Payment models will continue to shift while policy makers, regulators, and commercial entities search for value-based solutions to the cost of care dilemma. CIN accreditation fosters a viable and sustainable system-based, practical, data-driven response to the changing environment that utilizes clinical and financial integration, performance measurement and reporting transparency to advance an organization's mission and goals. Using this model, greater value can be delivered to the consumer and providers will find their work more rewarding and sustainable.

CHAPTER 9 DISCUSSION QUESTIONS

Discussion questions are provided for team building or class exercises. Answers for all questions are provided in Appendix C.

Question Number	Question
1	How does clinical integration assist providers to thrive in a value-based market?
2	What are the essential goals of clinically integrated network providers?
3	How does the process of becoming accredited assist providers to develop successful networks?
4	What are the goals of care coordination in a CIN?
5	How does development of health information technology capabilities facilitate value generation within a clinically integrated organization?

CHAPTER 9 HIGHLIGHTS

✓ As the healthcare industry begins to migrate into a new era of healthcare delivery based on value and accountability, clinical integration will be a crucial ingredient for creating a sustainable and value generating entity.

✓ To achieve true clinical integration, an entity must standardize its practices and operate under one cohesive set of policies and procedures.

✓ While regulatory compliance is not guaranteed, accreditation for a clinically integrated network entails that the entity is operating under the most-up-to-date best practices available.

✓ A would-be clinically integrated CIN must be aware of, and plan precisely for, a combination of broad arrangements and key details for disparate providers to attain integration goals.

✓ Accreditation takes organizations through a rigorous, comprehensive, transparent process to examine whether an applicant meets standards for efficiency, coordination and legal conduct.

✓ An accreditation process can both guide an aspiring clinically integrated network toward a workable structure and refine the structure of an established network.

✓ Four pillars of integration in any network, and rigorously examined in accreditation, are leadership and governance, organizational alignment, coordinated care, and technology infrastructure.

✓ Accreditation standards are comprehensive but not rigid, reflecting wide variety of possible arrangements based on service emphasis, geography and patient demographics.

CHAPTER 9 REFERENCES

Department of Justice and Federal Trade Commission. (1996). Statements of Antitrust Enforcement Policy in Health Care. Retrieved from http://www.justice.gov/atr/public/guidelines/0000.htm

Institute for Healthcare Improvement. (2014). Triple Aim Initiative. Retrieved from http://www.ihi.org/Engage/Initiatives/TripleAim/pages/default.aspx

National Transitions of Care Coalition. (2008, May). Improving Transitions of Care (pp. 20-23). Retrieved from http://www.ntocc.org/Portals/0/PDF/Resources/PolicyPaper.pdf

Justice Department Consent Decrees with Danbury, Connecticut and St. Joseph, Missouri PHOs Set Forth Antitrust Rules for the Formation and Operation of Multiprovider Networks," *The Health Lawyer*, Mid-Winter 1996, p. 14.

Letter from Markus H. Meier, Assistant Director, Health Care Division, Bureau of Competition to Michael E. Joseph, Esq., McAfee & Taft, Concerning Norman PHO's Proposal to Create a "Clinically Integrated" Network, dated February 13, 2013.

Federal Trade Commission. (2013, February 13). Letter from Markus H. Meier, Assistant Director, Health Care Division, Bureau of Competition to Michael E. Joseph, Esq., McAfee & Taft, Concerning Norman PHO's Proposal to Create a "Clinically Integrated" Network. Retrieved from http://www.ftc.gov/sites/default/files/documents/advisory-opinions/norman-physician-hospital-organization/130213normanphoadvltr_0.pdf

Marx, D. (1995). Justice Department Consent Decrees with Danbury, Connecticut and St. Joseph, Missouri PHOs Set Forth Antitrust Rules for the Formation and Operation of Multiprovider Networks. *Health Law*, 8, 14.

Peterson, M., & et. al. (2014, June). Growth and Dispersion of Accountable Care, 2014 Update. Leavitt Partners.

Chapter 10. Technology Solutions for the 21st Century

Holton Walker | Ken Yale

...IT must play a central role in the redesign of the health care system if a substantial improvement in health care quality is to be achieved during the coming decade. (Institute of Medicine and Committee on Quality of Health Care in America 2001)

Institute of Medicine
2001 Report. Crossing the Quality Chasm

CHAPTER 10 LEARNING OBJECTIVES

✓ What health care technology capabilities are required to support value-based purchasing programs?

✓ What role does EHR interoperability play in facilitating population health management?

✓ How does Health Information Exchange support improvements in quality of care?

✓ In what ways can predictive analytics impact population health?

✓ How can providers use technology to engage patients and families?

Introduction

The health care industry is in the midst of an unprecedented transformation, with health information technology (HIT) taking a lead role. Federal government legislation, policies, and programs of the last five years have invigorated the health care information technology community in an unprecedented way. Using a multipronged approach, characterized by significant investment in technology, technical standards, certification programs, and incentives, government policy and legislation is attempting to guide the industry towards an HIT capability that supports interoperability, clinical integration, and population health management on a grand scale. The national policy framework that guides HIT development and deployment today respond to policy thinking that has developed over an extended time in response to mounting concerns around escalating health care costs and quality issues. The actual path of healthcare information technology is following a less certain journey of innovation and expectation, fueled by government mandates, venture speculation, and entrepreneurial dedication.

In the early days of health care computerization, information technology was typically confined to health care organizations with large-scale operations, whose size and scope allowed funding and development of IT systems and infrastructure. Capital expenditure was driven mainly by economic considerations, with a projected return on investment (ROI) from the automation of business processes. As a result, early automation efforts focused predominantly on the development of business systems supporting operational concerns such as finance and administration. As computer technology became less costly and more widely deployed, health care leadership began to believe that information technology could play a larger role in addressing quality, safety, and cost concerns.

Government Mandate

In 1991, following a decade which saw the widespread introduction of personal computers to the home and business environments, and the advent of networked computing, the Institute of Medicine (IOM) issued a report *The Computer-Based Patient Record: An Essential Technology for Health Care.* (Institute of Medicine, Dick et al. 1991, Institute of Medicine and Committee on Improving the Patient Record 1997) That report advocated comprehensive adoption of automated systems by the United States health care industry with broad objectives for improvement in quality of care, productivity, adaptability, support for research, and security. The report also envisioned:

...a national transportation system for patient data. The transportation system will require an infrastructure (e.g., networks) and standards for connectivity and security but will retain a substantial amount of flexibility.

In 1997, the IOM issued a revised version of the report. In the intervening six years, there was broad evolution in technology, health care, and legislation (including introduction of the 1996 Health Information Portability and Accountability Act (HIPAA) and the Healthcare Effectiveness Data and Information Set (HEDIS)), development of the World Wide Web portion of the Internet, an eightfold increase in computing capacity, and the failed Clinton health reform legislation. The revised report noted that the health information technology industry's attention was shifting from administrative systems to clinical management and the availability of vendor clinical systems was expanding. But the report also noted challenges in areas such as interoperable clinical messaging and clinical coding standards, and pointed out that health information technology adoption in the United States was advancing at a rate slower than hoped and was surpassed by certain western European countries, such as the Netherlands and the United Kingdom. As a summary conclusion on what was needed to stimulate adoption of clinical information systems, the report asserted:

> Technological advances aside, progress toward CPRs [computer patient records] as envisioned in this report has been slower than anticipated. The IOM committee expressed its strong belief that the early phase of CPR's activities should be federally initiated and funded. A major coordinated national effort with federal funding and strong advisory support from the private sector is needed to accelerate the pace of change in the United States. Health care is a public good and many of the barriers to widespread implementation of CPR systems require national mandates, policy changes, or, in some cases, new legislation. Leadership in government and the private sector must be galvanized to make sweeping changes where possible (e.g., a national UHI, confidentiality legislation) and to instigate, motivate, and provide incentives to accelerate development of solutions to other impediments (e.g., terminology standards). (Institute of Medicine and Committee on Improving the Patient Record 1997)

In 2000 and 2001, the IOM issued two additional reports: *To Err Is Human: Building a Safer Health System* (Institute of Medicine, Kohn et al. 2000) and *Crossing the Quality Chasm: A New Health System for the 21st Century.* (Institute of Medicine and Committee on Quality of Health Care in America 2001) Taken together, the two reports articulated a crisis in patient safety, and set forth a framework of recommendations for re-organizing health care, including recommendations for deployment of information technology in a central role to reengineer care processes, manage the burgeoning clinical knowledge base, coordinate patient care across clinicians and settings and over time, support multidisciplinary team functioning, and facilitate performance and outcome measurements for improvement and accountability. (ibid) as well as development and support of evidence based medicine and clinical decision support tools.

In 2004, the Office of the National Coordinator for Health Information Technology (ONCHIT) was established within the Department of Health and Human Service by Presidential executive order (The White House, 2004) initiating the modern era of HIT standards. The ONCHIT was given responsibility to "develop, maintain, and direct the implementation of a strategic plan to guide the nationwide implementation of interoperable health information technology in both the public and private health care sectors that will reduce medical errors, improve quality, and produce greater value for health care expenditures". (The White House 2004) The ONCHIT and its subsidiary committees set about establishing and identifying key clinical use cases or scenarios to be addressed, and technical standards that could be applied to support those use cases. To that end, the committees began identifying specific standards that were deemed best in class in support of functionality required for each use case. Rather than authoring new standards, the preferred approach was to identify existing standards that had been defined by Standards Development Organizations (SDO) that could be leveraged to the benefit of the program.

ARRA and HITECH

In 2009, the Health Information Technology for Economic and Clinical Health (HITECH) Act was enacted as a component of the American Recovery and Reinvestment Act (ARRA). HITECH established congressionally appropriated funding for ONCHIT (renamed the Office of the National Coordinator, or ONC for short), and development and deployment of health care information technology in several categories. Some key programs included:

Federal Advisory Committees

The ONC was formally established in federal law, under the U.S. Department of Health and Human Services, which was given the authority to establish programs to promote HIT, health care quality, efficiency and safety.

The HIT Policy and Standards Committees were established to make recommendations on national HIT policy, standards implementation criteria, and certification criteria for the exchange and use of health information.

Health Information Exchange (HIE) Advancement

Development of HIE capabilities throughout the United States was mandated by HITECH and ARRA, including $548 million dollars awarded and distributed to 56 states and territories of the United States, as well as qualified State Designated Entities, to support deployment of HIE capabilities. An additional $16 million in Health Information Exchange Challenge grants has been awarded to "stimulate innovation."

Beacon Community Program

The ONC was authorized to provid $259 million to 17 select communities with established HIE capabilities to build on their experience, and translate "investments into improvements in cost, quality, and population health."(Department of Health and Human Services 2013)

Regional Extension Centers

Each state had funding for at least one regional extension center, for a total of 62 throughout the country. Regional Extension Centers were tasked to assist providers in navigating the implementation and adoption of electronic health records (EHRs) from vendor selection through implementation and Meaningful Use Certification.

Workforce Development

The Workforce Development program provided funding to universities, community colleges and institutions of higher education to develop and deliver education, training and certification programs to help develop the skilled workforce required to support HIT as it is deployed across the country.

Meaningful Use

One of the most significant, and perhaps controversial, components of the HITECH Act is the Meaningful Use (MU) of EHRs program. The Meaningful Use program provided incentives to eligible professionals, eligible hospitals, and critical access hospitals for adoption and use of EHR technology. The program also levies penalties in the form of reduced Medicare and Medicaid payments for providers who are eligible but do not participate. The program is administered by the Centers for Medicare and Medicaid Services (CMS) with participation by the ONC. Eligible Professionals (EPs) could receive up to $44,000 in incentive payments over 5 consecutive years via the Medicare program and up to $63,750 over 6 years via the Medicaid program. While Eligible Professionals had to pick either the Medicare or Medicaid program,(Centers for Medicare and Medicaid Services 2013) most hospitals could receive payments from both. Depending on several factors, such as the number of discharged patients and the schedule of EHR adoption, each hospital could receive financial incentive payments ranging from $2 million to approximately $6.3 million. (Centers for Medicare and Medicaid Services 2013) Table 10-1 illustrates the historical and forecasted payments from the program.

Table 1. EHR Meaningful Use Program Incentive Schedule

($s in 000)

	Fall 2010	2011	2012	2013	2014	2015	2016	2017	2018	2019	2020	2021	Max. Pmts.
		Stage 1											
				Stage 2									
						Stage 3							
Medicare Incentive Payments		$18K	$12K	$8K	$4K	$2K							$44K
			$18K	$12K	$8K	$4K	$2K						$44K
				$15K	$12K	$8K	$4K						$39K
					$12K	$8K	$4K						$24K
Medicaid Incentive Payments		$21K	$8.5K	$8.5K	$8.5K	$8.5K	$8.5K						$63.8K
			$21K	$8.5K	$8,500	$8.5K	$8.5K	$8.5K					$63.8K
				$21K	$8.5K	$8.5K	$8.5K	$8.5K	$8.5K				$63.8K
					$21K	$8.5K	$8.5K	$8.5K	$8.5K	$8.5K			$63.8K
						$21K	$8.5K	$8.5K	$8.5K	$8.5K	$8.5K		$63.8K
							$21K	$8.5K	$8.5K	$8.5K	$8.5K	$8.5K	$63.8K

Impact of Meaningful Use

The impact of the HITECH Act and Meaningful Use on the advancement of EHR adoption and interoperability capabilities in the United States cannot be overstated. As of October 2013, 90% of eligible hospitals and 80% of eligible professionals had registered for Medicare or Medicaid EHR incentive programs. Of those registered, 85% of eligible hospitals had received a Medicare or Medicaid EHR incentive payment. (Reider and Tagalicod December 6, 2013)

Medicare Shared Savings Program Accountable Care Organization (MSSP-ACO) quality measures include an EHR adoption measure based on meaningful use of a certified EHR. To emphasize the importance of the measure, it is double weighted in the MSSP-ACO scoring paradigm. In commercial ACOs and CINs as well, the adoption of performant EHR technology is an enabling factor in the organization's ability to meet their objectives.

Meaningful Use is divided into three stages:

Stage 1 - Data capture and sharing, (i.e. the creation of information);

Stage 2 - Advance clinical processes and interoperability;

Stage 3 – Improvement of outcomes.

The Medicare EHR incentive program began in 2011 with Stage 1. In order to receive incentive payments, Meaningful Use participants must obtain certification on specific Meaningful Use (MU) objectives for each stage. For Stage 1, Eligible Professionals must qualify on 15 core objectives and 5 additional objectives drawn from a menu set of 10. Eligible Hospitals and Critical Access Hospitals (CAHs) must qualify for 14 required core objectives; and an additional 5 objectives may be chosen from a menu set of 10.

On August 23, 2012, the federal government released the final rules for MU Stage 2, which is effective for program participants starting in 2014. The final rule contains 20 measures for physicians, of which 17 are core and 3 of 6 are menu, and 19 measures for hospitals, of which 16 are core and 3 of 6 are menu.

In December 2013, CMS and the ONC proposed an extension of the MU Stage 2 timeline, allowing EHR technology vendors more time to develop and bring MU Stage 2 capable, certified EHR technology to market. CMS and ONC will also have greater opportunity to review and respond to the experience of MU Stage 2 stakeholders; observe the recorded results of MU Stage 2 adoption and measures; and consider the content of MU Stage 3 measures.

In May 2014, HHS issued a new proposed rule that extended the timelines for MU Stage 2. The proposed rule offered eligible providers the option of continuing to use MU Stage 1 objectives and measures to provide MU attestation throughout 2014 instead of the MU Stage 2 capabilities that were previously required. The proposed rule also included a provision to extend MU Stage 2 through 2016 and begin MU Stage 3 in 2017. The extension recognized that it was taking longer than anticipated for EHR technology vendors to develop and gain certification for MU Stage 2 compliant products, which was subsquently making it difficult for eligible providers to implement those products and attest to their use in accordance with the original timeline.

Proposed rules for MU Stage 3 are anticipated to be released in the fall of 2014, followed by Final Stage 3 rules scheduled for the first half of 2015. For Medicare, following at least two years of participation in MU Stage 2, Eligible Professionals will be able to begin MU Stage 3 in January 2017 under the proposed timeline. Eligible Hospitals and CAHs would begin Stage 3 in October 2016. This represents an extension of approximately two years over the original timelines that were conceived for the overall Meaningful Use / EHR Certification timeline for Medicare, which was anticipated to last approximately two years per Stage (six years overall), concluding in 2016.

In order to qualify for Medicare MU incentive payments, participating providers and organizations must continue to certify throughout the three stages of the program, and the payment incentives are spread out throughout the three stages accordingly. Also, eligible participants who join the MU program in later years receive smaller incentive payments.

The MU certification timeline and payment schedule for Medicaid is structured somewhat differently than Medicare in that Medicaid Incentive payments do not diminish over time because Medicaid participants receive payments over six years of participation as compared to five years for Medicare participants. Also, unlike the Medicare program, which is administered centrally by CMS, the Medicaid program is administered by 46 participating states. As a result, details of each program vary according to individual state policy. In the case of both the Medicare and Medicaid MU programs, eligible providers who do not participate are subject to reduced payments.

MU Certification Process

The Meaningful Use program employs a two-tiered certification approach whereby EHR vendors obtain certification from the ONC under the ONCHIT Certification Program. Provider organizations then obtain and deploy the certified technology in support of MU objectives. If providers possess existing EHR capability that meets ONC criteria for EHR functional capabilities, providers are able to obtain equivalent certification for that technology as qualifying for MU incentives.

ACOs and Reimbursement Reform

At this point, the reader may be wondering how all this information and technology is related to, and impacts, CIN, ACO, PCMH, or any other acronym you might envision. First, let's review the purpose of ACOs and healthcare reform, to put this in context.

Reimbursement reform seeks to guide the industry away from fee-for-service reimbursement, and towards a payment model that rewards for better value as represented by improved quality, improved health and outcomes, and lower costs. In other words, reform seeks to change the economic incentives and context in which a healthcare provider operates. Through the application of shared savings and key quality measures, ACO programs reward clinical organizations for quality improvement and cost reductions across a defined population. As of December 2013, CMS is sponsoring three different kinds of ACO programs, each having different qualifications for admittance; and different reimbursement approaches. (Centers for Medicare and Medicaid Services 2013)

Medicare Shared Savings Program (MSSP) ACO

The MSSP-ACO Program seeks to "facilitate coordination and cooperation among providers to improve the quality of care for Medicare Fee-For-Service (FFS) beneficiaries and reduce unnecessary costs."(Centers for Medicare and Medicaid Services 2013) MSSP promotes accountability for the overall care of the Medicare patients served by the ACO through the use of quality measures, requires coordinated care for all Medicare patients attributed to the ACO, and shares savings accrued from any reduction in the projected cost of care.

Advance Payment Model

The Advance Payment ACO Model was developed in response to stakeholder input regarding the proposed rule for MSSP. It offers up-front and ongoing payments to selected organizations to assist in the costs associated with establishing and administering the ACO.

Pioneer ACO Model

The Pioneer ACO Program is open to organizations considered early adopters of coordinated care. It is characterized by higher savings and risk than the MSSP-ACO program in the first two years. In year three the ACO has an opportunity to transition to a population-based reimbursement arrangement.

ACO Technology Requirements

Value-based reimbursement models such as ACO are based on achieving specific quality measures and shared cost savings. ACO quality measures help ensure that the provider focuses on proactively managing the overall health of patients, rather than just limiting utilization as a means to improve savings. To score well on quality measures, providers are required to review their patient population on an ongoing basis, identify patient needs, and intervene or make recommendations to patients to drive better quality, cost, patient experience and outcomes.

From a technology perspective this creates a need to augment core EHR capabilities with population health management and patient engagement functionality, as well as supporting analytics. It is interesting to note that the HITECH and ARRA legislation mandating HIT activities (i.e., HIE and EHR) do not provide a pathway for these technologies, and in fact compliance with these two laws can be counter productive to population health managvement and patient engagement efforts. Without diminishing the importance of the worthy policy objectives of government mandated health information technology interoperability, or the many activities that constitute clinical practice, new technologies are required that specifically focus on population health management. Patient engagement is another arena necessary for health and care to succeed, but nothing in reform legislation suggests how this is best accomplished. Fortunately, venture speculation, and entrepreneurial dedication has continued in spite of government mandates and there have been significant new activities underway since the early 2000s to develop technologies and tools enabling population health management and enhancing patient engagement. We shall briefly cover some of these innovations at the end of this chapter.

Figure 10-1 Population Health Management Technology Foundations

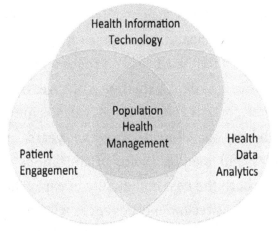

The path to incorporating population health management and patient engagement into a practice setting varies according to the population being managed, and the size, breadth, and technology foundation of the organization. EHR systems that fulfill the comprehensive needs of a clinical setting may possess some of the features of population health management that support Meaningful Use certification. At a practice level, for example, these features may include a patient registry, medication reconciliation, secure messaging, referrals and clinical data exchange. These are features key to managing basic clinical processes at the practice level. Broader clinical integration objectives required by ACOs, CINs and similar initiatives require additional technologies and workflows, such as the ability to aggregate patient information and population management processes across the potential continuum of care. It is therefore necessary to think of these capabilities as operating at a broad level that encompasses the integrated care continuum available to the population of patients being managed. Simply put, EHR, HIE, and meaningful use only get you so far, much more is needed to aggregate data across the entire continuum of care and make it useful for population health management and engaging consumers and patients.

Population Health Management Technology

Population health management capabilities are necessary to meet clinical quality improvements and cost efficiencies required by ACOs and CINs. By executing on population health management goals the organization performs well against quality measures and cost saving goals, and advances the Triple Aim: improved patient experience of care, better health for the population, and lower costs. Table 10-2 describes some population health management capabilities developed over the years, mainly by health insurance companies and managed care organizations who have always been accountable for both the cost and quality of care. These tools are used in a variety of ways, and as technology advances we may see some diminish in importance, especially with the growth of distributed technologies, such as smart phones, that make it easier to integrate the consumer and patient into the clinical workflow. We shall further describe how technology can facilitate population health management later in this chapter.

Table 10-2. Population Health Management Technology Capabilities

Population Health Management	Feature
Population Health Management	The ability to mine and analyze data about a specific population assigned to a provider, who is accountable for the quality and cost of care, and identify opportunities for medical and utilization management, care coordination, and other activities designed to improve quality and affordability
Registry	A list of patients and their associated diseases and conditions, sometimes also giving gaps in care, clinical pathways, and necessary procedures
Interactive patient registries	Patient registries integrated into population health management software and the ability to directly impact clinician workflow and outreach.
Coordinate care and workflow across all settings	Using secure messaging and application integration, support seamless workflow between the Physicians, Care Managers and Patient.
Support multiple care programs	Support multiple care management programs such as wellness, utilization management, case and disease management, and chronic condition management.
Support attribution and referrals	Identify and maintain relationship of patient to physician and care managers. Support referrals to appropriate clinical and non-clinical resources.
Reference material and evidence-based medicine	Provide reference material to guide clinical pathways and protocols, best practice and evidence-based medicine. Provide ability to send reference material to patients.
Secure messaging	Send and receive secure messaging among providers and with patients, and compatible with interoperability requirements.
Data integration	Normalize claims and/or clinical data, aggregated from diverse sources, to provide a comprehensive clinical

Population Health Management	Feature
	record from all settings.
Clinical decision support	Provide evidence-based medicine at appropriate points in the clinical pathway, identify evidence based gaps in care, alerts and best practice recommendations for care using aggregated data.

Patient Engagement Technologies

Patient engagement is a key component of population health management. We cover this topic in greater detail in Chapter 13. Here, we review one element of patient engagement- patient portals- recognized by HITECH and ARRA. The field of patient engagement, however, is much broader and richer, and has benefitted from advancements in sociology, psychology, and technology – some of which is covered in Chapter 13.

Patient portals are a key tool for population health management, according to the federal government (see HITECH and ARRA), as they help engage patients in their own health. Patient portals are usually web-based tools accessible to patients, or in some cases EHR components, that are specifically designed to offer patients a secure capability to access their medical information, may have biderctional communication with the provider, and sometimes offer other capabilities such as prescription renewal and appointment scheduling. Patient portals provide a key pivot point supporting the patient's active participation in their own care. Portals allow the patient to actively interact with physicians and care managers and provide relevant input. Allowing access to information and participation for patients and consumers, however, is just the starting point. Their active involvement cannot be guaranteed unless additional steps are taken to make the information relevant and accessible at the right time, place, and format. Predictive analytics is paving the way to understand patient preferences, and engage patients in ways that ensure their involvement and participation. These requirements shall be further explored later in this chapter.

Table 10-3. Patient Engagement Technology Capabilities

Patient Engagement	Feature
Patient Portal	Website accessible to patients, or in some cases EHR components, that offer patients a secure capability to access their medical information, care plans, wellness programs, health recommendations, and other useful information
Health trackers and device integration	The ability to track a persons current medical condition using remote automated devices as well as directly, and integrate the data generated into other software applications.
Health risk assessment	Evaluation of a persons current medical situation, based on responses to questions. Typically involves some kind of scoring mechanism (e.g. algorithm) and treatment recommendation. May also involve integration with health information technology and generating information appropriate to the practice setting or consumer context.
View health records	The ability for a patient to view an aggregated health record drawn from diverse sources.
Care plans and recommendations	Present clinical care plans and care recommendations appropriate to the patient.
Secure messaging	Messaging between clinicians and patients that is technically and physically secure.
Prescription refill	Support prescription refill requests by either the patient or clinician.
Scheduling	Allowing the patient to schedule or request appointments.
Blue Button	Enable Blue Button clinical record export. First deployed by the U.S. Department of Veterans Affairs (VA) in 2010, Blue Button offers patients the ability to download their medical records in a human readable form.

Patient Engagement	Feature
Wellness program	Provide a gateway, usually through a patient portal, to wellness programs that offer preventive services such as nutrition, exercise, tobacco counseling, substance abuse, weight loss counseling, etc.
Mobile	Support use on mobile device platforms, such as smart phones.
Referrals	Provide a list of elgibile clinicians among in-network clinicians and services, and the ability to connet the patient with the appropriate care setting.
Multi-modal communication	Use of multiple strategies to engage the patient through diverse channels, such as: voice, email, patient portals, mobile platforms, webinars, family caregivers, pharmacies, nurse care managers, social media, etc.
Descriptive Analytics	Data mining to produce descriptive reports of what happened to a patient or population in the past.
Predictive Analytics	Data mining and use of predictive algorithms and other statistical methods to mine past and current data to predict what will happen to a patient or population in the future.
Prescriptive Analytics	Data mining, machine learning, use of predictive algorithms and information about the health and care of individuals to create a care plan that prescribes specific activities to improve healthcare in an affordable and effective manner. (Miner L. et al, 2014)

Analytic Technologies

Analytic technology refers to any number of tools used to mine and analyze data. Traditionally this has included financial spreadsheets, insurance risk assessment and adjustment, clinical quality measurement, supply chain management, and patient registries. With greater computational power, and growing volumes of different varieties of data, advanced analytic technologies such as Predictive Analytics are starting to be used. As noted in

Table 10-3, these technologies are already in use to better engage patients and consumers.

Analytic technologies are also critical to meet the clinical and financial objectives of the ACO/CIN. Analysis of aggregated clinical and operational data allows the clinically integrated organization to have the internal visibility and external transparency necessary to successfully pursue a strategy of continuous improvement and return on investment. Analytics must be timely and include the clinical organization and individual patient needs for optimal effect.

Table 10-4. Analytic Technology Capabilities

Analytic Technology	Feature
Quality measures	Aggregate and analyze data, and report quality metrics across the network as close to real time as possible. Use aggregated data from diverse care settings to provide accurate measures. Support export of quality measure reports.
Clinical decision Support	Support real time clinical decision support using aggregated data.
Operations and clinical reporting	Report on clinical, administrative and financial performance metrics as appropriate to the practice setting.
Risk stratification	Retrospectively identify and stratify patients according to clinical risk. Identify risk-stratified patients whose conditions can be impacted.
Descriptive Analytics	Data mining to produce descriptive reports of what happened to a patient or population in the past. Typically used in traditional health insurance, managed care, or older patient registries.

Analytic Technology	Feature
Predictive analytics	Data mining and use of predictive algorithms to mine past and current data to predict what will happen to a patient or population in the future. May involve some, or all, of the following: Prospective identification of predicted utilization of services. Optimize patient communication vehicles and engagement effectiveness. Identify factors related to negatively trending cost factors. Identify factors related to negatively trending clinical conditions. Develop predictive models that allow automation of certain services. Prescriptive analytics giving information about the health and care of individuals to create a care plan that prescribes specific activities to improve healthcare in an affordable and effective manner.
Prescriptive Analytics	Data mining, machine learning, use of predictive algorithms and information about the health and care of individuals to create a care plan that prescribes specific activities to improve healthcare in an affordable and effective manner. (Miner L. et al, 2014)

Clinically Integrated Networks

CIN creation requires a focus on enhanced value, as demonstrated by improved quality of care and reduced costs; improvements the CIN is able to offer more efficiently than operation of its physicians in independent practices that are not integrated. CIN participants commit to enhanced quality of care and value through the use of common evidence based guidelines, integrated reporting, performance measures, and coordination throughout the continuum of care, among other things. The CIN usually uses medical and care management programs addressing population health concerns focused on the needs of specific population segments such as pediatrics, chronic disease such as Diabetes or Hypertension (HTN), or other ancillary services such as tobacco or substance abuse counseling, depending on the goals of the CIN and demographics of the populations served.

ACOs and CINs face common challenges in overcoming barriers that impede interoperability and data aggregation. In contrast to the Medicare ACO, which is required to adhere to CMS standard Quality Measures, CINs are able to select measures that are meaningful within the context of the CIN goals, based on local market needs and negotiated contracts. Through the strength of their clinical programs and compliance with Federal Trade Commission (FTC) guidelines, the CIN may have the capability to negotiate value-based reimbursement programs with payers. These value-based agreements may include incentives for improved care and lower cost achieved through reduced readmissions and emergency room (ER) visits. To achieve these goals, CINs must use population health management and patient engagement techniques.

Data Aggregation, Interoperability and Clinical Integration

ACOs and CINs need to gather data from the broad range of care settings encompassed by the organization. As technology innovation progresses, especially outside of government-mandated HIT, data outside the healthcare system is increasingly important to allow providers access to, and treatment during, the majority of the time patients experience conditions and diseases – while outside the healthcare system. Both internal and external (aka "exogenous") data can assist both with compilation of a comprehensive patient record and to allow treatment of patients, when, where, and how they wish. (Yale, K. 2014)

Physicians, nurses and other clinical service practitioners benefit from access to comprehensive patient records in several ways. By augmenting the existing EHR records in their current practice with clinical records from other care settings and exogenous sources, and leveraging interoperability, physicians improve care through:

- Avoidance of duplicate procedures based on access to existing results and orders;
- Avoidance of contraindicated procedures and medications;

- Sound, evidence-based clinical judgment and care paths based on a complete patient clinical history;
- Wireless telemetry of home devices inform physicians and care managers of adherence and effectiveness;
- Secure Communication with care coordinators and the patient; and
- Secure communication between physician and patient.

Care Coordinators and Care Managers benefit similarly from:

- Up to date and comprehensive clinical histories, including discharge plan, problem lists, medications, results and functional status;
- Accurate and up to date clinical notes and care plans;
- Access to risk stratification and evidence based recommendations based on complete clinical history, known as clinical decision support; and
- Access to Patient health risk assessment and health tracking.

Patients may benefit by:

- The ability to obtain clinical records electronically (an MU2 requirement);
- Secure communication with the physician and care coordinator / care manager;
- Gaining increased confidence and involvement in personal care through engagement with the care coordinator and communication with physicians;
- Obtaining timely recommendations for health and wellness, when, where, and how they wish; and
- Improved quality of care and access, at a lower cost.

Figure 10-2 illustrates four elements needed to achieve data aggregation and interoperability.

Figure 10-2. Data Aggregation and Interoperability

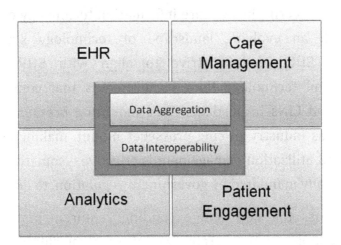

ACOs and CINs also benefit from clinical content originating outside the boundaries of the individual facility. Even among ACOs that possess a strong market presence encompassing ambulatory and inpatient services, patients seek services outside the ACO facilities. The ACO/CIN therefore benefits from acquisition of data from outside sources in several ways, not the least of which are records of inpatient and Emergency Department (ED) admittance, repetitive procedures (for purposes of avoidance), prescription fill history, and clinical history. ACOs with a strong bias towards ambulatory practice, for example, benefit from integration with hospitals in their service area.

Clinical Integration Strategies

As a result of demanding technology requirements that have arisen from the federal government over the last five years, pressure on health care information technology departments has never been higher. Health care IT organizations are burdened by a 'perfect storm' of regulatory compliance requirements in the 2013-2014 timeframe, including the International Classification of Diseases and Related Health Problems, 10th Revision (ICD-10) implementation (October 2015), Meaningful Use Stage 2 (attestation began Q4 2013), and the HIPAA Omnibus rule, as well as additional systems development work that may be required to support ACO or CIN operations. Adding to their concerns, health care information technology organizations are faced with an evolving landscape of technology standards and capabilities as EHR vendors strive to align with EHR certification requirements and technology floor requirements that continue to rise. Finally, ACOs and CINs in particular face mounting pressures to manage care and costs as industry pricing pressures mount, making it imperative that medical and utilization management is effective – something HIT is not prepared, or legally mandated by government regulation, to do.

Looking across the new and expanding requirements for HIT and ACOs/CINs, the topic of interoperability between organizations and systems looms large. ONC defines interoperability as, "the ability of two or more systems or components to exchange information and to use the information that has been exchanged."(Centers for Medicare and Medicaid Services 2013) FTC, on the other hand, defines clinical integration as collaborations of otherwise competing providers, organized in a way that improves efficiencies in care delivery (including quality improvement and cost reduction) for the benefit of consumers that outweigh any potential anticompetitive effects.

From a systems perspective, the implication of the ONC definition is that integration between health care systems must not only support access to data in another care setting, (i.e., the ability to view it), but must also include the ability to "use" the information. The definition of use for ONC/CMS is purposely vague. Here we focus on the ONC requirement for HIT interoperability, which helps lay the infrastructure foundation, realizing more is needed to to achieve quality improvements and cost reductions and incorporate data into the health system's operations in a meaningful way.

The simplest approach (from a technical perspective) to effecting interoperability of existing clinical assets is deployment of a single vendor enterprise EHR system. While not without its issues, which may include high cost and competition for vendor resources in a demanding market, this approach is a viable solution for interoperability within a single health system and the practice settings to which its systems are available. To the extent that connectivity is required between the Enterprise EHR and external entities, such as in a multi-provider ACO or CIN, interfaces need to be constructed. Such connectivity typically involves connections to other clinical organizations, clinical services and HIEs and is usually required to meet the overall ACO/CIN business goals.

Alternatively, organizations may possess multiple clinical information systems that serve specific aspects of their information technology needs, (i.e., a "Best of Breed" approach). In this model, the organization deploys separate application systems that provide optimum capabilities for specific areas of focus (e.g. Emergency Department, Radiology, Cardiology, Primary Care, Intensive Care Unit (ICU), etc.) In this case, where health systems have worked at developing diverse clinical information management capabilities over time, they have built up an organizational investment in technology assets that are desirable to carry forward. Those assets may consist of vendor systems or, in some cases, custom developed applications.

Organizations using best of breed or custom developed software are charged with the responsibility of managing their technology portfolios in a way that enables them to provide technology improvements in a cost efficient and effective fashion. Volumes of material have been devoted to this topic over 60 years of information technology literature, so we shall not address it here. Suffice it to say that it is not simple and requires skill, foresight and planning on multiple levels. Furthermore, the technology portfolio can become complicated by acquisitions and mergers of additional organizational units with divergent technology capabilities of varying strength. Such mergers and acquisitions are becoming common in the fast evolving healthcare environment. Thus, a well-managed application portfolio can offer a cost effective platform for continuing evolution of HIT capabilities.

Supporting interoperability between health care information technology assets requires implementing data exchange capabilities between each system. In the past, accomplishing this objective has been handled using interfaces built around HL7 V2 and ANSI X12 transactions as well as custom interfaces. Interaction between providers and payers is a particularly robust and widespread example of this architecture, focusing on verification of patient eligibility and claims processing. Other transactions in common use within health systems include Admission, Discharge and Transfer (ADT), Orders and Results (radiology, lab, cardiology), electronic Rx, notes and other transactions required to move clinical records between systems that are used in the operating units of a large medical center. Specialized health care message broker technology provides essential support in the movement of data between health care applications, supporting easy manipulation of industry specific messages along with flexible message routing and distribution capabilities.

Moving forward, ACOs and CINs look to engage practices and partners that external to health systems. As noted previously, ACOs and CINS benefit from clinical content originating outside the boundaries of the organization in many ways. Having complete clinical history that is inclusive of records from outside care settings supports improved quality and care coordination as well as cost reductions.

While some ACOs operate under the single technology umbrella of an enterprise EHR, other ACOs as well as CINs consist of independent facilities operating heterogeneous technical platforms. From a technology perspective, this creates a need for interoperability and data integration among those independent systems. Where hospitals have previously been concerned about internal sharing of data (i.e., orders and lab results), now the point of concern becomes exchange of data with network participants that may include ambulatory practices, other hospitals, networks and HIEs outside the hospital. Conversely, independent ambulatory practices in a CIN need to be connected to hospitals and HIEs as well as other ambulatory practices.

MU Stage 2 standards specify that clinical data will be exchanged using Extensible Markup Language (XML) content models developed by HL7 and elaborated by ONC sponsored work groups. In abbreviated form, the standardized format is called the CCDA. More on this below, in the discussion of standards.

Health Information Exchange

Health Information Exchange (HIE) technology is a key enabler for sharing data between clinical organizations. In addition, the federal government ONC believes, "HIE is fundamental to realizing the full potential of meaningful use of electronic health records and health information technology that can lead to improved coordination, quality, and efficiency of health care." (The Office of the National Coordinator for Health IT February 17, 2011)

While there are notable early examples of successful HIEs from the late 1990s, such as HealthBridge in Cincinnati, Ohio, the current wave of HIE growth began following establishment of the ONC and associated standards development in 2004.

HIEs leverage clinical data exchange standards to provide a clinical data sharing capability between constituent provider organizations. Clinical organizations participating in an HIE typically share a common geography or health system relationship. HIE participating organizations may include hospitals, ambulatory practices, community health centers, long term care facilities, home care services, laboratory testing services, private payers, and behavioral health facilities. HIEs can be either public organizations, sponsored by a state or other government entity, or private organizations. Most publicly funded HIEs usually receive fees and revenue from their participating provider organizations. Alternatively, HIEs can also be private organizations set up to share data within a specific health system, group medical practice, ACO or CIN. The private HIE may also connect to other private and public HIEs in order to obtain patient records those other organizations may have received.

HIEs gather clinical content from participating organizations and transform the data received into a consistent format that can be served up as an aggregated patient record. HIEs also typically provide user interfaces through which providers can view clinical data. In order to respond to external requests, HIEs also possess record locator services that enable participating organizations to query for records using patient demographics or identifiers and retrieve the related patient records.

To date, exchange of clinical data through HIE or direct transmission have rarely been fully interoperable in the sense of the ONC's adopted definition. Most exchanges of data using HIE technology are designed to present data for view, but not for incorporation into the EHR data or medical management functions. The following case study gives an example of the benefits of a fully interoperable HIE, and may shed light on gaps in current HIE.

Case Study

One of the challenges physicians face is being able to see what all the members of the patient's care team are doing across the care continuum from visits to other practitioners and specialists, to trips to emergency rooms and urgent care centers. This case study (names are changed) illustrates the complexities of a typical cross-provider scenario, and how it can be addressed through interoperable HIE.

Mr. Johnson is a 59-year-old construction worker with a long history of diabetes. He has documented early retinopathy and hypertension but no evidence of other end-organ changes from his chronic diabetes. He presents to his primary care physician, Dr. Clark, with fever, acute shortness of breath, and rales and wheezing in the left lower lobe. Dr. Clark diagnoses Mr. Johnson with acute pneumonia (confirmed on a chest x-ray) and admits him to Metro Community Hospital (MCH).

In the hospital, Mr. Johnson is newly diagnosed with renal disease (elevated serum creatinine, proteinuria, and mild acidosis). At discharge, he is placed in an intensive home care program for strict monitoring of sodium and protein intake along with diabetes monitoring. He is discharged to the MCH home care agency to be seen by a visiting RN. His discharge medications include insulin, oral antibiotic, and two new medications—a brand-name diuretic and a new angiotensin-converting-enzyme (ACE) inhibitor for renal disease and hypertension.

During the visiting RN's third visit to Mr. Johnson, she becomes concerned by his rising blood pressure, weight gain, and general lethargy. She calls Dr. Clark to order new laboratory tests, which she then draws and delivers to the lab herself. The nurse questions Mr. Johnson, who insists he is compliant with his medication program.

Because MCH, the home care agency, Dr. Clark's practice, the local laboratory, and Bayside Pharmacy, which fills Mr. Johnson's prescriptions, all belong to an ACO, their clinical findings on Mr. Johnson are published in a common electronic community health record. This community health record features an innovative patient management "dashboard" displayed electronically to all authenticated members of Mr. Johnson's care team.

The home care nurse consults the dashboard and notices the list of medications from the MCH discharge summary does not reconcile with the list from Bayside Pharmacy. During further discussions with Mr. Johnson, she learns that he filled the inexpensive generic prescriptions but not the expensive new diuretic and ACE inhibitor. With the recent decline in the construction business, Mr. Johnson's income has been severely reduced and he admits he cannot afford to take the two medications for his renal disease.

The nurse also receives Mr. Johnson's recent laboratory test results via the dashboard. The results show a deterioration of renal function with increased serum creatinine levels and electrolytes, suggesting a recurrence of metabolic acidosis. She contacts Dr. Clark, who switches Mr. Johnson to an alternative generic medication for his renal disease. Dr. Clark then sends an electronic referral to a new nephrologist to see Mr. Johnson emergently so that he can receive more intensive evaluation of his worsening renal disease.

Because the visiting RN and Dr. Clark are part of an ACO/CIN with active and interoperable HIE technology that supports high-quality care and efficient practice, they were able to intervene quickly with use of real-time and accurate patient health data to prevent another admission to the hospital. Without the collaborative capabilities provided by the technology framework and active exchange infrastructure, such a successful outcome would be in doubt and probably less efficient and more expensive.

HIE helps to improve the quality and coordination of care across the different practice settings. It enables care collaboration across multiple providers and organizations and is an important element of the ACO or CIN's clinical integration and population health management strategy. Technology solutions needed to support such continuity of care and enhanced provider collaboration include:

- A unified view of the patient across organizations and care locations;

- Data and workflow integration across disparate information systems and settings;

- Aggregation and gathering of data from outside of the health system to supplement the strength of the clinical record;

- Real-time updates from participating entities and alerts of such updates to ensure timely care synchronization across all accountable parties; and

- Medical and utilization management, predictive analytics and clinical decision support for real-time alerts and treatment recommendations.

Master Patient Index - A Unified Patient View

A common challenge faced by HIEs involves patient identification. Each provider organization that subscribes to the HIE possess their own administrative systems in which they record patient registrations. Since each of those systems assigns its own unique patient identifier, there is no shared identifier that can be used to locate an individual patient's records that may exist across the multiple practices. Put another way, there is no straightforward way to identify that records belonging to Patient John Doe at a Community Hospital, are the same John Doe found at his Allergist practice and another John Doe at his Internal Medicine practice.

Since one of the core objectives of HIE is to support coordinated care by presenting aggregated patient records, HIEs address the patient matching problem through the deployment of Master Patient Index (MPI) functionality. MPIs use sophisticated data algorithms to match patient records together using demographic information and any other shared information that may be available. Through the use of the MPI, HIEs are able to link together patient records from multiple sources to construct a single aggregate view.

Data and Workflow Integration

While the HIE represents a key resource as a repository of aggregated clinical information, the manner in which physician and care manager access the technology can impact clinician effectiveness and satisfaction. If clinicians are required to log into multiple user interfaces, the clinical experience suffers from lost time and the need to maintain additional security credentials. It is preferable to integrate HIE with EHR and medical management systems using "Single Sign On" technology that shares common security credentials. Ideally, the integration also maintains patient context so the patient viewed in the EHR or medical management system can be automatically displayed in the HIE as well. This approach supports a seamless clinician experience that promotes more frequent use of the HIE application.

External Data Sources

Just as ACOs and CINs benefit from access to clinical records from outside practice settings, they also benefit from additional clinical content in the form of administrative claims data from private payers as well as government payers (such as CMS) and exogenous data from consumer data aggregators.

Private payer claims can usually be obtained with accompanying pharmacy claims and laboratory results, providing a well-rounded view of patient activity across all settings. Payers also provide patient attribution records that indicate assignment of patients to primary care providers. These records are essential to calculating ACO and CIN quality measures and bonus payments.

Exogenous data from consumer data aggregators are another, emerging source of valuable consumer and patient data. This information is typically gathered from credit card vendors, retail merchants, federal and state governments, and other sources. The data is rich with information on lifestyle and behaviors, and can help inform care management activities and assist with patient engagement. A few clinical decision support and medical management vendors regularly use this information to assist with patient engagement, however the data is quite large and requires advanced predictive analytics capabilities and algorithms to make it useful for outreach, engagement, and treatment purposes. As patient engagement activities improve from this rich data source, more organizations will use the data to improve quality of care delivered and affordability of services. (Yale, 2014)

The EHR/HIE Interoperability Workgroup

The EHR/HIE Interoperability Workgroup is a consortium of 19 states, 22 HIE vendors and 21 EHR vendors that was formed in February 2011 to advance consistency and standards for interoperability between HIE platforms and their internal and external stakeholders. Initially founded by the New York eHealth Collaborative, the EHR/HIE Interoperability Workgroup works in partnership with HealtheWay and the eHealth Exchange, and also has a cooperative agreement with the ONC. The organization seeks to lower barriers to interoperability by clarifying standards and adopting common certification testing and procedures. Through the inclusion of both EHR and HIE vendors, alignment with MU requirements, and a commitment to consensus specifications, the workgroup seeks to move towards a "plug and play" capability that enables clinical organizations to easily connect to HIEs as well as enabling HIEs to connect to each other.

The Direct Project

The Direct Project was launched in March 2010 as part of the Nationwide Health Information Netwok (NwHIN). Noting that the technical standards set forth as of that date were designed for robust health information interaction, it was the workgroup's recommendation that additional specifications be developed for "simple, direct, secure standards for point-to-point messages."(The Direct Project 2010) Up until that time, forward looking standards for health data transmission were defined around profiles intended primarily for use by Health Information Exchange (HIE) organizations such as Regional Health Information Organizations (RHIO); and the complexity of the specifications was observed to be a barrier to adoption for use in simpler scenarios that could pertain outside of an HIE environment, such as transmission of records between providers in support of a referral, or transmission of data to a patient.

As noted, the Direct Project is focused on point-to-point exchange of data. As a simple solution to that need, it employs the straightforward address and transport protocols utilized by email systems (i.e., the Simple Mail Transfer Protocol (SMTP)), fortified with the security and privacy protocols required to support confidentiality. In support of legacy applications, and HIE implementations using more robust community architectures, Direct also supports point to point protocols based on HIE Web Services.

Administration of Direct data exchange is assisted by DirectTrust, (www.directtrust.org) under a cooperative agreement with the ONC.

Blue Button

Blue Button is a federal government initiative designed to allow patients access to their summarized health information. This initiative was first deployed as a government program by the U.S. Department of Veterans Affairs (VA) in 2010. Through a simple invocation of the"Button," patients are able to download their medical records in simple, human readable digital form. Since that time, Blue Button has been embraced by insurers, governmental agencies (e.g., CMS, DOD) and private sector organizations such as Aetna, United HealthCare, and Iatric Systems, Inc. In response to the surge of interest in Blue Button, responsibility for encouraging Blue Button's rollout and enhancement of its technical standards was transferred to the ONC in 2012. Blue Button+ constitutes a new specification incorporating structured data that supports MU2 requirements for View, Download and Transmit of patient health summaries.

Data Aggregation, Business Intelligence, and Quality Measures

Despite the value that HIE and EHR interoperability provide for information exchange, different solutions are required for quality measurement, performance reporting, medical and utilization management, and cost reduction. From the standpoint of performance reporting and quality measures, data analytics and business intelligence systems are essential to the ACO or CIN's ability to meet performance and reporting requirements.

There are several approaches to quality measures that are guided by organizational context. In the simplest scenario, clinical organizations receive certain, limited information from using an EHR receiving comprehensive certification (i.e., certification that indicates that the EHR meets the criteria of basic EHR capabilities plus all criteria associated with Meaningful Use). Criteria for that level of certification include the ability to produce quality measures meeting Meaningful Use program requirements. This capability is required for organizations of varying size, from ambulatory practice to health system. CINs and ACOs usually need to report many more quality measures in addition to Meaningful Use, such as MSSP-ACO measures, population-specifc metrics negotiated by a CIN, pay-for-performance metrics negotiated with each individual health plan, and metrics required by government regulation (e.g., CMS and state regulatory agencies). Availability of supporting data, information systems, analytics, and reporting systems required for gathering, monitoring, and calculation of those measures should be verified.

To calculate measures needed by CIN and ACO, data integration needs to span multiple contributing sources, and typically a data warehouse solution needs to be put in place that serves as an aggregation vehicle for the diverse sources of data required for managing the enterprise's reporting needs. Even in large organizations employing an enterprise EHR, a data warehouse reporting solution is recommended to meet reporting needs that are specific to an organization's needs.

Aggregated data also provides the basis for enhanced clinical decision support, risk stratification, and predictive analytics. Combining data from multiple sources offers the ability to transition clinical decision support from an analysis of local patient records resident only in the provider EHR, to comprehensive analysis of the consolidated patient record from multiple, internal and external sources.

Clinical data warehouse solutions are available commercially off-the-shelf as well as custom developed. They are characterized by multiple layers of data ingest and organization where:

- An interface layer collects data from interfacing systems;
- A transformation process standardizes the data into formats that can be handled in a consistent way despite diverse sources; and
- The data is aggregated into a data structure that supports efficient and accurate report production.

Patient Portals

A patient portal is a key vehicle for connecting with patients and their families. It may also engage patients in their care in several ways. Through secure messaging between physicians, care managers and patients, a portal offers a vehicle for involving patients in the decisions and course of their treatment, particularly chronic condition management.

In addition to traditional services, such as medication refills, appointment scheduling, and bill payment, patient portals can also offer reminders and recommendations and education material filtered to the specific patient's clinical profile. Other features can include portal sponsored gateways to lifestyle, fitness, and nutritional educational materials and coaching programs. Engagement of patients in wellness programs offers an opportunity for ongoing engagement via returns to the portal application with easy access provided by mobile interfaces – which are becoming a common feature.

Provider patient portals also help providers meet MU2 requirements for patients to receive clinical summaries and secure messaging. Many portals also offer Blue Button functionality, giving patients a downloadable copy of their clinical record.

HIT Standards

Under the guidance of the ONC, national HIT standards have been developed. HIT standards focus on three basic categories:

- Content, including structure, vocabulary and code sets
- Transport
- Security and privacy

While recognizing that transport, security and privacy are critically important elements of a nationwide health data exchange infrastructure, content definition captures our interest from an interoperability perspective.

In 2004, the ONC work groups selected HL7 Clinical Document Architecture Release 2 (CDA R2) as the foundation of clinical data expression. CDA R2 is an Extensible Markup Language (XML) based standard designed to express clinical content in a rich and nuanced way, particularly coded content. As a markup standard, CDA R2 is extremely flexible. This offers benefits as it is capable of carrying data appropriate to an extremely broad range of clinical situations. The negative of that flexibility is that trading partners would not necessarily know what content to expect in each transmission because of the wide diversity of content potential expressed in each transaction. The solution to the flexibility issue is to define different document profiles, each of which are still expressed in CDA R2, but each of which carries certain assumptions as to the data that it will contain.

From 2005 until recently most HIE data exchange has focused on utilization of the C32 Clinical Summary/ Continuity of Care Document (CCD) defined by the Health Information Technology Standards Panel (HITSP). HL7 initially worked with ASTM to define the content of the CCD to correspond with the content of the well-regarded clinical summary format supported by ASTM: the Continuity of Care Record (CCR). The CCR provided a strong definition of clinical content that included sections of clinical data defining the following topics:

Payer	Advanced Directives
Support	Functional Status
Problems	Family History
Social History	Allergies
Medications	Medical Equipment
Immunizations	Vital Signs
Results	Procedures
Encounters	Plan of Care

Beginning in 2011, the Standards and Interoperability Workgroup HIT Standards Committee defined a new framework of standards that leverages the work done with the C32. The new framework is Consolidated Clinical Document Architecture (CCDA). CCDA identifies nine templates deemed to be commonly used CCDA documents:

CCDA Clinical Document Templates

Consultation Note - According to CMS evaluation and management guidelines, a Consultation Note must be generated as a result of a physician or non-physician practitioner's (NPP) request for an opinion or advice from another physician or NPP.

Continuity of Care Document (CCD) - The CCD is a core data set of the most relevant administrative, demographic, and clinical information facts about a patient's healthcare, covering one or more healthcare encounters. CCD was defined from the ASTM Continuity of Care Record (CCR) standard.

Diagnostic Imaging Report (DIR) - A Diagnostic Imaging Report (DIR) is a document that contains a consulting specialist's interpretation of image data.

Discharge Summary - The discharge summary is a document that is a synopsis of a patient's admission to a hospital; it provides pertinent information for the continuation of care following discharge but also includes the hospital course and details of events that may not be pertinent to continuity of patient care. The discharge summary template is defined to meet Joint Commission requirements for discharge summaries.

History and Physical Note (H&P) - A History and Physical (H&P) note is a medical report that documents the current and past conditions of the patient to determine a patient's health status. The H&P Note is typically used upon admission to a hospital or prior to an operative procedure.

Operative Note - The operative note is created immediately following a surgical procedure and records the pre- and post-surgical diagnosis, pertinent events of the procedure, as well as the condition of the patient following the procedure.

Procedure Note - The procedure note is created immediately following a non-operative procedure and records the indications for the procedure and, when applicable, post-procedure diagnosis, pertinent events of the procedure, and the patient's tolerance of the procedure.

Progress Note - A progress note documents a patient's clinical status during a hospitalization or outpatient visit; thus, it is associated with an encounter. The Progress Note is not intended to be a re-evaluation note for Medicare requirements.

Unstructured Document - Used when the patient record is captured in an unstructured format, such as a word or PDF document, that is encapsulated within an image file or as unstructured text in an electronic file. Use of unstructured documents is prohibited in MU Stage 2.

(Office of the National Coordinator for Health IT 2013)

The Movement towards Interoperable Rigor

One of the chief intents of MU Stage 2 from a technology perspective is to advance EHR capabilities to interoperate in a seamless way. MU Stage 2 EHR certification requirements for Transitions of Care require the incorporation and electronic reconciliation of medications, medication allergies, and problem lists. (Office of the National Coordinator for Health IT 2013) The MU Stage 2 final rule has incorporated guidelines to assist the industry towards realizing this goal.

Thus, we believe it is necessary to clarify for EHR technology developers that in all instances where we have adopted a vocabulary standard in §170.207 the accompanying section template implemented must be done so using the section-template with required structured data, coded entries required. (U.S. Health and Human Services Department 2012)

Figure 10–3. The Progression of Interoperability in Meaningful Use

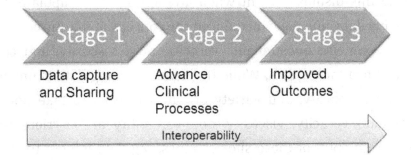

By focusing on stricter definitions of the CCDA document templates, the intent is to provide a more consistent implementation than was possible with previous specifications. As they have in the past, the standards and certification criteria for CCDA specify code sets to be used for each clinical data section. What has changed with the MU Stage 2 certification guidelines are new requirements that bind the certification to use of the code sets, and additional rules restricting the use of uncoded content. Since all related content will be tested and certified by the National Institute of Standards and Technology (NIST), the hope and expectation is that the common validation process will support common interoperability success.

Big Data and Analytics

Big data has become the latest "fad" in healthcare, and the the world of "information technology" in general. Big data has been commonly referred to as the "three Vs" of massive volumes, increasing velocity, and wide variety of data starting to appear as society becomes more digital and organizations are faced with accumulating and attempting to make sense of it. This is no less for healthcare, as the traditionally large amounts of claims data are enhanced with clinical data from EMR and HIE, and new information from patient lifestyle, behavior, and consumer data. In chapter 13 we shall review one use of big data to improve patient engagement.

As of the writing of this chapter, however, big data has been replaced at the peak of the Gartner "Hype Cycle" by a new craze, called the "Internet of Things," and is headed for the "trough of disillusionment." (Gartner Hype Cycle for Emerging Technologies, 2014). The authors have first-hand experienced this disillusionment when attempting to manipulate, analyze and utilize big data, and have introduced the concept of the "three Vs" of big data disillusionment: questionable veracity, poor viscosity, and constant variability of healthcare data. While the quantity of big data is undeniable, as the volume, velocity, and variety of data cause us to take notice, the quality of data veracity, viscosity, and variability are barriers to their practical use. In spite of these shortcomings, big data is here to stay, and new analytic capabilities are being created and used to extract value from this data deluge.

When we think about analytics, it's often within the context of technology, computers and spreadsheets. However, predictive and prescriptive analytics (PA) has the power to analyze big data, predict the future, identify problems before they happen, and recommend specific actions and interventions to avoid problems. (Siegel 2013) For example, analytics can predict how a patient will respond to a given treatment. As a result, adoption of advanced PA benefits all healthcare stakeholders. (Siegel 2013)

The healthcare industry has lagged behind many other sectors — including retail and banking — in the adoption and leveraging of PA to improve efficiencies and services. Recently though, healthcare has seen increased interest in this approach as new payment models and reform initiatives require greater internal visibility to clinical and business intelligence and external transparency for performance and payment. In addition, only recently has technology and data become available allowing people to truly analyze what is going on, and make improvements in how we approach health and care management. The demand for greater efficiency, effectiveness and quality in care creates a need for data-driven strategies that empower physicians, engage individuals and enhance organizational ability to deliver on the triple aim of improved population health, patient experience and affordability. PA is designed to do all this and more.

The volume and variety of data now available through claims, clinical, and exogenous consumer sources along with the exponential growth of computing velocity, are making PA and data mining more important. These developments require organizations to change their approach in order to transform Big Data into actionable insight. Unlocking the power of the massive amounts and different kinds of data require new data science capabilities that will bring incredible value to care delivery. (Miner, et al 2014)

New Technologies

Financial analytics have been used by healthcare for decades, mainly to manage a practice or hospital. These practice management systems are still in use but focus on business matters such as billing and payment. Financial analytics used by third party payers (such as the federal government (Medicare), state governments (Medicaid), health insurance companies, and managed care organizations started in the 1990s, (Winkelman and Mehmud 2007) but the technology focused on financial risk management of populations and did not provide a complete clinical picture of the individual. As these technologies evolved, they helped payers better understand the financial impact and risk of populations, but not quality in clinical practice, nor care of the individual.

New technologies predict risk better, identify individual-level medical needs, enhance care coordination, and help improve outcomes for the ihe individual as well as populations. Now, clinical and PA technology proactively learn from data, aide in predicting future clinical outcomes, and go far beyond current population-based financial approaches to predict the actions of an individual, also known as a "market of one," and recommend specific interventions and actions to improve care and outcomes. Clinical predictive analytics capabilities have been around for more than a dozen years, used mainly be health insurance companies to identify gaps in care and make specific clinical recommendations to improve care and outcomes. Recently these same analytics have been redesigned for the CIN and ACO environment (Yale, 2014).

Best Practices from Other Industries

These examples just scratch the surface in terms of the potential for PA in healthcare. If we look at the new capabilities from other industries, highly-advanced algorithms are now being used in "recommendation engines" built by major retailers, especially those with a large online presence. These engines filter through vast amounts of data to identify and correlate the most important factors influencing consumer preferences and behavior. As this same approach is applied to healthcare, engines can filter out irrelevant information and pinpoint the most important data that should be used to influence care recommendations. For example, advanced algorithms can scour through a patient's medical history, health conditions, phenotype, genotype, lifestyle and other variables. Based on only the most impactful information, data engines can then identify an optimal treatment plan. (McNeill and Davenport 2013)

While many opportunities for the application of PA in healthcare still have yet to be discovered, there are three areas in particular where PA are currently used: clinical risk stratification and identification, financial risk stratification, and identification of patient interests and engagement.

Clinical Risk Stratification

Using the breadth of available clinical information, including problems, details of medications, vital signs, test results, health risk assessment results, etc, predictive analytics can be applied to stratify patient populations according to their degree of illness, and establish probabilities of their capacity to respond to treatment. It can then recommend specific actions necessary to avoid further clinical problems, improve clinical care and outcomes, and reduce costs. This predictive analytic approach is extremely useful in guiding the activities of care managers to the most needy segment of the population. It is more useful, from a clinical perspective, than financial risk stratification as it goes beyond the simple financial information and identifies clinical impactability and specific actions and interventions that yield improved care and lower cost. (Yale, 2013)

Financial Risk Stratification

Financial risk stratification looks at past costs, and projects future potential costs based on experience with similar patients. Financial profiles can be coupled with utilization patterns and fee schedules to establish predictive models around cost and reimbursement trends. As discussed in Chapter 13, this data has very low predictability due to the various exogenous and clinical factors impacting cost and quality of care that are not included in a financial analysis. Recent research and development combining financial and clinical data has the ability to greatly increase predictability, and the authors are involved in research and development to greatly enhance the predictive power of financial analytics by combining it with clinical predictive analytics. (Wei, 2014)

Patient Engagement

Given the diffuse array of communication channels available in today's wired world, predictive models are being developed that enhance the ability to outreach and initially engage patients, maintain patient engagement over time, and intervene to improve clinical care and outcomes. These models discern patterns within clinical and financial data as well as demographic population segments and consumer behavior data, and seek to predict methods of outreach that may be most successful for given profiles, as well as establishing a self correcting capability to revise outreach strategies based on patient behavior. (Yale, 2014)

Future Directions

The last few years have seen technology advancements in EHR adoption and interoperability, big data analytics, population management, patient engagement, and clinical and predictive analytics software. Stimulated by federal incentives and value-based reimbursement arrangements, providers have moved to adopt related technologies and establish programs leading to improved quality and lower costs. Research and development by new ventures and entrepreneurs are creating predictive analytic algorithms that greatly improve the ability to manage risk, care, individual outcomes and population health.

Given the high impact of the current regulatory environment on the health care information technology community, the direction taken by future federal HIT laws and regulations will be an important determinant of future investment and innovation. The jury of providers has not yet weighed in on its ability to accomplish interoperability goals set forth by MU Stage 2, and further refinements are likely in MU Stage 3. If successful, interoperability will play an increasingly important role. As the technology becomes more standardized, barriers to communication will diminish and the costs of interoperability will fall, enabling a more fluid flow of clinical information between parties.

The population health management capabilities that have been developed and brought to market have established a new standard for care quality. Regardless of what path is taken at the federal government level, it seems plausible that value-based reimbursement and the associated benefits in cost and quality will continue to generate interest in the private payer market place as the capabilities of ACOs and CINs continue to advance.

Last, the velocity, variety, and volume at which clinical, financial, and exogenous data is accumulating continues to accelerate. In an expanding marketplace, this creates a fertile opportunity for development of new insights and interventions through the expansion and development of clinical and predictive analytics. Predictive analytics and "Big Data" have the potential to disruptive health care and bring greater value to individual consumers, physicians, hospitals, and payers.

CHAPTER 10 DISCUSSION QUESTIONS

Discussion questions are provided for team building or class exercises. Answers for all questions are provided in Appendix C.

Question Number	Question
1	How does Meaningful Use affect ACOs and CINs, now and in the future?
2	What are key technology capabilities required to support an ACO or CIN?
3	How does interoperability and health information exchange assist quality of care?
4	What is the value of aggregating data from diverse sources?
5	What is predictive analytics and how does it help with population health management and individual care?

CHAPTER 10 HIGHLIGHTS

✓ Technology support for health care quality has been a long-term goal of health care leadership.

✓ Federal legislation and policy initiatives have stimulated significant expansion of health care technology adoption and capabilities.

✓ Significant work has been accomplished in defining federal standards supporting health data exchange.

✓ Health care information technology organizations and technology vendors are struggling to keep up with the demands of health information technology regulatory compliance requirements.

✓ EHR vendors are facing key interoperability capability challenges as part of Meaningful Use Stage 2.

✓ Aggregation of data from diverse sources is an important driver of health care quality and value.

✓ Predictive analytics offers the opportunity to create new insights and intervention opportunities for CINs and ACOs.

CHAPTER 10 REFERENCES

Centers for Medicare and Medicaid Services (2013). Accountable Care Organizations. Retrieved from http://www.cms.gov/Medicare/Medicare-Fee-for-Service-Payment/ACO/

Centers for Medicare and Medicaid Services (2013). Center for Medicare and Medicaid and ONC Response to Public Comments with Interoperability Principles and Strategy. Retrieved from http://www.cms.gov/ehealth/ListServ_InteroperabilityPrinciples_Strategy.html

Centers for Medicare and Medicaid Services (2013). EHR Incentive Program for Medicare Hospitals: Calculating Payments. Baltimore, MD, Centers for Medicare and Medicaid Services.

Centers for Medicare and Medicaid Services (2013). EHR Incentive Programs. Retrieved from http://www.cms.gov/Regulations-and-Guidance/Legislation/EHRIncentivePrograms/index.html?redirect=/ehrincentiveprograms/

Centers for Medicare and Medicaid Services (2013). Shared Savings Program. Retrieved from http://www.cms.gov/Medicare/Medicare-Fee-for-Service-Payment/sharedsavingsprogram/index.html

Department of Health and Human Services (2013). Office of the National Coordinator for Health Information Technology. Health IT Adoption Programs. Retrieved from http://www.healthit.gov/policy-researchers-implementers/beacon-community-program

Gartner (2014). Gartner's 2014 Hype Cycle for Emerging Technologies Maps the Journey to Digital Business. Retrieved from http://www.gartner.com/newsroom/id/2819918

HealtheWay (2013). Current eHealth Exchange Participants. Retrieved from http://healthewayinc.org/index.php/exchange/participants

HealtheWay (2013). eHealth Exchange. Retrieved from http://healthewayinc.org/index.php/exchange

Institute of Medicine and Committee on Improving the Patient Record (1997). *Commentary. Conclusion. The computer-based patient record* (p. 17). Washington, DC: National Academies Press.

Institute of Medicine and Committee on Quality of Health Care in America (2001). Chapter 7. Using Information Technology. *Crossing the quality chasm. A new health system for the 21st century* (p. 165). Washington, DC: National Academies Press.

Institute of Medicine and Committee on Quality of Health Care in America (2001). *Crossing the quality chasm: A new health system for the 21st century*. Washington, DC: National Academies Press.

Institute of Medicine. (1991). *The computer-based patient record: An essential technology for health care*. Washington, DC: National Academies Press.

Institute of Medicine, et al. (2000). *To err is human: building a safer health system*. Washington, DC: National Academies Press.

McNeill, D. and T. H. Davenport (2013). Analytics in Healthcare and the Life Sciences: Strategies, Implementation Methods, and Best Practices, Pearson Education.

Miner, L., Bolding, P., Hilbe, J., Goldstein, M., Hill, T., Nisbet, R.,Miner, G. (2014). *Practical Predictive Analytics and Decisioning Systems for Medicine: Informatics Accuracy and Cost-Effectiveness for Healthcare Administration and Delivery Including Medical Research*, Waltham, MA: Academic Press.

Mostashari, F. (2012). HealthITBuzz - Meaningful Use Stage 2: a Giant Leap in Data Exchange. Retrieved from http://www.healthit.gov/buzz-blog/meaningful-use/meaningful-use-stage-2/

Office of the National Coordinator for Health IT (2013). Companion Guide to Consolidated CDA for MU2. Retrieved from http://wiki.siframework.org/file/view/Companion_Guide_to_CCDA_for_MU2_r0.docx/390 200714/Companion_Guide_to_CCDA_for_MU2_r0.docx

Office of the National Coordinator for Health IT (2013). Test Procedure for §170.314 (b)(1) Transitions of care – receive, display and incorporate transition of care/referral summaries. Retrieved from http://www.healthit.gov/sites/default/files/170.314b1receive_display_incorporate_2014_approved_tp_v1.6.pdf

Reider, M. J. and Tagalicod, R. (2013, December 6). Progress on Adoption of Electronic Health Records. Retrieved from http://www.healthit.gov/buzz-blog/electronic-health-and-medical-records/progress-adoption-electronic-health-records/

Siegel, E. (2013). *Predictive analytics: the power to predict who will click, buy, lie, or die.* Hoboken, NJ: John Wiley & Sons.

The Direct Project (2010). The Direct Project Overview. Retrieved August 8, 2014, from http://wiki.directproject.org/file/view/DirectProjectOverview.pdf.

The Office of the National Coordinator for Health IT (2011, February 17). Get the Facts about State Health Information Exchange Program. Retrieved from http://www.healthit.gov/sites/default/files/get-the-facts-about-state-hie-program-2.pdf

The White House (2004). Executive Order: Incentives for the Use of Health Information Technology and Establishing the Position of the National Health Information Technology Coordinator. Washington, DC: U.S. Government.

US Health and Human Services Department (2012). Health Information Technology: Standards, Implementation Specifications, and Certification Criteria for Electronic Health Record Technology, 2014 Edition; Revisions to the Permanent Certification Program for Health Information Technology." Retrieved from https://http://www.federalregister.gov/articles/2012/09/04/2012-20982/health-information-technology-standards-implementation-specifications-and-certification-criteria-for

Wei, H. (2014, November 15). *Prediction vs. Intervention.* Presentation to The Predictive Modeling Summit 2014, Washington, DC.

Winkelman, R. and S. Mehmud (2007). A comparative analysis of claims-based tools for health risk assessment. *Society of Actuaries*, 1-70.

Yale, K. (in press). Advanced Analytics: The Foundation for Transforming Care Delivery. *Health Management Technology.*

Yale, K. (2014, January). *Predictive Analytics and Patient Behavior*. Presentation to Data Stratification & Analytics Conference, Phoenix, AZ.

Yale, K., et al. (2014, June). *R For Improved Consumer Engagement and Health Outcomes*. Presentation to The 'R' User Conference 2014, University of California at Los Angeles, Los Angeles, CA.

Yale, K. (2014, September) MIT Chief Data Officer Forum West, Palo Alto, CA. http://chiefdataofficerforum.org/mit-2014-cdo-forum-west-agenda/

Yale, K. (2014, October). *Significant Improvements in Population Health Management.* presentation to Predictive Analytics World Healthcare, Boston, MA.

Chapter 11. Non-Traditional Mental Health and Substance Use Disorder Services as a Core Part of Health in CINs and ACOs

Roger Kathol | Susan Sargent |

Steve Melek | Lee Sacks | Kavita K. Patel

After you've done a thing the same way for two years, look it over carefully. After five years, look at it with suspicion. And after ten years, throw it away and start all over.

Alfred Edward Perlman
1902-1983
President, Penn Central Transportation Company

CHAPTER 11 LEARNING OBJECTIVES

✓ To understand the frequency and interaction of behavioral health (BH) with general medical conditions.

✓ To summarize the way that BH services are currently delivered.

✓ To clarify the effect of currently siloed behavioral health payment practices on care delivery and patient outcomes.

✓ To review the clinical and cost impact of untreated behavioral health conditions in the medical setting.

✓ To describe models of value-added non-traditional behavioral health services to consider when building a CIN or ACO.

✓ To discuss the opportunity cost of behavioral health exclusion / marginalization when setting up a CIN or ACO.

Introduction

Mental health (MH) and substance use disorders (SUD), hereafter referred to as "behavioral health" (BH) conditions, present as emotional, behavioral, or cognitive disturbances, which interfere with a person's ability to function optimally while symptoms are present. Over eighty percent of patients with BH conditions present only or primarily in the primary or specialty medical/surgical setting, hereafter called "medical" setting (Figure 11-1). (Regier et al., 1993; Reilly et al., 2012; P. S. Wang et al., 2006) Of these, sixty to seventy percent receive no treatment for their BH conditions. (Kessler et al., 2005; P. S. Wang et al., 2007; P. S. Wang, Demler, & Kessler, 2002; P. S. Wang, Lane, et al., 2005) Fewer than one in nine of those who do receive treatment in the medical setting are exposed to a BH intervention that would be expected to improve symptoms or return a person to productive, psychological health. (P. S. Wang et al., 2002; P. S. Wang, Lane, et al., 2005)

Figure 11-1. Most BH Patients are Seen in the Medical Setting

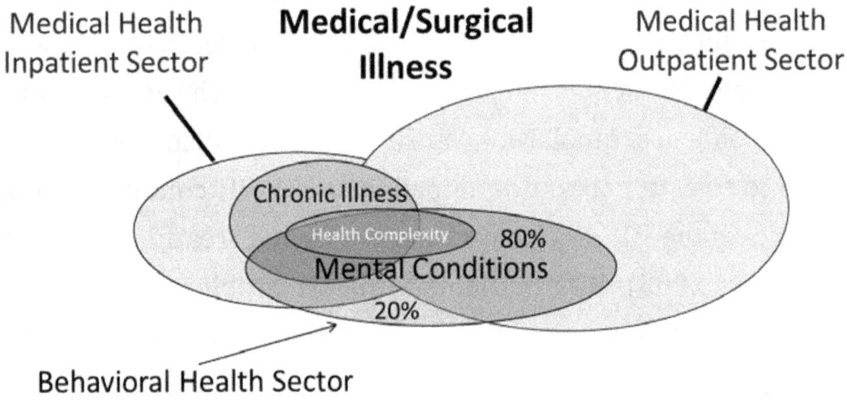

This Chapter will describe how BH services are delivered in today's health system; the influence that current payment practices have on how and where clinical services are delivered and where BH professionals practice; the impact of isolated BH service delivery on the quality and cost of care within national, health plan, and clinic systems; the BH delivery system changes needed to improve health and cost outcomes of untreated

BH conditions in the medical setting; and the opportunities associated with BH service implementation as a part of Clinically Integrated Networks (CINs) and/or Accountable Care Organizations (ACOs).

We posit that advanced CINs, such as those taking risk for total health and cost outcomes of populations of patients, including those developing ACOs, and many basic CINs that are providing integrated service delivery for targeted populations, will not be successful in an environment of increasing competition and cost pressures unless they include "value-added" BH services and professionals as core CIN/ACO services and providers.

Today's BH Service Delivery

Over ninety-five percent of BH professionals practice almost exclusively in standalone inpatient (IP) and outpatient (OP) BH settings. (Franz et al., 2010) This is where the majority of evidence-based BH interventions are delivered. (P. S. Wang et al., 2007; P. S. Wang, Lane, et al., 2005) Specialty BH settings are designed to support treatment for patients with mild to serious BH conditions but especially cater to the delivery of services for those with serious and persistent primary BH disorders, such as schizophrenia, substance dependence, bipolar illness, serious eating disorders, autism, etc. Only fifteen to twenty percent of all patients with BH conditions, however, choose to access the BH sector for assessment and treatment. (P. S. Wang, Berglund, et al., 2005) Most patients with BH problems are seen in the physical health sector where few BH practitioners are present to assist primary and specialty medical clinicians in the delivery of outcome changing BH care. This we refer to as the BH specialist-BH patient mismatch (Figure 11-2).

Figure 11-2. BH Specialist-BH Patient Mismatch

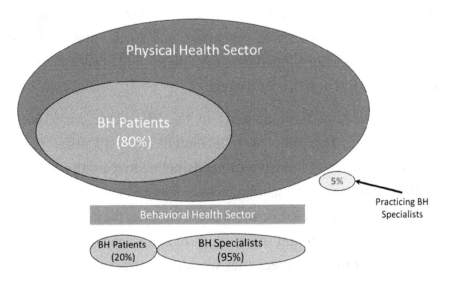

The original intent in creating a standalone BH sector was to maximize delivery of evidence-based care to patients in most need of BH interventions in settings designed for such. Unfortunately, few of those who need BH services have been or are willing to access treatment in independent BH service locations. This includes the majority of patients with serious and persistent behavioral conditions, albeit with the possible exception of patients with schizophrenia. Those who do choose to seek assistance for their BH conditions in the BH sector find that there are often delays of six or more weeks before initial appointments can be made due to personnel shortages. (Cunningham, 2009) Timely follow-up can pose a challenge for the same reason. Hindered access is particularly problematic for those with limited financial resources or those in public programs.

BH Sector Delivery of Care

The BH sector provides services in a different way than all other specialty medical settings. First, it is supported through funding streams segregated from all other medical disciplines (to be covered later). Separate payment procedures sometimes create the requirement to place service locations at a distance from other general medical and specialty services. This occurs either directly, as a part of participation rules, or indirectly by decrements in the amount paid for services or the complicated procedures needed to obtain permission to provide them. These BH service locations are governed by an independent set of regulatory and fiscal rules that create challenges in delivering coordinated care to patients, and especially to those with concurrent medical and BH conditions.

Second, clinicians that treat patients in the BH sector participate in networks of providers that may be independent from all other medical providers. Thus, they are responsive to needs delineated by the BH sector service locations (and payers), including where services can be delivered, to whom, and with what type of BH professionals. Further, they often maintain independent record keeping and quality improvement systems even when colleagues from other medical specialties working for the same hospital and clinic system also see the patients for whom they care. Communication among medical and BH practitioners can be difficult and in some situations impossible. In addition, independent record keeping prevents analysis of total health outcomes for patients with both medical and BH care needs.

Finally, despite the frequency with which patients with concurrent medical and BH conditions are seen, in many cases the BH sector is designed only for the delivery of BH care, often to the exclusion of any medical interventions other than the most basic. Conversely, the medical setting avoids delivery of BH services since they are considered the responsibility of professionals in the BH sector (and paid through a separate budget). This creates significant problems in medical and BH emergency rooms (ERs), in acute medical and BH settings (hospitals), in post-acute care settings (nursing home and assisted living facilities), and in medical and BH outpatient clinics.

Five to ten percent of "medical" ER visits are for patients with primary BH conditions. (Larkin, Claassen, Emond, Pelletier, & Camargo, 2005) Additionally, up to 40% of patients with a primary medical reason for their ER visits have a BH comorbidity contributing to the patient's health need, such as substance abuse associated with auto accidents and falls.

(Richmond et al., 2007) Despite these statistics, medical ERs typically do not have psychiatrist coverage, virtually the only allopathic medical specialty overlooked for ER participation. Likewise, standalone BH emergency assessment facilities, primarily accessible in standalone psychiatric facilities, have no medical service capabilities. Such segregation of services is associated with up to 25% higher BH-related admission rates to both medical and BH units and a high use of ambulances to transport patients from BH to medical ERs, and vice versa, for cross-disciplinary assessments.

In acute general hospital (GH) settings, consistently 25% to 35% of general medical admissions have BH comorbidity (Table 11-1). One would expect that such a high frequency would necessitate support for inpatient BH services access; however, BH specialists and clinical settings with medical and BH capabilities are the exception rather than the rule. Medical and psychiatric units, even if located in the same GH, are configured for discipline-specific care. Psychiatric units cannot handle acute medical problems and medical units address BH comorbidity only if it becomes flagrant, requiring physical or chemical restraints, one-on-one supervision, or transfer for close observation in the intensive care unit. Even then, cross-disciplinary patient treatment is not part of the equation in either setting. Transfers or safety measures prior to transfer are most typically provided.

Table 11-1. General Hospital Medical Admissions* with BH Comorbidity

Core Delivery Systems	Number of Hospitals	Total Adm/Yr	% BH	Longer BH vs. non-BH ALOS	Higher BH vs. non-BH Readmits	Sitter Use
System 1	>10	135,000+	26%	1.1	30%	$6.0M
System 2	1	19,000+	36%	1.2	40%	$3.1M
System 3	4	34,500+	29%	1.3	70%	$.42M
System 4	5	40,000+	26%	1.8	30%	$2+M
System 5	1	16,000+	23%	0.6	45%	

*Medical and surgical admissions to five general hospital systems in the United States, excluding neonate and primary psychiatric admissions.

Separation of medical and BH services even occurs in post-acute settings. BH providers build support services at selected nursing facilities that are independent of medical services, even for patients in whom both medical and BH issues contribute to challenges in assisting them with health needs. This limits the ability of post-acute settings to accept comorbid patients from acute care settings. Even though acute medical and BH conditions have stabilized enough for discharge, post-acute cross-disciplinary needs can lead to extended delays in placement to lower levels of care.

The last disconnect in medical and BH service is in outpatient clinics. Half of patients with serious mental illness have one or more chronic medical condition,(Druss & Walker, 2011) whereas BH comorbidity is present in 30% of medical outpatients. (Druss & Walker, 2011) As in the GH setting, access to coordinated outpatient medical and BH care is typically not available in either the primary medical or BH setting. The disconnect in medical and BH service coordination is now becoming a recognized area of potential growth due to the high clinical and economic cost of comorbidity. Neither the medical nor the BH settings have found ways to effectively introduce outcome changing, value-added, cross-disciplinary services because of funding challenges.

As a result, low cost BH professionals, such as counselors and social workers, are hired to assist with BH issues in medical settings because budget work arounds can often support their addition. However, they have limited assessment and intervention capabilities, especially for high cost patients with complex health conditions, including treatment resistant BH issues. Use of low cost BH professionals is not associated with either improved long-term clinical or fiscal outcomes. (Bower, Knowles, Coventry, & Rowland, 2011) On the reverse side, medical pract itioners added to BH settings find that they are limited in their medical assessments since simple and available ancillary medical testing and procedures are not possible in BH settings devoted to delivery of targeted BH services.

This mismatch of patients, providers, and settings is associated with well-documented adverse health outcomes. Medical patients with largely untreated comorbid BH conditions are: (1) medical ilness treatment resistant, (2) experience persistent medical symptoms and more chronic illness complications, (3) report greater impairment, (4) use more disability days, and (5) have doubling of total health care costs when compared to medical patients without BH comorbidity. (R. Kathol et al., 2005; W. J. Katon & Seelig, 2008; Prince et al., 2007; Seelig & Katon, 2008) Unfortunately, parity laws do not improve access to BH services in the medical setting nor does the ACA. They merely state that BH services should be "available" and paid *on par* with similar medical services. Nothing assures where and how they should be delivered, such as in the medical setting.

The Effect of Siloed Payments for BH Services on Medical and BH Care Delivery

Most non-BH clinicians and medical administrators are unaware of the effect that segregated payment for BH services has on their patients' access to evidence-based BH and medical care. Even medical health plan executives do not understand that "carving-out" or "carving-in" BH benefits from their medical insurance products significantly limits the ability of medical and BH practitioners to deliver coordinated care.

Segregated BH Payment Practices

Prior to passage of the ACA, health plans and the purchasers of their products were the primary organizations at risk for the total cost of care in covered populations. Further, while capitated contracts were occasionally used, the majority of contracts for medical care were based on fee-for-service business practices (i.e., volume-based). Thus, health plans and self-insured employers attempted to create payment practices designed to support delivery of services while controlling costs. Using volume-based models, payment practices often fostered delivery of unnecessary services while preventing delivery of value-added services, especially to those with complex health conditions and exceedingly high health care service use.

The ACA has created a new dynamic in the marketplace. Networks of treating clinicians (e.g., doctors) have become fiscally accountable for the quality and cost-effective delivery of value-added services. They are expected to use their understanding of health and health care delivery to develop coordinated delivery approaches that improve the patient experience, lead to better health, and save money to help meet the Triple Aim objective of the Medicare Shared Savings Program (MSSP). As a part of the ACA MSSP initiative, networks of providers (e.g., ACOs) in alliance with various other stakeholders in the health care delivery system (e.g., health plans, employers, government agencies, hospitals and clinics), are building new delivery approaches and payment practices to foster efficient and effective care. If successful, and quality thresholds are met, treatment providers can share in associated savings. Importantly, some of these networks are also at-risk for negative health and cost outcomes. This new "pay-for-performance" model we refer to as the "ACO World."

Under the historic fee-for-service model of care delivery and payment, health plans and payers instituted various utilization management initiatives in an attempt to monitor and reduce risk, thereby controlling costs. Among these initiatives has been the establishment of managed care organizations (MCOs) and separate managed behavioral health organizations (MBHOs). In these situations, separate medical and BH funding pools independently pay for medical and BH professional services and facility costs, which persists even after passage of the ACA (Figure 11-3).

Figure 11-3. Siloed Payment for Medical and BH Services Even in the ACO World

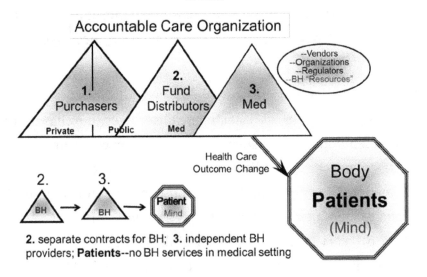

When a MCO "owns" its own BH business, funding for BH care uniformly comes from a BH subsidiary of the MCO plan. This BH subsidiary is known as a MBHO "carve-in." Alternatively, a medical health plan can choose to buy management of their BH business from an independent MBHO vendor. This is known as an MBHO "carve-out." Regardless of whether BH business is carved-in or carved-out, budgets for BH care are distinct from those for medical care. Importantly, the medical and BH budgets may compete with each other so that each can maximize profits from the populations they serve, even if the populations are the same.

While conceptually, one would think that carve-ins would be more supportive of BH services delivery, in fact, many carve-ins are more aggressive in managing (or minimizing) BH services utilization than some carve-outs. Both carve-ins and carve-outs have a vested interest in channeling payment for BH services from their budgets to their medical payment counterparts, especially when non-network "medical" providers in medical settings provide them. While the opportunity is present for carve-ins to look at the interaction of medical and BH costs for the same covered patients, this rarely happens since patient identifiers are separate, claims adjudication often occurs in discrete servers, and few understand the important impact that concurrent medical and BH conditions have on clinical outcomes and total health care costs. Furthermore, MBHOs benefit by isolating the BH payment system. They have no incentive to integrate benefits or services.

Independent budgets carry with them an additional feature. Since BH coverage is separate from all other medical services, purchasers of health care for selected populations, such as employers or government programs, can choose to purchase medical and BH care for their enrollees from different vendors. Thus, an employer could contract with Health Plan A to pay for medical services for its employees and with MBHO B (a carved-out MBHO) for BH services. This creates a disconnection for patients and providers. Medical practitioners paid through Health Plan A's contract benefits may work in the same care facilities as BH providers who are paid through MBHO B. Since BH providers are not contracted with Health Plan A's MBHO, Health Plan A's BH carve-in, it is necessary for medical practitioners to find BH practitioners outside their own system to service their patient's needs.

Disconnects such as this are common and lead to the need for medical providers to suggest that patients call a "1-800" number to access a BH professional rather than sending the patient down the hall to a known BH in-network colleague, as commonly occurs with pulmonary, surgical, or pediatric colleagues in the same "network" of providers. The situation becomes even more complicated when independent medical and BH payers cover patients needing medical and BH care. When a patient has medical coverage for services in one health system, but BH coverage for network services in a competing health system, both patients and practitioners suffer from the necessary disconnect. Alternatively, the patient can absorb additional costs of non-network treatment. More often, however, the patient and medical practitioner merely choose to ignore the BH condition with the resultant outcomes noted above.

Practices of BH in an Independent Payment System

Independent payment for BH and medical services shows up at multiple levels within the health care system (Table 11-2). First, it creates a competitive environment between medical and BH care delivery since each system is responsible for supporting services while maximizing profits from the discipline-specific services for which they are responsible. It does not matter that the BH budget for direct BH care constitutes only two to seven percent of the total health care spend (discussed below). Each looks to the most efficient use of its own resources, concentrating exclusively on those for which it is accountable.

Table 11-2. Effect of Independent Medical and BH Payment on Health System, Insurer, and Clinical Care Factors

	Factors	Effects
Health System	Interaction of medical and BH systems	Little communication, including EHR
Insurers	Patient identifiers	Two identifiers
	Payment pool	Two buckets
	Contract benefit descriptions	Disparate coverage and rules
	Network of providers	Separate medical and BH
	Member and provider support	Separate call-in numbers
	Approval process	Separate rules & approaches
	Case & utilization management	Discipline-specific
	Coding, billing, claims adjudication	Separate payment rules and billing forms
	Data warehousing & actuarial analysis	Separate & discrete
	Quality improvement programs	Discipline-specific
Clinical Care	Practice locations	Paid independently; necessarily separate
	Services delivery	Segregated
	Clinician collaboration and communication	Rare

Second, a separate budget for BH services necessitates duplication of health plan administrative divisions, such as those listed in Table 11-2. Carve-outs do this naturally since they are independent companies and are required to support their insurance products through appropriate business practices. Interestingly, however, the same completely segregated divisions and work processes are also necessary for carve-ins, though owned by a single company. Thus, separate medical and BH budgets are also associated with considerably higher total health plan administrative costs.

Just like carve-outs, many carve-ins sell their BH products independent of the medical products sold by the same insurer. Thus, they require separate actuarial projections, patient identifiers, and a detached network of providers. Discrete benefit descriptions, member and provider support services, insurance approval processes, denial and appeals procedures, case and utilization management practices, and quality improvement programs follow from these. Since medical and BH budgets are isolated, then coding, billing, and claims adjudication disconnected from medical are also necessary. Logically, accumulated data from services supported by each would flow into segregated data warehouses, contributing to independently analyzed discipline-specific performance assessment and quality improvement programs.

Third, and perhaps most important, independent payment drives where and how BH services are delivered. The independent network of BH providers allows MBHOs to target payment only to those with credentials to provide BH services. Since facility fees are also generated as a part of the care delivery process, MBHOs typically require that BH services be provided in locations discrete from medical services. This not only focuses BH funds for BH care, but also prevents the potential for inadvertent payment for direct or ancillary medical services delivered to the same patients, who often have concurrent medical conditions.

Thus, while a separate payment system for BH conditions seems innocuous, in fact, it has pervasive effects on the ability of BH clinicians to practice in the medical setting. MBHOs are rigorous about making sure that their dollars go to BH care. The best and most financially successful means to do this is to ensure segregation of medical from BH services. It is these business practices that are associated with the "traditional" approach to BH care delivery described below. One can only imagine what our health care would look like if similar practices were used in the medical setting (i.e., managed pulmonary organizations (MPOs) or managed surgical organizations (MSOs) that independently handled service support and payment for patients with lung or surgical disease).

Clinical and Economic Consequences of Siloed Medical and Behavioral Health Payment Practices

Few stakeholders participating in the development of CINs and ACOs give much thought to the inclusion of BH practitioners and services as they build their integrated programs. Both MH and SUD services have traditionally been considered outside the purview of the rest of medical care. This perception, and the stigma that accompanies it, is perpetuated by the way that it is handled in the current medical environment. In fact, a recent survey of ACOs indicates that less than half have any BH providers as part of their clinician network and only 14% include BH programs. (Lewis et al., 2014)

Patients with BH conditions are treated in separate clinical locations. BH providers are members of separate networks of clinicians. Separate payers adjudicate payment for BH services. Treatment outcomes and costs are analyzed separately from medical outcomes and costs. Some even continue to think that BH conditions are not "real" illnesses; that those with BH disorders bring it on themselves, such as with SUDs; and that BH treatments are ineffective and unnecessarily costly.

Even for those who recognize the importance of BH comorbidity in medical patients on health and cost outcomes and the advances in BH treatment that lead to comparable outcomes as found in the medical setting, critical factors inhibit implementation of integrated BH and medical care as a part of CINs and ACOs. The most important factor is the siloed payment system described above. Unless this is changed, the integration of medical and BH services will, at best, be piecemeal with corresponding adverse consequences for the patient. The question is whether there is good reason for developing CINs, and especially those anticipating entering the full risk market, such as ACOs, to go to the effort to include BH providers and services as a core component of their clinical operations.

The best place to start addressing this question is by taking a look at the financial impact that patients with BH conditions have on health care spending. In a recent report produced for the American Psychiatric Association, Melek et al. (Melek, Norris, & Paulus, 2013) at Milliman, Inc. used available commercial, Medicare, and Medicaid health care databases to assess health care costs for individuals with and without BH comorbidity covered by these three insurance vehicles. Consistent with other literature, their report confirmed that at a national level, the total cost of care for patients with BH conditions was 2.5 to 3.5 times that of those with no BH condition. Medicaid BH patients had 3.4 times the cost of those without (per member per month [PMPM] $1,301 versus $381). BH patients covered by commercial insurance or Medicare were 2.8 and 2.4 times more expensive, respectively (PMPM $940 versus $340 and $1,404 versus $582, respectively).

Also consistent with the literature, the majority of what's spent for BH patients was for medical services, with a range of 71% (Medicaid) to 92% (Medicare). In fact, if one compares the total spend for BH services in those with BH conditions to the "medical" spend (Table 11-3), the medical spend is nearly five times higher than the BH spend. This finding is magnified if one considers that nearly half of the BH spend for commercial and Medicaid patients was for BH medications (data not available for Medicare patients). Primary care physicians, not psychiatrists, write most BH prescriptions.

Table 11-3. Is BH the "Bottomless Pit"?

	Total Population Served	% of Pop. with BH Claims	Total Annual Spend	BH* Spend	Total Medical Claims Incurred by BH Pop. (% of Medical Claims
Commercial	198.8M	14%	$1.0T	$42.9B	$275B (28.7%)
Medicare/ Medicaid	91.8M	9%/20%	$0.67T	$49.0B	$169B (26.3%)
Total	290.6M	14%	$1.7T	$91.9B	$444B (27.5%)

*Includes BH meds for commercial and Medicaid but not Medicare.

Health plan claims data confirms that the addition of BH comorbidity in patients with medical conditions increases the total annual cost of care. This is readily evident in a consolidation of claims data on a nationally representative population of nearly six million patients covered by public and private insurance products performed by Cartesian Solutions, Inc.™ (Table 11-4). In this Table, the presence of a chronic medical illness doubles the annual cost of care compared to the entire population. In the thirty to forty percent with concurrent BH conditions and a chronic medical illness, annual cost of care more than doubles again.

Table 11-4. Health and Cost Impact of BH Comorbidity in Patients with Chronic Medical Conditions

Patient Groups	Annual Cost of Care	Illness Prevalence	% with Comorbid BH Condition*	Annual Cost with BH Condition	% Increase with BH Condition
All insured	$2,920		15%		
Arthritis	$5,220	6.6%	36%	$10,710	94%
Asthma	$3,730	5.9%	35%	$10,030	169%
Cancer	$11,650	4.3%	37%	$18,870	62%

Patient Groups	Annual Cost of Care	Illness Prevalence	% with Comorbid BH Condition*	Annual Cost with BH Condition	% Increase with BH Condition
Diabetes	$5,480	8.9%	30%	$12,280	124%
CHF	$9,770	1.3%	40%	$17,200	76%
Migraine	$4,340	8.2%	43%	$10,810	149%
COPD	$3,840	8.2%	38%	$10,980	186%

Cartesian Solutions, Inc.™--consolidated health plan claims data
*Approximately 10% receive evidence-based mental condition treatment.

These national findings are also reflected in what is experienced at the care delivery system level. Table 11-1 indicates that the 25% to 35% of patients admitted to medical and surgical units in general hospitals with comorbid BH conditions, excluding those admitted for primary psychiatric conditions, had longer average lengths of stay and higher readmission rates, both indicators of high total health care costs. The predominance of high medical versus BH costs in medical patients with comorbid BH conditions is further clarified in a Truven MarketScan database analysis where employees and their covered dependents with diabetes mellitus and alcoholism had PMPM costs of care 2.2 times higher than those without (Table 11-5). Ninety-one percent of the costs for those with comorbid alcoholism were for medical services and non-BH medications. These findings are similar to another population of patients with diabetes and depression.

Table 11-5. Diabetes – The Impact of Alcoholism

Chronic Medical Condition: DIABETES	Annual Episode Rate per 1,000	Average Number of Services Per Episode	Annual Utilization Rate per 1,000	Average Allowed Cost per Unit	Average Paid Cost per Unit	Paid Cost Per Member Per Month
with Alcoholism						
IP Facility-BHV	187.34	4.63	868.12	$757.63	$665.92	$48.17
IP Facility-MED	607.39	6.62	4,021.93	$1,475.13	$1,453.99	$487.32
PHP/IOP	187.82	7.48	1,405.02	$233.21	$206.46	$24.17
Hosp ER/Lab/Rad/Oth	2,481.24	17.65	43,784.51	$195.99	$168.01	$613.00
OP Professional-BHV	320.60	11.23	3,599.94	$82.11	$61.66	$18.50
Prof/Other Medical	8,082.01	8.11	65,570.54	$90.54	$78.80	$430.56
RX Behavioral			11,843.22	$88.74	$73.99	$73.02
RX Medical			30,931.70	$88.96	$72.99	$188.13
TOTAL	**166.84**	**13.65**	**2,278.06**	**$157.60**	**$139.45**	**$1,882.88**
w/o Alcoholism						
IP Facility-BHV	3.99	6.79	27.09	$659.62	$548.08	$1.24
IP Facility-MED	178.46	6.07	1,083.34	$1,392.35	$1,335.05	$120.53
PHP/IOP	7.56	4.57	34.55	$185.84	$157.01	$0.45
Hosp ER/Lab/Rad/Oth	1,536.06	12.22	18,773.11	$199.65	$169.82	$265.67
OP Professional BHV	61.57	8.36	514.55	$83.72	$59.49	$2.55
Prof/Other Medical	7,315.85	5.88	43,007.41	$83.95	$68.88	$246.88
RX Behavioral	-	-	4,443.18	$84.12	$68.79	$25.47

Chronic Medical Condition: DIABETES	Annual Episode Rate per 1,000	Average Number of Services Per Episode	Annual Utilization Rate per 1,000	Average Allowed Cost per Unit	Average Paid Cost per Unit	Paid Cost Per Member Per Month
RX Medical	-	-	31,317.00	$92.58	$74.33	$193.99
TOTAL	11,302.64	10.90	123,164.27	$123.06	$103.64	$856.77

The data analyses performed by Melek et al and Cartesian Solutions, Inc.™ provide robust support for the fact that BH comorbidity is associated with high health care service use. The majority of this is for medical, not BH service. In fact, earlier sections in this Chapter on the delivery of BH care indicate that BH care has limited availability in the medical setting and that patients with BH conditions seen in the medical setting don't accept referral to the BH sector. This is consistent with findings in the literature that most with BH conditions seen in the medical setting go untreated. (P. S. Wang et al., 2007; P. S. Wang, Lane, et al., 2005)

The lack of treatment for BH conditions in the medical setting is associated not only with poor BH outcomes, but it also predicts that patients, such as those with diabetes and depression, will have more symptoms. Patients will respond worse to treatment, will have worse medical illness control and more complications, will have less satisfaction with medical care, will be more disabled, and will have higher mortality than patients with medical illness alone. (Chang et al., 2011; Druss, Zhao, Von Esenwein, Morrato, & Marcus, 2011) Untreated BH conditions in medical patients have more than just cost consequences. They are also associated with greater impairment and persistent, poorly treated medical illness.

Thus, we come back to the comments at the beginning of this section. Does it make sense that BH services and providers should become core members of CINs as they are conceptualized and built? Since CINs or ACOs are tasked with putting together services that will lead to health improvement and conservation of health resources, then inclusion of BH providers and services as essential features seems reasonable. This, however, is only true if the addition of BH providers in the medical setting add value by improving health and cost outcomes.

Further, current payment practices and resultant care delivery processes do nothing to encourage greater consideration for the inclusion of BH services and professionals as core participants in CINs and ACOs. For instance, BH providers are paid exclusively by MBHOs. This necessarily creates a challenge for organizations setting up CINs and ACOs since they would then be required to set up payment work arounds that allow BH providers to deliver services to medical patients with BH comorbidity. The next sections discuss strategies to support value-added, non-traditional BH services through CINs and ACOs while transitioning from segregated to integrated medical and BH benefit contracting.

Models of Value-Added BH Care

The United States currently lives in a world of what we will call "traditional" BH service delivery. As discussed in the Section on BH Sector Delivery of Care, above, traditional BH services are almost exclusively provided in the BH sector. While this can help BH patients willing to avail themselves of treatment there, it is of no use to the seventy to eighty percent of BH patients seen exclusively or primarily in the medical sector. Restricting treatment to the BH setting also limits communication between BH providers and medical providers, an important aspect of coordinated care since medical and BH illnesses interact.

If BH professionals practicing in the BH sector are characteristic of traditional BH, then "non-traditional" BH may be characterized by delivery of BH services in the medical setting. The first attempt to do this was to add BH care to primary and specialty medical physicians' list of tasks for which they were responsible. It is no wonder that this path of least cost has not succeeded. Primary care physicians are already burdened with a 150% time commitment in a 100% time world just to provide for preventive, acute and chronic medical care needs. (Ostbye et al., 2005; Yarnall, Pollak, Ostbye, Krause, & Michener, 2003) Specialty medical physicians, also busy, are encumbered by limited interest in becoming involved in emotions, cognitions, and behavior when their preferred attention targets their chosen specialty area. To time and interest constraints, there is also the fact that primary and specialty medical physicians have limited training in evidence-based application of BH interventions, especially in medical patients with chronic and complex illness.

In order for the introduction of BH services in the primary and specialty medical setting to succeed, it is necessary for BH specialists with skills, time, and interest in the area to join medical teams and contribute to the holistic care of patients. It is unlikely, however, that the ninety-plus percent of BH practitioners working in the BH sector are going to put on their marching shoes and move to the medical sector to practice. They still get paid for providing services in the traditional BH setting, and this is unlikely to change soon.

An alternative would be for primary care and specialty medical system profits to pay for BH specialists to treat patients in the medical setting. This scenario is an equally unlikely possibility since primary care practices also have financial challenges. Specialty medical services are reluctant for both economic and perceptual reasons. They, after all, are primarily accountable only for specialty service outcomes.

Even if there were a way to pay for low cost counselors or social workers, would this be a value-added addition in the primary and specialty medical setting? A recent Cochrane review of counselor use in the UK, i.e., professionals who provide similar services to counselors and social workers in the United States, suggests not. While there was short-term satisfaction, there were no improved long-term clinical outcomes or cost savings,(Bower et al., 2011; Bower, Rowland, & Hardy, 2003) even after 40 years of implementation adjustments and outcome assessments.

Value-Added BH

For purposes of this Chapter, we use the term "value-added" to denote clinical services that have the potential to improve health and lower cost when delivered to a population of patients. This concept is core to the development of CINs and ACOs and should be no different for BH services than other decisions being made when setting up a CIN and/or ACO.

If traditional BH services are not an option for adding value for patients, since they do not target patients in the medical setting nor coordinate medical and BH service delivery, what about non-traditional BH services? During the past twenty years, there are a number of non-traditional approaches to BH care that show substantial promise (Table 11-6). Some have irrefutable data showing that when they are introduced, predictable improvements in health and cost occur.

Table 11-6. Examples of Value-Added Non-Traditional BH and Medical Services

(Improves Outcomes and Lowers Cost)

Category	Description
Depression and diabetes	2 months fewer days of depression/year; project $2.9 million/year lower total health costs/100,000 diabetic members[1]
Panic disorder in PC	2 months fewer days of anxiety/year; project $1.7 million/year lower total health costs/100,000 diabetic members[2]
Substance use disorders with medical compromise	14% increase in abstinence; $2,050 lower annual health care cost/patient in integrated program[3]
Delirium prevention programs	30% lower incidence of delirium; projected $16.5 million/year reduction in IP costs/30,000 admissions[4]
Unexplained physical complaints	no increase in missed general medical illness or adverse events; 9% to 53% decrease in costs associated with increased healthcare service utilization[5]
Health complexity	halved depression prevalence; statistical improvement of quality of life, perceived physical and mental health; 7% reduction in new admissions at 12 months[6]
Proactive psychiatric consultation	doubled psychiatric involvement with .92 shorter ALOS and 4:1 to 14:1 return on investment[7]

Notes: 1. Katon et al, *Diab Care* 29:265-270, 2006; 2. Katon et al, *Psychological Med* 36:353-363, 2006; 3. Parthasarathy et al, *Med Care* 41:257-367, 2003; 4. Inouye et al, Arch Int Med 163:958-964, 2003; 5. summary of 8 experimental/control outcome studies; 6. Stiefel et al, *Psychoth Psychosom* 77:247, 2008; 7. Desan et al, P*sychosom* 52:513, 2011.

Perhaps the best studied is the collaborative care model for depression identification and treatment in medical patients. (W. Katon et al., 2012; W. J. Katon et al., 2010; Unutzer et al., 2012; Unutzer et al., 2008; Woltmann et al., 2012) Over seventy randomized trials now confirm that a stepped approach to the care of depression in the primary care setting will improve depression and lower total cost of care in those exposed. Cost savings accrue for up to five years after exposure to the intervention and can be associated with millions of dollars in savings for populations as small as 100,000. More recent studies, in which the care managers who previously focused on support for depression treatment expanded their assistance to include concurrent medical conditions, now show that clinical improvement of associated chronic medical conditions can also occur with augmented depression outcomes in what is now called TEAMCare. (W. J. Katon et al., 2010)

While less well studied, there are also a number of non-traditional models of BH delivery that have initial data and significant promise since inpatient care is so much more expensive than outpatient care (Table 11-7). The two models with the best data are delirum prevention programs and proactive psychiatric consultation services. In the former, a BH team works with medical hospitalist clinicians to identify and correct anticedents to the development of delirium in at-risk patients. Several studies show that delirium prevention programs can decrease the occurance of delirium by one-third. Since delirium is associated with doubling of hospitalization days, both decreased morbidity and cost savings can be expected.

Table 11-7. Examples of Value-Added Non-Traditional Programs

Examples
• Inpatient and outpatient--complexity-based integrated care/case management
• Inpatient   o General hospital emergency room psychiatrist coverage and treatment

Examples
capability
o   Proactive psychiatry consultation teams
o   Delirium prevention and treatment programs
o   Standardized protocols for common BH situations in medical settings
o   Constant observation (sitter/security guard) review
o   Complexity Intervention Units (CIUs) with PH and BH capabilities in general hospitals
• Outpatient
o   Onsite TEAMCare services--includes all medical and BH conditions for complex patients
o   Functional symptom training and support
o   Substance use disorder assessment and treatment programs, including buprenorphine and SBIRT
• Post-acute care--nursing homes with medical and BH coverage & capabilities

The proactive psychiatric consultation model assigns members of a BH team, led by a psychiatrist, to work with admitting hospitalists from the day of a patient's medical admission. These proactive consultants identify BH comorbidities that prevent improvement in patients' medical conditions or are associated with extended hospit al stays. (Desan, Zimbrean, Weinstein, Bozzo, & Sledge, 2011) Using this model, it has been shown that average length of stay (ALOS) for affected patients can be reduced by one to three days depending on how patients are targeted and assistance is given. Again, this is a model with promise.

Other less well studied models of non-traditional BH care, include the introduction of psychiatrists in medical emergency rooms,(Little-Upah et al., 2013; Lucas et al., 2009) the development of Complexity Intervention Units,(R. G. Kathol et al., 2009) delirium treatment programs,(Akunne, Murthy, & Young, 2012; Chen et al., 2011; Inouye, Bogardus, Williams, Leo-Summers, & Agostini, 2003; W. Wang et al., 2012) development of common BH problem protocols (e.g., substance withdrawal, agitation/delirium) for use in medical settings, review of sitter (one-on-one patient supervision) use, and adding integrated case managers to support treatment for complex patients. (R. Kathol, Perez, & Cohen, 2010) Each of these has sufficient preliminary data to support their serious consideration as value-added programs are introduced into medical settings.

When to Introduce Value-Added BH Programs in CINs and ACOs

The first question to consider when deciding whether BH professionals should participate as core members of a CIN or ACO relates to the population served and the impact that BH conditions might have on health and cost outcomes. Virtually all advanced CINs, also called ACOs, would benefit from BH professional participation as full network member providers. ACOs may be at full-risk for total health outcomes and costs of the populations that they serve. Only by including BH professionals in their network will they have the opportunity to capture savings by decreasing unnecessary medical service use as BH conditions come under control.

By having BH providers as part of the CIN/ACO network, the BH providers will have the same expectations as all other network providers. They will attend the same indoctrination sessions; utilize the same clinical documentation, communication, and outcome recording approaches; implement the same quality care guidelines; follow the same referral and network program use parameters; have performance judged by the same outcome metrics as other providers in the ACO, and have their outcomes analyzed within consolidated medical and BH findings. Most importantly, however, network BH providers will adopt the primary goals of the ACO (i.e., to maximize total health outcomes and efficient use of resources for patients treated among the populations served). They would also be incented to apply effective and efficient medical practices, similar to other network providers, in order to share in ACO profits (or losses).

Since thirty to forty percent of medical patients served by an ACO have high health costs associated with comorbid BH conditions, in-network BH professionals, deployed in value-added BH programs in the medical setting, can work as health care team members with medical providers to improve health and thereby attenuate cost. If BH providers are not ACO members, on the other hand, either the ACO would have to create economic incentives for the BH providers to work in the medical setting or the BH providers would be forced to continue to provide traditional BH services paid on a siloed, fee-for-service basis, which bring no value to the ACO where the BH need is greatest.

The need for BH specialists to participate in more basic CINs (i.e., those delivering focused health services for a target population, such as a CIN of cardiologists or gastroenterologists, a CIN for pain management, a CIN specializing in rehabilitation, or a large primary care group practice CIN), would depend on the degree to which BH issues would contribute to health and cost outcomes for the target population. For instance, a targeted pain management CIN would serve a population with a high number of patients in whom untreated substance use disorders and depression predictably affects health and cost outcomes. BH specialists would logically contribute to improving health and lowering cost. BH issues would be less central to treatment in a cardiology CIN though a case for BH CIN provider participation could still be made since depression is now a known predictor of cardiac morbidity and mortality post-myocardial infarction.

After a decision is made about the need to include in-network BH professionals as core CIN providers, then the question arises about how to initiate the process (i.e., build or buy). The only BH purchase option in the market today is for traditional standalone BH services. Current BH providers only know this method of care delivery because it is the only one that allows fiscal (albeit marginal) solvency. To buy BH professionals and their services from existing vendors, even the ones that say they do "integrated care," therefore, will necessarily involve expansion of standalone BH care, a model consistent with the poor health and cost outcomes described above. Thus, the better option is to build the type of BH services that will bring the CIN/ACO value as it transitions to population-based risk contracting characteristic of health reform.

Building value-added BH services makes clinical and economic sense. By doing so, the CIN can hire and deploy BH professional teams configured to maximize clinical outcomes for medical patients with concurrent BH conditions, which lead to cost savings. Since the majority of patients are not currently receiving BH services in the medical setting, they will experience a better treatment encounter (patient centered approach). They will have improved health outcomes, presuming that evidence-based approaches to BH professional introduction are used. And, deployed correctly, they should decrease the additional medical spend, which is where the majority of waste is present in their care.

So how does one initially build a value-added BH program in a CIN/ACO?

Strategy to Introduce Value-Added BH Programs in CINs and ACOs

As documented above, the prevalence of BH conditions in the medical setting is significant. Few, if any, care delivery systems have the resources necessary to support the introduction of the number of BH professionals needed to address all patients' needs, especially when 30% or more of any population is affected. Further, there are few BH providers practicing in the medical setting and even fewer that would know how to deliver value-added services. Thus, if a system did have the resources to retain the necessary BH expertise, recruitment and retention of the necessary personnel would be challenging. Nor would medical health plans be likely to expand reimbursement to cover all BH care in the medical setting, especially since management and payment of BH services is typically siloed elsewhere.

Thus, it becomes important that non-traditional integrated BH services be implemented in a way that maximizes benefit to the most needy and costly patients while establishing value-added programs that produce the best outcomes. Results from early efforts can guide program expansion. For this reason, strategic introduction of non-traditional BH "teams" to deliver value-added services described above *for targeted high risk, high cost medical patients* is best. By doing this, it is possible to support and surpass unmet salary requirements for the additional BH professionals from savings achieved by the reduction of total medical service use, thus providing justification through a return on investment.

At-risk patients can be identified through predictive modeling tools, claims databases, registries, or developed clinical algorithms. This should start with chronic and complex patients seen in various medical settings. (Parenthetically, there are also high risk, high cost primary BH patients in traditional BH settings who could be similarly targeted with successful health improvement and reduction in total cost of care, but the scope of this Chapter does not allow elaboration on this topic.) Once identified, such patients could then be served by the value-added, non-traditional BH services described above.

Implementation of Integrated BH Services

Figure 11-4 summarizes the current state of ACO development as it relates to use of BH services; the impacts of current-state care delivery procedures on patients, outcomes, and costs; and the recommended transition process to a value-added future state. While each CIN/ACO will design a future state gauged to its mission, vision, and goals; ultimately, the desired outcome is the creation of a CIN/ACO that maximizes health while conserving delivery system resources in a patient-friendly system. It is necessary, however, to stage the transition in a way that financially supports health systems going from fee-for-service contracting to risk-based global contracting for services. We will discuss one approach that can be taken.

Figure 11-4. BH ACO Service Delivery

(Current to Future State)

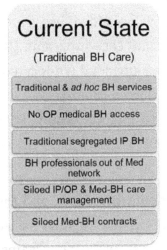
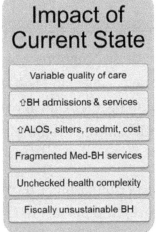
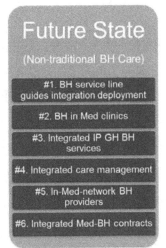

Current State (Traditional BH Care)	Impact of Current State	Future State (Non-traditional BH Care)
Traditional & *ad hoc* BH services	Variable quality of care	#1. BH service line guides integration deployment
No OP medical BH access	⬆BH admissions & services	#2. BH in Med clinics
Traditional segregated IP BH	⬆ALOS, sitters, readmit, cost	#3. Integrated IP GH BH services
BH professionals out of Med network	Fragmented Med-BH services	#4. Integrated care management
Siloed IP/OP & Med-BH care management	Unchecked health complexity	#5. In-Med-network BH providers
Siloed Med-BH contracts	Fiscally unsustainable BH	#6. Integrated Med-BH contracts

The first step (#1 in Figure 11-4) for many organizations will entail the development of a non-traditional BH Service Line. For instance, one medical and one BH thought leader within an organization could co-chair a cross-disciplinary, multi-professional task force charged with designing and deploying standardized BH service in the medical setting. Specifically, CIN leadership of the BH Service Line will want to:

- Design a clear vision for medical/BH integration;

- Identify/quantify existing barriers to achieving that vision;

- Determine the consequences of <u>not</u> making the necessary changes, i.e., doing nothing;

- Design the optimal service complement and degree of integration;

- Prioritize the services, providers, and populations to be addressed by the integration efforts;

- Design the implementation plan, including analytics for tracking successes and areas in need of strengthening;

- Design the provider payment plan, including medical and BH clinicians;

- Oversee the implementation of the plan.

This cross-disciplinary leadership team will initiate the chore of formulating the introduction of non-traditional, value-added integrated outpatient, emergency room, inpatient, and post-acute care programs (#2 and #3; Figure 11-4). All of these programs will be embedded (co-located) in medical settings (e.g., Patient-Centered Medical Homes (PCMH), medical specialty clinics, general hospital ERs, and inpatient medical units). They will have a functional relationship to traditional BH services but will be distinct in their operation.

In order to maximize the value brought to patients, providers, and the health system, integrated care/case managers (#4) will identify and assist, in collaboration with treating clinicians, the patients with the greatest complexity. (R. Kathol et al., 2010) This is the population present in all clinical settings that take the most clinical and administrative time, are the most challenging to treat, and use the most health care resources. Since 60% to 80% of these patients have comorbid BH problems,(Barnett et al., 2012) which if untreated predictably leads to poor outcomes, BH assessment and intervention, as a part of the care management process, is as important as medical.

BH professions providing services in the medical setting do not and will not meet salary demands in the current payment environment. In order to incentivize BH professionals to move to the medical setting and contribute to altering outcomes in complex comorbid patients, the best strategy is to include BH clinicians as part of the CIN/ACO network of providers (#5). By doing so, it will allow them to maximize the outcome changing BH expertise they bring as they integrate service delivery with other medical care. Perhaps more importantly, they can be supported in the service they provide under the guidance of the CIN/ACO rather than falling back on BH payment driven priorities. This will allow them to cover salary shortfalls via the savings generated through value-added care (covered below).

Finally, it is unsatisfactory and inappropriate for BH professionals contributing to better health outcomes and lower total costs of the population they serve to continue to have shortfalls in payment for services. To rectify this inequity, the final strategy for developing CINs/ACOs is to systematically move to contracting with medical health plans so that BH services delivered to the CIN/ACO network patients (#6; Figure 11-5) become a part of medical benefits. In essence, standalone contracts for BH payment by MBHOs, whether carve-ins or carve-outs, will sunset and will be picked up by the medical health plan. Such a transition is possible within three years of notification of intent to change contracting terms.

Figure 11-5. Recommended BH Strategy for BH Inclusion during ACO Formation

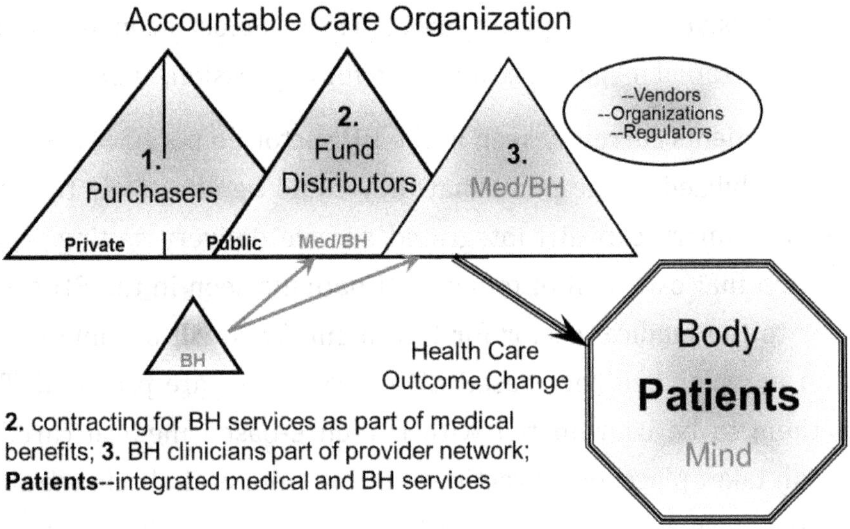

Accountable Care Organization

2. contracting for BH services as part of medical benefits; 3. BH clinicians part of provider network; **Patients**--integrated medical and BH services

Traditional BH Services

The strategic inclusion of BH services by emerging CINs/ACOs described above focuses on building non-traditional BH service capabilities, but says little about how traditional BH providers and services will coordinate with them. Traditional BH service locations currently provide the majority of outcome changing services available to patients with BH disorders. Thus, this group of professionals will serve as an initial resource to newly developing non-traditional BH delivery capabilities. It is likely, however, that many of those presently working in tradtional settings will be re-deployed to medical settings where application of their expertise can bring greater value to needy and high cost BH patients and to the health system.

Only approximately 20% of BH patients are seen in the specialty BH setting. Many, but not most, of these have serious and persistent mental illnesses (SMIs) that require specialty BH services to meet their clinical needs. Traditional BH services in a specialty BH sector will, therefore, remain the primary service location for these patients. The specialty BH sector will also be a resource to BH patients increasingly treated in the medical sector for specialized BH treatments not likely to be available in many non-traditional BH locations (e.g., dialectical behavioral therapy (DBT), intensive outpatient programs (IOPs), electroconvulsive therapy (ECT), transcranial magnetic stimulation for depression, etc.).

Many patients currently seen in the BH sector do not have a SMI or their SMI has stabilized to the point that they could be effectively treated in an expanded primary care-BH integrated service delivery setting. Thus, it is anticipated that over half of today's BH patients seen in the BH sector will transfer to the medical sector for treatment. This will become the default location in which evidence-based BH interventions are provided. This will allow them to be coordinated with evidence-based medical care. As this transition takes place, best practices coming from each discipline should be incorporated, such as the "recovery" approach used in the BH sector(Pratt, MacGregor, Reid, & Given, 2012) and cross-disciplinary integrated case management technology, which assists with medical, BH, and non-clinical barriers to improvement without patient handoffs. (R. Kathol, Lattimer, Gold, Perez, & Gutteridge, 2011) Core components of the expanded non-traditional BH services are covered in a recent publication. (R.G. Kathol, deGruy, & Rollman, in press)

Ultimately, traditional BH services will be incorporated into non-tradtional BH work processes, both clinically and financially. A smaller and focused specialty BH sector will service the needs of difficult to control SMI and non-SMI patients. It will provide specialty expertise and capabilities only possible in a specialty BH service sector. The specialty BH sector, however, will have become a part of the medical delivery system. (Manderscheid & Kathol, in press) Benefits will be paid by medical insurance companies. BH providers will be part of medical networks, including CINs and ACOs. They will use common documentation systems and have the same expectations for proving delivery of outcome changing care. Further, medical services will be as available in specialty BH settings as in medical settings and paid from the same funding pool.

Most importantly, when SMI and challenging non-SMI patients stabilize, they will transfer back to the integrated non-traditional setting for continued care. In essence, non-traditional BH will decompress the backlog of patients having difficulty in accessing specialized services because less severe BH patients will be treated and followed in the primary care medical sector. It will be a collaborative relationship.

Opportunity Costs Related to BH Services in CINs/ACOs or the Costs of Doing Nothing

The authors of this Chapter have been working with employers, government agencies, health plans, and care delivery systems for the past twenty years. They have helped them explore the impact that BH conditions have on total health outcomes and cost. Until the ACA, however, there has been little interest in addressing the thorny issue of how to better handle BH care. Care delivery systems saw no need to become more efficient and effective in BH care delivery as long as they maintained financial stability or growth.

Interestingly, it is not the ACA but rather projections of national insolvency due to unbridaled medical costs that drive the need for change. The ACA is just the current vehicle being used to try to accomplish cost control while maintaining quality health. During the next decade, the U.S. health system will be expected to reign in medical inflation, which has consistently been two percentage points higher than the gross domestic product. Part of the solution will include changing the way that BH services are delivered and paid.

To date, there has been a disincentive for the health system to change the way that BH is supported and delivered. First, most consider that it represents only 2% to 7% of the total health care budget. This is hardly enough to require a revamp. Second, there are few health care professionals with either medical or BH administrative and clinical expertise that have a vision of what a revamped system would look like. Yet, it is clear that expanded traditional BH will bring little value.

Third, evidence indicates that untreated or ineffectively treated BH conditions, particularly in those with chronic medical conditions, leads to increased health service use (i.e., more admissions, longer lengths of stay, more ancillary testing, greater medication use, and increased numbers of specialty medical consultations). These are all areas of medicine that lead to financial success for stakeholders in delivering traditional, fee-for-service reimbursed care.

Health plans can demand higher premiums due to high service use. Hospitals and clinics can fill beds and clinic appointments. Pharmaceutical companies can sell more drugs. Device manufactures can sell more appliances. The only losers in the process are the purchasers of health care services and the patients. Interestingly, government purchasers are bigger losers than commercial insurers and large businesses since those with BH comorbidity are more likely to lose commercial coverage due to persistent health reasons and end up in public programs.

Population health, as a central component of the ACA, is now turning what used to be profitable areas of care delivery in the fee-for-service world, such as radiology departments, cardiac cath labs, orthopedic surgical suites, and long in-hospital stays, into cost centers. In order for CINs/ACOs taking risk to successfully compete for market share as a part of future risk-based contracting, care delivery systems must demonstrate the ability to reduce unnecessary service use, especially in specialty areas with high margins, and to document high quality care.

Thus, the emphasis is shifting to prevention and maximizing long-term outcomes for patients with high cost and unnecessary service use. It will no longer be advantageous for care delivery systems forming CINs and ACOs to ignore the negative impact that untreated or ineffectively treated BH comorbidity has on health and cost. They must learn ways to mitigate these negative effects so that fewer of their patients end up in what used to be their most profitable areas of service delivery.

The best way to start looking at the value that revamping BH service delivery would have on total health costs for populations served in a CIN/ACO is by reviewing the opportunity costs associated with the current tradtitional BH system (i.e., doing nothing). At a national level, more than $290 billion annually for additional medical costs in patients with BH disorders can be expected (Table 11-3). This is an unwieldy number, but doesn't tell us much about what happens at the care delivery level that leads to this number.

Table 11-5 gives a glimpse of where the extra spend for untreated or poorly treated BH patients in the medical setting occurs (i.e., in the medical inpatient and outpatient settings, in pharmaceutical use, and in ancillary medical service use). The amount spent for "BH services" in BH patients is one fifth the medical spend. Therefore, to the extent that expanded non-traditional BH services can efficiently and effectively reverse medical service use, CINs/ACOs can better compete as health reform progresses.

This is where "value-added" services come into play. Extra admissions, longer lengths of stay, professional fees, and ancillary services and medication use can be translated into dollars and cents (Table 11-8), as can the salary expense for strategically deployed non-traditional BH professionals. The trick is to customize BH professional deployment to the population served by each health system and geographic location so that delivery capabilities lead to population health and total health care cost reduction.

Table 11-8. ACO BH Transition Options

Options	Health Outcome	Cost Outcome
Do Nothing	• Poor BH access • Retarded medical illness improvement due to untreated BH comorbidity	• Unfavorable BH finances • Comorbid medical patients: ~1 day longer ALOS, >$M+ for sitters, ~30% higher 30-day readmissions; ~$M+ in extra service delivery costs
Traditional Standalone BH Expansion (Buy)	• ↑ BH access • Small impact on medical sector outcomes	• More unfavorable BH finances • Similar cost outcomes to above since value-added BH not possible in medical setting
BH Service Expansion into General Medical Service Area	• BH access in medical setting • Medical/BH provider communication; patient satisfaction • ↑ inpatient and outpatient care coordination and medical and BH outcomes	• Better payment for BH services from medical benefits • Gap closure on ALOS, sitter use, 30-day readmissions, cost/net margin for general medical patients with BH comorbidity

Table 11-6 shares calculations of documented cost savings or return on investment from published articles on value-added BH services introduced into the medical setting. If one uses these and other published articles or reported experiences in clinical settings to calculate the savings potential for health systems choosing to introduce non-traditional BH services into their CINs/ACOs, it becomes apparent that savings for medical health systems can far exceed the cost of the personnel providing improved BH services, perhaps even significantly.

Some targeted areas are easier to predict cost savings than others. For instance, introduction of collaborative care into medical outpatient clinics can be expected to reduce total cost of care for program participants by 5%

to 15%. While these savings typically do not appear in the first year of the program since this is the health stabilization period, savings that run in the millions of dollars for populations as small as 100,000 have been documented to accrue for up to five years after program participation.

Real savings are also easily documented when psychiatrist-led teams of BH professionals become members of general medical hospitalist teams and assist with concurrent treatment of BH disorder from day one of general hospital admission. This is associated with shorter hospital stays of 0.9 to 3 days and a net return on investment in hospitals with very high censuses and/or a high percentage of at-risk payer arrangements (e.g., DRGs). As a result, general hospital early adopters nationally are subsidizing proactive BH consultation as a means of reducing total health costs, enhancing the quality of care, and improving hospital bottom lines for comorbid medical admissions when these patients are uninsured, underinsured, or insured on a fee per case basis.

During comprehensive evaluations of health systems encompassing 2 to more than 10 hospitals and often hundreds of corresponding medical clinics, it has been possible to estimate millions in annual net savings in a world of population risk-based contracting. The projected savings often allow inclusion/expansion of BH services even when available data is insufficiently developed to support BH service introduction on the basis of actual hospital system analytics (e.g., pediatric and child BH programs).

Doing nothing will predictably be associated with high costs of unnecessary care and declining fee-for-service bases, an unacceptable scenario for systems wishing to increase market share in the future. Thus, informed systems recognize this shortfall as an area of opportunity for improving health and cost management. They grapple with the decision of buying or building a solution. In today's world, buying is really not an option since few, if any, BH organizations deliver BH services effectively in the medical setting. Therefore, several health systems are now in the process of building non-traditional value-added services because they have run their own numbers.

Future Directions

When health systems are developing CINs/ACOs, little thought is given to the inclusion of BH services as a part of core CIN/ACO provider participation and service delivery. For those who do consider BH inclusion, siloed BH payment and independent service delivery procedures quickly drive decision-making leadership to exclude active BH participation due to the logistical challenges.

In this Chapter we make the case that BH comorbidity in the medical setting is associated with medical treatment resistance, especially in complex high cost patients, and large increases in total health care spending, especially for medical services in patients with comorbid BH conditions. Since the primary goal of CINs/ACOs is to improve health and decrease cost, without the inclusion of BH professionals and services as core members and activities in ACOs and many focused CINs, Federal Trade Commission and Department of Justice requirements will not be met. This is particularly true when one considers that there are now models of non-traditional integrated medical and BH care delivery that predicably attenuate the health and cost consequences of BH conditions in medical settings.

This Chapter recognizes that the inclusion of BH professionals and services in CINs/ACOs creates several challenges for those that are developing them. Therefore, it provides a roadmap that will allow those willing to maximize the effectiveness of their CIN/ACO to achive the Triple Aim. (Berwick, Nolan, & Whittington, 2008)

CHAPTER 11 DISCUSSION QUESTIONS

Discussion questions are provided for team building or class exercises. Answers for all questions are provided in Appendix C.

Question Number	Question
1	The expected total cost of care for patients with a chronic illness and a concurrent behavioral health condition compared to a general population of medical patients will be: a. About the same b. Twice as much c. Three to four times as much d. Five to six times as much
2	The majority of increased cost of care for patients with behavioral health conditions is for: a. Medical treatment b. Psychiatric hospitalization c. Psychotropic medication d. Residential care
3	"Carve-out" and "carve-in" managed behavioral health organizations: a. Are owned by the medical insurer that covers medical benefit payments. b. Use payment practices that encourage delivery of behavioral health services in the medical setting. c. Manage networks of behavioral health providers separate and apart from medical providers. d. Use the same claims adjudication procedures as for medical benefits.
4	CINs/ACOs in which behavioral health providers are contracted professional resources but not network members can be expected to: a. Provide easily accessible behavioral health services for high cost, complex network patients. b. Improve clinical outcomes and lower cost in the

Question Number	Question
	majority of network patients with behavioral health comorbidity.
	c. Follow CIN/ACO policies and procedures (referral use, documentation, formularies, clinical guidelines) just as medical specialty network providers.
	d. None of the above
5	What percentage of patients with behavioral health conditions is seen and receives the majority of their BH treatment in the behavioral health sector? a. 10-20% b. 30-50% c. 60-80% d. 90-100%
6	On average, the length of stay for medical/surgical inpatients with behavioral health comorbidity is: a. 1 day shorter due to psychiatric hospital transfer b. The same c. 1 day longer d. 4 days longer
7	7. On average, the thirty-day readmission rate for medical/surgical inpatient discharges with behavioral health comorbidity is: a. >30% higher than those without b. 20%-30% higher than those without c. 10%-20% higher than those without d. 5%-10% higher than those without

CHAPTER 11 HIGHLIGHTS

✓ Eighty percent of patients with BH conditions are seen in the medical sector.

✓ BH comorbidity in general medical patients is common, especially in complex high cost patients.

✓ Untreated, poorly treated BH conditions in general medical patients doubles medical service use and result in a spend four times greater than the spend on BH care.

✓ The siloed medical and BH payment systems obviates the opportunities for interdisciplinary care coordination and delivery of effective, efficient integrated care.

✓ Studies of value-added models of integrated medical and BH services delivery demonstrate health improvement, patient satisfaction, and cost reduction.

✓ CINs without BH network providers delivering BH services in the general medical setting can expect ongoing treatment resistance and high health care costs in comorbid general medical and BH patients.

CHAPTER 11 REFERENCES

Akunne, A., Murthy, L., & Young, J. (2012). Cost-effectiveness of multi-component interventions to prevent delirium in older people admitted to medical wards. *Age and Ageing*, 41(3), 285-291. doi: 10.1093/ageing/afr147

Barnett, K., Mercer, S. W., Norbury, M., Watt, G., Wyke, S., & Guthrie, B. (2012). Epidemiology of multimorbidity and implications for health care, research, and medical education: a cross-sectional study. *Lancet*, 380(9836), 37-43. doi: 10.1016/S0140-6736(12)60240-2

Berwick, D. M., Nolan, T. W., & Whittington, J. (2008). The triple aim: care, health, and cost. *Health Affairs*, 27(3), 759-769. doi: 10.1377/hlthaff.27.3.759

Bower, P., Knowles, S., Coventry, P. A., & Rowland, N. (2011). Counselling for mental health and psychosocial problems in primary care. *Cochrane Database of Systematic Reviews*, (9), CD001025. doi: 10.1002/14651858.CD001025.pub3

Bower, P., Rowland, N., & Hardy, R. (2003). The clinical effectiveness of counselling in primary care: a systematic review and meta-analysis. *Psychological Medicine*, 33(02), 203-215.

Chang, C. K., Hayes, R. D., Perera, G., Broadbent, M. T., Fernandes, A. C., Lee, W. E., . . . Stewart, R. (2011). Life expectancy at birth for people with serious mental illness and other major disorders from a secondary mental health care case register in London. *PloS One*, 6(5), e19590. doi: 10.1371/journal.pone.0019590

Chen, C. C., Lin, M. T., Tien, Y. W., Yen, C. J., Huang, G. H., & Inouye, S. K. (2011). Modified hospital elder life program: effects on abdominal surgery patients. *Journal of American College Surgeons*, 213(2), 245-252. doi: 10.1016/j.jamcollsurg.2011.05.004

Cunningham, P. J. (2009). Beyond parity: primary care physicians' perspectives on access to mental health care. *Health Affairs*, 28(3), w490-501. doi: hlthaff.28.3.w490 [pii]10.1377/hlthaff.28.3.w490

Desan, P. H., Zimbrean, P. C., Weinstein, A. J., Bozzo, J. E., & Sledge, W. H. (2011). Proactive psychiatric consultation services reduce length of stay for admissions to an inpatient medical team. *Psychosomatics*, 52(6), 513-520. doi: 10.1016/j.psym.2011.06.002

Druss, B. G., & Walker, E. R. (2011). Mental disorders and medical comorbidity. *The Synthesis project. Research synthesis report*, (21), 1-26.

Druss, B. G., Zhao, L., Von Esenwein, S., Morrato, E. H., & Marcus, S. C. (2011). Understanding excess mortality in persons with mental illness: 17-year follow up of a nationally representative US survey. *Medical Care*, 49(6), 599-604. doi: 10.1097/MLR.0b013e31820bf86e

Franz, C. E., Barker, J. C., Kim, K., Flores, Y., Jenkins, C., Kravitz, R. L., & Hinton, L. (2010). When help becomes a hindrance: mental health referral systems as barriers to care for primary care physicians treating patients with Alzheimer's disease. *American Journal of Geriatric Psychiatry*, 18(7), 576-585.

Inouye, S. K., Bogardus, S. T., Jr., Williams, C. S., Leo-Summers, L., & Agostini, J. V. (2003). The role of adherence on the effectiveness of nonpharmacologic interventions: evidence from the delirium prevention trial. *Archives of Internal Medicine*, 163(8), 958-964.

Kathol, R., Lattimer, C., Gold, W., Perez, R., & Gutteridge, D. (2011). Creating clinical and economic "wins" through integrated case management. Lessons for physicians and health system administrators. *Journal of Ambulatory Care Management*, 34(2), 140-151.

Kathol, R., McAlpine, D., Kishi, Y., Spies, R., Meller, W., Bernhardt, T., Gold, W. (2005). General medical and pharmacy claims expenditures in users of behavioral health services. *Journal of General Internal Medicine*, 20(2), 160-167.

Kathol, R., Perez, R., & Cohen, J. (2010). *The Integrated Case Management Manual: Assisting Complex Patients Regain Physical and Mental Health* (1st ed.). New York City: Springer Publishing.

Kathol, R. G., deGruy, F., & Rollman, B. L. (2014). Value-based financially sustainable behavioral health components for patient-centered medical homes. *Annal of Family Medicine*, 12(2), 172-175. doi: 10.1370/afm.1619

Kathol, R. G., Kunkel, E. J., Weiner, J. S., McCarron, R. M., Worley, L. L., Yates, W. R., Huyse, F. J. (2009). Psychiatrists for the medically complex: bringing value at the physical health & mental health substance use disorder interface. *Psychosomatics*, 50(March-April), 93-107. doi: 10.1176/appi.psy.50.2.93

Katon, W., Russo, J., Lin, E. H., Schmittdiel, J., Ciechanowski, P., Ludman, E., .Von Korff, M. (2012). Cost-effectiveness of a multicondition collaborative care intervention: a randomized controlled trial. *Archives of General Psychiatry*, 69(5), 506-514. doi: 10.1001/archgenpsychiatry.2011.1548

Katon, W. J., Lin, E. H., Von Korff, M., Ciechanowski, P., Ludman, E. J., Young, B., McCulloch, D. (2010). Collaborative care for patients with depression and chronic illnesses. *New England Journal of Medicine*, 363(27), 2611-2620. doi: 10.1056/NEJMoa1003955

Katon, W. J., & Seelig, M. (2008). Population-based care of depression: team care approaches to improving outcomes. *Journal of Occupational Environtal Medicine*, 50(4), 459-467. doi: 10.1097/JOM.0b013e318168efb7

Kessler, R. C., Demler, O., Frank, R. G., Olfson, M., Pincus, H. A., Walters, E. E., Zaslavsky, A. M. (2005). Prevalence and treatment of mental disorders, 1990 to 2003. *New England Journal of Medicine*, 352(24), 2515-2523.

Larkin, G. L., Claassen, C. A., Emond, J. A., Pelletier, A. J., & Camargo, C. A. (2005). Trends in U.S. emergency department visits for mental health conditions, 1992 to 2001. *Psychiatric Services*, 56(6), 671-677.

Lewis, V. A., Colla, C. H., Tierney, K., Van Citters, A. D., Fisher, E. S., & Meara, E. (2014). Few ACOs pursue innovative models that integrate care for mental illness and substance abuse with primary care. *Health Affairs*, 33(10), 1808-1816. doi: 10.1377/hlthaff.2014.0353

Little-Upah, P., Carson, C., Williamson, R., Williams, T., Cimino, M., Mehta, N., Kisiel, S. (2013). The Banner psychiatric center: a model for providing psychiatric crisis care to the community while easing behavioral health holds in emergency departments. *The Permanente Journal*, 17(1), 45-49. doi: 10.7812/TPP/12-016

Lucas, R., Farley, H., Twanmoh, J., Urumov, A., Evans, B., & Olsen, N. (2009). Measuring the opportunity loss of time spent boarding admitted patients in the emergency department: a multihospital analysis. *Journal of Healthcare Management*, 54(2), 117-124; discussion 124-115.

Manderscheid, R., & Kathol, R. G. (2014). Fostering sustainable, integrated medical and behavioral health services in medical settings. *Annals of Internal Medicine*, 160(1), 61-65. doi: 10.7326/M13-1693

Melek, S., Norris, D. T., & Paulus, J. (2013). *Economic impact of integrated medical-behavioral healthcare: implications for psychiatry*. In A. P. Press (Ed.). Arlington VA: American Psychiatric Assoication.

Ostbye, T., Yarnall, K. S., Krause, K. M., Pollak, K. I., Gradison, M., & Michener, J. L. (2005). Is there time for management of patients with chronic diseases in primary care? *Annals of Family Medicine*, 3(3), 209-214. doi: 10.1370/afm.310

Pratt, R., MacGregor, A., Reid, S., & Given, L. (2012). Wellness Recovery Action Planning (WRAP) in self-help and mutual support groups. *Psychiatric Rehabilitation Journal*, 35(5), 403-405. doi: 10.1037/h0094501

Prince, M., Patel, V., Saxena, S., Maj, M., Maselko, J., Phillips, M. R., & Rahman, A. (2007). No health without mental health. *Lancet*, 370(9590), 859-877. doi: S0140-6736(07)61238-0 [pii]

10.1016/S0140-6736(07)61238-0

Regier, D. A., Narrow, W. E., Rae, D. S., Manderscheid, R. W., Locke, B. Z., & Goodwin, F. K. (1993). The de facto US mental and addictive disorders service system. Epidemiologic catchment area prospective 1-year prevalence rates of disorders and services. *Archives of General Psychiatry*, 50(2), 85-94.

Reilly, S., Planner, C., Hann, M., Reeves, D., Nazareth, I., & Lester, H. (2012). The role of primary care in service provision for people with severe mental illness in the United Kingdom. *PloS One*, 7(5), e36468. doi: 10.1371/journal.pone.0036468

Richmond, T. S., Hollander, J. E., Ackerson, T. H., Robinson, K., Gracias, V., Shults, J., & Amsterdam, J. (2007). Psychiatric disorders in patients presenting to the Emergency Department for minor injury. *Nursing Research*, 56(4), 275-282. doi: 10.1097/01.NNR.0000280616.13566.84

Seelig, M. D., & Katon, W. (2008). Gaps in depression care: why primary care physicians should hone their depression screening, diagnosis, and management skills. *Journal of Occupational Environmental Medicine*, 50(4), 451-458. doi: 10.1097/JOM.0b013e318169cce4

U.S. Department of Justice, & Federal Trade Commission. (1996). Statements of Antitrust Enforcement Policy in Health Care. Retrieved from http://www.justice.gov/atr/public/guidelines/0000.htm

Unutzer, J., Chan, Y. F., Hafer, E., Knaster, J., Shields, A., Powers, D., & Veith, R. C. (2012). Quality improvement with pay-for-performance incentives in integrated behavioral health care. *American Journal of Public Health*, 102(6), e41-45. doi: 10.2105/AJPH.2011.300555

Unutzer, J., Katon, W. J., Fan, M. Y., Schoenbaum, M. C., Lin, E. H., Della Penna, R. D., & Powers, D. (2008). Long-term cost effects of collaborative care for late-life depression. *American Journal of Manag Care*, 14(2), 95-100. doi: 7019 [pii]

Wang, P. S., Aguilar-Gaxiola, S., Alonso, J., Angermeyer, M. C., Borges, G., Bromet, E. J., Wells, J. E. (2007). Use of mental health services for anxiety, mood, and substance disorders in 17 countries in the WHO world mental health surveys. *Lancet*, 370(9590), 841-850. doi: 10.1016/S0140-6736(07)61414-7

Wang, P. S., Berglund, P., Olfson, M., Pincus, H. A., Wells, K. B., & Kessler, R. C. (2005). Failure and delay in initial treatment contact after first onset of mental disorders in the National Comorbidity Survey Replication. *Archives of General Psychiatry*, 62(6), 603-613.

Wang, P. S., Demler, O., & Kessler, R. C. (2002). Adequacy of treatment for serious mental illness in the United States. *American Journal of Public Health*, 92(1), 92-98.

Wang, P. S., Demler, O., Olfson, M., Pincus, H. A., Wells, K. B., & Kessler, R. C. (2006). Changing profiles of service sectors used for mental health care in the United States. *American Journal of Psychiatry*, 163(7), 1187-1198. doi: 10.1176/appi.ajp.163.7.1187

Wang, P. S., Lane, M., Olfson, M., Pincus, H. A., Wells, K. B., & Kessler, R. C. (2005). Twelve-month use of mental health services in the United States: results from the National Comorbidity Survey Replication. *Archives of General Psychiatry*, 62(6), 629-640.

Wang, W., Li, H. L., Wang, D. X., Zhu, X., Li, S. L., Yao, G. Q., Zhu, S. N. (2012). Haloperidol prophylaxis decreases delirium incidence in elderly patients after noncardiac surgery: a randomized controlled trial*. *Critical Care Medicine*, 40(3), 731-739. doi: 10.1097/CCM.0b013e3182376e4f

Woltmann, E., Grogan-Kaylor, A., Perron, B., Georges, H., Kilbourne, A. M., & Bauer, M. S. (2012). Comparative effectiveness of collaborative chronic care models for mental health conditions across primary, specialty, and behavioral health care settings: systematic review and meta-analysis. *American Journal of Psychiatry*, 169(8), 790-804. doi: 10.1176/appi.ajp.2012.11111616

Yarnall, K. S., Pollak, K. I., Ostbye, T., Krause, K. M., & Michener, J. L. (2003). Primary care: is there enough time for prevention? *American Journal of Public Health*, 93(4), 635-641.

Chapter 12. Improving Future Care Through Comparative Effectiveness Research

Ken Yale

Comparative effectiveness research provides important guidance for health care innovations and patient treatment decisions based on quality outcomes and value.

Ronald A. Williams, MD, Chairman and CEO, Aetna, Inc.
"Addressing Insurance Reform,"
Testimony before the United States Senate, March 24, 2009

CHAPTER 12 LEARNING OBJECTIVES

✓ Understand the importance of comparative effectiveness research to healthcare, CINs and ACOs.

✓ Recognize the difference between clinical efficacy and comparative effectiveness.

✓ Know what types of organizations conduct CER and their reasons for engaging in it.

✓ Describe the establishment of the Patient Centered Outcomes Research Institute (PCORI) and the work this organization conducts.

✓ Know what federal government funding for CER came through ARRA and its intended purposes.

✓ Identify what organization was the pioneer in CER.

✓ Understand why health plans are interested in CER.

✓ Know what the Medicare National Coverage Process is and how it is used.

✓ Recognize the differences between randomized controlled trials and observational studies.

✓ Discuss some of the ways that health information technology is helping CER.

Comparative effectiveness research (CER) evaluates different medical therapies to determine what works best in healthcare. (Concato et al.,

2010)* Health information technology could play a significant role in CER activities. In fact, government policy makers and legislators recognize the link between greater availability of data through health information technology and potential improvements in CER. (Department of Health and Human Services Recovery Funding Page, 2011) Various technology tools are needed to conduct CER, including technology for sharing data sets that will be transformed into value-adding knowledge in the research infrastructure. (Navathe & Conway, 2010) To meet the needs of CER proposed by the federal government, significant resources will be needed, and they may include the use of electronic health records (EHRs) and other clinical databases to compile source data and information for CER studies and evidence compilation. (Etheredge, 2010)

So what does CER mean for Clinically Integrated Networks (CINs) and Accountable Care Organizations (ACOs)? That is an issue that we will explore in this chapter. If a provider-based organization is accountable or at-risk for a population of patients, there may be greater interest on the part of hospitals and physicians to identify which treatments are more effective and efficient. Comparative effectiveness research may provide some clues, but there are other methods more widely used in practice to identify effective treatments such as comparisons with evidence-based medicine that takes evidence-based consensus guidelines, which may be enhanced with comparative effectiveness and other medical research to develop best practice protocols. Gaps in care may be identified and corrected when clinical practice is compared to these best practice protocols. This application of evidence-based medicine is one of the practical results of medical research, and is widely used to improve the quality and affordability of care.

---

* CER may also compare different delivery models, such as primary care physician compared to hospitalist care, or clinically integrated networks versus patient centered medical homes, but the main focus of this chapter is on comparison of therapies.

Who performs comparative effectiveness research, how the research is conducted, and the use of the results are questions being asked as the field of comparative effectiveness research grows in visibility and importance. In addition, established methodologies comparing present physician practices to evidence-based medicine and identifying gaps in care will expand as providers become more accountable for care and seek out best practices.

Introduction

CER is generally used to refer to any work that compares different medical devices, drugs, and treatment methods to determine which are more effective in treating a disease or condition. Essentially, CER attempts to determine "what works best" in healthcare by comparing different therapies meant to treat the same disease or condition. (Concato et al., 2010) There is an established medical research infrastructure and a growing part of that infrastructure looks at the relative effectiveness of different treatments. The field of comparative effectiveness research has received increasing attention with the burgeoning availability of new medical technologies and the increasing cost of healthcare. Practical application of comparative effectiveness research includes use of evidence-based medicine and best-practice protocols. Patient preferences and preferred outcomes are also becoming increasingly important considerations.

The term comparative effectiveness research currently encompasses a wide range of activities and is almost as diverse as the universe of medical therapies being studied.[*] Payers, consumers, patients, providers, and other caregivers are increasingly interested in the technologies that provide the greatest value. Value may be defined as the technologies, medicines, or treatment techniques that are most effective at treating diseases and disorders that provide the greatest benefits while causing the least clinical

---

[*] Private discussion with Sean Tunis, Director, Center for Medical Technology Policy, May 2011.

harm, and provide them at the lowest economic cost. With reforms in the finance and delivery of healthcare, and perspectives brought by such new players as the Patient-Centered Outcomes Research Institute, the field of comparative effectiveness is growing and becoming increasingly important.

Comparative effectiveness may examine relative clinical benefits or harms (therapeutic effectiveness), and may include discovery of relative cost-effectiveness. There is ongoing debate among industry observers and policy makers as to whether cost-effectiveness should be included when comparing different treatments, especially for government-funded research—in part because of concerns about restricting the availability of costly treatments that benefit only a subpopulation or have marginal benefits over existing treatments. Restrictions on services with marginal clinical benefits and higher costs may satisfy government budget examiners, but clinicians and patients who see some benefit might object. There seems to be a general consensus among health services researchers about the importance of pursuing clinical comparative effectiveness while and leaving cost considerations to those in government and the private sector responsible for making decisions on how best to finance care. (Wilensky, 2009) As CINs and ACOs continue to advance as new models of care delivery, their interest in CER will increase as the benefits and drawbacks of specific treatment options are identified. CER may become even more important as models of performance evaluation continue to shift toward quality of care and value thus affecting reimbursement and compensation.

Clinical efficacy is sometimes confused with comparative effectiveness, but they are different activities with different purposes. Efficacy, according to the Food and Drug Administration (FDA), is a measure of whether a device or drug works better than doing nothing. Efficacy is usually determined through tightly structured and controlled clinical trials that compare a new drug or device to a placebo, although in some situations comparison may be made to existing treatments (such as pre-market notification for certain medical devices). Comparison to a placebo is a low threshold to meet and is not intended to compare different medical therapies that treat the same disease or condition. The FDA also weighs clinical benefits and risks of a new drug or device to determine its safety. Safety and efficacy must be proven before a drug or device is allowed by the FDA to be marketed and made available to the public. (Tunis, Stryer, & Clancy, 2003) Once safety and efficacy are established to the satisfaction of the FDA, the drug or device may be marketed to the public, even if the long-term effects of the treatment are unknown. This is a potentially fertile area for CER studies that can follow treatments after they are marketed, especially by using such health information technologies as EHR, and identify side effects not evident in the narrowly focused clinical trials used for FDA approval.

The 2009 American Recovery and Reinvestment Act (ARRA) and the 2010 Patient Protection and Affordable Care Act (ACA) created new CER programs with substantial increases in funding. Different approaches to CER, the wide range of activities related to comparative effectiveness, and confusion between efficacy and cost-effectiveness led to a need to define CER. The Institute of Medicine (IOM) Committee on Comparative Effectiveness Research Prioritization defined comparative effectiveness research as:

> ...the generation and synthesis of evidence that compares the benefits and harms of alternative methods to prevent, diagnose, treat, and monitor a clinical condition or to improve the delivery of care. The purpose of CER is to assist consumers, clinicians, purchasers, and policy makers to make informed decisions that will improve health care at both the individual and population levels. (Institute of Medicine & Committee on Comparative Effectiveness Research Prioritization, 2009c)

It is not insignificant that the definition of CER adopted by the IOM does not specifically mention cost-effectiveness, because of the sensitivities of focusing on cost at the expense of quality. (Wilensky, 2009) Moreover, legislation increasing federal government funding has specifically mandated that findings of federally funded research cannot be used for coverage decisions. (Department of Health and Human Services, 2010e) It remains to be seen how long federally funded CER can be kept separate from economic effectiveness considerations in federal government health care programs (e.g. Medicare and Medicaid, etc.). In addition, the IOM definition favors applied research, rather than basic research. This emphasis reflects Congressional interest in care delivery and wide dissemination of research findings that could directly inform consumer and provider clinical decision-making. (Department of Health and Human Services, 2010b)

Because of the lack of emphasis on cost-effectiveness, government-funded CER initiatives may not be immediately useful to new provider care models that focus on the financial impact of clinical actions, such as CINs and ACOs. All CER research findings, however, can help increase the body of knowledge of evidence-based medicine, improve best practice protocols and quality, and be used to strengthen clinical decision support for physician and patient benefit. It is unlikely that an individual hospital or physician will have the resources necessary to conduct research that compares different medical therapies. Nevertheless, new and more accountable provider organizations will make decisions on appropriate care, and look to reduce inappropriate care. As the ACOs and CINs models evolve and these organizations gradually assume greater degrees of risk essentially operating more like health insurance payers, they may become more involved in medical coverage decisions, benefit design, and appeals of decisions about care provided. These decisions require an understanding of both therapeutic effectiveness and cost-effectiveness. Fortunately, there is a large body of work in this field and other organizations have developed evidence-based medical protocols and clinical decision support tools useful to ACOs and CINs as they face these decisions. (Javitt, Rebitzer, & Reisman, 2008; Javitt et al., 2005)

History of Comparative Effectiveness Research

Research into the comparative effectiveness of medical drugs, devices, and treatment methodologies has been performed by a wide range of organizations and individuals for many different reasons. (Congressional Budget Office, December 2007f) Life science companies (manufacturers of drugs and medical devices), health plans, healthcare providers, and other private sector organizations perform a variety of CER-related programs. Independent, private organizations have also been established to organize, support, or conduct such research.[*] Governments may compare different treatments for a variety of purposes, including basic scientific research to increase knowledge; identify the highest-value product or service (best outcome and quality for the cost) for government reimbursement; or fulfill legislative fiat. Increasingly, federal government policy makers are looking to patients as the ultimate judges of value, and to patients' preferences as an important consideration in comparative effectiveness research.

Research into comparative effectiveness in the United States has been limited for a number of reasons. First, research is expensive to conduct, especially randomized, controlled trials that are believed to be more accurate and valid but are also very expensive to organize. An organization would have to see a return or benefit for the investment made, such as a manufacturer of a drug or device who may benefit directly from a study's positive findings. If an organization does benefit--or worse, if the results show harm--the results may be proprietary and kept confidential, limiting the value to society of such research. Second, once results of CER are in the public domain, they may benefit other organizations that did not pay for the research and eliminate any return on the investment anticipated by the organization originally funding the research. Furthermore, advances in healthcare may cause the technology or medicine being researched to become obsolete before effectiveness can be compared or established, especially for more costly but potentially more valid research

---

[*] For example, the Center for Medical Technology Policy, Cochrane Collaboration, Drug Effectiveness Review Project, ECRI Institute, Hayes, Inc., Institute for Clinical and Economic Review, Technology Evaluation Center at BCBS Association, ActiveHealth Management, and Tufts Medical Center Cost-Effectiveness Analysis Registry.

methodologies that take years to complete. For these and other reasons, CER is thought to be a public good, requiring government funding. (Congressional Budget Office, December 2007e)

The federal government has conducted CER but only sporadically. The National Center for Health Care Technology was created in 1978 to research and compare health care technologies. It evaluated a number of technologies and made coverage recommendations to the Medicare program, but was controversial and no longer received funding after 1981. At the same time the Congressional Office of Technology Assessment evaluated the costs and benefits of a variety of technologies but lost funding in 1995. (Congressional Budget Office, December 2007d)

As of 2011 a number of federal government agencies support or perform some form of CER, including the AHRQ), National Institutes of Health (NIH), CMS, FDA, Centers for Disease Control and Prevention (CDC), Department of Defense (DOD), and Department of Veterans Affairs (VA). Each agency has its own legislative requirements for conducting research, which is usually tied to its core mission. (Institute of Medicine & Committee on Comparative Effectiveness Research Prioritization, 2009a) For example, the VA compares various treatment options for recipients of Veterans Health Affairs services. This specification helps ensure that veterans receive proper treatments that are cost-effective and within budget limits. The NIH has a broad mandate to fund basic research and has occasionally sponsored research to compare treatments. CMS has funded research comparing different treatments but usually to determine clinical effectiveness or whether to pay the same amount for two different treatments. It is outside the legislative authority of CMS to look at cost-effectiveness. A vast number of activities and resources are available from the federal government related to comparative effectiveness. (National Library of Medicine, 1994)

ARRA increased total federal government funding for CER by an additional $1.1 billion. The funding was divided among AHRQ ($300 million), NIH ($400 million), and the Office of the Secretary of DHHS ($500 million). The amount given to the Office of the Secretary of DHHS is discretionary funding that can be used for a variety of comparative effectiveness programs. The ARRA funds were targeted to CER within the government (intramural) or outside government (extramural). In addition, $268 million of the funds were required to be used to encourage development and use of "clinical registries, clinical data networks, and other forms of electronic health data that can be used to generate or obtain outcomes data." This financial support to develop and use health information technology to generate and capture data in CER programs demonstrates the importance of new technologies to the future of CER and the importance of coordinating with other government health information technology programs. (Department of Health and Human Services Recovery Funding Page, 2011) ARRA also funded the IOM to consult with stakeholders and report on priorities for comparative effectiveness research. (Institute of Medicine & Committee on Comparative Effectiveness Research Prioritization, 2009b)

AHRQ has the broadest mandate for comparative effectiveness studies; however, until 2009 only $15 million of the entire $300 million AHRQ budget was targeted to programs related to comparative effectiveness. Before 2009 AHRQ had run a national clearinghouse for medical guidelines, helped fund a number of "evidence-based practice centers," sponsored an "Effective Health Care" program, and funded private sector research. ARRA's funding increase to AHRQ doubled the entire AHRQ annual budget thereby strengthening substantially its emphasis on CER. Programs created or expanded by the new funding include "horizon scanning" for new and emerging issues: synthesis of evidence to compare effectiveness of medical treatments; identification of gaps in research; translation and dissemination of CER findings; coordination and prioritization of comparative effectiveness projects; training and career development; and a program to formally engage stakeholders. (Department of Health and Human Services, 2010a) As these new initiatives gain momentum at the same time ACO and

CIN programs are maturing in the coming years, opportunities to leverage insights will materialize to help provider improve patient care.

Government agencies are subject to Congressional and public scrutiny, so great caution is exercised by these organizations to mitigate controversial actions or initiatives. In fact, AHRQ lost funding in the mid-1990s when research into back surgery resulted in controversial guidelines that were opposed by orthopedic surgeons. (Gray, Gusmano, & Collins, 2003) Concern about the effect of CER, and the potential to use such information to make reimbursement decisions, has led to restrictions on the use of CER results. For example, the ACA established a tax-exempt, private nonprofit organization called the Patient Centered Outcomes Research Institute (PCORI). PCORI is separate from the government to reduce the potential for political intervention and manipulation. In addition, PCORI research findings may "not be construed as mandates for practice guidelines, coverage recommendations, payment, or policy recommendations," nor may they be used for coverage or reimbursement decisions by "any public or private payer."(Department of Health and Human Services, 2010d)

The Patient Protection and Affordable Care Act of 2010

PCORI was created by the ACA to identify priorities for comparative effectiveness research and fund research comparing "health outcomes and clinical effectiveness, risks, and benefits of two or more medical treatments, services, or items."(Department of Health and Human Services, 2010c) PCORI takes a patient-centered approach, and is designed to improve the interaction between patient and provider by increasing the availability of valid evidence-based medical information to enable meaningful discussion between patient and the clinician. The "patient preference" approach is central as some policy makers believe most of medical decisions fall somewhere between 25 percent of care that is based on evidence and 10 percent of procedures that should never be done. It is this middle 65 percent, according to industry observers, where information can be applied to better inform patient preference. According to a governing board member, PCORI expects to bring about a new era in which both patients and their caregivers have access to the best information, and the tools to turn that information into knowledge allowing both patient and clinician to make the best decisions.

The PCORI website describes the organization as:

> ...an independent organization created to help patients, clinicians, purchasers and policy makers make better informed health decisions. PCORI will commission research that is responsive to the values and interests of patients and will provide patients and their caregivers with reliable, evidence-based information for the health care choices they face. (Patient Centered Outcomes Research Institute, 2009)

The description is decidedly focused on patients and decision making, which may limit the ability of the organization to fund or participate in basic research that increases scientific knowledge unless there is a connection with consumer health decisions. Of course, the argument can be made that all basic research increasing scientific knowledge should be related to consumer health decisions. In addition, PCORI may not "mandate coverage, reimbursement, or other policies for any public or private payer,"(Department of Health and Human Services, 2010b) limiting the organization's ability to keep from being involved in considerations of cost-effectiveness--a concern for organizations paying the costs of care, such as government health programs, employers, health insurance companies, and partially capitated CINs, or ACOs. Nevertheless, the output of PCORI will add to medical knowledge, and if valid the results will be used by healthcare stakeholders.

PCORI is required to establish and carry out a research agenda that focuses on "priority areas" of research. It is governed by a board of governors appointed by the U.S. Government Accountability Office from public nominations, and must appoint advisory panels and a methodology committee. PCORI does not itself perform research; rather it supports research through a variety of activities, including funding, collaborating with other government agencies, establishing a peer-review process for primary research, adopting research priorities, standards, processes and protocols, and disseminating and publishing research findings. PCORI is required to submit annual reports to Congress, the Administration, and the public; and there are a number of requirements that increase the transparency of the work performed by PCORI--which helps to increase the validity of the process and projects funded). (Department of Health and Human Services, 2010e)

Funding for PCORI comes from a new Patient-Centered Outcomes Research Trust Fund that receives monies from several sources, including Medicare trust funds, private sector health plans, self-insured plans, pharmaceutical companies, and general funds of the federal government. While funding will slowly increase from 2010 to 2019, it is expected to rise to $500 million by 2014. The amount of funding available to PCORI depends on a complex set of formulas tied to the number of persons covered by public and private health care. (Clancy & Collins, 2010) Some believe PCORI annual funding could be as much as $650 million, depending on the amount brought in by the health coverage surtax, and total $3 billion over 10 years. (Leonard, April 2010)

National Institute for Health and Clinical Excellence

A number of organizations in other countries sponsor or perform comparative effectiveness research. This factor is important as it not only shows that comparative effectiveness is a global issue but also because it provides lessons learned from comparative effectiveness activities in other countries. In the United Kingdom (UK) the National Institute for Health and Clinical Excellence (NICE) is widely recognized as a pioneer in comparative effectiveness research. NICE was created in 1999 by the government of the United Kingdom to evaluate the clinical and cost effectiveness of various drugs, devices, and procedures. Part of the UK National Health Service (NHS), NICE organizes systematic reviews of existing comparative effectiveness research (meta-analyses), and develops cost effectiveness models to arrive at cost-benefit conclusions. It does not fund primary research, nor does it directly decide which treatments to cover or how much to pay. If a drug, device, or methodology is approved by NICE as effective, it must be covered for reimbursement by the NHS health program. But the NHS decides how much to pay, and if a medical therapy is not approved by NICE it is not automatically rejected by the NHS. With a staff of 200 and a budget of approximately $60 million, NICE does not have extensive resources and it takes awhile to develop studies and produce results. NICE has published about 250 recommendations on procedures, over 100 studies on specific technologies, and 60 treatment guidelines. It is up to local government authorities to make coverage decisions on treatment technologies and methodologies that are not studied by NICE. Australia, Canada, France, and Germany have government agencies similar to NICE. All of these countries have some form of centralized government-funded and controlled health care finance and delivery system, perhaps making NICE and similar organizations not directly applicable to the U.S. healthcare system.

Commercial Comparative Effectiveness Research

A number of private sector comparative effectiveness programs currently operate in the United States. Life science companies, such as drug and device manufacturers, commission CER to determine the effectiveness of their products to gain a competitive advantage, identify improved uses for their products, and potential new uses. As reimbursement becomes more restrictive and the market becomes more competitive, life science companies may find it increasingly important to engage in comparative effectiveness studies to understand cost and benefits of their products. Health plans, self-insured employers, and government payers are interested in CER to determine the quality of drugs, devices, and procedures, and to better understand their overall value to patients. Hospitals and health systems review treatment methodologies in their pharmacy and therapeutic committees and quality committees to assist with quality and risk management, determine pharmacy formularies, and make capital allocation for new devices. As integrated delivery networks, physician-hospital organizations, and physician groups assume increased risk and greater responsibility for quality and cost in such new provider organizations such as CINs and accountable care arrangements, CER and evidence-based medicine will increase in importance. (Miller, 2011) In addition as this shift occurs the federal government may re-examine regulations governing the use of comparative effectiveness studies to better align with such reformed delivery entities as ACOs, CINs, and other new models of care delivery.

Medical drug and device manufacturers are required by the FDA to conduct clinical trials in developing their products to demonstrate safety and efficacy, and in some cases to show how one device compares to another. These studies focus on safety and efficacy, but not relative clinical or cost effectiveness. Manufacturers are beginning to study clinical and cost effectiveness through CER and application of pharmacoeconomics mainly to inform the design and content of package inserts but also to determine how their products compare with competitors as they prepare to go to market and help identify differentiators in the marketplace. This activity will become more critical as drugs and devices lose their patent protections and the protected drug and device portfolios of large companies shrink. In addition, the FDA is beginning to use the results of CER in the regulation of products. Comparative effectiveness is also becoming more critical for manufacturers, as payers increasingly perform comparative studies to find drugs and devices that provide greater value. Providers, consumers, health plans, self-funded employers, governments, CINs and ACOs are interested in proof that a more costly drug or device results in a commensurate increase in clinical benefit for patients. (Institute of Medicine & Committee on Comparative Effectiveness Research Prioritization, 2009e)

Health insurance plans have an interest in CER as they strive to improve quality and affordability. Health insurance plans at risk not only for the cost of care, they are also legally accountable for the quality of care, required to justify coverage decisions, and must work with patients or physicians who challenge these decisions and adjudicate their appeals. Health plans also use the results of CER to increase their knowledge of evidence-based medicine, develop best practice clinical protocols, and provide clinical decision support tools and technologies to physicians, nursing care managers, and patients. These technologies are used for predictive modeling and risk stratification, care management, disease management, total population registries, quality measurement, specific care recommendations, and personal health records, (Juster, 2005) Many of these technologies and tools may be leveraged by CINs and ACOs as the industry evolves and these organizations are increasingly interested in evidence-based medicine.

While CINs and ACOs will assume more accountability and risk for the outcomes of care, and pay-for-performance programs are taking greater responsibility for care the reality is that in most areas of the country today, health plans are the predominant bearers of risk and have the greatest experience and largest array of tools for risk mitigation and care management. As a result, health insurance plans are at the forefront of researching the quality and effectiveness of various medical drugs, devices, and procedures, and they have sophisticated infrastructure for reviewing the findings of medical research and making decisions. (Kongstvedt, 2007) The result has been identification of optimal treatment methodologies and processes that assist patients and physicians in understanding appropriateness of different treatment options. (Javitt et al., 2005) Many health plans publish the results of their research as medical coverage policies.[*] As the market expands around risk-sharing between providers and health insurance plans, observers anticipated that many of these risk mitigation and care management strategies and tools may be shared with providers. (Aetna Corporate, 2011) As CINs and ACOs become more experienced in managing and improving care outcomes, they may become key players in the U.S. healthcare system's larger framework of comparative effectiveness capabilities.

---

[*] For example, see Aetna Clinical Policy Bulletins, which are detailed, technical documents explaining how decisions are made: http://www.aetna.com/healthcare-professionals/policies-guidelines/clinical_policy_bulletins.html

Many of the provider organizations noted in Figure 3-3 in Chapter 3 use comparative effectiveness techniques to assist with quality and risk management, determine pharmacy formularies, and make capital allocations. Such new business models for healthcare delivery and finance as medical homes, CINs, and ACOs require providers to take greater clinical and financial responsibility and risk in the process of ensuring that optimal care is delivered for their patients. As these organizations refine their business practices, their perspective on clinical effectiveness may become broader, looking not only at the quality of care but affordability as well. Managing these new models of care delivery will require providers to have greater awareness of the relative benefit and harm of different treatment methodologies. This information will increase the importance of and demand for CER and related evidence-based medicine and clinical decision support services. (Miller, 2011)

Life science companies, provider organizations, health plans, and other commercial entities also support such broader efforts in CER, as the government-funded PCORI, which focuses on increasing the ability of patients and physicians to make better informed treatment decisions and improve overall quality and affordability. Government policy makers maintain that the current health finance and delivery system allows treatments with marginal clinical benefit relative to their cost. They see the current situation as contributing to unsustainable cost growth requiring greater information and transparency on clinical effectiveness and cost of care to address this national problem. It is therefore natural that a wide range of stakeholders support such organizations as PCORI and other private sector efforts to obtain up-to-date, objective, and credible information on the effectiveness and value of health care services.

Comparative Effectiveness and Coverage Decisions

Organizations with the responsibility and burden of risk for clinical and financial outcomes of care have an interest in comparing both clinical and cost effectiveness. These comparisons are used to determine benefit design and decide which therapies are covered in the benefit package. Coverage decisions are made by all organizations accountable for care of a defined population, including government agencies that fund health programs (e.g. Medicare, Medicaid, state indigent care and children's health programs, Veterans Health Administration, and the like.), unions, self-insured employers, health insurance plans, and ACOs. All these organizations have developed a wide range of activities to determine which treatments provide the best clinical outcomes for the resources expended.

A variety of comparative effectiveness services have been created to assist with decisions on clinical and cost effectiveness. The Blue Cross and Blue Shield Association has operated the Technology Evaluation Center whose clients include many of the Blue Plans and the CMS. (Wilensky, 2009) Other organizations that support or perform clinical effectiveness research include the Center for Medical Technology Policy, Cochrane Collaboration, Drug Effectiveness Review Project, ECRI Institute, Hayes, Inc., Institute for Clinical and Economic Review, and Tufts Medical Center Cost-Effectiveness Analysis Registry. (Congressional Budget Office, December 2007e; Institute of Medicine & Committee on Comparative Effectiveness Research Prioritization, 2009d)

CMS is the largest payer of health care services and products in the United States, with a total budget for fiscal year 2011 of $782 billion. Given the size of its budget, and continued growth of its programs administered, funded, and regulated by CMS (e.g. Medicare, Medicaid, State Children's Health plans, and the new health insurance exchanges), CMS has a substantial interest in CER. (Wilensky, 2009) An example of a coverage decision-making process, which includes comparative effectiveness input from external technology assessment resources is shown in Figure 12-1. (Jacques, 2011) The Medicare National Coverage decision-making process illustrates the level of complexity in evaluating medical therapies for coverage decisions.

Figure 12-1. Medicare National Coverage Process[*]

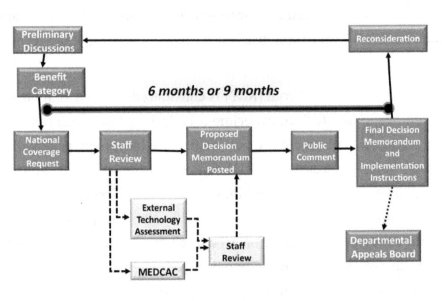

Source: Center for Medicare and Medicaid Services

Decisions rendered through this process are for items and services required for the diagnosis and treatment of an illness or injury covered by Medicare. The underlying methodology and program is run as an evidence-based process that allows opportunities for public participation. (Centers for Medicare and Medicaid Services, 2011) As CINs and ACOs continue to grow in their tolerance of clinical and financial risk and acceptance of responsibility, they will be more attuned to the decisions made by such payer organizations such as CMS in their national and local coverage processes, and may even begin to adopt these coverage determinations.

Comparative Effectiveness Research Methods

A variety of methods are used to research the effectiveness of medical therapies, and arrive at conclusions about the best treatment for a

---

[*] From "Evidence for Decisionmaking, A Medicare Perspective" presentation by Louis B Jacques, MD, Director, Coverage & Analysis Group, Centers for Medicare and Medicaid Services, third DEcIDE Methods Symposium: Methods for Developing and Analyzing Clinically Rich Data for Patient-Centered Outcomes Research, Monday June 6, 2011, Rockville, MD.

condition. Each method has strengths and weaknesses and requires different levels of rigor and validity. Here we look at two different categories of research methods--randomized controlled trials and observational studies--and their usefulness in comparative effectiveness research.

The randomized controlled trial (RCT) is considered the gold standard of research methods. In an RCT, an experiment is designed in which research subjects are chosen and randomly assigned to a treatment group or a control group, with the assignment unbeknown to the observer, and the effects of treatment are then isolated and observed. The research subjects are chosen to minimize differences in their health status, and all other aspects of the study are controlled or accounted for as well as possible so that the only difference between the two groups is the treatment provided. By controlling as many variables as possible in the study, researchers attempt to isolate the cause-effect relationship between the treatment given and outcome recorded. (Agency for Healthcare Research and Quality, 2011)

Observational studies include a variety of research designs in which no experiment is set up in advance with random assignment or controls. Observational studies may be used in situations in which a controlled experiment may not be possible. Controlled trials are not possible, for example, where ethical standards prohibit the use of human subjects (e.g., effects of radon gas or cigarette smoking), or when setting up an RCT is difficult (e.g., rare occurrence of side effects, or lack of resources to get a large enough experimental population). Observational studies make conclusions about the effects of the treatment in question based on educated guesses (inferences) from the data. (ClinicalTrials.gov Protocol Registration System, 2011) Observational studies include cohort studies, case-controlled studies, case series, and case reports. (Akobeng, 2005) Figure 12-2 illustrates progression through a hierarchy of evidence. (Akobeng, 2005)

Figure 12-2. Hierarchy of Evidence for Intervention or Treatment Effectiveness

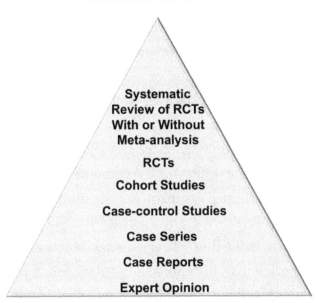

The RCT is considered the most rigorous and valid research design as it attempts to reduce errors, eliminate bias and extraneous effects (also known as confounding variables) by controlling the study as much as possible. A systematic review of a set of randomized controlled trials using meta-analysis may provide additional validity as it assembles results of many RCT and can cover larger populations and filter out weaknesses of individual trials.

There are weaknesses to RCT, however, especially in situations in which decisions that impact a large group of persons must be made quickly, such as coverage decisions that must be implemented in the short-term for a large population in a health plan, CIN/ACO, or clinical formulary decisions by one of these organizations. To begin, RCTs are more expensive to conduct and take much longer to set up, implement, and provide results--in many cases it takes years and millions of dollars. Second, because the population is controlled, the results apply to a defined population and may not be generally applicable. Finally, because the procedures used in a RCT are controlled and the experiment is carried out under optimal conditions, it may be difficult to replicate or implement in a regular clinical setting. (Concato et al., 2010)

Observational studies have been criticized as more prone to error as they are perceived to be less rigorous or valid than a RCT. Perhaps not as rigorous as RCTs, observational studies can be designed to reduce errors and improve their validity. The lack of ability to rigorously control the situation and the potential for extraneous variables to affect the results leads to a need for adjustments to observational studies. Once these adjustments are made, the effects of treatment can more reliably be determined. (ClinicalTrials.gov Protocol Registration System, 2011) Such techniques as propensity scoring and instrumental variables are used to correct for errors by adjusting observational studies to more closely replicate RCT experiments. Recent studies have shown that properly adjusted observational studies are almost as good as RCTs. (Horwitz, Viscoli, Clemens, & Sadock, 1990)

Observational studies have important advantages for application of CER. Because they are less expensive and may use data already collected, they can be completed more rapidly. In addition, observational studies are usually done in real-world clinical settings on actual patients using real interventions rather than strict experimental controls. (Concato et al., 2010) Thus, the results can be obtained and applied more easily, which is important in situations in which decisions must be made quickly. Future improvements in observational study design will increase the availability of information on better medical therapies, help organizations with decision making on what works best, including which treatments should be used in clinical settings. The selection of one research methodology over another involves a number of issues. Table 12-1 below provides a summary of some myths regarding each of these methodologies. (Concato et al., 2010)

Table 12-1. Myths and Evidence on RCTs and Observational Studies

Issue	Myth	Evidence
Gold standard	Randomized, controlled trials are always the gold standard in research design	Randomized trials on the same topic often contradict each other
Unknown confounders	Unknown confounders undermine all observational studies	If a factor is unknown, treatment will not be influenced and confounding is unlikely
Designed to Replicate RCT	Novel strategies in designing and analyzing observational studies can replicate randomization	Purported benefits of new strategies to design and analyze are often conceptual rather than actual
Design vs. Details	Study design matters more than specific details and attributes	Details of patients, interventions, and outcomes are highly relevant

Pragmatic randomized clinical trials (PCTs) have been proposed to combine the validity of RCT with the practical applicability of observational studies. In a PCT the study design is set up specifically to address clinical quality and cost issues of interest to decision makers. (Tunis et al., 2003) The Center for Medical Technology Policy has pioneered PCTs as a way to get provide valid information to all decision makers, including patients, physicians, providers, policy-makers, payers and health care administrators. (Center for Medicare Technology Policy, 2011a) PCTs are designed to be more applicable and useful in real world situations because they recruit a diverse set of participants from a wide variety of real-world clinical practices and focus on comparing specific medical therapies while collecting a wide range of outcomes. (Center for Medicare Technology Policy, 2011b)

It is important for CINs and ACOs to understand the implications of these different research methodologies. As the use of CER expands, study results can benefit the patients and providers by bringing new intelligence into the shared decision-making process. This new information will improve patients' quality of care and ultimately their quality of life.

Health Information Technology and CER

The increasing availability of health information technology is creating tremendous new opportunities to advance knowledge and evidence while strengthening the healthcare industry's ability to study and compare the effectiveness of medical interventions. ARRA recognized the importance of the health information technology data infrastructure in advancing the national CER agenda and allocated $268 million to data infrastructure development. (Department of Health and Human Services Recovery Funding Page, 2011) In addition to such existing clinical study methods as RCT and observational studies, health information technology has created opportunities for new analyses by combining such traditional data sources as administrative claims, with clinical information from electronic medical records, registries, and other clinical databases. These new combinations of data and information will enhance CER studies and medical evidence compilation. (Etheredge, 2010)

Claims data brings a number of advantages to comparative effectiveness studies. There is a large body of literature describing ways to analyze the data, and established methods (such as propensity scoring) to adjust for potential errors. All health plans and self-insured employers have used claims data for years to analyze and improve the quality and affordability of healthcare. As discussed previously, health plans include claims data in their analyses of different treatment options when they develop medical coverage policies. Claims data is also used for a variety of quality, performance improvement, clinical decision support, and care management purposes. Some organizations have taken additional steps to develop sophisticated predictive models and advanced clinical decision support algorithms that yield accurate models of patients and their needed care. These systems are used to improve quality by scanning both claims and clinical data to detect and correct errors in the care delivery process and deviations from best medical practices. (Javitt et al., 2005) If you combine a clinical trial with subsequent claims data, you can also create a longitudinal record for a patient and continue to follow his or her progress even after the trial is completed. Use of such a longitudinal record could take trials out of the clinic and into daily life, identifying both beneficial and harmful effects in real-life situations.

There are disadvantages to only using claims data as the data may be specific to an episode of care, and lack information necessary to understand the patient's full health status. Without additional information about the patient, it is difficult to identify similar patients or populations and compare the effectiveness of different medical therapies. (Congressional Budget Office, December 2007c)

Clinical information from such health information technology as electronic health records, personal health records and medical registries, can fill in the elements missing in administrative claims data, providing a more complete picture of a patient or population, and result in a more robust data set for CER. These technologies can provide such important data as medical histories, measures of health status, laboratory test results, and treatment outcomes. (Congressional Budget Office, December 2007b) The additional data can give sufficient detail to allow proper research methodologies to compare medical therapies, to be compared. Incorporating clinical data with claims data has been described as the "holy grail" of CER, but issues of federal government research priorities, privacy concerns, lack of information technology standardization, and difficulty in aggregating data are roadblocks to such integration. (Congressional Budget Office, December 2007a; Navathe & Conway, 2010)

The private sector has advanced its comparative effectiveness research agenda and methodologies at a faster pace than the federal government. It is already aggregating and integrating administrative claims data with clinical-level data from health information technology. These efforts in time will allow ACOs and CINs to combine quality measures from clinical data with financial performance goals in their claims systems so they can monitor their performance against targets and annual goals in real time. (Medicity, September 2010)

Comparative Effectiveness and Clinical Decision Support

Clinical decision support (CDS) refers to any methodical process used to assist clinicians or patients with medical decisions. Computer-based CDS is further defined as the use of computers to bring relevant knowledge to bear on decisions about patients' healthcare and well-being. (Greenes, 2007) Knowledge relevant to clinical care includes patient data, medical and pharmaceutical claims, clinical data, evidence-based guidelines, the most recent medical literature, personal values, and any other information that could help clinicians and patients make decisions and improve the quality of care. CER is part of the medical literature that goes into CDS.

Basic computer-based CDS technology combines data from a variety of sources, such as medical claims, pharmacy claims, and clinical data from EMRs and translates those data into information and knowledge applied by physicians, other clinicians, and multi-disciplinary caregiver teams to improve the quality of care. The translation of data and resulting conclusions is often accomplished by comparing patient treatments to evidence-based guidelines and identifying gaps in care and sometimes given recommendations on appropriate care according to the evidence-based guidelines used. Comparing treatment recommendations to guidelines is a form of practical comparative effectiveness but has shortcomings.

Many EHRs have basic CDS, which was a nominal requirement for achieving meaningful use under the CMS Meaningful Use of EHRs incentive program.* The CMS meaningful use regulations require "one clinical decision support to improve performance on high-priority health conditions" in "Stage 1" implementations, and "...5 clinical decision support interventions related to 4 or more clinical quality measures" in "Stage 2" implementations.**

One rule may be appropriate to prove the concept of delivering CDS, but is inadequate for ongoing decision support across a broad spectrum of diseases and conditions if you are looking for improved outcomes. In addition, studies have shown that current EHRs do not deliver the features needed to improve patient care. Additional technologies are needed for EHRs to be effective, including registries, personal health records, and clinical decision support. (Bates & Bitton, 2010) A recent study the use of clinical decision support in EHRs from 2005 to 2007 showed "no consistent association between EHRs and CDS and better quality."

Clearly, something is missing; additional clinical information from medical literature and CER is needed to improve and strengthen CDS. Advanced CDS technology is starting to become available, and it addresses the shortcomings of current EHR-based basic CDS by including a variety of additional data, tools, and techniques to improve decision support and care results. Advanced CDS is of great interest to ACOs and CINs as it is more accurate in identifying appropriate care, and allowing providers to mitigate and manage their risk and responsibility for clinical and economic outcomes.

---

* Fed. Reg. Vol. 75, No. 144, II(A)(2)(c). Stage 1 Criteria for Meaningful Use. p. 44350. CMS defines CDS in the context of meaningful use, as "HIT functionality that builds upon the foundation of an EHR to provide persons involved in care processes with general and person-specific information, intelligently filtered and organized, at appropriate times, to enhance health and health care."

** .Office of the National Coordinator for Health IT. How to Implement EHRs. Step 5: Achieve Meaningful Use Stage 2. Clinical Decision Support Rule. Accessed online November 2, 2014 at http://www.healthit.gov/providers-professionals/achieve-meaningful-use/core-measures-2/clinical-decision-support-rule.

Additional data not currently available to clinically focused EHRs but used in advanced CDS include pharmacy data, claims data, health risk assessments, patient-reported data, disability data, and other medical and demographic information. These additional elements help to provide a more complete picture of the patient, including medical history and future health risk.

Another feature of advanced CDS is the use of more recent medical findings, such as the results of CER. Basic CDS takes clinical information and compares it to evidence-based guidelines. By definition, evidence-based guidelines are consensus standards developed at a given point in time, using the medical literature then available. Industry experts recognize that medical research is constantly advancing, and that "no physician can keep up with the literature and changing medical advances simply with intuition and top-of-mind memory."(Miller, 2011) Advanced CDS technologies, on the other hand, bring the capability to search the latest medical literature; present the latest medical findings identified by a team of experts; and update the evidence in real time––presenting evidence-based medicine practices at the point of care. (Jenrette & Yale, November 19, 2010) One drawback of some CDS is the level of effort and cost of human-intensive expert system techniques. (Greenes, 2007)

A systematic review of studies of clinical decision support technologies identified specific features of CDS correlated with significant improvements in patient care. These features include: information that fits into clinician workflow; specific care recommendations; information at the point of care; periodic performance feedback; sharing recommendations with patients; and requesting documentation of reasons for not following recommendations. (Kawamoto, Houlihan, Balas, & Lobach, 2005) Advanced CDS tools and techniques build in all these features by using real-time care recommendations at the point of care, allowing bidirectional information sharing with the treating clinician and utilizing such patient-facing tools, as personal health records to allow patient self-management. (Jenrette & Yale, November 19, 2010)

Comparative Effectiveness and New Provider Organizations

Given current restrictions on government-funded CER, its research results may not be directly useful to such new care models as CINs and ACOs. All CER findings, however, increase general medical knowledge and evidence-based medicine used by these organizations for decision support. Whether directly or indirectly improvements in medical knowledge improve best practice protocols. Thus even government-funded CER with its restrictions increases the body of medical knowledge, indirectly helping physicians and patients make more informed decisions about treatment options that improve patient care and quality of life.

CINs and ACOs do have commercially available advanced CDS tools to assist decision-making on appropriate care. As these new provider organizations accept greater responsibility for clinical and financial outcomes, they will find themselves making medical coverage decisions including benefit design, and responding to appeals of care decisions. Fortunately, there is a large body of work in this field and many tools on the market that allow providers to access this information. (Javitt et al., 2008; Javitt et al., 2005)*

The success of such new provider organizations as ACOs and CINs will depend heavily on continued advancements in health information technology. Many organizations are strengthening their clinical integration in order to have the infrastructure necessary to operate in the new environment. Consider this possibility: properly established CINs and ACOs operating with appropriate health information technology and advanced CDS, and actively exchanging and aggregating data, may contribute to a "rapid-learning health system." Such a system would combine evidence

---

* A description of one such service and results obtained, can be found at the two referenced Javitt papers.

from clinical and comparative effectiveness research with individual patients' information from electronic medical records to determine what works best for a patient. (Etheredge, 2010)

Another form of CER is comparing different healthcare finance and delivery models. For example, different ACO models (both public and private) could be evaluated and compared as they emerge, their operations become established, and their results and outcomes tested.

This kind of initiative would focus on the effectiveness of variations in administrative systems, payment reforms, and related compensation models that would tie into opportunities for improving benchmarks to ensure comparability of results and savings achieved against targets. Ideally different health finance and delivery models could be compared, and help advance the study of health care quality, accessiblity and affordability.

Future Directions

The field of CER covers a broader spectrum that includes federally funded programs and private sector initiatives. While federally funded CER holds promise, it brings challenges to the industry in terms of limits on the use of federal funds and maximizing the utilization of results and findings. Private sector CER studies and programs, such as those funded through the pharmaceutical and biotechnology industry, provide results more quickly, but are usually proprietary and may not be widely publicized. In addition, there may be an element of bias in pharmaceutical and biotechnology CER, especially when the studies are performed for marketing purposes. CER associated with health insurance plans can be more specifically targeted to both clinical and economic outcomes, but may not be readily available to providers unless there is a preexisting relationship.

Finally, health information technology brings additional challenges. New technologies are arriving at a rapid pace, and often faster than industry can keep up with them. There are inherent risks in the development and implementation of new technologies, called "technology-related adverse events" by the Joint Commission's 2008 Sentinel Event Report Number 42. (The Joint Commission, 2008)

EMRs, EHRs, and registries used in CER can pose such risks, as the ability of society to develop new technologies may exceed the capacity of clinicians to use them safely and effectively.

Some of the most important challenges for CINs and ACOs involve effective and permissible use of CER study results to support improvements in the quality of patient care. It remains to be seen whether restrictions on the use of government-funded CER will persist. In addition, providers must consider whether it is worthwhile and economically viable to support CER. As both CER and new provider models continue to shape the future of healthcare services, new challenges will emerge and stakeholders will find ways to meet them for the benefit of providers, patients, and the organizations that fund healthcare.

We need to take medicine from empirical to evidence-based, and not just broad guidelines, but patient-specific medicine.

Janet Woodcock, MD,
Director, Food and Drug Administration,
Center for Drug Evaluation and Research

CHAPTER 12 DISCUSSION QUESTIONS

Discussion questions are provided for team building or class exercises. Answers for all questions are provided in Appendix C.

Question Number	Question
1	What is comparative effectiveness research (CER)?
2	Why should CINs and ACOs be interested in comparative effectiveness research?
3	What types of organizations have conducted CER in the past, and why?
4	What type of work does PCORI perform?
5	Why are health plans interested in CER?
6	How is health information technology benefiting CER?

CHAPTER 12 HIGHLIGHTS

✓ Comparative effectiveness research is an applied research methodology that gained funding and support through the 2009 American Recovery and Reinvestment Act (ARRA) and the 2010 Patient Protection and Affordable Care Act.

✓ Three benefits of comparative effectiveness research findings include:

✓ Help increase the body of knowledge of evidence-based medicine,

✓ Improve best practice protocols and quality, and

✓ Be used to strengthen clinical decision support for physician and patient benefit.

✓ The ARRA appropriated $1.1B in funds for CER that was distributed to AHRQ ($300 million), NIH ($400 million), and the Office of the Secretary of DHHS ($500 million).

✓ The ACA established the Patient-Centered Outcomes Research Institute (PCORI) and funding for PCORI comes from the Patient-Centered Outcomes Research Trust Fund.

✓ The National Institute for Health and Clinical Excellence (NICE) by the government of the United Kingdom (UK) and is widely recognized as the pioneer in comparative effectiveness research. NICE was created in 1999 to evaluate the clinical and cost effectiveness of various drugs, devices, and procedures.

✓ Randomized controlled trials (RCTs) and observational studies are two types of research methods that have been and can be applied in conducting CER studies.

✓ Health information technology has significantly strengthened CER capabilities but is bringing new challenges such as "technology related adverse events."

✓ The field of CER has a bright future but is mixed in purpose and focus depending on the organizations conducting studies (e.g., government vs. private sector).

CHAPTER 12 REFERENCES

Aetna Corporate. (2011). Aetna and Carilion Clinic Announce Plans to Collaborate on Accountable Care Organization. Retrieved from http://www.aetna.com/news/newsReleases/2011/0310_Aetna_and_Carilion.html

Agency for Healthcare Research and Quality. (2011). Glossary of Terms, definition of randomized controlled trials. Retrieved from http://www.effectivehealthcare.ahrq.gov/index.cfm/glossary-of-terms/?pageaction=showterm&termid=101

Akobeng, A. K. (2005). Understanding randomised controlled trials. *Archives of Disease in Childhood*, 90(8), 840-844.

Bates, D. W., & Bitton, A. (2010). The future of health information technology in the patient-centered medical home. *Health Affairs*, 29(4), 614-621. doi: 10.1377/hlthaff.2010.0007

Center for Medicare Technology Policy. (2011a). Issue Brief: Pragmatic/Practical Randomized Controlled Trials. Retrieved from http://www.cmtpnet.org/comparative-effectiveness/PCT_issue_brief_11-26-08.pdf

Center for Medicare Technology Policy. (2011b). Pragmatic Clinical Trials, Center for Medical Technology Policy. Retrieved from http://www.cmtpnet.org/comparative-effectiveness/pragmatic-trials

Centers for Medicare and Medicaid Services. (2011). Overview of Medicare Coverage Determination Process. Retrieved from https://http://www.cms.gov/DeterminationProcess/

Clancy, C., & Collins, F. S. (2010). Patient-centered outcomes research institute: the intersection of science and health care. Science *Translational Medicine*, 2(37), 37cm18-37cm18. doi: 10.1126/scitranslmed.3001235

ClinicalTrials.gov Protocol Registration System. (2011). Protocol Data Element Definitions (DRAFT), definition of observational studies. Retrieved from http://prsinfo.clinicaltrials.gov/definitions.html

Concato, J., Lawler, E. V., Lew, R. A., Gaziano, J. M., Aslan, M., & Huang, G. D. (2010). Observational methods in comparative effectiveness research. *The American Journal of Medicine*, 123(12), e16-e23. doi: 10.1016/j.amjmed.2010.10.004

Congressional Budget Office. (2007a, December). Research on the Comparative Effectiveness of Medical Treatments. Publication 2975 (pp. 22). Washington, DC: Congressional Budget Office.

Congressional Budget Office. (2007b, December). Research on the Comparative Effectiveness of Medical Treatments. Publication 2975 (pp. 22-23). Washington, DC: Congressional Budget Office.

Congressional Budget Office. (2007c, December). Research on the Comparative Effectiveness of Medical Treatments. Publication 2975 (pp. 21-22). Washington, DC: Congressional Budget Office.

Congressional Budget Office. (2007d, December). Research on the Comparative Effectiveness of Medical Treatments. Publication 2975 (pp. 9). Washington, DC: Congressional Budget Office.

Congressional Budget Office. (2007e, December). Research on the Comparative Effectiveness of Medical Treatments. Publication 2975 (pp. 8). Washington, DC: Congressional Budget Office.

Congressional Budget Office. (2007f, December). Research on the Comparative Effectiveness of Medical Treatments. Publication 2975 (pp. 7-9). Washington, DC: Congressional Budget Office.

Department of Health and Human Services. (2010a). American Recovery and Reinvestment Act. Agency for Healthcare Research and Quality: Comparative Effectiveness Research Program Summary. Retrieved from http://www.hhs.gov/recovery/reports/plans/pdf20100610/AHRQ CER June 2010.pdf

H.R. 3590, Patient Protection and Affordable Care Act, §937(a)(1), Dissemination and Building Capacity for Research. p. 621. (2010) (2010b).

H.R. 3590, Patient Protection and Affordable Care Act, §6301(a)(2)(A), Comparative Clinical Effectiveness Research; Research. (2010) (2010c).

H.R. 3590, Patient Protection and Affordable Care Act, §6301(d)(8), Release of Research Findings. §6301(i). Rules. (2010) (2010d).

H.R. 3590, Patient Protection and Affordable Care Act, §6301(i) and (j), Patient-centered Outcomes Research . Rules and Rules of Construction. p. 620. (2010). (2010e).

Department of Health and Human Services. (2011). Fed. Reg. Vol. 76, No. 67. April 7, 2011. I(4)(b). Competition and Quality of Care. p. 19630.

Department of Health and Human Services Recovery Funding Page. (2011). Comparative Effectiveness Research. Retrieved from http://www.hhs.gov/recovery/programs/cer/index.html

Etheredge, L. M. (2010). Creating a high-performance system for comparative effectiveness research. *Health Affairs*, 29(10), 1761-1767. doi: 10.1377/hlthaff.2010.0608

Gray, B. H., Gusmano, M. K., & Collins, S. R. (2003). AHCPR and the changing politics of health services research. *Health Affairs*, 22(3; SUPP), W3-283.

Greenes, R. A. (2007). Clinical decision support: the road ahead. Maryland Heights, MD: Academic Press.

Horwitz, R. I., Viscoli, C. M., Clemens, J. D., & Sadock, R. T. (1990). Developing improved observational methods for evaluating therapeutic effectiveness. *The American Journal of Medicine*, 89(5), 630-638.

Institute of Medicine, & Committee on Comparative Effectiveness Research Prioritization. (2009a). Initial National Priorities for Comparative Effectiveness Research. Washington, DC: National Academies Press.

Institute of Medicine, & Committee on Comparative Effectiveness Research Prioritization. (2009b). Initial National Priorities for Comparative Effectiveness Research. Washington, DC: National Academies Press.

Institute of Medicine, & Committee on Comparative Effectiveness Research Prioritization. (2009c). Initial National Priorities for Comparative Effectiveness Research. Washington, DC: National Academies Press.

Institute of Medicine, & Committee on Comparative Effectiveness Research Prioritization. (2009d). Initial National Priorities for Comparative Effectiveness Research. Washington, DC: National Academies Press.

Institute of Medicine, & Committee on Comparative Effectiveness Research Prioritization. (2009e). Initial National Priorities for Comparative Effectiveness Research. Washington, DC: National Academies Press.

Jacques, L. B. (2011, June 6). The Stakeholder Perspective, presentation at the third DEcIDE Symposium on Comparative Effectiveness Research Methods.

Javitt, J. C., Rebitzer, J. B., & Reisman, L. (2008). Information technology and medical missteps: evidence from a randomized trial. *Journal of Health Economics*, 27(3), 585-602. doi: 10.1016/j.jhealeco.2007.10.008

Javitt, J. C., Steinberg, G., Locke, T., Couch, J. B., Jacques, J., Juster, I., & Reisman, L. (2005). Using a claims data-based sentinel system to improve compliance with clinical guidelines: results of a randomized prospective study. *American Journal of Managed Care*, 11(2), 93-102.

Jenrette, J., & Yale, K. (2010, November 19). *ACO Technologies: Performance and Reporting Tools.* Presented at ACO West Conference, San Diego, CA.

Juster, I. A. (2005). Technology-driven interactive care management identifies and resolves more clinical issues than a claims-based alerting system. *Disease Management*, 8(3), 188-197.

Kawamoto, K., Houlihan, C. A., Balas, E. A., & Lobach, D. F. (2005). Improving clinical practice using clinical decision support systems: a systematic review of trials to identify features critical to success. *BMJ*, 330(7494), 765.

Kongstvedt, P. (2007). *Essentials of managed health care.* Sudbury, MA: Jones & Bartlett Publishers.

Leonard, D. (2010, April). Time for PCORI's implementation.   Retrieved from http://www.npcnow.org/commentary/commentaryemployers-are-focusing-improving-health-outcomes

Medicity. (2010, September). Technology Fundamentals for Realizing ACO Success. Retrieved from http://www.himss.org/content/files/Medicity_ACO_Whitepaper.pdf

Miller, J. (2011). Aetna Manages Cancer Care. *Managed Healthcare Executive*, 21(7), 18-21.

National Library of Medicine. (1994). Health Services/Technology Assessment Texts (HSTAT). Bethesda, MD: National Library of Medicine.

Navathe, A. S., & Conway, P. H. (2010). Optimizing health information technology's role in enabling comparative effectiveness research. *The American Journal of Managed Care*, 16(12 Suppl HIT), SP44-47.

Patient Centered Outcomes Research Institute. (2009). Home Page. Organizational Description. Retrieved from http://www.pcori.org/home.html

The Joint Commission. (2008). Safely implementing health information and converging technologies. (42).

Tunis, S. R., Stryer, D. B., & Clancy, C. M. (2003). Practical clinical trials: increasing the value of clinical research for decision making in clinical and health policy. *The Journal of the American Medical Association*, 290(12), 1624-1632.

Wilensky, G. R. (2009). The policies and politics of creating a comparative clinical effectiveness research center. *Health Affairs*, 28(4), w719-w729. doi: 10.1377/hlthaff.28.4.w719

Chapter 13. Motivation, Patient Engagement and Self-Management

Ewa Matuszewski | Thomas A. Raskauskas

Ken Yale

Progress is impossible without change, and those who cannot change their minds cannot change anything.

George Bernard Shaw

CHAPTER 13 LEARNING OBJECTIVES

✓ Identify the Principles of the Patient Centered Medical Home as they relate to patient engagement.

✓ Describe the Chronic Care Model relationship to patient engagement.

✓ Explain the Transtheoretical Model of Change (TTM) concept by Prochaska and DiClemente.

✓ Review the 5 A's behavior change model which supports self-management.

✓ Illustrate the Readiness to Change Ruler.

✓ Discuss challenges in traditional patient engagement initiatives, and new developments allowing more accurate understanding of consumers, their needs, and how to engage them better.

Introduction

The World Health Organization (WHO) reports that non-communicable diseases (NCDs) are the leading causes of death globally, and account for over 75% of all deaths. (Riley & Cowan, July 2014) In 2008, 36 million deaths were attributed to NCDs, which were mainly cardiovascular disease, cancers, injury, diabetes and chronic lung diseases. About one fourth of the deaths took place before the age of 60. On a smaller scale, similar statistics are found in the United States. According to the Centers for Disease Control and Prevention's (CDC) preliminary 2011 mortality reports, seven of the top 10 all-cause death rates are in line with the WHO statistics.

With these startling numbers one would think people would be lining up outside physician offices, wanting to know what to do to prevent or reverse a chronic condition. But such is not the case. In spite of efforts to reduce and prevent chronic illnesses, including insurmountable research and education on the necessity of living a healthier lifestyle (such as a low-fat diet, regular exercise, not smoking, and decreasing stress) people are reluctant to change and/or lack the motivation, education or skills to adopt healthy lifelong habits to slow the progression of disease. Health care providers and health systems have traditionally been geared (and reimbursed) toward managing acute conditions, not these chronically ill patients requiring life-long care. Numerous interventions are employed by organizations such as health insurance plans and Clinically Integrated Networks (CINs) to assist these patients, including: population health management, disease management, health coaching, guilt or shame tactics. Yet, fewer than three percent of persons in a typical population engaged with these interventions show improvement in outcomes. (Frazee, Kirkpatrick, Fabius, & Chimera, 2007)

One key strategy to engage patients is self-management. Self-management involves empowerment of the individual with techniques and tools, including self-management support by health care providers, so the person is able to care for their condition on their own to achieve healthier lifestyles and outcomes. Self-management is one of eight essential elements the WHO has defined as necessary to reduce the threats chronic conditions pose to countries, their citizens, their health care systems, and their economies. In the 2002 WHO global report, *Innovative Care for Chronic Conditions*, element six states:

> Because the management of chronic conditions requires lifestyle and daily behavior change, emphasis must be upon the patient's central role and responsibility in health care…..At present, systems relegate the patient to passive recipient of care, missing the opportunity to leverage what he or she can do to promote personal health. Health care for

chronic conditions must be re-oriented around the patient and family. (World Health Organization, 2002)

Self-management teaches problem solving skills. It allows patients/individuals to identify their problems and provides techniques to help them make decisions, take appropriate actions, and alter these actions as they encounter changes in circumstances or disease. Numerous tools and education methods have been developed for self-management based on the premise that all patients know about their disease or health, and all they need to do is follow provider instructions and expectations, but this is not always the case. People must *want* to change. For health care providers and CINs operating in a patient-centered care environment, they must meet the patient where he/she is right now, not where providers want or expect them to be.

Two pieces of the puzzle have not been easily integrated into self-management: patient engagement and motivation to change. Assessing a patient's level of engagement (or activation), and motivation to change has been studied for more than 20 years. A review of the literature demonstrates it takes almost a decade for widespread implementation of guidelines that are recommended as evidence based. (Yuan et al., 2010) This is no less true for self-management and motivational theory, which was developed years ago in the fields of psychology and behavior medicine. Only since the patient-centered care movement began, and providers started becoming more accountable for care, has self-management started to take a firm foothold in practices. Likewise, motivational theory has only recently received widespread interest in healthcare.

Patient engagement is generally defined as "involving patients in their own care," (James, 2013) and includes methods, such as motivational interviewing, to gauge the patient's knowledge, skills and confidence needed to self-manage their health and disease. There are several tools available to measure patient engagement. The most widely tested and used, the Patient Activation Measure (PAM), was developed by Dr. Judith Hibbard and Dr. Bill Mahoney, while at the University of Oregon. (Insignia Health, 2014) Measuring a patient's engagement can be useful in tailoring interventions toward self-management.

As for motivation to change behavior towards healthy choices, sustaining the change in behavior is more effective when motivation comes from internal desire, rather than imposed by external forces. (Rollnick et al., 2005) This perspective is novel in a healthcare system that has traditionally taken a paternalistic, top-down and directive approach towards patients and their care.

To understand and meet patients at their current level of engagement, it is important to intertwine the behavioral science of readiness to change. The Transtheoretical Model of Change (TTM), developed by James Prochaska and Carlos DiClemente in the late 1970's, states that people move through five stages of change in modifying health-related behaviors: precontemplation, contemplation, preparation, action and maintenance. These stages will be developed later in this chapter. People do not move behaviorally on a longitudinal scale but rather through a cyclic continuum, as relapses or new health challenges can occur. Self-management interventions can be targeted to patients depending on which stage of change they are in.

Patient engagement, self-management, and motivational theory have seen a renaissance in the past decade, as psychology and behavioral medicine have found increasing application in medical practice. Implementation of these activities, however, has not been a panacea as evidenced by the continuing problems of chronic disease permeating society. New developments in predictive analytics and incentives have proven effective, in some cases doubling the engagement rate, and hold the promise of helping patients when, where, and how they prefer – and in the process injecting a consumer and retail approach into health and care. At the end of the chapter we cover the latest of these innovations in predictive analytics, consumer micro-segmentation, and incentives. These innovations could radically change the way we approach consumers and usher in a new approach, alternatively described as "personalized, predictive healthcare" and "personal health management."™ (Miner et al., 2014)

A Patient Centered Medical Home and Self-management Scenario

The United States (U.S.) healthcare system's traditional model of medical care is based on treating and paying for acute episodes of care. Typically, the patient gets sick or experiences a new symptom or complaint (whether a chronic or acute condition) and he/she makes an appointment to see the doctor. For example, a patient that develops a sudden onset of knee pain and stiffness that is not going away makes an appointment to see a doctor for the first time. After seeing the primary care physician, who thinks the patient has osteoarthritis, an x-ray is ordered, a prescription for stronger pain relief is provided, advice on what to do or not do is given, and the visit ends. On rare occasions, a one page educational handout on knee osteoarthritis and lifestyle adaptations may be provided, without regard to the patient's understanding or comprehension. Final advice includes calling if symptoms continue or worsen. The current, acute symptoms may have been addressed as a discrete episode, but their historical causation and context or future, long-term progression may not.

In the patient centered medical home (PCMH) model of care, the visit would be quite different. In addition to the patient receiving a prescription and an order for the x-ray, a member of the care team may ask more detailed questions about physical health and current habits, exercise/activity regimen and family support. Questions may entail assessing the pain level and a more detailed history of pain tolerance with activities and how often and what type medications or treatments have been tried with or without pain relief. These questions might allow the patient to give their perspective for the current situation, and potentially their needs and desires – all important context to understand motivation and determine how best to engage the person, for self-management or provider led medical management. But the questioning is more clinically focused, rather than motivationally attuned, and does not go far enough to elicit personal needs and motivations.

The primary care physician (PCP) remarks how the weight has gone up 20 pounds since the last visit, adding stress to joints and increasing risks for other illnesses. In reviewing other aspects of the patient's health not directly related to the acute event, bloodwork is ordered to evaluate risks for development of chronic conditions and compare results to those ordered a few years previously. Upon leaving the office, but before even getting to the car, the patient decides to get the knee x-ray, but not the lab work. This is because there are no symptoms perceived by the patient that would indicate a condition eliciting the doctor's concerns; the knee pain is the current concern.

Fortunately, the doctor follows up with the x-ray result confirming osteoarthritis. He/she asks about pain control and if the prescribed meds are working, whether leg strengthening exercises are helping, and recommends diet changes including starting a low-fat diet to lose weight. He reminds the patient to have the lab work done, which the patient grudgingly does two weeks later. A member of the care team calls and wants the person to come in to discuss abnormal results. Evidence of abnormal lipids and glucose has been discovered, and the doctor connects the patient to a member of the care team, such as a wellness coach, to discuss lifestyle changes in more detail. At that meeting, there is joint discussion between the patient and the wellness coach to create an action plan to eat a healthier low-fat diet, and some simple ideas to incorporate more exercise into the daily routine, such as parking further from the office. Routine follow up 6 months later is arranged.

Beyond the greater attention and potentially improved care provided in the second scenario, the patient fails in follow up for the next visit. What was missing from this encounter with the patient? There was a visit for acute-onset knee pain which resulted in discovering the patient had high cholesterol and is overweight. Educational materials were provided, and a wellness coach helped devise an action plan for some lifestyle changes. The patient seemed to understand the information, asking few questions, and even scored themselves as an "8" on the confidence interval. So why did he miss the next six-month check-up and not return a phone call to reschedule?

A healthcare provider's primary role has evolved to helping patients stay well, and when they are ill helping them get better. This is achieved mainly through evaluation, education, ordering tests, following up, and consulting specialists and other ancillary providers to assist the physician and patient in attaining expert opinion and guidance. Well intentioned care plans and adherence to evidence based guidelines can be done to the best of the provider's ability, but fall short on execution due to one element - the patient. If the patient is not motivated, unwilling, or unable to change, all the evidence-based care provided do just that – give care that looks great on review of paper or in the electronic health record (EHR), but are not effective due to lack of patient motivation, engagement and follow through, all of which ultimately affect the outcome.

Most chronic illnesses are lifestyle induced, rather than acute situations (the latter being an immediate sign or symptom of a worsening chronic condition). As a result, clinicians need a new approach to manage patients with chronic conditions (such as diabetes, cardiovascular disease, pain management, asthma and obesity) that addresses lifestyle and environmental issues, rather than immediate, episodic and acute matters. The Chronic Care Model (CCM), devised by Ed Wagner, MD and his colleagues (at Group Health Cooperative in Washington state), is one such approach that helps meet the demand of chronic care by transforming practices to focus on the patient as the center of all interactions. The core concepts of the CCM include health system organization, clinical information systems, self-management support, community resources and policies, delivery system design, and decision support. These elements are brought to bear by the prepared, proactive practice team to enhance their relationship with the patient and produce an informed and activated patient, which results in improved outcomes.

According to Wagner,

> ...the evidence is substantial that structured self-management and behavioral change programs improve important outcomes in diabetes, hypertension, arthritis, coronary heart disease and other chronic diseases. (Wagner, Austin, & Michael Von, 1996)

In the patient case scenario above, self-management support was offered to the patient who cooperated with it while in the doctor office. Once the patient left the practice, however, things fell apart. To help address this deficiency, this chapter offers a missing piece of the puzzle to self-management support (SMS), the equally important concept of assessing the motivation and readiness to change.

Readiness to Change Theory

For more than 20 years, much research has been done in the field of behavior change. The underlying questions researchers have asked are: "Why do people change?" and "What can we do to help?"(Butterworth, 2008)

James Prochaska and Carlos DiClemente have delved into those questions and more over the past 30 years and developed a model that offers an integrative framework for understanding and intervening with intentional behavior changes. (J. Prochaska, DiClemente, & Norcorss, 1992) The TTM, also known as the Stages of Change (SOC), is a set of theories that helps clinicians and patients understand readiness to make changes, barriers to change and help patients anticipate relapse. The SOC model has been tested, mainly in smoking cessation and other addictive behaviors, but also applied to disease management, chronic care management, contraceptive use, dietary habits, weight loss, and stress management, with equally significant results.

The SOC moves along a cyclic continuum, recognizing that change is a process moving over time. There are five stages people move through: pre-contemplation, contemplation, preparation, action, and maintenance, which are briefly described here:

Pre-contemplation – In this first phase there is no intention to change behavior in the foreseeable future. People are in denial or unaware they have a problem. "Ignorance is bliss."

Contemplation – People are aware that a problem exists and are thinking about changing, but no firm commitment is made. People can stay stuck in this stage for long periods, even years. "I have a problem and I think I should work on it."

Preparation – In this phase, people intend to take action, generally in the next month. Problem behaviors may be decreased and haven't quite reached the action stage, but the person has made a commitment to abstain from bad behaviors or adopt good behaviors.

Action – People make the commitment to modify their behavior, including use of experiences or environment to overcome their problems. This period can last from one day to 6 months.

Maintenance – People are actively working to prevent relapse. They have abstained from the problem behavior (or endorsed a new healthier behavior) for six months or longer. Stabilizing behavior change and avoiding relapse are key elements of maintenance.

(J. Prochaska et al., 1992; University of Rhode Island Cancer Prevention Research Center, 2014a)

Roughly 20% of a population at risk for serious illness or problem behaviors is ready to take action on an issue at any point in time. (Norcross, Krebs, & Prochaska, 2011) Therefore, action-oriented advice given in the pre-contemplative or contemplative stages can be a disservice and not be a motivator for change. (Norcross et al., 2011)

A second major dimension of the SOC Model that further explains how shifts in behavior occur within the stages is the "processes of change."(J. Prochaska et al., 1992) The first five processes are classified as experiential and used primarily in the early stages of transition. The latter five are considered behavioral and useful in latter stages of change.

Processes of Change - Experiential

<u>Consciousness Raising</u> – increased awareness about the causes, consequences and cures for a specific problem behavior.

<u>Dramatic Relief</u> – increased emotional experiences followed by reduced affect if appropriate action can be taken.

<u>Environmental Reevaluation</u> – combines both affective and cognitive assessments of how the presence or absence of a personal habit effects one's social environment.

<u>Social Liberation</u> – an increase in social opportunities or alternatives especially for people who are relatively deprived or oppressed

<u>Self Reevaluation</u> – combines both cognitive and affective assessments of one's self-image with, and without, a particular unhealthy habit.

Processes of Change—Behavioral

<u>Stimulus Control</u> - removes cues for unhealthy habits and adds prompts for healthier alternatives.

<u>Helping Relationship</u> – combine caring, trust, openness and acceptance as well as support for the healthy behavior change.

<u>Counter Conditioning</u> – the learning of healthier behaviors that can substitute for problem behaviors.

<u>Reinforcement Management</u> – consequences for taking steps in a particular direction. Reinforcements are emphasized, since a philosophy of the stage model is to work in harmony with how people change naturally,

<u>Self Liberation</u> - the belief that one can change and the commitment and recommitment to act on that belief.

(University of Rhode Island Cancer Prevention Research Center, 2014b)

When undergoing behavior change, most people will progress gradually over time, moving forward and backward through these stages, as relapses may occur. It is important for health care providers to know and assess in which stage or process people are currently, in order to initiate interventions targeted to that stage. Utilizing these processes with strategies will help people adopt and maintain change.

The third major dimension in the SOC Model involves decisional balance, self-efficacy and temptation. Decisional balance can best be described as balancing the advantages (pros) and disadvantages (cons) of the behavior in question. This can occur in any of the stages discussed previously, and the impact varies depending on the stage. In the pre-contemplative stage, for example, people usually judge whether the pros of their problem behavior outweigh the cons. (J.O. Prochaska et al., 1994) During the action and maintenance stages, the opposite usually occurs. (J.O. Prochaska et al., 1994) Assigning a level of importance to the advantages and disadvantages of the behavior in question opens the door to a person's motivation to change. How important and what value does one place on this behavior? When the pros of new, healthier behavior outweigh the cons, people will be better prepared to take action.

Self-efficacy is defined as the confidence or sense of mastery in managing the new behavior or current illness. (Wagner et al., 1996) A deficiency in either the level of importance or self-efficacy can lead to a person's lack of motivation to change.

Temptation is the urge to engage in a specific habit or revert to a behavior a person is trying to change while undergoing difficult situations. In self-management when setting action plans this is identified as a barrier or challenge that could keep the person from accomplishing a stated goal.

Tools for Assessing Readiness to Change

A number of tools can be used to assess patients' readiness to change assist the clinician to determine which stage the person may be in, and therefore which approach to take to facilitate self-management to modify behavior. The Readiness to Change Ruler, for example, is used in primary care to assess patient's motivational state to change a single problem behavior or make a new change (such as taking a medication). (Zimmerman, Olsen, & Bosworth, 2000) Using a straight line or drawing of a ruler on a piece of paper, an individual marks their current position in the change process. The left side indicates "not prepared to change" and the right side of the ruler indicates "already changing."(Adult Meducation & Zimmerman, n.d.) See Chapter 13 Appendix B for example. Use of motivational interviewing techniques when discussing the results is helpful to elicit internal responses for motivation to change and exploring ambivalence. (Butterworth, 2008)

Patient Activation and Engagement

The goal of the CCM, as presented earlier, is a prepared practice team working in cohort with an informed, activated patient to achieve improved outcomes. According to Julia James, the concept of an activated patient,

> ...refers to a patient's knowledge, skills, ability and willingness to manage his or her own health and care. Patient engagement is a broader concept that combines patient activation with interventions designed to increase activation and promote positive patient behavior such as obtaining preventive care or exercising regularly. (James, 2013)

Studies have shown that activated patients experience better health outcomes at lower costs. (James, 2013) In one large study of over 25,000 patients, Hibbard and colleagues found that patients with the lowest activation scores incurred costs 8-21% higher, on average, than the patient with the highest activation levels. (Greene & Hibbard, 2012)

Activation must be measureable in order to assist patients in self-management and becoming an active participant in his or her health. Judith Hibbard and Bill Mahoney, both of the University of Oregon, developed a Patient Activation Measure® (PAM), which scores the extent of an individual's perception of their ability to manage their own health. The PAM tool is comprised of 13 statements on confidence, beliefs, knowledge and skills about managing one's health. It is a uni-dimensional, Guttman-like scale that reflects a developmental model of activation. The PAM was developed in two versions targeted at people with or without chronic disease. It has been tested in numerous studies and settings, including hospitals during transitions of care. The PAM score reflects the four different levels patients move through, from passive recipient to greater activation:

Level 1 - patients are overwhelmed and unprepared to play an active role in their own health,

Level 2 - lack of knowledge and confidence to self-manage,

Level 3 - beginning to take action; still lack confidence and skill to support positive behaviors, and

Level 4 - Adoption of behavior to support their health but may relapse when under stress.

(Hibbard, Stockard, Mahoney, & Tusler, 2004)

Some of the conclusions drawn from a 25-study summary of evidence to determine whether 1) the levels of PAM reflect the degree of engagement; 2) interventions designed to empower patients lead to increased PAM levels; 3) use of PAM leads to increased understanding of care; and 4) PAM scores relate to socio-demographic and health status characteristics, are summarized here. Higher PAM scores correlate with: increased patient participation in positive self-care and self-management behaviors; better health and lower doctor visits, emergency room (ER) visits and hospital nights; healthy behaviors routinely exhibited; improved adherence to treatment; and increased levels of activation with self-management interventions. (Mukoro, May 2012)

Once a patient is assessed using the PAM, and a score assigned, it allows the practice team to better understand the patient and employ intervention techniques aimed at engaging the patient. This creates a collaborative environment to address patients' priorities, circumstances and goals. (Simmons, Baker, Schaefer, Miller, & Anders, 2009)

Self-management Support

As mentioned earlier, a patient's readiness to change and activation level are key elements when preparing to work with patients on any level and for any health issue, whether addiction, chronic conditions, or just adopting healthier habits in the absence of disease. The most successful approaches are ones that assess the patient's behavior, readiness to change, self-efficacy, personalized improvement plans, feedback, and teaching skills to manage daily symptoms, including the psychosocial issues of the condition. (Wagner et al., 1996)

Kate Lorig and her colleagues at Stanford University are leaders in the field of self-management, especially in the field of chronic care. Rather than only measure effect of patient education on outcomes, their research has led to the concept of self-efficacy – the confidence that one can manage their own illness, improved disease states, and facilitate behavior change to become a more active participant in their care. (Wagner et al., 1996) Stanford's Chronic Disease Self-Management Program is based on self-efficacy and taught mainly by peer instructors. It emphasizes problem solving, decision-making, peer interaction and support, and confidence building. (Lorig, Sobel, Ritter, & Hobbs, 2001) Incorporating tools to measure patient readiness to change and/or engagement prior to initiating self-management is the driver needed to pull patients and clinicians into more patient-centric, quality driven care.

The best, tested strategy to date to support self-management employs the 5A's model – assessment, advice, agree, assist and arrange. Clinicians can use the 5 A's format in any clinical setting, and it interfaces with all levels of both the stages of change and patient activation models of patient engagement. The 5 A's behavior change model is also part of the self-management and action plan approaches utilized in the CCM. Its components are summarized here:

Assessment - Assess the knowledge, beliefs and behavior related to the condition or behavior that needs to change. It is important to understand more about what patients' value and what they do.

Advise - Provide specific information about health risks and benefits of change

Agree - Collaboratively set goals based on patient's interest and confidence in their ability to change the behavior

Assist - Identify personal barriers, strategies, problem-solving techniques and social/environmental support

Arrange - Specify plan for follow-up (e.g., visits, phone calls, mailed reminders) including utilizing internal and community resources to provide ongoing self-management support to patients.

(Improving Chronic Illness Care, 2002)

Here are some examples using the 5A's and applying self-management to the different stages of change and the four levels (in parentheses) of patient activation:

Pre-contemplation - Validate patient lack of readiness; encourage self-exploration, for example, asking what they like about smoking and have they ever thought about not smoking. (Level 1)

Contemplation - Encourage patient to evaluate the pros and cons of behavior change, such as, "When you used to exercise, what was your favorite activity to do? Write down on a piece of paper the advantages of doing (named activity) again and the disadvantages of doing (named activity). What day next week can I call you to discuss this?" (Level 2)

Preparation - Identify and assist in problem solving barriers and obstacles. Encourage small initial steps. "You mentioned that you like to walk in the morning but don't like to go alone. Is there a neighbor or friend you could ask?" (Level 3)

<u>Action</u> - Bolster self-efficacy for dealing with obstacles. Reiterate long-term goals. "You've been walking for 2 months now. How do you feel compared to 6 months ago?" or "There is a community 5K walk for diabetes next month. How would you like to be on our team?" (Level 3 or 4)

<u>Maintenance</u> - Continuous follow up support; discuss coping with relapse; reinforce internal rewards. Self-efficacy and the willingness or desire to change is personal. (Level 4)

(University of Rhode Island Cancer Prevention Research Center, 2014a)

Experience and Evolution

Patient engagement, self-management, the Stages of Change model, and motivational theory have been incorporated in many care and disease management programs over the past decade. They have met with some success, especially if they are used in combination and in concert with population health management tools such as clinical stratification and patient identification. These tools allow an organization to better understand their entire population of consumers, identify those who are patients, learn which patients can be impacted, and direct resources to individuals with the greatest need.

Most stratification and identification efforts, however, have focused on the cost of care and especially the cost of episodic care (using episode treatment groupers and similar devices to try and get a broader picture of treatment), rather than clinical insight. As a result, the ability to identify individuals with impactable clinical conditions is limited. One study, by the Society of Actuaries in 2007, showed that less than one-third of a population could be reliably identified by most of the commercially available risk stratification tools, with the best tool only able to predict risk of future health problems for 27.6 percent of the population as shown in Figure 13-1. (Winkelman & Mehmud, 2007)

Figure 13-1. Predictive Modeling Health Risk: Low Predictability[*]

TABLE I.1	R-Squared and MAPE for Prospective Nonlagged - Offered vs. Optimized (Recalibrated, with Prior Cost, 250k Claim Truncation)		Offered Models		Optimized Models w/ Prior Costs	
Risk Adjuster Tool	Developer	Inputs	R-2	MAPE %	R-2	MAPE %
ACG	Johns Hopkins	Diag	19.2%	89.9%	23.0%	86.2%
CDPS	Kronick / UCSD	Diag	14.9%	95.3%	24.6%	85.6%
Clinical Risk Groups	3M	Diag	17.5%	90.9%	20.5%	86.6%
DxCG DCG	DxCG	Diag	20.6%	87.5%	26.5%	82.5%
DxCG RxGroups	DxCG	Rx	20.4%	85.3%	27.1%	80.7%
Ingenix PRG	Ingenix	Rx	20.5%	85.8%	27.4%	80.9%
MedicaidRx	Gilmer / UCSD	Rx	15.8%	89.6%	26.3%	81.9%
Impact Pro	Ingenix	Med+Rx+Use	24.4%	81.8%	27.2%	80.6%
Ingenix ERG	Ingenix	Med+Rx	19.7%	86.4%	26.5%	81.2%
ACG w/ Prior Cost	Johns Hopkins	Diag+$Rx	22.4%	85.6%	25.4%	82.1%
DxCG UW Model	DxCG	Diag+$Total	27.4%	80.4%	29.1%	78.3%
Service Vendor		Inputs	R-2	MAPE	R-2	MAPE
MEDai	MEDai	All	N/A	N/A	32.1%	75.2%

[*] The offered MEDai model was not tested in the study.

One of the results of the inability to predict future health status is that patient engagement rates are low because you don't know who to contact. In addition, another study showed that even if you can identify persons at risk for future health events who are eligible for additional, focused services, many times it is difficult or impossible to contact them. (Lynch, Chen, Bender, & Edington, 2006) The study showed that of the population eligible for additional disease management services, only half could be contacted through standard procedures, such as nurse disease manager telephone calling. After they are contacted, according to the study, only 40 percent of those decide to participate in additional services designed to improve their health or condition, and only half of those who participate actually show changes in behavior leading to improvement in their condition or outcomes. Clearly patient engagement is not working in these

[*] Winkelman, R., & Mehmud, S. (2007). A comparative analysis of claims-based tools for health risk assessment. Society of Actuaries, 1-70.

situations, and that has been the industry norm for some time as illustrated in Figure 13-2. (Lynch et al., 2006)

Figure 13-2. Patient Engagement Low Rates[*]

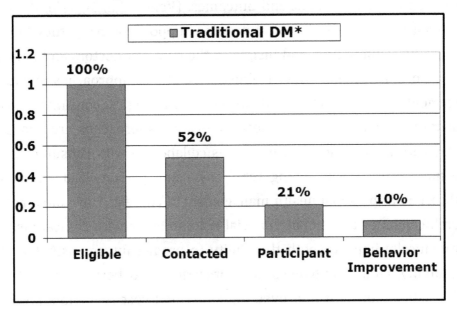

Since this study came out, a number of organizations have been working hard to increase the ability to outreach and engage patients and improve outcomes. This has become even more important in the era of accountable care, when additional payment depends on improved outcomes. Fortunately, new technology and data has become available, allowing clinical insights and predictive analysis to better understand patients, and improve engagement and medical management.

One organization, ActiveHealth Management, pioneered the use of data to measure gaps in care, stratify consumers according to their clinical and financial risk for further health issues, identify persons who are

---

[*] Lynch, W. D., Chen, C.-Y., Bender, J., & Edington, D. W. (2006). Documenting participation in an employer-sponsored disease management program: selection, exclusion, attrition, and active engagement as possible metrics. Journal of occupational and environmental medicine, 48(5), 447-454.

"impactible" (greater likelihood of an impact from health inferventions), identify opportunities to improve health and care, generate prescriptive analytics output, utilize the latest motivational interviewing techniques, and improve patient engagement and outcomes. (Vemireddi, M, Yale, K, et al., 2014) As a research-based clinical decision support company, they believe putting clinical knowledge and insight in the hands of doctors and patients can transform lives. Their story is illustrative of new approaches to patient engagement using predictive and prescriptive analytics, consumer micro-segmentation, and incentives. These innovative approaches are changing the way care management organizations collaborate with consumers, and show how healthcare is "going retail" by using personalized, predictive healthcare in a "personal health management"™ context. Their most recent research combines traditional financial risk modeling with clinical insights to dramatically improve both the ability to predict future costs, but also impactability, clinical outcomes, and prescribe who best to contact and specific actions for both improved outcomes and cost reduction. (Wei, H., 2014)

Predictive Analytics for Personal Health

The low engagement rate for disease management, mentioned previously, was an industry average that caused many to wonder if medical management services worked at all. Although engagement rates were better at ActiveHealth, they were still looking for ways to improve outreach and engagement.

Most of the traditional ways to improve engagement had already been implemented, including clinical stratification and identification, predictive auto-dialing using interactive voice-response systems, advanced telephone number search services, physician office coordination and others (see Figure 13-3). In addition, ActiveHealth® was already using every data source available in healthcare to both identify and engage patients, and ensure proper care plan and provider coordination. Data sources already used included medical and pharmacy claims, lab values, health risk assessment, patient reported information in personal health records, nurse care manager reported information, evidence-based guidelines, daily evidence-based medical literature updates, government agency health recommendations (e.g., FDA, CDC, CMS, etc.), university medical center review of protocols, electronic health records, electronic medical records, and other sources.

These data were aggregated and used by ActiveHealth for a variety of clinical decision support activities, including medical management, utilization management, provider care management, and patient self-management. But that was not enough, with new technologies, more could be done.

Figure 13-3. Care Management Process

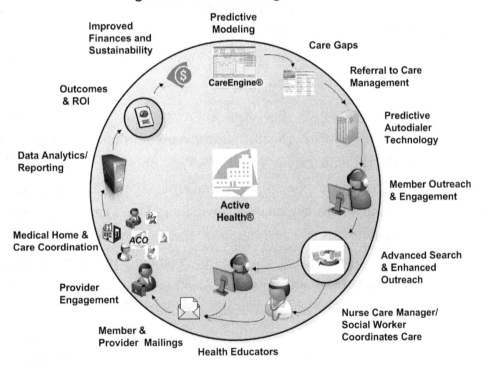

To find new ways to improve consumer outreach and engagement, ActiveHealth turned to Big Data and predictive analytics. Predictive analytics has been used by commercial marketing firms for years to better define the needs and interests of consumers. (Nisbet, Elder IV, & Miner, 2009) ActiveHealth had also used predictive analytics to stratify and identify patients through financial and clinical data. But new data sources, such as consumer purchasing patterns and lifestyle information (exogenous to healthcare) could be used to define much better the personal needs and interests of patients outside the healthcare context, separate populations of patients into homogenous "micro-segments," and identify opportunities to better engage patients by better understanding their personal preferences. (Miner et al., 2014)

As a research-based, advanced clinical decision support and care management organization, however, ActiveHealth wanted to be sure predictive analytics would work before adding the service to their existing operations. Using advanced predictive analytics techniques, they micro-segmented a specific population using generally available consumer data, then set up a controlled trial to measure how micro-segmentation might improve outreach and engagement.

Using a rigorous study protocol, ActiveHealth combined existing financial (claims), clinical (health improvement opportunities), and personal (health risk assessment, etc.) data. They obtained exogenous data (household information, personal behaviors, lifestyles, and other demographics) and micro-segmented the population. The specific group used for the analytic work was randomly drawn from an existing client patient population with permission. The new segments identified from the data showed remarkable homogeneity, indicating the new segments were not only valid, but consistent. ActiveHealth then set up a randomized "A/B" test to see if the additional information made any difference. The results were stunning: the "lift" obtained over previously used techniques was almost double, resulting in more persons engaged using the new segmentation techniques. (Yale 2014) This showed the effectiveness of identifying specific interests of individuals, and improving engagement by appealing to those specific interests - getting to that elusive "market-of-one," as commercial marketing and predictive analytics professionals have described. (Siegel, 2013) Using these and other findings, ActiveHealth is improving their operations across all patients and health plan members, and continue to advance the science of patient engagement with further studies in incentives (Yale 2014), motivation, outreach, engagement, and outcomes. (Vemireddy et. al., 2014)

Summary and Future Direction

Self-management support is an essential element in managing a chronic condition. As CINs continue to evolve their medical management, care coordination, provider-patient communications, and patient engagement strategies, tailoring interventions based on an individual's activation level or stage of change is an approach that warrants application in clinical practice. Numerous tools and published studies have validated their usefulness and validity. As Big Data and predictive analytics are increasingly used in healthcare, new tools and methods are beginning to accelerate and improve the ability to outreach and engage consumers in their own care.

The whole premise of self-management support is to empower patients and prepare them to manage their health and health care. Effective self-management support strategies include assessment, goal-setting, action planning, problem-solving, and follow-up. Evidence now strongly suggests that to achieve optimal outcomes in most chronic illness, we must improve the patients' ability and interest in managing their own condition.

Herein is the challenge – meeting the patient where they are at any given moment in time with the appropriate questions and available resources to engage them - necessary for effective patient communications, clinical decision-making, self-management, and improved outcomes. The patient is the expert on their life. Our role as health care providers is to act as advocates, educators and coaches to guide individuals along the path with tools and techniques that will hopefully lead to empowerment and positive changes. This must be done with the individual's perspective, levels of engagement and motivation firmly in mind. This approach takes time, skill-building and patience for both clinicians and patients. The end result of an engaged, informed patient and practice team will help attain the Triple Aim - improved population health, lower costs, and improved patient's experience of care, create a new model to meet the new demands for care delivery, and allow CINs and ACOs to meet their overarching goals of improving quality and affordability across the United States.

Predictive and prescriptive analytics may present the best opportunity to meet this challenge, with new ways that allow payers and providers to engage patients at the right time and place, with the right intervention. As a group of data scientists recently demonstrated, it is only a matter of time and data before we are able to truly personalize healthcare to the individual, allowing "personalized, predictive and prescriptive healthcare." (Miner et al., 2014) The chart in Figure 13-4 shows this evolution, from reactive medicine to proactive health and care. (Davenport & Harris, 2007)

Figure 13-4. Predictive Analytics Enables Proactive Care[*]

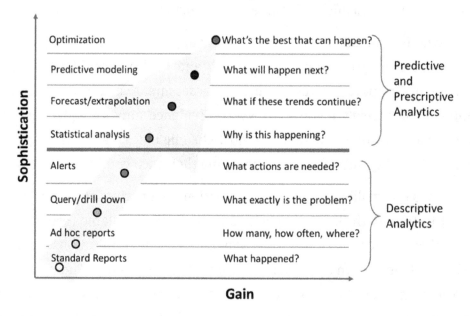

[*] Davenport, T. H., & Harris, J. G. (2007). *Competing on Analytics: The New Science of Winning.* Watertown, MA: Harvard Business Press.

CHAPTER 13. APPENDIX A: CASE STUDIES

The following three case studies feature utilization of Readiness to Change Measurement Tools.

Case Study #1*

Three teenage individuals were referred to the R-Team™ for weight management. The R-Team ("Reshaping Thru Exercise, Attitudes and Meals) is a fun and educational group available to children and teens along with their parents/guardians. Group sessions last 90 minutes and are held every other week for three months, totaling 10 sessions, with the final session occurring six months from the first group session. Prior to starting the group sessions, individual assessments are completed to identify the participant's readiness to change, life satisfaction, and knowledge.

The **"Readiness to Change Assessment"** identifies participant readiness to start making various lifestyle changes prior to beginning the program and at program completion. Readiness to change was assessed in parent and child based on a scale of 1-10 (1 = not ready/pre-contemplative, 5 = somewhat ready/contemplative, 10 = already doing it/action). Each variable was assessed on an individual basis and compiled as an average readiness score. The average score reflects readiness pertaining to nutrition, exercise, and general healthy lifestyle changes.

The **"Life Satisfaction Survey"** identifies satisfaction pertaining to relationships, lifestyle habits, and self-esteem prior to beginning the program and at program completion. Life satisfaction was assessed in parent and child based on a scale of 1-5 (1= never, 5 = almost always). Each variable was combined for a total satisfaction score.

---

* Case Study #1 submitted by Erin Olsen, BS, Pediatric Program Coordinator, Certified Wellness Practitioner.

The **"Healthy Habits Knowledge Assessment"** identifies knowledge pertaining to exercise, nutrition, and emotional wellness prior to beginning the program and at program completion. The knowledge check was distributed to parent and child separately and scored on a percentage scale.

Participant A: 15 year old male

Participant A began the program in the contemplative/preparation stage of change; assessed by a multidisciplinary team and the readiness to change assessment tool. Participant A scored an initial average of 6.67 out of 10 on the readiness to change assessment. Scores were the lowest for: decreasing screen time, and feeling he had family support to make lifestyle changes. His diet included minimal fruit and vegetable intake; 1-2 servings a day on average. Sneak eating presented as a consistent problem throughout the week; often binge eating after his mom went to bed. Throughout the program, the multidisciplinary team worked with participant A in a group educational setting reinforcing self-management through weekly action plans and journaling. Weekly action plans were presented as "Take Home Challenges" and were used to help reinforce the topics discussed in group for each session and increase accountability.

Participant A worked with the clinicians to set SMART goals in addition to the take-home challenges. Motivational interviewing was used to identify motivators for change and aid the participant in discovering what goals were priorities for that week. Participant A had two weeks in between sessions to work on the take home challenge as well as his specific SMART goal. Successes and barriers were shared in a group setting; with advanced issues being discussed on an individual level. Through discussion, it was discovered that participant A was not eating enough in the evening; which led to binge eating late at night. By working with a Dietitian, a meal plan was created. By adding an additional healthy snack between dinner and bedtime, the late night binge eating was no longer an issue.

Four months into the program, the participant worked his way from contemplation/preparation to actively making healthy lifestyle changes discussed. By providing the participant with multiple tools, identifying motivators, and brainstorming solutions to barriers, the participant presented with a new sense of confidence and motivation to change. Participant A had increased his fruit and vegetable intake, increased his activity and decreased weight by 14.2 pounds. His readiness to change score increased from a 6.67 to 9.67 out of 10. Scores for decreasing screen time and feeling he had family support had doubled; likely due to the family involvement component of the program. Additional assessments showed life satisfaction increased by 7% and his knowledge increased by 10%.

Participant B: 15 year old female

Participant B was referred by her primary care physician for childhood obesity. She began the program in-between the pre-contemplative and contemplative stage of change; assessed by a multidisciplinary team as well as the readiness to change assessment tool. Participant B scored a five out of ten on the readiness to change assessment. The participant was difficult to engage during the initial consultation; playing on her phone and stating her mom was making her come to the program. Participant reported consuming fast food and other convenience store snacks five days a week, less than one serving of fruits and vegetables daily, spending approximately seven or more hours on the computer, and not participating in any physical activity other than walking to class. Although the participant was hesitant to attend the program, she was able to identify losing weight as a motivator to making changes.

Throughout the program, the multidisciplinary team worked with participant B in a group educational setting reinforcing self-management through weekly action plans and journaling. Weekly action plans were presented as "Take Home Challenges" and were used to help reinforce the topics discussed in group for each session. "Take Home Challenges" helped to increase accountability to the discussed healthy lifestyle changes; giving the participant two weeks in-between sessions to work on the specific challenge. She was encouraged to utilize the healthy lifestyle journal to document progress and identify challenges in-between sessions.

Clinicians utilized motivational interviewing skills to help the participant identify first steps in making changes. Small changes were encouraged by setting SMART goals in addition to the take home challenges to decrease feeling overwhelmed. During the first month of working with the clinicians, participant B remained in the pre-contemplative stage of change displaying resistance to change and not completing goals set. Successes and barriers were shared in a group setting; participants along with clinicians brainstormed solutions to the barriers discussed. Instruction on how to set rewards to increase motivation was given to engage participant B in making changes. As a family decision, purchasing songs on "iTunes" was the reward put in place if goals were met.

During the second month of the program, participant B continued to have minimal variety in her diet however; she started to incorporate more fruits and whole grains which resulted in a four pound weight decrease. Participant B presented with a stronger motivation to change after weight decrease was seen and as a result was adhering to nutrition goals set on a regular basis. During the third month, the participant maintained weight decrease of 4.8 pounds likely due to trying new fruits, decreasing milk to ½ percent, and choosing healthier breakfast options.

Motivational interviewing was used to brainstorm physical activities that may be of interest to her to begin adding exercise into her daily regimen. Four months into the program, participant B reported an increased readiness to change by .83 points. Although her subjective readiness to change remained low, the participant reported an increased frequency and duration of physical activity; exercising most days of the week for at least 45 minutes and was continuing to try new fruits. At the end of four months, she maintained a 9.1 pound weight decrease, a 21.42 percent increase in life satisfaction, and a 20 percent increase in her healthy lifestyle knowledge. She still continued to struggle with adding vegetables into her diet. The healthy plate was reviewed and multiple recipes were provided on different ways to add vegetables into meals.

Participant C: 15 year old female

Participant C was referred by her primary care physician for childhood obesity and asthma. She attended the program with her mother and her two sisters who were also referred for childhood obesity. She began the program in-between the preparation and action stage of change; assessed by the readiness to change tool and a multidisciplinary team made up of a Registered Dietitian, Exercise Specialist, Wellness Coach, and Registered Nurse. Her initial average readiness score was 8.5 out of 10 on the readiness to change assessment.

Participant C was starting to make changes to her dietary habits and incorporating exercise into her regimen; however she was hesitant on increasing her exercise frequency and was resistant to eating three balanced meals a day; often skipping breakfast and lacking vegetable intake. She presented with low self- esteem and self-reported feelings of depression, which she identified as barriers to her success. On her initial life satisfaction score, participant C answered "never" in response to feeling satisfied with her "inside" and "outside" self. To aid in overcoming this barrier, clinicians addressed self-esteem and body image throughout the program through interactive and educational games.

Motivational interviewing was used and SMART goals were set with this participant; focusing on attitude and increasing self-efficacy. Participant C identified her personal appearance and wanting to lose weight as motivators for change. Her overall goal was to learn how to lose weight in a healthy way and maintain the weight loss. The multidisciplinary team worked toward this goal by providing nutritional counseling on serving sizes, portion control, and building a balanced meal as well as educating on all areas of fitness; providing specific exercise regimens. Self-management was reinforced through action plans and weekly journaling of food intake and exercise.

Clinicians collected the journal each session and made positive comments on where improvement was seen and encouraging comments on what areas needed more attention. Weekly action plans were presented as "Take Home Challenges" and were used to help reinforce the topics discussed in group for each session and increase accountability. Participant C made progress with eating breakfast throughout the program, however, had relapses pertaining to this goal. Clinicians continually brainstormed solutions; however, participant did not appear ready to incorporate this specific change at this time. Education and tools were provided for future goal setting on this topic.

As a result of providing the participant with multiple tools, identifying motivators, brainstorming solutions to barriers, and emphasizing the importance of family involvement; the participant presented an increased readiness to change and life satisfaction. Her readiness to change score increased from an 8.5 to a 9.83 out of 10 and her life satisfaction increased by 5%. Post scores reflecting how satisfied she felt with her "inside" self drastically increased from "never" to "almost always". She achieved her overall goal of wanting to lose weight and maintain the weight loss; steadily averaging a reduction of three pounds every two weeks and maintaining the weight loss for a total of 16.8 pounds throughout a six month span. Success could also be attributed to an increased family involvement; with mom decreasing weight by 35 pounds in six months with her own readiness to change score increasing from a 6.33 to 9.17 out of 10.

*Case Studies #2 and #3**

The following cases are examples of two adults engaged in self-management for transitions of care at a large family practice based in southeast Michigan.

Patient #1

---

*Case Studies #2 and #3 submitted by Angela Siegmon, R.N., BSN, Hybrid Care Manager.

Mr. B (not his real name) is a 61 year old male with a diagnosis of atrial fibrillation, pulmonary hypertension, diabetes, and colitis. He was recently hospitalized for exacerbation of his medical conditions. Mr. B has been in case management and the RN care manager (CM) has met with the patient in person, and Mr. B agreed to care management services. Mr. B rarely answers the phone and when reached by phone in the evening, both Mr. B and his spouse will be on the call. All patients in the clinic receive follow-up phone calls from the nurse care manger after an inpatient stay. The goal of the call is to ensure a smooth transition from hospital to home.

The call was made two days post-discharge from the hospital.

The phone conversation took place with Mr. B's spouse. The RN care manager did try Mr. B's phone initially but after no answer and unable to leave a message contacted the wife on her phone. She said Mr. B was on track with all medications and voiced no concerns. The patient himself was not on the call. During the phone call, the RN CM completed medication reconciliation, reviewed current signs and symptoms, educated on worsening symptoms and promoting early action, along with answering any questions or concerns. Mr. B's long term goal: "I like to be with my grandkids. I enjoy my time with them."

The goals for this week/month are: Appointments with the following physicians:

- PCP and nurse care manager visit one week post-discharge;
- Specialist visits two weeks post-discharge, including:
    - o Pulmonary Hypertension Clinic,
    - o Hepatologist appointment;, and
    - o Ongoing maintenance of fluid restrictions.

Goal attainment dates for physician follow up appointments were established, and daily monitoring of fluid intake and symptoms for fluid retention.

There are no current barriers observed at this time that would make it hard to reach these goals. Family is supportive, the spouse and patient have a good understanding of disease processes, early signs and symptoms to report, and when to call 911 -- as evidenced by education & teach back. Some of the challenges that need a plan to overcome are: maintaining fluid restriction of 1.5 liters daily by measuring fluid, following up with nurse CM, PCP and specialists. Nurse CM contact information provided to both spouses. Good understanding of monitoring cardiac and respiratory symptoms. Good communication between specialists and PCP, as evidenced by a call to specialists from the care manager, and updates/reports faxed to PCP.

On a scale of 1-10, 1 being not ready and 10 extremely ready, to reach goals: spouse rated Mr. B a 10.

When asked how confident the wife was that goals can be done, on a scale of 1-10, with 1 being not confident to 10 extremely confident: spouse rated Mr. B a 10.

When asked how well do you understand the information discussed today, on a scale of 1 not well to 10 extremely well: spouse rated Mr. B a 10.

During a scheduled care manager visit, the RN CM met face to face with Mr. B as planned. The PCP was pleased with his progress. There was one medication adjustment, no other changes. The action plan was updated to include a coaching call with the dietitian. An RN follow-up coaching call for care management was schedule. The progress evidenced in this care management visit, which took place one week after hospital discharge, illustrates the immediate progress that can be made when patient engagement and self-management activities are properly initiated.

Patient #2:

Mrs. D (not her real name) is an 85 year-old female diagnosed with dementia and referred to care management by the PCP to assess long term care. Mrs. D's current living arrangements alternate at a grandson's house and her daughter's house. Goal setting was done with the daughter, who is the primary caregiver and is in the process of applying for guardianship. A phone call was placed by the nurse care manager to the daughter to discuss care management, current living assessment, advance care planning and community resources. Community resources provided include Life Alert® (info and phone number provided) and also Area Agency on Aging services. Advance Directives (AD) were discussed with the daughter. Mrs. D does not have an AD in place, so forms were mailed to the family along with an information packet called "Planning for your Piece of Mind, a Guide to Medical and Legal Decisions". There was no resistance to any information about the Advance Directives, or any other information provided.

The long term goals discussed were safety and memory care, and completing an Advance Directive. Short term goals for the next week: daughter to call Area Agency on Aging and Services for the Aging. Information provided to obtain safety services from LifeLine Alert. The daughter states she will make calls to agencies and for the Lifeline Alert and will reach this goal within the week. When asked, "What might make it hard to reach this goal?" the daughter responded that the patient does not wish to relinquish certain activities. The plan to overcome challenges is for the daughter to investigate obtaining guardianship. Mrs. D is invited to participate and plan for events. When asked by the nurse care manager how ready the daughter was to do this, and rate it on a scale of 1 (not ready) to 10 (extremely ready), the daughter rated it a 10.

When asked how confident the daughter was that goals can be done, on a scale of 1-10, with 1 being not confident to 10 extremely confident, the daughter rated it an 8 (very confident). When asked how well she understands the information discussed today, on a scale of 1 not well to 10 extremely well, the daughter rated it a 10. All this was verified with teach back.

The daughter stated she was taking notes during the conversation with the nurse care manager. The care manager will do a follow up coaching call in one week to discuss the care plan, community resources, AD, and any other updates. Nurse care manager contact information was given to the daughter, and the case was later discussed with Mrs. D's PCP.

This case study illustrates many of the patient engagement and self-management steps used in an actual case, and in a typical elderly patient situation. Notice the family care giver (daughter) is the person directly engaged by the nurse care manager, presumably because of some cognitive issue with the mother (Mrs. D). This is a summary of an actual exchange between a nurse care manager and a patient's guardian, and alludes to the empathy that is shown by the nurse throughout the interaction, which takes considerable time over a phone conversation. This is critical for good communication, understanding the perspective of the patient and her guardian, and arriving at a realistic and achievable care plan and follow-up steps.

CHAPTER 13. APPENDIX B: READINESS SUPPLEMENT[*]

READINESS RULER

Below, mark where you are now on this line that measures your change in _____.

Are you not prepared to change, already changing or somewhere in the middle?

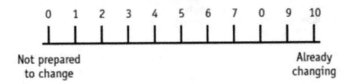

| 0 | 1 | 2 | 3 | 4 | 5 | 6 | 7 | 0 | 9 | 10 |

Not prepared   Already
to change   changing

---

[*] Appendix B material from Adult Meducation, & Zimmerman, G. L. (n.d.). Readiness-to-Change Ruler Retrieved from http://www.adultmeducation.com/AssessmentTools_3.html

READINESS-TO-CHANGE RULER

The Readiness-to-Change Ruler is used to assess a person's willingness or readiness to change, determine where they are on the continuum between "not prepared to change" and "already changing", and promote identification and discussion of perceived barriers to change. The ruler represents a continuum from "not prepared to change" on the left, to "already changing" on the right.

The Readiness-to-Change Ruler can be used as a quick assessment of a person's present motivational state relative to changing a specific behavior, and can serve as the basis for motivation-based interventions to elicit behavior change. Readiness to change should be assessed regarding a very specific activity such as taking medications, following a diet, or exercising, since persons may differ in their stages of readiness to change for different behaviors.

ADMINISTRATION

1. Indicate the specific behavior to be assessed on the Readiness-to-Change Ruler form. Ask the person to mark on a linear scale from 0 to 10 their current position in the change process. A 0 on the left side of the scale indicates "not prepared for change" and a 10 on the right side of the scale indicates "already changing".

2. Question the person about why he or she did not place the mark further to the left, which elicits motivational statements.

3. Question the person about why he or she did not place mark further to the right, which elicits perceived barriers.

4. Ask the person for suggestions about ways to overcome identified barriers and actions that might be taken.

SCORING

A score above 5 shows that the person is willing to consider change and should be supported and encouraged.

Source: adultmeducation.com

CHAPTER 13 DISCUSSION QUESTIONS

Discussion questions are provided for team building or class exercises. Answers for all questions are provided in Appendix C.

Question Number	Question
1	Identify one essential element to reduce the threats of chronic conditions.
2	What are the two elements that have not been easily integrated into patient self-management?
3	What is a method used to gauge a patient's knowledge, skills and confidence needed to self-manage their health?
4	What are the core concepts of Wagner's Chronic Care Model?
5	What is the Transtheoretical Model (TTM)?
6	What are the four different levels patients move through?

CHAPTER 13 HIGHLIGHTS

✓ Introduced the Transtheoretical Model (TTM) also known as the Stages of Change (SOC), as a concept that can help clinicians and patients understand readiness to make changes, barriers to change and help patients anticipate relapse.

✓ Discussed the Chronic Care Model (CCM) and how it can meet the demand of chronic illness care by transforming practices to focus on the patient as the center of all interactions.

✓ Reviewed the importance of a prepared practice team working in cohort with an informed activated patient.

✓ Recognized that self-management is necessary to reduce the threats chronic conditions pose to patients, health care systems and economies.

✓ Explained the Readiness to Change Ruler and how it has been used in primary care to assess patient's motivational state to change a single problem behavior or make a new change (such as taking a medication).

✓ Restated why activation must be measureable in order to assist patients in becoming an active participant in his or her health.

✓ Presented three case examples featuring utilization of Readiness to Change Measurement Tools.

✓ Introduced predictive analytics as an innovative way to use exogenous data, combined with traditional healthcare data, to improve patient identification, outreach, and engagement.

✓ Demonstrated how Big Data and predictive analytics holds the promise of enabling patient engagement and "personal health management"™

CHAPTER 13 REFERENCES

Adult Meducation, & Zimmerman, G. L. (n.d.). Readiness-to-Change Ruler. Retrieved from http://www.adultmeducation.com/AssessmentTools_3.html

Butterworth, S. W. (2008). Influencing patient adherence to treatment guidelines. *Journal of Managed Care Pharmacy*, 14(6 Suppl B), 21-24.

Davenport, T. H., & Harris, J. G. (2007). *Competing on analytics: the new science of winning*. Watertown, MA: Harvard Business Press.

Frazee, S. G., Kirkpatrick, P., Fabius, R., & Chimera, J. (2007). Leveraging the trusted clinician: documenting disease management program enrollment. *Disease Management*, 10(1), 16-29.

Greene, J., & Hibbard, J. H. (2012). Why does patient activation matter? An examination of the relationships between patient activation and health-related outcomes. *Journal of General Internal Medicine*, 27(5), 520-526. doi: 10.1007/s11606-011-1931-2

Hibbard, J., H., Stockard, J., Mahoney, E., R., & Tusler, M. (2004). Development of the patient activation measure (PAM): conceptualizing and measuring activation in patients and consumers. *Health Services Research*, 39(4p1), 1005-1026.

Improving Chronic Illness Care. (2002). *The 5 A's behavior change model adapted for self-management support improvement.* Retrieved from http://www.improvingchroniccare.org/downloads/3.5_5_as_behaviior_change_model.pdf

Insignia Health. (2014). Insignia Health. PAM Development & Validation. Retrieved from www.insigniahealth.com.

James, J. (2013). Health policy brief: patient engagement. *Health Affairs*, 1-6.

Javitt, J. C., Steinberg, G., Locke, T., Couch, J. B., Jacques, J., Juster, I., & Reisman, L. (2005). Using a claims data-based sentinel system to improve compliance with clinical guidelines: results of a randomized prospective study. *American Journal of Managed Care*, 11(2), 93-102.

Lorig, K. R., Sobel, D. S., Ritter, P. L., & Hobbs, M. (2001). Effect of a self-management program on patients with chronic disease. *Effective Clinical Practice*, 4(6), 256-262.

Lynch, W. D., Chen, C.-Y., Bender, J., & Edington, D. W. (2006). Documenting participation in an employer-sponsored disease management program: selection, exclusion, attrition, and active engagement as possible metrics. *Journal of Occupational and Environmental Medicine*, 48(5), 447-454.

Miner, L., Bolding, P., Hilbe, J., Goldstein, M., Hill, T., Nisbet, R.,Miner, G. (2014). *Practical Predictive Analytics and Decisioning Systems for Medicine: Informatics Accuracy and Cost-Effectiveness for Healthcare Administration and Delivery Including Medical Research*, Waltham, MA: Academic Press.

Mukoro, F. (May 2012). *Summary of the evidence on performance of the patient activation measure.* Retrieved from http://selfmanagementsupport.health.org.uk/media_manager/public/179/SMS_resource-centre_publications/PatientActivation-1.pdf

Nisbet, R., Elder IV, J., & Miner, G. (2009). *Handbook of statistical analysis and data mining applications*. Waltham, MA: Academic Press.

Norcross, J. C., Krebs, P. M., & Prochaska, J. O. (2011). Stages of change. *Journal of Clinical Psychology*, 67(2), 143-154. doi: 10.1002/jclp.20758

Prochaska, J., DiClemente, C., & Norcorss, J. (1992). In search of how people change: applications to addictive behaviours. *American Psychologist*, 47(9), 1102-1114.

Prochaska, J. O., Velicer, W. F., Rossi, J. S., Goldstein, M. G., Marcus, B. H., Rakowski, W., Rosenbloom, D. (1994). Stages of change and decisional balance for 12 problem behaviors. *Health Psychology*, 13(1), 39.

Riley, L., & Cowan, M. (July 2014). Non-communicable diseases by country profiles, 2014. World Health Organization. Retrieved from http://apps.who.int/iris/bitstream/10665/128038/1/9789241507509_eng.pdf

Rollnick, S., Butler, C. C., McCambridge, J., Kinnersley, P., Elwyn, G., & Resnicow, K. (2005). Consultations about changing behaviour. *BMJ*, 331(7522), 961-963.

Siegel, E. (2013). *Predictive analytics: the power to predict who will click, buy, lie, or die*. Hoboken, NJ: John Wiley & Sons.

Simmons, L., Baker, N. J., Schaefer, J., Miller, D., & Anders, S. (2009). Activation of patients for successful self-management. *The Journal of Ambulatory Care Management*, 32(1), 16-23.

University of Rhode Island Cancer Prevention Research Center. (2014a). Detailed overview of the transtheoretical model. Retrieved from www.uri.edu/research/cprc

University of Rhode Island Cancer Prevention Research Center. (2014b). *Transtheoretical model processes of change*. Retrieved from http://www.uri.edu/research/cprc/TTM/ProcessesOfChange.htm

Vemireddy, M., et. al. (2014). *Promoting healthy behaviors: A five-year study on the impact of incentives*. ActiveHealth Management White Paper. Retrieved from http://go.activehealth.com/IncentivesWhitePaper_WhitePaperRequest.html

Vemireddy, M., Yale, K., et. al. (2014). *CareEngine: Advancing the Cause of Evidence-Based Care*. New York, NY.

Wagner, E. H., Austin, B. T., & Michael Von, K. (1996). Organizing care for patients with chronic illness. *The Milbank Quarterly*, 74(4), 511-544. doi: 10.2307/3350391.

Wei, H. (2014, November, 15). *Prediction vs. Intervention*. Presentation to National Predictive Modeling Summit 2014, Washington, DC.

Winkelman, R., & Mehmud, S. (2007). *A comparative analysis of claims-based tools for health risk assessment*. Society of Actuaries, 1-70.

World Health Organization. (2002). *Innovative care for chronic conditions: building blocks for actions: global report*. p. 5.

Yale, K., (2014, September 7). *Promoting Healthy Behaviors: Exploring Five Years of Data on Incentives*. Presentation to Stanford University MedicineX Conference, Palo Alto, CA, Retrieved from http://medicinex.stanford.edu/conf/a/medx2014/conference/event/384

Yale, K. (2014, October). *Significant Improvements in Population Health Management*. Presentation to Predictive Analytics World Healthcare, Boston, MA.

Yuan, C. T., Nembhard, I. M., Stern, A. F., Brush, J. E., Krumholz, H. M., Bradley, E. H., & Fund, C. (2010). *Blueprint for the dissemination of evidence-based practices in health care.* New York, NY: Commonwealth Fund.

Zimmerman, G. L., Olsen, C. G., & Bosworth, M. F. (2000). A'stages of change'approach to helping patients change behavior. *American Family Physician*, 61(5), 1409-1416.

Chapter 14. Clinical Integration: A Bridge to Improved Population Health and Care

Ken Yale | Thomas A. Raskauskas

Joanne Bohn | Colin Konschak

Once we see this fundamentally open quality of the universe, it immediately opens us up to the potential for change; we see that the future is not fixed, and we shift from resignation to a sense of possibility. (Jaworski, 1996)

Joseph Jaworski, JD
Chairman, Generon International
Founder, American Leadership Forum

CHAPTER 14 LEARNING OBJECTIVES

✓ Describe the strategic lens applied for provider environment monitoring.

✓ How many commercial and public ACOs are in the United States as of Deccember 5, 2014?

✓ What are some of the tennets for a "Community-accountable health development system" as identified by Halfon and colleagues?

✓ Identify some of the health insurance mandate related Sections from the ACA and describe their implications for CINs and ACOs.

✓ Describe the dimensions of integrated delivery in healthcare today.

✓ Understand the concluding recommendations for future CIN and ACO leaders.

American Healthcare is embroiled in a period of transformational and institutional change. For those that embrace change, there are challenges to overcome but rewards for improving the health of individuals, communities and the nation. As Jaworkski's quote from his seminal work on leadership alludes, when we remain open to the potential for change, the possibilities to make greater progress are endless. American Healthcare and Medicine have evolved as organizational fields, and from the sociological study of institutional change a few general characteristics at the macro level were noted in 2010 by Richard Scott, PhD, Professor of Sociology, Emeritus, Stanford University, including,

- A focus on the interdependence of and interactions between organized units at multiple levels;
- Awareness of the effects of non-local, as well as local factors; and
- An awareness that processes may produce convergence of procedures and forms but also promote diversity and the emergence of new types of social behavior and novel systems. (Scott, 2010)

Clinically Integrated Networks (CINs) along with commercial, private, and publicly funded Accountable Care Organizations (ACOs) are evolutionary structures that have emerged and taken hold as the institution of American Healthcare has evolved through the technological changes and managed care eras of the past 50 years. Innovations across industry sectors are being tested anew, adopted, and implemented at a faster pace than ever before by both commercial and public payers. Such innovations can be seen as new enabling tools and resources for CINs and ACOs to improve the health of populations. Resistance to change is diminishing as organizations, policy makers, healthcare leaders, and care delivery teams realize the opportunity to make both incremental improvements and quantum leaps in improving the health of populations. Ultimately with a goal of achieving the Triple Aim: better care for individuals, reducing the cost of care, and better health for populations. (Berwick, Nolan, & Whittington, 2008; Mosquera, January 27, 2012) To do this, it is important for leaders of CINs and ACOs to keep a strategic view of the road ahead. Figure 14-1 offers a set of lenses to apply in monitoring the environment.

Figure 14-1. Strategic Lenses for CIN/ACO Environment Monitoring

Economic	Legal	Technology/ Infrastructure	Population Health
Salary and compensation structure	FTC/DOJ state antitrust	Data governance	Medical / disease / care / utilization management
Insurance and public payer reimbursement	CMS reimbursements	HIE/data interoperability	Regulatory requirements
Risk management	Tax law impacts on not-for-profits and consumers	Big Data / predictive analytics / artificial intelligence / machine learning	Local market needs
Cost of care and elimination of waste	Medicaid expansion / Medicare changes	Design thinking / human-computer interface	Medicaid unique requirements
Cost/risk shifting (payers-providers-patients)	Health insurance exchanges	Adopting enabling and emerging technologies	Medicare / Baby Boomer unique needs
Infrastructure costs	HIE/EHR and Meaningful Use	Ubiquitous use of social media and mobile platforms	Care coordination / integration challenges
Local economic/market environment	Contractual obligations	HIPAA and consumer protection	Social determinants of health

Several issues are identified under each of these lenses: economic, legal, technology/infrastructure, and population health. The environment for healthcare is rapidly evolving, so staying abreast of emergent issues gives opportunities to take action and positively impact the health of both the bottom line and the community. Additionally, partnering among CINs/ACOs and payers (public and commercial) is testing and instituting new and innovative models for payment reform and care. In order to meet the challenges identified through environmental monitoring, collaborative leadership, strong project management, and flexible participation is needed by all stakeholders.

What We Have Learned

The previous 13 chapters covered a spectrum of critical issues for CINs, ACOs, and Patient-Centered Medical Homes (PCMHs). Chapter 1 introduced the transformation to today's Care Revolution Era and touched on key regulatory requirements for clinical integration. Chapters 2 and 3 raised the importance of primary care in the changing health delivery paradigm, new innovations in strengthening primary care in CINs, and leadership needed to help these organizations function at a high level. Chapter 4 discussed the evolution of the network and 10 core elements foundational for every CIN and ACO. Chapter 5 provided an update on the complex legal and regulatory issues that serve as guardrails for CINs and ACOs to operate. Chapters 6-9 covered key operational topics of quality, finance, new URAC standards for CINs and ACOs, and the increasingly important issue of care coordination within and outside of a provider organization. Chapter 10 gave an update on several technology-related developments, and Chapter 11 provided a new, in depth look at the importance of integrating behavioral health as part of CINs and ACOs. Chapter 12 covered the field of comparative effectiveness research (CER) and Chapter 13 gave us a fresh look at the role and increasing importance of patient engagement for providers and their CINs and ACOs.

Collectively, these chapters provided insights on how to address situations and challenges that many healthcare leaders and practitioners are facing today. This final chapter covers some important topics not yet addressed and serves as a conclusion to a collection of writings intended to aid leaders, practitioners, policy makers, patients, and students in the continued transformation of American Healthcare.

The Future for Accountable Care Organizations

The emergence of new care delivery and finance models, and the underlying innovations to support the transition to value-based care, is occurring both in the United States (U.S.) and abroad. (Barnes, Unruh, Chukmaitov, & van Ginneken, 2014; de Bakker et al., 2012; Hildebrandt, Schulte, & Stunder, 2012) In the United States, two years after the launch of the Medicare Shared Savings Program (MSSP) and with over 600 commercial and public ACOs operating in the market (e.g., including 287 commercial ACOs) the Center for Medicare and Medicaid Services (CMS) proposed new rules for the MSSP. (Evans, December 1, 2014; Petersen & Muhlestein, May 30, 2014) While it will be several months before these rules are final, a key proposed provision granted an additional three years for participating ACOs to reach targeted goals before they were hit with penalties. After year six, however, these ACOs would be assessed penalties if they did not achieve agreed-upon performance goals. (Evans, December 1, 2014) In addition, recognizing the importance of health IT adoption to the success of the MSSP participants, a few related proposed requirements include,

- Promotion and use of enabling technologies for improving care coordination" in all ACO applications, "population health management and data aggregation and analytic tools", "telehealth services" and health information exchange.

- Description of partnering plans for the ACO with "long-term and post-acute care providers to improve care coordination", and

- Provide a defined plan that it will "submit major milestones or performance targets" annually on its progress for adoption of these enabling technologies.

(Centers for Medicare and Medicaid Services, 2014)

In light of the rapidly changing environment, the Brookings Institute's ACO Learning Network provides the industry valuable resources that support leaders of ACOs and CINs. One tool they provide lists ACOs recognized by insurers, illustrated in Figure 14-2.

Figure 14-2. ACO Map from Brookings ACO Learning Network

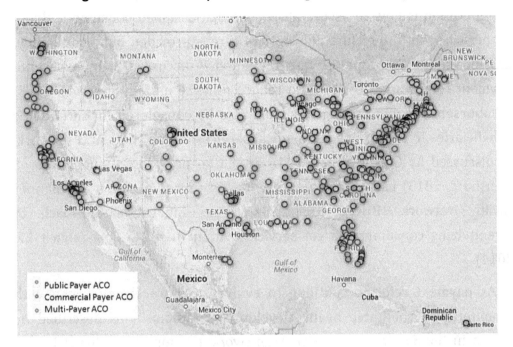

Source: Map courtesy of the Brookings ACO Learning Network ACO Tracking Database (http://www.acolearningnetwork.org/database/). Not publicly accessible and received December 5, 2014.*

The ACO map provides a visual topology showing the geographic density of three types of ACOs: public, commercial, and multi-payer. The Brookings Institute's ACO Learning Network is led by Mark McClellan, MD, PhD and Elliot Fisher, MD, MPH and was started in 2007. The organization, "...is a member-driven network that provides participating organizations with the tools and knowledge necessary to successfully implement accountable care, and delivers national guidance on practical policy steps."(Brookings Instute, 2014)

As public (MSSP and Medicaid), private, and multi-payer ACOs continue to proliferate and become an increasingly important part of the

---

* At the time of this book's publication, CMS has announced an additional 89 MSSP ACOs to start in January 2015.

reimbursement strategy for CINs, there are a few things to consider. One consideration is how to assure all parties that assigned consumers obtain proper care, both to ensure appropriate care is provided but also to allow provider to obtain proper payment. Chapter 7 discussed many aspects of payment reform used by ACOs to reduce reliance on fee-for-service (FFS) reimbursements, but strategies should also be considered for incentiving beneficiaries to obtain needed medical services within their ACO network, as discussed by Ginsburg in a 2013 article on provider payment reform. (Ginsburg, 2013) Later we shall present a case study of Aetna and Banner Health Network (BHN), which shows an innovative approach to incentivizing consumers to get services within BHN. (Coplin, August 27, 2014)

As payment reforms continue to evolve, a future is envisioned with "Community-accountable health development systems" as described by Halfon in the *3.0 Transformation Framework*. (Halfon et al., 2014) Halfon describes the expansion of CINs, fading of the cottage industry of medicine, and emergence of ACOs and PCMHs. This community-level model embraces the movement toward integrated care delivery, envisions a continued strengthening of the population focus as enabling technologies continue to mature, and foresees the growing importance of multi-sectoral collaboration at the community level.

While this paints a promising future for ACOs as part of the overall CIN strategy, there are other challenges to address. These include ethical issues, such as monitoring for equitable resource use and fair decision making processes; maintaining the right-size medical staff as ACO beneficiary populations change; and the industry wide need for greater health IT interoperability. (DeCamp et al., 2014; Pearl, August 14, 2014) The future seems bright for the continued evolution of ACOs and CINs, but physician leaders, policy makers and researchers will need to recognize unanticipated and unintended consequences, such as unintentional underutilization of needed medical care, that are certain to emerge and present challenges in the future.

Health Insurance Reform - Impact on Consumers and the Care Delivery Ecosystem

With enactment of the 2010 Patient Protection and Affordable Care Act (ACA) came the first health insurance coverage mandate for all Americans. The rollout of this law started in 2010 and will continue to be implemented over the coming years. While the entire impact of this law can't be covered in this short section, we will discuss some of the health insurance mandate sections, and their implications for CINs and ACOs.

Table 14-1 shows a list of some of the health insurance mandate Sections (Sec.) in the ACA. (111th Congress, 2010) This is a sample of Sections that have direct and indirect impacts on consumers and care delivery stakeholders such as CINs and ACOs.

Table 14-1. Select Programmatic Sections of the ACA

ACA Section	Title / Description
Title I, Subtitle A—Immediate Improvements in Health Care Coverage for All Americans	
Sec. 1001: Sec. 2711	No lifetime or annual limits,
Sec. 1001: Sec. 2713	Established new coverage of preventive services
Sec. 1001: Sec. 2714	Extended dependent coverage age to 26 years old
Title I, Subtitle B—Immediate Access to Preserve and Expand Coverage	
Sec. 1101	Grants access to health insurance for uninsured and those with pre-existing conditions
Title I, Subtitle D—Available Coverage Choices for All Americans Part I- Establishment of Qualified Health Plans	
Sec. 1301	Defining of qualified health plans
Sec. 1302	Establishment of essential health benefits
Title I, Subtitle F- Shared Responsibility for Health Care Part I- Individual Responsibility	

ACA Section	Title / Description
Sec. 1501	Requirement to maintain minimum essential coverage
Sec. 1502	Reporting of health insurance coverage
Title II, Subtitle A- Improved Access to Medicaid	
Sec. 2001	Medicaid coverage for the lowest income populations

The Sections in Table 14-1 represent some of the historic changes in the accessibility and affordability of health insurance for American consumers. Our intent is not to judge these sections, but to provide insight on their impact for CINs, ACOs, and Federally Qualified Health Centers (FQHCs).

Elimination of lifetime limits on coverage and ending denial of coverage to persons with pre-existing conditions represent two of the major changes implemented by the ACA. As Joseph Swedish, Chief Executive Officer of Trinity Healthcare in Michigan, noted in a September 2013 article, this change ended a long-standing industry restriction on the annual and lifetime benefits that in some cases would leave patients exposed to potential financial ruin from catastrophic events. (Swedish, 2010) Additionally, the pre-existing condition exclusion had long kept many Americans from being able to obtain health insurance coverage for needed medical services. (Thaler, January 22, 2011) This issue impacted the lives of millions of consumers and put healthcare providers (e.g., CINs, physician practices, free-standing hospitals, etc.) in the position of providing additional charity care and/or seeking payment for large medical service bills that, in some cases, could be challenging for consumers to repay.

Section 1501 is perhaps one of the most significant sections, as it requires U.S. citizens to maintain health insurance coverage or be subject to an annual penalty (assessed through annual income tax reporting to the Internal Revenue Service (IRS)). 2014 was the first year requiring health insurance enrollment, and while there were significant problems with federal and state insurance market place exchanges when they launched in 2013, ultimately it was reported that over 7 million previously uninsured people obtained health insurance coverage by late spring 2014. (Currie, 2014; Goodnough & Abelson, November 12, 2013; Sun & Wilson, October 21, 2013). Enrollments in states that expanded Medicaid availability have seen the greatest decreases in uninsured. For example, in Baltimore, MD saw an 8.7 percent decline in uninsured persons as Maryland expanded Medicaid, versus Miami, FL where 25 percent of the population were still uninsured at the end of 2013, as Florida had not yet expanded Medicaid coverage. (McGill, 2014) Florida and other states were being cautious due to the drop in federal subsidies for Medicaid expansion, and the potential large unfunded budget shortfalls projected if more persons were enrolled in an unfunded entitlement program mandating coverage. The states that did not accept the initial Medicaid expansion were re-evaluating this optional expansion.

The Congressional Budget Office, in February 2014, forecasted that due to the ACA, by 2015 there would be 20 million fewer "nonelderly people" (i.e., persons with either private or public coverage not in Medicare) with health insurance, with this number forecasted to increase to 25 million in 2024. (Congressional Budget Office, February 2014) Although this number seems large, it represents roughly half of the uninsured persons in the United States.

For CINs, and public or privately funded ACOs, this expansion in both commercial insurance and Medicaid coverage has both upside and downside potential. In general, increased coverage is certain to increase the demand for healthcare services. As a CIN provider this could mean increasing volume of patients, but it may or may not result in higher reimbursement. If the higher volume of patients are Medicaid reimbursed, there may be a decrease in payment due to elimination of the "Disproportionate Share Hospital" payment (Rudowitz, November 18, 2013) and other government subsidies that used to be given for uncompensated care, but were eliminated by the ACA. If, on the other hand, the higher volume of patients are newly insured under the ACA, through health insurance exchanges, but purchased the lower cost "high deductible" plans, much of the initial coverage may be uncompensated due bad debt from individual patients with high deductible health plans who may be unable to pay their share of out-of-pocket costs. Because of the decline in funds going to hospitals and physicians, also resulting from elimination of "cost shifting" from public payers to private payers, most providers were seeing higher costs but lower payments by the beginning of 2014. (Green, August 23, 2014; Staff, August 25, 2014)

For the commercial ACO market, the results are mixed as well. As noted in the previous section, there are over 287 commercial ACOs. These organizations, by definition, are responsible for both the quality and cost of care. If they are fully at-risk for the costs of care, they have essentially taken on responsibility for financial risk of the covered population, essentially the function of health insurance companies. While they may receive the full insurance "premium" payment, they also are obliged to cover the costs of care. For previously uninsured persons who buy coverage from health insurance exchanges, by law and practical experience, there is no experience from which to learn how much these patients have cost in the past and therefore no way to predict the future liability. This could cause large financial pressures on "at-risk" ACOs. While Medicaid ACOs are the fewest in numbers, they may have the highest financial liabilities as Medicaid disabled populations tend to have the highest costs. Of course, they will have the benefit of taking best practices from Medicare and Commercial ACOs to help with their efforts in achieving savings while improving quality of care. (Petersen & Muhlestein, May 30, 2014; Sandberg et al., 2014) But this may not be enough to keep them financially solvent. Ultimately there will also be several million Americans who go uninsured, even with the ACA, and there will be uneven effects experienced by hospitals and physicians based on their financial health, and ultimately, as noted by David Orentlicher, MD, JD,

> We can make educated guesses about the impact of the ACA, but we will not be able to make reliable judgments until we have hard data. By measuring actual outcomes, we will be able to sort out disagreements among experts regarding the likely effects of the ACA's various provisions. (Orentlicher, 2014)

For the CINs, ACOs and other care providers, the new law is clearly a mixed blessing. The insurance mandate brings more options for individual access to minimum health benefits (Sec. 1302) than was available in the past. But changes in reimbursement, and greater financial risk and clinical performance requirements will result in higher costs and lower margins for profit or error. At this stage in the game, healthcare leaders must press on with implementation, hoping that new innovations intended to improve quality of life and health of populations they serve will ultimately result in at least "break-even" for the persons they employ.

Thoughts on the Future of Health Care

As CINs and ACOs take shape, other organizations across the healthcare ecosystem will continue to evolve as part of our care delivery system. As summarized in a December 2014 *World Health Organization Bulletin*,

> The relatively high costs and poor outcomes that characterize the performance of the United States' health system are the result of many factors....poverty, a lack of universal health coverage, a general lack of focus on primary care and public health, high rates of accidents, violence and teenage pregnancy, and poor health behaviors—e.g. poor diets and an overreliance on automobiles for travel – that lead to obesity and lack of fitness. (Rice et al., December 2014)

This summary shows that even with health reform, social determinants of health and individual behaviors may be largely responsible for the condition of our healthcare system. This may also show that a partnership is needed between providers and patients, to overcome the wide range of individual factors that influence health, care, and outcomes, even when patients are fully engaged (see also Chapter 13). Social determinants of health play a direct role in many of these challenges as "unequal distribution of power, income, goods, and services" coupled with individual preference and structural aspects of communities people live and work in can directly impact choices they make. (Marmot, Friel, Bell, Houweling, & Taylor, 2008) These factors impact the operations of CINs, ACOs, and other care providers as they find themselves more "at-risk" for building services and programs to care for consumers without the traditional financial "back stop" provided by health insurance companies, managed care organizations, and public payers such as CMS and state Medicaid departments.

ACO and CIN Examples

An example illustrates a successful partnership between a health insurance company and a provider to create an ACO that builds on each organizations' strengths.

Aetna and Banner Health Network. Excellence in ACO Development and Achievements

A number of commercial payers have led the way for the emergence of commercial shared savings programs and ACOs. In 2011 Aetna launched a commercial ACO partnership with Banner Health Network (BHN) in Phoenix, AR. In August 2014, Aetna announced that their accountable care collaboration resulted in "shared savings of approximately $5 million on Aetna Whole Health fully-insured commercial membership in 2013 and a five percent decline in average medical cost on the members."(Coplin, August 27, 2014)

With the right care model, incentives and technology in place, Aetna and BHN believe they can achieve better care at a better price. This partnership is proving that benefits from an ACO go beyond their attributed lives. In addition to the financial savings for the commercial ACO, Aetna's Whole Health Plan members served by BHN had improved cancer screening rates, better blood sugar management in diabetic members, reduction in use of radiology services, and fewer avoidable hospital admissions. In addition, tools, best practices, and lessons learned were later leveraged in BHN's Medicare Pioneer ACO that launched in 2012. Per CMS's reported results for Year 1 and Year 2 for all 19 of the Pioneer ACOs, BHN achieved 2.8 percent improvement and $15.5 million in gross savings. (Centers for Medicare and Medicaid Services & CMS Innovation Center, October 2014)

For the Aetna and BHN partnership, Chuck Lehn, BHN's Chief Executive Officer said, "Aetna and BHN have a collaborative relationship that is to the benefit of

Aetna and Banner Health Network. Excellence in ACO Development and Achievements

our members and employers." In addition, BHN's "relationship with Aetna" has provided the critical patient and population health-level data needed to identify opportunities for improved care delivery and quality. For both the commercial and Pioneer ACO ventures, BHN is supported in its information technology infrastructure by Aetna's Accountable Care Solutions clinical analytics for population health management, care coordination and patient engagement applications. (Aetna Accountable Care Solutions, 2014)

In 2014, Aetna had over 554 "value-based health care arrangements". (Aetna, August 27, 2014)

Aetna and BHN's partnership serves as an excellent example of "revolutionary collaboration" that is positively impacting an ACO, its commercial members, and its Medicare ACO members. (Aetna, August 27, 2014) Building on this venture and many other value-based care initiatives, Aetna is part of the new Health Care Transformation Task Force in collaboration with some of the top health care payer and provider organizations in the United States, "...to find better ways to improve the health of people and communities," according to Fran Soistman, Executive Vice President of Government Services, Aetna. (Aetna, January 28, 2015)

Reflecting on this example, there are a variety of opportunities for CINs and ACOs to improve their care delivery. One way to look at this example is to view each integrated delivery organization as operating within four dimensions: as CIN, provider, patient, and community. Each dimension has a direct impact on CINs. There are certainly other dimensions, such as regulatory, technological, and financial, but these four involve key innovations and major changes in the way care is delivered and financed, and therefore provide a framework for a final discussion (see Figure 14-3).

Figure 14-3. Dimensions of Integrated Delivery

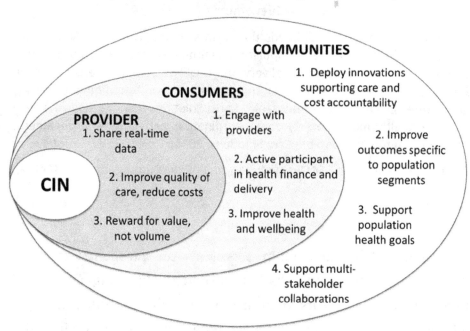

CINs Central to the Ecosystem

For every CIN there are key aspects of their operation that must be developed and maintained to support their mission and serve their community. They have a responsibility to maintain interdependence with affiliated providers across their network, and communication with a broader set of providers (both affiliated and non-affiliated) in accordance with Federal Trade Commission (FTC) / Department of Justice (DOJ) antitrust requirements. Second, coordinating care and monitoring performance, especially in the age of shared savings programs for commercial and public ACOs, is a required high priority. Third, staying abreast of the needs of their providers, patients and their community was emphasized through the strategic lenses model in Figure 14-1 at the beginning of this chapter.

One example of a key industry challenge and patient need being addressed by the CIN is care transitions. The following case vignette highlights a key challenge being dealt with and the approach used to addressing it.

St. Vincent's Health Partners, Inc. Addressing the Challenge of Care Transitions

As the health care system currently exists, individual settings are highly fragmented (Cebul et al, 2008; Strange, 2009). Post-acute care has often functioned largely separate from primary and acute care, and communication and transitions between these three settings rarely exist. With changes in payment models and the shift away from fee-for-service, it becomes crucial to identify the various inefficiencies in the process and to work proactively and collaboratively to address them.

To address this issue, a clinically integrated network should bring together key providers from different specialties within a single network to facilitate in-network communication. In depth process mapping (see Figure 14-4) and discussions will bring to light the various challenges that Post-acute care faces, such as inconsistent referral practices and paperwork lags. This type of venue allows providers to air their issues and work collaboratively to resolve them. One CIN took hold of this concept and now holds biweekly transitions-of-care meetings with multiple stakeholders from both acute and post-acute care settings. This practice allows them to discover challenges to better efficiency and improved practice, and understand the reasoning behind the need for timely paperwork and improved care transitions.

With this knowledge, they were able to take steps to remedy the issue. For example, the hospital case management supervisor sent direct contact information for all weekend case managers to each of the network facilities each Friday, to ensure they could reach someone immediately should issues arise over the weekend. This eased the challenges of weekend transitions from the hospital to the post-acute care facilities. Discussions such as this can inform future transitions and best practices.

Figure 14-4. Skilled Nursing Facility Care Transitions Example

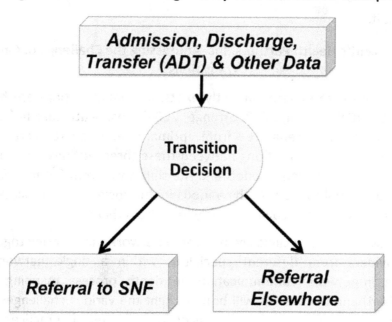

Underlying this care transitions example in Figure 14-4 are some critical actions to support the care transition. First at the point of "Admission, Discharge, Transfer (ADT) & Other Data" and leading into the Transition Decision:

- In-person evaluator reviews medical record and obtains additional information regarding demographics, immunizations, insurance, cost out medications, isolation, medication reconciliation, social services, etc. that have a bearing on the decision of how, and where to refer the patient,

- Centralized transitions office reviews insurance, obtains/reviews authorization, checks provider availability, and

- Clinically complex cases are reviewed by appropriate staff for appropriate referral.

- Care manager or transition navigator decides whether to send the patient (outplacement) or not to admit the patient (in placement).

Then the decision process leads to either a "Referral to SNF" or "Referral Elsewhere." This decision reflects the transitions of care purpose and decision – to refer appropriately, and it may be to a SNF, ALF, other step-down facility, homecare, hospice, primary care physician for follow up, specialist, etc.

Throughout this process it is important to remember a few *"Transition Pain Points"* that can impact the process for CINs, ACOs, and their step-down operations:

- Medication reconciliation is a priority, as the patient cannot be counted upon to communicate all the outpatient, over-the-counter, inpatient, and other medications they have taken, are currently taking, and may resume in the future,

- Communication is key. For example, education of patient is the primary function of the transition team, including self-management until they reach their next care setting, and warning signs indicating worsened conditions and the need for immediate or emergent contact with the transition coordinator,

- Coaching on the transition, including what to tell the physician or nurse, can help assure a successful placement,

- Multiple admissions scheduled after 3pm to one floor can lead to delayed assessments and low customer service, and

- Information not received from the hospital can lead to workflow inefficiencies including: peripherally inserted central catheter (PICC) line placement, discharge (d/c) summary, diet, inaccurate medication lists, wrong patient W-10, lengthy paper work that is not reader friendly, etc.

The importance of having an integrated, highly coordinated care team that has continuous communications starting with admissions, running through nursing and physician care, and continuing through discharge and even to post-discharge transitions cannot be overstated.

Provider Dimension

As illustrated here, three key takeaways are: sharing real-time data among providers to effect better care; improving quality and reducing costs both for the benefit of consumers but also the efficiency and effectiveness of providers; and being rewarded for delivering care services based on the value and quality of outcomes, instead of volume of patient encounters.

Real-time data sharing includes clinical, pharmacy, laboratory, billing, and clinician/patient reported data. Claims data may also be useful, as there is an entire body of knowledge that has been built over the years to interpret, extrapolate, and interpolate claims data to make it directly useful for predictive modeling and patient care. Claims data, however, is usually not available real-time, thus the need to use billed charges. The issue with billed charges is that it may be altered in the billing cycle, therefore adjudicated claims are "cleaner," but again they are delayed. Thus we shall focus on the other data as primary sources for actionable information and insights.

As providers continue to adopt health information technology, the ability to utilize medical and population health management (PHM), as insurance companies have done for years, will accelerate. Adopting and utilizing these tools is critical, and new health information technologies, such as electronic medical records, health information exchanges, and personal health records shall enable more real-time availability.

PHM tools are established technologies that have been used by health insurance companies and managed care organizations to understand and better manage care. Their use by providers are in their infancy, mainly because in a "pay-for-procedure" world the providers had no interest in managing care, that was "someone else's job." Now that hospitals and physicians are increasingly being paid for their performance, or accepting health insurance risk, they have a keen interest in these tools. Thus, partnerships between companies like Aetna and BHN have become commonplace as providers seek to understand and adopt health insurance and managed care tools. As Cassidy noted in a 2013 *Journal of AHIMA* article, key attributes that need to be in place for PHM tools,

> Some of the first things that must be understood when launching a PHM program is what a population of healthy people looks like, how clinical risk is defined, how financial risk is measured, and what will be the metrics used to analyze how sick patients with chronic disease do and do not get sicker. PHM programs also track and trend inpatient, ambulatory, and emergency department patients. (Cassidy, 2013)

Having real-time applications that support medical management, utilization management, care coordination, patient engagement, chronic disease management, performance monitoring, and payer information flow will help providers and CINs meet their clinical and business needs to improve population health in ways that improve care and lower costs – the second dimension listed in the Provider dimension in Figure 14-3.

Improving quality of care and reducing costs to benefit consumers must be an overarching goal for otherwise independent providers to collaborate in a CIN structure, and is a requirement of FTC and DOJ to avoid antitrust prosecution. Beyond regulatory requirements, improving quality and reducing costs also helps providers by focusing on outcomes and eliminating waste and redundancy. This is critical in the current environment, where traditional hospital cost shifting that increases insurer and employer expenses to pay for losses in government programs is no longer a viable option. Creation of Health Insurance Exchanges, inevitable decreases in commercial employer/insurer volume, and increased government volume are ending this traditional cost shift. Health care reform accelerates this trend as more employers drop health coverage, more individuals obtain coverage from Health Insurance Exchanges, creating enormous pricing pressures on hospitals and physician offices and forcing dramatic change,(Avalere Health, 2010) Reducing costs, eliminating waste and inefficiency has become a survival tactic for most hospitals.

Improving quality and focusing on outcomes also helps both patient and provider. All providers want to give the best care, but until now most providers have been rewarded for every procedure performed. By rewarding for performance, hospitals and physicians are freed to focus on care management and coordination, improving clinical pathways and protocols, and ultimately benefitting patients with quality outcomes.

This focus on performance allows providers to be rewarded for the quality of patient outcomes achieved, instead of the volume of patient encounters, which is the third point of our Provider dimension in Figure 14-3. Moving away from fee-for-service reimbursement is a massive undertaking riddled with organizational and cultural complexities. A few of these complexities and challenges were summarized by Conrad and colleagues in their 2014 article entitled, *Emerging Lessons from Regional and State Innovation in Value-Based Payment Reform: Balancing Collaboration and Disruptive Innovation*. Those barriers include,

> ...incompatible information systems, technical difficulties and transaction costs of altering existing billing and payment systems,...providers' limited experience with risk-bearing payment models, and failure to align care delivery models with the form of payment. (Conrad, Grembowski, Hernandez, Lau, & Marcus-Smith, 2014)

In order to overcome these challenges there will be a "co-evolution of organization and payment."(Miller, 2009) This co-evolution will include changes to organizational structures as they exist today and payment reforms that move toward bundled payment models and other innovative means of compensating based on achievement of positive quality outcomes.

Consumer Dimension

The Consumer dimension is the newest, and perhaps most unfamiliar of the dimensions covered in Figure 14-3. Hospitals and physicians are used to treating patients in acute care settings. With the advent of ACOs, they also must learn to engage them as consumers before they need to access the healthcare system, identify their risk for future illness, and intervene before they require expensive emergent or acute care.

Health Insurance Exchanges, with their requirement that past history of health and care cannot be provided, has had the unintended consequence of limiting the ability of insurance companies, managed care organizations, ACOs, CINs, PCMHs, hospitals, health systems, physicians, nurses, or anyone in the care team to figure out what the consumer needs, and even whether or not the person is or should be a patient. With time, and experience, this should be less of a problem, but it has very real consequences for the health and care of the individual. As a result, it is imperative the consumer engages with the provider, in order to benefit from coverage and care available.

Becoming an active participant in health care, finance, and delivery is becoming a reality with the internet and mobile health. Mobile health (mHealth) applications help fuel patient's knowledge gaps on health related issues and accessibility to information when needed. (Konschak, Levin, & Morris, 2013) As more people are enrolled in consumer directed and high-deductible health plans, whether through choice or directive, the individual becomes more responsible for their own care and the ability to actively engage with the healthcare system is both a financial and clinical imperative.

From a consumer perspective, there is increasing value in having information and knowledge about health issues, impact of lifestyle and behavioral choices, and the quality of services offered by different care providers. This knowledge will help sculpt the future landscape and the competitive environment for healthcare services and products. The sharing of a consumer's health data will continue to be a concern as more providers, vendors, and payers seek access to more and more insights on patient-centric issues—who owns such data and what people with access to it will do with it in the future will continue to evolve. (Kahn, October 7, 2014)

Retail consumerism is the next big frontier in healthcare. As Health Insurance Exchanges and mHealth capabilities become entrenched parts of our culture, the healthcare services delivered to consumers will (and already are in many ways) strive to meet the consumer's new sense of needs and increasing demands.

Consumers are also gaining more insights from transparency about the quality of services delivered by care providers, which is enhancing their decision-making about needed and elective services and which insurance products to choose. As the health insurance market and exchanges continue to take shape, a few changes that should benefit consumers were noted by Kingsdale in a 2014 article:

- "Promote enrollment and national consumer choice,
- Enhance "health" competition among insurers."(Kingsdale, 2014)

A more transparent insurance marketplace should increase access to care, but only time will tell whether ACA reforms result in improved efficiency and quality of care. In any case, the demands of retail consumers for improved health and wellbeing will need to be addressed by providers and members of the care team on the front lines of healthcare if consumer expectations are to be met.

Community Dimension

For CINs, ACOs, and their physicians, improving health of their populations, rather than increasing the number of procedures, is rapidly becoming the highest priority. As ACOs and shared savings programs become more main stream, it will only fuel innovations that base reimbursement on performance, taking a community perspective that works on improving population health. These innovations require a different approach and perspective on the practice of medicine. As George Isham, co-chair of the Institute of Medicine Roundtable for Population Health Improvement, noted in 2014,

> Population health outcomes, such as improved life expectancy and quality of life, are shaped by interdependent social, economic, environmental, genetic, behavioral, and health care factors and will

require robust national and community-based policies and dependable resources to accomplish them...(Roundtable on Population Health Improvement & Institute of Medicine, 2014)

These interdependent factors will, over time, help providers build better strategies and tactics to engage patients. These new approaches must address the spectrum of factors that impact patients' lives on a daily basis in order to effect the quality of health they experience and demonstrate improvements in outcomes and performance.

Innovation is the heart of change. But getting innovations adopted to improve the health of a population, rather than falling back on traditional increases in procedure, can be a challenge. As Christensen noted in *The Innovator's Prescription: A Disruptive Solution for Healthcare*, sustaining disruptive innovations is very difficult because incumbents nearly always win due to their relationships with customers and fear of disruption. Throughout history, however, disruption in business models (e.g., ACO and CIN) has been the dominant way to make products and services more affordable and accessible, and to generate economic growth. (Christensen, 2008) Thus, disruptive innovations may be our best hope for sustainable reform, making healthcare more accessible and affordable and giving providers new avenues for economic growth. Identifying, testing and implementing disruptive innovations requires an organizational culture that is agile, flexible, and adaptable to change. CINs and ACOs such as Geisinger Health System in Pennsylvania, Advocated Healthcare in Illinois, Banner Health in Arizona, BayCare Health System in Florida, and St. Vincent's in Connecticut serve as examples. They have the culture, operational processes, leadership, and flexibility to evaluate and deploy new innovations that are helping improve quality and reduce the cost of care. But to deploy innovations that improve outcomes and support population health goals, ACOs also require collaboration with all parties involved. These multi-stakeholder collaborations must include payers, providers, patients, and populations in order for healthcare organizations to move forward and evolve into the future.

Lessons Learned

The road for providers to implement new population health strategies and tactics is complex. Organizations are struggling with where to start in the process. The authors experience with establishing successful CINs and ACOs contributes to the following guidance and lessons learned.

We encourage starting with a small framework, then adding elements of population health as political hurdles are overcome (both internal to the organization and external within the provider network), providers become more engaged, and there is better understanding of all the components necessary to manage health and the "total costs of care" (to use a health insurance industry phrase).

Encourage providers to engage early and often. The CIN or ACO cannot over communicate its goals, both organizationally and by individual physician. Not only is this strategically important, but from a tactical perspective the federal FTC requires every physician to demonstrate commitment to operationalize the goals of the organization and understand their individual responsibilities. From a practical perspective too, the more engaged the provider network is, the more successes it will achieve.

Be aware of change fatigue. Providers in practice are seeing more new delivery systems and models of reimbursement, along with regulatory components, impacting their practices and diminishing their income. The more assistance the CIN can provide the practice, the greater the success.

Be open to many models of care, and don't be afraid to discard those that don't work. However, implement the models uniformly, give them sufficient time to take hold and work, identify and understand problems as they arise, and be sure you are improving processes and diminishing variations in care.

New skill sets need to be developed by physicians, staff, and physician leaders. Having everyone practice at the top of their license, and taking non-clinical items off the provider's plate, increases job satisfaction as well as improving operational processes and flow.

Embrace population health. The ability of providers to comprehend population health analytics is developing, as is the Information Technology necessary to implement predictive analytics. Encourage physician leaders to seek out new skills to tackle the new tasks required to run the CIN.

Conclusion: Recommendations for Tomorrow's CIN and ACO Leaders

Throughout this book a number of concepts, approaches and ideas have been provided to further practical action, policy change, and continued mobilization of CINs and ACOs. It can serve as a guide to learning in the field of work and in the classroom, for both seasoned healthcare professionals and persons just entering the field. In the opening chapter we introduced the idea of a paradigm shift to the Care Revolution Era. In this new era, continued shifts in risk sharing, movement toward value and outcome-driven care, and a population management focus are seen as dominant. As Wilson and Nesbitt noted in the concluding chapter of *Population Health. Management, Policy and Technology*, a special focus on change will be needed, "In order to change the trajectory of our health outcomes it is imperative that we change the way we address health."(Wilson & Nesbitt, 2014)

One way CINs and ACOs are changing how they address health is integrating primary care with other disciplines brought together in CINs and PCMHs, as discussed in Chapter 2. As Providers continues to adopt predictive analytics and other analytic tools, they will better understand the social determinants and behavioral choices that impact the health of populations. Changes such as these can bring about structural change in American medicine, healthcare, and the broader society served.

Norbert Elias, German Sociologist, wrote in his 1939 classic, *The Civilizing Process*, of how, "...two main directions of structural changes of societies may be distinguished: those tending toward increased differentiation and integration and those tending toward decreased differentiation and integration."(Elias, 1939, 1969)

In healthcare, for the last five decades, the movement has been on the path toward greater fragmentation and differentiation. With the emergence of CINs and ACOs, our industry is moving more towards integration, with its social structure of networked organizations, harnessing the power of technology, and recognizing the importance of standardizing processes of care and greater collaboration among stakeholders to improve care. The movement to care for patients at the population level, developed by health insurance companies and managed care organizations for the past two decades, is becoming a necessity for CINs and ACOs that are evaluated on performance, including quality outcomes and cost reductions. In light of the need to achieve even greater integration of clinical resources and capabilities, Table 14-2 offers a set of recommendations.

Table 14-2. Recommended Actions for CIN and ACO Future Leaders

Category	Action
Coordination of Care	Ensure that "continuous communication" is used to connect all medical professionals through enabling technologies and processes that continuously improve performance and reach patients when and where they need it most.
Payment Reform	Implement innovative payment and compensation programs, and recognize blended payment programs may be needed to gradually shift the organization away from FFS reimbursements. Understand the implications of health insurance market reforms as they directly effect provider revenue cycle and reimbursements.
Performance Measurement	Establish a proactive performance measurement and review program to ensure all key staff are aware of key regulatory, CIN, and ACO performance metrics.
Lead Collaboratively	Institute a collaborative leadership approach that engages all staff and physicians in cross-functional efforts focused on population health improvement.
Embrace Innovation	Strive to test and adopt new innovations that bring potential for positive change.

Category	Action
Standards	For CINs, understand industry standards (e.g., URAC) for clinical integration programs and accountable care, and what your organization should do to attain accreditation.
Community Engagement	Participate in multi-stakeholder collaboration efforts to ensure communication, understanding and adoption.
Volume to Value-Driven Transition	Recognize the significance of structural changes, and incremental steps necessary, to achieve a value and outcomes-driven culture.

These eight recommendations are certainly not all inclusive, but they are intended to serve as a set of guideposts and a reframing mechanism for the ecosystem of clinical, technical, administrative, business, and human capital considerations that form the foundation of every new, provider healthcare business model, whether CIN, ACO, PCMH, retail clinic, other provider entities. Success for CINs and ACOs will in part be influenced by their evolving ability to understand the existing and new PHM tools that can be leveraged to better manage needed care and the choices people make that impact their health and wellbeing.

Clayton Christensen and colleagues in their book, *The Innovator's Prescription: A Disruptive Solution for Healthcare*, brought us the concept of disruption in healthcare through the enablement of a "new value network",

> Disruption means that many distinctly different business models will provide care. But this reflects an important step in all of the disruptive transformations we have studied: the benefits of these focused models will be a dramatic reduction in overhead costs and improvements in quality grounded in better integration. (Christensen, Grossman, & Hwang, 2009)

Just as the vision of Elias (Elias, 1939, 1969), on grander scale, described the foretelling journey of movement toward greater integration, Christensen and colleagues emphasize the power of disruptive ideas and innovations that are helping shape the new value network that is embodying the U.S. and broader global healthcare systems. Big Data, PHM tools, and predictive analytics promise to bolster the power of health information technology and better enable physicians, care teams, and patients to improve clinical decision making. These enabling technologies are improving patient-provider communications and care as the industry continues to shift from intuitive medicine to personalized and population medicine making greater use of the vast arrays of clinical, claims, genetic, demographic, environmental, and other exogenous data being made available for better clinical decision support, diagnosis, and treatment. (Mega, Sabatine, & Antman, 2014)

The future is ripe with challenges for CINs, ACOs, and other healthcare providers as the United States works to achieve the Triple Aim of better care for individuals, reducing the cost of care, and better health for populations. (Berwick et al., 2008) The industry continues to strengthen the bridges between consumers, providers, payers, government agencies, healthcare organizations, populations, and communities on the road to improving clinical integration in American Healthcare. The next step is up to each of us in contributing to the establishment of healthier populations today and for generations to come.

CHAPTER 14 DISCUSSION QUESTIONS

Discussion questions are provided for team building or class exercises. Answers for all questions are provided in Appendix C.

Question Number	Question
1	What are the four strategic lenses for ACO/CIN environment monitoring?
2	What are three characteristics of institutional change as referred to from Richard Scott, PhD?
3	What are the four dimensions of an integrated delivery organization that help conceptualize ways to improve care delivery?
4	What section of the ACA eliminated the denial of pre-existing conditions for consumers to get health insurance coverage?
5	From the Aetna and Banner Health Network commercial ACO partnership what were some of the initial benefits achieved?
6	From the Recommendations for Future ACO and CIN Leaders what are the key elements of the Care Coordination and Community Engagement recommendations?

CHAPTER 14 HIGHLIGHTS

✓ The Strategic Lenses for CIN/ACO Environmental Monitoring in Figure 14-1 can serve as an enabling framework for healthcare leaders to stay abreast of key developments across the industry landscape that affect their organizations today and in the future.

✓ New regulatory changes for the MSSP in 2015 will have operational and strategic effects on the future of the ACO entities in operation today and those that enter the market in the future.

✓ The Brookings Institute's ACO Learning Network is serving as a national hub for "guidance and practical policy steps" as ACOs continue to evolve.

✓ The health insurance reforms are having a transformative effect on consumer's lives and on the cost, quality and availability of health benefits across the United States. Table 14-1 highlighted some of the select programmatic sections from the ACA.

✓ The Aetna and Banner Health Network case study highlighted the benefits that can be achieved in both private payer and public payer ACO initiatives.

✓ The St. Vincent's Health Partners case study highlighted the importance of addressing the challenge of care transitions.

✓ The Dimensions of Care identify key initiatives to be considered as priorities for the CIN at the provider, consumer, and community dimension.

✓ Lessons learned for those working to lead and implement efforts in CINs were noted as encouraging providers to engage early and often, be aware of change fatigue, remain open to emergent models of care, and recognize the need to continuously develop new skill sets in physicians, staff and physician leaders.

✓ CINs and ACOs have emerged as part of the social structure of networked organizations throughout the healthcare industry. Understanding the processes that are enabling and inhibiting strategic and structural change will continue to help make improvements in the quality, cost and delivery of care.

✓ The eight recommendations for CIN and ACO leaders provide a set of guideposts to help organizational leaders and their staff institute and monitor core initiatives that critical to the success of every CIN.

CHAPTER 14 REFERENCES

111th Congress. (2010). Patient Protection and Affordable Care Act. (Public Law 111-148).

Aetna. (2014, August 27). Infographic: Quality of care versus quantity of service. *Aetna Health Section.* Retrieved from https://news.aetna.com/quality-quantity-core-value-based-care/

Aetna. (2015, January 28). Insurers and health systems agree: Pay for health care quality, not quantity. *Aetna Health Section.* Retrieved from http://news.aetna.com/insurers-and-health-systems-agree-pay-for-health-care-quality/

Aetna Accountable Care Solutions. (2014). Collaboration Profiles. *Aetna Accountable Care Solutions.* Retrieved from http://www.aetnaacs.com/collaboration-profiles

Avalere Health. (2010). Analysis of American Hospital Association Annual survey data, 2010, for community hospitals.

Barnes, A. J., Unruh, L., Chukmaitov, A., & van Ginneken, E. (2014). Accountable care organizations in the USA: Types, developments and challenges. *Health Policy.*

Berwick, D. M., Nolan, T. W., & Whittington, J. (2008). The triple aim: care, health, and cost. *Health Affairs, 27*(3), 759-769. doi: 10.1377/hlthaff.27.3.759

Brookings Instute. (2014). ACO Learning Network Home Page. Retrieved from http://www.acolearningnetwork.org/

Cassidy, B. (2013). The next HIM frontier. Population health information management presents a new opportunity for HIM. *Journal of AHIMA/American Health Information Management Association, 84*(8), 40-46.

Medicare Program; Medicare Shared Savings Program: Accountable Care Organizations. Proposed Rule. , RIN 0938-AS06 C.F.R. § II(B)8. (b)(c) Accelerating Health Information Technology and Proposed Revisions (2014).

Centers for Medicare and Medicaid Services, & CMS Innovation Center. (2014, October). Medicare Pioneer ACO Model Performance Year 1 and Performance Year 2 Financial Results. *CMS Innovation Center Reports.* Retrieved from http://innovation.cms.gov/Files/x/PioneerACO-Fncl-PY1PY2.pdf

Christensen, C., Grossman, J. H., & Hwang, J. (2009). Introduction *The Innovator's Prescription. A Disruptive Solution for Healthcare* (pp. xxix). New York, NY: McGraw Hill.

Congressional Budget Office. (2014, February). Budget and Economic Outlook 2014-2014. Appendix B: Updated Estimates of the Insurance Coverage Provisions of the Affordable Care Act. Retrieved from http://www.cbo.gov/sites/default/files/cbofiles/attachments/45010-breakout-AppendixB.pdf

Conrad, D., A., Grembowski, D., Hernandez, S., E., Lau, B., & Marcus-Smith, M. (2014). Emerging Lessons From Regional and State Innovation in Value-Based Payment Reform: Balancing Collaboration and Disruptive Innovation. *Milbank Quarterly, 92*(3), 568-623. doi: 10.1111/1468-0009.12078

Coplin, A. (2014, August 27). Lower Costs, More Proactive Care in Aetna and Banner Health Network Accountable Care Collaboration. *Aetna News Release.* Retrieved from https://news.aetna.com/news-releases/lower-costs-more-proactive-care-in-aetna-and-banner-health-network-accountable-care-collaboration/

Currie, D. (2014). Success in Affordable Care Act enrollment 'just the beginning'. *Nation's Health, 44*(5), 6-6.

de Bakker, D. H., Struijs, J. N., Baan, C. B., Raams, J., de Wildt, J. E., Vrijhoef, H. J., & Schut, F. T. (2012). Early results from adoption of bundled payment for diabetes care in the Netherlands show improvement in care coordination. *Health Affairs, 31*(2), 426-433. doi: 10.1377/hlthaff.2011.0912

DeCamp, M., Farber, N. J., Torke, A. M., George, M., Berger, Z., Keirns, C. C., & Kaldjian, L. C. (2014). Ethical challenges for accountable care organizations: A Structured Review. *Journal of General Internal Medicine*, 1-8. doi: 10.1007/s11606-014-2833-x

Elias, N. (1939, 1969). Postscript (1968) *The Civilizing Process* (pp. 450). Malden, MA: Blackwell Publishers, Ltd.

Evans, M. (2014, December 1). Draft Medicare ACO rules would allow more time with less risk. *Modern Healthcare.* Retrieved from http://www.modernhealthcare.com/article/20141201/NEWS/312019943?utm_source=AltURL&utm_medium=email&utm_campaign=am%3Fmh

Ginsburg, P., B,. (2013). Achieving health care cost containment through provider payment reform that engages patients and providers. *Health Affairs, 32*(5), 929-934.

Goodnough, A., & Abelson, R. (2013, November 12). Some state insurance exchanges continue to battle technical problems. *New York Times.* Retrieved from http://www.nytimes.com/2013/11/13/us/some-state-insurance-exchanges-continue-to-battle-technical-problems.html?_r=0

Green, J. (2014, August 23). Health care reform targets hospitals for savings. *Crain's Detroit News.* Retrieved from http://www.crainsdetroit.com/article/20140722/BLOG010/140729950/health-care-reform-targets-hospitals-for-savings

Halfon, N., Long, P., Chang, D. I., Hester, J., Inkelas, M., & Rodgers, A. (2014). Applying A 3.0 Transformation framework to guide large-scale health system reform. *Health Affairs, 33*(11), 2003-2011. doi: 10.1377/hlthaff.2014.0485

Hildebrandt, H., Schulte, T., & Stunder, B. (2012). Triple Aim in Kinzigtal, Germany: Improving population health, integrating health care and reducing costs of care–lessons for the UK? *Journal of Integrated Care, 20*(4), 205-222. doi.org/10.1108/14769011211255249

Jaworski, J. (1996). Chapter 24. Creating the Future *Synchronicity. The Inner Path of Leadership* (pp. 183). San Francisco, CA: Berrett-Koehler Publishers, Inc.

Kahn, A. (2014, October 7). What is the future of health care? *US News HEALTH.* Retrieved from http://health.usnews.com/health-news/hospital-of-tomorrow/articles/2014/10/07/what-is-the-future-of-health-care

Kingsdale, J. (2014). After the false start—what can we expect from the new health insurance marketplaces? *New England Journal of Medicine, 370*(5), 393-396. doi: 10.1056/NEJMp1315956

Konschak, C., Levin, D., & Morris, W. (2013). *mHealth: The Coming* Revolution *mHealth. Global Opportunities and Challenges* (pp. 6-37). Virginia Beach, VA: Convurgent Publishing.

Marmot, M., Friel, S., Bell, R., Houweling, T. A., & Taylor, S. (2008). Closing the gap in a generation: health equity through action on the social determinants of health. *The Lancet, 372*(9650), 1661-1669. doi: 10.1016/S0140-6736(08)61690-6

McGill, N. (2014). Rate of uninsured Americans continues to drop, data show: Bigger decreases yet to come, experts say. *The Nation's Health, 44*(9), 1-18.

Mega, J. L., Sabatine, M. S., & Antman, E. M. (2014). Population and personalized medicine in the modern era. *Journal of the American Medical Association, 312*(19), 1969. doi: 10.1001/jama.2014.15224

Miller, H. D. (2009). From volume to value: better ways to pay for health care. *Health Affairs, 28*(5), 1418-1428. doi: 10.1377/hlthaff.28.5.1418

Mosquera, M. (2012, January 27). Triple aim' is priority for Tavenner and CMS. *Healthcare Finance News.* Retrieved from http://www.healthcarefinancenews.com/news/triple-aim-priority-tavenner-and-cms

Orentlicher, D. (2014). The future of the Affordable Care Act: protecting economic health more than physical health? *Houston Law Review, 51*(4).

Pearl, R. (2014, August 14). The 4 biggest obstacles ACOs face. *Forbes.* Retrieved from http://www.forbes.com/sites/robertpearl/2014/08/14/the-4-biggest-obstacles-acos-face/print/

Petersen, M., & Muhlestein, D. (2014, May 30). ACO results: what we know so far. *Health Affairs Blog.* Retrieved from http://healthaffairs.org/blog/2014/05/30/aco-results-what-we-know-so-far/

Rice, T., Unruh, L. Y., Rosenau, P., Barnes, A. J., Saltmane, R. B., & van Ginnekenf, E. (2014, December). Challenges facing the United States of America in implementing universal coverage. *Bulletin of the World Health Organization, 92,* 894-902. doi: http://dx.doi.org/10.2471/BLT.14.141762

Roundtable on Population Health Improvement, & Institute of Medicine. (2014). Chapter 6. Reaction and Discussion *The Role and Potential of Communities in Population Health Improvement* (pp. 43). Washington, DC: National Academies Press.

Rudowitz, R. (2013, November 18). How do Medicaid Disproportionate Share Hospital (DSH) payments change under the ACA? *The Henry J. Kaiser Family Foundation.* Retrieved from http://kff.org/medicaid/issue-brief/how-do-medicaid-disproportionate-share-hospital-dsh-payments-change-under-the-aca/

Sandberg, S. F., Erikson, C., Owen, R., Vickery, K. D., Shimotsu, S. T., Linzer, M., . . . DeCubellis, J. (2014). Hennepin Health: A Safety-Net Accountable Care Organization For The Expanded Medicaid Population. *Health Affairs, 33*(11), 1975-1984. doi: 10.1377/hlthaff.2014.0648

Scott, W. R. (2010). Reflections: The past and future of research on institutions and institutional change. *Journal of Change Management, 10*(1), 5-21. doi: 10.1080/14697010903549408

Staff, M. H. (2014, August 25). Hospitals see more paying patients, but there's a hitch. *Crain's Detroit Business.* Retrieved from http://www.crainsdetroit.com/article/20140825/NEWS/140829968/hospitals-see-more-paying-patients-but-theres-a-hitch#

Sun, L. H., & Wilson, S. (2013, October 21). Health insurance exchange launched despite signs of serious problems. *Washington Post*. Retrieved from http://www.washingtonpost.com/national/health-science/health-insurance-exchange-launched-despite-signs-of-serious-problems/2013/10/21/161a3500-3a85-11e3-b6a9-da62c264f40e_story.html

Swedish, J. (2010). A step forward. *Modern Healthcare, 40*(17), 20-20.

Thaler, R. (2011, January 22). Adding clarity to health care reform. *New York Times*. Retrieved from http://www.nytimes.com/2011/01/23/business/23view.html?scp=1&sq=thaler%20economic%20view&st=cse

Wilson, R., & Nesbitt, L. S. (2014). Chapter 14. The Future of Population Health: Moving Forward with Networks, Policies and Innovations *Population Health. Management, Policy, and Technology, First Edition* (pp. 499). Virginia Beach, VA: Convurgent Publishing.

Appendix A: Glossary

Accountable Care Organization - Accountable Care Organizations (ACOs) are collaborations between physicians, hospitals, and other providers of clinical services that will be clinically and financially accountable for the cost and quality of care, usually for a designated patient populations in a defined geographic market. The ACO is typically (and by Medicare standards) "physician-led" with a focus on population-based care management, and may provide services to patients under both public and private payer programs.

Antitrust Rule - In the context of a Clinically Integrated Nettwork, the FTC regulations and guidelines that pertain to any activities between competitors, such as physicians who practice as separate and independent business entities in the same market, that involve setting or "fixing" prices, that could potentially restrain trade, increase costs to consumers, or result in some form of monopoly situation. Unless FTC guidance is followed, such activities may be in violation of antitrust laws and coule be, by definition, ("per se") illegal.

Antitrust Safety Zone - An economic model established by the Department of Justice (DOJ) and Federal Trade Commission (FTC) that allows for a percentage of shared common services within a designated primary service area, that could otherwise raise antitrust issues but will not draw antitrust scrutiny. For ACOs that fall within a safety zone, they are unlikely to raise antitrust competitive concerns and not be challenged except in the case of improper conduct.

Behavioral Health Conditions - Emotional, behavioral, or cognitive disturbances, which interfere with a person's ability to function optimally while symptoms are present.

Baby Boomers - The largest demographic cohort in the United States, born between 1946 and 1964.

Balanced Scorecard - The balanced scorecard is a "methodology that converts an organization's vision and strategy into a comprehensive set of linked performance and action measures that provide the basis for sound strategic measurement and management."

Big Data - The collection of data found throughout an industry, much of which may not currently be used but all of which has intrinsic value, requiring innovative processing and tools to aggregate, mine, and generate insights to support decision making.

Care Coordination - The foundation of medical management that oversees the entire population, or a specific population subset, cared for by an organization. This function within each clinically integrated network (CIN) and ACO focuses attention on care management to assure efficient and effective patient care among providers and sites of care, and meeting the medical care requirements for both chronic and preventative care.

Chronic Care Model - An evidence-based model created by Dr. Ed Wagner in the 1990s that focuses on the delivery of planned, proactive, population-based care rather than acute episodic care for patients with chronic diseases. The six components of this model include: 1) self-management support, 2) delivery system design, 3) decision support, 4) clinical information systems, 5) community resources, and 6) organization of the health system.

Chronic Disease - A complex illness that persists for an extended period of time and is difficult to cure or often not able to be totaly cured.

Clinically Integrated Network - Collections of physicians and hospitals working together as an integrated unit to achieve economies of scale in care delivery, enable joint contracting with insurers, and launch programs designed to increase the quality and coordination of patient care while reducing the cost of that care for the benefit of consumers.

Comparative Effectiveness Research - As defined by the Institute of Medicine (IOM) Committee on Comparative Effectiveness Research, comparative effectiveness research (CER) is, "...the generation and synthesis of evidence that compares the benefits and harms of alternative methods to prevent, diagnose, treat, and monitor a clinical condition or to improve the delivery of care. The purpose of CER is to assist consumers, clinicians, purchasers, and policy makers to make informed decisions that will improve health care at both the individual and population levels."

Descriptive Analytics - Data mining to produce descriptive reports of what happened to a patient or population in the past.

Electronic Health Record - Electronic health records (EHRs) are records in electronic format that document health and medical information, and because of federal government regulations most are capable of being shared across multiple care settings and organizations. They may include data on each patient's demographics, medical history, medications and allergies, laboratory test results, radiology results, vital signs, and other information.

Electronic Medical Record- A health information technology system that includes a clinical data repository, clinical decision support (CDS), controlled medical vocabulary, computerized provider order entry, pharmacy order entry, and clinical documentation applications. These systems warehouse patient's personal health data for both inpatient and outpatient environments in use by physicians and clinicians to document, monitor, and manage health care delivery.

Fee-for-Service - A reimbursement model that compensates providers based on individual procedures or patient encounters.

FTC and DOJ Joint Statements - The federal regulatory framework that serves as guidance on collaborative arrangements between and among hospitals and physicians.

Health Information Exchange - Health information exchange (HIE) can be defined as a noun or a verb. As a noun, HIE refers to an organization formed to enable information sharing of patient information among multiple healthcare organizations. As a verb, HIE is the activity of exchanging patient health records across disparate systems and locations.

Indicia of Clinical Integration - Required elements for any clinically integrated network to fall under guidelines jointly identified by the DOJ and the FTC. They include: a) staff for care coordination and case management, 2) use of EHRs and other health information technology (HIT) to ensure patient data exchange, 3) development and adoption of practice standards and protocols, and 4) staff to monitor standards and protocols.

Managed Behavioral Health Organizations (MBHOs) - Either a "carved-in" subsidiary of a medical insurer or a "carved-out" subcontracted external vendor, which uses a segregated funding pool to pay for behavioral health services separate from all other delivered medical services.

Meaningful Use of EHRs Program - The Meaningful Use program (administered by the Centers for Medicare and Medicaid Services (CMS)) provides incentives to eligible professionals, eligible hospitals, and critical access hospitals for adoption and use of EHR technology that specifically meets meaningful use standards, as promulgated by CMS. The incentives were available the first few years of the program. After the first years of the program, it levies penalties in the form of reduced Medicare and Medicaid payments for providers who are eligible but do not adopt and use EHR technology meeting meaningful use standards.

Non-traditional Behavioral Health Service Delivery - Behavioral health (BH) services delivered in consolidated medical and BH service locations, which are coordinated with medical services and ultimately paid from a single benefit funding pool.

Parity Laws - Enacted legislation in 2008, which aims to ensure that when *coverage* for mental health and substance use conditions is provided, it is generally comparable to coverage for medical and surgical care (mandated in contracts through the 2010 Patient Protection and Affordable Care Act). Do not address issues created by a segregated delivery system.

Patient-Centered Medical Home - The Patient-Centered Medical Home (PCMH) is a foundational philosophy for primary care model originally mentioned in 1967 by the American Academy of Pediatrics (AAP). The PCMH model is one of the organizing constructs around which CINs and ACOs can succeed and establish primary care operations.

Patient-Centered Outcomes Research Institute (PCORI) - PCORI is, "...an independent organization created to help patients, clinicians, purchasers and policy makers make better informed health decisions. PCORI will commission research that is responsive to the values and interests of patients and will provide patients and their caregivers with reliable, evidence-based information for the health care choices they face."

Patient Engagement - Patient engagement is defined as getting patients involved in the management of their own health care decisions and activities including evaluating their abilities to self-manage their health and disease conditions.

Patient Portal - A patient-centric, web-based tool accessible to patients that offers a secure capability to access their medical information, care plans, wellness programs, health recommendations, and other useful information. It provides a key vehicle for engaging patients and their families through secure messaging between physicians, care managers and patients, record of treatments, and serves as a vehicle for involving patients in the decisions and course of their treatment, particularly as pertains to chronic condition management.

Population Health - The health outcomes of a group of individuals, including the distribution of such outcomes within the group.

Population Health Management - The technical field of endeavor which utilizes a variety of individual, organizational and cultural interventions to help improve the morbidity patterns (i.e., the illness and injury burden) and the health care use behavior of defined populations, with the goals of improving care, access, and affordability.

Predictive Analytics - Statistical techniques and tools used to analyze facts to make predictions and identify problems before they happen. In population health it is a tool that can help predict patients or populations at-risk for a health or medical event, when and how a patient or population may be afflicted with a condition, or how a patient or population of patients may respond to a given treatment.

Prescriptive Analytics - Data mining, machine learning, use of predictive algorithms and information about the health and care of individuals to create a care plan that prescribes specific activities to improve healthcare in an affordable and effective manner.

Primary Care - Primary care is a component of healthcare systems that can effectively address the majority of medical needs for common conditions among people of all ages with the ability to provide a means to improving and sustaining the health status of a community or population.

Randomized Controlled Trial - Considered the gold standard of research methods, randomized controlled trials (RCTs), are an experimental design in which research subjects are chosen and randomly assigned to a treatment group or a control group, and the effects of treatment are then isolated and observed.

Relationship-Centered Care - Relationship-Centered Care (RCC) is a humanistic approach toward patient care that has a foundation of the bio-psycho-social model of healthcare for individals in a social context and a socio-cultural-ecologic model for population health. RCC leverages complementary approaches from medical, technological and social aspects of population health.

Resource-Based Relative Value Scale - The Resource-Based Relative Value Scale (RBRVS), is a system, created and implemented originally by the Health Care Financing Administration (now CMS) that consolidated and standardized physician payments by assigning relative value units (RVUs) for all professional services.

Social Determinants of Health - Living conditions and social circumstances – such as the inequitable distribution of wealth or power – that contribute to differences in health status for individuals and populations.

Specialty BH Settings (Sector) - Clinical delivery settings that support treatment for patients with mild to serious BH conditions but especially cater to the delivery of services for those with serious and persistent primary BH disorders.

Stark Law - Also known as the physician self-referral law, is a civil statute that prohibits physicians from making referrals for "designated health services" reimbursable by Medicare or Medicaid, including hospital services, to entities with which they or their immediate family members have a financial relationship, unless a specific exception to the referral prohibition applies.

Traditional Behavioral Health Service Delivery - BH services delivered in clinical locations separate from medical services by BH providers paid to work in independent BH specialty locations.

URAC- URAC is a nonprofit, independent accreditation agency that provides a nationally and internationally recognized accreditation seal of approval that distinguishes organizations as having met a standard of excellence. URAC works with healthcare industry stakeholders to benchmark URAC standards against key organizational structures and business functions.

"Value-added" Clinical Services - Delivery of clinical care that predictably leads to improved population health while conserving health care resources and comparatively lowering cost.

Appendix B: Author Biographies

Joanne Bohn, MBA, is a published author, book designer, and corresponding editor on contemporary healthcare topics, and principal for KMI Communications, LLC. Bohn is a PhD candidate in Public Health Sciences with a specialization in Health Management at the University of Louisville School of Public Health and Information Sciences.

Kylanne Green is president and CEO of URAC, a national accreditation leader. A Registered Nurse and Adult Nurse Practitioner by background, Ms. Green has more than 40 years of experience in healthcare delivery and insurance strategy and operations. Most recently, she served as Executive Vice President and CEO of Care Management and Health Plan Operations for Inova Health System. While at Inova, Ms. Green was the chief architect of a 50/50 joint venture with Aetna, establishing the first of its kind collaboration between a health system and an insurer. In addition, she oversaw the purchase and subsequent operations of a 60,000 member Virginia Medicaid MCO. Ms. Green served as the Chief Operating Officer of the Health Insurance Association of America, Chief Operating Officer of Aetna Health Plans of the Mid-Atlantic, and held various leadership positions at Kaiser Permanente, where she spent the first 16 years of her career. She also serves on a number of academic, community service and private industry boards, and is a past member of the Council on Graduate Medical Education.

Michael G. Hunt, DO, graduated from the University of Osteopathic Medicine and Health Sciences, Des Moines, Iowa and completed his internship and residency in Pediatrics at William Beaumont Army Medical Center in 1994. After residency, he held several leadership positions including Chief of Medicine and Chief of Pediatrics. In 2005 he joined Mercy, Oklahoma City, to grow his pediatric practice. He advocated for the system to implement an EMR. His participation as physician champion and CMIO helped the organization to implement EPIC in 29 hospitals and 200 ambulatory offices representing more than 50 medical specialties.

Dr. Hunt completed his Masters in Medical Informatics at Northwestern University in 2012, and is an associate professor of informatics at St. Louis University. He is Board Certified in Pediatrics, and is an Assistant Professor of Pediatrics at St. Vincent's Hospital and Medical Center and the Frank H. Netter MD School of Medicine at Quinnipiac University. In addition to his current role as CMO/CMIO of St. Vincent's Health Partners, Inc, Dr. Hunt continues to see patients at St. Vincent's Family Health Center.

St. Vincent's Health Partners, a Physician Hospital Organization in Connecticut, is soon to be nationally recognized as a clinically integrated network by URAC Accreditation. St. Vincent's Health Partners' (SVHP) membership consists of more than 350 providers, and St. Vincent's Medical Center. The organization's mission is to be the leader in healthcare reform, provide patients with high quality cost-effective patient-centric care, and celebrate and reinforce the patient-physician relationship while respecting each participating member's desire to remain independent.

Roger G. Kathol, MD, is president of Cartesian Solutions, Inc., is a health care consultant who assists employers, government agencies, health plans, hospitals and clinics, and care management vendors develop integrated medical and behavioral health programs for patients with high cost health complexity. Dr. Kathol is board certified in internal medicine, psychiatry, and medical management with extensive experience gained during 22 years as a physician/teacher/researcher at the University of Iowa and 16 years as an international health complexity and integrated health solutions, which improve care quality, augment outcomes, and lower total health care and health-related costs. Clients include: general hospitals and clinics, accountable care organizations; general medical health plans; case management programs and vendors; and employers and government agencies. Dr. Kathol is an adjunct professor of internal medicine and psychiatry at the University of Minnesota and has published over 165 peer reviewed articles and 25 book chapters.

Colin Konschak, MBA, FACHE, FHIMSS, is the managing partner and CEO of the Virginia Beach, Va.-based management consulting firm, Divurgent. Divurgent provides services related to Clinical and Revenue Cycle Transformation, as well as Strategic Planning services to providers, payers, and healthcare focused vendors.

Ewa Matuszewski, Ewa Matuszewski is the CEO of MedNetOne Health Solutions (formerly Medical Network One). A champion of innovative primary care and chronic care initiatives, including the award-winning Community Care Travel Team, Ms. Matuszewski has guided MedNetOne Health Solutions (MNOHS) since its founding in 1981 as a traditional physician's organization. Today, MNOHS is not only a P.O., but a healthcare management organization serving the infrastructure and clinical support needs of private practice physicians and behavior health specialists as well as providing broad-base primary care initiatives such as the Patient-Centered Medical Home and Patient-Centered Medical Home Neighborhood, and the High Intensity Care Management (HICM) model for the chronically ill.

Ms. Matuszewski is also thefounding Principal of the Michigan-based, IACET-accredited health care learning organization, Practice Transformation Institute (PTI), which designs, develops and delivers educational programs introducing the twenty-first century model of medicine to the health care community and medical practice teams. She has consulted with medical societies; and state, local, national and international health care organizations and has been a frequent speaker on the management of innovation and primary care based chronic disease programs.

Throughout her many experiences in leading physicians and their practice teams through change, Ms. Matuszewski has promoted a vision of patient-centered medicine and a culture of organizational excellence. Her areas of expertise are health policy analysis, physician workforce strategies, physician practice environment, primary care team leadership, and primary care practice management-governance interface.

She is a member of the Patient Centered Primary Care Collaborative (MPCC), BCBSM Stewardship Council, BCBSM Organized Systems of Care Workgroup, BCBSM High Intensity Care Management Workgroup, Advocates Michigan Osteopathic Association, American College of Physician Executives, and the Michigan Primary Care Consortium. Steering Committee of the Michigan Primary Care Consortium; MPCC Population Registry Task Force; and the Michigan IPIP (Improving Performance in Practice) Steering Committee. She served on the URAC Patient-Centered Health Care Home (PCHCH) Advisory Group.

Steve Melek, is principal and consulting actuary with the Denver Health practice of Milliman. Steve's areas of expertise include healthcare product development, management, and financial analyses. He has worked extensively in the behavioral healthcare specialty field. He has worked with many managed behavioral healthcare organizations, parity issues and cost analyses, mental health utilization and costs in primary care settings, psychotropic drug treatment patterns, and strategic behavioral healthcare system design. He has experience with plan design, pricing, capitation and risk analysis, provider reimbursement analysis and strategies, healthcare revenue distribution, and utilization management analysis. He has completed valuations and projections of healthcare businesses and product lines, profitability and experience analysis, reinsurance analysis, pricing model and strategy development, and actuarial liability determination.

John H. Morse, MBA, is currently Assistant to the Executive Vice President for Health Affairs at the University of Louisville Health Sciences Center. He is currently acting as a loaned executive to the University's Department of Family and Geriatric Medicine, serving as Chief Development Officer for the Department. Prior to joining the Health Sciences Center at the University of Louisville in 1999, Mr. Morse served for four years as the Secretary of the Cabinet for Health Services for the Commonwealth of Kentucky. As such, he was responsible for the Departments of Public Health, Medicaid Services, and Mental Health and Mental Retardation, and the Offices of Licensure and Regulation, Aging Services and Certificate of Need. Prior to serving in Kentucky state government,

Mr. Morse held various executive positions over a 24-year career in the health care industry. He has been a hospital chief executive, a corporate officer with a major managed care company, and president of a start-up physician practice management company.Mr. Morse received his undergraduate degree from the United States Naval Academy and his MBA from the Wharton School of the University of Pennsylvania.

Isaac J. Myers, II, MD, began his healthcare administration career as a family practitioner in 1991 and in 1996 he begins a 20-year career in administrative roles. His extensive experience spans all aspects of healthcare delivery, including a physician hospital organization, management service organization and health insurance companies. His also was an executive leader at Wishard Health Services, one of America's five largest safety net health systems, and was an adjunct faculty member for Indiana University in Indianapolis, teaching Healthcare IT in the Health Care Administration master's program. Dr. Myers joined Baptist's health in February of 2014 as the president of the Baptist Health Medical Group and in October 2014 he was named Baptist's Chief Health Integration Officer. In this role he will lead Baptist's population health strategy, health plan, managed care contracting and employer solutions.Each of Dr. Myers' administrative positions has provided opportunities for him to create efficiencies while consistently improving quality. In addition, he has extensive information technology (IT) experience in integrating electronic health records and designing IT platforms for the health care industry. A New York City native, Dr. Myers holds a bachelor's degree from Hope College in Holland, Mich., and a medical degree from Wayne University in Detroit, completing his family practice residency at Indiana University Hospital.

Brian Nichols, JD, MBA, is a member of Robinson+Cole's Health Law Group, where he represents hospitals, physician groups, nursing homes, community providers, and other provider entities. Mr. Nichols provides legal counsel on a full range of transactional and regulatory health law issues, including contracting, fraud and abuse, tax exemption, licensure, government investigations, medical staff, joint ventures, affiliations, physician recruitment, reimbursement, and privacy of medical information. He also counsels clients on risk management issues. Prior to joining Robinson+Cole, Mr. Nichols worked for eight years in various industries, including aerospace/defense, electric utilities, and health insurance.

Kavita K. Patel, MD, MS, is a Fellow and Managing Director in the Engelberg Center for Health Care Reform at the Brookings Institution where she leads research on delivery system reforms, healthcare cost, physician payment and healthcare workforce productivity. Dr. Patel is, in addition, a practicing primary care physician at Johns Hopkins Medicine and a clinical instructor at UCLA's Geffen School of Medicine. Dr. Patel was previously a Director of Policy for The White House under President Obama and a senior advisor to the late Senator Edward Kennedy. Her prior research in healthcare quality and community approaches to mental illness have earned national recognition and she has published numerous papers and book chapters on healthcare reform and health policy. She has testified before Congress several times and she is a frequent guest expert on CBS, NBC and MSNBC as well as serving on the editorial board of the journal Health Affairs.

Thomas Raskauskas, MD, is CEO of President of St. Vincent's Health Partners, Inc. (SVHP), a physician hospital organization in southwestern Connecticut. He graduated from Georgetown University School of Medicine in Washington, D.C. in 1985, and is a Board Certified Obstetrician Gynecologist. He started his career in private practice in Salem, Massachusetts, and has held teaching appointments through the Medical Schools at Harvard University, Brown University, Michigan State University and Quinnipiac University. Dr. Raskauskas has been a medical director overseeing a multispecialty multi-site clinic, and a Chief Medical Officer for a multi-state Medicaid managed care plan in the Midwest. He served in the United States Navy as a Medical Officer. He has been involved in health reform projects at the state level in both Michigan and Connecticut through the CMS Innovation Center.

Lee Sacks, MD, is Executive Vice President, Chief Medical Officer for Advocate Healthcare and is responsible for health outcomes, safety, clinical transformation, information systems, risk management/insurance, research and medical education and clinical laboratory services at Advocate Health Care. He also serves as Chief Executive Officer of Advocate Physician Partners (APP), the clinically integrated network with 4,500 physicians serving 610,000 attributable lives. Modern Health Care recognized APP as the nation's largest ACO in 2013 and 2014. He serves as Chair of the ACL Lab Operating Committee, the joint venture that provides laboratory services to the Advocate and Aurora systems.

Susan C. Sargent, MBA, is president of Sargent Healthcare Management Advisors, LLC. Ms. Sargent has provided strategic planning, marketing, operations, and management assistance to healthcare providers nationally for over 25 years with a focus on bringing best practice medicine to best practice program and facility design. As such, she has worked with acute care general hospitals, multi-hospital systems, academic medical centers, and specialized civil, forensic and veterans' behavioral health facilities, contributing currency and fluency in the treatment, management, and operational issues facing providers. Sargent HMA is registered with the Central Contractor Registry (CCR) as a small business and a woman-owned business, and is certified as a woman business enterprise (WBE) in Pennsylvania, Delaware, and Virginia.

Deborah S. Smith, MN, RB-BC, is is the Product Development Principal at URAC. Prior to joining the URAC staff she spent 25 years as a consultant for healthcare providers on compliance with accreditation and regulatory requirements, quality improvement, hospital operations, case management and nursing systems. She has a long history of working with URAC on standards development as a volunteer and consultant. Deborah holds both a BSN and MN from UCLA and is board certified by ANCC in Case Management and Advanced Nursing Administration.

Robert Steiner, MD, PhD, is professor of health management and system sciences in the University of Louisville School of Public Health and Information Sciences. Dr. Steiner received his medical degree from the University of Louisville, his PhD in epidemiology from the University of North Carolina at Chapel Hill, and a master's degree in public health from the School of Public Health at the University of North Carolina at Chapel Hill. Dr. Steiner previously served as associate professor in the Department of Family and Community Medicine of the School of Medicine, University of Louisville; deputy director and liaison for the University of Louisville and the Jefferson County Health Department in Louisville; and director of the Healthy Communities Constanta Partnership for Women's Health in Romania. He is a Fellow of the American Board of Preventive Medicine and the American Academy of Family Physicians.

Colleen Swedberg MSN, RN, CNL, obtained her undergraduate nursing degree at the University of Calgary in Alberta, Canada, and Master of Science in Nursing at

Fairfield University in Fairfield, CT. She is certified as a Clinical Nurse Leader (CNL) with the American Association of Colleges of Nursing (AACN). She worked in surgical trauma in Calgary and surgical oncology at Tulane Medical Center in New Orleans as well as community health with Tulane's hospital based home care agency, primarily in the 9th ward of New Orleans. From 1989 to 1996 Colleen worked in rural and urban programs in Haiti primarily in women and children's health including providing technical assistance to an immunization outreach project, reviewing child survival activities funded by a U.S. government grant (micronutrients, diarrhea, health education, immunizations) and with Save the Children Federation, developing the reproductive health subsector with local government and agency medical staff. In the U.S. Colleen became team leader of a VNS maternal child health program in CT, coordinating home-based skilled care to antenatal, postpartum, premature and normal maternal/newborn duos, working to improve access of a medically underserved population to community health services. In 2004, Colleen joined the team of the first Connecticut branch of a national home health care agency, Bayada Home Health Care, progressing to the clinical lead in 2007 of over 30 multidisciplinary field staff providing skilled services to acutely ill patients at home. Currently Colleen serves as Director for Care Coordination and Integration at St. Vincent's Health Partners in Bridgeport, CT. SVHP is a physician-hospital organization representing more than 350 physicians and providers, and a community medical center. SVHP is supporting the efforts of the member medical professionals and institutions to realize the Triple Aim: provide quality care that exceeds patient expectation, improve the health of the patient population, and reduce the cost-of-care. Redefining the roles of care coordination and case management and integrating the use of an organizational Playbook are key strategies to effectively provide health management of the population.

Holton Walker has over 30 years experience in software development, integration and consulting with numerous leadership positions in healthcare, government, and the insurance, and telecommunications industries. He has previously held positions of Executive Director of Technology Solutions at DMR Consulting Group, Principal at BDO Seidman, and Vice President at Marsh, Inc. Holton has been engaged in the development and deployment of healthcare information technology standards since 2008 with a focus on integration architecture and interoperability. Holton has led his own consulting company, Langdon Moore, Inc. since 1999. He has a long-term consultative relationship with ActiveHealth Management where he supports the company's enterprise architecture and client integration solutions.

Ken Yale, DDS, JD, is a senior executive with a track record of creating new products, establishing new markets, and growing innovative healthcare businesses through start-up, capital raising, mergers, acquisitions, and liquidity events. Dr. Yale has extensive prior and current work experience in care and disease management, health information technology, and physician and patient engagement. He is a clinician and business professional with expertise in law, science, and medicine - and experience with government regulation, data science, and health care.

Dr. Yale created a number of health system innovations, including the first Provider Sponsored Network (ACO 1.0) in 2000, led the team that set up Medicare Subvention - now called TRICARE for Life, and ran several Medicare demonstration projects that evolved into the current Medicare Shared Savings Program ACO. He has been an advisor to corporate boards on the future of healthcare and digital health strategies.

Dr. Yale is currently Vice President of Clinical Solutions at ActiveHealth Management, where he is involved in business development, new market creation, and new product innovation. His work focuses on advanced clinical decision support, clinical and financial integration, big data, predictive analytics, and patient engagement. He also holds a teaching appointment in predictive analytics in healthcare with the University of California.

Previously he founded and built innovative health companies in medical management, data analytics, and patient engagement, including Advanced Health Solutions, EduNeering, CorSolutions, Matria Healthcare, UnitedHealth AmeriChoice MSO, and Health Solutions Network. Before building innovative health businesses, he was Chief of Staff of the White House Office of Science and Technology, Special Assistant to the President and Executive Director of the White House Domestic Policy Council (DPC), legislative counsel in the U.S. Senate, and a commissioned officer in the U.S. Public Health Service.

Appendix C: Answers to Chapter Questions

CHAPTER 1

1. What was a central focus of the ACA noted in the chapter?

ANSWER:

Improving population health through the "Triple Aim."

2. What are the six elements of the Care Revolution Era?

ANSWER:

The six elements of the Care Revolution Era include: risk sharing, value seeking, quality focus, population management, technology, and collaborative care.

3. What is one industry shift that results from the Baby Boomer demographic segment's influence on health services?

ANSWER:

The Baby Boomers have contributed to a shift to prevention and chronic care. There will be a ripple effect over future decades requiring new technologies, new services, and emergent care delivery relationships to meet the needs of this segment.

4. What are some of the factors included in the social determinants of health and what is one strategy that CINs may take to address their effect on community and population health?

ANSWER:

Social determinants of health include factors such as housing, income, access to healthy foods, social support networks, education level, behavioral risk factors, and stigma and discrimination. CINs and ACOs should acknowledge and understand social determinants, and engage with community partners to drive medical care and preventive services in a community. Identifying and delivering the most effective treatment plans for patients based on the broader spectrum of needs, taking into account social determinant factors, have been a challenge but one that CINs, ACOs and other care provider organizations can work toward improving over time.

5. What is one novel approach noted in the chapter being piloted in some communities as a way to improve collaboration and population health?

ANSWER:

Accountable care communities emerged in 2013 with a pilot program in Akron, OH. In this pilot, there is a collaborative, multidisciplinary effort among health care delivery organizations, community partners, faith-based organizations, and public health service providers with a focus on solving some aspects of the social determinant challenges that impact population health.

6. What are the four areas that help illustrate the changing environment in the Care Revolution Era?

ANSWER:

The four areas of change fueling the Care Revolution Era include: healthcare reform, technology innovation, social determinants of health, and population demographics.

CHAPTER 2

1. Name and discuss at least four characteristics of primary care.

ANSWER:

Starfield suggested the following characteristics for primary care:

- First-contact for care;
- Continuity of care over time;
- Comprehensiveness of care, including concern for the whole person rather than one disease or one physiologic system; and

- Coordination of care with other parts of the health care system.

2. How are the concepts of chronic care model, insurance reform and healthcare financing reform related to the development of PCMH?

ANSWER:

The Chronic Care Model is designed to enable primary care clinical teams to interact with patients in a social context to minimize symptoms and maximize functional status and quality of life. Insurance reform is the essence of ACA, providing increased access to medical insurance coverage, especially cost-effective primary care, for those who are currently un-insured or under-insured. Healthcare financing reform is designed to increase payments to primary care physicians and better balance the demand for specialty medical services. Changing to value-based outcomes and reimbursements, rather than fee-for-service payments, will aid in this transition. All three of these concepts use the primary care team, and specifically PCMH, as a foundation on which to build.

3. Why are HIT and EMR important for the development of PCMH, ACO and CIN?

ANSWER:

HIT and EMR are sources of information for clinical decision-making, necessary for PCMH, ACO, and CIN to meet both their clinical and financial goals and objectives

4. What is the Triple Aim? How is it related to PCMH?

ANSWER:

The Triple Aim is a short-hand way, coined by Dr. Donald Berwick (former head of CMS), to reference actions needed to reform healthcare, and includes improved population health, lower costs, and improved patient's experience of care. These principles are common to many new models of care, such as the PCMH.

5. How do the topics of complexity in management and relationship-centered care relate to PCMH?

ANSWER:

Complexity is a new perspective, representing a new paradigm for relationship-centered care, inter-dependence, network sciences, and socio-ecologic context. Both interpersonal relationships and technical skills are necessary for optimal outcomes in patient care. Complexity typically involves bottom-up and shared methods for decision-making in primary care arenas, more so than hierarchical or top-down directives that are more common in emergency situations and tertiary specialty care, although the two methods are not mutually exclusive. Complexity depends upon the availability and qualities of local resources, and the values that are present within the local communities and office settings where clinical care will be offered. There is no standard strategy to approach the transformation of primary care to the PCMH model, and both complexity and relationship-centered care can help in making the transformation. Indeed, the culture-of-care in any setting is an emergent property, and depends on the diverse interactions between people in their social environments.

CHAPTER 3

1. What are the six types of ACO models listed in the chapter?

ANSWER:

a) IPA-directed, b) MSPG-directed, c) PHO-directed, d) IDN-directed, e) private payer directed, and f) private payer partnership.

2. What are three styles of leadership discussed in the chapter?

ANSWER:

The three styles of leadership discussed include:

a) Situational - adaptable to specific situations and understands the need for worker empowerment.

b) Transformational - facilitates team growth and influences subordinates to move toward ethically inspired goals.

c) Servant - engages in active listening, engages in empathy, and creates a community in the workplace.

3. What are 'Relational Connectors' and how does Malcolm Gladwell's "*The Tipping Point*" fit in to the concept?

ANSWER:

Relational Connectors is identified as one of the Building Blocks for CIN and ACO Leaders. Relational connector leaders operate as connectors for their organizations and in their communities. In Malcolm Gladwell's 2001 classic, *The Tipping Point: How Little Things Can Make a Big Difference*, Gladwell emphasized relational connectors' "...ability to span many different worlds is a function of something intrinsic to their personality." When applying this notion to CIN or ACO leaders, we see leaders who can recognize all the nodes in the community ecosystem that can benefit from CIN and ACO goals, such as improving patient outcomes, increasing access to care, and lowering the cost of care for their communities.

4. What are the four elements necessary for effective ACO governance according to the AMA?

ANSWER:

The four elements are a) medical decisions should be made by physicians; b) governance should be by a board of directors elected by the ACO's professionals; c) Physician leadership should be licensed in the state in which the ACO operates and licensed for the active practice of medicine in the ACO's service area and d) the ACO's governing board should be separate from and independent of the hospital's board of directors (when a hospital is part of the ACO entity).

5. What is the Accountable Care Network (ACN) concept? Where was it first cited?

ANSWER:

An Accountable Care Network (ACN) is a new concept comprised of three or more separate business entities, such as a physician group, hospital, and insurer, with a formal shared vision, mission, network strategy, and network governance structure. This conceptual operating model focuses heavily on patient engagement using innovative health information technologies. It was first cited in the book *Accountable Care. Bridging the Health Information Technology Divide, First Edition.*

6. What are the two pillars of the Building Blocks for CIN and ACO Leaders (found in Figure 3-1)?

ANSWER:

The two pillars of the Building Blocks for CIN and ACO Leaders are Shared Purpose and Shared Culture. Shared Purpose is a core trait, and means establishing a common bond and positive motivating force to help an organization achieve their goals and engage and drive collaborative multidisciplinary teams. Shared Culture is comprised of three key elements—mission, values, and engagement. Any CIN or ACO leader must be able to communicate the mission and the vision of the organization and be able to drive positive engagement of clinical and administrative staff to accomplish that mission and vision.

CHAPTER 4

1. What are two essential elements of culture for a CIN or ACO as discussed in the chapter?

ANSWER:

The two essential elements of culture addressed in the chapter are how the culture is created, and the importance of consistant actions, including a heedful focus on mission critical systems and striving to improve patient safety.

2. What is a "takeaway" from the St. Vincent's Health Partners CIN Development Workplan case example in the four figures illustrated in the chapter?

ANSWER:

One "takeaway" is that the work plan should be developed and then revisited periodically to update progress of the CIN.

3. What are the five key initiatives in the CIN/ACO Start-up Planning Framework? How might you apply these initiatives to your own organization?

ANSWER:

The five key intiatives in the CIN/ACO Start-up Planning Framework include: establishing the mission and vision; situational awareness of the business environement of the CIN/ACO stakeholders; understanding weaknesses of the organization and internal threats that can weaken the organization; developing an intelligence network that feeds off agents and interactions among individuals and organizations to identify changes needed to support organizational advancement; and systematic innovation to create new and improved services.

4. Regarding physician/provider relations, what is the key transition that has taken place with the shift from a provider-centric focus in the industry to a patient-centric focus (as noted in the chapter)?

ANSWER:

The key transition that has taken place with the shift from a provider centric to patient centered focus is leaving behind autonomy and control and moving toward collaboration, empowerment of others, and performance based upon data driven analysis and evidence.

5. Patient engagement was noted as one of the essential elements and building blocks in the evolution of any network. What are some key considerations for patient engagement (and patient experience as a part of patient engagement) as discussed in the chapter?

ANSWER:

Key components include: measuring patient engagement, focusing on evaluation of specific events, patient surveys focusing on "patint-provider interactions," and ensuring timely assessment of the patient's experience of care received.

CHAPTER 5

1. How can an ACO take advantage of the pre-participation waiver?

ANSWER:

An ACO can take advantage of the pre-participation waiver if the ACO is engaged in a good- faith, diligent process to submit an application for participation in the MSSP and has an arrangement that contributes to the goals of the MSSP. The ACO's governing body must make and duly authorize a bona fide determination that the start-up arrangement is reasonably related to the purposes of the MSSP. The documentation of the arrangement must be made at the same time that the arrangement is entered into and must describe the steps being taken to participate in the MSSP. A description of the arrangement must be made public on the ACO's website.

2. Can an ACO member provide electronic health records software to physician participants in the ACO?

ANSWER: Members of ACOs can take advantage of the pre-participation waiver and/or the participation waiver to "donate" electronic health records software to ACO participants without having to comply with the requirements of the Anti-kickback Statute or Stark Law.

3. Do the MSSP Waivers apply to ACOs participating in private payer arrangements?

ANSWER:

No. Commercial ACOs cannot take advantage of the Waivers as they only apply to the MSSP.

4. What are four innovation areas identified in the second edition that still hold merit for CINs and ACOs to develop closer integration within the construct of antitrust regulations?

ANSWER:

Four innovation areas, identified in the second edition and carried over here to the third edition, for CINs and ACOs to continue to develop tighter integration include:

a. Formation and ongoing management of the joint venture;
b. Regulatory monitoring, especially in the formative stages of the organization;
c. Clinical and financial integration; and
d. Compliance with FTC, DOJ, DHHS, CMS, IRS, and other government regulations.

5. What guidance did the IRS issue in 2011 regarding involvement of tax-exempt hospitals or other healthcare organizations in the Medicare Shared Savings Program?

ANSWER:

In summary, the guidance indicated that participation in an ACO through the MSSP, in accordance with the rules and regulations relating to the proper creation and maintenance of such MSSP or ACO, will not, in and of itself, affect the tax consequences for a tax-exempt participant.

6. What conditions must be met for the Stark Law to be waived with respect to arrangements in an ACO?

ANSWER:

In order for the Stark Law to be waived for the participants in an ACO the following conditions must be met:

a. The ACO has entered into a participation agreement with CMS and remains in good standing;
b. The ACO satisfies requirements regarding governance, leadership and management of the ACO;

c.   The ACO's governing body must make and duly authorize a bona fide determination that the arrangement is reasonably related to the purposes of the MSSP;

d.   The documentation of the arrangement must be contemporaneous with the establishment of the arrangement, the authorization, and with the diligent steps; and

e.   Public disclosure of the arrangement.

(see chapter details in Stark Law section for additional details)

7. What are the three landmark laws that form the framework for antitrust law enforcement?

ANSWER:

The three landmark laws that create the framework for antitrust regulations are: the Sherman Act of 1890, the Federal Trade Commission Act of 1914, and the Clayton Act of 1914.

8. What types of conduct should be avoided by CINs and ACOs to reduce the likelihood of antitrust investigation?

ANSWER:

Five types of conduct were noted in the Federal Register in 2011 to be avoided by CINs and ACOs in order to reduce the likelihood of antitrust investigations:

a.   Taking actions to keep commercial payers from directing or incentivizing patients to choose certain providers;

b.   Implicit or explicit linkage of sales (through pricing policy) of ACO services to commercial payers' purchase of other services from providers outside the ACO including providers affiliated with an ACO participant;

c.   Except for primary care physicians, "contracting with other ACO physician specialists, hospitals, ambulatory service centers, or other providers on an exclusive basis, thus preventing or discouraging them from contracting outside the ACO, either individually or through other ACOs or provider networks";

d. "Restricting a commercial payer's ability to make available to its health plan enrollees cost, quality, efficiency, and performance information to aid enrollees in evaluating and selecting providers in the health plan..."; and

e. "Sharing among the ACO's provider participants competitively sensitive pricing or other data that they could use to set prices or other terms for services they provide outside the ACO."

CHAPTER 6

1. What are the six dimensions of quality and how do you think they might be measured?

ANSWER:

The six dimensions of quality are:

Dimension	Description
Safe	Avoiding injuries to patients from the care that is intended to help them.
Effective	Providing services based on scientific knowledge to all who could benefit and refraining from providing services to those not likely to benefit (avoiding underuse and overuse).
Patient Centered	Providing care that is respectful of and responsive to individual patient preferences, needs, and values and ensuring that patient values guide all clinical decisions.
Timely	Reducing waiting times and harmful delays for both those who receive and those who give care.
Efficient	Avoiding waste, in particular waste of equipment, supplies, ideas, and energy.
Equitable	Providing care that does not vary in quality because of personal characteristics such as gender, ethnicity,

Dimension	Description
	geographic location, and socioeconomic status.

Possible measures could include:

Category	Measure
Safe	# documented injuries per inpatient day; % patients in a population documented as injured; # and % of types of errors / injuries reported; % of errors occurring during transitions of care.
Effective	% practitioners in a group demonstrating compliance with selected care guidelines; % of patients in a population with a specific identified condition who met targeted outcomes (eg: BMI, HA1c; LDL; use of rescue inhaler rate); % of patients in a population with a specific identified condition who met self-management goals; mortality rates.
Patient Centered	% of health records documenting patient/family/caregiver involvement in decision making; patient satisfaction / experience of care scores; patient complaint rates related to patient-centered values (respect, responsiveness, preferences, needs, personal values); quality of life outcomes.
Timely	% of requests for same day appointments fulfilled on the day requested; % of hospital discharge / transition of care plan documents sent to / received by the next provider within 24 hours of discharge; % of diagnostic study results available at time of next office visit.
Efficient	% reduction in avoidable hospitalization and/or ED visit rates; cost reductions from efficient use of resources.
Equitable	Disparity of care reductions in a contracted population; closure rates for gaps in care of under-served populations.

2. What metrics would you choose to evaluate achievement of the three aspects of the Triple Aim using process measures?

ANSWER:

Aspect of the Triple Aim	Process Measure
Improving patient experience of care;	% of patients assessed for self-management ability; % of patients whose records demonstrate involvement in decision-making.
Improving the health of populations;	% of eligible consumers engaged in a disease management program
Reducing per capita cost of care	Resource use (e.g. # inpatient days; # ED visits; cost of pharmaceuticals)

3. What metrics would you choose to evaluate achievement of the three aspects of the Triple Aim using outcome measures?

ANSWER:

Aspect of the Triple Aim	Outcome Measure
Improving patient experience of care;	% of patients reporting overall satisfaction at the highest level of the scale; % of patients reporting satisfaction with their provider at the highest level of the scale.
Improving the health of populations;	Changes in functional status, morbidity (eg: BMI, HA1c; LDL; use of rescue inhaler rate); mortality rates.
Reducing per capita cost of care	Comparison over time of per capita cost of care in actual $ spent.

4. Why is transparency of data the gold standard?

ANSWER:

Transparency of data is the gold standard because it is most consistent with the demands of accountability. Level of accountability can be seen as directly related to degree of transparency and the audiences to whom a practice discloses its performance data.

5. Why is measurement and reporting accountability important to practice transformation?

ANSWER:

Practice transformation depends not only on improvements in workflow processes and patient-centeredness, but also on the ability to modify practice patterns and improve population health. Measurement announces progress or failure on these latter two variables. Practitioners participating in value-based accountable organizations and networks must have comparative feedback to gauge their individual and collective performance to enable rewards distribution and/or course corrections.

CHAPTER 7

1. What are some points to consider in developing a plan for managing increasing risk for the CIN/ACO while working in a largely fee-for-service oriented market?

ANSWER:

There are several points to consider in developing a plan for managing risk, starting with a risk tolerance assessment, which can be a continuous monitoring activity or functional evaluation at critical decision making points. A transition plan from fee for service to other reimbursement models needs to be mapped out. Total cost of care actuarial and accounting capabilities need to be developed. Curriculum at academic medical centers is needed in this field to provide proper skills for future physician leaders. Finally, the risk sharing distribution model needs to be developed.

2. What are the five elements of a financial roadmap for CINs and ACOs discussed in the chapter?

ANSWER:

The five elements of a financial road map discussed in this chapter include a risk tolerance assessment, engaging in revenue cycle management, developing physician compensation models, internal audit capabilities to ensure the integrity of the organization, and financial capital management.

3. How is the four-stage learning system model (from the IOM's 2001 *Crossing the Quality Chasm* report) applied to payment model evolution?

ANSWER:

The four stage learning system model, going from highly fragment to a highly adaptive learning system, can help organizations develop pathways that lead from a fee-for-service model to interim reimbursement models the allow an institution to fund tomorrow's delivery of care financed by today's reimbursement. Having a mix of models that transition away from fee-for-service and adapt to quality-based payment structures helps the organization develop into a clinically integrated network.

4. What are global payments for CINs and ACOs and what is one of the most important benefits from their use and adoption?

ANSWER:

Global payments for CINs and ACOs provide a single payment to cover all the costs of care for a person's treatment during a specific period of time regardless of the number of patient episodes experienced. They are intended to contain costs and reduce the use of unnecessary services, at the same time encouraging integration and coordination of services across the care continuum.

5. What are the four categories of bundled payment models from CMS's bundled payment demonstration?

ANSWER:

The four categories of bundled payment models from the CMS demonstration on bundled payments are:

Model 1- the episode of care is defined as the inpatient stay in the acute care hospital. Medicare will pay the hospital a discounted amount based on the payment rates established under the Inpatient Prospective Payment System used in the original Medicare program. Medicare will continue to pay physicians separately for their services under the Medicare Physician Fee Schedule. Under certain circumstances, hospitals and physicians will be permitted to share gains arising from the providers' care redesign efforts;

Model 2- the episode-based payment is retrospective. Medicare continues to make fee-for-service (FFS) payments to providers and suppliers furnishing services to beneficiaries in Model 2 episodes, after which the total payment for a beneficiary's episode is reconciled against a bundled payment amount (the target price) predetermined by CMS. Retrospective, acute care hospital stay for an episode will include all services up to 30, 60 or 90 days post inpatient discharge. Participants select up to 48 different clinical condition episodes;

Model 3- the episode-based payment is retrospective. Medicare continues to make fee-for-service (FFS) payments to providers and suppliers furnishing services to beneficiaries in Model 3, after which the total payment for a beneficiary's episode is reconciled against a bundled payment amount (the target price) predetermined by CMS. The episode includes post-acute care following an inpatient acute care hospital stay and all related care covered under Medicare Part A and Part B within 30, 60, or 90 days following initiation of post-acute services;

Model 4- the episode-based payment is prospective. CMS makes a single, predetermined bundled payment to the Episode Initiator (an acute care hospital) instead of an Inpatient Prospective Payment System (IPPS) payment. The bundled payment includes all Medicare Part A and Part B covered services furnished during the inpatient stay by the hospital, physicians, and nonphysician practitioners, as well as any related readmissions that occur within 30 days after discharge.

CHAPTER 8

1. The fishbone diagram demonstrates the most common challenges facing an organization. How do you use the fishbone to meet the ever-changing organizational stressors that prevent high quality patient care?

ANSWER:

The fishbone may be used to establish a baseline of the known contributing stressors to care coordination unique to the organization. The fishbone has four major components: Provider, Structure, Patients, and Quality Relationships. Within each of those components, or 'bones,' are issues or processes that require organizational attention to achieve patient-centered, timely, safe, effective, efficient, and equitable care. Use the fishbone to clarify the cause and effect status of the challenges to care coordination unique to the organization. Opportunities for improvement can then be identified. Improvement work can proceed depending on decision making based on the organization's resources and priorities. This process provides a logical and sustainable strategy for continuous improvement.

2. What are the actionable features of the proposed care coordination model? How does it answer the Triple Aim?

ANSWER:

The Triple Aim is improved population health, lower costs, and improved patient's experience of care. The care coordination model empowers every health care provider (irrespective of specialty) to provide coordinate case management directly with patients. and enhance the provider-patient relationship. Care Coordination focuses on the population using evidence-based guidelines. Care coordination allows the provider to identify patients with risk, care gaps, and those who are high resource utilizers. Care

Coordination "empowers" case managers and provider staff to manage individual patients. When quality follows national care guidelines and information is shared between providers, efficient use of medical resources occurs. Efficient use of medical resources lowers costs. Patients engaged in purposeful care coordination will have the opportunity to participate in development of their care plans and consequently have a personal stake in their care resulting in greater patient satisfaction.

3. Describe how the proposed care coordination model contributes to the goals of clinical integration.

ANSWER:

The goals of clinical integration (according to the URAC definition) include providers working together to share clinical data within a framework, rendering necessary care to patients in an efficient manner with the best possible outcomes. Successful clinical integration requires collaboration and coordination at all levels of the network, thus the care coordination model contributes to the goals of clinical integration.

4. Describe the difference between case management and care coordination.

ANSWER:

Care coordination is performed primarily at the enterprise level while case management is delivered patient-by-patient at the local level. Case management directly engages the patient with their care and services, educates the patient about disease management, facilitates solutions, and overcomes barriers that inhibit effective care. Case managers assist with discharge follow-up, and tailor medical service referrals to reflect the individual's needs. Care coordination, on the other hand, reinforces the culture of the integrated network and the inherent linkages instilled amongst physicians, hospitals, skilled nursing facilities and ambulatory settings. Care coordinators, based at the corporate/enterprise level, do not necessarily have direct patient contact. Instead, they utilize patient-specific and population level medical data to constantly oversee the attributed patients of the organization and ensure gaps of care are closed. A common operational issue that distinguishes case management from care coordination is that once a patient is discharged the case manager no longer works with the individual, or continued contact is narrowly focused to the exclusion of other chronic diseases or healthcare issues, whereas with care coordiantion, the patient is always being evaluated for care gaps. (See Table 8.1)

CHAPTER 9

1. How does clinical integration assist providers to thrive in a value-based market?

ANSWER:

Clinically integrated networks are collaborative, provider-led ventures based on the goal of financial sustainability in a value-based market environment. Successful CINs develop the infrastructure to make improvements in quality, utilization and cost and demonstrate progress in management of the health of their population via measurement and reporting. Alignment of business interests with integrated clinical practice leads to opportunities for rewarding provider network participation, medical neighborhood formation, and sustainable practice in a value-based market.

2. What are the essential goals of clinically integrated network providers?

ANSWER:

Essential goals of CIN providers are financial sustainability and clinical transformation. Everything flows from these goals, including the objectives of clinical quality, health outcomes, and cost efficiency. At its core, the CIN is market driven, thus the focus on financial and clinical goals. Because of federal government (FTC) regulations, the driving business model is wedded to consumer interests. As a result, CIN leadership must be provider dominated with strong philosophical cohesion among providers aligning together for both clinical and financial integration in a way that ultimately benefits the consumer.

3. How does the process of becoming accredited assist providers to develop successful networks?

ANSWER:

Accreditation programs are the health care industry's mechanisms to advance the adoption of systems, processes and performance requirements according to predetermined criteria and consistent agreed-upon national standards. Standards provide clarity to principles required to function as a clinically integrated entity. The roadmap found in accreditation standards are enabling and validating pathways for successful integration and accountability. URAC standards are formed in ways that capture sound business practices for whatever type of venture is seeking accreditation.

4. What are the goals of care coordination in a CIN?

ANSWER:

The goals of coordination are streamlined care facilitated by effective communication. Clinical integration demands the capability of rendering high-quality, coordinated care services to the network's designated population. Coordination is expected throughout the medical neighborhood among all providers. Successful CIN leaders, management and providers understand the ability of a CIN to achieve cost-reduction and quality-improvement objectives is dependent on the daily execution of integrated, collaborative activity.

5. How does development of health information technology capabilities facilitate value generation within a clinically integrated organization?

ANSWER:

Demonstrating and documenting quality in a CIN are among the critical capabilities vested in the construction and intelligent implementation of information systems and infrastructure. For governance to create, communicate and align incentives, and for clinicians to play their roles in a coordinated system, there has to be a unifying and accessible information network readily available. Technology and infrastructure, when sophisticated and ubiquitous, supports decision-making, record-keeping, population management and performance assessment – all critical functions of a CIN. The accreditation process acknowledges the essential role of technology in the success of a CIN by emphasizing core standards that encourage planning for technology acquisition over time. Reporting requirements are more easily met in organizations having some level of automation.

CHAPTER 10

1. How does Meaningful Use affect ACOs and CINs, now and in the future?

ANSWER:

Medicare ACO quality measures include an EHR adoption measure based on meaningful use of a certified EHR. To emphasize the importance of the measure, it is double weighted in the Medicare ACO scoring paradigm. In commercial ACOs and CINs, the adoption of EHR technology is an enabling factor in the organization's ability to meet their objectives, however meaningful use is not as important and may be replaced by other, more advanced technologies and processes.

2. What are key technology capabilities required to support an ACO or CIN?

ANSWER:

Throughout the chapter a number of key technology capabilities were noted as critical to develop and operate an ACO or CIN. They include: patient portals, technology standards, health information exchange, interoperability, Meaningful Use, EHR functional capacity, data exchange, flexible message routing and distribution, and population health management.

3. How does interoperability and health information exchange assist quality of care?

ANSWER:

Achieving interoperability and health information exchange assists in improving the quality of care delivered by ACOs and CINs in a variety of ways. For example, physicians, nurses and other clinical service providers benefit from access to comprehensive patient records that inform them of clinical, quality, and financial metrics. By leveraging interoperability and health information exchange, clinicians improve care and quality through:

- Avoidance of duplicate procedures based on access to existing results and orders;

- Avoidance of contraindicated procedures and medications;

- Sound evidence-based clinical judgment and care paths based on a complete patient clinical history;

- Wireless telemetry of home devices informing physicians and care managers of adherence and effectiveness;

- Secure communication with care coordinators and the patient; and

- Performance monitoring, reporting, and feedback.

4. What is the value of aggregating data from diverse sources?

ANSWER:

The value of aggregating data from diverse sources is to provide a more comprehensive clinical record and patient view from data obtained from a variety of sources.

5. What is predictive analytics and how does it help with population health management and individual care?

ANSWER:

Predictive analytics includes disciplines such as data mining, machine learning, and use of predictive algorithms and other statistical methods to mine past and current data to predict what will happen to a patient or population in the future.

CHAPTER 11

1. The expected total cost of care for patients with a chronic illness and a concurrent behavioral health condition compared to a general population of medical patients will be:

a) About the same

b) Twice as much

c) Three to four times as much

d) Five to six times as much

ANSWER:

Answer C. Three to four times as much.

2. The majority of increased cost of care for patients with behavioral health conditions is for:

a) Medical treatment

b) Psychiatric hospitalization

c) Psychotropic medication

d) Residential care

ANSWER:

Answer A. Medical treatment.

3. "Carve-out" and "carve-in" managed behavioral health organizations:

a) Are owned by the medical insurer that covers medical benefit payments.

b) Use payment practices that encourage delivery of behavioral health services in the medical setting.

c) Manage networks of behavioral health providers separate and apart from medical providers.

d) Use the same claims adjudication procedures as for medical benefits.

ANSWER: Answer C. Manage networks of behavioral health providers separate and apart from medical providers.

4. CINs/ACOs in which behavioral health providers are contracted professional resources but not network members can be expected to:

a) Provide easily accessible behavioral health services for high cost, complex network patients.
b) Improve clinical outcomes and lower cost in the majority of network patients with behavioral health comorbidity.
c) Follow CIN/ACO policies and procedures (referral use, documentation, formularies, clinical guidelines) just as medical specialty network providers.
d) None of the above

ANSWER:

Answer D. None of the above.

5. What percentage of patients with behavioral health conditions is seen and receives the majority of their BH treatment in the behavioral health sector?

a) 10-20%
b) 30-50%
c) 60-80%
d) 90-100%

ANSWER:

Answer A. 10-20%

6. On average, the length of stay for medical/surgical inpatients with behavioral health comorbidity is:

a) 1 day shorter due to psychiatric hospital transfer
b) The same
c) 1 day longer
d) 4 days longer

ANSWER:

Answer C. 1 day longer.

7. On average, the thirty-day readmission rate for medical/surgical inpatient discharges with behavioral health comorbidity is:

a) >30% higher than those without
b) 20%-30% higher than those without
c) 10%-20% higher than those without
d) 5%-10% higher than those without

ANSWER:

Answer A. >30% higher than those without.

CHAPTER 12

1. What is comparative effectiveness research (CER)?

ANSWER:

Applied research that compares different medical devices, drugs, and treatment methods to determine which are more effective in treating a disease or condition. CER attempts to determine "what works best" in healthcare by comparing different therapies meant to treat the same disease or condition. Also defined by the IOM as,

> ...the generation and synthesis of evidence that compares the benefits and harms of alternative methods to prevent, diagnose, treat, and monitor a clinical condition or to improve the delivery of care. The purpose of CER is to assist consumers, clinicians, purchasers, and policy makers to make informed decisions that will improve health care at both the individual and population levels.

2. Why should CINs and ACOs be interested in comparative effectiveness research?

ANSWER:

CINs and ACOs are responsible for the cost and quality of care for a given population. As a result, these organizations have a growing interest in what works and which treatments are more effective. Interest from CINs and ACOs in CER is increasing as they are at greater risk for the cost and quality of care, and they see the clinical and financial benefits and drawbacks of specific treatment options. As the ACO and CIN models evolve they will become more involved in medical coverage decisions, benefit design, and appeals of decisions about care they provide, all of which benefit from a greater understanding of both therapeutic and cost-effectiveness provided by CER.

3. What types of organizations have conducted CER in the past, and why?

ANSWER:

Life science and pharmaceutical companies, health plans, healthcare providers, and other private sector organizations perform different types of CER-related initiatives. Private organizations have also been established solely to organize, support, or conduct CER. Governments may compare different treatments for a variety of purposes, including basic scientific research to: a) increase knowledge, b) identify the highest-value product or service for government reimbursement, and c) to meet legislative needs for therapeutic or cost effectiveness research.

4. What type of work does PCORI perform?

ANSWER:

PCORI was created to Identify priorities for comparative effectiveness research and fund research comparing "health outcomes and clinical effectiveness, risks, and benefits of two or more medical treatments, services, or items." PCORI takes a patient-centered approach, and is designed to improve the interaction between patient and provider by increasing the availability of valid evidence-based medical information to enable meaningful discussion between patient and the clinician.

5. Why are health plans interested in CER?

ANSWER:

Because they are at risk for the cost of care, legally accountable for the quality of care, required to justify coverage decisions, and must work with patients or physicians who challenge these decisions and adjudicate their appeals. They can use the results of CER to increase knowledge of evidence-based medicine, develop best practice clinical protocols, and provide clinical decision support tools and technologies to physicians, nursing care managers, and patients.

6. How is health information technology benefiting CER?

ANSWER:

Health information technology (HIT) is being used in a number of CER approaches and is deeply engrained in the advancement of CER. ARRA designated $268 million for data infrastructure development and HIT, intended to facilitate new opportunities for analysis of claims data and clinical records from electronic health record systems – both activities that can be used in CER.

CHAPTER 13

1. Identify one essential element to reduce the threats of chronic conditions.

ANSWER:

Self-management is one of eight essential elements the World Health Organization (WHO) has defined as necessary to reduce the threats chronic conditions pose to their citizens, their healthcare systems and their economies.

2. What are the two elements that have not been easily integrated into patient self-management?

ANSWER:

Two elements that have not been easily integrated into self-management are patient engagement and motivation to change.

3. What is a method used to gauge a patient's knowledge, skills and confidence needed to self-manage their health?

ANSWER:

Motivational interviewing is a method to gauge the patient's knowledge, skills and confidence needed to self-manage their health and disease.

4. What are the core concepts of Wagner's Chronic Care Model?

ANSWER:

The core concepts include health system organization, clinical information systems, self-management support, community resources and policies, delivery system design, and decision support – all of which is designed to produce an informed, activated patient interacting with a prepared pro-active, practice team.

5. What is the Transtheoretical Model (TTM)?

ANSWER:

The Transtheoretical Model (TTM), also known as the Stages of Change (SOC), is a concept that can help clinicians and patients understand readiness to make changes in behavoir, barriers to change, and help patients anticipate relapse.

6. What are the four different levels patients move through?

ANSWER:

The Patient Activation Measure (PAM) score reflects the four different levels patients move through, from passive recipient to greater activation:

Level 1 – patients are overwhelmed and unprepared to play an active role in their own health,

Level 2 – lack of knowledge and confidence to self-manage,

Level 3 – beginning to take action; still lack confidence and skill to support positive behaviors,

Level 4 – Adoption of the behavior to support their health but may relapse when under stress.

CHAPTER 14

1. What are the four strategic lenses for ACO/CIN environment monitoring?

ANSWER:

The four lenses are: economic, legal, technology/infrastructure, and population health. The healthcare environment is rapidly changing, so physician, nursing, ancillary, and administrative leaders need to stay abreast of emergent issues that can lead to opportunities to positively impact the bottom line for the organization and the health of the community's population.

2. What are three characteristics of institutional change, as described by Richard Scott, PhD?

ANSWER:

Three characteristics of institutional change include:

- "A focus on the interdependence of, and interactions between, organized units at multiple levels;

- Awareness of the effects of non-local, as well as local factors; and

- An awareness that processes may produce convergence of procedures and forms but also promote diversity and the emergence of new types of social behavior and novel systems."

(Scott, 2010)

3. What are the four dimensions of an integrated delivery organization that help conceptualize ways to improve care delivery?

ANSWER:

The four dimensions of an integrated delivery organization that help conceptualize ways to improve care delivery are the CIN, providers, consumers, and communities.

4. What section of the ACA eliminated the denial of pre-existing conditions for consumers to get health insurance coverage?

ANSWER:

Section 1101 (access to health insurance for uninsured and those with pre-existing conditions). This section eliminated the practice of prohibiting consumers from getting health insurance due to pre-existing conditions. This factor has long kept many Americans from being able to obtain health insurance coverage.

5. From the Aetna and Banner Health Network commercial ACO partnership what were some of the initial benefits achieved?

ANSWER:

The partnership between Aetna and BHN achieved improvements in their rates of cancer screenings, diabetes control, and reduction in use of radiology services in the first few months of operation.

6. From the Recommendations for Future ACO and CIN Leaders what are key elements of the Care Coordination and Community Engagement recommendations?

ANSWER:

For Care Coordination a key element is to ensure that "continuous communication" is used to connect all medical professionals through enabling technologies and processes that continuously improve performance and reach patients when and where they need it most. For Community Engagement a key element is to drive participation in multi-stakeholder collaborations to ensure communication, understanding and adoption.

Index

CPSIA information can be obtained
at www.ICGtesting.com
Printed in the USA
LVHW021648080822
725445LV00004B/26

Prealgebra

Third Edition

Marvin L. Bittinger

Indiana University—Purdue University
at Indianapolis

David J. Ellenbogen

Community College of Vermont

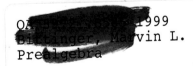
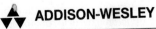 ADDISON-WESLEY

An imprint of Addison Wesley Longman, Inc.

Reading, Massachusetts • Menlo Park, California • New York • Harlow, England
Don Mills, Ontario • Sydney • Mexico City • Madrid • Amsterdam

Publisher	Jason A. Jordan
Project Manager	Ruth Berry
Assistant Editor	Susan Connors Estey
Managing Editor	Ron Hampton
Production Supervisor	Kathleen A. Manley
Production Coordinator	Jane DePasquale
Design Direction	Susan Carsten
Text Designer	Rebecca Lloyd Lemna
Editorial and Production Services	Jennifer Bagdigian
Copy Editor	Martha Morong/Quadrata, Inc.
Art Editor	Janet Theurer
Photo Researcher	Naomi Kornhauser
Marketing Managers	Craig Bleyer and Laura Rogers
Illustrators	Scientific Illustrators, Gayle Hayes, and Rolin Graphics
Compositor	The Beacon Group
Cover Designer	Jeannet Leendertse
Cover Photographs	© Photodisc, 1998; © Navaswan/FPG International
Prepress Buyer	Caroline Fell
Manufacturing Coordinator	Evelyn Beaton

LIBRARY OF CONGRESS CATALOGING-IN-PUBLICATION DATA

Bittinger, Marvin L.
    Prealgebra/Marvin L. Bittinger, David J. Ellenbogen.—3rd ed.
        p. cm.
    Includes index.
    ISBN 0-201-34024-0
    1. Mathematics. I. Ellenbogen, David. II. Title.
QA39.2.B585 1999
513'.14—dc21
                                    99-26893
                                       CIP

Annotated Instructor's Edition 0-201-64602-1

1 2 3 4 5 6 7 8 9 10—VH—02010099

In Memory of Saul Ellenbogen,
Whose Love of Art and Mathematics
Served as Inspiration

Contents

3 Fractional Notation: Multiplication and Division   143

4 Fractional Notation: Addition and Subtraction   205

Developmental Units   619

Preface

This text is the first in a series of texts that includes the following:

Bittinger: *Basic Mathematics*, Eighth Edition

Bittinger: *Introductory Algebra*, Eighth Edition

Bittinger: *Intermediate Algebra*, Eighth Edition

Bittinger/Beecher: *Introductory and Intermediate Algebra: A Combined Approach*

Bittinger/Ellenbogen: *Elementary Algebra: Concepts and Applications*, Fifth Edition

Bittinger/Ellenbogen: *Intermediate Algebra: Concepts and Applications*, Fifth Edition

Bittinger/Ellenbogen/Johnson: *Elementary and Intermediate Algebra: Concepts and Applications—A Combined Approach*, Second Edition

Prealgebra, Third Edition, is a significant revision of the Second Edition, particularly with respect to design, art program, pedagogy, features, and supplements package. Its unique approach, which has been developed and refined over three editions, continues to blend the following elements in order to bring students success:

- *Writing style.* The authors write in a clear, easy-to-read style that helps students progress from concepts through examples and margin exercises to section exercises.

- *Problem-solving approach.* The basis for solving problems and real-data applications is a five-step process (*Familiarize, Translate, Solve, Check,* and *State*) introduced early in the text and used consistently throughout. This problem-solving approach provides students with a consistent framework for solving applications. (See pages 61, 258, 335, and 338.)

- *Real data.* Real-data applications aid in motivating students by connecting the mathematics to their everyday lives. Extensive research was conducted to find new applications that relate mathematics to the real world.

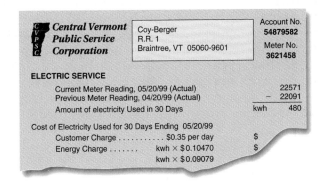

Bicycle Color Preferences

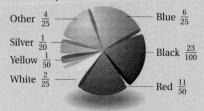

Other $\frac{4}{25}$ Blue $\frac{6}{25}$

Silver $\frac{1}{20}$

Yellow $\frac{1}{50}$ Black $\frac{23}{100}$

White $\frac{2}{25}$

Red $\frac{11}{50}$

Source: Bicycle Market Research Institute

- ***Art program.*** The art program has been expanded to improve the visualization of mathematical concepts and to enhance the real-data applications.

- ***Reviewer feedback.*** The authors solicit feedback from reviewers and students to help fulfill student and instructor needs.

- ***Accuracy.*** The manuscript is subjected to an extensive accuracy-checking process to eliminate errors.

- ***Supplements package.*** All ancillary materials are closely tied with the text and have been created by members of the author team to provide a complete and consistent package for both students and instructors.

What's New in the Third Edition?

The style, format, and approach have been strengthened in this new edition in a number of ways.

Updated Applications   Extensive research has been done to make the applications in the Third Edition even more up-to-date and realistic. A large number of the applications are new to this edition, and many are 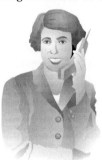 drawn from the fields of business and economics, life and physical sciences, social sciences, and areas of general interest such as sports and health. To encourage students to understand the relevance of mathematics, many applications are enhanced by graphs and drawings similar to those found in today's newspapers and magazines. Many applications are also titled for quick and easy reference, and use real-data applications. (See pages 61, 256, 336, 354, 365, and 399.) Often applications are credited with a source line.

New Art and Design   To enhance the greater emphasis on real data and applications, we have extensively increased the number of pieces of technical and situational art (see pages 3, 333, and 341). Color has been used in a methodical and precise manner so that its use carries a consistent meaning, which enhances the readability of the text. *Prealgebra* now appears in full color, so virtually every page looks more inviting to the reader.

World Wide Web Integration   In an effort to encourage students to benefit from the resources that are available on the Addison Wesley Longman MathMax Web site (see description of the Web site later in this preface), we have added Web site icons to a number of key locations throughout the book. The Web site icons are intended to communicate to students that they will find additional related content on the Web site. For example, students can further explore the subject of the chapter opening applications (see icons on pages 83, 205, and 273) or seek additional practice exercises (see icons on pages 15, 175, and 259) on the MathMax *Prealgebra* Web site. In addition, students can visit the Web site to access InterAct Math exercises, extensive Chapter Reviews, and other helpful resources.

Collaborative Learning Features An icon ⟨Collaborative Learning Manual⟩ located at the end of an exercise set signals the existence of a Collaborative Learning Activity correlating to that section in Irene Doo's *Collaborative Learning Activities Manual* (see pages 72, 230, and 496). Please contact your Addison Wesley Longman sales consultant for details on ordering this supplement.

Exercises The deletion of answer lines in the exercise sets has allowed us to include more exercises in the Third Edition. Exercises are paired, meaning that each even-numbered exercise is very much like the odd-numbered one that precedes it. This gives the instructor several options: If an instructor wants the student to have answers available, the odd-numbered exercises are assigned; if an instructor wants the student to practice (perhaps for a test) with no answers available, then the even-numbered exercises are assigned. In this way, each exercise set actually serves as two exercise sets. Answers to all odd-numbered exercises, with the exception of the Thinking and Writing exercises, and *all* Skill Maintenance exercises appear at the back of the text.

Skill Maintenance Exercises The Skill Maintenance exercises have been enhanced by the inclusion of 60% more exercises in this edition. These exercises review important skills and concepts from earlier chapters of the book. Section and objective codes now appear next to each Skill Maintenance exercise for easy reference (see pages 110, 212, and 318). Answers to all Skill Maintenance exercises appear at the back of the book.

Synthesis Exercises These exercises now appear in every exercise set, Summary and Review, Chapter Test, and Cumulative Review. Synthesis exercises help build critical thinking skills by challenging students to synthesize or combine learning objectives from the section being studied as well as preceding sections in the book.

Thinking and Writing Exercises Each Synthesis exercise section begins with two or three exercises that require written answers that aid in comprehension, critical thinking, and conceptualization. These exercises are designated with the icon ◈ and have been written with all students in mind—not just those looking for a challenge. Answers to the writing exercises are not given at the back of the book because some instructors may collect answers to these exercises, and because correct answers will vary from student to student (see pages 152, 230, and 332). In response to user feedback, the number of Thinking and Writing Exercises has been increased by 50%.

Content We have made the following improvements to the content of *Prealgebra*.

- It is more important than ever for students to be statistically literate. To address this need, the Third Edition of *Prealgebra* expands the coverage of statistics first introduced in the Second Edition. Specifically, increased use of bar graphs and averages appears throughout the text (see pages 61, 240, 258, 304, and 393). New material on the basics of interpolation, extrapolation, and probability is also now included (see pages 399–406).

- The incorporation of algebraic concepts has always been emphasized in *Prealgebra*. In keeping with this emphasis and in response to user feedback, the Third Edition includes a new section devoted solely to solving a mix of equations that involve either addition or multiplication (see pages 131–136). This introduction is then reinforced throughout the text (see pages 195, 225, 231, and 326). New emphasis is placed on distinguishing between equivalent expressions and equivalent equations (see pages 131, 231, and 325).

- Geometry is a topic that has always been an important part of *Prealgebra*. In the Third Edition, coverage has been expanded to integrate more work with circles, angles, and circle graphs (see pages 337 and 545).

- ▦ Calculator exercises and "spotlights" appeared in the Second Edition and, in response to user and reviewer feedback, have been expanded in this edition. Several new Calculator Spotlights now appear, and nearly all exercise sets now include at least one pair of synthesis exercises designed to provide practice using a scientific calculator (see pages 112, 130, 258, and 438). Answers to all Calculator Spotlight exercises appear at the back of the text.

- To impove the flow of topics in Chapter 5, material on estimation now follows rather than precedes the section titled "More with Fractional Notation and Decimal Notation."

- Beginning in Section 6.5, the word "mean" is used in place of "average."

- Chapter 10, Polynomials, now includes the use of FOIL when multiplying two binomials, as well as improved coverage of negative exponents (see pages 599 and 604).

- Approximately once per chapter, a mini-lesson, Improving Your Math Study Skills, appears. (See pages 6, 100, and 322.) These features are referenced in the Table of Contents and can be covered in their entirety at the beginning of the course or as they arise in the text. These features can also be used in conjunction with the authors' "Math Study Skills" Videotape. Please see your Addison Wesley Longman sales consultant for details on how to obtain this videotape.

Learning Aids

Interactive Worktext Approach   The pedagogy of this text is designed to provide an interactive learning experience between the student and the exposition, annotated examples, art, margin exercises, and exercise sets. This approach provides students with a clear set of learning objectives, involves them with the development of the material, and provides immediate and continual reinforcement and assessment.

Section objectives are keyed by letter not only to section subheadings, but also to exercises in the exercise sets and Summary and Review, and to the answers to the Pretest, Chapter Test, and Cumulative Review questions. This enables students to find appropriate review material easily if they need help with a particular exercise.

Throughout the text, students are directed to numerous *margin exercises,* which provide immediate reinforcement of the concepts covered in each section.

Review Material   The Third Edition of *Prealgebra* continues to provide many opportunities for students to prepare for final assessment.

Now in a two-column format, a *Summary and Review* appears at the end of each chapter and provides an extensive set of review exercises. Reference codes beside each exercise or direction line direct the student to the specific subsection being reviewed (see pages 137, 265, and 447).

Also included at the end of every chapter but Chapters 1 and 10 is a *Cumulative Review*, which reviews material from all preceding chapters. At the back of the text are answers to all Cumulative Review exercises, together with section and objective references, so that students know exactly what material to study if they need help with a review exercise (see pages 141, 349, and 451). A final examination follows Chapter 10.

For Extra Help   Many valuable study aids accompany this text. Below the list of objectives found at the beginning of each section are references to appropriate videotape, tutorial software, and CD-ROM programs to make it easy for the student to find the correct support materials.

Testing   The following assessment opportunities exist in the text.

The *Diagnostic Pretest,* provided at the beginning of the text, helps place students in the appropriate chapter for their skill level by identifying familiar material and specific trouble areas (see page xxi).

Chapter Pretests can then be used to place students in a specific section of the chapter, allowing them to concentrate on topics with which they have particular difficulty (see pages 84, 206, and 418).

Chapter Tests allow students to review and test comprehension of skills developed in each chapter (see pages 139, 269, and 411).

Answers to all Diagnostic Pretest, Chapter Pretest, and Chapter Test questions are found at the back of the book, along with appropriate section and objective references.

Supplements for the Instructor

Annotated Instructor's Edition
0-201-64602-1

The Annotated Instructor's Edition is a specially bound version of the student text with answers to all margin exercises, exercise sets, and chapter tests printed in blue near the corresponding exercises.

Instructor's Solutions Manual
by Judith A. Penna
ISBN 0-201-64603-X

This manual contains brief, worked-out solutions to all even-numbered exercises in the text's exercise sets and answers to all Thinking and Writing exercises.

Printed Test Bank/Instructor's Resource Guide
by Laura Hurley
ISBN 0-201-64604-8

The test-bank section of this supplement contains the following:

- Two alternate test forms for each chapter modeled after the Chapter Tests in the text
- Two alternate test forms for each chapter, with questions presented in the same topical order as the chapter objectives
- Two alternate test forms for each chapter designed for a 50-minute class period

---

Objectives

[a]   Add using mixed numerals.

[b]   Subtract and combine using mixed numerals.

[c]   Solve applied problems involving addition and subtraction with mixed numerals.

[d]   Add and subtract using negative mixed numerals.

For Extra Help

TAPE 8   MAC   CD-ROM
                WIN

- Two multiple-choice test forms for each chapter
- Two cumulative review tests for each chapter, with the exception of Chapters 1 and 10
- Six alternate test forms of the final examination: two with questions organized by chapter, two with questions scrambled, and two with multiple-choice questions
- Answers for the chapter tests and final examinations

The Instructor's Resource Manual section contains the following:

- Extra practice exercise sheets and answers for several of the most challenging topics in the text
- A conversion guide from the Second Edition to the Third Edition
- A videotape index for the "Steps to Success" video series that accompanies the text
- Black-line masters of grids and number lines for transparency masters or test preparation

Collaborative Learning Activities Manual
by Irene Doo
ISBN 0-201-66198-5

The Collaborative Learning Activities Manual, written by Irene Doo of Austin Community College, features group activities that are tied graphically to sections of the textbook via an icon. This manual also provides instruction on the setup and administration of a collaborative classroom environment.

TestGen-EQ/QuizMaster-EQ CD-ROM
ISBN 0-201-64607-2

This powerful test-generation software is provided on a dual-platform Windows/Macintosh CD-ROM. TestGen-EQ's friendly graphical interface enables instructors to easily view, edit, and add questions, transfer questions to tests, and print tests in a variety of fonts and forms. Search and sort features help the instructor locate questions quickly and arrange them in a preferred order. Several question formats are available, including short-answer, true/false, multiple-choice, essay, matching, and bimodal (a bimodal question is one that can be saved in either multiple-choice or short-answer form). A built-in question editor allows the instructor to create graphs, import graphics, and insert variable numbers, text, and mathematical symbols and templates. Computerized test banks include algorithmically defined problems organized according to the textbook table of contents. Instructors can create and export practice tests as HTML for use on the World Wide Web.

Using QuizMaster-EQ, instructors can post tests and quizzes created in TestGen-EQ to a computer network so that students can take them on-line. Instructors can set preferences for how and when tests are administered. QuizMaster automatically grades the exams and allows the instructor to view or print a variety of reports for individual students, classes, or courses.

InterAct Math Plus Instructor's Package
ISBN 0-201-63555-0 (Windows), ISBN 0-201-64805-9 (Macintosh)

Used in conjunction with the InterAct Math Tutorial Software for students (0-201-64609-9), this networkable software provides instructors with full course management capabilities for tracking and reporting student use of the tutorial software. Instructors can create and administer on-line tests, summarize student results, and monitor student progress in the software.

Instructors should also review the list of supplements for students that follows.

Supplements for the Student

Student's Solutions Manual
by Judith A. Penna
ISBN 0-201-34026-7

This manual provides completely worked-out solutions with step-by-step annotations for all odd-numbered exercises except the Thinking and Writing exercises. It may be purchased by students from Addison Wesley Longman.

"Steps to Success" Videotapes
ISBN 0-201-64807-5

This videotape series features an engaging team of mathematics instructors, including your authors, presenting comprehensive coverage of each section of the text in a student-interactive format. The lecturers' presentations include examples and problems from the text and support an approach that emphasizes visualization and problem solving. A video icon ▣ at the beginning of each section references the appropriate videotape number.

InterAct Math Tutorial Software
ISBN 0-201-64609-9

The InterAct Math Tutorial Software, provided on a dual-platform Windows/Macintosh CD-ROM has been developed by professional software engineers working closely with a team of experienced developmental mathematics instructors. This software includes exercises that are linked one-to-one to the odd-numbered exercises in the text; the InterAct Math exercises require the same computational and problem-solving skills as their companion exercises in the book. Each exercise is accompanied by an example and an interactive guided solution designed to involve students in the solution process and help them identify precisely where they are having trouble. For each section of the text, the software tracks student activity and scores, which can be printed out in summary form. An InterAct Math icon ⟁ InterAct math at the beginning of each section identifies section coverage.

MathMax Multimedia CD-ROM for *Prealgebra*
ISBN 0-201-64806-7

This dual-platform Windows/Macintosh CD-ROM provides an interactive environment using graphics, animations, and audio narration to build on some of the unique and proven features of the MathMax series. The content of the CD is tightly and consistently integrated with the text, highlighting key concepts and referencing the *Prealgebra* numbering scheme so that students can move smoothly between the CD and other supplements. The CD includes narrated animations that provide step-by-step explanations of many of the examples in the text, and the narrations are accompanied by multiple-choice exercises. Also included are interactive chapter reviews, multimedia study skills presentations, InterAct Math exercises for every section of the text, and a glossary of key terms. A CD-ROM icon ◑ at the beginning of each section indicates section coverage.

An Addison Wesley Longman sales consultant can arrange for a demonstration of the *Prealgebra* MathMax CD-ROM.

World Wide Web Supplement (www.mathmax.com)

This on-line supplement provides additional practice and reinforcement for students through detailed chapter review material, extra practice worksheets, and expanded chapter openers. In addition, students can download a plug-in for Addison Wesley Longman's InterAct Math exercises that allows them to access tutorial problems directly through their Web browser. The site also provides teaching tips and information for instructors about all the MathMax supplements available from Addison Wesley Longman.

MathPass, Version 2.0 for Windows
ISBN 0-201-66192-6

MathPass helps students succeed in their developmental mathematics courses by creating customized study plans based on diagnostic test results from ACT, Inc.'s Computer-Adaptive Placement Assessment and Support System (COMPASS®). MathPass pinpoints topics where the student needs in-depth study or targeted review and correlates these topics with the student's textbook and related supplements (such as videos, student's solutions manuals, Web sites, tutorial software, and multimedia CD-ROMs). The MathPass Learning System provides diagnostic assessment, focused instruction, and exit placement all in one package. Contact your local Addison Wesley Longman sales consultant for more information about MathPass.

MathXL
ISBN 0-201-68154-4
(*Prealgebra* bundled with the MathXL coupon package)

MathXL is a Web-based testing and tutorial system that allows students to take practice tests similar to the chapter tests in their book. MathXL generates a personalized study plan that indicates students' strengths and pinpoints topics where they need more practice. The program then provides the practice and instruction students need to improve their skills. Test scores and practice sessions are tracked by the program so that students can monitor their progress throughout the semester. The MathXL Web site requires each student to purchase a user ID and password.

"Math Study Skills for Students" Videotape
ISBN 0-201-88039-3

Designed to help students make better use of their math study time, this videotape helps students improve retention of concepts and procedures taught in classes from basic mathematics through intermediate algebra. Through carefully crafted graphics and comprehensive on-camera explanation, author Marvin L. Bittinger helps viewers focus on study skills that are commonly overlooked.

Overcoming Math Anxiety, Second Edition
by Randy Davidson and Ellen Levitov
ISBN 0-321-06918-8

Written to help students succeed with college-level mathematics coursework, this book includes step-by-step guidelines to problem solving, note taking, and word problems. This book helps students discover the reasons behind math anxiety, learn relaxation techniques, build better math skills, and improve learning strategies for math.

Spanish Glossary
ISBN 0-321-01647-5

This pocket-sized glossary includes concise, easy-to-understand English-to-Spanish translations for key mathematical terms.

Math Tutor Center
ISBN 0-201-66352-X
(*Prealgebra* bundled with Math Tutor Center registration)

The Addison Wesley Longman Math Tutor Center provides FREE tutoring to students enrolled in courses ranging from developmental mathematics through calculus. Assisted by qualified mathematics instructors via phone, fax, or e-mail, students can receive tutoring on examples, exercises, and problems contained in their Addison Wesley Longman math textbooks. Upon request, each new book can be bundled with a free registration number that provides the student with a 6-month subscription to the service. The Math Tutor Center is open Sunday through Thursday from 3 pm to 10 pm Eastern Standard Time. Contact your local Addison Wesley Longman sales consultant for more information about the Math Tutor Center.

Acknowledgments

We would like to express our appreciation to the many people who helped make this book possible. Judy Penna deserves special thanks for her preparation of the *Student's Solution Manual*, the *Instructor's Solutions Manual*, and her careful checking of the manuscript. Laura Hurley deserves special thanks for her preparation of the *Printed Test Bank/Instructor's Resource Manual* and her careful checking of page proofs and compilation of the answers. Sincere thanks to Irene Doo for her outstanding work on the *Collaborative Learning Activities Manual*. Heartfelt thanks also to Professor Susan McAuliffe of the University of Vermont, Tracy Psaute and Thomas Schicker of the Community College of Vermont, and Vincent Koehler for their thorough inspection of the typeset pages and answers.

Martha Morong again showed why she's the best copyeditor in the business, and Jenny Bagdigian provided superb stewardship skills in juggling many different tasks at once, while preserving the high quality that we all consider essential. Thanks also to Janet Theurer for her fine work as art editor and to Kathy Manley for her work as production supervisor and for reworking numerous pages of manuscript. A big thank you to Ruth Berry for her fine work as project manager, and we also thank Tricia Mescall for supervising the production of our videotape series. Finally, a big thank you to Jason Jordan, our most trusted and talented publisher, for making sound decisions and providing us with the freedom we need to do our jobs right.

In addition, we thank the following professors for their thoughtful reviews, suggestions, and comments.

Kenneth Benson, *University of Illinois at Urbana-Champaign*
Timmy G. Bremer, *Prestonburg Community College*
Beverly R. Broomell, *Suffolk Community College*
Debra Bryant, *Tennessee Technological University*
Jean-Marie Magnier, *Springfield Technical Community College*
Tom Carson, *Midlands Technical College*
Mary Jane Cordon
Katherine Creery, *University of Memphis*
Carol Flakus, *Lower Columbia College*
Linda Galloway, *Macon Sate College*
Kay Haralson, *Austin Peay State University*
Celeste Hernandez, *Richland College*
Courtney Hubbell, *Nicholls State University*
Marilyn Jacobi, *Gateway Community-Technical College*
Nancy Johnson, *Broward Community College, North Campus*
Steve Kahn, *Anne Arundel Community College*
Joanne Kelly, *Palm Beach Community College*
Theodore Lai, *Hudson County Community College*

Nancy Lehmann, *Austin Community College*
Bob Maynard, *Tidewater Community College*
Frank Miller, *Orange Coast College*
Gary Nelson, *Asheville-Buncombe Technical Community College*
David Newell, *Pierce College / Cypress College*
Patricio A. Rojas, *Albuquerque Technical Vocational Institute*
Mickey Sargent, *Ranger College*
Sally Sestini, *Cerritos College*
David Swarbrick, *St. Edwards University / Austin Community College*
Sharon Testone, *Onondaga Community College*
David E. Thielk, *Port Townsend High School*
Victor Thomas, *Holyoke Community College*
Peter Wursthorn, *Capitol Community Tech College*
Kevin Yokoyama, *College of the Redwoods*

Diagnostic Pretest

Chapter 1

1. Add: $549 + 3764$.

2. Solve: $43 + x = 71$.

3. Multiply:
$$\begin{array}{r} 4\ 5\ 3 \\ \times\ \ \ 3\ 7 \\ \hline \end{array}$$

4. A vat contains 140 oz of hot sauce. How many 6-oz bottles can be filled from the vat? How many ounces will be left over?

Chapter 2

5. Evaluate $6x^2$ for $x = -5$.

6. Find the opposite, or additive inverse, of -17.

Compute and simplify.

7. $-8 + (-5)$

8. $-20 + 17$

9. $-5 - 12$

10. $-4 - (-9)$

11. $(-6)(-9)$

12. $10 \div (-5) + 3^2$

13. Find the perimeter of a 20-ft by 15-ft garden.

14. Combine like terms: $9 - 3x + 4 + 10x$.

15. Solve: $3 + t = -14$.

16. Solve: $-6x = -24$.

Chapter 3

17. Multiply and simplify: $-\dfrac{6}{7} \cdot \dfrac{21}{12}$.

18. Solve: $\dfrac{3}{5}x = -24$.

19. Find another name for $\frac{7}{8}$, but with 40 as the denominator.

20. A group of 5 diners shares $\frac{3}{4}$ of a pie equally. How much of the pie does each person receive?

Chapter 4

21. Solve: $x + \dfrac{4}{5} = \dfrac{9}{10}$.

22. Divide and simplify: $3\dfrac{1}{2} \div \dfrac{3}{4}$.

23. Find the average: $3\dfrac{1}{2}$, 5, $1\dfrac{1}{4}$.

24. Solve: $\dfrac{11}{5} = \dfrac{8}{5} + \dfrac{5}{4}a$.

Chapter 5

Perform the indicated operation.

25. $3.95 + 5.026$

26. $152.7 \div (-1.5)$

27. Combine like terms: $8.2x - 9.4y - 5.7x + 2.1y$.

28. Solve: $1.5t + 4.2 = 7.8$.

Chapter 6

29. Graph: $x + 2y = -6$.

30. Find the mean, the median, and the mode:

$$9,\ 12,\ 12,\ 14,\ 18,\ 19.$$

Chapter 7

31. The ratio of the number of adults to the number of children at the Wildflower Daycare Center cannot be less than 1 to 8. If there are 30 children at the center, how many adults must be present?

32. How tall is a street sign that casts a 12-ft shadow at the same time that a 5-ft woman casts an 8-ft shadow?

Chapter 8

33. Find percent notation: $\dfrac{5}{8}$.

34. Find decimal notation: 2.4%.

35. The price of a bicycle helmet was reduced from $45 to $36. Find the percent of decrease in price.

36. A principal of $2000 earned 4.5% simple interest for one year. How much was in the account at the end of the year?

Chapter 9

Complete.

37. 2 yd = _____ in.

38. 4 cm = _____ km

39. 64 oz = _____ lb

40. 5 mg = _____ g

41. 2 yd^2 = _____ ft^2

42. 10 qt = _____ gal

43. Find the area and the circumference of a circle with a diameter of 12 cm. Leave answers in terms of π.

44. Each side of a cube is 5 m long. Find the volume of the cube.

Chapter 10

45. Add: $(5x^3 + 4x^2 - 9) + (3x^3 - 7x^2 - 1)$.

46. Subtract: $(7x^4 - 8x^3 + 5) - (3x^4 + x^2 + 7)$.

47. Multiply: $(2x - 1)(x + 3)$.

48. Factor: $10x^5 + 8x^4 - 12x^3$.

49. Evaluate $(2x + 3)^0$ for $x = 7$.

50. Simplify: $(5a^{-3}b)(2a^7b^4)$.

Using a Scientific Calculator

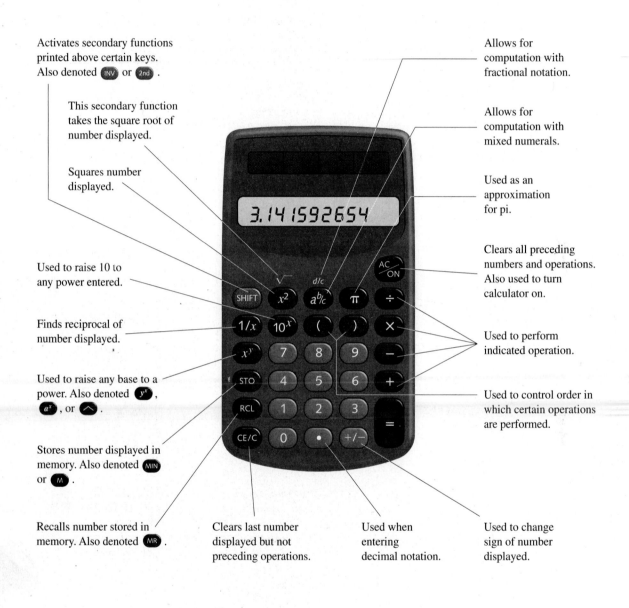

Activates secondary functions printed above certain keys. Also denoted INV or 2nd .

This secondary function takes the square root of number displayed.

Squares number displayed.

Used to raise 10 to any power entered.

Finds reciprocal of number displayed.

Used to raise any base to a power. Also denoted y^x, a^x, or ⌃ .

Stores number displayed in memory. Also denoted MIN or M .

Recalls number stored in memory. Also denoted MR .

Clears last number displayed but not preceding operations.

Used when entering decimal notation.

Used to change sign of number displayed.

Allows for computation with fractional notation.

Allows for computation with mixed numerals.

Used as an approximation for pi.

Clears all preceding numbers and operations. Also used to turn calculator on.

Used to perform indicated operation.

Used to control order in which certain operations are performed.

1

Operations on the Whole Numbers

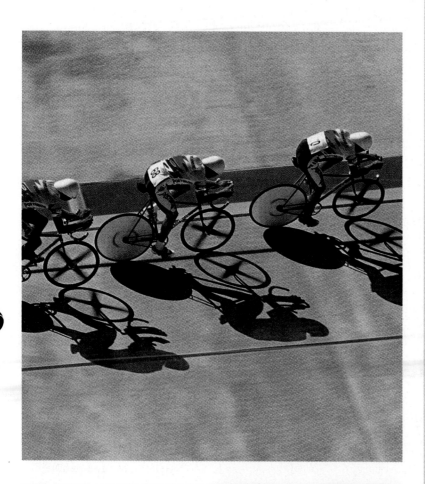

An Application	The Mathematics
Total sales, in millions of dollars, of bicycles and related sporting supplies were \$3534 in 1993, \$3470 in 1994, \$3435 in 1995, and \$3356 in 1996. (**Source**: National Sporting Goods Association.) Find the total sales for the entire four-year period.	We let $T =$ the total sales, in millions of dollars. Since we are combining sales, addition can be used. We translate the problem to the equation
This problem appears as Exercise 4 in Exercise Set 1.8.	$$3534 + 3470 + 3435 + 3356 = T.$$ This is how addition can occur in applications and problem solving.

World Wide Web   For more information, visit us at www.mathmax.com

Pretest: Chapter 1

1. Write a word name: 3,078,059.

2. Write in expanded notation: 6987.

3. Write in standard notation: Two billion, forty-seven million, three hundred ninety-eight thousand, five hundred eighty-nine.

4. What does the digit 6 mean in 2,967,342?

5. Round 956,449 to the nearest thousand.

6. Estimate the product $594 \cdot 126$ by first rounding the numbers to the nearest hundred.

7. Add.

$$\begin{array}{r} 7\ 3\ 1\ 2 \\ +\ 2\ 9\ 0\ 4 \\ \hline \end{array}$$

8. Subtract.

$$\begin{array}{r} 7\ 0\ 1\ 2 \\ -\ 2\ 9\ 0\ 4 \\ \hline \end{array}$$

9. Multiply: $359 \cdot 64$.

10. Divide: $23{,}149 \div 46$.

Use either $<$ or $>$ for ▧ to form a true sentence.

11. 346 ▧ 364

12. 54 ▧ 45

Solve.

13. $326 \cdot 17 = m$

14. $y = 924 \div 42$

15. $19 + x = 53$

16. $34 \cdot n = 850$

Solve.

17. Anna weighs 121 lb and Kari weighs 109 lb. How much more does Anna weigh?

18. How many 12-jar cases are needed for 1512 jars of spaghetti sauce?

19. *Population.* The population of Illinois is 11,830,000. The population of Ohio is 11,151,000. (**Source**: U.S. Bureau of the Census.) What is the total population of Illinois and Ohio?

20. A rectangular lot measures 48 ft by 54 ft. A pool that is 15 ft by 20 ft is constructed on the lot. How much area is left over?

Evaluate.

21. 5^2

22. 4^3

Simplify.

23. $8^2 \div 8 \cdot 2 - (2 + 2 \cdot 7)$

24. $108 \div 9 - \{4 \cdot [18 - (5 \cdot 3)]\}$

1.1 Standard Notation

We study mathematics in order to be able to solve problems. In this chapter, we learn how to use operations on the whole numbers. We begin by studying how numbers are named.

a | From Standard Notation to Expanded Notation

To answer questions such as "How many?", "How much?", and "How tall?", we use whole numbers. The set, or collection, of **whole numbers** is

0, 1, 2, 3, 4, 5, 6, 7, 8, 9, 10, 11, 12, ...

The set goes on indefinitely. There is no largest whole number, and the smallest whole number is 0. Each whole number can be named using various notations. The set 1, 2, 3, 4, 5, ..., without 0, is called the set of **natural numbers**.

As examples, we use data from the bar graph shown here.

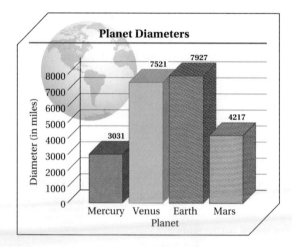

Planet Diameters

Note that the diameter of Mars is 4217 miles (mi). **Standard notation** for this number is 4217. We find **expanded notation** for 4217 as follows:

4217 = 4 thousands + 2 hundreds + 1 ten + 7 ones.

Example 1 Write expanded notation for 3031 mi, the diameter of Mercury.

3031 = 3 thousands + 0 hundreds + 3 tens + 1 one

Example 2 Write expanded notation for 54,567.

54,567 = 5 ten thousands + 4 thousands
+ 5 hundreds + 6 tens + 7 ones

Do Exercises 1 and 2 (in the margin at the right).

Objectives

a | Convert from standard notation to expanded notation.

b | Convert from expanded notation to standard notation.

c | Write a word name for a number given standard notation.

d | Write standard notation for a number given a word name.

e | Given a standard notation like 278,342, tell what 8 means, what 3 means, and so on; identify the hundreds digit, the thousands digit, and so on.

For Extra Help

TAPE 1

MAC WIN

CD-ROM

Write in expanded notation.

1. 1805

1 thousand + 8 hundreds +
0 tens + 5 ones, or
1 thousand + 8 hundreds +
5 ones

2. 36,223

3 ten thousands + 6 thousands +
2 hundreds + 2 tens + 3 ones

Answers on page A-1

Write in expanded notation.

3. 3210

3 thousands + 2 hundreds + 1 ten

4. 2009

2 thousands + 9 ones

5. 5700

5 thousands + 7 hundreds

Write in standard notation.

6. 5 thousands + 6 hundreds +
8 tens + 9 ones

5689

7. 8 ten thousands +
7 thousands + 1 hundred +
2 tens + 8 ones

87,128

8. 9 thousands + 3 ones

9003

Write a word name.

9. 57

Fifty-seven

10. 29

Twenty-nine

11. 88

Eighty-eight

Answers on page A-1

Example 3   Write expanded notation for 3400.

$$3400 = 3 \text{ thousands} + 4 \text{ hundreds} + 0 \text{ tens} + 0 \text{ ones}, \quad \text{or}$$
$$3 \text{ thousands} + 4 \text{ hundreds}$$

Do Exercises 3–5.

b   From Expanded Notation to Standard Notation

Example 4   Write standard notation for 2 thousands + 5 hundreds + 7 tens + 5 ones.

Standard notation is 2575.

Example 5   Write standard notation for 9 ten thousands + 6 thousands + 7 hundreds + 1 ten + 8 ones.

Standard notation is 96,718.

Example 6   Write standard notation for 2 thousands + 3 tens.

Standard notation is 2030.

Do Exercises 6–8.

c   Word Names

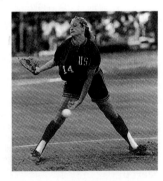

"Three," "two hundred one," and "forty-two" are **word names** for numbers. When we write word names for two-digit numbers like 42, 76, and 91, we use hyphens. For example, U.S. Olympic softball pitcher Michelle Granger can pitch a softball at a speed of 72 miles per hour (mph). A word name for 72 is "seventy-two."

Examples   Write a word name.

7. 43   Forty-three   **8.** 91   Ninety-one

Do Exercises 9–11.

For large numbers, digits are separated into groups of three, called **periods**. Each period has a name: *ones, thousands, millions, billions,* and so on. When we write or read a large number, we start at the left with the largest period. The number named in the period is followed by the name of the period; then a comma is written and the next period is named. Recently, the U.S. national debt was $5,103,040,000,000. We can use a **place-value** chart to illustrate how to use periods to read the number 5,103,040,000,000.

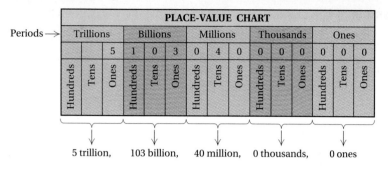

PLACE-VALUE CHART														
Periods →	Trillions			Billions			Millions			Thousands			Ones		
			5	1	0	3	0	4	0	0	0	0	0	0	0
	Hundreds	Tens	Ones	Hundreds	Tens	Ones	Hundreds	Tens	Ones	Hundreds	Tens	Ones	Hundreds	Tens	Ones

5 trillion,   103 billion,   40 million,   0 thousands,   0 ones

The U.S. debt was five trillion, one hundred three billion, forty million dollars.

Example 9   Write a word name for 46,605,314,732.

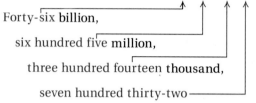

Forty-six billion,

six hundred five million,

three hundred fourteen thousand,

seven hundred thirty-two

The word "and" *should not* appear in word names for whole numbers. Although we commonly hear such expressions as "two hundred *and* one," the use of "and" is not, strictly speaking, correct in word names for whole numbers. In decimal notation, we will find it appropriate to use "and" for the decimal point. For example, 317.4 is read as "three hundred seventeen *and* four tenths."

Do Exercises 12–15.

d │ From Word Names to Standard Notation

Example 10   Write in standard notation.

Five hundred six million,

three hundred forty-five thousand,

two hundred twelve

Standard notation is 506,345,212.

Do Exercise 16.

e │ Digits

A **digit** is a number 0, 1, 2, 3, 4, 5, 6, 7, 8, or 9 that names a place-value location.

Examples   What does the digit 8 mean in each case?

11. 278,342   8 thousands
12. 872,342   8 hundred thousands
13. 28,343,399,223   8 billions

Do Exercises 17–20.

Write a word name.
12. 204

Two hundred four

13. 79,204

Seventy-nine thousand, two hundred four

14. 1,879,204

One million, eight hundred seventy-nine thousand, two hundred four

15. 22,301,879,204

Twenty-two billion, three hundred one million, eight hundred seventy-nine thousand, two hundred four

16. Write in standard notation.

Two hundred thirteen million, one hundred five thousand, three hundred twenty-nine

213,105,329

What does the digit 2 mean in each case?
17. 526,555

2 ten thousands

18. 265,789

2 hundred thousands

19. 42,789,654

2 millions

20. 24,789,654

2 ten millions

Answers on page A-1

Golf Balls. On an average day, Americans buy 486,574 golf balls. In 486,574, what digit tells the number of:

21. Thousands?   6

22. Ten thousands?   8

23. Ones?   4

24. Hundreds?   5

Example 14 *Dunkin Donuts.* On an average day, about 2,739,626 Dunkin Donuts are served in the United States. In 2,739,626, what digit tells the number of:

a) Hundred thousands?   7

b) Thousands?   9

Do Exercises 21–24.

Improving Your Math Study Skills

Tips for Using This Textbook

Throughout this textbook, you will find a feature called "Improving Your Math Study Skills." Some students find it helpful to read all of these early in the course. Each topic title is listed in the table of contents beginning on p. v.

One of the most important ways to improve your math study skills is to learn the proper use of the textbook. Here we highlight a few points that we consider most helpful.

- **Be sure to note the special symbols** a , b , c , **and so on, that correspond to the objectives you are to be able to perform.** They appear in many places throughout the text. The first time you see them is in the margin at the beginning of each section. The second time is in the subheadings of each section, and the third time is in the exercise set. You will also find them next to the skill maintenance exercises in each exercise set and in the review exercises at the end of each chapter, as well as in the answers to the chapter tests, pretests, and cumulative reviews. These objective symbols allow you to refer to the appropriate section whenever you need to review a topic.

- **Note the symbols in the margin under the list of objectives at the beginning of each section.** These refer to the many distinctive study aids that accompany the book.

- **Read and study each step of each example.** The examples include important side comments that explain each step. These carefully chosen examples and comments prepare you for success in the exercise set.

- **Stop and do the margin exercises as you study a section.** When our students come to us troubled about how they are doing in the course, the first question we ask is "Are you doing the margin exercises when directed to do so?" This is one of the most effective ways to enhance your ability to learn mathematics from this text. Don't deprive yourself of its benefits!

- **When you study the book, don't mark the points that you think are important, but mark the points you do not understand!** This book includes many design features that highlight important points. Use your efforts to mark where you are having trouble. Then when you go to class, a math lab, or a tutoring session, you will be prepared to ask questions that pertain to your difficulties rather than spend time going over what you already understand.

- **If you are having trouble, consider using the** *Student's Solutions Manual,* **which contains worked-out solutions to the odd-numbered exercises in the exercise sets.**

- **Try to keep one section ahead of your syllabus.** If you study ahead of your lectures, you can concentrate on what is being explained in them, rather than try to write everything down. You can then take notes only of special points or of questions related to what is happening in class.

Answers on page A-1

Exercise Set 1.1

Always review the objectives before doing an exercise set. See page 3. Note how the objectives are keyed to the exercises.

a Write in expanded notation.

1. 5742

    5 thousands +
7 hundreds +
4 tens + 2 ones

2. 3897

    3 thousands +
8 hundreds +
9 tens + 7 ones

3. 27,342

    2 ten thousands +
7 thousands + 3 hundreds +
4 tens + 2 ones

4. 93,986

    9 ten thousands +
3 thousands +
9 hundreds +
8 tens + 6 ones

5. 5609

    5 thousands +
6 hundreds + 9 ones

6. 9990

    9 thousands +
9 hundreds + 9 tens

7. 2300

    2 thousands +
3 hundreds

8. 7020

    7 thousands +
2 tens

b Write in standard notation.

9. 2 thousands + 4 hundreds + 7 tens + 5 ones

    2475

10. 7 thousands + 9 hundreds + 8 tens + 3 ones

    7983

11. 6 ten thousands + 8 thousands + 9 hundreds + 3 tens + 9 ones

    68,939

12. 1 ten thousand + 8 thousands + 4 hundreds + 6 tens + 1 one

    18,461

13. 7 thousands + 3 hundreds + 0 tens + 4 ones

    7304

14. 8 thousands + 0 hundreds + 2 tens + 0 ones

    8020

15. 1 thousand + 9 ones

    1009

16. 2 thousands + 4 hundreds + 5 tens

    2450

c Write a word name.

17. 85

    Eighty-five

18. 48

    Forty-eight

19. 88,000

    Eighty-eight thousand

20. 45,987

    Forty-five thousand, nine hundred eighty-seven

21. 123,765

    One hundred twenty-three thousand, seven hundred sixty-five

22. 111,013

    One hundred eleven thousand, thirteen

23. 7,754,211,577

    Seven billion, seven hundred fifty-four million, two hundred eleven thousand, five hundred seventy-seven

24. 43,550,651,808

    Forty-three billion, five hundred fifty million, six hundred fifty-one thousand, eight hundred eight

Write a word name for the number in each sentence.

25. *NBA Salaries.* In a recent year, the average salary in the National Basketball Association was $1,867,000.

    One million, eight hundred sixty-seven thousand

26. *Oceanography.* The area of the Pacific Ocean is about 64,186,000 square miles.

    Sixty-four million, one hundred eighty-six thousand

27. *Population.* The population of South Asia is about 1,583,141,000.

    One billion, five hundred eighty-three million, one hundred forty-one thousand

28. *Monopoly.* In a recent Monopoly game sponsored by McDonald's restaurants, the odds of winning the grand prize were estimated to be 467,322,388 to 1.

    Four hundred sixty-seven million, three hundred twenty-two thousand, three hundred eighty-eight

| d | Write in standard notation. |

29. Two million, two hundred thirty-three thousand, eight hundred twelve

2,233,812

30. Three hundred fifty-four thousand, seven hundred two

354,702

31. Eight billion

8,000,000,000

32. Seven hundred million

700,000,000

Write standard notation for the number in each sentence.

33. *Light Distance.* Light travels nine trillion, four hundred sixty billion kilometers in one year.

9,460,000,000,000

34. *Pluto.* The distance from the sun to Pluto is three billion, six hundred sixty-four million miles.

3,664,000,000

35. *Area of Greenland.* The area of Greenland is two million, nine hundred seventy-four thousand, six hundred square kilometers.

2,974,600

36. *Memory Space.* On computer hard drives, one gigabyte is actually one billion, seventy-three million, seven hundred forty-one thousand, eight hundred twenty-four bytes of memory.

1,073,741,824

| e | What does the digit 5 mean in each case? |

37. 235,888

5 thousands

38. 253,888

5 ten thousands

39. 488,526

5 hundreds

40. 500,346

5 hundred thousands

In 89,302, what digit tells the number of:

41. Hundreds?

3

42. Thousands?

9

43. Tens?

0

44. Ones?

2

47. All 9's as digits. Answers may vary. For an 8-digit readout, it would be 99,999,999. This number has three periods.

Synthesis

Exercises designated as *Synthesis exercises* will challenge you to combine two or more objectives at once. The icon ◈ denotes synthesis exercises that are writing exercises. Writing exercises are meant to be answered in one or more complete sentences and are usually less challenging than other synthesis exercises. Because answers to writing exercises may vary, they are not listed at the back of the book. Exercises marked with a ▦ are meant to be solved using a calculator.

45. ◈ Write an English sentence in which the number 260,000,000 is used.

46. ◈ Explain why we use commas when writing large numbers.

47. ▦ What is the largest number that you can name on your calculator? How many digits does that number have? How many periods? Answers vary.

48. How many whole numbers between 100 and 400 contain the digit 2 in their standard notation? 138

1.2 Addition and Perimeter

a Addition and the Real World

Addition of whole numbers corresponds to combining or putting things together. Let's look at various situations in which addition applies.

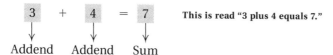

The addition that corresponds to the figure above is

$$3 + 4 = 7.$$

The number of objects in a set can be found by counting. We count and find that the two sets have 3 members and 4 members, respectively. After combining, we count and find that there are 7 objects. We say that the **sum** of 3 and 4 is 7. The numbers added are called **addends**.

$$\underset{\text{Addend}}{3} \; + \; \underset{\text{Addend}}{4} \; = \; \underset{\text{Sum}}{7}$$

This is read "3 plus 4 equals 7."

Example 1 Write an addition sentence that corresponds to this situation.

Kelly has $3 and earns $10 more. How much money does she have?

An addition that corresponds is $3 + $10 = $13.

Do Exercises 1 and 2.

Addition also corresponds to combining distances or lengths.

Example 2 Write an addition sentence that corresponds to this situation.

A car is driven 44 mi from San Francisco to San Jose. It is then driven 42 mi from San Jose to Oakland. How far is it from San Francisco to Oakland along the same route?

$$44 \text{ mi} + 42 \text{ mi} = 86 \text{ mi}$$

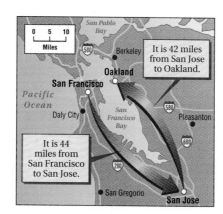

Do Exercises 3 and 4.

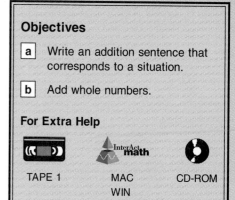

Objectives

a Write an addition sentence that corresponds to a situation.

b Add whole numbers.

For Extra Help

TAPE 1   MAC WIN   CD-ROM

Write an addition sentence that corresponds to each situation.

1. John has 8 music CD-ROMs in his backpack. Then he buys 2 educational CD-ROMs at the bookstore. How many CD-ROMs does John have in all?

   8 + 2 = 10

2. Sue earns $45 in overtime pay on Thursday and $33 on Friday. How much overtime pay does she earn altogether on the two days?

   $45 + $33 = $78

Write an addition sentence that corresponds to each situation.

3. A car is driven 100 mi from Austin to Waco. It is then driven 93 mi from Waco to Dallas. How far is it from Austin to Dallas along the same route?

   100 mi + 93 mi = 193 mi

4. A coaxial cable 5 feet (ft) long is connected to a cable 7 ft long. How long is the resulting cable?

   5 ft + 7 ft = 12 ft

Answers on page A-1

Write an addition sentence that corresponds to each situation.

5. Find the perimeter of (distance around) the figure.

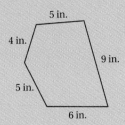

4 in. + 5 in. + 9 in. + 6 in. + 5 in. = 29 in.

6. Find the perimeter of (distance around) the figure.

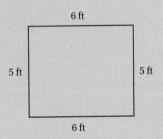

5 ft + 6 ft + 5 ft + 6 ft = 22 ft

Write an addition sentence that corresponds to each situation.

7. The front parking lot of Sparks Electronics contains 30,000 square feet (sq ft) of parking space. The back lot contains 40,000 sq ft. What is the total area of the two parking lots?

30,000 sq ft + 40,000 sq ft = 70,000 sq ft

8. You own a small rug that contains 8 square yards (sq yd) of fabric. You buy another rug that contains 9 sq yd. What is the area of the floor covered by both rugs?

8 sq yd + 9 sq yd = 17 sq yd

Answers on page A-1

When we find the sum of the distances around an object, we are finding its **perimeter.**

Example 3 Write an addition sentence that corresponds to this situation.

A computer salesperson travels the following route to visit various electronics stores. How long is the route?

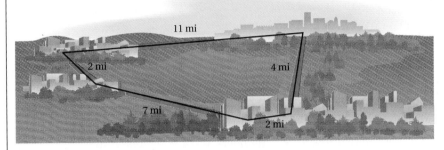

2 mi + 7 mi + 2 mi + 4 mi + 11 mi = 26 mi

Do Exercises 5 and 6.

Addition also corresponds to combining areas.

Example 4 Write an addition sentence that corresponds to this situation.

The area of a standard large index card is 40 square inches (sq in.). The area of a standard small index card is 15 sq in. Altogether, what is the total area of a large and a small card?

The area of the large index card is 40 sq in.	The area of the small index card is 15 sq in.	The total area of the two cards is 55 sq in.
40 sq in.	+ 15 sq in.	= 55 sq in.

Do Exercises 7 and 8.

Addition corresponds to combining volumes as well.

Example 5 Write an addition sentence that corresponds to this situation.

Two trucks haul dirt to a construction site. One hauls 5 cubic yards (cu yd) and the other hauls 7 cu yd. Altogether, how many cubic yards of dirt have they hauled to the site?

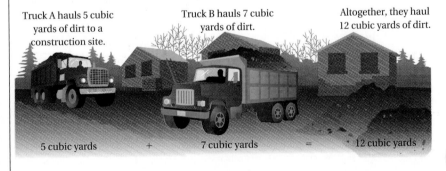

5 cu yd + 7 cu yd = 12 cu yd

Do Exercises 9 and 10.

b | Addition of Whole Numbers

To add numbers, we add the ones digits first, then the tens, then the hundreds, and so on.

Example 6   Add: 7312 + 2504.

Place values are lined up in columns.

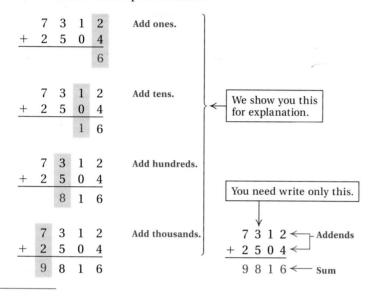

```
  7 3 1 2     Add ones.
+ 2 5 0 4
        6
```

```
  7 3 1 2     Add tens.
+ 2 5 0 4
      1 6
```
We show you this for explanation.

```
  7 3 1 2     Add hundreds.
+ 2 5 0 4
    8 1 6
```
You need write only this.

```
  7 3 1 2     Add thousands.
+ 2 5 0 4
  9 8 1 6
```

```
  7 3 1 2  ←── Addends
+ 2 5 0 4  ←──
  9 8 1 6  ←── Sum
```

Do Exercise 11.

Example 7   Add: 6878 + 4995.

```
      1
  6 8 7 8
+ 4 9 9 5
        3
```
Add ones. We get 13 ones, or 1 ten + 3 ones. Write 3 in the ones column and 1 above the tens. This is called *carrying*, or *regrouping*.

```
    1 1
  6 8 7 8
+ 4 9 9 5
      7 3
```
Add tens. We get 17 tens, or 1 hundred + 7 tens. Write 7 in the tens column and 1 above the hundreds.

```
  1 1 1
  6 8 7 8
+ 4 9 9 5
    8 7 3
```
Add hundreds. We get 18 hundreds, or 1 thousand + 8 hundreds. Write 8 in the hundreds column and 1 above the thousands.

```
  1 1 1
  6 8 7 8
+ 4 9 9 5
1 1 8 7 3
```
Add thousands. We get 11 thousands.

Do Exercises 12 and 13.

Write an addition sentence that corresponds to each situation.

9. Two trucks haul sand to a construction site to use in a driveway. One hauls 6 cu yd and the other hauls 8 cu yd. Altogether, how many cubic yards of sand are they hauling to the site?

6 cu yd + 8 cu yd = 14 cu yd

10. A football fan drives to all college football games using a motor home. On one trip the fan buys 80 gallons (gal) of gasoline and on another, 56 gal. How many gallons were bought in all?

80 gal + 56 gal = 136 gal

11. Add.
```
  6 2 0 3
+ 3 5 4 2
```
9745

Add.
12.
```
  7 9 6 8
+ 5 4 9 7
```
13,465

13.
```
  9 8 0 4
+ 6 3 7 8
```
16,182

Answers on page A-1

Add from the top.

14.   9
          9
          4
        + 5
       —————
         27

15.   8
          6
          9
          7
        + 4
       —————
         34

16. Add from the bottom.
          9
          9
          4
        + 5
       —————
         27

Answers on page A-1

How do we do an addition of three numbers, like 2 + 3 + 6? We do so by adding 3 and 6, and then 2. We can show this with parentheses:

$$2 + (3 + 6) = 2 + 9 = 11.$$ **Parentheses tell what to do first.**

We could also add 2 and 3, and then 6:

$$(2 + 3) + 6 = 5 + 6 = 11.$$

Either way we get 11. It does not matter how we group the numbers. This illustrates the **associative law of addition,** $a + (b + c) = (a + b) + c$. We can also add whole numbers in any order. That is, $2 + 3 = 3 + 2$. This illustrates the **commutative law of addition,** $a + b = b + a$. Together the commutative and associative laws tell us that to add more than two numbers, we can use any order and grouping we wish.

Example 8   Add from the top.

          8
          9
          7
        + 6

We first add 8 and 9, getting 17; then 17 and 7, getting 24; then 24 and 6, getting 30.

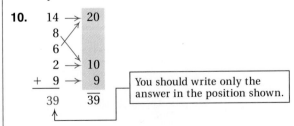

```
   8
   9  ──→  17
   7         7  ──→  24
 + 6                   6  ──→  30
 ————
  30  ←————————————————  You write only this.
```

Do Exercises 14 and 15.

Example 9   Add from the bottom.

```
   8                          8  ──→  30
   9                 9  ──→  22
   7  ──→  13
 + 6
 ————
  30  ←——  You still write the answer here.
```

Do Exercise 16.

Sometimes it is easier to look for pairs of numbers whose sums are 10 or 20 or 30, and so on.

Examples   Add.

10.
```
   14  ──→  20
    8
    6
    2  ──→  10
 +  9  ──→   9        You should write only the
 ————      ————       answer in the position shown.
   39        39
```

11. $23 + 19 + 7 + 21 + 4 = 74$

$$30 + 40 + 4$$
$$74$$

Do Exercises 17–19.

Example 12 Add: $2391 + 3276 + 8789 + 1498$.

$$
\begin{array}{r}
^{2} \\
2\ 3\ 9\ 1 \\
3\ 2\ 7\ 6 \\
8\ 7\ 8\ 9 \\
+\ 1\ 4\ 9\ 8 \\
\hline
4
\end{array}
$$

Add ones: We get 24, so we have 2 tens + 4 ones. Write 4 in the ones column and 2 above the tens.

$$
\begin{array}{r}
^{3}\ ^{2} \\
2\ 3\ 9\ 1 \\
3\ 2\ 7\ 6 \\
8\ 7\ 8\ 9 \\
+\ 1\ 4\ 9\ 8 \\
\hline
5\ 4
\end{array}
$$

Add tens: We get 35 tens, so we have 30 tens + 5 tens, or 3 hundreds + 5 tens. Write 5 in the tens column and 3 above the hundreds.

$$
\begin{array}{r}
^{1}\ ^{3}\ ^{2} \\
2\ 3\ 9\ 1 \\
3\ 2\ 7\ 6 \\
8\ 7\ 8\ 9 \\
+\ 1\ 4\ 9\ 8 \\
\hline
9\ 5\ 4
\end{array}
$$

Add hundreds: We get 19 hundreds, or 1 thousand + 9 hundreds. Write 9 in the hundreds column and 1 above the thousands.

$$
\begin{array}{r}
^{1}\ ^{3}\ ^{2} \\
2\ 3\ 9\ 1 \\
3\ 2\ 7\ 6 \\
8\ 7\ 8\ 9 \\
+\ 1\ 4\ 9\ 8 \\
\hline
1\ 5\ 9\ 5\ 4
\end{array}
$$

Add thousands: We get 15 thousands.

Do Exercise 20.

Add. Look for pairs of numbers whose sums are 10, 20, 30, and so on.

17.
$$
\begin{array}{r}
1\ 5 \\
7 \\
5 \\
3 \\
+\ 8 \\
\hline
38
\end{array}
$$

18. $6 + 12 + 14 + 8 + 7$

47

19. $27 + 8 + 13 + 2 + 11$

61

20. Add.

$$
\begin{array}{r}
1\ 9\ 3\ 2 \\
6\ 7\ 2\ 3 \\
9\ 8\ 7\ 8 \\
+\ 8\ 9\ 4\ 1 \\
\hline
27,474
\end{array}
$$

To the instructor and the student: This section presented a review of addition of whole numbers. Students who are successful should go on to Section 1.3. Those who have trouble should study developmental unit A near the back of this text and then repeat Section 1.2.

Answers on page A-1

Improving Your Math Study Skills

Getting Started in a Math Class:
The First-Day Handout or Syllabus

There are many ways in which to improve your math study skills. We have already considered some tips on using this book (see Section 1.1). We now consider some more general tips.

- **Textbook.** On the first day of class, most instructors distribute a handout that lists the textbook and other materials needed in the course. If possible, call the instructor or the department office before the term begins to find out which textbook you will be using and visit the bookstore to pick it up. This way, you can be ready to begin studying as soon as class starts. Delay in obtaining a copy of the textbook may cause you to fall behind in your homework.

- **Attendance.** The handout may also describe the attendance policy for your class. Some instructors take attendance at every class, while others use different methods to track students' attendance. Regardless of the policy, you should plan to attend class every time. Missing even one class can cause you to fall behind. If attendance counts toward your course grade, find out if there is a way to make up for missed days. In general, missing a class is not catastrophic if you put in the effort to catch up by studying the material on your own.

  If you do miss a class, call the instructor as soon as possible to find out what material was covered and what was assigned for the next class. If you have a study partner, call this person; ask if you can make a copy of his or her notes and find out what the homework assignment was. It is a good idea to meet with your instructor in person to clarify any concepts that you do not understand. This way, when you do return to class, you will be able to follow along with the rest of the group.

- **Homework.** The first-day handout may also detail how homework is handled. Find out when, and how often, homework will be assigned, whether homework is collected or graded, and whether there will be quizzes on the homework material.

  If the homework will be graded, find out what part of the final grade it will determine. Also, ask what the policy is for late homework and the format in which homework should be submitted. If you do miss a homework deadline, be sure to do the assigned homework anyway, as this is the best way to learn the material.

- **Grading.** The handout may also provide information on how your grade will be calculated at the end of the term. Typically, there will be tests during the term and a final exam at the end of the term. Frequently, homework is counted as part of the grade calculation, as are the quizzes. Find out how many tests will be given, if there is an option for make-up tests, or if any test grades will be dropped at the end of the term.

  Some instructors keep the class grades on a computer. If this is the case, find out if you can receive current grade reports throughout the term. This will help you focus on what is needed to obtain the desired grade in the course. Although a good grade should not be your only goal in this class, most students find it motivational to know what their grade is at any time during the term.

- **Get to know your classmates.** It can be a big help in a math class to get to know your fellow students. You might consider forming a study group. To do so, simply exchange phone numbers and schedules with other group members so that you can coordinate study time for homework or tests.

- **Get to know your instructor.** It can, of course, help immensely to get to know your instructor. Trivial though it may seem, get basic information like his or her name, how he or she can be contacted outside of class, and where the office is.

  Learn about your instructor's teaching style. Does he or she use an overhead projector or the board? Will there be frequent in-class questions? Try to adjust to your instructor's style.

Exercise Set 1.2

a Write an addition sentence that corresponds to each situation.

1. Isabel receives 7 e-mail messages on Tuesday and 8 on Wednesday. How many e-mail messages did she receive altogether on the two days?

7 + 8 = 15

2. At a construction site, there are two gasoline containers to be used by earth-moving vehicles. One contains 400 gal and the other 200 gal. How many gallons do both contain altogether?

400 gal + 200 gal = 600 gal

3. A builder buys two parcels of land to build a housing development. One contains 500 acres and the other 300 acres. What is the total number of acres purchased?

500 acres + 300 acres = 800 acres

4. During March and April, Deron earns extra money doing income taxes part time. In March he earned $220, and in April he earned $340. How much extra did he earn altogether in March and April?

$220 + $340 = $560

Find the perimeter of (distance around) each figure.

5.

114 mi

6.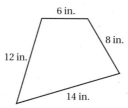

40 in.

7.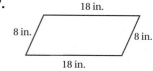

52 in.

8.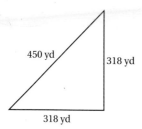

1086 yd

9.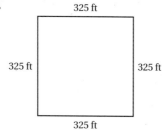

1300 ft

10.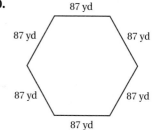

522 yd

b Add.

11.
```
  3 6 4
+   2 3
```
387

12.
```
  1 5 2 1
+   3 4 8
```
1869

13.
```
  1 7 0 6
+ 3 4 8 2
```
5188

14.
```
  7 5 0 3
+ 2 6 8 3
```
10,186

15.
```
   8 6
 + 7 8
```
164

16.
```
   7 3
 + 6 9
```
142

17.
```
   9 9
 +   1
```
100

18.
```
   9 9 9
 +    1 1
```
1010

19. 789 + 111

900

20. 839 + 386

1225

21. 909 + 101

1010

22. 707 + 909

1616

23. 8113 + 390

8503

24. 271 + 3338

3609

25. 356 + 4910

5266

26. 280 + 34,702

34,982

27. 3870 + 92 + 7 + 497   4466

28. 10,120 + 12,989 + 5738   28,847

29.
```
   5 0 9 3
 + 3 2 1 7
```
8310

30.
```
   3 6 5 4
 + 2 7 0 0
```
6354

31.
```
   4 8 2 5
 + 1 7 8 3
```
6608

32.
```
   6 7 7 5
 + 1 4 3 2
```
8207

33.
```
   9 9 9 9
 + 6 7 8 5
```
16,784

34.
```
   4 5,8 7 9
 + 2 1,7 8 6
```
67,665

35.
```
   2 3,4 4 3
 + 1 0,9 8 9
```
34,432

36.
```
   6 7,6 5 4
 + 9 8,7 8 6
```
166,440

37.
```
   7 7,5 4 3
 + 2 3,7 6 7
```
101,310

38.
```
   4 4,6 5 4
 +   4,7 6 5
```
49,419

39.
```
   9 9,9 9 9
 +      1 0 2
```
100,101

40.
```
   1 2 7,5 5 6
 +   6 8,7 6 6
```
196,322

Add from the top. Then check by adding from the bottom.

41.
```
   7
   9
   4
 + 8
  28
```

42.
```
   4
   3
   9
   1
 + 8
  25
```

43.
```
   8
   6
   2
   3
 + 7
  26
```

44.
```
   9
   4
   7
   8
 + 7
  35
```

Add. Look for pairs of numbers whose sums are 10, 20, 30, and so on.

45.
```
    7
  1 8
    3
  3 7
 +  2
   67
```

46.
```
  2 3
  1 6
  1 1
  1 8
 +1 9
   87
```

47.
```
  4 5
  2 5
  3 6
  4 4
 +8 0
  230
```

48.
```
  3 8
  2 7
  3 2
  1 4
 +7 6
  187
```

Add.

49.
```
  2 3
  6 2
 +4 5
  130
```

50.
```
  4 3
  1 1
 +3 7
   91
```

51.
```
  4 5 1
    3 6
 +8 6 2
  1349
```

52.
```
    3 1
  7 5 3
 +9 2 4
  1708
```

53.
```
   2,6 0 3
  2 8,2 1 4
 +  6,1 0 9
   36,926
```

54.
```
  9 3,2 4 9
     1,2 6 8
 +7 4,8 2 3
  169,340
```

55.
```
  1 2,0 7 0
     2,9 5 4
 +   3,4 0 0
   18,424
```

56.
```
  4 2,4 8 7
  8 3,1 4 1
 +3 6,7 1 2
  162,340
```

57.
```
  3 2 7
  4 2 8
  5 6 9
  7 8 7
 +2 0 9
  2320
```

58.
```
  9 8 9
  5 6 6
  8 3 4
  9 2 0
 +7 0 3
  4012
```

59.
```
  4 8 3 5
    7 2 9
  9 2 0 4
  8 9 8 6
 +7 9 3 1
  31,685
```

60.
```
      5,9 4 6
        8 3 4
    1 2,9 5 6
  9 2 8,3 4 2
    3 4,9 0 1
 +  5 6,0 0 0
  1,038,979
```

61.
```
  2 0 3 7
  4 9 2 3
  3 4 7 1
+ 1 2 4 8
```
11,679

62.
```
  4 5 6 7
  1 0 2 3
  4 8 2 1
+ 3 6 8 3
```
14,094

63.
```
  3 4 2 0
  8 7 1 9
  4 3 1 2
+ 6 2 0 3
```
22,654

64.
```
  2 0 0 3
    1 4 9
      5 8
+ 3 4 2 6
```
5636

65.
```
  5,6 7 8,9 8 7
  1,4 0 9,3 1 2
    8 9 8,8 8 8
+ 4,7 7 7,9 1 0
```
12,765,097

66.
```
  7 8,8 9 9,3 1 1
   6,7 8 4,1 7 0
  1 1,5 4 1,9 1 3
+     1 0 0,8 1 7
```
97,326,211

68. Nine hundred twenty-four million, six hundred thousand

Skill Maintenance

The exercises that follow begin an important feature called *skill maintenance exercises.* These exercises provide an ongoing review of any preceding objective in the book. You will see them in virtually every exercise set. It has been found that this kind of extensive review can significantly improve your performance on a final examination.

67. Write standard notation for 7 thousands + 9 hundreds + 9 tens + 2 ones. [1.1b] 7992

68. Write a word name for the number in the following sentence: [1.1c]

Recently, the National Basketball Association's gross revenue was $924,600,000 (**Source:** *Wall Street Journal*).

69. What does the digit 8 mean in 486,205? [1.1e]

8 ten thousands

70. Write in standard notation: [1.1d]

Twenty-three million. 23,000,000

Synthesis

71. ◆ Describe a situation that corresponds to the addition 80 sq ft + 140 sq ft. (See Examples 2–5.)

72. ◆ Explain in your own words what the associative law of addition means.

Add.

73. ▦ 5,987,943 + 328,959 + 49,738,765 56,055,667

74. ▦ 39,487,981 + 8,709,486 + 989,765 49,187,232

75. A fast way to add all the numbers from 1 to 10 inclusive is to pair 1 with 9, 2 with 8, and so on. Use a similar approach to add all the numbers from 1 to 100 inclusive. 1 + 99 = 100, 2 + 98 = 100,..., 49 + 51 = 100.
Then 49 · 100 = 4900 and 4900 + 50 + 100 = 5050.

1.3 Subtraction

a | Subtraction and the Real World: Take Away

Subtraction of whole numbers corresponds to two kinds of situations. The first one is called "take away."

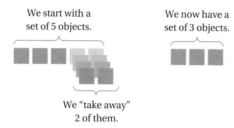

We start with a set of 5 objects.

We now have a set of 3 objects.

We "take away" 2 of them.

The subtraction that corresponds to the figure above is as follows.

5 − 2 = 3   This is read "5 minus 2 equals 3."

Minuend   Subtrahend   Difference

A **subtrahend** is the number being subtracted. A **difference** is the result of subtracting one number from another. That is, it is the result of subtracting the subtrahend from the **minuend**.

Examples Write a subtraction sentence that corresponds to each situation.

1. Juan goes to a music store and chooses 10 CDs to take to the listening station. He rejects 7 of them, but buys the rest. How many CDs did Juan buy?

There are 10 CDs to begin with.

He rejects 7 of them.

He buys the remaining 3.

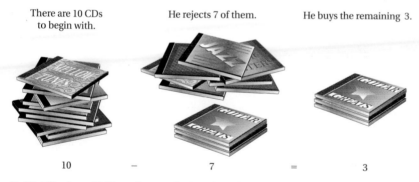

10   −   7   =   3

2. Kaitlin has $300 and spends $85 for office supplies. How much money is left?

Amount to begin with

Amount spent for office supplies

Amount left

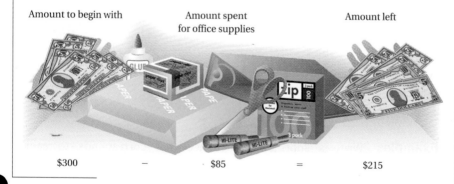

$300   − $85   = $215

Do Exercises 1 and 2.

Write a subtraction sentence that corresponds to each situation.

1. A contractor removes 5 cu yd of sand from a pile containing 67 cu yd. How many cubic yards of sand are left in the pile?

67 cu yd − 5 cu yd = 62 cu yd

2. Sparks Electronics owns a field next door that has an area of 20,000 sq ft. Deciding they need more room for parking, the owners have 12,000 sq ft paved. How many square feet of field are left unpaved?

20,000 sq ft − 12,000 sq ft = 8000 sq ft

Answers on page A-2

Write a related addition sentence.

3. $7 - 5 = 2$

$7 = 2 + 5$, or $7 = 5 + 2$

4. $17 - 8 = 9$

$17 = 9 + 8$, or $17 = 8 + 9$

Write two related subtraction sentences.

5. $5 + 8 = 13$

$5 = 13 - 8; 8 = 13 - 5$

6. $11 + 3 = 14$

$11 = 14 - 3; 3 = 14 - 11$

---

b | Related Sentences

Subtraction is defined in terms of addition. For example, $5 - 2$ is that number which when added to 2 gives 5. Thus for the subtraction sentence

$5 - 2 = 3$,   Taking away 2 from 5 gives 3.

there is a *related addition* sentence

$5 = 3 + 2$.   Putting back the 2 gives 5 again.

In fact, we know answers to subtractions are correct only because of the related addition, which provides a handy way to check a subtraction.

Example 3   Write a related addition sentence: $8 - 5 = 3$.

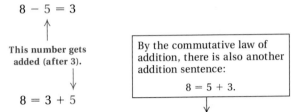

The related addition sentence is $8 = 3 + 5$.

Do Exercises 3 and 4.

Example 4   Write two related subtraction sentences: $4 + 3 = 7$.

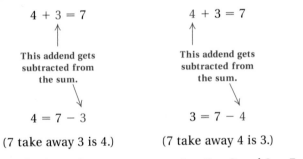

(7 take away 3 is 4.)   (7 take away 4 is 3.)

The related subtraction sentences are $4 = 7 - 3$ and $3 = 7 - 4$.

Do Exercises 5 and 6.

c | How Much More?

The second kind of situation to which subtraction corresponds is called "how much more?". We need the concept of a missing addend for "how-much-more" problems. From the related sentences, we see that finding a *missing addend* is the same as finding a *difference*.

Missing addend   Difference

$12 = 3 + \blacksquare$ $12 - 3 = \blacksquare$

Examples   Write a subtraction sentence that corresponds to each situation.

5. A student has $47 and wants to buy a graphing calculator that costs $89. How much more is needed to buy the calculator?

To find the subtraction sentence, we first consider addition.

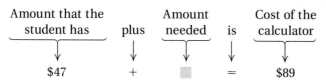

Amount that the student has	plus	Amount needed	is	Cost of the calculator
$47	+	▓	=	$89

Now we write a related subtraction sentence:

$$47 + ▓ = 89$$

$$▓ = 89 - 47.$$ **The addend 47 gets subtracted.**

6. Cathy is reading *True Success: A New Philosophy of Excellence,* by Tom Morris, as part of her philosophy class. It contains 288 pages. She has read 126 pages. How many more pages must she read?

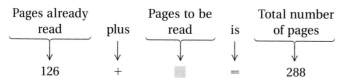

Pages already read	plus	Pages to be read	is	Total number of pages
126	+	▓	=	288

Now we write a related subtraction sentence:

$$126 + ▓ = 288$$

$$▓ = 288 - 126.$$ **126 gets subtracted.**

Do Exercises 7 and 8.

d | Subtraction of Whole Numbers

To subtract numbers, we subtract the ones digits first, then the tens, then the hundreds, and so on.

Example 7 Subtract: $9768 - 4320$.

```
   9 7 6 8      Subtract ones.
 - 4 3 2 0
         8
```

```
   9 7 6 8      Subtract tens.
 - 4 3 2 0
       4 8
```

```
   9 7 6 8      Subtract hundreds.
 - 4 3 2 0
     4 4 8
```

```
   9 7 6 8      Subtract thousands.
 - 4 3 2 0
   5 4 4 8
```

> This is for explanation.

```
   9 7 6 8
 - 4 3 2 0
   5 4 4 8
```

> You should write only this.

Do Exercise 9.

Write an addition sentence and a related subtraction sentence corresponding to each situation. You need not carry out the subtraction.

7. It is 348 mi from Miami to Jacksonville. Alice has driven 67 mi from Miami to West Palm Beach on the way to Jacksonville. How much farther does she have to drive to get to Jacksonville?

$67 + ▉ = 348;$ $▉ = 348 - 67$

8. A bricklayer estimates that it will take 1200 bricks to complete the side of a building but has only 800 bricks on the job site. How many more bricks will be needed?

$800 + ▉ = 1200;$ $▉ = 1200 - 800$

9. Subtract.

$$\begin{array}{r} 7\,8\,9\,3 \\ -\,4\,0\,9\,2 \\ \hline \end{array}$$

3801

Answers on page A-2

Subtract. Check by adding.

10.
```
  8 6 8 6
- 2 3 5 8
```
6328

11.
```
  7 1 4 5
- 2 3 9 8
```
4747

Subtract.

12.
```
    7 0
  - 1 4
```
56

13.
```
    5 0 3
  - 2 9 8
```
205

Subtract.

14.
```
  7 0 0 7
- 6 3 4 9
```
658

15.
```
  6 0 0 0
- 3 1 4 9
```
2851

16.
```
  9 0 3 5
- 7 4 8 9
```
1546

To the instructor and the student: This section presented a review of subtraction of whole numbers. Students who are successful should go on to Section 1.4. Those who have trouble should study developmental unit S near the back of this text and then repeat Section 1.3.

Answers on page A-2

Sometimes we need to borrow.

Example 8   Subtract: 6246 − 1879.

```
        3 16
  6 2 4̶ 6̶
- 1 8 7 9
          7
```
We cannot subtract 9 ones from 6 ones, but we can subtract 9 ones from 16 ones. We borrow 1 ten to get 16 ones.

```
      13
    1 3̶ 16
  6 2̶ 4̶ 6̶
- 1 8 7 9
        6 7
```
We cannot subtract 7 tens from 3 tens, but we can subtract 7 tens from 13 tens. We borrow 1 hundred to get 13 tens.

```
    11 13
  5 1̶ 3̶ 16
  6̶ 2̶ 4̶ 6̶
- 1 8 7 9
  4 3 6 7
```
We cannot subtract 8 hundreds from 1 hundred, but we can subtract 8 hundreds from 11 hundreds. We borrow 1 thousand to get 11 hundreds.

We can always check the answer by adding it to the number being subtracted.

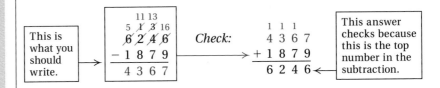

This is what you should write.

```
    11 13
  5 1̶ 3̶ 16
  6̶ 2̶ 4̶ 6̶
- 1 8 7 9
  4 3 6 7
```

Check:

```
  1 1 1
  4 3 6 7
+ 1 8 7 9
  6 2 4 6
```

This answer checks because this is the top number in the subtraction.

Do Exercises 10 and 11.

Example 9   Subtract: 902 − 477.

```
  8 9 12
  9̶ 0̶ 2̶
- 4 7 7
  4 2 5
```
We cannot subtract 7 ones from 2 ones. We have 9 hundreds, or 90 tens. We borrow 1 ten to get 12 ones. We then have 89 tens.

Do Exercises 12 and 13.

Example 10   Subtract: 8003 − 3667.

```
  7 9 9 13
  8̶ 0̶ 0̶ 3̶
- 3 6 6 7
  4 3 3 6
```
We have 8 thousands, or 800 tens.
We borrow 1 ten to get 13 ones. We then have 799 tens.

Examples

11. Subtract: 6000 − 3762.

```
  5 9 9 10
  6̶ 0̶ 0̶ 0̶
- 3 7 6 2
  2 2 3 8
```

12. Subtract: 6024 − 2968.

```
        11
    5 9 1̶ 14
  6̶ 0̶ 2̶ 4̶
- 2 9 6 8
  3 0 5 6
```

Do Exercises 14−16.

Exercise Set 1.3

a Write a subtraction sentence that corresponds to each situation. You need not carry out the subtraction.

1. Jeanne has $1260 in her college checking account. She spends $450 for her food bill at the dining hall. How much is left in her account?

$1260 − $450 = ■

2. *Frozen Yogurt.* A dispenser at a frozen yogurt store contains 126 ounces (oz) of strawberry yogurt. A 13-oz cup is sold to a customer. How much is left in the dispenser?

126 oz − 13 oz = ■

3. A host pours 5 oz of salsa from a jar containing 16 oz. How many ounces are left?

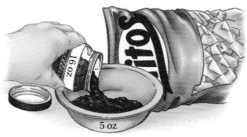

16 oz − 5 oz = ■

4. *Chocolate Cake.* One slice of chocolate cake with fudge frosting contains 564 calories (cal). One cup of hot cocoa made with skim milk contains 188 calories. How many more calories are in the cake than in the cocoa?

564 cal − 188 cal = ■

b Write a related addition sentence.

5. 7 − 4 = 3

7 = 3 + 4, or
7 = 4 + 3

6. 12 − 5 = 7

12 = 7 + 5, or
12 = 5 + 7

7. 13 − 8 = 5

13 = 5 + 8, or
13 = 8 + 5

8. 9 − 9 = 0

9 = 0 + 9, or
9 = 9 + 0

9. 23 − 9 = 14

23 = 14 + 9, or
23 = 9 + 14

10. 20 − 8 = 12

20 = 12 + 8, or
20 = 8 + 12

11. 43 − 16 = 27

43 = 27 + 16, or
43 = 16 + 27

12. 51 − 18 = 33

51 = 33 + 18, or
51 = 18 + 33

Write two related subtraction sentences.

13. 6 + 9 = 15

6 = 15 − 9;
9 = 15 − 6

14. 7 + 9 = 16

7 = 16 − 9;
9 = 16 − 7

15. 8 + 7 = 15

8 = 15 − 7;
7 = 15 − 8

16. 8 + 0 = 8

8 = 8 − 0;
0 = 8 − 8

17. 17 + 6 = 23

17 = 23 − 6;
6 = 23 − 17

18. 11 + 8 = 19

11 = 19 − 8;
8 = 19 − 11

19. 23 + 9 = 32

23 = 32 − 9;
9 = 32 − 23

20. 42 + 10 = 52

42 = 52 − 10;
10 = 52 − 42

c Write an addition sentence and a related subtraction sentence corresponding to each situation. You need not carry out the subtraction.

21. *Kangaroos.* There are 32 million kangaroos in Australia and 17 million people. How many more kangaroos are there than people?

17 + ■ = 32; ■ = 32 − 17

22. *Interstate Speeds.* Recently, speed limits on interstate highways in many western states were raised from 65 mph to 75 mph. By how many miles per hour were they raised?

65 + ■ = 75; ■ = 75 − 65

23. A set of drapes requires 23 yards (yd) of material. The decorator has 10 yd of material in stock. How much more must be ordered?

10 + ■ = 23; ■ = 23 − 10

24. Marv needs to bowl a score of 223 in order to beat his opponent. His score with one frame to go is 195. How many pins does Marv need in the last frame to beat his opponent?

195 + ■ = 223; ■ = 223 − 195

d Subtract.

25.
```
  1 6
−   4
```
12

26.
```
  8 6
− 1 3
```
73

27.
```
  6 5
− 2 1
```
44

28.
```
  8 7
− 3 4
```
53

29.
```
  8 6 6
− 3 3 3
```
533

30.
```
  5 2 6
− 3 2 3
```
203

31.
```
  4 5 4 7
− 3 4 2 1
```
1126

32.
```
  6 8 7 5
− 2 1 1 1
```
4764

33. 86 − 47

39

34. 73 − 28

45

35. 625 − 327

298

36. 726 − 509

217

37. 835 − 609

226

38. 953 − 246

707

39. 981 − 747

234

40. 887 − 698

189

41.
```
  7 7 6 9
− 2 3 8 7
```
5382

42.
```
  6 4 3 1
− 2 8 9 6
```
3535

43.
```
  3 9 8 2
− 2 4 8 9
```
1493

44.
```
  7 6 5 0
− 1 7 6 5
```
5885

45.
```
  5 0 4 6
− 2 8 5 9
```
2187

46.
```
  6 3 0 8
− 2 6 7 9
```
3629

47.
```
  7 6 4 0
− 3 8 0 9
```
3831

48.
```
  8 0 0 3
−   5 9 9
```
7404

49.
```
  1 2,6 4 7
-    4,8 9 9
```
7748

50.
```
  1 6,2 2 2
-    5,8 8 8
```
10,334

51.
```
  4 6,7 7 1
- 1 2,9 7 7
```
33,794

52.
```
  9 5,6 5 4
- 4 8,9 8 5
```
46,669

53. 10,002 − 7834

2168

54. 23,048 − 17,592

5456

55. 90,237 − 47,209

43,028

56. 84,703 − 298

84,405

57.
```
  8 0
- 2 4
```
56

58.
```
  4 0
- 3 7
```
3

59.
```
  9 0
- 5 4
```
36

60.
```
  9 0
- 7 8
```
12

61.
```
  1 4 0
-   5 6
```
84

62.
```
  4 7 0
- 1 8 8
```
282

63.
```
  6 9 0
- 2 3 6
```
454

64.
```
  8 0 3
- 4 1 8
```
385

65.
```
  9 0 3
- 1 3 2
```
771

66.
```
  6 4 0 8
-   2 5 8
```
6150

67.
```
  2 3 0 0
-   1 0 9
```
2191

68.
```
  3 5 0 6
- 1 2 9 3
```
2213

69.
```
  6 8 0 8
- 3 0 5 9
```
3749

70.
```
  7 8 4 0
- 3 0 2 7
```
4813

71.
```
  8 0 9 2
- 1 0 7 3
```
7019

72.
```
  6 0 0 7
- 1 5 8 9
```
4418

73. 5843 − 98

5745

74. 10,002 − 398

9604

75. 101,734 − 5760

95,974

76. 15,017 − 7809

7208

77. 10,008 − 19

9989

78. 21,043 − 8909

12,134

79. 83,907 − 89

83,818

80. 311,568 − 19,394

292,174

81.
```
  7 0 0 0
− 2 7 9 4
```
4206

82.
```
  8 0 0 1
− 6 5 4 3
```
1458

83.
```
  4 8,0 0 0
− 3 7,6 9 5
```
10,305

84.
```
  1 7,0 4 3
− 1 1,5 9 8
```
5445

85. 7 ten thousands   **86.** Six million, three hundred seventy-five thousand, six hundred two

Skill Maintenance

85. What does the digit 7 mean in 6,375,602?   [1.1e]

86. Write a word name for 6,375,602.   [1.1c]

87. Write standard notation for 2 ten thousands + 9 thousands + 7 hundreds + 8 ones.   [1.1b]   29,708

88. Add: 9807 + 12,885.   [1.2b]   22,692

Synthesis

89. ◈ Is subtraction commutative (is there a commutative law of subtraction)? Why or why not?

90. ◈ Describe a situation that corresponds to the subtraction $20 − $17. (See Examples 2 and 5.)

Subtract.

91. ▦ 3,928,124 − 1,098,947   2,829,177

92. ▦ 21,431,206 − 9,724,837   11,706,369

93. Fill in the missing digits to make the equation true:
9,▮48,621 − 2,097,▮81 = 7,251,140.   3; 4

1.4 Rounding and Estimating; Order

a | Rounding

We round numbers in various situations if we do not need an exact answer. For example, we might round to check if an answer to a problem is reasonable or to check a calculation done by hand or on a calculator. We might also round to see if we are being charged the correct amount in a store.

To understand how to round, we first look at some examples using number lines, even though this is not the way we normally do rounding.

Example 1 Round 47 to the nearest ten.

Here is a part of a number line; 47 is between 40 and 50.

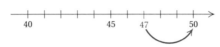

Since 47 is closer to 50 than it is to 40, we round up to 50.

Example 2 Round 42 to the nearest ten.

42 is between 40 and 50.

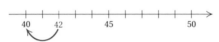

Since 42 is closer to 40 than it is to 50, we round down to 40.

Do Exercises 1–4.

Example 3 Round 45 to the nearest ten.

45 is halfway between 40 and 50.

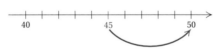

We could round 45 down to 40 or up to 50. We agree to round up to 50.

> ▶ When a number is halfway between rounding numbers, round up.

Do Exercises 5–7.

Here is a rule for rounding.

> To round to a certain place:
> a) Locate the digit in that place.
> b) Consider the next digit to the right.
> c) If the digit to the right is 5 or higher, round up; if the digit to the right is 4 or lower, round down.
> d) Change all digits to the right of the rounding location to zeros.

Objectives

a | Round to the nearest ten, hundred, or thousand.

b | Estimate sums and differences by rounding.

c | Use < or > for ▒ to write a true sentence in a situation like 6 ▒ 10.

For Extra Help

TAPE 1   InterAct **math**   CD-ROM
             MAC
             WIN

Round to the nearest ten.

1. 37

40

2. 52

50

3. 73

70

4. 98

100

Round to the nearest ten.

5. 35

40

6. 75

80

7. 85

90

Answers on page A-2

Round to the nearest ten.

8. 137

140

9. 473

470

10. 235

240

11. 295

300

Round to the nearest hundred.

12. 641

600

13. 759

800

14. 750

800

15. 9325

9300

Round to the nearest thousand.

16. 7896

8000

17. 8459

8000

18. 19,843

20,000

19. 68,500

69,000

Answers on page A-2

Example 4   Round 6485 to the nearest ten.

a) Locate the digit in the tens place.

6 4 8 5
   ↑

b) Consider the next digit to the right.

6 4 8 5
   ↑

c) Since that digit is 5 or higher, round 8 tens up to 9 tens.

d) Change all digits to the right of the tens digit to zeros.

6 4 9 0 ← This is the answer.

Example 5   Round 6485 to the nearest hundred.

a) Locate the digit in the hundreds place.

6 4 8 5
 ↑

b) Consider the next digit to the right.

6 4 8 5
  ↑

c) Since that digit is 5 or higher, round 4 hundreds up to 5 hundreds.

d) Change all digits to the right of hundreds to zeros.

6 5 0 0 ← This is the answer.

Example 6   Round 6485 to the nearest thousand.

a) Locate the digit in the thousands place.

6 4 8 5
↑

b) Consider the next digit to the right.

6 4 8 5
 ↑

c) Since that digit is 4 or lower, round down, meaning that 6 thousands stays as 6 thousands.

d) Change all digits to the right of thousands to zeros.

6 0 0 0 ← This is the answer.

CAUTION!   7000 is not a correct answer to Example 6. It is incorrect to round from the ones digit over, as follows:

6485,   6490,   6500,   7000.

Do Exercises 8–19.

There are many methods of rounding. For example, in computer applications, the rounding of 8563 to the nearest hundred might be done using a different rule called **truncating**, meaning that we simply change all digits to the right of the rounding location to zeros. Thus, 8563 would round to 8500, which is not the same answer that we would get using the rule discussed in this section.

b | Estimating

Estimating is used to simplify a problem so that it can then be solved easily or mentally. Rounding is used when estimating. There are many ways to estimate.

Example 7   Michelle earned $21,791 as a consultant and $17,239 as an instructor in a recent year. Estimate Michelle's yearly earnings.

There are many ways to get an answer, but there is no one perfect answer based on how the problem is worded. Let's consider two methods.

METHOD 1.   Round each number to the nearest thousand and then add.

$$
\begin{array}{r}
2\ 1,7\ 9\ 1 \\
+\ 1\ 7,2\ 3\ 9 \\
\end{array}
\qquad
\begin{array}{r}
2\ 2,0\ 0\ 0 \\
+\ 1\ 7,0\ 0\ 0 \\
\hline
\$\ \ 3\ 9,0\ 0\ 0 \leftarrow \text{Estimated answer}
\end{array}
$$

METHOD 2.   We might use a less formal approach, depending on how specific we want the answer to be. We note that both amounts are close to $20,000, and so the total is close to $40,000. In some contexts, such as retirement planning, this might be sufficient.

The point to be made is that estimating can be done in many ways and can have many answers, even though in the problems that follow we ask you to round in a specific way.

Example 8   Estimate this sum by first rounding to the nearest ten:

78 + 49 + 31 + 85.

We round each addend to the nearest ten. Then we add.

$$
\begin{array}{r}
7\ 8 \\
4\ 9 \\
3\ 1 \\
+\ 8\ 5 \\
\end{array}
\qquad
\begin{array}{r}
8\ 0 \\
5\ 0 \\
3\ 0 \\
+\ 9\ 0 \\
\hline
2\ 5\ 0 \leftarrow \text{Estimated answer}
\end{array}
$$

Do Exercise 20.

Example 9   Estimate this sum by first rounding to the nearest hundred:

850 + 674 + 986 + 839.

We have

$$
\begin{array}{r}
8\ 5\ 0 \\
6\ 7\ 4 \\
9\ 8\ 6 \\
+\ 8\ 3\ 9 \\
\end{array}
\qquad
\begin{array}{r}
9\ 0\ 0 \\
7\ 0\ 0 \\
1\ 0\ 0\ 0 \\
+\ \ \ 8\ 0\ 0 \\
\hline
3\ 4\ 0\ 0
\end{array}
$$

Do Exercise 21.

20. Estimate the sum by first rounding to the nearest ten. Show your work.

$$
\begin{array}{r}
7\ 4 \\
2\ 3 \\
3\ 5 \\
+\ 6\ 6 \\
\hline
\end{array}
$$

200

21. Estimate the sum by first rounding to the nearest hundred. Show your work.

$$
\begin{array}{r}
6\ 5\ 0 \\
6\ 8\ 5 \\
2\ 3\ 8 \\
+\ 1\ 6\ 8 \\
\hline
\end{array}
$$

1800

Answers on page A-2

22. Estimate the difference by first rounding to the nearest hundred. Show your work.

$$\begin{array}{r} 9\ 2\ 8\ 5 \\ -\ 6\ 7\ 3\ 9 \\ \hline \end{array}$$

2600

23. Estimate the difference by first rounding to the nearest thousand. Show your work.

$$\begin{array}{r} 2\ 3,2\ 7\ 8 \\ -\ 1\ 1,6\ 9\ 8 \\ \hline \end{array}$$

11,000

Use < or > for ▮ to form a true sentence. Draw a number line if necessary.

24. 8 ▮ 12   <

25. 12 ▮ 8   >

26. 76 ▮ 64   >

27. 64 ▮ 76   <

28. 217 ▮ 345   <

29. 345 ▮ 217   >

Answers on page A-2

Example 10   Estimate the difference by first rounding to the nearest thousand: 9324 − 2849.

We have

$$\begin{array}{r} 9\ 3\ 2\ 4 \\ -\ 2\ 8\ 4\ 9 \\ \end{array} \qquad \begin{array}{r} 9\ 0\ 0\ 0 \\ -\ 3\ 0\ 0\ 0 \\ \hline 6\ 0\ 0\ 0 \end{array}$$

Do Exercises 22 and 23.

The sentence $7 - 5 = 2$ says that $7 - 5$ is the same as 2. Later we will use the symbol $\approx$ when rounding. This symbol means **"is approximately equal to."** Thus, when 687 is rounded to the nearest ten, we may write

$$687 \approx 690.$$

c | Order

We know that 2 is not the same as 5. This can be written $2 \neq 5$. In fact, 2 is less than 5. We can see this order on a number line: 2 is to the left of 5. The number 0 is the smallest whole number.

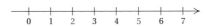

> For any whole numbers a and b:
>
> **1.** $a < b$ (read "a is less than b") is true when a is to the left of b on a number line.
>
> **2.** $a > b$ (read "a is greater than b") is true when a is to the right of b on a number line.
>
> We call < and > **inequality symbols.**

Example 11   Use < or > for ▮ to form a true sentence: 7 ▮ 11.

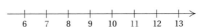

Since 7 is to the left of 11, we write $7 < 11$.

Example 12   Use < or > for ▮ to form a true sentence: 92 ▮ 87.

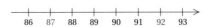

Since 92 is to the right of 87, we write $92 > 87$.

A sentence like $8 + 5 = 13$ is called an **equation**. A sentence like $7 < 11$ is called an **inequality**. The sentence $7 < 11$ is a true inequality. The sentence $23 > 69$ is a false inequality.

Do Exercises 24–29.

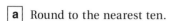

Exercise Set 1.4

a Round to the nearest ten.

1. 48
50

2. 17
20

3. 67
70

4. 99
100

5. 731
730

6. 532
530

7. 895
900

8. 798
800

Round to the nearest hundred.

9. 146
100

10. 874
900

11. 957
1000

12. 650
700

13. 9079
9100

14. 4645
4600

15. 32,850
32,900

16. 198,402
198,400

Round to the nearest thousand.

17. 5876
6000

18. 4500
5000

19. 7500
8000

20. 2001
2000

21. 45,340
45,000

22. 735,562
736,000

23. 373,405
373,000

24. 6,713,855
6,714,000

b Estimate each sum or difference by first rounding each addend to the nearest ten. Show your work.

25.   7 8
        + 9 7

        180

26.   6 2
           9 7
           4 6
        + 8 8

        300

27. 8 0 7 4
        − 2 3 4 7

        5720

28.   6 7 3
        −   2 8

        640

Estimate each sum by first rounding each addend to the nearest ten. Do any of the given sums seem to be incorrect when compared to the estimate? Which ones?

29.   4 5
           7 7
           2 5
        + 5 6

        3 4 3

        220; incorrect

30.   4 1
           2 1
           5 5
        + 6 0

        1 7 7

        180

31.   6 2 2
             7 8
             8 1
        + 1 1 1

          9 3 2

        890; incorrect

32.   8 3 6
          3 7 4
          7 9 4
        + 9 3 8

        3 9 4 7

        2940; incorrect

Estimate each sum or difference by first rounding to the nearest hundred. Show your work.

33.   7 3 4 8
        + 9 2 4 7

        16,500

34.   5 6 8
          4 7 2
          9 3 8
        + 4 0 2

        2400

35.   6 8 5 2
        − 1 7 4 8

        5200

36.   9 4 3 8
        − 2 7 8 7

        6600

Estimate each sum by first rounding the addends to the nearest hundred. Do any of the given sums seem to be incorrect when compared to the estimate? Which ones?

37.
```
   2 1 6
     8 4
   7 4 5
+ 5 9 5
―――――
   1 6 4 0
```
1600

38.
```
     4 8 1
     7 0 2
     6 2 3
+ 1 0 4 3
―――――
   1 8 4 9
```
2800; incorrect

39.
```
   7 5 0
   4 2 8
     6 3
+ 2 0 5
―――――
   1 4 4 6
```
1500

40.
```
   3 2 6
   2 7 5
   7 5 8
+ 9 4 3
―――――
   2 3 0 2
```
2300

Estimate each sum or difference by first rounding to the nearest thousand. Show your work.

41.
```
   9 6 4 3
   4 8 2 1
   8 9 4 3
+ 7 0 0 4
```
31,000

42.
```
   7 6 4 8
   9 3 4 8
   7 8 4 2
+ 2 2 2 2
```
27,000

43.
```
   9 2,1 4 9
 − 2 2,5 5 5
```
69,000

44.
```
   8 4,8 9 0
 − 1 1,1 1 0
```
74,000

c Use < or > for ▓ to form a true sentence. Draw a number line if necessary.

45. 0 ▓ 17

<

46. 32 ▓ 0

>

47. 34 ▓ 12

>

48. 28 ▓ 18

>

49. 1000 ▓ 1001

<

50. 77 ▓ 117

<

51. 133 ▓ 132

>

52. 999 ▓ 997

>

53. 460 ▓ 17

>

54. 345 ▓ 456

<

55. 37 ▓ 11

>

56. 12 ▓ 32

<

Skill Maintenance

Add. [1.2b]

57.
```
   6 7,7 8 9
+ 1 8,9 6 5
```
86,754

58.
```
   9 0 0 2
+ 4 5 8 7
```
13,589

Subtract. [1.3d]

59.
```
   6 7,7 8 9
− 1 8,9 6 5
```
48,824

60.
```
   9 0 0 2
− 4 5 8 7
```
4415

Synthesis

61. ◆ When rounding 748 to the nearest hundred, a student rounds to 750 and then to 800. What mistake is the student making?

62. ◆ Explain how estimating and rounding can be useful when shopping for groceries.

63.–66. ▦ Use a calculator to find the sums or differences in Exercises 41–44. Since you can still make errors on a calculator—say, by pressing the wrong buttons—you can check your answers by estimating.

63. 30,411 **64.** 27,060 **65.** 69,594 **66.** 73,780

1.5 Multiplication and Area

a | Multiplication and the Real World

Multiplication of whole numbers corresponds to two kinds of situations.

Repeated Addition

The multiplication 3×5 corresponds to this repeated addition:

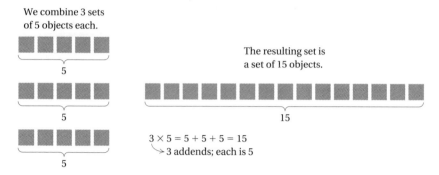

We combine 3 sets of 5 objects each.

5

5

5

The resulting set is a set of 15 objects.

15

$3 \times 5 = 5 + 5 + 5 = 15$

↘ 3 addends; each is 5

We say that the *product* of 3 and 5 is 15. The numbers 3 and 5 are called *factors*.

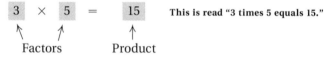

$$3 \quad \times \quad 5 \quad = \quad 15 \qquad \text{This is read "3 times 5 equals 15."}$$

Factors   Product

The numbers that we multiply can be called **factors**. The result of the multiplication is a number called a **product**.

Rectangular Arrays

The multiplication 3×5 corresponds to this rectangular array:

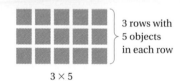

3 rows with 5 objects in each row

3×5

When you write a multiplication sentence corresponding to a real-world situation, you should think of either a rectangular array or repeated addition. In some cases, it may help to think both ways.

We have used an "×" to denote multiplication. A dot "·", as in $3 \cdot 5 = 15$, is also commonly used. (Use of the dot is attributed to the German mathematician Gottfried Wilhelm von Leibniz in 1698.) Parentheses are also used to denote multiplication—for example, $(3)(5) = 15$, or $3(5) = 15$.

Objectives

a | Write a multiplication sentence that corresponds to a situation.

b | Multiply whole numbers.

c | Estimate products by rounding.

For Extra Help

TAPE 2   InterAct math   CD-ROM
                MAC
                WIN

Write a multiplication sentence that corresponds to each situation.

1. Marv practices for the U.S. Open bowling tournament. He bowls 8 games each day for 7 days. How many games does he bowl altogether for practice?

8 · 7 = 56

2. A lab technician pours 75 milliliters (mL) of acid into each of 10 beakers. How much acid is poured in all?

10 · 75 = 750 mL

3. *Checkerboard.* A checkerboard consists of 8 rows with 8 squares in each row. How many squares in all are there on a checkerboard?

8 · 8 = 64

Answers on page A-2

Examples Write a multiplication sentence that corresponds to each situation.

1. It is known that Americans drink 24 million gal of soft drinks per day (*per day* means *each day*). What quantity of soft drinks is consumed every 5 days?

We draw a picture in which 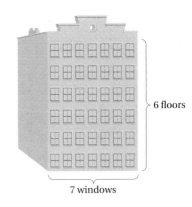 = 1 million gallons or we can simply visualize the situation. Repeated addition fits best in this case.

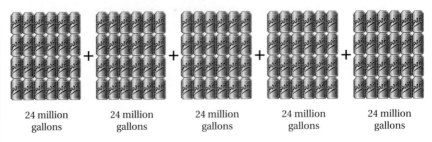

| 24 million gallons | 24 million gallons | 24 million gallons | 24 million gallons | 24 million gallons |

5 · 24 million gallons = 120 million gallons

2. One side of a building has 6 floors with 7 windows on each floor. How many windows are there on that side of the building?

We have a rectangular array and can easily draw a sketch.

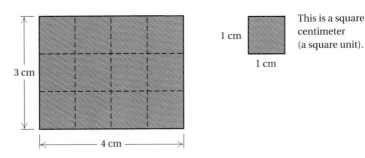

6 floors

7 windows

6 · 7 = 42

Do Exercises 1–3.

Area

The area of a rectangular region is often considered to be the number of square units needed to fill it. Here is a rectangle 4 cm (centimeters) long and 3 cm wide. It takes 12 square centimeters (sq cm) to fill it.

3 cm

4 cm

1 cm

1 cm

This is a square centimeter (a square unit).

In this case, we have a rectangular array. The number of square units is 3 · 4, or 12. The total area is 12 sq cm.

Once exponents are introduced in Section 1.9, we will often abbreviate square centimeters as cm², square feet as ft², and so on.

Example 3 Write a multiplication sentence that corresponds to this situation.

A rectangular room is 10 ft long and 8 ft wide. Find its area.

We draw a picture.

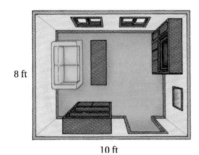

8 ft

10 ft

If we think of filling the rectangle with square feet, we have a rectangular array. The length $l = 10$ ft, and the width $w = 8$ ft. The area A is given by the formula

$$A = l \cdot w = 10 \cdot 8 = 80 \text{ sq ft.}$$

Do Exercise 4.

b | Multiplication of Whole Numbers

Let's find the product

$$\begin{array}{r} 5\,4 \\ \times\,3\,2 \\ \hline \end{array}$$

To do this, we multiply 54 by 2, then 54 by 30, and then add.

$$\begin{array}{r} 5\,4 \\ \times\quad 2 \\ \hline 1\,0\,8 \end{array} \qquad \begin{array}{r} {}^{1}\\ 5\,4 \\ \times\quad 3\,0 \\ \hline 1\,6\,2\,0 \end{array}$$

Since we are going to add the results, let's write the work this way.

$$\begin{array}{r} 5\,4 \\ \times\,3\,2 \\ \hline 1\,0\,8 \\ 1\,6\,2\,0 \\ \hline 1\,7\,2\,8 \end{array}$$

   Multiplying 54 by 2

   Multiplying 54 by 30

   Adding to obtain the product

The fact that we can do this is based on a property called the **distributive law.** It says that to multiply a number by a sum, $a \cdot (b + c)$, we can multiply each part by a and then add like this: $(a \cdot b) + (a \cdot c)$. Thus, $a \cdot (b + c) = (a \cdot b) + (a \cdot c)$. Applied to the example above, the distributive law gives us

$$54 \cdot 32 = 54 \cdot (30 + 2) = \underbrace{(54 \cdot 30)}_{} + \underbrace{(54 \cdot 2)}_{}$$
$$= \quad 1620 \quad + \quad 108$$
$$= 1728.$$

4. What is the area of this pool table?

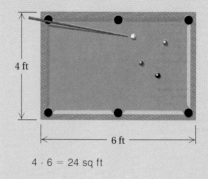

4 ft

6 ft

$4 \cdot 6 = 24$ sq ft

Answer on page A-2

Multiply.

5.
```
    4 5
  × 2 3
─────────
  1 0 3 5
```

6. 48 × 63

3024

Multiply.

7.
```
    7 4 6
  ×   6 2
─────────
  46,252
```

8. 245 × 837

205,065

Example 4   Multiply: 43 × 57.

```
        2
    5   7
  × 4   3
─────────
  1 7   1          Multiplying 57 by 3
```

```
        2
        2
    5   7
  × 4   3
─────────
  1 7   1          Multiplying 57 by 40 (We write a 0
2 2 8   0          and then multiply 57 by 4.)
```

You may have learned that such a 0 does not have to be written. You may omit it if you wish. If you do omit it, remember, when multiplying by tens, to put the answer in the tens place.

```
        2
        2
    5   7
  × 4   3
─────────
  1 7   1
2 2 8   0
─────────
2 4 5   1          Adding to obtain the product
```

Do Exercises 5 and 6.

Example 5   Multiply: 457 × 683.

```
      5   2
    6 8   3
  × 4 5   7
───────────
  4 7 8   1        Multiplying 683 by 7
```

```
      4   1
      5   2
    6 8   3
  × 4 5   7
───────────
  4 7 8   1
3 4 1 5   0        Multiplying 683 by 50
```

```
      3   1
      4   1
      5   2
    6 8     3
  × 4 5     7
─────────────
    4 7 8   1
  3 4 1 5   0
2 7 3 2 0   0      Multiplying 683 by 400
─────────────
3 1 2 , 1 3 1      Adding
```

Do Exercises 7 and 8.

Zeros in Multiplication

Example 6 Multiply: 306×274.

Note that $306 = 3$ hundreds $+ 6$ ones.

```
        2 7 4
      × 3 0 6
      1 6 4 4      Multiplying 274 by 6
    8 2 2 0 0      Multiplying 274 by 3 hundreds (We write 00
                   and then multiply 274 by 3.)
    8 3,8 4 4      Adding
```

Do Exercises 9–11.

Example 7 Multiply: 360×274.

Note that $360 = 3$ hundreds $+ 6$ tens.

```
        2 7 4  ┌ Multiplying by 6 tens (We write 0
      ×   3 6 0 └ and then multiply 274 by 6.)
      1 6 4 4 0 ◄─ Multiplying by 3 hundreds (We write 00
    8 2 2 0 0 ◄─  and then multiply 274 by 3.)
    9 8,6 4 0      Adding
```

Do Exercises 12–15.

Note the following.

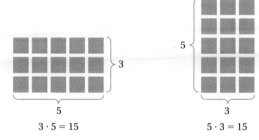

$$3 \cdot 5 = 15 \qquad\qquad 5 \cdot 3 = 15$$

If we rotate the array on the left, we get the array on the right. The answers match. This illustrates the **commutative law of multiplication.** It says that we can multiply two numbers in any order, $a \cdot b = b \cdot a$, and still get the same answer.

Do Exercise 16.

Multiply.

9.
```
    4 7 2
  × 3 0 6
  144,432
```

10. 408×704

287,232

11.
```
    2 3 4 4
  × 6 0 0 5
  14,075,720
```

Multiply.

12.
```
    4 7 2
  × 8 3 0
  391,760
```

13.
```
    2 3 4 4
  × 7 4 0 0
  17,345,600
```

14. 100×562

56,200

15. 1000×562

562,000

16. a) Find $23 \cdot 47$.

1081

b) Find $47 \cdot 23$.

1081

c) Compare your answers from parts (a) and (b).

Same

Answers on page A-2

Multiply.

17. $5 \cdot 2 \cdot 4$

40

18. $5 \cdot 1 \cdot 3$

15

19. Estimate the product twice: first by rounding to the nearest ten and then by rounding to the nearest hundred. Show your work.

$$\begin{array}{r} 8\ 3\ 7 \\ \times\ 2\ 4\ 5 \\ \hline \end{array}$$

210,000; 160,000

To multiply three or more numbers, we usually group them so that we multiply two at a time. Consider $2 \cdot (3 \cdot 4)$ and $(2 \cdot 3) \cdot 4$. The parentheses tell what to do first:

$$2 \cdot (3 \cdot 4) = 2 \cdot (12) = 24. \qquad \text{We multiply 3 and 4, then that result and 2.}$$

We can also multiply 2 and 3, then that result and 4:

$$(2 \cdot 3) \cdot 4 = (6) \cdot 4 = 24.$$

Either way we get 24. It does not matter how we group the numbers. This illustrates that **multiplication is associative**: $a \cdot (b \cdot c) = (a \cdot b) \cdot c$. Together the commutative and associative laws tell us that to multiply more than two numbers, we can use any order and grouping we wish.

CAUTION! Do not confuse the associative law with the distributive law. To multiply $2 \cdot (3 \cdot 4)$, each number is used twice. To multiply $2 \cdot (3 + 4)$, the 2 is used twice: $2 \cdot 3 + 2 \cdot 4$.

Do Exercises 17 and 18.

c | Rounding and Estimating

Example 8 Estimate the following product twice: first by rounding to the nearest ten and then by rounding to the nearest hundred: 683×457.

Nearest ten	*Nearest hundred*	*Exact*
$\begin{array}{r} 6\ 8\ 0 \\ \times\ \ \ 4\ 6\ 0 \\ \hline 4\ 0\ 8\ 0\ 0 \\ 2\ 7\ 2\ 0\ 0\ 0 \\ \hline 3\ 1\ 2\ 8\ 0\ 0 \end{array}$	$\begin{array}{r} 7\ 0\ 0 \\ \times\ \ \ 5\ 0\ 0 \\ \hline 3\ 5\ 0\ 0\ 0\ 0 \end{array}$	$\begin{array}{r} 6\ 8\ 3 \\ \times\ \ \ 4\ 5\ 7 \\ \hline 4\ 7\ 8\ 1 \\ 3\ 4\ 1\ 5\ 0 \\ 2\ 7\ 3\ 2\ 0\ 0 \\ \hline 3\ 1\ 2\ 1\ 3\ 1 \end{array}$

Note in Example 8 that the estimate, having been rounded to the nearest ten, is

312,800.

The estimate, having been rounded to the nearest hundred, is

350,000.

Note how the estimates compare to the exact answer,

312,131.

Do Exercise 19.

Answers on page A-2

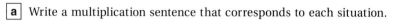

Exercise Set 1.5

a Write a multiplication sentence that corresponds to each situation.

1. The *Los Angeles Sunday Times* crossword puzzle is arranged rectangularly with squares in 21 rows and 21 columns. How many squares does the puzzle have altogether?

21 · 21 = 441

2. *Pixels.* A computer screen consists of small rectangular dots called *pixels.* How many pixels are there on a screen that has 600 rows with 800 pixels in each row?

600 · 800 = 480,000

3. A new soft drink beverage carton contains 8 cans, each of which holds 12 oz. How many ounces are there in the carton?

8 · 12 oz = 96 oz

4. There are 7 days in a week. How many days are there in 18 weeks?

18 · 7 = 126

Find the area of each region.

5.
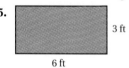
3 ft
6 ft

18 sq ft

6.
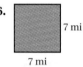
7 mi
7 mi

49 sq mi

7.
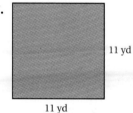
11 yd
11 yd

121 sq yd

8.
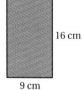
16 cm
9 cm

144 sq cm

9.
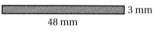
3 mm
48 mm

144 sq mm

10.
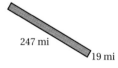
247 mi
19 mi

4693 sq mi

b Multiply.

11. $\begin{array}{r} 8\ 7 \\ \times\ 1\ 0 \\ \hline \end{array}$

870

12. $\begin{array}{r} 1\ 0\ 0 \\ \times\ \ \ \ 9\ 6 \\ \hline \end{array}$

9600

13. $\begin{array}{r} 2\ 3\ 4\ 0 \\ \times 1\ 0\ 0\ 0 \\ \hline \end{array}$

2,340,000

14. $\begin{array}{r} 8\ 0\ 0 \\ \times\ \ \ \ 7\ 0 \\ \hline \end{array}$

56,000

15. $\begin{array}{r} 6\ 5 \\ \times\ \ \ 8 \\ \hline \end{array}$

520

16. $\begin{array}{r} 8\ 7 \\ \times\ \ \ 4 \\ \hline \end{array}$

348

17. $\begin{array}{r} 9\ 4 \\ \times\ \ \ 6 \\ \hline \end{array}$

564

18. $\begin{array}{r} 7\ 6 \\ \times\ \ \ 9 \\ \hline \end{array}$

684

19. $\begin{array}{r} 6\ 5\ 2 \\ \times 1\ 0\ 0 \\ \hline \end{array}$

65,200

20. $\begin{array}{r} 6\ 5\ 2 \\ \times\ \ \ 1\ 0 \\ \hline \end{array}$

6520

21. $\begin{array}{r} 4\ 3\ 7\ 1 \\ \times 1\ 0\ 0\ 0 \\ \hline \end{array}$

4,371,000

22. $\begin{array}{r} 4\ 3\ 7\ 1 \\ \times\ \ \ 1\ 0\ 0 \\ \hline \end{array}$

437,100

23. $3 \cdot 509$

1527

24. $7 \cdot 806$

5642

25. 7(9229)

64,603

26. 4(7867)

31,468

27. 90(53)

4770

28. 60(78)

4680

29. (47)(85)

3995

30. (34)(87)

2958

31. $\begin{array}{r} 6\ 4\ 0 \\ \times\ \ \ 7\ 2 \\ \hline \end{array}$

46,080

32. $\begin{array}{r} 6\ 6\ 6 \\ \times\ \ \ 6\ 6 \\ \hline \end{array}$

43,956

33. $\begin{array}{r} 4\ 4\ 4 \\ \times\ \ \ 3\ 3 \\ \hline \end{array}$

14,652

34. $\begin{array}{r} 5\ 0\ 9 \\ \times\ \ \ 8\ 8 \\ \hline \end{array}$

44,792

Chapter 1   Operations on the Whole Numbers

35. 509
    ×408
  207,672

36. 432
    ×375
  162,000

37. 853
    ×936
  798,408

38. 346
    ×650
  224,900

39. 489
    ×340
  166,260

40. 7080
    × 160
  1,132,800

41. 4378
    ×2694
  11,794,332

42. 8007
    × 480
  3,843,360

43. 6428
    ×3224
  20,723,872

44. 8928
    ×3172
  28,319,616

45. 3482
    × 104
  362,128

46. 6408
    ×6064
  38,858,112

47. 5006
    ×4008
  20,064,048

48. 6789
    ×2330
  15,818,370

49. 5608
    ×4500
  25,236,000

50. 4560
    ×7890
  35,978,400

51. 876
    ×345
  302,220

52. 355
    ×299
  106,145

53. 7889
    ×6224
  49,101,136

54. 6501
    ×3449
  22,421,949

55. 555
    × 55
  30,525

56. 888
    × 88
  78,144

57. 734
    ×407
  298,738

58. 5080
    × 302
  1,534,160

c Estimate each product by first rounding to the nearest ten. Show your work.

59. 4 5
  $\times$ 6 7

50 · 70 = 3500

60. 5 1
  $\times$ 7 8

50 · 80 = 4000

61. 3 4
  $\times$ 2 9

30 · 30 = 900

62. 6 3
  $\times$ 5 4

60 · 50 = 3000

Estimate each product by first rounding to the nearest hundred. Show your work.

63. 8 7 6
  $\times$ 3 4 5

900 · 300 = 270,000

64. 3 5 5
  $\times$ 2 9 9

400 · 300 = 120,000

65. 4 3 2
  $\times$ 1 9 9

400 · 200 = 80,000

66. 7 8 9
  $\times$ 4 3 4

800 · 400 = 320,000

Estimate each product by first rounding to the nearest thousand. Show your work.

67. 5 6 0 8
  $\times$ 4 5 7 6

6000 · 5000 =
30,000,000

68. 2 3 4 4
  $\times$ 6 1 2 3

2000 · 6000 =
12,000,000

69. 7 8 8 8
  $\times$ 6 2 2 4

8000 · 6000 =
48,000,000

70. 6 5 0 1
  $\times$ 3 4 4 9

7000 · 3000 =
21,000,000

Skill Maintenance

71. Add. [1.2b]

     2 0
     8 5 0
  $+$ 3 5 0 0   4370

72. Subtract. [1.3d]

     6 0 0 3
  $-$ 2 8 9 4

3109

73. Round 2345 to the nearest ten, to the nearest hundred, and to the nearest thousand. [1.4a]

   2350; 2300; 2000

Synthesis

74. ◈ Explain in your own words what it means to say that multiplication is commutative.

75. ◈ Describe a situation that corresponds to the multiplication 4 · $150. (See Examples 1 and 2.)

76. ▦ An 18-story office building is box-shaped. Each floor measures 172 ft by 84 ft with a 20-ft by 35-ft rectangular area lost to an elevator and a stairwell. How much area is available as office space?   247,464 sq ft

1.6 Division

a | Division and the Real World

Division of whole numbers corresponds to two kinds of situations. In the first, consider the division $20 \div 5$, read "20 divided by 5." We can think of 20 objects arranged in a rectangular array. We ask "How many rows, each with 5 objects, are there?"

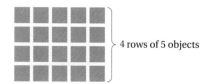

> 4 rows of 5 objects

Since there are 4 rows of 5 objects each, we have

$20 \div 5 = 4.$ **This is read "20 divided by 5 equals 4."**

In the second situation, we can ask, "If we make 5 rows, how many objects will there be in each row?"

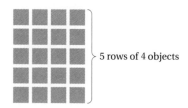

> 5 rows of 4 objects

Since there are 4 objects in each of the 5 rows, we have

$20 \div 5 = 4.$

We say that the **dividend** is 20, the **divisor** is 5, and the **quotient** is 4.

$$\underset{\text{Dividend}}{20} \quad \div \quad \underset{\text{Divisor}}{5} \quad = \quad \underset{\text{Quotient}}{4}$$

The *dividend* is what we are dividing into. The result of the division is the *quotient*.

We also write a division such as $20 \div 5$ as

$$20/5 \quad \text{or} \quad \frac{20}{5} \quad \text{or} \quad 5\overline{)20}.$$

Example 1 Write a division sentence that corresponds to this situation.

A parent gives $24 to 3 children, with each child getting the same amount. How much does each child get?

We think of an array with 3 rows. Each row will go to a child. How many dollars will be in each row?

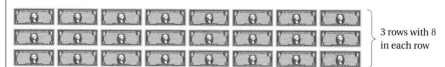

> 3 rows with 8 in each row

$24 \div 3 = 8$

Objectives

a Write a division sentence that corresponds to a situation.

b Given a division sentence, write a related multiplication sentence; and given a multiplication sentence, write two related division sentences.

c Divide whole numbers.

For Extra Help

TAPE 2

MAC WIN

CD-ROM

Write a division sentence that corresponds to each situation. You need not carry out the division.

1. There are 112 students in a college band, and they are marching with 14 in each row. How many rows are there?

   112 ÷ 14 = ■

2. A college band is in a rectangular array. There are 112 students in the band, and they are marching in 8 rows. How many students are there in each row?

   112 ÷ 8 = ■

Example 2   Write a division sentence that corresponds to this situation. You need not carry out the division.

How many mailboxes that cost $45 each can be purchased for $495?

We think of an array with 45 one-dollar bills in each row. The money in each row will buy a mailbox. How many rows will there be?

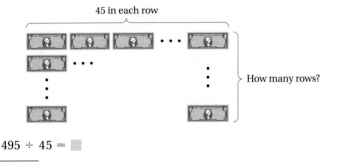

495 ÷ 45 = ■

▶ Whenever we have a rectangular array, we know the following:

(The total number) ÷ (The number of rows) = (The number in each row).

Also:

(The total number) ÷ (The number in each row) = (The number of rows).

Do Exercises 1 and 2.

b | Related Sentences

By looking at rectangular arrays, we can see how multiplication and division are related. The following array shows that 4 · 5 = 20.

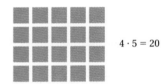

4 · 5 = 20

The array also shows the following:

20 ÷ 5 = 4   and   20 ÷ 4 = 5.

Division is actually defined in terms of multiplication. For example, 20 ÷ 5 is defined to be the number that when multiplied by 5 gives 20. Thus, for every division sentence, there is a related multiplication sentence.

20 ÷ 5 = 4   Division sentence

20 = 4 · 5   Related multiplication sentence

To get the related multiplication sentence, we use

Dividend = Quotient · Divisor.

Example 3 Write a related multiplication sentence: $12 \div 6 = 2$.

We have

$$12 \div 6 = 2 \qquad \text{Division sentence}$$

$$12 = 2 \cdot 6. \qquad \text{Related multiplication sentence}$$

The related multiplication sentence is $12 = 2 \cdot 6$.

By the commutative law of multiplication, there is also another multiplication sentence: $12 = 6 \cdot 2$.

Do Exercises 3 and 4.

For every multiplication sentence, we can write related divisions, as we can see from the preceding array.

Example 4 Write two related division sentences: $7 \cdot 8 = 56$.

We have

$$7 \cdot 8 = 56 \qquad\qquad 7 \cdot 8 = 56$$

This factor becomes a divisor.   This factor becomes a divisor.

$$7 = 56 \div 8. \qquad\qquad 8 = 56 \div 7.$$

The related division sentences are $7 = 56 \div 8$ and $8 = 56 \div 7$.

Do Exercises 5 and 6.

c Division of Whole Numbers

Multiplication can be thought of as repeated addition. Division can be thought of as repeated subtraction. Compare.

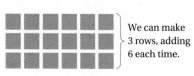

We can make 3 rows, adding 6 each time.

If we take away 6 objects at a time, we can do so 3 times.

$$18 = 6 + 6 + 6 \qquad\qquad 18 - 6 - 6 - 6 = 0$$

3 additions   3 subtractions

$$= 3 \cdot 6 \qquad\qquad\qquad 18 \div 6 = 3$$

Write a related multiplication sentence.

3. $15 \div 3 = 5$

$15 = 5 \cdot 3$, or $15 = 3 \cdot 5$

4. $72 \div 8 = 9$

$72 = 9 \cdot 8$, or $72 = 8 \cdot 9$

Write two related division sentences.

5. $6 \cdot 2 = 12$

$6 = 12 \div 2$; $2 = 12 \div 6$

6. $7 \cdot 6 = 42$

$6 = 42 \div 7$; $7 = 42 \div 6$

Answers on page A-2

7. $54 \div 9$

6; $6 \cdot 9 = 54$

8. $61 \div 9$

6 R 7; $6 \cdot 9 = 54$,
$54 + 7 = 61$

9. $53 \div 12$

4 R 5; $4 \cdot 12 = 48$,
$48 + 5 = 53$

10. $157 \div 24$

6 R 13; $6 \cdot 24 = 144$,
$144 + 13 = 157$

Answers on page A-2

To divide by repeated subtraction, we keep track of the number of times we subtract.

Example 5   Divide by repeated subtraction: $20 \div 4$.

$$
\begin{array}{r}
2\ 0 \\
-\quad 4 \longrightarrow \\
\hline
1\ 6 \\
-\quad 4 \longrightarrow \\
\hline
1\ 2 \\
-\quad 4 \longrightarrow \\
\hline
8 \\
-\quad 4 \longrightarrow \\
\hline
4 \\
-\quad 4 \longrightarrow \\
\hline
0
\end{array}
$$

We subtracted 5 times, so $20 \div 4 = 5$.

Example 6   Divide by repeated subtraction: $23 \div 5$.

$$
\begin{array}{r}
2\ 3 \\
-\quad 5 \longrightarrow \\
\hline
1\ 8 \\
-\quad 5 \longrightarrow \\
\hline
1\ 3 \\
-\quad 5 \longrightarrow \\
\hline
8 \\
-\quad 5 \longrightarrow \\
\hline
3 \longrightarrow
\end{array}
$$

We subtracted 4 times.

We have 3 left. This number is called the *remainder*.

We write

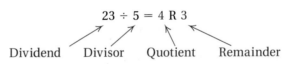

$$23 \div 5 = 4 \text{ R } 3$$

Dividend   Divisor   Quotient   Remainder

CHECKING DIVISIONS.   To check a division, we multiply. Suppose we divide 98 by 2 and get 49:

$$98 \div 2 = 49.$$

To check, we think of the related multiplication sentence $49 \cdot 2 = \blacksquare$. We multiply 49 by 2 and see if we get 98.

If there is a remainder, we add it after multiplying.

Example 7   Check the division in Example 6.

We found that $23 \div 5 = 4 \text{ R } 3$. To check, we multiply 5 by 4. This gives us 20. Then we add 3 to get 23. The dividend is 23, so the answer checks.

Do Exercises 7–10.

When we use the process of long division, we are doing repeated subtraction, even though we are going about it in a different way.

To divide, we start from the digit of highest place value in the dividend and work down to the lowest place value through the remainders. At each step we ask if there are multiples of the divisor in the quotient.

Example 8 Divide and check: $3642 \div 5$.

```
         ?
      _____
   5 ) 3 6 4 2
      ←
```

1. We start with the thousands digit in the dividend. Are there any thousands in the thousands place of the quotient? No; $5 \cdot 1000 = 5000$, and 5000 is larger than 3000.

```
          7
      _____
   5 ) 3 6 4 2
       3 5 0 0
         1 4 2
```

2. Now we go to the hundreds place in the dividend. Are there any hundreds in the hundreds place of the quotient? Think of the dividend as 36 hundreds. Estimate 7 hundreds. Write 7 in the hundreds place, multiply 700 by 5, write the answer below 3642, and subtract.

No!

```
         7 3
      _____
   5 ) 3 6 4 2
       3 5 0 0
       _____
         1 4 2    Can't
         1 5 0 ← subtract
```

3. a) We go to the tens place of the first remainder. Are there any tens in the tens place of the quotient? To answer the question, think of the first remainder as 14 tens. Estimate 3 tens. When we multiply, we get 150, which is too large.

b) We lower our estimate to 2 tens. Write 2 in the tens place, multiply 20 by 5, and subtract.

```
         7 2
      _____
   5 ) 3 6 4 2
       3 5 0 0
       _____
         1 4 2
         1 0 0
       _____
           4 2
```

4. We go to the ones place of the second remainder. Are there any ones in the ones place of the quotient? To answer the question, think of the second remainder as 42 ones. Estimate 8 ones. Write 8 in the ones place, multiply 8 by 5, and subtract.

```
         7 2 8
      _____
   5 ) 3 6 4 2
       3 5 0 0
       _____
         1 4 2
         1 0 0
       _____
           4 2
           4 0
       _____
             2
```

You may have learned to divide like this, not writing the extra zeros. You may omit them if desired.

```
         7 2 8
      _____
   5 ) 3 6 4 2
       3 5 ↓  |
       ___   |
         1 4 |
         1 0 ↓
         ___
           4 2
           4 0
         ___
             2
```

The answer is 728 R 2. To check, we multiply the quotient 728 by the divisor 5. This gives us 3640. Then we add 2 to get 3642. The dividend is 3642, so the answer checks.

Do Exercises 11–13.

We can summarize our division procedure as follows.

> To do division of whole numbers:
> **a)** Estimate.
> **b)** Multiply.
> **c)** Subtract.

Divide and check.

11. 4) 2 3 9

59 R 3

12. 6) 8 8 5 5

1475 R 5

13. 5) 5 0 7 5

1015

Answers on page A-2

Divide.

14. 4 5) 6 0 3 0

134

15. 5 2) 3 2 8 8

63 R 12

Sometimes rounding the divisor helps us find estimates.

Example 9   Divide: 8904 ÷ 42.

We mentally round 42 to 40.

$$\begin{array}{r} 2 \\ 4\,2\overline{\smash{)}\,8\ 9\ 0\ 4} \\ 8\ 4\ 0\ 0 \\ \hline 5\ 0\ 4 \end{array}$$ ← *Think*: 89 hundreds ÷ 40.
Estimate 2 hundreds, but write
2 × 42 = 84.

$$\begin{array}{r} 2\ 1 \\ 4\,2\overline{\smash{)}\,8\ 9\ 0\ 4} \\ 8\ 4\ 0\ 0 \\ \hline 5\ 0\ 4 \\ 4\ 2\ 0 \\ \hline 8\ 4 \end{array}$$ ← *Think*: 50 tens ÷ 40.
Estimate 1 ten, but write
1 × 42 = 42.

$$\begin{array}{r} 2\ 1\ 2 \\ 4\,2\overline{\smash{)}\,8\ 9\ 0\ 4} \\ 8\ 4\ 0\ 0 \\ \hline 5\ 0\ 4 \\ 4\ 2\ 0 \\ \hline 8\ 4 \\ 8\ 4 \\ \hline 0 \end{array}$$ ← *Think*: 84 ones ÷ 40.
Estimate 2 ones, but write
2 × 42 = 84.

> *CAUTION*!   Be careful to keep
> the digits lined up correctly.

The answer is 212. *Remember*: If after estimating and multiplying you get a number that is larger than the divisor, you cannot subtract, so lower your estimate.

Do Exercises 14 and 15.

Calculator Spotlight

Calculators usually provide division answers in decimal notation. (Decimal notation will be considered in Chapter 5.) There are calculators that give quotients and remainders directly. One such calculator, the *TI Math Explorer*, uses a special division key INT÷ . An I indicator is displayed when INT÷ is pressed. Then a [Q] and an [R] in brackets indicate the quotient and the remainder.

Example   Divide: 3642 ÷ 5.

Press	Display
3642 INT÷	I 3642
5 =	728 2
	[Q] [R]

The quotient is 728 and the remainder is 2.

Exercises

Use a calculator that finds quotients and remainders to do the following divisions.

1. 8855 ÷ 6   1475 R 5   **2.** 9724 ÷ 27   360 R 4
3. 44,847 ÷ 56   800 R 47   **4.** 6030 ÷ 45   134

Answers on page A-2

Zeros in Quotients

Example 10   Divide: $6341 \div 7$.

```
         9
    7 ) 6 3 4 1        ←  Think: 63 hundreds ÷ 7.
        6 3 0 0           Estimate 9 hundreds.
            4 1
```

```
         9 0
    7 ) 6 3 4 1
        6 3 0 0
            4 1        ←  Think: 4 tens ÷ 7. There are no tens
                          in the quotient (other than the tens in 900).
                          We write a 0 to show this.
```

```
         9 0 5
    7 ) 6 3 4 1
        6 3 0 0
            4 1        ←  Think: 41 ones ÷ 7.
            3 5           Estimate 5 ones.
               6
```

The answer is 905 R 6.

Do Exercises 16 and 17.

Example 11   Divide: $8889 \div 37$.

We mentally round 37 to 40.

```
            2
   3 7 ) 8 8 8 9      ←  Think: 37 ≈ 40; 88 hundreds ÷ 40.
         7 4 0 0          Estimate 2 hundreds, but write
         1 4 8 9          2 × 37 = 74.
```

```
            2 4
   3 7 ) 8 8 8 9
         7 4 0 0
         1 4 8 9      ←  Think: 148 tens ÷ 40.
         1 4 8 0          Estimate 4 tens, but write
               9          4 × 37 = 148.
```

```
            2 4 0
   3 7 ) 8 8 8 9
         7 4 0 0
         1 4 8 9
         1 4 8 0
               9     ←  Think: 9 ones ÷ 40.
                        There are no ones in the quotient.
```

The answer is 240 R 9.

Do Exercises 18 and 19.

Divide.

16. 6) 4 8 4 6

807 R 4

17. 7) 7 6 1 6

1088

Divide.

18. 2 7) 9 7 2 4

360 R 4

19. 5 6) 4 4,8 4 7

800 R 47

To the instructor and the student: This section presented a review of division of whole numbers. Students who are successful should go on to Section 1.7. Those who have trouble should study developmental unit D near the back of this text and then repeat Section 1.6.

Answers on page A-2

Improving Your Math Study Skills

Homework

Before Doing Your Homework

• **Setting.** Consider doing your homework as soon as possible after class, before you forget what you learned in the lecture. Research has shown that after 24 hours, most people forget about half of what is in their short-term memory. To avoid this "automatic" forgetting, you need to transfer the knowledge into long-term memory. The best way to do this with math concepts is to perform practice exercises repeatedly. This is the "drill-and-practice" part of learning math that comes when you do your homework. It cannot be overlooked if you want to succeed in your study of math.

Try to set a specific time for your homework. Then choose a location that is quiet and free from interruptions. Some students find it helpful to listen to music when doing homework. Research has shown that classical music creates the best atmosphere for studying: Give it a try!

• **Reading.** Before you begin doing the homework exercises, you should reread the assigned material in the textbook. You may also want to look over your class notes again and rework some of the examples given in class.

You should not read a math textbook as you would a novel or history textbook. Math texts are not meant to be read passively. Be sure to stop and do the margin exercises when directed. Also be sure to reread any paragraphs as you see the need.

While Doing Your Homework

• **Study groups.** For some students, forming a study group can be helpful. Many times, two heads are better than one. Also, it is true that "to teach is to learn again." Thus, when you explain a concept to your classmate, you often gain a deeper understanding of the concept yourself. If you do study in a group, resist the temptation to waste time by socializing.

If you work regularly with someone, be careful not to become dependent on that person. Work on your own some of the time so that you do not rely heavily on others and are able to learn even when they are not available.

• **Notebook.** When doing your homework, consider using notebook paper in a spiral or three-ring binder. You want to be able to go over your homework when studying for a test. Therefore, you need to be able to easily access any problem in your homework notebook. Write legibly in your notebook so you can check over your work. Label each section and each exercise clearly, and show all steps. Your clear writing will also be appreciated by your instructor should your homework be collected. Most tutors and instructors can be more helpful if they can see and understand all the steps in your work.

When you are finished with your homework, check the answers to the odd-numbered exercises at the back of the book or in the *Student's Solutions Manual* and make corrections. If you do not understand why an answer is wrong, draw a star by it so you can ask questions in class or during your instructor's office hours.

After Doing Your Homework

• **Review.** If you complete your homework several days before the next class, review your work every day. This will keep the material fresh in your mind. You should also review the work immediately before the next class so that you can ask questions as needed.

Exercise Set 1.6

a Write a division sentence that corresponds to each situation. You need not carry out the division.

1. *Canyonlands.* The trail boss for a trip into Canyonlands National Park divides 760 pounds (lb) of equipment among 4 mules. How many pounds does each mule carry?

$760 \div 4 = \blacksquare$

2. *Surf Expo.* In a swimwear showing at Surf Expo, a trade show for retailers of beach supplies, each swimsuit test takes 8 minutes (min). If the show runs for 240 min, how many tests can be scheduled?

$240 \div 8 = \blacksquare$

3. A lab technician pours 455 mL of sulfuric acid into 5 beakers, putting the same amount in each. How much acid is in each beaker?

$455 \div 5 = \blacksquare$

4. A computer screen is made up of a rectangular array of pixels. There are 480,000 pixels in all, with 800 pixels in each row. How many rows are there on the screen?

$480,000 \div 800 = \blacksquare$

b Write a related multiplication sentence.

5. $18 \div 3 = 6$
$18 = 3 \cdot 6$, or
$18 = 6 \cdot 3$

6. $72 \div 9 = 8$
$72 = 9 \cdot 8$, or
$72 = 8 \cdot 9$

7. $22 \div 22 = 1$
$22 = 22 \cdot 1$, or
$22 = 1 \cdot 22$

8. $32 \div 1 = 32$
$32 = 1 \cdot 32$, or
$32 = 32 \cdot 1$

9. $54 \div 6 = 9$
$54 = 6 \cdot 9$, or
$54 = 9 \cdot 6$

10. $40 \div 8 = 5$
$40 = 8 \cdot 5$, or
$40 = 5 \cdot 8$

11. $37 \div 1 = 37$
$37 = 1 \cdot 37$, or
$37 = 37 \cdot 1$

12. $28 \div 28 = 1$
$28 = 28 \cdot 1$, or
$28 = 1 \cdot 28$

Write two related division sentences.

13. $9 \times 5 = 45$
$9 = 45 \div 5$;
$5 = 45 \div 9$

14. $2 \cdot 7 = 14$
$2 = 14 \div 7$;
$7 = 14 \div 2$

15. $37 \cdot 1 = 37$
$37 = 37 \div 1$;
$1 = 37 \div 37$

16. $4 \cdot 12 = 48$
$4 = 48 \div 12$;
$12 = 48 \div 4$

17. $8 \times 8 = 64$
$8 = 64 \div 8$

18. $9 \cdot 7 = 63$
$9 = 63 \div 7$;
$7 = 63 \div 9$

19. $11 \cdot 6 = 66$
$11 = 66 \div 6$;
$6 = 66 \div 11$

20. $1 \cdot 43 = 43$
$1 = 43 \div 43$;
$43 = 43 \div 1$

c Divide.

21. $277 \div 5$

55 R 2

22. $699 \div 3$

233

23. $864 \div 8$

108

24. $869 \div 8$

108 R 5

25. $4\overline{)1228}$

307

26. $3\overline{)2124}$

708

27. $6\overline{)4521}$

753 R 3

28. $9\overline{)9110}$

1012 R 2

29. $297 \div 4$

74 R 1

30. $389 \div 2$

194 R 1

31. $738 \div 8$

92 R 2

32. $881 \div 6$

146 R 5

33. $5\overline{)8515}$

1703

34. $3\overline{)6027}$

2009

35. $9\overline{)8888}$

987 R 5

36. $8\overline{)4139}$

517 R 3

37. $127{,}000 \div 10$

12,700

38. $127{,}000 \div 100$

1270

39. $127{,}000 \div 1000$

127

40. $4260 \div 10$

426

41. $70\overline{)3692}$

52 R 52

42. $20 \overline{)5798}$

289 R 18

43. $30 \overline{)875}$

29 R 5

44. $40 \overline{)987}$

24 R 27

45. $852 \div 21$

40 R 12

46. $942 \div 23$

40 R 22

47. $85 \overline{)7672}$

90 R 22

48. $54 \overline{)2729}$

50 R 29

49. $111 \overline{)3219}$

29

50. $102 \overline{)5612}$

55 R 2

51. $8 \overline{)843}$

105 R 3

52. $7 \overline{)749}$

107

53. $5 \overline{)8047}$

1609 R 2

54. $9 \overline{)7273}$

808 R 1

55. $5 \overline{)5036}$

1007 R 1

56. $7 \overline{)7074}$

1010 R 4

57. $1058 \div 46$

23

58. $7242 \div 24$

301 R 18

59. $3425 \div 32$

107 R 1

60. $48 \overline{)4899}$

102 R 3

61. $24 \overline{)8880}$

370

62. $36 \overline{)7563}$

210 R 3

63. $2\,8\,)\,\overline{1\,7,0\,6\,7}$

609 R 15

64. $3\,6\,)\,\overline{2\,8,9\,2\,9}$

803 R 21

65. $8\,0\,)\,\overline{2\,4,3\,2\,0}$

304

66. $9\,0\,)\,\overline{8\,8,5\,6\,0}$

984

67. $2\,8\,5\,)\,\overline{9\,9\,9,9\,9\,9}$

3508 R 219

68. $3\,0\,6\,)\,\overline{8\,8\,8,8\,8\,8}$

2904 R 264

69. $4\,5\,6\,)\,\overline{3,6\,7\,9,9\,2\,0}$

8070

70. $8\,0\,3\,)\,\overline{5,6\,2\,2,6\,0\,6}$

7002

Skill Maintenance

71. Write expanded notation for 7882. [1.1a]

7 thousands + 8 hundreds + 8 tens + 2 ones

72. Use < or > for ▓ to write a true sentence: [1.4c]

888 ▓ 788. >

Write a related addition sentence. [1.3b]

73. $21 - 16 = 5$ $21 = 16 + 5$, or $21 = 5 + 16$

74. $56 - 14 = 42$ $56 = 14 + 42$, or $56 = 42 + 14$

Write two related subtraction sentences. [1.3b]

75. $47 + 9 = 56$ $47 = 56 - 9$; $9 = 56 - 47$

76. $350 + 64 = 414$ $350 = 414 - 64$; $64 = 414 - 350$

Synthesis

77. ◈ Describe a situation that corresponds to the division $1180 \div 295$. (See Examples 1 and 2.)

78. ◈ Is division associative? Why or why not?

79. A group of 1231 college students is going to take buses for a field trip. Each bus can hold only 42 students. How many buses are needed? 30

80. ▦ Fill in the missing digits to make the equation true:

$34,584,132 \div 76\,▓ = 4\,▓,386.$ 2; 5

1.7 Solving Equations

a | Solutions by Trial

Let's find a number that we can put in the blank to make this sentence true:

$$9 = 3 + \boxed{}.$$

We are asking "9 is 3 plus what number?" The answer is 6.

$$9 = 3 + \boxed{6}$$

Do Exercises 1 and 2.

A sentence with = is called an **equation**. A **solution** of an equation is a number that makes the sentence true. Thus, 6 is a solution of

$$9 = 3 + \boxed{} \quad \text{because} \quad 9 = 3 + \boxed{6} \text{ is true.}$$

However, 7 is not a solution of

$$9 = 3 + \boxed{} \quad \text{because} \quad 9 = 3 + \boxed{7} \text{ is false.}$$

Do Exercises 3 and 4.

We can use a letter instead of a blank. For example,

$$9 = 3 + x.$$

We call x a **variable** because it can be replaced by a variety of numbers.

> A **solution** is a replacement for the variable that makes the equation true. When we find all the solutions, we say that we have **solved** the equation.

Example 1 Solve $x + 12 = 27$ by trial.

We replace x with several numbers.

If we replace x with 13, we get a false equation: $13 + 12 = 27$.
If we replace x with 14, we get a false equation: $14 + 12 = 27$.
If we replace x with 15, we get a true equation: $15 + 12 = 27$.

No other replacement makes the equation true, so the solution is 15.

Examples Solve.

2. $7 + n = 22$
(7 plus what number is 22?)
The solution is 15.

3. $8 \cdot 23 = y$
(8 times 23 is what?)
The solution is 184.

Note, as in Example 3, that when the variable is alone on one side of the equation, the other side shows us what calculations to do in order to find the solution.

Do Exercises 5–8.

Objectives

a Solve simple equations by trial.

b Solve equations like $t + 28 = 54$, $28 \cdot x = 168$, and $98 \div 2 = y$.

For Extra Help

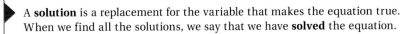

TAPE 2   MAC   CD-ROM
                WIN

Find a number that makes the sentence true.

1. $8 = 1 + \boxed{}$ 7

2. $\boxed{} + 2 = 7$ 5

3. Determine whether 7 is a solution of $\boxed{} + 5 = 9$.

No

4. Determine whether 4 is a solution of $\boxed{} + 5 = 9$.

Yes

Solve by trial.

5. $n + 3 = 8$

5

6. $x - 2 = 8$

10

7. $45 \div 9 = y$

5

8. $10 + t = 32$

22

Answers on page A-3

Solve.

9. $346 \times 65 = y$

22,490

10. $x = 2347 + 6675$

9022

11. $4560 \div 8 = t$

570

12. $x = 6007 - 2346$

3661

Solve.

13. $x + 9 = 17$

8

14. $77 = m + 32$

45

Answers on page A-3

b ## Solving Equations

We now begin to develop more efficient ways to solve certain equations. When an equation has a variable alone on one side, it is easy to see the solution or to compute it. For example, the solution of

$$x = 12$$

is 12. When a calculation is on one side and the variable is alone on the other, we can find the solution by carrying out the calculation.

Example 4 Solve: $x = 245 \times 34$.

To solve the equation, we carry out the calculation.

$$
\begin{array}{r}
2\ 4\ 5 \\
\times\ \ \ 3\ 4 \\
\hline
9\ 8\ 0 \\
7\ 3\ 5\ 0 \\
\hline
8\ 3\ 3\ 0
\end{array}
$$

The solution is 8330.

Do Exercises 9–12.

Look at the equation

$$x + 12 = 27.$$

We can get x alone on one side of the equation by writing a related subtraction sentence:

$$x = 27 - 12 \qquad \text{12 is subtracted to find the related subtraction sentence.}$$
$$x = 15. \qquad \text{Doing the subtraction}$$

It is useful in our later study of algebra to think of this as "subtracting 12 *on both sides.*" Thus,

$$x + 12 - 12 = 27 - 12 \qquad \text{Subtracting 12 on both sides}$$
$$x + 0 = 15 \qquad \text{Carrying out the subtraction}$$
$$x = 15.$$

> To solve $x + a = b$, subtract a on both sides.

Note that $x = 15$ is easier to solve than $x + 12 = 27$. This is because we see easily that when x is replaced with 15, we get a true equation: $15 = 15$. The solution of $x = 15$ is 15, which is also the solution of $x + 12 = 27$. When two equations have the same solution(s), the equations are said to be **equivalent**. Thus, $x = 15$ and $x + 12 = 27$ are equivalent.

Example 5 Solve: $t + 28 = 54$.

We have

$$t + 28 = 54$$
$$t + 28 - 28 = 54 - 28 \qquad \text{Subtracting 28 on both sides}$$
$$t + 0 = 26$$
$$t = 26.$$

The solution is 26.

Do Exercises 13 and 14.

Example 6   Solve: $182 = 65 + n$.

We have

$$182 = 65 + n$$
$$182 - 65 = 65 + n - 65 \qquad \text{Subtracting 65 on both sides}$$
$$117 = 0 + n \qquad \text{65 plus } n \text{ minus 65 is } 0 + n.$$
$$117 = n.$$

The solution is 117.

Do Exercise 15.

Example 7   Solve: $7381 + x = 8067$.

We have

$$7381 + x = 8067$$
$$7381 + x - 7381 = 8067 - 7381 \qquad \text{Subtracting 7381 on both sides}$$
$$x = 686.$$

The solution is 686.

Do Exercises 16 and 17.

We now learn to solve equations like $8 \cdot n = 96$. Look at

$$8 \cdot n = 96.$$

We can get n alone by writing a related division sentence:

$$n = 96 \div 8 = \frac{96}{8} \qquad \text{96 is divided by 8.}$$
$$= 12. \qquad \text{Doing the division}$$

Note that $n = 12$ is equivalent to $8 \cdot n = 96$ but easier to solve.

It is useful in our later study of algebra to think of "dividing by the same number on both sides to form an equivalent equation." Thus,

$$\frac{8 \cdot n}{8} = \frac{96}{8} \qquad \text{Dividing by 8 on both sides}$$
$$n = 12. \qquad \text{8 times } n \text{ divided by 8 is } n.$$

▶ To solve $a \cdot x = b$, divide by a on both sides.

15. Solve: $155 = t + 78$.

77

Solve.

16. $4566 + x = 7877$

3311

17. $8172 = h + 2058$

6114

Answers on page A-3

Solve.

18. $8 \cdot x = 64$

8

19. $144 = 9 \cdot n$

16

20. Solve: $5152 = 8 \cdot t$.

644

21. Solve: $18 \cdot y = 1728$.

96

22. Solve: $n \cdot 48 = 4512$.

94

Answers on page A-3

Example 8 Solve: $10 \cdot x = 240$.

We have

$$10 \cdot x = 240$$
$$\frac{10 \cdot x}{10} = \frac{240}{10} \qquad \text{Dividing by 10 on both sides}$$
$$x = 24.$$

The solution is 24.

Do Exercises 18 and 19.

Example 9 Solve: $5202 = 9 \cdot t$.

We have

$$5202 = 9 \cdot t$$
$$\frac{5202}{9} = \frac{9 \cdot t}{9} \qquad \text{Dividing by 9 on both sides}$$
$$578 = t.$$

The solution is 578.

Do Exercise 20.

Example 10 Solve: $14 \cdot y = 1092$.

We have

$$14 \cdot y = 1092$$
$$\frac{14 \cdot y}{14} = \frac{1092}{14} \qquad \text{Dividing by 14 on both sides}$$
$$y = 78.$$

The solution is 78.

Do Exercise 21.

Example 11 Solve: $n \cdot 56 = 4648$.

We have

$$n \cdot 56 = 4648$$
$$\frac{n \cdot 56}{56} = \frac{4648}{56} \qquad \text{Dividing by 56 on both sides}$$
$$n = 83.$$

The solution is 83.

Do Exercise 22.

Exercise Set 1.7

a Solve by trial.

1. $x + 0 = 14$
14

2. $x - 7 = 18$
25

3. $y \cdot 17 = 0$
0

4. $56 \div m = 7$
8

b Solve.

5. $13 + x = 42$
29

6. $15 + t = 22$
7

7. $12 = 12 + m$
0

8. $16 = t + 16$
0

9. $3 \cdot x = 24$
8

10. $6 \cdot x = 42$
7

11. $112 = n \cdot 8$
14

12. $162 = 9 \cdot m$
18

13. $45 \times 23 = x$
1035

14. $23 \times 78 = y$
1794

15. $t = 125 \div 5$
25

16. $w = 256 \div 16$
16

17. $p = 908 - 458$
450

18. $9007 - 5667 = m$
3340

19. $x = 12,345 + 78,555$
90,900

20. $5678 + 9034 = t$
14,712

21. $3 \cdot m = 96$
32

22. $4 \cdot y = 96$
24

23. $715 = 5 \cdot z$
143

24. $741 = 3 \cdot t$
247

25. $10 + x = 89$
79

26. $20 + x = 57$
37

27. $61 = 16 + y$
45

28. $53 = 17 + w$
36

29. $6 \cdot p = 1944$
324

30. $4 \cdot w = 3404$
851

31. $5 \cdot x = 3715$
743

32. $9 \cdot x = 1269$
141

33. $47 + n = 84$
37

34. $56 + p = 92$
36

35. $x + 78 = 144$
66

36. $z + 67 = 133$
66

37. $165 = 11 \cdot n$

15

38. $660 = 12 \cdot n$

55

39. $624 = t \cdot 13$

48

40. $784 = y \cdot 16$

49

41. $x + 214 = 389$

175

42. $x + 221 = 333$

112

43. $567 + x = 902$

335

44. $438 + x = 807$

369

45. $18 \cdot x = 1872$

104

46. $19 \cdot x = 6080$

320

47. $40 \cdot x = 1800$

45

48. $20 \cdot x = 1500$

75

49. $2344 + y = 6400$

4056

50. $9281 = 8322 + t$

959

51. $8322 + 9281 = x$

17,603

52. $9281 - 8322 = y$

959

53. $234 \times 78 = y$

18,252

54. $10,534 \div 458 = q$

23

55. $58 \cdot m = 11,890$

205

56. $233 \cdot x = 22,135$

95

Skill Maintenance

57. Write two related subtraction sentences:
$7 + 8 = 15$. [1.3b] $7 = 15 - 8$; $8 = 15 - 7$

58. Write two related division sentences: $6 \cdot 8 = 48$.
[1.6b] $6 = 48 \div 8$; $8 = 48 \div 6$

Use > or < for ▨ to write a true sentence. [1.4c]

59. 123 ▨ 789 <

60. 342 ▨ 339 >

Divide. [1.6c]

61. $1283 \div 9$ 142 R 5

62. $1\,7\,\overline{)\,5\,6\,8\,9}$ 334 R 11

Synthesis

63. ◆ Describe a procedure that can be used to convert any equation of the form $a + b = c$ to a related subtraction equation.

64. ◆ Describe a procedure that can be used to convert any equation of the form $a \cdot b = c$ to a related division equation.

Solve.

65. ▦ $23,465 \cdot x = 8,142,355$ 347

66. ▦ $48,916 \cdot x = 14,332,388$ 293

1.8 Applications and Problem Solving

a   Applications and problem solving are the main uses of mathematics. To solve a problem using the operations on the whole numbers, we first look at the situation. We try to translate the problem to an equation. Then we solve the equation. We check to see if the solution of the equation is a solution of the original problem. Thus we are using the following five-step strategy.

Objective

a   Solve applied problems involving addition, subtraction, multiplication, or division of whole numbers.

For Extra Help

TAPE 2   InterAct math   MAC WIN   CD-ROM

> ▶ **FIVE STEPS FOR PROBLEM SOLVING**
>
> 1. *Familiarize* yourself with the situation. If it is described in words, as in a textbook, *read carefully*. In any case, think about the situation. Draw a picture whenever it makes sense to do so. Choose a letter, or *variable*, to represent the unknown quantity to be solved for.
> 2. *Translate* the problem to an equation.
> 3. *Solve* the equation.
> 4. *Check* the answer in the original wording of the problem.
> 5. *State* the answer to the problem clearly with appropriate units.

Example 1   *Minivan Sales.* Recently, sales of minivans have stabilized. The bar graph at right shows the number of Chrysler Town & Country LXi minivans sold in recent years. Find the total number of minivans sold during those years.

1. **Familiarize.** We can make a drawing or at least visualize the situation.

$$50{,}733 \;+\; 84{,}828 \;+\; 76{,}653 \;+\; 71{,}981 \;=\; n$$

in 1995   in 1996   in 1997   in 1998   Total sold

Since we are combining objects, addition can be used. First we define the unknown. We let n = the total number of minivans sold.

2. **Translate.** We translate to an equation:

$$50{,}733 + 84{,}828 + 76{,}653 + 71{,}981 = n.$$

3. **Solve.** We solve the equation by carrying out the addition.

```
    1 3 1 1
  5 0,7 3 3
  8 4,8 2 8
  7 6,6 5 3
+ 7 1,9 8 1
  ─────────
2 8 4,1 9 5
```

Thus, $284{,}195 = n$, or $n = 284{,}195$.

4. **Check.** We check 284,195 in the original problem. There are many ways in which this can be done. For example, we can repeat the calculation. (We leave this to the student.) Another way is to check the reasonableness of the answer by noting that it is larger than the sales in any of the individual years. We can also estimate by rounding. Here, we round to the nearest thousand:

$$50{,}733 + 84{,}828 + 76{,}653 + 71{,}981$$
$$\approx 51{,}000 + 85{,}000 + 77{,}000 + 72{,}000$$
$$= 285{,}000.$$

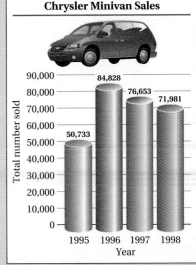

Chrysler Minivan Sales

Source: Chrysler Corporation

1. *Teacher needs in 2005.* The data in the table show the estimated number of new jobs for teachers in the year 2005. The reason is an expected boom in the number of youngsters under the age of 18. Find the total number of new jobs available for teachers in 2005.

Type of Teacher	Number of New Jobs
Secondary	386,000
Aide	364,000
Childcare worker	248,000
Elementary	220,000
Special education	206,000

Source: Bureau of Labor Statistics

1,424,000

2. *Checking Account.* You have $756 in your checking account. You write a check for $387 to pay for a sound system for your campus apartment. How much is left in your checking account?

$369

Answers on page A-3

Since $284{,}195 \approx 285{,}000$, we have a partial check. If we had an estimate like 236,000 or 580,000, we might be suspicious that our calculated answer is incorrect. Since our estimated answer is close to our calculation, we are further convinced that our answer checks.

5. State. The total number of Town and Country minivans sold during these years is 284,195.

Do Exercise 1.

Example 2 *Hard-Drive Space.* The hard drive on your computer has 572 megabytes (MB) of storage space available. You install a software package called Microsoft® Office, which uses 84 MB of space. How much storage space do you have left after the installation?

1. Familiarize. We first make a drawing or at least visualize the situation. We let M = the amount of space left.

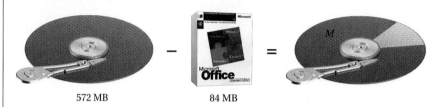

572 MB   84 MB

2. Translate. We see that this is a "take-away" situation. We translate to an equation.

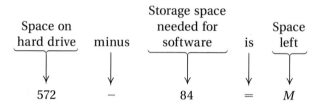

Space on hard drive	minus	Storage space needed for software	is	Space left
572	−	84	=	M

3. Solve. This sentence tells us what to do. We subtract.

$$
\begin{array}{r}
{}^{16}\\
{}^{4}\;{}^{6}\;{}^{12}\\
\cancel{5}\,\cancel{7}\,\cancel{2}\\
-\quad 8\;4\\
\hline
4\;8\;8
\end{array}
$$

Thus, $488 = M$, or $M = 488$.

4. Check. We check our answer of 488 MB by repeating the calculation. We note that the answer should be less than the original amount of memory, 572 MB, which it is. We can also add the difference, 488, to the subtrahend, 84: $84 + 488 = 572$. We can also estimate:

$$572 - 84 \approx 600 - 100 = 500 \approx 488.$$

5. State. There are 488 MB of memory left.

Do Exercise 2.

In the real world, problems may not be stated in written words. You must still become familiar with the situation before you can solve the problem.

Example 3 *Travel Distance.* Vicki is driving from Indianapolis to Salt Lake City to work during summer vacation. The distance from Indianapolis to Salt Lake City is 1634 mi. She travels 1154 mi to Denver. How much farther must she travel?

1. **Familiarize.** We first make a drawing or at least visualize the situation. We let $x =$ the remaining distance to Salt Lake City.

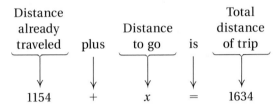

2. **Translate.** We see that this is a "how-much-more" situation. We translate to an equation.

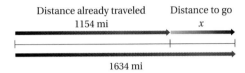

$$1154 \quad + \quad x \quad = \quad 1634$$

3. **Solve.** We solve the equation.

$$1154 + x = 1634$$
$$1154 + x - 1154 = 1634 - 1154 \quad \textbf{Subtracting 1154 on both sides}$$
$$x = 480$$

$$
\begin{array}{r}
{\scriptstyle 5\ 13} \\
1\ \cancel{6}\ \cancel{3}\ 4 \\
-\ 1\ 1\ 5\ 4 \\
\hline
4\ 8\ 0
\end{array}
$$

4. **Check.** We check our answer of 480 mi in the original problem. This number should be less than the total distance, 1634 mi, which it is. We can add the difference, 480, to the subtrahend, 1154: $1154 + 480 = 1634$. We can also estimate:

$$1634 - 1154 \approx 1600 - 1200$$
$$= 400 \approx 480.$$

The answer, 480 mi, checks.

5. **State.** Vicki must travel 480 mi farther to Salt Lake City.

Do Exercise 3.

3. *Calculator Purchase.* Bernardo has $76. He wants to purchase a graphing calculator for $94. How much more does he need?

$18

Answer on page A-3

4. *Total Cost of Laptop Computers.* What is the total cost of 12 laptop computers with CD-ROM drive and printer if each one costs $3249?

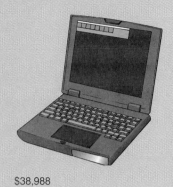

$38,988

Example 4 *Total Cost of VCRs.* What is the total cost of 5 four-head VCRs if each one costs $289?

1. **Familiarize.** We first make a drawing or at least visualize the situation. We let n = the cost of 5 VCRs. Repeated addition works well here.

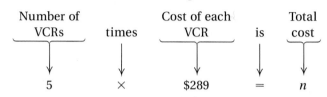

2. **Translate.** We translate to an equation.

Number of VCRs	times	Cost of each VCR	is	Total cost
↓	↓	↓	↓	↓
5	×	$289	=	n

3. **Solve.** This sentence tells us what to do. We multiply.

$$\begin{array}{r} \overset{4\ 4}{2\ 8\ 9} \\ \times\quad\ 5 \\ \hline 1\ 4\ 4\ 5 \end{array}$$

Thus, $n = 1445$.

4. **Check.** We have an answer that is much larger than the cost of any individual VCR, which is reasonable. We can repeat our calculation. We can also check by estimating:

$$5 \times 289 \approx 5 \times 300 = 1500 \approx 1445.$$

The answer checks.

5. **State.** The total cost of 5 VCRs is $1445.

Do Exercise 4.

Answer on page A-3

Example 5 *Bed Sheets.* The dimensions of a sheet for a king-size bed are 108 in. by 102 in. What is the area of the sheet? (The dimension labels on sheets list width × length.)

1. **Familiarize.** We first make a drawing. We let A = the area.

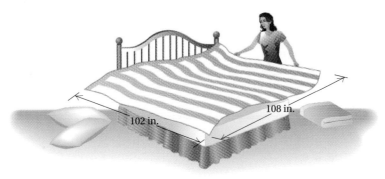
108 in.
102 in.

2. **Translate.** Using a formula for area, we have

$$A = \text{length} \cdot \text{width} = l \cdot w = 102 \cdot 108.$$

3. **Solve.** We carry out the multiplication.

```
      1 0 8
  ×   1 0 2
      2 1 6
  1 0 8 0 0
  1 1 0 1 6
```

Thus, $A = 11{,}016$.

4. **Check.** We repeat our calculation. We also note that the answer is larger than both the length and the width, which it should be. (This would not be the case if we were using numbers smaller than 1.) The answer checks.

5. **State.** The area of a king-size bed sheet is 11,016 sq in.

Do Exercise 5.

Example 6 *Diet Cola Packaging.* Diet Cola has become popular in the quest to control weight. A bottling company produces 2203 cans of cola. How many 8-can packages can be filled? How many cans will be left over?

1. **Familiarize.** We first draw a picture. We let n = the number of 8-can packages to be filled.

8 in each row

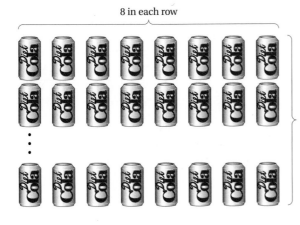

How many rows?

5. *Bed Sheets.* The dimensions of a sheet for a queen-size bed are 90 in. by 102 in. What is the area of the sheet?

9180 sq in.

Answer on page A-3

6. *Diet Cola Packaging.* The bottling company also uses 6-can packages. How many 6-can packages can be filled with 2269 cans of cola? How many cans will be left over?

378 packages; 1 can left over

2. Translate. We can translate to an equation as follows.

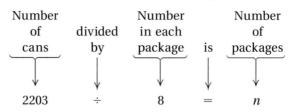

Number of cans	divided by	Number in each package	is	Number of packages
2203	÷	8	=	n

3. Solve. We solve the equation by carrying out the division.

```
          2 7 5
    8 ) 2 2 0 3
        1 6 0 0
          6 0 3
          5 6 0
            4 3
            4 0
              3
```

4. Check. We can check by multiplying the number of packages by 8 and adding the remainder, 3:

$$8 \cdot 275 = 2200, \qquad 2200 + 3 = 2203.$$

5. State. Thus, 275 8-can packages can be filled. There will be 3 cans left over.

Do Exercise 6.

Example 7 *Automobile Mileage.* The Chrysler Town & Country LXi minivan featured in Example 1 gets 18 miles to the gallon (mpg) in city driving. How many gallons will it use in 4932 mi of city driving?

1. **Familiarize.** We first make a drawing. It is often helpful to be descriptive about how you define a variable. In this example, we let g = the number of gallons (g comes from "gallons").

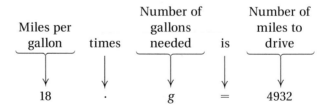

18 mi   18 mi   18 mi   · · ·   18 mi

4932 mi to drive

2. **Translate.** Repeated addition applies here. Thus the following multiplication corresponds to the situation.

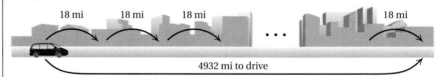

Miles per gallon	times	Number of gallons needed	is	Number of miles to drive
18	·	g	=	4932

Answer on page A-3

3. Solve. To solve the equation, we divide by 18 on both sides.

$$18 \cdot g = 4932$$

$$\frac{18 \cdot g}{18} = \frac{4932}{18}$$

$$g = 274$$

```
        2 7 4
  1 8 ) 4 9 3 2
        3 6 0 0
        1 3 3 2
        1 2 6 0
            7 2
            7 2
             0
```

4. Check. To check, we multiply 274 by 18: $18 \cdot 274 = 4932$.

5. State. The minivan will use 274 gal.

Do Exercise 7.

Multistep Problems

Sometimes we must use more than one operation to solve a problem, as in the following example.

Example 8 *Weight Loss.* Many Americans exercise for weight control. It is known that one must burn off about 3500 calories in order to lose one pound. The chart shown here details how many calories are burned by certain activities. How long would an individual have to run at a brisk pace in order to lose one pound?

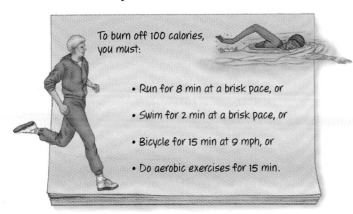

To burn off 100 calories, you must:

• Run for 8 min at a brisk pace, or

• Swim for 2 min at a brisk pace, or

• Bicycle for 15 min at 9 mph, or

• Do aerobic exercises for 15 min.

1. Familiarize. We can first make a chart.

ONE POUND			
3500 calories			
100 cal 8 min	100 cal 8 min	. . . . . .	100 cal 8 min

2. Translate. Repeated addition applies here. Thus the following multiplication corresponds to the situation. We must find out how many 100's there are in 3500. We let x = the number of 100's in 3500.

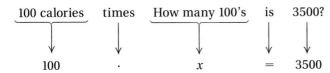

100 calories	times	How many 100's	is	3500?
100	·	x	=	3500

7. *Automobile Mileage.* The Chrysler Town & Country LXi minivan gets 24 miles to the gallon (mpg) in highway driving. How many gallons will it use in 888 mi of highway driving?

37 gal

Answer on page A-3

8. *Weight Loss.* Using the chart for Example 8, determine how long an individual must swim in order to lose one pound.

70 min, or 1 hr, 10 min

9. *Bones in the Hands and Feet.* There are 27 bones in each human hand and 26 bones in each human foot. How many bones are there in all in the hands and feet?   106

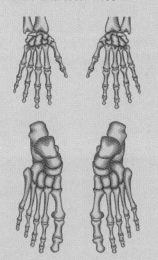

3. Solve.   To solve the equation, we divide by 100 on both sides.

$$100 \cdot x = 3500$$

$$\frac{100 \cdot x}{100} = \frac{3500}{100}$$

$$x = 35$$

$$
\begin{array}{r}
35 \\
100\,\overline{)\,3500} \\
3000 \\
\hline
500 \\
500 \\
\hline
0
\end{array}
$$

We know that running for 8 min will burn off 100 calories. To do this 35 times will burn off one pound, so you must run for 35 times 8 minutes in order to burn off one pound. We let t = the time it takes to run off one pound.

$$35 \times 8 = t$$
$$280 = t$$

$$
\begin{array}{r}
35 \\
\times\ \ 8 \\
\hline
280
\end{array}
$$

4. Check.   Suppose you run for 280 min. Every 8 minutes you burn 100 calories. If we divide 280 by 8, we get 35, and 35 times 100 is 3500, the number of calories it takes to lose one pound.

5. State.   It will take 280 min, or 4 hr, 40 min, of running to lose one pound.

Do Exercises 8 and 9.

As you consider the following exercises, here are some words and phrases that may be helpful to look for when you are translating problems to equations.

Addition:	sum, total, increase, altogether, plus
Subtraction:	difference, minus, how much more?, how many more?, decrease, deducted, how many left?
Multiplication:	given rows and columns, how many in all?, product, total from a repeated addition, area, of
Division:	how many in each row?, how many rows?, how many pieces?, how many parts in a whole?, quotient, divisible

Answers on page A-3

Exercise Set 1.8

a Solve.

1. During the first four months of a recent year, Campus Depot Business Machine Company reported the following sales:

January $3572
February $2718
March $2809
April $3177

What were the total sales over this time period?

$12,276

2. A family travels the following miles during a five-day trip:

Monday   568
Tuesday   376
Wednesday   424
Thursday   150
Friday   224

How many miles did they travel altogether?

1742 mi

Bicycle Sales. The bar graph below shows the total sales, in millions of dollars, for bicycles and related supplies in recent years. Use this graph for Exercises 3–6.

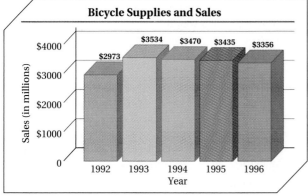

Bicycle Supplies and Sales

Sales (in millions): $4000, $3000, $2000, $1000, 0

$2973 (1992), $3534 (1993), $3470 (1994), $3435 (1995), $3356 (1996)

Year

Source: National Sporting Goods Association

3. What were the total sales for 1993 and 1994?

$7,004,000,000

4. What were the total sales for 1993 through 1996?

$13,795,000,000

5. How much more were the sales in 1993 than in 1994? $64,000,000

6. How much more were the sales in 1994 than in 1992? $497,000,000

7. *Longest Rivers.* The longest river in the world is the Nile, which has a length of 4145 mi. It is 138 mi longer than the next longest river, which is the Amazon in South America. How long is the Amazon?

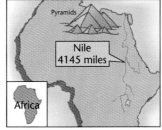

Amazon ?

Coffee beans

South America

Pyramids

Nile 4145 miles

Africa

4007 mi

8. *Largest Lakes.* The largest lake in the world is the Caspian Sea, which has an area of 317,000 square kilometers (sq km). The Caspian is 288,900 sq km larger than the second largest lake, which is Lake Superior. What is the area of Lake Superior?

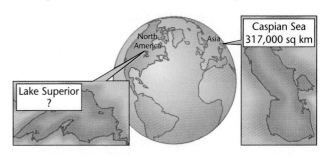

North America   Asia

Caspian Sea 317,000 sq km

Lake Superior ?

28,100 sq km

9. *Sheet Perimeter.* The dimensions of a sheet for a queen-size bed are 90 in. by 102 in. What is the perimeter of the sheet?   384 in.

10. *Sheet Perimeter.* The dimensions of a sheet for a king-size bed are 108 in. by 102 in. What is the perimeter of the sheet?   420 in.

11. *Paper Quantity.* A ream of paper contains 500 sheets. How many sheets are in 9 reams?

4500

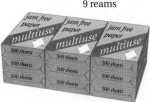

9 reams

500 sheets in each

12. *Reading Rate.* Cindy's reading rate is 205 words per minute. How many words can she read in 30 min?

6150

13. *Elvis Impersonators.* When Elvis Presley died in 1977, there were already 48 professional Elvis impersonators (**Source:** *Chance Magazine* 9, no. 1, Winter 1996). In 1995, there were 7328. How many more were there in 1995?

7280

14. *LAV Vehicle.* A fully-loaded U.S. Light Armed Vehicle 25 (LAV-25) weighs 3930 lb more than its empty curb weight. The loaded LAV-25 weighs 28,400 lb. (**Source:** *Car & Driver* 42, no. 1, July 1996: 153–155) What is its curb weight? ·

24,470 lb

15. Dana borrows $5928 for a used car. The loan is to be paid off in 24 equal monthly payments. How much is each payment (excluding interest)? $247

16. A family borrows $4824 to build a sunroom on the back of their house. The loan is to be paid off in equal monthly payments of $134 (excluding interest). How many months will it take to pay off the loan?   36

17. *Cheers Episodes.* *Cheers* is the longest-running comedy in the history of television, with 271 episodes created. A local station picks up the syndicated reruns. If the station runs 5 episodes per week, how many full weeks will pass before it must start over with past episodes? How many episodes will be left for the last week?

54 weeks; 1 episode left over

18. A lab technician separates a vial containing 70 cubic centimeters (cc) of blood into test tubes, each of which contains 3 cc of blood. How many test tubes can be filled? How much blood is left over?

23 test tubes; 1 cc left over

19. There are 24 hours (hr) in a day and 7 days in a week. How many hours are there in a week?

168 hr

20. There are 60 min in an hour and 24 hr in a day. How many minutes are there in a day?

1440 min

21. You have $568 in your checking account. You write checks for $46, $87, and $129. Then you deposit $94 back in the account upon the return of some books. How much is left in your account? $400

22. The balance in your checking account is $749. You write checks for $34 and $65. Then you make a deposit of $123 from your paycheck. What is your new balance? $773

23. *NBA Court.* The standard basketball court used by college and NBA players has dimensions of 50 ft by 94 ft (*Source:* National Basketball Association).

   a) What is its area?   4700 sq ft
   b) What is its perimeter?   288 ft

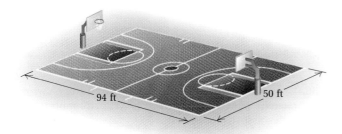

24. *High School Court.* The standard basketball court used by high school players has dimensions of 50 ft by 84 ft.

   a) What is its area? What is its perimeter?
   b) How much larger is the area of an NBA court than a high school court? (See Exercise 23.)

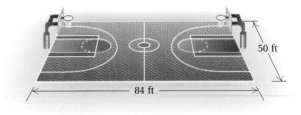

(**a**) 4200 sq ft; 268 ft; (**b**) 500 sq ft

25. Sixteen-ounce bottles of catsup are generally shipped in cartons containing 12 bottles each. How many cartons are needed to ship 528 bottles of catsup?

44

26. Copies of this book are generally shipped from the warehouse in cartons containing 24 books each. How many cartons are needed to ship 840 books?

35

27. Copies of this book are generally shipped from the warehouse in cartons containing 24 books each. How many cartons are completely filled when shipping 1355 books? How many books are left over?

56 cartons; 11 books left over

28. Sixteen-ounce bottles of catsup are generally shipped in cartons containing 12 bottles each. How many cartons are completely filled when shipping 1033 bottles of catsup? How many bottles are left over?

86 cartons; 1 bottle left over

29. *Map Drawing.* A map has a scale of 64 mi to the inch. How far apart *in reality* are two cities that are 25 in. apart on the map? How far apart *on the map* are two cities that, in reality, are 1728 mi apart?

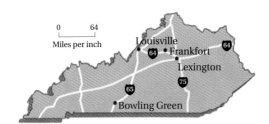

1600 mi; 27 in.

30. *Map Drawing.* A map has a scale of 25 mi to the inch. How far apart *on the map* are two cities that, in reality, are 2200 mi apart? How far apart *in reality* are two cities that are 13 in. apart on the map?

88 in.; 325 mi

31. A carpenter drills 216 holes in a rectangular array in a pegboard. There are 12 holes in each row. How many rows are there?

18

32. Lou works as a CPA. He arranges 504 entries on a spreadsheet in a rectangular array that has 36 rows. How many entries are in each row?

14

33. Elaine buys 5 video games at $44 each and pays for them with $10 bills. How many $10 bills does it take?

22

34. Lowell buys 5 video games at $44 each and pays for them with $20 bills. How many $20 bills does it take?

11

35. Before going back to college, David buys 4 shirts at $59 each and 6 pairs of pants at $78 each. What is the total cost of this clothing?

$704

36. Ann buys office supplies at Office Depot. One day she buys 8 boxes of paper at $24 each and 16 pens at $3 each. How much does she spend?

$240

37. *Weight Loss.* Use the information from the chart on page 67. How long must you do aerobic exercises in order to lose one pound?

525 min, or 8 hr, 45 min

38. *Weight Loss.* Use the information from the chart on page 67. How long must you bicycle at 9 mph in order to lose one pound?

525 min, or 8 hr, 45 min

39. *Index Cards.* Index cards of dimension 3 in. by 5 in. are normally shipped in packages containing 100 cards each. How much writing area is available if one uses the front and back sides of a package of these cards?

3000 sq in.

40. An office for adjunct instructors at a community college has 6 bookshelves, each of which is 3 ft long. The office is moved to a new location that has dimensions of 16 ft by 21 ft. Is it possible for the bookshelves to be put side by side on the 16-ft wall?

No

Skill Maintenance

Round 234,562 to the nearest: [1.4a]

41. Hundred. 234,600

42. Thousand. 235,000

Estimate each computation by rounding to the nearest thousand. [1.4b]

43. 2783 + 4602 + 5797 + 8111 22,000

44. 28,430 − 11,977 16,000

Estimate each product by rounding to the nearest hundred. [1.5c]

45. 787 · 363 320,000

46. 887 · 799 720,000

Synthesis

47. ◈ Of the five problem-solving steps listed at the beginning of this section, which is the most difficult for you? Why?

48. ◈ Write a problem for a classmate to solve. Design the problem so that the solution is "The driver still has 329 mi to travel."

49. ▦ *Speed of Light.* Light travels about 186,000 miles per second (mi/sec) in a vacuum as in outer space. In ice it travels about 142,000 mi/sec, and in glass it travels about 109,000 mi/sec. In 18 sec, how many more miles will light travel in a vacuum than in ice? in glass? 792,000 mi; 1,386,000 mi

50. Carney Community College has 1200 students. Each professor teaches 4 classes and each student takes 5 classes. There are 30 students and 1 teacher in each classroom. How many professors are there at Carney Community College? 50

Collaborative
Learning Manual

Make a budget for a road trip to your favorite destination.

1.9 Exponential Notation and Order of Operations

a | Exponential Notation

Consider the product $3 \cdot 3 \cdot 3 \cdot 3$. Such products occur often enough that mathematicians have found it convenient to create a shorter notation, called **exponential notation,** explained as follows.

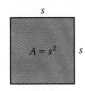

$3 \cdot 3 \cdot 3 \cdot 3$ is shortened to $3^4 \leftarrow$ exponent

4 factors $\qquad$ base

We read 3^4 as "three to the fourth power," 5^3 as "five to the third power," or "five cubed," and 5^2 as "five squared." The latter comes from the fact that a square of side s has area A given by $A = s^2$.

s

$A = s^2$ s

Example 1 Write exponential notation for $10 \cdot 10 \cdot 10 \cdot 10 \cdot 10$.

Exponential notation is 10^5.   5 is the *exponent.*
10 is the *base.*

Example 2 Write exponential notation for $2 \cdot 2 \cdot 2$.

Exponential notation is 2^3.

Do Exercises 1–4.

b | Evaluating Exponential Notation

We evaluate exponential notation by rewriting it as a product and computing the product.

Example 3 Evaluate: 10^3.

$10^3 = 10 \cdot 10 \cdot 10 = 1000$

Example 4 Evaluate: 5^4.

$5^4 = 5 \cdot 5 \cdot 5 \cdot 5 = 625$

Caution! 5^4 does not mean $5 \cdot 4$.

Do Exercises 5–8.

Objectives

a Write exponential notation for products such as $4 \cdot 4 \cdot 4$.

b Evaluate exponential notation.

c Simplify expressions using the rules for order of operations.

d Remove parentheses within parentheses.

For Extra Help

TAPE 2   MAC   CD-ROM
              WIN

Write in exponential notation.

1. $5 \cdot 5 \cdot 5 \cdot 5$

   5^4

2. $5 \cdot 5 \cdot 5 \cdot 5 \cdot 5$

   5^5

3. $10 \cdot 10$

   10^2

4. $10 \cdot 10 \cdot 10 \cdot 10$

   10^4

Evaluate.

5. 10^4

   10,000

6. 10^2

   100

7. 8^3

   512

8. 2^5

   32

Answers on page A-3

Simplify.

9. $93 - 14 \cdot 3$ 51

10. $104 \div 4 + 4$ 30

11. $25 \cdot 26 - (56 + 10)$ 584

12. $75 \div 5 + (83 - 14)$

     84

Simplify and compare.

13. $64 \div (32 \div 2)$ and
     $(64 \div 32) \div 2$ 4; 1

14. $(28 + 13) + 11$ and
     $28 + (13 + 11)$ 52; 52

Answers on page A-3

c   Simplifying Expressions

Suppose we have a calculation like the following:

$$3 + 4 \cdot 8.$$

How do we find the answer? Do we add 3 to 4 and then multiply by 8, or do we multiply 4 by 8 and then add 3? In the first case, the answer is 56. In the second, the answer is 35. We agree to compute as in the second case.
    Consider the calculation

$$7 \cdot 14 - (12 + 18).$$

What do the parentheses mean? To deal with these questions, we must make some agreement regarding the order in which we perform operations. The rules are as follows.

RULES FOR ORDER OF OPERATIONS

1. Do all calculations within parentheses ( ), brackets [ ], or braces {} before operations outside.

2. Evaluate all exponential expressions.

3. Do all multiplications and divisions in order from left to right.

4. Do all additions and subtractions in order from left to right.

    It is worth noting that these are the rules that a computer uses to do computations. In order to program a computer, you must know these rules.

Example 5   Simplify: $16 \div 8 \times 2$.

There are no parentheses or exponents, so we start with the third step.

$$16 \div 8 \times 2 = 2 \times 2 \qquad \text{Doing all multiplications and divisions in order from left to right}$$
$$= 4$$

Example 6   Simplify: $7 \cdot 14 - (12 + 18)$.

$$7 \cdot 14 - (12 + 18) = 7 \cdot 14 - 30 \qquad \text{Carrying out operations inside parentheses}$$
$$= 98 - 30 \qquad \text{Doing all multiplications and divisions}$$
$$= 68 \qquad \text{Doing all additions and subtractions}$$

Do Exercises 9–12.

Example 7   Simplify and compare: $23 - (10 - 9)$ and $(23 - 10) - 9$.

We have

$$23 - (10 - 9) = 23 - 1 = 22;$$
$$(23 - 10) - 9 = 13 - 9 = 4.$$

We can see that $23 - (10 - 9)$ and $(23 - 10) - 9$ represent different numbers. Thus subtraction is not associative.

Do Exercises 13 and 14.

Example 8 Simplify: $7 \cdot 2 - (12 + 0) \div 3 - (5 - 2)$.

$$7 \cdot 2 - (12 + 0) \div 3 - (5 - 2) = 7 \cdot 2 - 12 \div 3 - 3 \qquad \text{Carrying out operations inside parentheses}$$

$$= 14 - 4 - 3 \qquad \text{Doing all multiplications and divisions in order from left to right}$$

$$= 7 \qquad \text{Doing all additions and subtractions in order from left to right}$$

Do Exercise 15.

Example 9 Simplify: $15 \div 3 \cdot 2 \div (10 - 8)$.

$$15 \div 3 \cdot 2 \div (10 - 8) = 15 \div 3 \cdot 2 \div 2 \qquad \text{Carrying out operations inside parentheses}$$

$$= 5 \cdot 2 \div 2 \qquad \text{Doing all multiplications and divisions in order from left to right}$$

$$= 10 \div 2$$

$$= 5$$

Do Exercises 16–18.

Example 10 Simplify: $4^2 \div (10 - 9 + 1)^3 \cdot 3 - 5$.

$$4^2 \div (10 - 9 + 1)^3 \cdot 3 - 5$$

$$= 4^2 \div (1 + 1)^3 \cdot 3 - 5 \qquad \text{Carrying out operations inside parentheses}$$

$$= 4^2 \div 2^3 \cdot 3 - 5 \qquad \text{Adding inside parentheses}$$

$$= 16 \div 8 \cdot 3 - 5 \qquad \text{Evaluating exponential expressions}$$

$$\left. \begin{array}{l} = 2 \cdot 3 - 5 \\ = 6 - 5 \end{array} \right\} \quad \text{Doing all multiplications and divisions in order from left to right}$$

$$= 1$$

Do Exercises 19–21.

Calculator Spotlight

Calculators often have an $\boxed{x^y}$, $\boxed{a^x}$, or $\boxed{\wedge}$ key for raising a base to a power. To find 3^5 with such a key, we press $\boxed{3}$ $\boxed{x^y}$ $\boxed{5}$ $\boxed{=}$. The result is 243.

1. Find 4^5.   1024   **2.** Find 7^9.   40,353,607   **3.** Find 2^{20}.   1,048,576

To determine whether a calculator is programmed to follow the rules for order of operations, press $\boxed{3}$ $\boxed{+}$ $\boxed{4}$ $\boxed{\times}$ $\boxed{2}$ $\boxed{=}$. If the result is 11, that particular calculator follows the rules. If the result is 14, the calculator performs operations as they are entered. To compensate for the latter case, we would press $\boxed{4}$ $\boxed{\times}$ $\boxed{2}$ $\boxed{=}$ $\boxed{+}$ $\boxed{3}$ $\boxed{=}$.

4. Find $84 - 5 \cdot 7$.   49   **5.** Find $80 + 50 \div 10$.   85

When a calculator has parentheses, $\boxed{(}$ and $\boxed{)}$, expressions like $5(4 + 3)$ can be found without first entering the addition. We simply press $\boxed{5}$ $\boxed{\times}$ $\boxed{(}$ $\boxed{4}$ $\boxed{+}$ $\boxed{3}$ $\boxed{)}$ $\boxed{=}$. The result is 35.

6. Find $9(7 + 8)$.   135   **7.** Find $8[4 + 3(7 - 1)]$.   176

---

15. Simplify:

$9 \times 4 - (20 + 4) \div 8 - (6 - 2)$.

29

Simplify.

16. $5 \cdot 5 \cdot 5 + 26 \cdot 71 - (16 + 25 \cdot 3)$ 1880

17. $30 \div 5 \cdot 2 + 10 \cdot 20 + 8 \cdot 8 - 23$

253

18. $95 - 2 \cdot 2 \cdot 2 \cdot 5 \div (24 - 4)$

93

Simplify.

19. $5^3 + 26 \cdot 71 - (16 + 25 \cdot 3)$

1880

20. $(1 + 3)^3 + 10 \cdot 20 + 8^2 - 23$

305

21. $95 - 2^3 \cdot 5 \div (24 - 4)$ 93

Answers on page A-3

22. *NBA Tall Men.* The heights, in inches, of several of the tallest players in the NBA are given in the bar graph below. Find the average height of these players.   87 in.

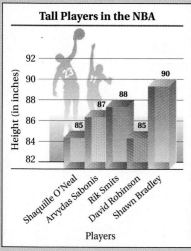

Tall Players in the NBA

Source: NBA

Simplify.

23. $9 \times 5 + \{6 \div [14 - (5 + 3)]\}$

46

24. $[18 - (2 + 7) \div 3]$
     $- (31 - 10 \times 2)$

4

Answers on page A-3

To find the **average** of a set of numbers, we first add the numbers and then divide by the number of addends.

Example 11 *Average Height of Waterfalls.* The heights of the four tallest waterfalls in the world are given in the bar graph at right. Find the average height of all four.

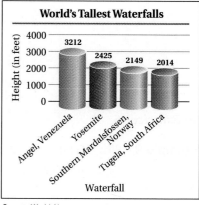

World's Tallest Waterfalls

Source: World Almanac

The average is given by

$$(3212 + 2425 + 2149 + 2014) \div 4.$$

To find the average, we carry out the computation using the rules for order of operations:

$$(3212 + 2425 + 2149 + 2014) \div 4 = 9800 \div 4$$
$$= 2450.$$

Thus the average height of the four tallest waterfalls is 2450 ft.

Do Exercise 22.

d | Parentheses Within Parentheses

When parentheses occur within parentheses, we can make them different shapes, such as [ ] (also called "brackets") and { } (also called "braces"). All of these have the same meaning. When parentheses occur within parentheses, computations in the innermost pair are to be done first.

Example 12 Simplify: $16 \div 2 + \{40 - [13 - (4 + 2)]\}$.

$16 \div 2 + \{40 - [13 - (4 + 2)]\}$

$= 16 \div 2 + \{40 - [13 - 6]\}$ Doing the calculations in the innermost parentheses first

$= 16 \div 2 + \{40 - 7\}$ Again, doing the calculations in the innermost parentheses

$= 16 \div 2 + 33$

$= 8 + 33$ Doing all multiplications and divisions in order from left to right

$= 41$ Doing all additions and subtractions in order from left to right

Example 13 Simplify: $[25 - (4 + 3) \times 3] \div (11 - 7)$.

$[25 - (4 + 3) \times 3] \div (11 - 7) = [25 - 7 \times 3] \div (11 - 7)$
$= [25 - 21] \div (11 - 7)$
$= 4 \div 4$
$= 1$

Do Exercises 23 and 24.

Exercise Set 1.9

a Write in exponential notation.

1. $3 \cdot 3 \cdot 3 \cdot 3$
3^4

2. $2 \cdot 2 \cdot 2 \cdot 2 \cdot 2$
2^5

3. $5 \cdot 5$
5^2

4. $13 \cdot 13 \cdot 13$
13^3

5. $7 \cdot 7 \cdot 7 \cdot 7 \cdot 7$
7^5

6. $10 \cdot 10$
10^2

7. $10 \cdot 10 \cdot 10$
10^3

8. $1 \cdot 1 \cdot 1 \cdot 1$
1^4

b Evaluate.

9. 7^2
49

10. 5^3
125

11. 9^3
729

12. 10^2
100

13. 12^4
20,736

14. 10^5
100,000

15. 11^2
121

16. 6^3
216

c Simplify.

17. $12 + (6 + 4)$
22

18. $(12 + 6) + 18$
36

19. $52 - (40 - 8)$
20

20. $(52 - 40) - 8$
4

21. $1000 \div (100 \div 10)$
100

22. $(1000 \div 100) \div 10$
1

23. $(256 \div 64) \div 4$
1

24. $256 \div (64 \div 4)$
16

25. $(2 + 5)^2$
49

26. $2^2 + 5^2$
29

27. $(11 - 8)^2 - (18 - 16)^2$
5

28. $(32 - 27)^3 + (19 + 1)^3$
8125

29. $16 \cdot 24 + 50$
434

30. $23 + 18 \cdot 20$
383

31. $83 - 7 \cdot 6$
41

32. $10 \cdot 7 - 4$
66

33. $10 \cdot 10 - 3 \cdot 4$
88

34. $90 - 5 \cdot 5 \cdot 2$
40

35. $4^3 \div 8 - 4$
4

36. $8^2 - 8 \cdot 2$
48

37. $17 \cdot 20 - (17 + 20)$
303

38. $1000 \div 25 - (15 + 5)$
20

39. $6 \cdot 10 - 4 \cdot 10$
20

40. $3 \cdot 8 + 5 \cdot 8$
64

41. $300 \div 5 + 10$
70

42. $144 \div 4 - 2$
34

43. $3 \cdot (2 + 8)^2 - 5 \cdot (4 - 3)^2$
295

44. $7 \cdot (10 - 3)^2 - 2 \cdot (3 + 1)^2$
311

45. $4^2 + 8^2 \div 2^2$
32

46. $6^2 - 3^4 \div 3^3$
33

47. $10^3 - 10 \cdot 6 - (4 + 5 \cdot 6)$

906

48. $7^2 + 20 \cdot 4 - (28 + 9 \cdot 2)$

83

49. $6 \cdot 11 - (7 + 3) \div 5 - (6 - 4)$

62

50. $8 \times 9 - (12 - 8) \div 4 - (10 - 7)$

68

51. $120 - 3^3 \cdot 4 \div (5 \cdot 6 - 6 \cdot 4)$

102

52. $80 - 2^4 \cdot 15 \div (7 \cdot 5 - 45 \div 3)$

68

53. Find the average of $64, $97, and $121. $94

54. Find the average of four test grades of 86, 92, 80, and 78.   84

$\boxed{d}$ Simplify.

55. $8 \times 13 + \{42 \div [18 - (6 + 5)]\}$ 110

56. $72 \div 6 - \{2 \times [9 - (4 \times 2)]\}$ 10

57. $[14 - (3 + 5) \div 2] - [18 \div (8 - 2)]$ 7

58. $[92 \times (6 - 4) \div 8] + [7 \times (8 - 3)]$ 58

59. $(82 - 14) \times [(10 + 45 \div 5) - (6 \cdot 6 - 5 \cdot 5)]$

544

60. $(18 \div 2) \cdot \{[(9 \cdot 9 - 1) \div 2] - [5 \cdot 20 - (7 \cdot 9 - 2)]\}$

9

61. $4 \times \{(200 - 50 \div 5) - [(35 \div 7) \cdot (35 \div 7) - 4 \times 3]\}$ 708

62. $\{[18 - 2 \cdot 6] - [40 \div (17 - 9)]\} + \{48 - 13 \times 3 + [(50 - 7 \cdot 5) + 2]\}$ 27

Skill Maintenance

Solve.   [1.7b]

63. $x + 341 = 793$ 452

64. $7 \cdot x = 91$ 13

Solve.   [1.8a]

65. *Colorado.* The state of Colorado is roughly the shape of a rectangle that is 270 mi by 380 mi. What is its area?   102,600 mi^2

66. On a long four-day trip, a family bought the following amounts of gasoline for their motor home:

23 gallons,   24 gallons,
26 gallons,   25 gallons.

How much gasoline did they buy in all?   98 gal

74. $(1 \cdot 2 \cdot 3) + (6 \cdot 7) - (4 \cdot 5) + (8 \cdot 9) = 100$; answers may vary

Synthesis

67. ◈ The expression $9 - (4 \times 2)$ contains parentheses. Are they necessary? Why or why not?

68. ◈ The expression $(3 \cdot 4)^2$ contains parentheses. Are they necessary? Why or why not?

Simplify.

69. ▦ $15(23 - 4 \cdot 2)^3 \div (3 \cdot 25)$ 675

70. ▦ $(19 - 2^4)^5 - (141 \div 47)^2$ 234

Each of the equations in Exercises 71–73 is incorrect. First find the correct answer. Then place as many parentheses as needed in the original equation in order to make the incorrect answer correct.

71. $1 + 5 \cdot 4 + 3 = 36$ 24; $1 + 5 \cdot (4 + 3) = 36$

72. $12 \div 4 + 2 \cdot 3 - 2 = 2$ 7; $12 \div (4 + 2)(3 - 2) = 2$

73. $12 \div 4 + 2 \cdot 3 - 2 = 4$ 7; $12 \div (4 + 2) \cdot 3 - 2 = 4$

74. Use the symbols $+$, $-$, $\times$, $\div$, and $(\ )$ and one occurrence each of 1, 2, 3, 4, 5, 6, 7, 8, and 9 to represent 100.

Collaborative
Learning Manual

Use the order of operations as a group to simplify expressions.

Summary and Review Exercises: Chapter 1

The review exercises that follow are for practice. Answers are given at the back of the book. If you miss an exercise, restudy the objective indicated in blue next to the exercise or direction line that precedes it.

Write in expanded notation. [1.1a]

1. 2793

2. 56,078

Write in standard notation. [1.1b]

3. 8 thousands + 6 hundreds + 6 tens + 9 ones

4. 9 ten thousands + 8 hundreds + 4 tens + 4 ones

Write a word name. [1.1c]

5. 67,819

6. 2,781,427

Write in standard notation. [1.1d]

7. Four hundred seventy-six thousand, five hundred eighty-eight

8. *San Francisco International.* The total number of passengers passing through San Francisco International Airport in a recent year was thirty-six million, two hundred sixty thousand, sixty-four.

9. What does the digit 8 mean in 4,678,952? [1.1e]

10. In 13,768,940, what digit tells the number of millions? [1.1e]

11. Write an addition sentence that corresponds to the situation. [1.2a]

Toni has $406 in her checking account. She is paid $78 for a part-time job and deposits that in her checking account. How much is then in the account?

12. Find the perimeter. [1.2a]

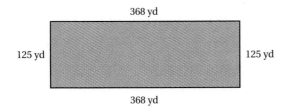

Add. [1.2b]

13. 7304 + 6968

14. 27,609 + 38,415

15. 2743 + 4125 + 6274 + 8956

16.
```
   9 1,4 2 6
+    7,4 9 5
```

Write a subtraction sentence that corresponds to each situation. [1.3a], [1.3c]

17. By exercising daily, you lose 12 lb in one month. If you weighed 151 lb at the beginning of the month, what is your weight now?

18. Natasha has $196 and wants to buy a fax machine for $340. How much more does she need?

19. Write a related addition sentence: [1.3b]
$$10 - 6 = 4.$$

20. Write two related subtraction sentences: [1.3b]
$$8 + 3 = 11.$$

Subtract. [1.3d]

21. 8045 − 2897

22. 8465 − 7312

23. 6003 − 3729

24.
```
   3 7,4 0 5
 − 1 9,6 4 8
```

Round 345,759 to the nearest: [1.4a]

25. Hundred.

26. Ten.

27. Thousand.

Estimate each sum, difference, or product by first rounding to the nearest hundred. Show your work. [1.4b], [1.5c]

28. 41,348 + 19,749

29. 38,652 − 24,549

30. 396 · 748

Use < or > for ▒ to form a true sentence. [1.4c]

31. 67 ▒ 56

32. 1 ▒ 23

33. Write a multiplication sentence that corresponds to the situation. [1.5a]

A farmer plants apple trees in a rectangular array. He plants 15 rows with 32 trees in each row. How many apple trees does he have altogether?

34. Find the area of the rectangle in Exercise 12.

Multiply. [1.5b]

35. $700 \cdot 600$

36. $7846 \cdot 800$

37. $726 \cdot 698$

38. $587 \cdot 47$

39.
$$\begin{array}{r} 8\ 3\ 0\ 5 \\ \times\ \ \ 6\ 4\ 2 \\ \hline \end{array}$$

Write a division sentence that corresponds to each situation. You need not carry out the division. [1.6a]

40. A cheese factory made 176 lb of Monterey Jack cheese. The cheese was placed in 4-lb boxes. How many boxes were filled?

41. A beverage company packed 222 cans of soda into 6-can cartons. How many cartons did they fill?

42. Write a related multiplication sentence: [1.6b]
$56 \div 8 = 7$.

43. Write two related division sentences: [1.6b]
$13 \cdot 4 = 52$.

Divide. [1.6c]

44. $63 \div 5$

45. $80 \div 16$

46. $7\ )\overline{6\ 3\ 9\ 4}$

47. $3073 \div 8$

48. $6\ 0\ )\overline{2\ 8\ 6}$

49. $4266 \div 79$

50. $3\ 8\ )\overline{1\ 7,1\ 7\ 6}$

51. $1\ 4\ )\overline{7\ 0,1\ 1\ 2}$

52. $52,668 \div 12$

Solve. [1.7b]

53. $46 \cdot n = 368$

54. $47 + x = 92$

55. $x = 782 - 236$

Solve. [1.8a]

56. An apartment builder bought 3 electric ranges at $299 each and 4 dishwashers at $379 each. What was the total cost?

57. *Lincoln-Head Pennies.* In 1909, the first Lincoln-head pennies were minted. Seventy-three years later, these pennies were first minted with a decreased copper content. In what year was the copper content reduced?

58. A family budgets $4950 for food and clothing and $3585 for entertainment. The yearly income of the family was $28,283. How much of this income remained after these two allotments?

59. A chemist has 2753 mL of alcohol. How many 20-mL beakers can be filled? How much will be left over?

60. Write in exponential notation: $4 \cdot 4 \cdot 4$. [1.9a]

Evaluate. [1.9b]

61. 10^4

62. 6^2

Simplify. [1.9c, d]

63. $8 \cdot 6 + 17$

64. $10 \cdot 24 - (18 + 2) \div 4 - (9 - 7)$

65. $7 + (4 + 3)^2$

66. $7 + 4^2 + 3^2$

67. $(80 \div 16) \times [(20 - 56 \div 8) + (8 \cdot 8 - 5 \cdot 5)]$

68. Find the average of 157, 170, and 168.

Synthesis

69. ◆ Write a problem for a classmate to solve. Design the problem so that the solution is "Each of the 144 bottles will contain 8 oz of hot sauce." [1.8a]

70. ◆ Is subtraction associative? Why or why not? [1.2b], [1.3d]

71. ▦ Determine the missing digit d. [1.5b]

$$\begin{array}{r} 9\ d \\ \times\ \ d\ 2 \\ \hline 8\ 0\ 3\ 6 \end{array}$$

72. ▦ Determine the missing digits a and b. [1.6c]

$$\begin{array}{r} 9\ a\ 1 \\ 2\ b\ 1\ )\overline{2\ 3\ 6,4\ 2\ 1} \end{array}$$

73. A mining company estimates that a crew must tunnel 2100 ft into a mountain to reach a deposit of copper ore. Each day the crew tunnels about 500 ft. Each night about 200 ft of loose rocks roll back into the tunnel. How many days will it take the mining company to reach the copper deposit? [1.8a]

Test: Chapter 1

1. Write in expanded notation: 8843.

   [1.1a] 8 thousands + 8 hundreds +
   4 tens + 3 ones

2. Write a word name: 38,403,277.

   [1.1c] Thirty-eight million, four hundred
   three thousand, two hundred seventy-seven

3. In the number 546,789, which digit tells the number of hundred thousands?

Add.

4.
```
   6 8 1 1
 + 3 1 7 8
```

5.
```
   4 5,8 8 9
 + 1 7,9 0 2
```

6.
```
   1 2
    8
    3
    7
 +  4
```

7.
```
   6 2 0 3
 + 4 3 1 2
```

Subtract.

8.
```
   7 9 8 3
 - 4 3 5 3
```

9.
```
   2 9 7 4
 - 1 9 3 5
```

10.
```
   8 9 0 7
 - 2 0 5 9
```

11.
```
   2 3,0 6 7
 - 1 7,8 9 2
```

Multiply.

12.
```
   4 5 6 8
 ×       9
```

13.
```
   8 8 7 6
 ×   6 0 0
```

14.
```
   6 5
 × 3 7
```

15.
```
   6 7 8
 × 7 8 8
```

Divide.

16. 15 ÷ 4

17. 420 ÷ 6

18. 8 9) 8 6 3 3

19. 4 4) 3 5,4 2 8

Solve.

20. *James Dean.* James Dean was 24 yr old when he died. He was born in 1931. In what year did he die?

21. A beverage company produces 739 cans of soda. How many 8-can packages can be filled? How many cans will be left over?

22. *Area of New England.* Listed below are the areas, in square miles, of the New England states (**Source:** U.S. Bureau of the Census). What is the total area of New England?

Maine	30,865
Massachusetts	7,838
New Hampshire	8,969
Vermont	9,249
Connecticut	4,845
Rhode Island	1,045

23. A rectangular lot measures 200 m by 600 m. What is the area of the lot? What is the perimeter of the lot?

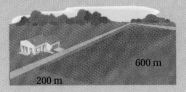

600 m

200 m

24. A sack of oranges weighs 27 lb. A sack of apples weighs 32 lb. Find the total weight of 16 bags of oranges and 43 bags of apples.

25. A box contains 5000 staples. How many staplers can be filled from the box if each stapler holds 250 staples?

Answers

1.

2.

3. [1.1e] 5

4. [1.2b] 9989

5. [1.2b] 63,791

6. [1.2b] 34

7. [1.2b] 10,515

8. [1.3d] 3630

9. [1.3d] 1039

10. [1.3d] 6848

11. [1.3d] 5175

12. [1.5b] 41,112

13. [1.5b] 5,325,600

14. [1.5b] 2405

15. [1.5b] 534,264

16. [1.6c] 3 R 3

17. [1.6c] 70

18. [1.6c] 97

19. [1.6c] 805 R 8

20. [1.8a] 1955

21. [1.8a] 92 packages; 3 cans left over

22. [1.8a] 62,811 mi²

23. [1.8a] 120,000 m²; 1600 m

24. [1.8a] 1808 lb

25. [1.8a] 20

Solve.

26. $28 + x = 74$ **27.** $169 \div 13 = n$ **28.** $38 \cdot y = 532$

Round 34,578 to the nearest:

29. Thousand.   **30.** Ten.   **31.** Hundred.

Estimate each sum, difference, or product by first rounding to the nearest hundred. Show your work.

32.   2 3,6 4 9
   + 5 4,7 4 6

33.   5 4,7 5 1
  − 2 3,6 4 9

34.   8 2 4
  × 4 8 9

Use < or > for ▒ to form a true sentence.

35. 34 ▒ 17   **36.** 117 ▒ 157

37. Write in exponential notation: $12 \cdot 12 \cdot 12 \cdot 12$.

Evaluate.

38. 7^3 **39.** 2^3

Simplify.

40. $(10 - 2)^2$ **41.** $10^2 - 2^2$ **42.** $(25 - 15) \div 5$

43. $8 \times \{(20 - 11) \cdot [(12 + 48) \div 6 - (9 - 2)]\}$ **44.** $2^4 + 24 \div 12$

45. Find the average of 97, 98, 87, and 86.

Synthesis

46. An open cardboard shoe box is 8 in. wide, 12 in. long, and 6 in. high. How many square inches of cardboard are used?

47. Cara spends $229 a month to repay her student loan. If she has already paid $9160 on the 10-yr loan, how many payments remain?

48. Jennie scores three 90's, four 80's, and a 74 on her eight quizzes. Find her average.

49. Use trials to find the single digit number a for which

$$359 - 46 + a \div 3 \times 25 - 7^2 = 339.$$

2

Introduction to Integers and Algebraic Expressions

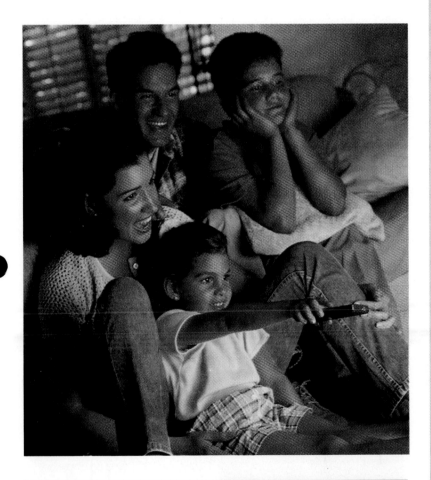

An Application

Midway through a movie, Lisa resets the counter on her VCR to 0. She then fast-forwards the tape 12 min and rewinds it 19 min. What does the counter now read?

This problem appears as Exercise 69 in Exercise Set 2.3.

The Mathematics

If we let *t* be the final counter reading, we have

$$\underbrace{12 + (-19)}_{} = t.$$

This is addition of integers.

World Wide Web For more information, visit us at www.mathmax.com

Pretest: Chapter 2

1. Tell which integers correspond to the following situation: Bill lost $35 in Atlantic City and Janet won $67 in Las Vegas.

Use either < or > for ▩ to form a true sentence.

2. -7 ▩ 0 3. -2 ▩ -17 4. -12 ▩ 7

Find the absolute value.

5. $|73|$ 6. $|-57|$

7. Find $-x$ when x is -32. 8. Find the opposite, or additive inverse, of -17.

Compute and simplify.

9. $-6 + (-12)$ 10. $15 + (-9)$ 11. $-19 + 10$ 12. $-13 + 13$

13. $-7 - 9$ 14. $-8 - (-10)$ 15. $7 - (-11)$ 16. $3 - 9$

17. $-37 \cdot 0$ 18. $-8 \cdot (-6)$ 19. $(-4)^3$ 20. $45 \div (-9)$

21. $(-33) \div (-3)$ 22. $\dfrac{-400}{5}$ 23. $\dfrac{0}{-7}$ 24. $10 \div 2 \cdot 5 - 5^2$

25. Evaluate $7a - b$ for $a = -2$ and $b = -1$.

Multiply.

26. $3(x + 5)$ 27. $7(2x - 3y - 1)$

Combine like terms.

28. $7a + 8a$ 29. $-9x + 7 - x + 8$

30. Find the perimeter of a 12-ft by 20-ft deck.

Solve.

31. $-3x = 54$ 32. $-5 + t = 17$ 33. $x \cdot 8 = 48$

2.1 Integers and the Number Line

In this section, we extend the set of whole numbers to form the set of *integers*.

Integers

To create the set of integers, we begin with the set of whole numbers, 0, 1, 2, 3, and so on. For each number 1, 2, 3, and so on, we obtain a new number to the left of zero on the number line:

> For the number 1, there will be an *opposite* number -1 (negative 1).
>
> For the number 2, there will be an *opposite* number -2 (negative 2).
>
> For the number 3, there will be an *opposite* number -3 (negative 3), and so on.

The **integers** consist of the whole numbers and these new numbers. We illustrate them on a number line as follows.

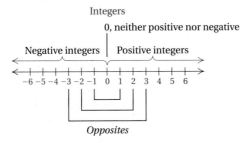

The integers to the left of zero are called **negative integers** and those to the right of zero are called **positive integers.** Zero is neither positive nor negative.

> The **integers**: $\ldots, -5, -4, -3, -2, -1, 0, 1, 2, 3, 4, 5, \ldots$

a | Integers and the Real World

Integers correspond to many real-world problems and situations. The following examples will help you get ready to translate problem situations to mathematical language.

Example 1 Tell which integer corresponds to this situation: The coldest temperature ever recorded in Vermont is 55° below zero Fahrenheit (F).

55° below zero is $-55°$.

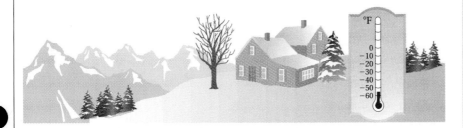

Objectives

a Tell which integers correspond to a real-world situation.

b Form a true sentence using < or >.

c Find the absolute value of any integer.

d Find the opposite of any integer.

For Extra Help

TAPE 3   MAC WIN   CD-ROM

Tell which integers correspond to each situation.

1. The halfback gained 8 yd on first down. The quarterback was sacked for a 5-yd loss on second down.

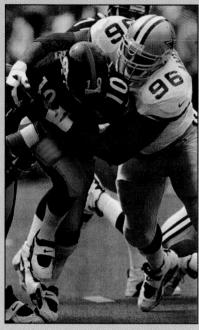

8; −5

2. The highest temperature ever recorded in the United States was 134° in Death Valley on July 10, 1913. The coldest temperature ever recorded in the United States was 80° below zero in Prospect Creek, Alaska, in January 1971.

134; −80

3. At 10 sec before liftoff, ignition occurs. At 148 sec after liftoff, the first stage is detached from the rocket.

−10; 148

4. Jacob owes $137 to the bookstore. Fortunately, he has $289 in a savings account.

−137; 289

Answers on page A-4

Example 2 Tell which integer corresponds to this situation: Death Valley is 280 feet below sea level.

The integer −280 corresponds to the situation. The elevation is −280 ft.

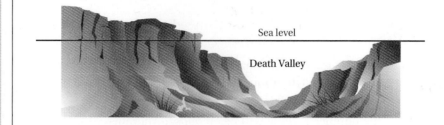

Sea level

Death Valley

Example 3 Tell which integers correspond to this situation: Elaine rewound the videotape in her VCR 17 min and then fast-forwarded it 25 min.

The integers −17 and 25 correspond to the situation. The integer −17 corresponds to the rewinding and 25 corresponds to the fast-forwarding.

Some common uses for negative integers are as follows:

Time:	Before an event;
Temperature:	Degrees below zero;
Money:	Amount lost, spent, owed, or withdrawn;
Elevation:	Depth below sea level;
Travel:	Motion in the backward (reverse) direction.

Do Exercises 1–4.

Calculator Spotlight

To enter a negative number on most calculators, we use the $\boxed{+/-}$ key. This key gives the opposite of whatever number is currently displayed. Thus, to enter −27, we press $\boxed{2}$ $\boxed{7}$ $\boxed{+/-}$. Some graphing calculators have a $\boxed{(-)}$ key. To enter −27 on such a graphing calculator, we simply press $\boxed{(-)}$ $\boxed{2}$ $\boxed{7}$.

Exercises

Press the appropriate keys so that your calculator displays each of the following numbers.

1. −9   2. −57   3. −1996

Keystrokes will vary by calculator.

b | Order on the Number Line

Numbers are named in order on the number line, with numbers increasing as we move to the right. For any two numbers on the line, the one to the left is *less than* the one to the right.

Since the symbol < means "is less than," the sentence −5 < 9 means "−5 is less than 9." The symbol > means "is greater than," so the sentence −4 > −8 means "−4 is greater than −8."

Examples Use either < or > for ▧ to form a true sentence.

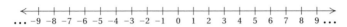

4. −9 ▧ 2   Since −9 is to the left of 2, we have −9 < 2.

5. 7 ▧ −13   Since 7 is to the right of −13, we have 7 > −13.

6. −19 ▧ −6   Since −19 is to the left of −6, we have −19 < −6.

Do Exercises 5–8.

c | Absolute Value

From the number line, we see that some integers, like 5 and −5, are the same distance from zero.

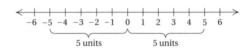

How far is 5 from 0? How far is −5 from 0? Since distance is never negative (it is "nonnegative," that is, either positive or zero), it follows that 5 is 5 units from 0 and −5 is also 5 units from 0.

> The **absolute value** of a number is its distance from zero on a number line. We use the symbol $|x|$ to represent the absolute value of a number x.

Examples Find the absolute value.

7. $|-3|$ The distance of −3 from 0 is 3, so $|-3| = 3$.

8. $|25|$ The distance of 25 from 0 is 25, so $|25| = 25$.

9. $|0|$ The distance of 0 from 0 is 0, so $|0| = 0$.

10. $|-17|$ The distance of −17 from 0 is 17, so $|-17| = 17$.

11. $|9|$ The distance of 9 from 0 is 9, so $|9| = 9$.

> To find a number's absolute value:
>
> **1.** If a number is positive or zero, use the number itself.
>
> **2.** If a number is negative, make the number positive.

Do Exercises 9–12.

Use either < or > for ▧ to form a true sentence.

5. 15 ▧ 7   >

6. 12 ▧ −3   >

7. −13 ▧ −3   <

8. −4 ▧ −20   >

Find the absolute value.

9. $|18|$ 18

10. $|-9|$ 9

11. $|-29|$ 29

12. $|52|$ 52

Answers on page A-4

In each case draw a number line, if necessary.

13. Find $-x$ when x is 1. -1

14. Find $-x$ when x is -2.   2

15. Evaluate $-x$ when x is 0.   0

Answers on page A-4

d | **Opposites, or Additive Inverses**

The set of integers is represented below on a number line.

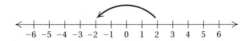

Given a number on one side of 0, we can get a number on the other side by *reflecting* the number across zero. For example, the *reflection* of 2 is -2.

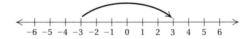

We can read -2 as "negative 2," "the opposite of 2," or "the additive inverse of 2." We read $-x$ as "the opposite of x."

> The **opposite** of a number x is written $-x$.

Example 12   If x is -3, find $-x$.

To find the opposite of x when x is -3, we reflect -3 to the other side of 0.

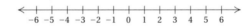

We have $-(-3) = 3$. The opposite of -3 is 3.

Example 13   Find $-x$ when x is 0.

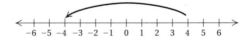

When we try to reflect 0 "to the other side of 0," we go nowhere:

$$-x = 0 \quad \text{when} \quad x \text{ is } 0.$$

In Examples 12 and 13, the variable was replaced with a number. When this occurs, we say that we are **evaluating** the expression.

Example 14   Evaluate $-x$ when x is 4.

To find the opposite of x when x is 4, we reflect 4 to the other side of 0.

We have $-(4) = -4$. The opposite of 4 is -4.

Do Exercises 13–15.

A negative number is sometimes said to have a "negative sign." A positive number is said to have a "positive sign." Replacing a number with its opposite, or additive inverse, is sometimes called *changing the sign.*

Examples Change the sign. (Find the opposite, or additive inverse.)

15. -6 $-(-6) = 6$

16. -10 $-(-10) = 10$

17. 0 $-(0) = 0$

18. 14 $-(14) = -14$

Do Exercises 16–19.

Note that when we change a number's sign twice, we return to the original number.

Example 19 If x is 2, find $-(-x)$.

We replace x with 2 and find $-(-2)$.

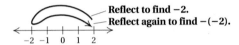
Reflect to find -2.
Reflect again to find $-(-2)$.

We see from the figure that $-(-2) = 2$.

Example 20 Evaluate $-(-x)$ for $x = -4$.

We replace x with -4 and find $-(-(-4))$.

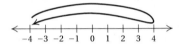

Reflecting -4 to the other side of 0 and then back again gives us -4. Thus, $-(-(-4)) = -(\ 4\ ) = -4$.

Do Exercises 20–23.

Change the sign. (Find the opposite, or additive inverse.)

16. -4 4

17. -13 13

18. 28 -28

19. 0   0

20. If x is 7, find $-(-x)$.   7

21. If x is 1, find $-(-x)$.   1

22. Evaluate $-(-x)$ for $x = -6$.
   -6

23. Evaluate $-(-x)$ for $x = -2$.
   -2

*To the student and the instructor:
Recall that the Skill Maintenance
Exercises, which occur at the end of
most exercise sets, review any skill that
has been studied before in the text.
Often skill maintenance exercises are
chosen to provide preparation for the
next section in the text.*

Answers on page A-4

Improving Your Math Study Skills

Learning Resources and Time Management

Two important topics to consider in enhancing your math study skills are learning resources and time management.

Learning Resources

- **Textbook supplements.** Are you aware of all the supplements that exist for this textbook? Many details are given in the Preface. Now that you are more familiar with the book, let's discuss them.

  1. The *Student's Solutions Manual* contains worked-out solutions to the odd-numbered exercises in the exercise sets. Consider obtaining a copy if you are having trouble. It should be your first choice if you can make an additional purchase.

  2. An extensive set of *videotapes* supplement this text. These may be available to you on your campus at a learning center or math lab. Check with your instructor.

  3. *Tutorial software* also accompanies the text. If not available in the campus learning center or lab, this software can be ordered by calling 1-800-322-1377.

  4. The Math Tutor Center is a free tutoring resource for students possessing a valid registration number. This service is available Sunday through Thursday from 3 PM to 10 PM eastern standard time. To receive help by phone, FAX, or Email with any odd-numbered exercise, simply dial 1-888-777-0463.

- **The Internet.** Our on-line World Wide Web supplement provides additional practice resources. If you have internet access, you can reach this site through the address:

  http://www.mathmax.com

  It contains many helpful ideas as well as many links to other resources for learning mathematics.

- **Your college or university.** Your own college or university probably has resources to enhance your math learning.

  1. For example, there may be a learning lab or tutoring center for drop-in tutoring.

  2. There may be special lab classes or group tutoring sessions tailored for the specific course you are taking.

  3. Perhaps there is a bulletin board or network where you can locate the names of experienced private tutors.

  4. Often classmates interested in forming a study group can be found.

- **Your instructor.** Although it may seem obvious, you should consider an often overlooked resource: your instructor. Find out your instructor's office hours and make it a point to visit when you need additional help.

Time Management

- **Juggling time.** Have reasonable expectations about the time you need to study math. Unreasonable expectations may lead to lower grades and increased frustrations. Working 40 hours per week and taking 12 hours of credit is equivalent to working two full-time jobs. Can you handle such a load? As a rule of thumb, your ratio of work hours to credit load should be about 40/3, 30/6, 20/9, 10/12, and 5/14. Budget about 2–3 hours of homework and studying per hour of class.

- **Daily schedule.** Make an hour-by-hour schedule of your typical week. Include work, college, home, personal, sleep, study, and leisure times. Be realistic about the amount of time needed for sleep and home duties. If possible, try to schedule study time for when you are most alert.

Other study tips appear on pages 50, 100, 150, 322, 368, and 596.

Exercise Set 2.1

a Tell which integers correspond to each situation.

1. Hewlett-Packard stock recently dropped 2 points. −2

2. Redbank, Montana, once recorded a temperature of 70° below zero. −70

3. The Dead Sea, between Jordan and Israel, is 1286 ft below sea level, whereas Mt. Everest is 29,028 ft above sea level. −1286; 29,028

4. The space shuttle stood ready, 3 sec before liftoff. Solid fuel rockets were released 128 sec after liftoff. −3; 128

5. Terry deposited $850 in a savings account. Two weeks later, she withdrew $432. 850; −432

6. Ben & Jerry's stock recently rose 3 points after having dropped 1 point. 3; −1

b Use either < or > for ▮ to form a true sentence.

7. 7 ▮ 0   >

8. 9 ▮ 0   >

9. −9 ▮ 5   <

10. 8 ▮ −8   >

11. −6 ▮ 6   <

12. 0 ▮ −7   >

13. −8 ▮ −5   <

14. −5 ▮ −3   <

15. −5 ▮ −11   >

16. −3 ▮ −4   >

17. −6 ▮ −5   <

18. −10 ▮ −14   >

c Find the absolute value.

19. |23| 23

20. |11| 11

21. |0| 0

22. |−4| 4

23. |−24| 24

24. |−36| 36

25. |53| 53

26. |54| 54

27. |−8| 8

28. |−79| 79

d Find $-x$ when x is each of the following.

29. −8   8

30. −6   6

31. −7   7

32. 6   −6

33. 0   0

34. −15   15

35. −19   19

36. 50   −50

37. 42   −42

38. −73   73

Change the sign. (Find the opposite, or additive inverse.)

39. −8   8

40. −7   7

41. 7   −7

42. 10   −10

43. −29   29

44. −14   14

45. −22   22

46. 0   0

47. 1   −1

48. −53   53

Evaluate $-(-x)$ when x is each of the following.

49. 3   3

50. -7 -7

51. -8 -8

52. 1   1

53. 2   2

54. 19   19

55. 0   0

56. -2 -2

57. -34 -34

58. -23 -23

Skill Maintenance

59. Add: $327 + 498$.   [1.2b]   825

60. Evaluate: 5^3.   [1.9b]   125

61. Multiply: $209 \cdot 34$.   [1.5b]   7106

62. Solve: $300 \cdot x = 1200$.   [1.7b]   4

63. Evaluate: 9^2.   [1.9b]   81

64. Multiply: $31 \cdot 50$.   [1.5b]   1550

Synthesis

65. ◆ Explain in your own words why $-(-x)$ is x.

66. ◆ Does $-x$ always represent a negative number? Why or why not?

67. ◆ Does $|x|$ always represent a positive number? Why or why not?

68. ▦ List the keystrokes needed to find the opposite of the sum of 972 and 589 on your calculator.

69. ▦ List the keystrokes needed to find the opposite of the product of 327 and 83 on your calculator.

Simplify.

70. $-|3|$ -3

71. $-|-8|$ -8

72. $-|-2|$ -2

73. $-|7|$ -7

Solve. Consider only integer replacements.

74. $|x| = 7$ $-7, 7$

75. $|x| < 2$ $-1, 0, 1$

76. Simplify $-(-x)$, $-(-(-x))$, and $-(-(-(-x)))$.

  $x, -x, x$

77. List these integers in order from least to greatest.

  2^{10}, -5, $|-6|$, 4, $|3|$, -100, 0, 2^7, 7^2, 10^2

  $-100, -5, 0, |3|, 4, |-6|, 7^2, 10^2, 2^7, 2^{10}$

68. [9] [7] [2] [+] [5] [8] [9] [=] [+/−] . Answers may vary.

69. [3] [2] [7] [×] [8] [3] [=] [+/−] . Answers may vary.

2.2 Addition of Integers

a | Addition

To explain addition of integers, we can use the number line.

> To do the addition $a + b$, we start at a, and then move according to b.
>
> a) If b is positive, we move to the right.
>
> b) If b is negative, we move to the left.
>
> c) If b is 0, we stay at a.

Example 1 Add: $2 + (-5)$.

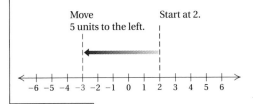

$2 + (-5) = -3$

Example 2 Add: $-1 + (-3)$.

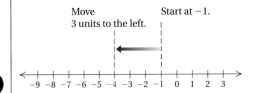

$-1 + (-3) = -4$

Example 3 Add: $-4 + 9$.

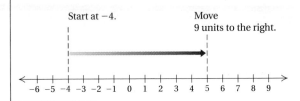

$-4 + 9 = 5$

Do Exercises 1–7.

You may have noticed a pattern in Example 2 and Margin Exercises 2 and 6. When two negative integers are added, the result is negative.

> To add two negative integers, add their absolute values and change the sign (making the answer negative).

Examples Add.

4. $-5 + (-7) = -12$ *Think:* Add the absolute values: $5 + 7 = 12$.
                            Make the answer negative, -12.

5. $-8 + (-2) = -10$

Do Exercises 8–11.

Add, using a number line.

1. $3 + (-4)$ -1

2. $-3 + (-5)$ -8

3. $-3 + 7$ 4

4. $-5 + 5$ 0

Write an addition sentence.

5. $4 + (-5) = -1$

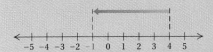

6. $-2 + (-4) = -6$

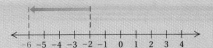

7. $-3 + 8 = 5$

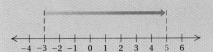

Add. Do not use a number line except as a check.

8. $-5 + (-6)$ -11

9. $-9 + (-3)$ -12

10. $-20 + (-14)$ -34

11. $-11 + (-11)$ -22

Answers on page A-4

Add. Do not use a number line except as a check.

12. $-4 + 6$ 2

13. $-7 + 3$ -4

14. $5 + (-7)$ -2

15. $10 + (-7)$ 3

16. $5 + (-5)$ 0

17. $-6 + 6$ 0

18. $-10 + 10$ 0

19. $89 + (-89)$ 0

Add.

20. $(-15) + (-37) + 25 + 42 + (-59) + (-14)$ -58

21. $42 + (-81) + (-28) + 24 + 18 + (-31)$ -56

22. $-35 + 17 + 14 + (-27) + 31 + (-12)$ -12

Answers on page A-4

When we add a positive integer and a negative integer, as in Examples 1 and 3, the answer is negative or positive, depending on which number has the greater absolute value.

> To add a positive integer and a negative integer, find the difference of their absolute values.
>
> a) If the negative integer has the greater absolute value, the answer is negative.
>
> b) If the positive integer has the greater absolute value, the answer is positive.

Examples   Add.

6. $3 + (-5) = -2$ *Think*: The absolute values are 3 and 5. The difference is 2. Since the negative number has the larger absolute value, the answer is *negative*, -2.

7. $11 + (-8) = 3$ *Think*: The absolute values are 11 and 8. The difference is 3. The positive number has the larger absolute value, so the answer is *positive*, 3.

8. $1 + (-5) = -4$ **9.** $-7 + 4 = -3$

10. $7 + (-3) = 4$ **11.** $-6 + 10 = 4$

We call $-a$ the *additive inverse* of a, because adding any number to its additive inverse always gives 0, the *additive identity*:

$$-8 + 8 = 0, \quad 14 + (-14) = 0, \quad \text{and} \quad 0 + 0 = 0.$$

> For any integer a,
> $$a + (-a) = -a + a = 0.$$
> (The sum of any number and its opposite is 0.)

Do Exercises 12–19.

Suppose we wish to add several numbers, positive and negative:

$$15 + (-2) + 7 + 14 + (-5) + (-12).$$

Because of the commutative and associative laws for addition, we can group the positive numbers together and the negative numbers together and add them separately. Then we add the two results.

Example 12   Add: $15 + (-2) + 7 + 14 + (-5) + (-12)$.

First add the positive numbers: $15 + 7 + 14 = 36$.

Then add the negative numbers: $-2 + (-5) + (-12) = -19$.

Finally, add the results: $36 + (-19) = 17$.

We can also add in any other order we wish, say, from left to right:

$$
\begin{aligned}
15 + (-2) + 7 + 14 + (-5) + (-12) &= 13 + 7 + 14 + (-5) + (-12) \\
&= 20 + 14 + (-5) + (-12) \\
&= 34 + (-5) + (-12) \\
&= 29 + (-12) \\
&= 17.
\end{aligned}
$$

Do Exercises 20–22.

Exercise Set 2.2

a Add, using a number line.

1. $-7 + 2$ -5 **2.** $2 + (-5)$ -3 **3.** $-9 + 5$ -4 **4.** $8 + (-3)$ 5 **5.** $-3 + 9$ 6

6. $5 + (-5)$ 0 **7.** $-7 + 7$ 0 **8.** $-8 + (-5)$ -13 **9.** $-3 + (-1)$ -4 **10.** $-2 + (-9)$ -11

Add. Use a number line only as a check.

11. $-4 + (-11)$ -15 **12.** $-3 + (-7)$ -10 **13.** $-6 + (-5)$ -11 **14.** $-10 + (-14)$ -24

15. $9 + (-9)$ 0 **16.** $10 + (-10)$ 0 **17.** $-2 + 2$ 0 **18.** $-3 + 3$ 0

19. $0 + 8$ 8 **20.** $7 + 0$ 7 **21.** $0 + (-8)$ -8 **22.** $-7 + 0$ -7

23. $-25 + 0$ -25 **24.** $-43 + 0$ -43 **25.** $0 + (-27)$ -27 **26.** $0 + (-19)$ -19

27. $17 + (-17)$ 0 **28.** $-13 + 13$ 0 **29.** $-25 + 25$ 0 **30.** $11 + (-11)$ 0

31. $8 + (-5)$ 3 **32.** $-7 + 8$ 1 **33.** $-4 + (-5)$ -9 **34.** $0 + (-3)$ -3

35. $0 + (-5)$ -5 **36.** $10 + (-12)$ -2 **37.** $14 + (-5)$ 9 **38.** $-3 + 14$ 11

39. $-11 + 8$ -3 **40.** $0 + (-34)$ -34 **41.** $-19 + 19$ 0 **42.** $-10 + 3$ -7

43. $-17 + 7$ -10 **44.** $-15 + 5$ -10 **45.** $-17 + (-7)$ -24 **46.** $-15 + (-5)$ -20

47. $11 + (-16)$ -5 **48.** $-7 + 15$ 8 **49.** $-15 + (-6)$ -21 **50.** $-8 + 8$ 0

51. $11 + (-9)$ 2 **52.** $-14 + (-19)$ -33 **53.** $-20 + (-6)$ -26 **54.** $19 + (-19)$ 0

55. $-15 + (-7) + 1$ -21 **56.** $23 + (-5) + 4$ 22 **57.** $30 + (-10) + 5$ 25 **58.** $40 + (-8) + 5$ 37

59. $-23 + (-9) + 15$ -17

60. $-25 + 25 + (-9)$ -9

61. $40 + (-40) + 6$ 6

62. $63 + (-18) + 12$ 57

63. $85 + (-65) + (-12)$ 8

64. $-35 + (-63) + (-27) + (-14) + (-59)$ -198

65. $-24 + (-37) + (-19) + (-45) + (-35)$ -160

66. $75 + (-14) + (-17) + (-5)$ 39

67. $28 + (-44) + 17 + 31 + (-94)$ -62

68. $27 + (-54) + (-32) + 65 + 46$ 52

Skill Maintenance

69. Write in expanded notation: 39,417.   [1.1a]
3 ten thousands + 9 thousands + 4 hundreds + 1 ten + 7 ones

70. Round to the nearest hundred: 746.   [1.4a]   700

71. Round to the nearest thousand: 32,831.   [1.4a]
33,000

72. Multiply: $42 \cdot 56$.   [1.5b]   2352

73. Divide: $288 \div 9$.   [1.6c]   32

74. Round to the nearest ten: 3496.   [1.4a]   3500

Synthesis

75. ◆ Why was the concept of absolute value introduced in Section 2.1?

76. ◆ Explain in your own words why the sum of two negative numbers is always negative.

77. ◆ A student states that -93 is "bigger than" -47. What mistake is the student making?

Add.

78. $-|27| + (-|-13|)$ -40

79. $|-32| + (-|15|)$ 17

80. ▦ $-3496 + (-2987)$ -6483

81. ▦ $497 + (-3028)$ -2531

82. For what numbers x is $x + (-7)$ positive?
All numbers greater than 7

83. For what numbers x is $-7 + x$ negative?
All numbers less than 7

Tell whether each sum is positive, negative, or zero.

84. If n is positive and m is negative, then $-n + m$ is
_____.   Negative

85. If $n = m$ and n is negative, then $-n + (-m)$ is
_____.   Positive

86. If n is negative and m is less than n, then $n + m$ is
_____.   Negative

87. If n is positive and m is greater than n, then $n + m$
is _____.   Positive

Add integers using a variety of methods.

2.3 Subtraction of Integers

a | Subtraction

We now consider subtraction of integers. Subtraction is defined as follows.

> The difference $a - b$ is the number that when added to b gives a.

For example, $45 - 17 = 28$ because $28 + 17 = 45$. Let's consider an example in which the answer is a negative number.

Example 1 Subtract: $5 - 8$.

Think: $5 - 8$ is the number that when added to 8 gives 5. What number can we add to 8 to get 5? The number must be negative. The number is -3:

$$5 - 8 = -3.$$

That is, $5 - 8 = -3$ because $5 = -3 + 8$.

Do Exercises 1–3.

The definition above does *not* provide the most efficient way to do subtraction. From that definition, however, a faster way can be developed. Look for a pattern in the following table.

Subtractions	Adding an Opposite
$5 - 8 = -3$	$5 + (-8) = -3$
$-6 - 4 = -10$	$-6 + (-4) = -10$
$-7 - (-10) = 3$	$-7 + 10 = 3$
$-7 - (-2) = -5$	$-7 + 2 = -5$

Do Exercises 4–7.

Perhaps you have noticed that we can subtract by adding the opposite of the number being subtracted. This can always be done.

> To subtract, add the opposite, or additive inverse, of the number being subtracted:
> $$a - b = a + (-b).$$

This is the method generally used for quick subtraction of integers.

Objectives

a Subtract integers and simplify combinations of additions and subtractions.

b Solve applied problems involving addition and subtraction of integers.

For Extra Help

TAPE 3

InterAct **math**

MAC
WIN

CD-ROM

Subtract.

1. $-6 - 4$

   Think: What number can be added to 4 to get -6?

   -10

2. $-7 - (-10)$

   Think: What number can be added to -10 to get -7?

   3

3. $-7 - (-2)$

   Think: What number can be added to -2 to get -7?

   -5

Complete the addition and compare with the subtraction.

4. $4 - 6 = -2$;
   $4 + (-6) = \underline{-2}$

5. $-3 - 8 = -11$;
   $-3 + (-8) = \underline{-11}$

6. $-5 - (-9) = 4$;
   $-5 + 9 = \underline{4}$

7. $-5 - (-3) = -2$;
   $-5 + 3 = \underline{-2}$

Answers on page A-4

Equate each subtraction with a corresponding addition. Then write the equation in words.

8. 3 − 10

3 − 10 = 3 + (−10); three minus ten is three plus negative ten.

9. 13 − 5

13 − 5 = 13 + (−5); thirteen minus five is thirteen plus negative five.

10. −12 − (−9)

−12 − (−9) = −12 + 9; negative twelve minus negative nine is negative twelve plus nine.

11. −12 − 10

−12 − 10 = −12 + (−10); negative twelve minus ten is negative twelve plus negative ten.

12. −14 − (−14)

−14 − (−14) = −14 + 14; negative fourteen minus negative fourteen is negative fourteen plus fourteen.

Subtract.

13. 2 − 8   −6

14. −6 − 10   −16

15. 14 − 9   5

16. −8 − (−11)   3

17. −8 − (−2)   −6

18. 5 − (−8)   13

Answers on page A-4

Examples Equate each subtraction with a corresponding addition. Then write the equation in words.

2. 3 − 7;

$$3 - 7 = 3 + (-7)$$ Adding the opposite of 7

Three minus seven is three plus negative seven.

3. −14 − (−23);

$$-14 - (-23) = -14 + 23$$ Adding the opposite of −23

Negative fourteen minus negative twenty-three is negative fourteen plus twenty-three.

4. −12 − 30;

$$-12 - 30 = -12 + (-30)$$ Adding the opposite of 30

Negative twelve minus thirty is negative twelve plus negative thirty.

5. −20 − (−17);

$$-20 - (-17) = -20 + 17$$ Adding the opposite of −17

Negative twenty minus negative seventeen is negative twenty plus seventeen.

Do Exercises 8–12.

Once the subtraction has been rewritten as addition, we add as in Section 2.2.

Examples Subtract.

6. 2 − 6 = 2 + (−6)   The opposite of 6 is −6. We change the subtraction to addition and add the opposite. Instead of subtracting 6, we add −6.

    = −4

7. 4 − (−9) = 4 + 9   The opposite of −9 is 9. We change the subtraction to addition and add the opposite. Instead of subtracting −9, we add 9.

    = 13

8. −3 − 8 = −3 + (−8)   We change the subtraction to addition and add the opposite. Instead of subtracting 8, we add −8.

    = −11

9. 10 − 7 = 10 + (−7)   We change the subtraction to addition and add the opposite. Instead of subtracting 7, we add −7.

    = 3

10. −4 − (−9) = −4 + 9   Instead of subtracting −9, we add 9.

    = 5   To check, note that 5 + (−9) = −4.

11. −5 − (−3) = −5 + 3   Instead of subtracting −3, we add 3.

    = −2   *Check*: −2 + (−3) = −5.

Do Exercises 13–18.

When several additions and subtractions occur together, we can make them all additions. The commutative law for addition can then be used.

Example 12 Simplify: $-3 - (-5) - 9 + 4 - (-6)$.

$$-3 - (-5) - 9 + 4 - (-6) = -3 + 5 + (-9) + 4 + 6 \quad \text{Adding opposites}$$
$$= -3 + (-9) + 5 + 4 + 6 \quad \text{Using a commutative law}$$
$$= -12 + 15$$
$$= 3$$

Do Exercises 19 and 20.

b   Applications and Problem Solving

Let's now see how we can use addition and subtraction of integers to solve applied problems.

Example 13 *Home-Run Differential.* In baseball the difference between the number of home runs hit by a team's players and the number given up by its pitchers is called the *home-run differential*, that is,

$$\text{Home run differential} = \frac{\text{Number of home}}{\text{runs hits}} - \frac{\text{Number of home}}{\text{runs allowed}}.$$

Teams strive for a positive home-run differential.

a) In a recent year, Atlanta hit 215 home runs and gave up 117. Find its home-run differential.

b) In a recent year, San Francisco hit 161 home runs and gave up 171. Find its home-run differential.

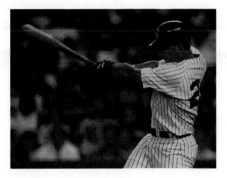

We solve as follows.

a) We subtract 117 from 215 to find the home-run differential for Atlanta:

Home-run differential $= 215 - 117 = 98$.

b) We subtract 171 from 161 to find the home-run differential for San Francisco:

Home-run differential $= 161 - 171 = -10$.

Do Exercises 21 and 22.

Simplify.

19. $-6 - (-2) - (-4) - 12 + 3$
  -9

20. $9 - (-6) + 7 - 11 - 14 - (-20)$ 17

21. *Home-Run Differential.* Complete the following table to find the home-run (HR) differentials (Diff) for all the National League baseball teams.

National League			
	HRs hit	HRs allowed	Diff.
Atlanta	215	117	98
St. Louis	223	151	72
Chicago	212	180	32
San Diego	167	139	28
Los Angeles	159	135	24
Houston	166	147	19
Colorado	183	174	9
Montreal	147	156	−9
San Francisco	161	171	−10
New York	136	152	−16
Arizona	159	188	−29
Cincinnati	138	170	−32
Milwaukee	152	188	−36
Pittsburgh	107	147	−40
Philadelphia	126	188	−62
Florida	114	182	−68

22. *Temperature Extremes.* In Churchill, Manitoba, Canada, the average daily low temperature in January is −31° Celsius (C). The average daily low temperature in Key West, Florida, is 19°C. How much higher is the average daily low temperature in Key West, Florida?   50°C

Answers on page A-4

Improving Your Math Study Skills

Studying for Tests and Making the Most of Tutoring Sessions

This math study skill feature focuses on the very important task of test preparation.

Test-Taking Tips

- **Make up your own test questions as you study.** You have probably become accustomed by now to the section and objective codes that appear throughout the book. After you have done your homework for a particular objective, write one or two questions on your own that you think might be on a test. This allows you to carry out a task similar to what a teacher does in preparing an exam. You will be amazed at the insight this will provide.

- **Do an overall review of the chapter focusing on the objectives and the examples.** This should be accompanied by a thorough review of any class notes you may have taken.

- **Do the review exercises at the end of the chapter.** Check your answers at the back of the book. If you have trouble with an exercise, use the objective symbol as a guide to go back for further study of that objective. These review exercises are very much like a sample test.

- **Do the chapter test at the end of the chapter.** This is like taking a second sample test. Check the answers and objective symbols at the back of the book.

- **Ask your instructor or former students for old exams.** Working such exams can be very helpful and allows you to see what your instructor thinks is important.

- **When taking a test, read each question carefully and try to do all the questions the first time through, but pace yourself.** Answer all the questions, and mark those to recheck if you have time at the end. Very often, your first hunch will be correct.

- **Try to write your test in a neat and orderly manner.** Very often, instructors try to award partial credit when grading an exam. If your test paper is sloppy and disorderly, it is difficult to verify the partial credit. Doing your work neatly can ease such a task for the instructor. Try using a pencil with soft lead or an erasable pen to make your writing darker and therefore more readable.

- **What about the student who says, "I could do the work at home, but on the test I made silly mistakes"?** Yes, all of us, including instructors, make silly computational mistakes in class, on homework, and on tests. But your instructor, if he or she has taught for some time, is probably aware that 90% of students who make such comments in truth do not have sufficient depth of knowledge of the subject matter. Silly mistakes often are a sign that the student has not mastered the material. There is no way we can make that analysis for you. It will have to be unraveled by some careful soul searching on your part or by a conference with your instructor.

Making the Most of Tutoring and Help Sessions

Often students find that a tutoring session would be helpful. The following comments may help you to make the most of such sessions.

- **Work on the topics before you go to the help or tutoring session. Do not go to such sessions viewing yourself as an empty cup and the tutor as a magician who will pour in the learning.** The primary source of your ability to learn is within you. We have seen many students over the years go to help or tutoring sessions with no advanced preparation. When students do this they waste time and, in many cases, money. Go to class, study the textbook, and mark trouble spots. Then use the help and tutoring sessions to work on these trouble spots efficiently.

- **Do not be afraid to ask questions in these sessions!** The more you talk to your tutor, the more the tutor can help you with your difficulties.

- **Try being a "tutor" yourself.** Explaining a topic to someone else—a classmate, your instructor—is often the best way to master that topic.

Exercise Set 2.3

a Subtract.

1. $4 - 7$ -3

2. $3 - 8$ -5

3. $0 - 8$ -8

4. $0 - 9$ -9

5. $-8 - (-4)$ -4

6. $-6 - (-8)$ 2

7. $-11 - (-11)$ 0

8. $-6 - (-6)$ 0

9. $12 - 17$ -5

10. $14 - 19$ -5

11. $20 - 27$ -7

12. $30 - 4$ 26

13. $-9 - (-5)$ -4

14. $-7 - (-9)$ 2

15. $-40 - (-40)$ 0

16. $-9 - (-9)$ 0

17. $7 - 7$ 0

18. $9 - 9$ 0

19. $7 - (-7)$ 14

20. $4 - (-4)$ 8

21. $8 - (-3)$ 11

22. $-7 - 4$ -11

23. $-6 - 8$ -14

24. $6 - (-10)$ 16

25. $-4 - (-9)$ 5

26. $-14 - 2$ -16

27. $1 - 8$ -7

28. $2 - 8$ -6

29. $-6 - (-5)$ -1

30. $-4 - (-3)$ -1

31. $8 - (-10)$ 18

32. $5 - (-6)$ 11

33. $0 - 10$ -10

34. $0 - 18$ -18

35. $-5 - (-2)$ -3

36. $-3 - (-1)$ -2

37. $-7 - 14$ -21

38. $-9 - 16$ -25

39. $0 - (-5)$ 5

40. $0 - (-1)$ 1

41. $-8 - 0$ -8

42. $-9 - 0$ -9

43. $7 - (-5)$ 12

44. $7 - (-4)$ 11

45. $2 - 25$ −23   **46.** $18 - 63$ −45   **47.** $-42 - 26$ −68   **48.** $-18 - 63$ −81

49. $-71 - 2$ −73   **50.** $-49 - 3$ −52   **51.** $24 - (-92)$ 116   **52.** $48 - (-73)$ 121

53. $-50 - (-50)$ 0   **54.** $-70 - (-70)$ 0   **55.** $-30 - (-85)$ 55   **56.** $-25 - (-15)$ −10

Simplify.

57. $7 - (-5) + 4 - (-3)$ 19   **58.** $-5 - (-8) + 3 - (-7)$ 13   **59.** $-31 + (-28) - (-14) - 17$ −62

60. $-43 - (-19) - (-21) + 25$
    22

61. $-34 - 28 + (-33) - 44$
    −139

62. $39 + (-88) - 29 - (-83)$
    5

63. $-93 - (-84) - 41 - (-56)$
    6

64. $84 + (-99) + 44 - (-18) - 43$
    4

65. $-5 - (-30) + 30 + 40 - (-12)$
    107

66. $14 - (-50) + 20 - (-32)$
    116

67. $132 - (-21) + 45 - (-21)$
    219

68. $81 - (-20) - 14 - (-50) + 53$
    190

b Solve.

69. Midway through a movie, Lisa resets the counter on her VCR to 0. She then fast-forwards the tape 12 min and rewinds it 19 min. What does the counter now read?   −7 min

70. Laura has a charge of $476.89 on her credit card, but she then returns a sweater that cost $128.95. How much does she now owe on her credit card?

    $347.94

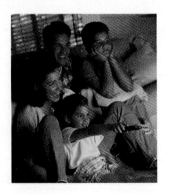

71. Jan is $120 in debt. How much money does Jan need to earn in order to raise her total assets to $350?
$470

72. Through exercise, Rod went from 8 lb above his "ideal" body weight to 9 lb below it. How many pounds did Rod lose?   17 lb

73. *Offshore Oil.* In 1993, the elevation of the world's deepest offshore oil well was −2860 ft. In 1998, the deepest well was 360 ft deeper. (**Source:** *New York Times,* 12/7/94, p. D1.) What was the elevation of the deepest well in 1998?   −3220 ft

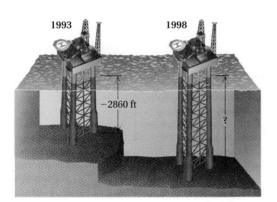

74. *Oceanography.* The deepest point in the Pacific Ocean is the Marianas Trench, with a depth of 11,033 m. The deepest point in the Atlantic Ocean is the Puerto Rico Trench, with a depth of 8648 m. What is the difference in the elevation of the two trenches?   2385 m

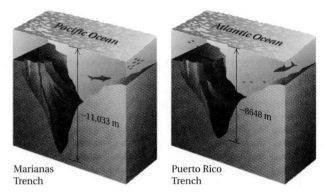

Marianas Trench

Puerto Rico Trench

Skill Maintenance

Evaluate.

75. 4^3 [1.9b]   64

76. 1^7 [1.9b]   1

77. How many 12-oz cans of soda can be filled with 96 oz of soda?   [1.8a]   8

78. A case of soda contains 24 bottles. If each bottle contains 12 oz, how many ounces of soda are in the case?   [1.8a]   288 oz

Simplify.

79. $5 + 4^2 + 2 \cdot 7$ [1.9c]   35

80. $45 \div (2^2 + 11)$ [1.9c]   3

Synthesis

81. ◆ Explain why the commutative law was used in Example 12.

82. ◆ If a negative number is subtracted from a positive number, will the result always be positive? Why or why not?

83. ◆ Write a problem for a classmate to solve. Design the problem so that the solution is "The temperature dropped to −9°F."

Subtract.

84. 🖩 123,907 − 433,789   −309,882

85. 🖩 23,011 − (−60,432)   83,443

Tell whether each statement is true or false for all integers a and b. If false, show why.

86. $a - 0 = 0 - a$ False; $3 - 0 \neq 0 - 3$

87. $0 - a = a$ False; $0 - 3 \neq 3$

88. If $a \neq b$, then $a - b \neq 0$.   True

89. If $a = -b$, then $a + b = 0$.   True

90. If $a + b = 0$, then a and b are opposites.   True

91. If $a - b = 0$, then $a = -b$.
False; $3 - 3 = 0$, but $3 \neq -3$.

92. Doreen is a stockbroker. She kept track of the changes in the stock market over a period of 5 weeks. By how many points (pts) had the market risen or fallen over this time?   Up 15 points

Week 1	Week 2	Week 3	Week 4	Week 5
Down 13 pts	Down 16 pts	Up 36 pts	Down 11 pts	Up 19 pts

93. *Blackjack Counting System.* The casino game of blackjack makes use of many card-counting systems to give players a winning edge if the count becomes negative. One such system is called *High–Low*, first developed by Harvey Dubner in 1963. Each card counts as −1, 0, or 1 as follows:

2, 3, 4, 5, 6   count as +1;
7, 8, 9   count as 0;
10, J, Q, K, A   count as −1.

(***Source:*** Patterson, Jerry L., *Casino Gambling*. New York: Perigee, 1982)

a) Find the final count on the sequence of cards

K, A, 2, 4, 5, 10, J, 8, Q, K, 5.   −2

b) Does the player have a winning edge?   Yes

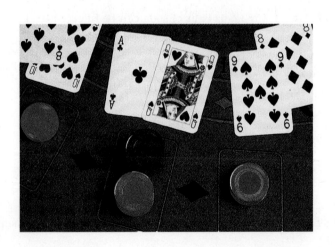

Subtract integers using tiles.

Collaborative
Learning Manual

2.4 Multiplication of Integers

a | Multiplication

Multiplication of integers is very much like multiplication of whole numbers. The only difference is that we must determine whether the answer is positive or negative.

Multiplication of a Positive Integer and a Negative Integer

To see how to multiply a positive integer and a negative integer, consider the pattern of the following.

This number decreases by 1 each time.

This number decreases by 5 each time.

$$4 \cdot 5 = 20$$
$$3 \cdot 5 = 15$$
$$2 \cdot 5 = 10$$
$$1 \cdot 5 = 5$$
$$0 \cdot 5 = 0$$
$$-1 \cdot 5 = -5$$
$$-2 \cdot 5 = -10$$
$$-3 \cdot 5 = -15$$

Do Exercise 1.

According to this pattern, it looks as though the product of a negative integer and a positive integer is negative. This leads to the first part of the rule for multiplying integers.

▶ To multiply a positive integer and a negative integer, multiply their absolute values and make the answer negative.

Examples Multiply.

1. $8(-5) = -40$

2. $50(-1) = -50$

3. $-7 \cdot 6 = -42$

Do Exercises 2–4.

Multiplication of Two Negative Integers

How do we multiply two negative integers? Again we look for a pattern.

This number decreases by 1 each time.

This number increases by 5 each time.

$$4 \cdot (-5) = -20$$
$$3 \cdot (-5) = -15$$
$$2 \cdot (-5) = -10$$
$$1 \cdot (-5) = -5$$
$$0 \cdot (-5) = 0$$
$$-1 \cdot (-5) = 5$$
$$-2 \cdot (-5) = 10$$
$$-3 \cdot (-5) = 15$$

Do Exercise 5.

Objective

a | Multiply integers.

b | Find products of three or more integers and simplify powers of integers.

For Extra Help

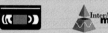 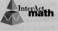

TAPE 3   MAC   CD-ROM
                 WIN

1. Complete, as in the example.

$$4 \cdot 10 = 40$$
$$3 \cdot 10 = 30$$
$$2 \cdot 10 =$$
$$1 \cdot 10 =$$
$$0 \cdot 10 =$$
$$-1 \cdot 10 =$$
$$-2 \cdot 10 =$$
$$-3 \cdot 10 =$$

20; 10; 0; −10; −20; −30

Multiply.

2. $-3 \cdot 6$ −18

3. $20 \cdot (-5)$ −100

4. $9(-1)$ −9

5. Complete, as in the example.

$$3 \cdot (-10) = -30$$
$$2 \cdot (-10) = -20$$
$$1 \cdot (-10) =$$
$$0 \cdot (-10) =$$
$$-1 \cdot (-10) =$$
$$-2 \cdot (-10) =$$
$$-3 \cdot (-10) =$$

−10; 0: 10; 20; 30

Answers on page A-5

Multiply.

6. $(-3)(-4)$ 12

7. $-16(-2)$ 32

8. $(-1)(-7)$ 7

Multiply.

9. $0 \cdot (-5)$ 0

10. $-23 \cdot 0$ 0

Answers on page A-5

According to the pattern, the product of two negative integers is positive. This leads to the second part of the rule for multiplying integers.

> To multiply two negative integers, multiply their absolute values. The answer is positive.

Examples Multiply.

4. $(-2)(-4) = 8$

5. $(-10)(-7) = 70$

6. $(-9)(-1) = 9$

Do Exercises 6–8.

The following is another way to state the rules for multiplication.

> To multiply two integers:
> **a)** Multiply the absolute values.
> **b)** If the signs are the same, the answer is positive.
> **c)** If the signs are different, the answer is negative.

Multiplication by Zero

No matter how many times 0 is added to itself, the answer is 0. This leads to the following result.

> For any integer a,
> $$a \cdot 0 = 0.$$
> (The product of 0 and any integer is 0.)

Examples Multiply.

7. $-19 \cdot 0 = 0$

8. $0(-7) = 0$

Do Exercises 9 and 10.

b | Multiplication of More Than Two Integers

Because of the commutative and the associative laws, to multiply three or more integers, we can group as we please.

Examples Multiply.

9. a) $-8 \cdot 2(-3) = -16(-3)$ **Multiplying the first two numbers**
$\qquad\qquad\qquad\quad = 48$ **Multiplying the results**

b) $-8 \cdot 2(-3) = 24 \cdot 2$ **Multiplying the negatives**
$\qquad\qquad\qquad = 48$ **The result is the same as above.**

10. $7(-1)(-4)(-2) = (-7)8$ **Multiplying the first two numbers**
$\qquad\qquad\qquad\quad = -56$ **and the last two numbers**

11. a) $-5 \cdot (-2) \cdot (-3) \cdot (-6) = 10 \cdot 18$ **Each pair of negatives gives a**
$\qquad\qquad\qquad\qquad\qquad\quad = 180$ **positive product.**

b) $-5 \cdot (-2) \cdot (-3) \cdot (-6) \cdot (-1) = 10 \cdot 18 \cdot (-1)$ **Making use of**
$\qquad\qquad\qquad\qquad\qquad\qquad\qquad = -180$ **Example 11(a)**

We can see the following pattern in the results of Examples 9–11.

> ▶ The product of an even number of negative integers is positive.
> The product of an odd number of negative integers is negative.

Do Exercises 11–13.

Powers of Integers

The result of raising a negative number to a power is positive or negative, depending on the exponent.

Examples Simplify.

12. $(-7)^2 = (-7)(-7) = 49$ **The result is positive.**

13. $(-4)^3 = (-4)(-4)(-4)$
$\qquad\quad = 16(-4)$
$\qquad\quad = -64$ **The result is negative.**

14. $(-3)^4 = (-3)(-3)(-3)(-3)$
$\qquad\quad = 9 \cdot 9$
$\qquad\quad = 81$ **The result is positive.**

15. $(-2)^5 = (-2)(-2)(-2)(-2)(-2)$
$\qquad\quad = 4 \cdot 4 \cdot (-2)$
$\qquad\quad = 16(-2)$
$\qquad\quad = -32$ **The result is negative.**

Perhaps you noted the following.

> When a negative number is raised to an even exponent, the result is positive.
> When a negative number is raised to an odd exponent, the result is negative.

Do Exercises 14–16.

We have seen that when an integer is multiplied by -1, the result is the opposite of that integer. That is, $-1 \cdot a = -a$, for any integer a.

Multiply.

11. $-2 \cdot (-5) \cdot (-4) \cdot (-3)$ 120

12. $(-4)(-5)(-2)(-3)(-1)$ -120

13. $(-1)(-1)(-2)(-3)(-1)(-1)$ 6

Simplify.

14. $(-2)^3$ -8

15. $(-9)^2$ 81

16. $(-1)^7$ -1

Answers on page A-5

17. Simplify: -5^2. -25

Example 16 Simplify: -7^2.

We first note that -7^2 lacks parentheses so the base is 7, not -7. Thus we regard -7^2 as $-1 \cdot 7^2$:

$$-7^2 = -1 \cdot 7^2$$
$$= -1 \cdot 7 \cdot 7 \qquad \text{The rules for order of operations tell us to square first.}$$
$$= -1 \cdot 49$$
$$= -49.$$

Compare Examples 12 and 16 and note that $(-7)^2 \neq -7^2$. In fact, the expressions $(-7)^2$ and -7^2 are not read the same way: $(-7)^2$ is read "negative seven squared," whereas -7^2 is read "the opposite of seven squared."

Do Exercises 17 and 18.

18. Write $(-8)^2$ and -8^2 in words.

Negative eight squared;
the opposite of eight squared

Calculator Spotlight

When using a calculator to calculate numbers like $(-39)^4$, it is important to use the correct sequence of keystrokes. On most scientific calculators, the appropriate keystrokes are

$$\boxed{3}\ \boxed{9}\ \boxed{+/-}\ \boxed{x^y}\ \boxed{4}\ \boxed{=}.$$

Note that in this instance the $\boxed{+/-}$ key is used to change a number's sign. To calculate -39^4, the following keystrokes are needed:

$$\boxed{1}\ \boxed{+/-}\ \boxed{\times}\ \boxed{3}\ \boxed{9}\ \boxed{x^y}\ \boxed{4}\ \boxed{=},$$

or

$$\boxed{3}\ \boxed{9}\ \boxed{x^y}\ \boxed{4}\ \boxed{=}\ \boxed{+/-}.$$

On many graphing calculators, $(-39)^4$ is found by pressing

$$\boxed{(}\ \boxed{(-)}\ \boxed{3}\ \boxed{9}\ \boxed{)}\ \boxed{\wedge}\ \boxed{4}\ \boxed{ENTER}$$

and -39^4 is found by pressing

$$\boxed{(-)}\ \boxed{3}\ \boxed{9}\ \boxed{\wedge}\ \boxed{4}\ \boxed{ENTER}.$$

You can either experiment or consult a user's manual if you are unsure of the proper keystrokes for your calculator.

Exercises

Use a calculator to determine each of the following.

1. $(-23)^6$ 148,035,889
2. $(-17)^5$ $-1,419,857$
3. $(-104)^3$ $-1,124,864$
4. $(-4)^{10}$ 1,048,576
5. -9^6 $-531,441$
6. -7^6 $-117,649$
7. -6^5 -7776
8. -3^9 $-19,683$

Answers on page A-5

Exercise Set 2.4

a Multiply.

1. $-3 \cdot 7$ -21

2. $-8 \cdot 2$ -16

3. $-9 \cdot 2$ -18

4. $-7 \cdot 6$ -42

5. $8 \cdot (-6)$ -48

6. $8 \cdot (-3)$ -24

7. $-10 \cdot 3$ -30

8. $-9 \cdot 8$ -72

9. $-2 \cdot (-5)$ 10

10. $-8 \cdot (-2)$ 16

11. $-9 \cdot (-2)$ 18

12. $(-8)(-9)$ 72

13. $-7 \cdot (-6)$ 42

14. $-8 \cdot (-3)$ 24

15. $-10(-3)$ 30

16. $-9(-8)$ 72

17. $12(-10)$ -120

18. $15(-8)$ -120

19. $-6(-50)$ 300

20. $-25(-8)$ 200

21. $(-72)(-1)$ 72

22. $41(-3)$ -123

23. $(-20)17$ -340

24. $(-1)43$ -43

25. $-23 \cdot 0$ 0

26. $-17 \cdot 0$ 0

27. $0(-14)$ 0

28. $0(-38)$ 0

b Multiply.

29. $3 \cdot (-8) \cdot 4$ -96

30. $(-3) \cdot (-4) \cdot (-5)$ -60

31. $7(-4)(-3)5$ 420

32. $9(-2)(-6)7$ 756

33. $-2(-5)(-7)$ -70

34. $(-2)(-5)(-3)(-5)$ 150

35. $(-5)(-2)(-3)(-1)$ 30

36. $-6(-5)(-9)$ -270

37. $(-15)(-29)0 \cdot 8$ 0

38. $19(-7)(-8)0 \cdot 6$ 0

39. $(-7)(-1)(7)(-6)$ -294

40. $(-5)6(-4)5$ 600

Simplify.

41. $(-5)^2$ 25

42. $(-8)^2$ 64

43. $(-5)^3$ −125

44. $(-2)^4$ 16

45. $(-10)^4$ 10,000

46. $(-1)^5$ −1

47. -2^4 −16

48. $(-2)^6$ 64

49. $(-3)^5$ −243

50. -10^4 −10,000

51. $(-1)^{12}$ 1

52. $(-1)^{13}$ −1

53. -3^6 −729

54. -2^6 −64

55. -5^3 −125

56. -2^5 −32

Write each of the following expressions in words.

57. -7^4

The opposite of seven
to the fourth power

58. $(-6)^8$

Negative six to the
eighth power

59. $(-9)^6$

Negative nine to the
sixth power

60. -5^4

The opposite of five
to the fourth power

Skill Maintenance

61. Round 532,451 to the nearest hundred. [1.4a]
532,500

62. Write standard notation for sixty million. [1.1d]
60,000,000

63. Divide: $2880 \div 36$. [1.6c] 80

64. Multiply: 75×34. [1.5b] 2550

65. A rectangular rug measures 5 ft by 8 ft. What is the
area of the rug? [1.8a] 40 sq ft

66. How many 12-egg cartons can be filled with
2880 eggs? [1.8a] 240

Synthesis

67. ◆ Explain in your own words why $(-8)^{12}$ is
positive.

68. ◆ Explain in your own words why $-7(-1)^3$ is the
opposite of −7.

69. ◆ Which number is larger, $(-3)^{79}$ or $(-5)^{79}$? Why?

Simplify.

70. $(-3)^5(-1)^{379}$ 243

71. $(-2)^3 \cdot [(-1)^{29}]^{46}$ −8

72. $(-2)^6(-1^8)$ 64

73. $-5^2(-1)^{29}$ 25

74. $|(-2)^5 + 3^2| - (3-7)^2$ 7

75. $|-12(-3)^2 - 5^3 - 6^2 - (-5)^2|$ 294

76. ▦ $-935(238 - 243)^3$ 116,875

77. ▦ $(-17)^4(129 - 133)^5$ −85,525,504

78. Jo wrote seven checks for $13 each. If she had a
balance of $68 in her account, what was her
balance after writing the checks? −$23

79. After diving 95 m below the surface, a diver rises at
a rate of 7 meters per minute for 9 min. What is the
diver's new elevation? −32 m

80. What must be true of m and n if $[(-5)^m]^n$ is to be
(a) negative? **(b)** positive?
(a) Both m and n must be odd. **(b)** At least one of m
and n must be even.

81. What must be true of m and n if $-mn$ is to be
(a) positive? **(b)** zero? **(c)** negative?

(a) m and n must have different signs. **(b)** At least one of m
and n must be zero. **(c)** m and n must have the same sign.

2.5 Division of Integers

We now consider division of integers. The definition of division results in rules for division that are the same as those for multiplication.

a | Division of Integers

> The quotient $\dfrac{a}{b}$ (or $a \div b$) is the number, if there is one, that when multiplied by b gives a.

Let's use the definition to divide integers.

Examples   Divide, if possible. Check each answer.

1. $14 \div (-7) = -2$ *Think*: **What number multiplied by −7 gives 14?**
The number is −2. *Check*: **(−2)(−7) = 14.**

2. $\dfrac{-32}{-4} = 8$ *Think*: **What number multiplied by −4 gives −32?**
The number is 8. *Check*: **8(−4) = −32.**

3. $\dfrac{-21}{7} = -3$ *Think*: **What number multiplied by 7 gives −21?**
The number is −3. *Check*: **(−3) · 7 = −21.**

4. $0 \div (-5) = 0$ *Think*: **What number multiplied by −5 gives 0?**
The number is 0. *Check*: **0(−5) = 0.**

The rules for division are the same as those for multiplication. We state them together.

> To multiply or divide two integers:
> a) Multiply or divide the absolute values.
> b) If the signs are the same, the answer is positive.
> c) If the signs are different, the answer is negative.

Do Exercises 1–6.

In Example 4, we divided *into* 0. Consider now division of a number *by* 0, as in $9 \div 0$. The expression $9 \div 0$ represents the number that when multiplied by 0 gives 9. But any number times 0 gives 0, not 9. For this reason, we say that $9 \div 0$ is **undefined**. This result is generalized as follows.

> Division by zero is undefined: $a \div 0$, or $\dfrac{a}{0}$, is undefined for all integers a.

Example 5   Divide, if possible: $-17 \div 0$.

$\dfrac{-17}{0}$ is undefined.   *Think*: **What number multiplied by 0 gives −17?**
There is no such number because the product of 0 and *any* number is 0.

Do Exercises 7–9.

Objectives

a   Divide integers.

b   Use the rules for order of operations with integers.

For Extra Help

TAPE 4   MAC   CD-ROM
                WIN

Divide.

1. $6 \div (-3)$ -2

Think: What number multiplied by −3 gives 6?

2. $\dfrac{-15}{-3}$ 5

Think: What number multiplied by −3 gives −15?

3. $-24 \div 8$ -3

Think: What number multiplied by 8 gives −24?

4. $\dfrac{0}{-4}$ 0

5. $\dfrac{30}{-5}$ -6

6. $\dfrac{-45}{9}$ -5

Divide, if possible.
7. $26 \div 0$ Undefined

8. $0 \div (-12)$ 0

9. $-52 \div 0$ Undefined

Answers on page A-5

Simplify.

10. $5 - (-7)(-3)^2$ 68

11. $(-2) \cdot |3 - 2^2| + 5$ 3

12. $\dfrac{(-5)(-9)}{1 - 2 \cdot 2}$ -15

Answers on page A-5

b Order of Operations

When several operations are to be done in a calculation or a problem, we apply the same rules that were used in Section 1.9. We repeat them here for review, now including absolute-value symbols.

RULES FOR ORDER OF OPERATIONS

1. Do all calculations within parentheses, brackets, braces, or absolute-value symbols. Simplify, if possible, above and below any fraction bars.
2. Evaluate all exponential expressions.
3. Do all multiplications and divisions in order from left to right.
4. Do all additions and subtractions in order from left to right.

Examples   Simplify.

6. $17 - 10 \div 2 \cdot 4$

There are no parentheses or powers so we begin with the third rule.

$$\left.\begin{aligned} 17 - 10 \div 2 \cdot 4 &= 17 - 5 \cdot 4 \\ &= 17 - 20 \end{aligned}\right\} \quad \begin{array}{l}\text{Carrying out all multipli-} \\ \text{cations and divisions in} \\ \text{order from left to right}\end{array}$$
$$= -3$$

7. $|(-2)^3 \div 4| - 5(-2)$

We first simplify within the absolute-value symbols.

$$|(-2)^3 \div 4| - 5(-2) = |-8 \div 4| - 5(-2) \quad \begin{array}{l}(-2)^3 = \\ (-2)(-2)(-2) = -8\end{array}$$
$$= |-2| - 5(-2) \quad \text{Dividing}$$
$$= 2 - 5(-2) \quad \begin{array}{l}\text{Finding the abso-} \\ \text{lute value of } -2\end{array}$$
$$= 2 - (-10) \quad \text{Multiplying}$$
$$= 12 \quad \begin{array}{l}\text{Subtracting by adding the opposite} \\ \text{of } -10\end{array}$$

A fraction bar is a grouping symbol. It separates any calculations in the numerator from those in the denominator.

Example 8   Simplify: $\dfrac{5 - (-3)^2}{-2}$.

$$\frac{5 - (-3)^2}{-2} = \frac{5 - 9}{-2} \quad \begin{array}{l}\text{Simplifying:} \\ (-3)^2 = (-3)(-3) = 9\end{array}$$
$$= \frac{-4}{-2} \quad \text{Subtracting}$$
$$= 2 \quad \text{Dividing}$$

Do Exercises 10–12.

Exercise Set 2.5

a Divide, if possible. Check each answer.

1. $28 \div (-4)$ -7

2. $\dfrac{35}{-7}$ -5

3. $\dfrac{28}{-2}$ -14

4. $26 \div (-13)$ -2

5. $\dfrac{18}{-2}$ -9

6. $-22 \div (-2)$ 11

7. $\dfrac{-48}{-12}$ 4

8. $-63 \div (-9)$ 7

9. $\dfrac{-72}{8}$ -9

10. $\dfrac{-50}{25}$ -2

11. $-100 \div (-50)$ 2

12. $\dfrac{-400}{8}$ -50

13. $-344 \div 8$ -43

14. $\dfrac{-128}{8}$ -16

15. $\dfrac{200}{-25}$ -8

16. $-651 \div (-31)$ 21

17. $\dfrac{-56}{0}$ Undefined

18. $\dfrac{0}{-5}$ 0

19. $\dfrac{88}{-11}$ -8

20. $\dfrac{-145}{-5}$ 29

21. $-\dfrac{276}{12}$ -23

22. $-\dfrac{217}{7}$ -31

23. $\dfrac{0}{-2}$ 0

24. $\dfrac{-13}{0}$ Undefined

25. $\dfrac{19}{-1}$ -19

26. $\dfrac{-17}{1}$ -17

27. $-41 \div 1$ -41

28. $23 \div (-1)$ -23

b Simplify, if possible.

29. $8 - 2 \cdot 3 - 9$ -7

30. $8 - (2 \cdot 3 - 9)$ 11

31. $8 - 2(3 - 9)$ 20

32. $(8 - 2)(3 - 9)$ -36

33. $16 \cdot (-24) + 50$ -334

34. $10 \cdot 20 - 15 \cdot 24$ -160

35. $40 - 3^2 - 2^3$ 23

36. $2^4 + 2^2 - 10$ 10

37. $4 \cdot (6 + 8)/(4 + 3)$ 8

38. $4^3 + 10 \cdot 20 + 8^2 - 23$ 305

39. $4 \cdot 5 - 2 \cdot 6 + 4$ 12

40. $5^3 + 4 \cdot 9 - (8 + 9 \cdot 3)$ 126

41. $\dfrac{9^2 - 1}{1 - 3^2}$ -10

42. $\dfrac{100 - 6^2}{(-5)^2 - 3^2}$ 4

43. $8(-7) + 6(-5)$ -86

44. $10(-5) \div 1(-1)$ 50

45. $20 \div 5(-3) + 3$ -9

46. $14 \div 2(-6) + 7$ -35

47. $8 \div 2 \cdot 0 \div 6$ 0

48. $9 \cdot 0 \div 5 \cdot 4$ 0

49. $4 \cdot 5^2 \div 10$ 10

50. $(2 - 5)^2 \div (-9)$ -1

51. $(3 - 8)^2 \div (-1)$ -25

52. $3 - 3^2$ -6

53. $12 - 20^3$ -7988 **54.** $20 + 4^3 \div (-8)$ 12 **55.** $2 \times 10^3 - 5000$ -3000 **56.** $-7(3^4) + 18$ -549

57. $6[9 - (3 - 4)]$ 60 **58.** $8[(6 - 13) - 11]$ -144 **59.** $-1000 \div (-100) \div 10$ 1 **60.** $256 + (-32) \div (-4)$
                                                                                                            264

61. $8 - |7 - 9| \cdot 3$ 2 **62.** $|8 - 7 - 9| \cdot 2 + 1$ 17 **63.** $9 - |7 - 3^2|$ 7 **64.** $9 - |5 - 7|^3$ 1

65. $\dfrac{(-5)^3 + 17}{10(2 - 6) - 2(5 + 2)}$ 2 **66.** $\dfrac{(3 - 5)^2 - (7 - 13)}{(2 - 5)3 + 2 \cdot 4}$ -10 **67.** $\dfrac{2 \cdot 4^3 - 4 \cdot 32}{19^3 - 17^4}$ 0 **68.** $\dfrac{-16 \cdot 28 \div 2^2}{5 \cdot 25 - 5^3}$
                                                                                                                                    Undefined

Skill Maintenance

69. Fabrikant Fine Diamonds ran a 4-in. by 7-in. advertisement in *The New York Times*. Find the area of the ad.   [1.8a]   28 sq in.

70. A classroom contains 7 rows of chairs with 6 chairs in each row. How many chairs are there in the classroom?   [1.8a]   42

71. A Ford Windstar gets 25 miles per gallon (mpg). How many gallons will it take to travel 350 mi? [1.8a]   14 gal

72. A Honda Passport gets 20 mpg. How many gallons will it take to travel 340 mi?   [1.8a]   17 gal

73. A 7-oz bag of tortilla chips contains 1050 calories. How many calories are in a 1-oz serving?   [1.8a]
150 calories

74. A 7-oz bag of tortilla chips contains 8 grams (g) of fat. How many grams of fat are in a carton containing 12 bags of chips?   [1.8a]   96 g

Synthesis

75. ◆ Explain in your own words why $23 \div 0$ is undefined.

76. ◆ Explain how multiplication can be used to justify why the quotient of two negative integers is a positive integer.

77. ◆ Explain how multiplication can be used to justify why a negative integer divided by a positive integer is a negative integer.

Simplify.

78. $\dfrac{(25 - 4^2)^3}{17^2 - 16^2} \cdot ((-6)^2 - 6^2)$ **79.** $\dfrac{(7 - 8)^{37}}{7^2 - 8^2} \cdot (98 - 7^2 \cdot 2)$ **80.** ▦ $\dfrac{19 - 17^2}{13^2 - 34}$ -2 **81.** ▦ $\dfrac{195 + (-15)^3}{195 - 7 \cdot 5^2}$
   0 0

Determine the sign of each expression if m is negative and n is positive. -159

82. $\dfrac{-n}{m}$ Positive   **83.** $\dfrac{-n}{-m}$ Negative   **84.** $-\left(\dfrac{-n}{m}\right)$ Negative   **85.** $-\left(\dfrac{n}{-m}\right)$ Negative   **86.** $-\left(\dfrac{-n}{-m}\right)$
                                                                                                               Positive

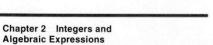

Use the order of operations as a group to simplify expressions.

Collaborative Learning Manual

2.6 Introduction to Algebra and Expressions

a   Algebraic Expressions

In arithmetic, we work with expressions such as

$$37 + 86, \quad 7 \times 8, \quad 19 - 7, \quad \text{and} \quad \frac{3}{8}.$$

In algebra, we use both numbers and variables and work with *algebraic expressions* such as

$$x + 86, \quad 7 \times t, \quad 19 - y, \quad \text{and} \quad \frac{a}{b}.$$

Expressions like these should be familiar from the equation and problem solving that we have already done.

When a letter can stand for various numbers, we call the letter a **variable**. A number or a letter that stands for just one number is called a **constant**. Let $c =$ the speed of light. Then c is a constant. Let $a =$ your age in years. Then a is a variable since the value of a changes every second.

An **algebraic expression** consists of variables, numerals, and operation signs. When we replace a variable with a number, we say that we are **substituting** for the variable. This process is called **evaluating the expression.**

Example 1   Evaluate $x + y$ for $x = 37$ and $y = 29$.

We substitute 37 for x and 29 for y and carry out the addition:

$$x + y = 37 + 29 = 66.$$

The number 66 is called the **value** of the expression.

Algebraic expressions involving multiplication can be written in several ways. For example, "8 times a" can be written as $8 \times a$, $8 \cdot a$, $8(a)$, or simply $8a$. Two letters written together without an operation symbol, such as ab, also indicates multiplication.

Example 2   Evaluate $3y$ for $y = -14$.

$$3y = 3(-14) = -42 \qquad \textbf{Parentheses are required here.}$$

Do Exercises 1–3.

Algebraic expressions involving division can also be written in several ways. For example, "8 divided by t" can be written as $8 \div t$, $8/t$, or $\dfrac{8}{t}$.

Example 3   Evaluate $\dfrac{a}{b}$ and $\dfrac{-a}{-b}$ for $a = 35$ and $b = 7$.

We substitute 35 for a and 7 for b:

$$\frac{a}{b} = \frac{35}{7} = 5; \qquad \frac{-a}{-b} = \frac{-35}{-7} = 5.$$

Note that $\dfrac{-a}{-b} = \dfrac{a}{b}$, as the rules for division would lead us to expect.

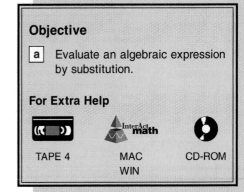
1. Evaluate $a + b$ for $a = 38$ and $b = 26$.   64

2. Evaluate $x - y$ for $x = 57$ and $y = 29$.   28

3. Evaluate $4t$ for $t = -15$.   −60

Answers on page A-5

For each number, find two equal expressions with negative signs in different places.

4. $\dfrac{-7}{x}$ $\quad -\dfrac{7}{x} ; \dfrac{7}{-x}$

5. $-\dfrac{m}{n}$ $\quad \dfrac{-m}{n} ; \dfrac{m}{-n}$

6. $\dfrac{r}{-4}$ $\quad \dfrac{-r}{4} ; -\dfrac{r}{4}$

7. Evaluate $\dfrac{a}{-b}, \dfrac{-a}{b}$, and $-\dfrac{a}{b}$ for $a = 28$ and $b = 4$. $-7; -7; -7$

8. Find the Fahrenheit temperature that corresponds to 10 degrees Celsius (see Example 5). 50

9. Evaluate $3x^2$ for $x = 4$ and $x = -4$. $48; 48$

10. Evaluate a^4 for $a = 3$ and $a = -3$. $81; 81$

11. Evaluate $(-x)^2$ and $-x^2$ for $x = 3$. $9; -9$

12. Evaluate $(-x)^2$ and $-x^2$ for $x = 2$. $4; -4$

13. Evaluate x^5 for $x = 2$ and $x = -2$. $32; -32$

Answers on page A-5

Example 4 Evaluate $-\dfrac{a}{b}, \dfrac{-a}{b}$, and $\dfrac{a}{-b}$ for $a = 15$ and $b = 3$.

We substitute 15 for a and 3 for b:

$$-\frac{a}{b} = -\frac{15}{3} = -5; \qquad \frac{-a}{b} = \frac{-15}{3} = -5; \qquad \frac{a}{-b} = \frac{15}{-3} = -5.$$

Note that $-\dfrac{a}{b}, \dfrac{-a}{b}$, and $\dfrac{a}{-b}$ all represent the same number.

Do Exercises 4–7.

Example 5 Evaluate $\dfrac{9C}{5} + 32$ for $C = 20$.

This expression can be used to find the Fahrenheit temperature that corresponds to 20 degrees Celsius:

$$\frac{9C}{5} + 32 = \frac{9 \cdot 20}{5} + 32 = \frac{180}{5} + 32 = 36 + 32 = 68.$$

Do Exercise 8.

Example 6 Evaluate $5x^2$ for $x = 3$ and $x = -3$.

The rules for order of operations specify that the replacement for x be squared first. That result is then multiplied by 5:

$$5x^2 = 5(3)^2 = 5(9) = 45;$$
$$5x^2 = 5(-3)^2 = 5(9) = 45.$$

Example 6 shows that when opposites are raised to an even power, the results are the same.

Do Exercises 9 and 10.

Example 7 Evaluate $(-x)^2$ and $-x^2$ for $x = 7$.

We have

$$(-x)^2 = (-7)^2 = (-7)(-7) = 49. \qquad \textbf{Substitute 7 for } x \textbf{. Then evaluate the power.}$$

To evaluate $-x^2$, recall from Section 2.4 that taking the opposite of a number is the same as multiplying that number by -1. Thus, $-x^2$ can be rewritten as $-1 \cdot x^2$. When x is replaced with 7, we will need to square first and then take the opposite or multiply by -1:

$$-x^2 = -1 \cdot x^2$$
$$= -1 \cdot 7^2$$
$$= -1 \cdot 49$$
$$= -49.$$

These steps emphasize that we find -7^2 by first squaring 7 and then finding the opposite.

CAUTION! Example 7 shows that
$$(-x)^2 \neq -x^2.$$

Do Exercises 11—13.

Exercise Set 2.6

a Evaluate.

1. $7t$, for $t = 2$
(The cost, in cents, of using a microwave for 2 hr) 14¢

2. $40t$, for $t = 2$
(The cost, in cents, of using an electric oven for 2 hr) 80¢

3. $\dfrac{x}{y}$, for $x = 9$ and $y = -3$ −3

4. $\dfrac{m}{n}$, for $m = 14$ and $n = 2$ 7

5. $\dfrac{3p}{q}$, for $p = 2$ and $q = 6$ 1

6. $\dfrac{5y}{z}$, for $y = 15$ and $z = -25$ −3

7. $\dfrac{x + y}{5}$, for $x = -10$ and $y = 20$ 2

8. $\dfrac{p - q}{2}$, for $p = 16$ and $q = -2$ 9

9. $3 + 5 \cdot x$, for $x = 2$ 13

10. $9 - 2 \cdot x$, for $x = 3$ 3

11. $2l + 2w$, for $l = 3$ and $w = 4$
(The perimeter, in feet, of a 3-ft by 4-ft rectangle) 14 ft

12. $3(a + b)$, for $a = 2$ and $b = 4$ 18

13. $2(l + w)$, for $l = 3$ and $w = 4$
(The perimeter, in feet, of a 3-ft by 4-ft rectangle) 14 ft

14. $3a + 3b$, for $a = 2$ and $b = 4$ 18

15. $7a - 7b$, for $a = 5$ and $b = 2$ 21

16. $4x - 4y$, for $x = 6$ and $y = 1$ 20

17. $7(a - b)$, for $a = 5$ and $b = 2$ 21

18. $4(x - y)$, for $x = 6$ and $y = 1$ 20

19. $16t^2$, for $t = 5$
(The distance, in feet, that an object falls in 5 sec) 400 ft

20. $\dfrac{49t^2}{10}$, for $t = 10$
(The distance, in meters, that an object falls in 10 sec) 490 m

21. $9m - m^2$, for $m = -4$ -52

22. $7n - n^2$, for $n = -5$ -60

23. $a + (b - a)^2$, for $a = 6$ and $b = 4$ 10

24. $(x + y)^2 - y$, for $x = 2$ and $y = 3$ 22

25. $a + b - a^2$, for $a = 6$ and $b = 4$ -26

26. $x + y^2 - y$, for $x = 2$ and $y = 3$ 8

27. $\dfrac{n^2 - n}{2}$, for $n = 9$

(For determining the number of handshakes possible among 9 people) 36

28. $\dfrac{5(F - 32)}{9}$, for $F = 50$

(For converting 50 degrees Fahrenheit to degrees Celsius) 10

For each expression, write two equal expressions with negative signs in different places.

29. $-\dfrac{3}{a}$ $\dfrac{-3}{a}; \dfrac{3}{-a}$

30. $\dfrac{7}{-x}$ $\dfrac{-7}{x}; -\dfrac{7}{x}$

31. $\dfrac{-n}{b}$ $\dfrac{n}{-b}; -\dfrac{n}{b}$

32. $-\dfrac{3}{r}$ $\dfrac{-3}{r}; \dfrac{3}{-r}$

33. $\dfrac{9}{-p}$ $\dfrac{-9}{p}; -\dfrac{9}{p}$

34. $\dfrac{-u}{5}$ $\dfrac{u}{-5}; -\dfrac{u}{5}$

35. $\dfrac{-14}{w}$ $\dfrac{14}{-w}; -\dfrac{14}{w}$

36. $\dfrac{-23}{m}$ $\dfrac{23}{-m}; -\dfrac{23}{m}$

Evaluate $\dfrac{-a}{b}, \dfrac{a}{-b}$, and $-\dfrac{a}{b}$ for the given values.

37. $a = 35, b = 7$ $-5; -5; -5$

38. $a = 40, b = 5$ $-8; -8; -8$

39. $a = 81, b = 3$ $-27; -27; -27$

40. $a = 56, b = 7$ $-8; -8; -8$

Evaluate.

41. $(-3x)^2$ and $-3x^2$, for $x = 7$ 441; −147

42. $(-2x)^2$ and $-2x^2$, for $x = 3$ 36; −18

43. $5x^2$, for $x = 2$ and $x = -2$ 20; 20

44. $2x^2$, for $x = 5$ and $x = -5$ 50; 50

45. x^3, for $x = 6$ and $x = -6$ 216; −216

46. x^6, for $x = 2$ and $x = -2$ 64; 64

47. x^6, for $x = 1$ and $x = -1$ 1; 1

48. x^5, for $x = 3$ and $x = -3$ 243; −243

49. a^7, for $a = 2$ and $a = -2$ 128; −128

50. a^7, for $a = 1$ and $a = -1$ 1; −1

51. $-m^2 + m$, for $m = -4$ −20

52. $-n^3 - n$, for $n = 5$ −130

53. $a - 3a^3$, for $a = -5$ 370

54. $x^3 - 5x$, for $x = -3$ −12

55. $x^2 + 5x \div 2$, for $x = -6$ 21

56. $6x \div x^2 - 2x$, for $x = 3$ −4

57. $m^3 - m^2$, for $m = 5$ 100

58. $a^6 - a$, for $a = -2$ 66

Skill Maintenance

59. Write a word name for 23,043,921.   [1.1c]

Twenty-three million, forty-three thousand, nine hundred twenty-one

60. Multiply: $17 \cdot 53$.   [1.5b]   901

61. Estimate by rounding to the nearest ten. Show your work.   [1.4b]

$\begin{array}{r} 5\ 2\ 8\ 3 \\ -\ 2\ 4\ 7\ 5 \end{array}$ $5280 - 2480 = 2800$

62. Divide: $2982 \div 3$.   [1.6c]   994

63. On January 6, it snowed 9 in., and on January 7, it snowed 8 in. How much did it snow altogether? [1.8a]   17 in.

64. On March 9, it snowed 12 in., but on March 10, the sun melted 7 in. How much snow remained?   [1.8a]

5 in.

Synthesis

65. ◆ Under what condition(s) will the expression ax^2 be nonnegative? Explain.

66. ◆ A student evaluates $a + a^2$ for $a = 5$ and gets 100 as the result. What mistake did the student probably make?

67. ◆ Does $-\dfrac{a}{b}$ always represent a negative number? Why or why not?

Evaluate.

68. ▦ $a - b^3 + 17a$, for $a = 19$ and $b = -16$ 4438

69. ▦ $x^2 - 23y + y^3$, for $x = 18$ and $y = -21$ -8454

70. $a^{1996} - a^{1997}$, for $a = -1$ 2

71. $x^{1492} - x^{1493}$, for $x = -1$ 2

72. $(m^3 - mn)^m$, for $m = 4$ and $n = 6$ 2,560,000

73. $5a^{3a-4}$, for $a = 2$ 20

Classify each statement as true or false. If false, write an example showing why.

74. For any choice of x, $x^2 = (-x)^2$.

True

75. For any choice of x, $x^3 = -x^3$.

False; $2^3 = 8$; but $-2^3 = -8$

76. For any choice of x, $x^6 + x^4 = (-x)^6 + (-x)^4$.

True

77. For any choice of x, $(-3x)^2 = 9x^2$.

True

2.7 Like Terms and Perimeter

Two of the most important topics in algebra are solving equations and forming *equivalent expressions*. In this section, we see how the *distributive law* can be used to form equivalent expressions.

a Equivalent Expressions and the Distributive Law

It is useful to know when two algebraic expressions will represent the same number.

Example 1 Evaluate $1 \cdot x$ for $x = 5$ and $x = -8$ and compare the results to x.

We substitute 5 for x:

$$1 \cdot x = 1 \cdot 5 = 5.$$

Next, we substitute -8 for x:

$$1 \cdot x = 1 \cdot (-8) = -8.$$

We see that $1 \cdot x$ and x represent the same number.

Do Exercises 1 and 2.

Example 1 and Margin Exercise 1 illustrate that the expressions $1 \cdot x$ and x represent the same number for any replacement of x. Because of this, $1 \cdot x$ and x are said to be **equivalent expressions.**

> Two expressions that have the same value for all allowable replacements are called **equivalent**.

In Section 2.6, we saw that the expressions $\dfrac{-a}{-b}$ and $\dfrac{a}{b}$ are equivalent but that the expressions $(-x)^2$ and $-x^2$ are *not* equivalent.

An important concept, known as the **distributive law,** is useful for finding equivalent algebraic expressions. The distributive law involves two operations: multiplication and either addition or subtraction.

To review how the distributive law works, consider the following:

```
    4 5
 ×    7
    3 5  ← This is 7 · 5.
  2 8 0  ← This is 7 · 40.
  3 1 5  ← This is the sum 7 · 40 + 7 · 5.
```

To carry out the multiplication, we actually added two products. That is,

$$7 \cdot 45 = 7(40 + 5) = 7 \cdot 40 + 7 \cdot 5.$$

Complete each table by evaluating each expression for the given values.

1.

	$1 \cdot x$	x
$x = 3$	3	3
$x = -6$	-6	-6
$x = 0$	0	0

2.

	$-1 \cdot x$	$-x$
$x = 2$	-2	-2
$x = -6$	6	6
$x = 0$	0	0

Answers on page A-5

Multiply.

3. $4(a + b)$ $4a + 4b$

4. $5(x + y + z)$ $5x + 5y + 5z$

Multiply.

5. $3(x - y)$ $3x - 3y$

6. $2(a - b + c)$ $2a - 2b + 2c$

The distributive law says that if we want to multiply a sum of several numbers by a number, we can either add within the grouping symbols and then multiply, or multiply each of the terms separately and then add.

> ▶ **THE DISTRIBUTIVE LAW**
> For any numbers a, b, and c,
> $$a(b + c) = ab + ac.$$

In the statement of the distributive law, we know that in an expression such as $ab + ac$, the multiplications are to be done first according to the rules for order of operations. This means that in $a(b + c)$, we cannot omit the parentheses. If we did we would have $ab + c$, which means $(ab) + c$.

To see that $a(b + c)$ and $ab + ac$ are equivalent, note that

$$3(4 + 2) = 3 \cdot 4 + 3 \cdot 2$$
$$3 \cdot \quad 6 \quad = \quad 12 \quad + \quad 6$$
$$18 = 18.$$

To see that $a(b + c) \neq ab + c$, note that

$$3(4 + 2) \neq 3 \cdot 4 + 2$$
$$3 \cdot \quad 6 \quad \neq \quad 12 \quad + 2$$
$$18 \neq 14.$$

Example 2   Multiply: $2(l + w)$.

We use the distributive law to write an equivalent expression:

$$2(l + w) = 2 \cdot l + 2 \cdot w$$
$$= 2l + 2w. \quad \text{Try to go directly to this step.}$$

Exercises 11 and 13 in Section 2.6 can serve as a check that $2(l + w)$ and $2l + 2w$ are equivalent.

Do Exercises 3 and 4.

Since subtraction can be regarded as addition of the opposite, it follows that the distributive law holds in cases involving subtraction.

Example 3   Multiply: $7(a - b)$.

$$7(a - b) = 7 \cdot a - 7 \cdot b$$
$$= 7a - 7b \quad \text{Try to go directly to this step.}$$

Exercises 15 and 17 in Section 2.6 can serve as a check that $7(a - b)$ and $7a - 7b$ are equivalent.

Do Exercises 5 and 6.

Answers on page A-5

In more complicated problems, it is sometimes helpful to write one or more middle steps.

Example 4 Multiply: **(a)** $9(x - 5)$; **(b)** $8(a + 2b - 7)$; **(c)** $-4(x - 2y + 3z)$.

a) $9(x - 5) = 9x - 9(5)$ Using the distributive law

$= 9x - 45$

b) $8(a + 2b - 7) = 8 \cdot a + 8 \cdot 2b - 8 \cdot 7$ Using the distributive law

$= 8a + 16b - 56$

c) $-4(x - 2y + 3z) = -4 \cdot x - (-4)(2y) + (-4)(3z)$ Using the distributive law

$= -4x - (-4 \cdot 2)y + (-4 \cdot 3)z$ Using an associative law (twice)

$= -4x - (-8y) + (-12z)$

$= -4x + 8y - 12z$ Try to go directly to this step.

Do Exercises 7–10.

b   Combining Like Terms

A **term** is a number, a variable, or a product of numbers and/or variables, or a quotient of numbers and/or variables. Terms are separated by addition signs. If there are subtraction signs, we can find an equivalent expression that uses addition signs.

Example 5 What are the terms of $3x - 4y + \dfrac{2}{z}$?

$3x - 4y + \dfrac{2}{z} = 3x + (-4y) + \dfrac{2}{z}$ Separating parts with + signs

The terms are $3x$, $-4y$, and $\dfrac{2}{z}$.

Example 6 What are the terms of $5xy + 3x^2 - 8$?

$5xy + 3x^2 - 8 = 5xy + 3x^2 + (-8)$ Separating parts with + signs

The terms are $5xy$, $3x^2$, and -8.

Do Exercises 11 and 12.

Multiply.

7. $3(x - 5)$ $3x - 15$

8. $5(x - y + 4)$ $5x - 5y + 20$

9. $-2(x - 3)$ $-2x + 6$

10. $-5(x - 2y + 4z)$
$-5x + 10y - 20z$

What are the terms of each expression?

11. $5x - 4y + 3$ $5x; -4y; 3$

12. $-4y - 2x + \dfrac{x}{y}$ $-4y; -2x; \dfrac{x}{y}$

Answers on page A-5

Identify the like terms.

13. $9a^3 + 4ab + a^3 + 3ab + 7$

$9a^3$ and a^3; $4ab$ and $3ab$

14. $3xy - 5x^2 + y^2 - 4xy + y$

$3xy$ and $-4xy$

Combine like terms.

15. $4a + 7a$ $11a$

16. $5x^2 - 9 + 2x^2 + 3$ $7x^2 - 6$

17. $4m - 2n^2 + 3 + n^2 + m - 7$

$5m - n^2 - 4$

Answers on page A-5

Terms in which the variable factors are exactly the same, such as $9x$ and $-4x$, are called **like**, or **similar, terms.** For example, $3y^2$ and $7y^2$ are like terms, whereas $5x$ and $6x^2$ are not.

Examples   Identify the like terms.

7. $7x + 5x^2 + 2x + 8 + 5x^3 + 1$

$7x$ and $2x$ are like terms;   8 and 1 are like terms.

8. $5ab + a^3 - a^2b - 2ab + 7a^3$

$5ab$ and $-2ab$ are like terms; a^3 and $7a^3$ are like terms.

Do Exercises 13 and 14.

When an algebraic expression contains like terms, an equivalent expression can be formed by **combining**, or **collecting, like terms.** To combine like terms, we rely on the distributive law even though that step is often not written out.

Example 9   Combine like terms: **(a)** $5x + 3x$;   **(b)** $6mn - 7mn$; **(c)** $7y - 5 - 3y + 8$; **(d)** $2a^5 + 9ab + 3 + a^5 - 7 - 4ab$.

a) $5x + 3x = (5 + 3)x$ Using the distributive law (in "reverse")

          $= 8x$ We usually go directly to this step.

b) $6mn - 7mn = (6 - 7)mn$ Try to do this mentally.

               $= -1mn$, or simply $-mn$

c) $7y - 5 - 3y + 8 = 7y + (-5) + (-3y) + 8$ Rewriting as addition

                    $= 7y + (-3y) + (-5) + 8$ Using a commutative law

                    $= 4y + 3$ Try to go directly to this step.

d) $2a^5 + 9ab + 3 + a^5 - 7 - 4ab$

   $= 2a^5 + 9ab + 3 + a^5 + (-7) + (-4ab)$

   $= 2a^5 + a^5 + 9ab + (-4ab) + 3 + (-7)$ Rearranging terms

   $= 3a^5 + 5ab + (-4)$ Think of a^5 as $1a^5$.

   $= 3a^5 + 5ab - 4$

As you gain more experience, you will perform several of these steps mentally.

Do Exercises 15–17.

c | Perimeter

> A **polygon** is a closed geometric figure with three or more sides. The **perimeter** of a polygon is the distance around it, or the sum of the lengths of its sides.

Example 10 Find the perimeter of this polygon.

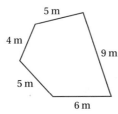

We add the lengths of the sides. Since all the units are the same, we are effectively combining like terms.

Perimeter = 6 m + 5 m + 4 m + 5 m + 9 m

= (6 + 5 + 4 + 5 + 9) m   **Using the distributive law**

= 29 m   **Try to go directly to this step.**

Do Exercises 18 and 19.

A **rectangle** is a polygon with four sides and four 90° angles. Opposite sides of a rectangle have the same measure. The symbol ⌐ indicates a 90° angle.

Example 11 Find the perimeter of a rectangle that is 3 cm by 4 cm.

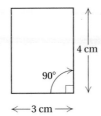

Perimeter = 3 cm + 3 cm + 4 cm + 4 cm

= (3 + 3 + 4 + 4) cm

= 14 cm

Do Exercise 20.

Note that the perimeter of the rectangle in Example 11 is 2 · 3 cm + 2 · 4 cm, or equivalently 2(3 cm + 4 cm). This can be generalized, as follows.

> The **perimeter P of a rectangle** of length l and width w is given by
> $$P = 2l + 2w, \quad \text{or} \quad P = 2 \cdot (l + w).$$
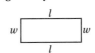

Find the perimeter of the polygon.

18.

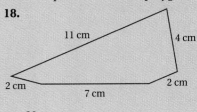

26 cm

19.

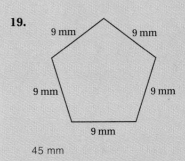

45 mm

20. Find the perimeter of a rectangle that is 2 cm by 4 cm.

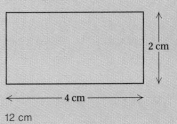

12 cm

Answers on page A-5

21. Find the perimeter of a 4-ft by 8-ft sheet of plywood.

24 ft

22. Find the perimeter of a square with sides of length 10 km.

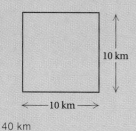

40 km

23. Find the perimeter of a square sandbox with sides of length 6 ft. 24 ft

Answers on page A-5

Example 12 Find the perimeter of a rectangular table that is 4 ft by 6 ft.

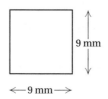

$$P = 2l + 2w$$ We could also use $P = 2(l + w)$.

$$= 2 \cdot 6 \text{ ft} + 2 \cdot 4 \text{ ft}$$

$$= (2 \cdot 6) \text{ ft} + (2 \cdot 4) \text{ ft}$$ Try to do this mentally.

$$= 12 \text{ ft} + 8 \text{ ft}$$

$$= 20 \text{ ft}$$

The perimeter of the table is 20 ft.

Do Exercise 21.

A **square** is a rectangle in which all sides have the same length.

Example 13 Find the perimeter of a square with sides of length 9 mm.

9 mm

←9 mm→

$$P = 9 \text{ mm} + 9 \text{ mm} + 9 \text{ mm} + 9 \text{ mm}$$

$$= (9 + 9 + 9 + 9) \text{ mm}$$

$$= 36 \text{ mm}$$

Do Exercise 22.

The **perimeter P of a square** is four times *s*, the length of a side:

$$P = s + s + s + s$$
$$= 4s.$$

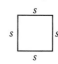

Example 14 Find the perimeter of a square garden with sides of length 12 ft.

$$P = 4s$$

$$= 4 \cdot 12 \text{ ft}$$

$$= 48 \text{ ft}$$

The perimeter of the garden is 48 ft.

Do Exercise 23.

Exercise Set 2.7

a Multiply.

1. $5(a + b)$ $5a + 5b$

2. $7(x + y)$ $7x + 7y$

3. $4(x + 1)$ $4x + 4$

4. $6(a + 1)$ $6a + 6$

5. $2(b + 5)$ $2b + 10$

6. $4(x + 3)$ $4x + 12$

7. $7(1 - t)$ $7 - 7t$

8. $4(1 - y)$ $4 - 4y$

9. $6(5x + 2)$ $30x + 12$

10. $9(6m + 7)$ $54m + 63$

11. $8(x + 7 + 6y)$ $8x + 56 + 48y$

12. $4(5x + 8 + 3p)$ $20x + 32 + 12p$

13. $-7(y - 2)$ $-7y + 14$

14. $-9(y - 7)$ $-9y + 63$

15. $-9(-5x - 6y + 8)$
$45x + 54y - 72$

16. $-7(-2x - 5y + 9)$
$14x + 35y - 63$

17. $-4(x - 3y - 2z)$
$-4x + 12y + 8z$

18. $8(2x - 5y - 8z)$
$16x - 40y - 64z$

19. $8(a - 3b + c)$
$8a - 24b + 8c$

20. $-6(a + 2b - c)$
$-6a - 12b + 6c$

21. $4(x - 3y - 7z)$
$4x - 12y - 28z$

22. $5(9x - y + 8z)$
$45x - 5y + 40z$

23. $5(4a - 5b + c - 2d)$
$20a - 25b + 5c - 10d$

24. $7(9a - 4b + 3c - d)$
$63a - 28b + 21c - 7d$

b Combine like terms.

25. $7a + 12a$ $19a$

26. $12x + 2x$ $14x$

27. $10a - a$ $9a$

28. $-16x + x$ $-15x$

29. $2x + 6z + 9x$ $11x + 6z$

30. $3a - 5b + 7a$ $10a - 5b$

31. $27a + 70 - 40a - 8$ $-13a + 62$

32. $42x - 6 - 4x + 2$ $38x - 4$

33. $23 + 5t + 7y - t - y - 27$

    $-4 + 4t + 6y$

34. $45 - 90d - 87 - 9d + 3 + 7d$

    $-39 - 92d$

35. $5x - 12x$

    $-7x$

36. $9t - 17t$

    $-8t$

37. $y - 17y$

    $-16y$

38. $3m - 9m + 4$

    $-6m + 4$

39. $-8 + 11a - 5b + 6a - 7b + 7$

    $-1 + 17a - 12b$

40. $8x - 5x + 6 + 3y - 2y - 4$

    $3x + 2 + y$

41. $8x + 3y - 2x$

    $6x + 3y$

42. $8y - 3z + 4y$

    $12y - 3z$

43. $11x + 2y - 4x - y$

    $7x + y$

44. $13a + 9b - 2a - 4b$

    $11a + 5b$

45. $a + 3b + 5a - 2 + b$

    $6a + 4b - 2$

46. $x + 7y + 5 - 2y + 3x$

    $4x + 5y + 5$

47. $6x^3 + 2x - 5x^3 + 7x$

    $x^3 + 9x$

48. $9a^2 - 4a + a - 3a^2$

    $6a^2 - 3a$

49. $3a^2 + 7a^3 - a^2 + 5 + a^3$

    $2a^2 + 8a^3 + 5$

50. $x^3 - 5x^2 + 2x^3 - 3x^2 + 4$

    $3x^3 - 8x^2 + 4$

51. $9xy + 4y^2 - 2xy + 2y^2 - 1$

    $7xy + 6y^2 - 1$

52. $7a^3 + 4ab - 5 - 7ab + 8$

    $7a^3 - 3ab + 3$

53. $8a^2b - 3ab^2 - 4a^2b + 2ab$

    $4a^2b - 3ab^2 + 2ab$

54. $9x^3y + 4xy^3 - 6xy^3 + 3xy$

    $9x^3y - 2xy^3 + 3xy$

55. $3x^4 - 2y^4 + 8x^4y^4 - 7x^4 + 8y^4$

    $-4x^4 + 6y^4 + 8x^4y^4$

56. $3a^6 - 9b^4 + 2a^6b^4 - 7a^6 - 2b^4$

    $-4a^6 - 11b^4 + 2a^6b^4$

c Find the perimeter of each polygon.

57.
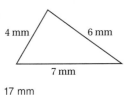
4 mm   6 mm
7 mm

17 mm

58.
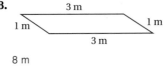
3 m
1 m   1 m
3 m

8 m

59.
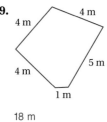
4 m
4 m   4 m
5 m
4 m
1 m

18 m

60.
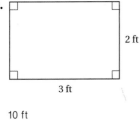
2 ft
3 ft

10 ft

61.
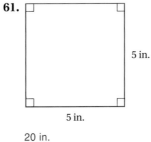
5 in.

5 in.

20 in.

62.
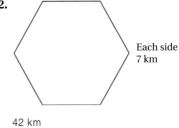
Each side
7 km

42 km

Soccer Field. A soccer field contains many rectangles. Use the diagram of a regulation soccer field (at right) to find the perimeter of each of the following rectangles.

63. The perimeter of the smallest possible regulation field   300 yd

64. The perimeter of the largest possible regulation field   460 yd

65. The perimeter of each penalty area   124 yd

66. The perimeter of each goal area   52 yd

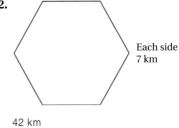

Goal
Goal line   Corner flag
Corner area   Goal area
Penalty area
Penalty spot
Touch line
Penalty arc
Optional flag
Center spot
Halfway line
10 yards
Center circle
Maximum 100 yds — Minimum 50 yds
Minimum 100 yds
Maximum 130 yds
44 yards
18 yards
6 yards   20 yards
8 yards

67. Find the perimeter of a 12-ft by 14-ft bedroom.
52 ft

68. Find the perimeter of a 3-ft by 7-ft screen door.
20 ft

69. Find the perimeter of a checkerboard that is 14 in. on each side.   56 in.

70. Find the perimeter of a square skylight that is 2 m on each side.   8 m

71. Find the perimeter of a square frame that is 75 cm on each side.   300 cm

72. Find the perimeter of a square garden that is 12 yd on each side.   48 yd

73. Find the perimeter of a 12-ft by 20-ft deck.   64 ft

74. Find the perimeter of a 40-ft by 35-ft backyard.
150 ft

Skill Maintenance

75. A box of Grand Union Corn Flakes contains 510 grams (g) of corn flakes. A serving of corn flakes weighs 30 g. How many servings are in one box?   [1.8a]   17

76. Estimate the difference by rounding to the nearest ten.   [1.4b]   210

$$\begin{array}{r} 7\ 0\ 4 \\ -\ 4\ 8\ 6 \end{array}$$

77. Multiply: $6 \cdot 529$.   [1.5b]   3174

78. Write a word name: 3,534,512.   [1.1c]
Three million, five hundred thirty-four thousand, five hundred twelve

79. Divide: $3549 \div 5$.   [1.6c]   709 R 4

80. Subtract: $3000 - 2189$.   [1.3d]   811

Synthesis

81. ◈ Explain in your own words what it means for two algebraic expressions to be equivalent.

82. ◈ Can the formula for the perimeter of a rectangle be used to find the perimeter of a square? Why or why not?

83. ◈ Why do you think the distributive law is introduced *before*, rather than after, the material on combining like terms.

Replace the blanks with $\boxed{+}$, $\boxed{-}$, $\boxed{\times}$, or $\boxed{\div}$ to make each statement true.

84. ▦ -32 ▨ $(88$ ▨ $29) = -1888$

85. ▦ 59 ▨ 17 ▨ 59 ▨ $8 = 1475$

86. ▦ 27 ▨ 18 ▨ 21 ▨ $18 = 864$

Simplify. (Multiply and then combine like terms.)

87. $5(x + 3) + 2(x - 7)$ $7x + 1$

88. $3(a - 7) + 7(a + 4)$ $10a + 7$

89. $2(3 - 4a) + 5(a - 7)$ $-29 - 3a$

90. $7(2 - 5x) + 3(x - 8)$
$-10 - 32x$

91. $-5(2 + 3x + 4y) + 7(2x - y)$
$-10 - x - 27y$

92. $3(4 - 2x) + 5(9x - 3y + 1)$
$17 + 39x - 15y$

93. In order to save energy, Andrea plans to run a bead of caulk sealant completely around each of 3 doors and 13 windows. Each door measures 3 ft by 7 ft, each window measures 3 ft by 4 ft, and each sealant cartridge covers 56 ft. If each cartridge costs $5.95, how much will it cost Andrea to seal the windows and doors? $29.75

94. Eric is attaching lace trim to small tablecloths that are 5 ft by 5 ft, and to large tablecloths that are 7 ft by 7 ft. If the lace costs $1.95 per yard, how much will the trim cost for 6 small tablecloths and 6 large tablecloths? $187.20

84. 32 $\boxed{\times}$ $(88$ $\boxed{-}$ $29) = -1888$ **85.** 59 $\boxed{\times}$ 17 $\boxed{+}$ 59 $\boxed{\times}$ 8 = 1475
86. 27 $\boxed{\times}$ 18 $\boxed{+}$ 21 $\boxed{\times}$ 18 = 864

2.8 Solving Equations

In Section 1.7, we learned to solve certain equations by writing a "related equation." We now formalize this approach in a manner that will be used throughout this book.

a | The Addition Principle

In Section 1.7, we learned to solve an equation like $x + 12 = 27$ by writing the related subtraction, $x = 27 - 12$, or $x = 15$. We can easily see that the solution of $x = 15$ is 15: Replacing x with 15, we get

$$15 = 15, \quad \text{which is true.}$$

You should check that the solution of $x + 12 = 27$ is also 15. Because their solutions are identical, $x = 15$ and $x + 12 = 27$ are said to be **equivalent equations.**

> Equations with the same solutions are called **equivalent equations.**

Note the difference between equivalent *expressions* and equivalent *equations*:

> $6a$ and $4a + 2a$ are equivalent expressions because, for any replacement of a, both expressions represent the same number.
>
> $3x = 15$ and $4x = 20$ are equivalent equations because any solution of one equation is also a solution of the other equation.

There are principles that enable us to begin with one equation and create an equivalent equation similar to $x = 15$, for which the solution is obvious. One such principle, the *addition principle*, is stated below.

Suppose that a and b stand for the same number and some number c is added to a. We get the same result if we add c to b, because a and b represent the same number.

> **THE ADDITION PRINCIPLE**
> For any numbers a, b, and c,
> $$a = b \quad \text{is equivalent to} \quad a + c = b + c.$$

Objectives

a Use the addition principle to solve equations.

b Use the division principle to solve equations.

c Decide which principle should be used to solve an equation.

For Extra Help

TAPE 4   MAC   CD-ROM
WIN

Solve.

1. $x - 5 = 19$ 24

2. $x - 9 = -12$ -3

Solve.

3. $42 = x + 17$ 25

4. $a + 8 = -6$ -14

Answers on page A-6

Example 1   Solve: $x - 7 = -2$.

We have

$$x - 7 = -2$$
$$x - 7 + 7 = -2 + 7 \qquad \text{Using the addition principle: adding 7 on both sides}$$
$$x + 0 = 5 \qquad \text{Adding 7 "undoes" the subtraction of 7.}$$
$$x = 5.$$

The solution appears to be 5. To be sure, we check in the original equation.

CHECK: $$\begin{array}{c} x - 7 = -2 \\ \hline 5 - 7 \; ? \; -2 \\ -2 \; | \qquad \text{TRUE} \end{array}$$

The solution is 5.

Do Exercises 1 and 2.

Recall from Section 2.3 that subtraction can be regarded as adding the opposite of the number being subtracted. Because of this, the addition principle allows us to subtract the same number on both sides of the equation.

Example 2   Solve: $23 = t + 7$.

We have

$$23 = t + 7$$
$$23 - 7 = t + 7 - 7 \qquad \text{Using the addition principle to add } -7 \text{ or to subtract 7 on both sides}$$
$$16 = t + 0 \qquad \text{Subtracting 7 "undoes" the addition of 7.}$$
$$16 = t.$$

The solution is 16. The check is left to the student.

To visualize the addition principle, think of a jeweler's balance. When both sides of the balance hold equal amounts of weight, the balance is level. If weight is added or removed, equally, on both sides, the balance remains level.

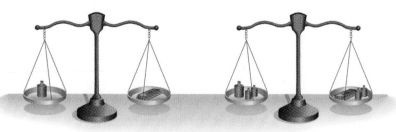

Do Exercises 3 and 4.

b | The Division Principle

In Section 1.7, we found that $8n = 96$ could be solved by dividing by 8 on both sides:

$$8 \cdot n = 96$$

$$\frac{8 \cdot n}{8} = \frac{96}{8} \qquad \text{Dividing by 8 on both sides}$$

$$n = 12. \qquad \text{8 times } n \text{, divided by 8, is } n. \; 96 \div 8 \text{ is 12.}$$

You can check that $8 \cdot n = 96$ and $n = 12$ are equivalent. We can divide an equation by any nonzero number in order to find an equivalent equation.

THE DIVISION PRINCIPLE

For any numbers a, b, and c ($c \neq 0$),

$$a = b \quad \text{is equivalent to} \quad \frac{a}{c} = \frac{b}{c}.$$

In Chapter 3, after we have discussed multiplication of fractions, we will use an equivalent form of this principle: the multiplication principle.

Example 3 Solve: $9x = 63$.

We have

$$9x = 63$$

$$\frac{9x}{9} = \frac{63}{9} \qquad \begin{array}{l} \text{Using the division principle to} \\ \text{divide by 9 on both sides} \end{array}$$

$$x = 7.$$

CHECK:
$$\begin{array}{r} 9x = 63 \\ \hline 9 \cdot 7 \; ? \; 63 \\ 63 \; | \qquad \text{TRUE} \end{array}$$

The solution is 7.

Do Exercises 5 and 6.

Solve.

5. $7x = 42$ 6

6. $-24 = 3t$ -8

Answers on page A-6

Solve.

7. $63 = -7n$ −9

8. $-6x = 72$ −12

Solve.

9. $-2x = -52$ 26

10. $-2 + x = -52$ −50

11. $x \cdot 7 = -28$ −4

Answers on page A-6

Example 4   Solve: $48 = -8n$.

It is important to distinguish between a negative sign, as we have in $-8n$, and a minus sign, as we had in Example 1. To undo multiplication by -8, we use the division principle:

$$48 = -8n$$

$$\frac{48}{-8} = \frac{-8n}{-8} \qquad \text{Dividing by } -8 \text{ on both sides}$$

$$-6 = n.$$

CHECK: $$\frac{48 = -8n}{48 \;?\; -8(-6)}$$
$$\qquad |\; 48 \qquad \text{TRUE}$$

The solution is -6.

Do Exercises 7 and 8.

c   Selecting the Correct Approach

It is important for you to be able to determine which principle should be used to solve a particular equation. In future chapters, you will need to use both principles together as well as individually.

Examples   Solve.

5. $39 = -3 + t$

To undo addition of -3, we subtract -3 or simply add 3 on both sides:

$$3 + 39 = 3 + (-3) + t \qquad \text{Using the addition principle}$$
$$42 = 0 + t$$
$$42 = t.$$

CHECK: $$\frac{39 = -3 + t}{39 \;?\; -3 + 42}$$
$$\qquad |\; 39 \qquad \text{TRUE}$$

The solution is 42.

6. $39 = -3t$

To undo multiplication of -3, we divide by -3 on both sides:

$$39 = -3t$$
$$\frac{39}{-3} = \frac{-3t}{-3} \qquad \text{Using the division principle}$$
$$-13 = t.$$

CHECK: $$\frac{39 = -3t}{39 \;?\; -3(-13)}$$
$$\qquad |\; 39 \qquad \text{TRUE}$$

The solution is -13.

Do Exercises 9–11.

Exercise Set 2.8

a Solve.

1. $x - 7 = 5$ 12

2. $x - 2 = 13$ 15

3. $x - 6 = -9$ −3

4. $x - 5 = -12$ −7

5. $t + 5 = 13$ 8

6. $a + 7 = 25$ 18

7. $x + 9 = -3$ −12

8. $x + 8 = -6$ −14

9. $17 = n - 6$ 23

10. $24 = t - 7$ 31

11. $-9 = x + 3$ −12

12. $-12 = x + 5$ −17

13. $-9 + t = 8$ 17

14. $-5 + a = 13$ 18

15. $3 = 17 + x$ −14

16. $9 = 14 + t$ −5

b Solve.

17. $3x = 24$ 8

18. $6x = 30$ 5

19. $-8t = 32$ −4

20. $-6t = 42$ −7

21. $-5n = -65$ 13

22. $-7n = -35$ 5

23. $64 = 8x$ 8

24. $72 = 3x$ 24

25. $81 = -3t$ −27

26. $55 = -5t$ −11

27. $-x = 83$ −83

28. $-x = 56$ −56

29. $n(-6) = -42$ 7

30. $n(-4) = -48$ 12

31. $-x = -475$ 475

32. $-x = -390$ 390

c Solve.

33. $t - 7 = -2$ 5

34. $3t = 48$ 16

35. $6x = -90$ −15

36. $x + 9 = -15$ −24

37. $8 + x = 43$ 35

38. $-40 = 10x$ −4

39. $18 = x - 27$ 45

40. $-33 = x(-11)$ 3

41. $35 = -5t$ -7 **42.** $9 + t = -19$ -28 **43.** $19x = -171$ -9 **44.** $-36 = x - 12$ -24

45. $19 + x = -171$ -190 **46.** $-36 = x(-12)$ 3 **47.** $-38 = t + 43$ -81 **48.** $-135 = -9t$ 15

Skill Maintenance

Simplify.   [1.9c]

49. $5 + 3 \cdot 2^3$ 29

50. $(9 - 7)^4 - 3^2$ 7

51. $12 \div 3 \cdot 2$ 8

52. $27 \div 3(2 + 1)$ 27

53. $15 - 3 \cdot 2 + 7$ 16

54. $30 - 4^2 \div 8 \cdot 2$ 26

Synthesis

55. ◈ Explain in your own words the difference between equivalent equations and equivalent expressions.

56. ◈ Debra decides to solve $x - 9 = -5$ by adding 5 on both sides of the equation. Is there anything wrong with her doing this? Why or why not?

57. ◈ James decides to solve $-3x = 15$ by adding 3 on both sides of the equation. Is there anything wrong with his doing this? Why or why not?

Solve.

58. $2x - 7x = -40$ 8

59. $9 + x - 5 = 23$ 19

60. $17 - 3^2 = 4 + t - 5^2$ 29

61. $(-9)^2 = 2^3 t + (3 \cdot 6 + 1)t$ 3

62. $(-7)^2 - 5 = t + 4^3$ -20

63. ▦ $(-17)^3 = 15^3 x$ $-\frac{4913}{3375}$

64. ▦ $x - (19)^3 = -18^3$ 1027

65. ▦ $23^2 = x + 22^2$ 45

66. $3x - 5 = 13$ 6

67. $4x + 3 = 31$ 7

68. $6 - 2x = -12$ 9

69. $8 + 3x = -22$ -10

Summary and Review: Chapter 2

Important Properties and Formulas

For any integers a, b, and c: $a + (-a) = 0$; $a - b = a + (-b)$;
$a \cdot 0 = 0$; $a(b + c) = ab + ac$

Perimeter of a Rectangle: $P = 2l + 2w$, or $P = 2(l + w)$
Perimeter of a Square: $P = 4s$

Review Exercises

1. Tell which integers correspond to this situation: [2.1a]

Bonnie has $527 in her savings account and Roger is $53 in debt.

Use either $<$ or $>$ for ▨ to form a true statement. [2.1b]

2. 0 ▨ -5 **3.** -7 ▨ 6 **4.** -4 ▨ -19

Find the absolute value.   [2.1c]

5. $|-39|$ **6.** $|12|$ **7.** $|0|$

8. Find $-x$ when $x = -53$.   [2.1d]

9. Find $-(-x)$ when $x = 29$.   [2.1d]

Compute and simplify.   [2.2a], [2.3a], [2.4a, b], [2.5a, b]

10. $-14 + 5$ **11.** $-5 + (-6)$

12. $14 + (-8)$ **13.** $0 + (-24)$

14. $15 - 24$ **15.** $9 - (-14)$

16. $-8 - (-7)$ **17.** $-3 - (-10)$

18. $-3 + 7 + (-8)$ **19.** $8 - (-9) - 7 + 2$

20. $-23 \cdot (-4)$ **21.** $7(-12)$

22. $2(-4)(-5)(-1)$ **23.** $15 \div (-5)$

24. $\dfrac{-55}{11}$ **25.** $\dfrac{0}{7}$

26. $7 \div 1^2 \cdot (-3) - 4$ **27.** $(-3)|4 - 3^2| - 5$

28. Evaluate $3a + b$ for $a = 4$ and $b = -5$. [2.6a]

29. Evaluate $\dfrac{-x}{y}$, $\dfrac{x}{-y}$, and $-\dfrac{x}{y}$ for $x = 20$ and $y = 5$.
[2.6a]

Multiply. [2.7a]

30. $4(5x + 9)$ **31.** $3(2a - 4b + 5)$

Combine like terms. [2.7b]

32. $5a + 13a$ **33.** $-7x + 13x$

34. $9m + 14 - 12m - 8$

35. Find the perimeter of a frame that is 8 in. by 10 in. [2.7c]

36. Find the perimeter of a square pane of glass that is 25 cm on each side. [2.7c]

Solve. [2.8a, b, c]

37. $x - 9 = -17$ **38.** $-4t = 36$ **39.** $x \cdot 7 = -42$

40. Write a word name for 386,451. [1.1c]

41. Estimate by rounding to the nearest ten. Show your work. [1.4b]

$$\begin{array}{r} 7\ 2\ 9\ 6 \\ -\ 2\ 7\ 4\ 1 \\ \hline \end{array}$$

42. Estimate by rounding to the nearest hundred. Show your work. [1.4b]

$2481 - 1729$

43. In 1998, Mark McGwire hit 70 home runs and Sammy Sosa hit 66. How many did they hit altogether that year? [1.8a]

Multiply. [1.5b]

44. $3 \cdot 8495$ **45.**

$$\begin{array}{r} 7\ 3\ 4 \\ \times\ \ \ \ 2\ 9 \\ \hline \end{array}$$

Synthesis

46. ◈ A classmate insists on reading $-x$ as "negative x." When asked why, the response is "because $-x$ is negative." What mistake is this student making? [2.1d]

47. ◈ Are $(a - b)^2$ and $(b - a)^2$ equivalent for all choices of a and b? Why or why not? Experiment with different replacements for a and b. [2.6a]

Simplify. [2.5b]

48. ▦ $87 \div 3 \cdot 29^3 - (-6)^6 + 1957$

49. ▦ $1969 + (-8)^5 - 17 \cdot 15^3$

50. ▦ $\dfrac{113 - 17^3}{15 + 8^3 - 507}$

51. For what values of x is $|x| > x$? [2.1b, c]

52. For what values of x will $8 + x^3$ be negative? [2.6a]

Test: Chapter 2

1. Tell which integers correspond to this situation: The Tee Shop sold 542 fewer tee-shirts than expected in January and 307 more than expected in February.

2. Use either $<$ or $>$ for ▊ to form a true statement.

$$-14 \; ▊ \; -21$$

3. Find the absolute value: $|-429|$.

4. Find $-(-x)$ when $x = -19$.

Compute and simplify.

5. $6 + (-17)$

6. $-9 + (-12)$

7. $-8 + 17$

8. $0 - 12$

9. $7 - 22$

10. $-5 - 19$

11. $-8 - (-27)$

12. $17 - (-3) - 5 + 9$

13. $(-4)^3$

14. $13(-10)$

15. $-9 \cdot 0$

16. $-72 \div (-9)$

17. $\dfrac{-56}{7}$

18. $8 \div 2 \cdot 2 - 3^2$

19. $29 - (3 - 5)^2$

Answers

20. [2.3b] 13°F

21. [2.6a] −3

22. [2.7a] 14x + 21y − 7

23. [2.7b] 4x − 17

24. [2.8b] 5

25. [2.8a] −12

26. [1.1c] Two million, three hundred eight thousand, four hundred fifty-one

27. [1.4b] 3200 − 1920 = 1280

28. [1.4b] 9200 − 2900 = 6300

29. [1.8a] 21

30. [1.5b] 5648

31. [1.5b] 20,536

32. [2.7c] 66 ft

33. [2.7a, b] 35x − 7

34. [2.7a, b] −24x − 57

20. On January 9, the temperature dropped from −2°F to −15°F. How many degrees did it drop?

21. Evaluate $\frac{a-b}{6}$ for $a = -8$ and $b = 10$.

22. Multiply: 7(2x + 3y − 1).

23. Combine like terms: 9x − 14 − 5x − 3.

Solve.

24. −7x = −35

25. a + 7 = −5

Skill Maintenance

26. Write a word name for 2,308,451.

27. Estimate by rounding to the nearest ten. Show your work.
$$3204$$
$$-1915$$

28. Estimate the difference by rounding to the nearest hundred. Show your work.
9247 − 2879

29. Maurice shoveled 9 driveways while Phyllis shoveled 12. How many driveways did they shovel between the two of them?

Multiply.

30. 8 · 706

31. 302×68

Synthesis

32. A carpenter plans to attach trim around a doorway and along the base of all walls in a 12-ft by 14-ft room. If the doorway is 3 ft by 7 ft, how many feet of trim are needed? (Only three sides of a doorway get trim.)

Simplify.

33. 9 − 5[x + 2(3 − 4x)] + 14

34. 15x + 3(2x − 7) − 9(4 + 5x)

Cumulative Review: Chapters 1–2

1. Write standard notation for the number in the following sentence: The earth travels five hundred eighty-four million, seventeen thousand, eight hundred miles around the sun.

2. Write a word name for 5,380,621.

Add.

3. $\begin{array}{r} 1\,4,8\,6\,2 \\ +\ \ 2,9\,3\,5 \\ \hline \end{array}$

4. $\begin{array}{r} 7\,9\,8\,9 \\ 7\,8\,9 \\ +\ \ \ \ 7\,9 \\ \hline \end{array}$

Subtract.

5. $\begin{array}{r} 5\,3\,7\,6 \\ -\ \ 4\,3\,0 \\ \hline \end{array}$

6. $\begin{array}{r} 2\,0\,0\,4 \\ -\ \ 5\,7\,9 \\ \hline \end{array}$

Multiply.

7. $\begin{array}{r} 6\,2\,1 \\ \times\ \ 2\,7 \\ \hline \end{array}$

8. $\begin{array}{r} 2\,5\,0\,5 \\ \times 3\,3\,0\,0 \\ \hline \end{array}$

9. $31 \cdot (-8)$

10. $-12(-6)$

Divide.

11. $19\,\overline{)4\,5\,8\,0}$

12. $62\,\overline{)3\,8\,4\,4}$

13. $0 \div (-32)$

14. $60 \div (-12)$

15. Round 427,931 to the nearest thousand.

16. Round 5309 to the nearest hundred.

Estimate each sum or product by rounding to the nearest hundred. Show your work.

17. $\begin{array}{r} 7\,4\,9,5\,5\,9 \\ +\,3\,0\,1,3\,6\,2 \\ \hline \end{array}$

18. $\begin{array}{r} 7\,4\,9 \\ \times 5\,3\,1 \\ \hline \end{array}$

19. Use < or > for ▦ to form a true sentence:
    −26 ▦ 19.

20. Find the absolute value: $|-279|$.

Simplify.

21. $35 - 25 \div 5 + 2 \times 3$

22. $\{17 - [8 - (5 - 2 \times 2)]\} \div (3 + 12 \div 6)$

23. $10 \div 1(-5) - 6^2$

24. 5^3

25. Evaluate $\dfrac{x + y}{5}$ for $x = 11$ and $y = 4$.

26. Evaluate $7x^2$ for $x = -2$.

Multiply.

27. $-2(x + 5)$

28. $6(3x - 2y + 4)$

Simplify.

29. $-12 + (-14)$

30. $-17 - 14$

31. $23 - 38$

32. $-12 - (-25)$

Solve.

33. $x + 8 = 35$

34. $-12t = 36$

35. $-6 + x = -9$

36. $384 \div 16 = n$

Solve.

37. The Barnes & Noble Bookstore in lower Manhattan is the world's largest, covering 154,250 sq ft. Although W. & G. Foyle Ltd. of London has the most titles in the world, it covers "only" 75,825 sq ft. (**Source**: *The Guinness Book of Records,* 1998). How much larger is the Barnes & Noble store?

38. Four of the largest hotels in the United States are in Las Vegas. One has 3174 rooms, the second has 2920 rooms, the third has 2832 rooms, and the fourth has 5005 rooms. What is the total number of rooms in these four hotels?

39. Amanda is offered a part-time job paying $3900 a year. How much is each weekly paycheck?

40. Eastside Appliance sells a refrigerator for $600 and $30 tax with no delivery charge. Westside Appliance sells the same model for $560 and $28 tax plus a $25 delivery charge. Which is the better buy?

41. Combine like terms: $-9 + 10x - 5 + 13x$.

Synthesis

42. A soft drink distributor has 142 loose cans of cola. The distributor wishes to form as many 24-can cases as possible and then, with any remaining cans, as many six-packs as possible. How many cases will be filled? How many six-packs? How many loose cans will remain?

43. Simplify: $a - \{3a - [4a - (2a - 4a)]\}$.

3

Fractional Notation: Multiplication and Division

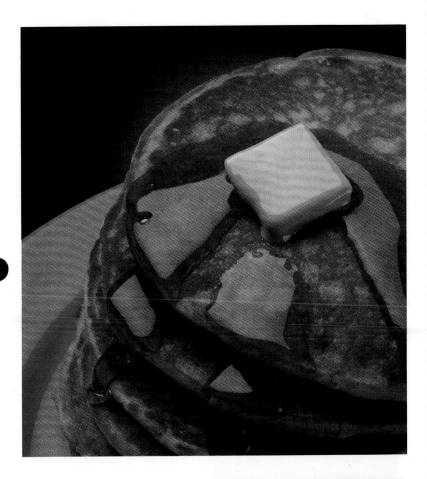

An Application

For their annual pancake breakfast, the Colchester Boy Scouts need $\frac{2}{3}$ cup of Bisquick® per person. If 135 people are expected, how much Bisquick do they need?

This problem appears as Example 5 in Section 3.6.

The Mathematics

We let n = the number of cups of Bisquick needed. The problem then translates to

$$n = 135 \cdot \frac{2}{3}.$$

Multiplication using fractional notation occurs often in problem solving.

Pretest: Chapter 3

1. Determine whether 165 is divisible by 3. Do not use long division.

2. Determine whether 1645 is divisible by 5. Do not use long division.

3. Determine whether 67 is prime, composite, or neither.

4. Find the prime factorization of 280.

Simplify.

5. $\dfrac{75}{75}$

6. $\dfrac{7x}{1}$

7. $\dfrac{0}{50}$

8. $\dfrac{-8}{32}$

9. $\dfrac{10a}{35a}$

10. Find an equivalent expression for $\dfrac{3}{7}$ with a denominator of 28.

Multiply and simplify.

11. $\dfrac{1}{3} \cdot \dfrac{18}{5}$

12. $\dfrac{5}{6} \cdot (-24)$

13. $\dfrac{2a}{5} \cdot \dfrac{25}{8}$

Find the reciprocal.

14. $\dfrac{7}{8}$

15. 11

Divide and simplify.

16. $15 \div \dfrac{5}{8}$

17. $\dfrac{2}{3} \div \left(-\dfrac{8}{9}\right)$

18. $\dfrac{14}{9} \div (7x)$

Solve.

19. $-\dfrac{8}{7} = 4x$

20. $\dfrac{7}{10} \cdot x = 21$

21. $\dfrac{5}{12} = \dfrac{2}{3} \cdot a$

Solve.

22. Heather earns $72 for working a full day. How much will she earn for working $\frac{3}{4}$ of a day?

23. A piece of twine $\frac{5}{8}$ m long is to be cut into 15 pieces of the same length. What is the length of each piece?

24. A triangular sign with a base of 3 ft and a height of 4 ft is cut from a 4-ft by 8-ft sheet of plywood. Find the area of the leftover plywood.

3.1 Multiples and Divisibility

In this chapter, we begin our work with fractions. Certain skills make this work easier. For example, in order to simplify fractions like

$$\frac{15}{40},$$

it will be useful to learn about *multiples* and *divisibility*.

a | Multiples

A **multiple** of a number is a product of it and some integer. For example, some multiples of 2 are:

2   (because $2 = 1 \cdot 2$);

4   (because $4 = 2 \cdot 2$);

6   (because $6 = 3 \cdot 2$);

8   (because $8 = 4 \cdot 2$);

10   (because $10 = 5 \cdot 2$).

We can also find multiples of 2 by counting by twos: 2, 4, 6, 8, and so on.

Example 1 Show that each of the numbers 3, 6, 9, and 15 is a multiple of 3.

We show that each of 3, 6, 9, and 15 can be expressed as a product of 3 and some integer:

$$3 = 1 \cdot 3; \quad 6 = 2 \cdot 3; \quad 9 = 3 \cdot 3; \quad 15 = 5 \cdot 3.$$

Do Exercises 1 and 2.

Example 2 Multiply by 1, 2, 3, and so on, to find ten multiples of 7.

$1 \cdot 7 = 7$	$6 \cdot 7 = 42$
$2 \cdot 7 = 14$	$7 \cdot 7 = 49$
$3 \cdot 7 = 21$	$8 \cdot 7 = 56$
$4 \cdot 7 = 28$	$9 \cdot 7 = 63$
$5 \cdot 7 = 35$	$10 \cdot 7 = 70$

Do Exercise 3.

> A number b is said to be **divisible** by another number a if b is a multiple of a.

Thus,

6 is divisible by 2 because 6 is a multiple of 2 ($6 = 3 \cdot 2$);

27 is divisible by 3 because 27 is a multiple of 3 ($27 = 9 \cdot 3$);

100 is divisible by 25 because 100 is a multiple of 25 ($100 = 4 \cdot 25$).

> A number b is divisible by another number a if division of b by a results in a remainder of zero. We sometimes say that a divides b "evenly."

Objectives

a   Find some multiples of a number, and determine whether a number is divisible by another number.

b   Test to see if a number is divisible by 2, 3, 5, 6, 9, or 10.

For Extra Help

TAPE 5   MAC WIN   CD-ROM

1. Show that each of the numbers 5, 45, and 100 is a multiple of 5.

   $5 = 1 \cdot 5$; $45 = 9 \cdot 5$; $100 = 20 \cdot 5$

2. Show that each of the numbers 10, 60, and 110 is a multiple of 10.

   $10 = 1 \cdot 10$; $60 = 6 \cdot 10$; $110 = 11 \cdot 10$

3. Multiply by 1, 2, 3, and so on, to find ten multiples of 5.

   5, 10, 15, 20, 25, 30, 35, 40, 45, 50

Answers on page A-7

4. Determine whether 16 is divisible by 2.

Yes

5. Determine whether 125 is divisible by 5.

Yes

6. Determine whether 125 is divisible by 6.

No

Answers on page A-7

Example 3   Determine whether 24 is divisible by 3.

We divide 24 by 3:

$$
\begin{array}{r}
8 \\
3\overline{)24} \\
\underline{24} \\
0
\end{array}
$$

The remainder of 0 indicates that 24 is divisible by 3.

Example 4   Determine whether 98 is divisible by 4.

We divide 98 by 4:

$$
\begin{array}{r}
24 \\
4\overline{)98} \\
\underline{8} \\
18 \\
\underline{16} \\
2 \longleftarrow \text{Not 0!}
\end{array}
$$

Since the remainder is not 0 we know that 98 is *not* divisible by 4.

Do Exercises 4–6.

Calculator Spotlight

Rather than list remainders, most calculators display quotients using decimal notation. Although decimal notation is not studied until Chapter 5, it is still possible for us to now check for divisibility using a calculator.

To see if a number, like 551, is divisible by another number, like 19, we simply press [5] [5] [1] [÷] [1] [9] [=] . If the resulting quotient contains no digits to the right of the decimal point, the first number is divisible by the second. Thus, since 551 ÷ 19 = 29, we know that 551 is divisible by 19. On the other hand, since 551 ÷ 20 = 27.55, we know that 551 is *not* divisible by 20.

Exercises

For each pair of numbers, determine whether the first number is divisible by the second number.

1. 731, 17   Yes

2. 1502, 79   No

3. 1053, 36   No

4. 4183, 47   Yes

b Tests for Divisibility

We now learn quick ways of checking for divisiblity by 2, 3, 5, 6, 9, or 10 without actually performing long division.

Divisibility by 2

You may already know the test for divisibility by 2.

> A number is divisible by 2 (is *even*) if it has a ones digit of 0, 2, 4, 6, or 8 (that is, it has an even ones digit).

To see why this test works, consider 354, which is

$$3 \text{ hundreds} + 5 \text{ tens} + 4 \text{ ones}.$$

Hundreds and tens are both multiples of 2. If the ones digit is a multiple of 2, then the entire number is a multiple of 2.

Examples Determine whether each of the following numbers is divisible by 2.

5. 355 *is not* divisible by 2; 5 is not even.

6. 4786 *is* divisible by 2; 6 is even.

7. 8990 *is* divisible by 2; 0 is even.

8. 4261 *is not* divisible by 2; 1 is not even.

Do Exercises 7–10.

Divisibility by 3

> A number is divisible by 3 if the sum of its digits is divisible by 3.

An explanation of why this test works is outlined in Exercise 52.

Examples Determine whether each of the following numbers is divisible by 3.

9. 18 $\quad 1 + 8 = 9$
10. 93 $\quad 9 + 3 = 12$
11. 201 $\quad 2 + 0 + 1 = 3$

All are divisible by 3 because the sums of their digits are divisible by 3.

12. 256 $\quad 2 + 5 + 6 = 13$

The sum is not divisible by 3, so 256 is not divisible by 3.

Do Exercises 11–14.

Divisibility by 6

A number divisible by 6 is a multiple of 6. But $6 = 2 \cdot 3$, so the number is also a multiple of 2 and 3. Thus a number is divisible by 6 if it is divisible by both 2 and 3.

> A number is divisible by 6 if its ones digit is even (0, 2, 4, 6, or 8) and the sum of its digits is divisible by 3.

Determine whether each of the following numbers is divisible by 2.

7. 84   Yes

8. 59   No

9. 998   Yes

10. 2225   No

Determine whether each of the following numbers is divisible by 3.

11. 111   Yes

12. 1111   No

13. 309   Yes

14. 17,216   No

Answers on page A-7

Determine whether each of the following numbers is divisible by 6.

15. 420   Yes

16. 106   No

17. 321   No

18. 444   Yes

Determine whether each of the following numbers is divisible by 9.

19. 16   No

20. 117   Yes

21. 930   No

22. 29,223   Yes

Examples   Determine whether each of the following numbers is divisible by 6.

13. 720

Because 720 is even, it is divisible by 2. Since $7 + 2 + 0 = 9$ and 9 is divisible by 3, we know that 720 is also divisible by 3. Since 720 is divisible by both 2 and 3, we know that 720 *is* divisible by 6.

720          $7 + 2 + 0 = 9$
↑   ↑
Even   Divisible by 3

14. 531

Because 531 is not divisible by 2, we know that 531 *is not* divisible by 6.

531
↑
Not even

15. 478

Because the sum of its digits is not divisible by 3, we know that 478 is not divisible by 3. Since 478 is not divisible by 3, we know that 478 *is not* divisible by 6.

$4 + 7 + 8 = 19$
↑
Not divisible by 3

Do Exercises 15–18.

Divisibility by 9

The test for divisibility by 9 is similar to the test for divisibility by 3. An explanation of why it works is outlined in Exercise 52.

> ▶ A number is divisible by 9 if the sum of its digits is divisible by 9.

Example 16   The number 6984 *is* divisible by 9 because

$6 + 9 + 8 + 4 = 27$

and 27 is divisible by 9.

Example 17   The number 322 *is not* divisible by 9 because

$3 + 2 + 2 = 7$

and 7 is not divisible by 9.

Do Exercises 19–22.

Answers on page A-7

Divisibility by 10

▶ A number is divisible by 10 if its ones digit is 0.

We know that this test works because the product of 10 and *any* number has a ones digit of 0.

Examples   Determine whether each of the following numbers is divisible by 10.

18. 3440   *is* divisible by 10 because its ones digit is 0.

19. 3447   *is not* divisible by 10 because its ones digit is not 0.

Do Exercises 23–26.

Divisibility by 5

▶ A number is divisible by 5 if its ones digit is 0 or 5.

Examples   Determine whether each of the following numbers is divisible by 5.

20.   220   *is* divisible by 5 because its ones digit is 0.

21.   475   *is* divisible by 5 because its ones digit is 5.

22. 6514   *is not* divisible by 5 because its ones digit is neither 0 nor 5.

Do Exercises 27–30.

To see why the test for 5 works, consider 7830:

$$7830 = 10 \cdot 783 = 5 \cdot 2 \cdot 783.$$

Since 7830 is a multiple of 10 and 10 is a multiple of 5, it follows that 7830 is divisible by 5.
 Next, consider 6325:

$$6325 = 632 \text{ tens} + 5 \text{ ones}.$$

Tens are multiples of 5, and the ones digit, 5, is as well. Thus, 6325 is a multiple of 5. Only if the ones digit is 0 or 5, as in 7830 or 6325, will the entire number be divisible by 5.

Divisibility by 4, 7, and 8

Although tests exist for divisibility by 4, 7, and 8, they are often more difficult to perform than the actual long division.

Determine whether each of the following numbers is divisible by 10.

23. 305   No

24. 300   Yes

25. 847   No

26. 8760   Yes

Determine whether each of the following numbers is divisible by 5.

27. 5780   Yes

28. 3427   No

29. 34,678   No

30. 7775   Yes

Answers on page A-7

Improving Your Math Study Skills

Classwork: Before and During Class

Before Class

Textbook

- Check your syllabus (or ask your instructor) to find out which sections will be covered during the next class. Then be sure to read, or at least skim, these sections *before* class. Although you may not understand all the concepts, you will at least familiarize yourself with the material. This will help you to understand the next lesson.

- This book makes use of color, shading, and design elements to highlight important concepts, so you do not need to highlight these. Instead, it is more productive for you to note trouble spots with either a highlighter or Post-It™ notes. Then use these marked points as possible questions for clarification by your instructor at the appropriate time. Be sure to always have a pencil or erasable pen in hand when reading this book.

Homework

- Review the previous day's homework just before class. This will refresh your memory on the concepts covered in the last class, and again provide you with possible questions to ask your instructor.

During Class

Class Seating

- If possible, choose a seat at the front of the class. In most classes, the more serious students tend to sit up front so you will probably be able to concentrate better if you do the same. You should also avoid sitting next to noisy or distracting students.

- If your instructor uses an overhead projector, select a seat that will give you an unobstructed view of the screen.

Taking Notes

- This textbook has been written and laid out so that it represents a quality set of notes at the same time that it teaches. Thus you might not need to take many notes in class. Just watch, listen, and ask yourself questions as the class moves along, rather than continually taking notes.

  However, if you still feel more comfortable taking your own notes, consider using the following two-column method. Divide your page in half vertically so that you have two columns side by side. Write down what is on the board or screen in the left column; then, in the right column, write clarifying comments or questions.

- If you have any difficulty keeping up with the instructor, use abbreviations to speed up your note-taking. Consider standard abbreviations like "Ex" for "Example," "$\approx$" for "approximately equal to," or "$\therefore$" for "therefore." Create your own abbreviations as well.

- Another shortcut for note-taking is to write only the beginning of a word, leaving space for the rest. Be sure you write enough of the word to know what it means later on!

- Some students find it helpful to follow lectures with their textbooks open so that they can see exactly which portion of the book is being discussed. These students write their notes directly in the margins of their book.

- Whatever approach you use for note-taking, be sure to review the notes that you write while they are still fresh in your mind. Sometimes you may need to insert corrections if you wrote too quickly or copied something incorrectly.

Other study tips appear on pages 50, 90, 100, 322, 368, and 596.

Exercise Set 3.1

a Multiply by 1, 2, 3, and so on, to find ten multiples of each number.

1. 6

6, 12, 18, 24,
30, 36, 42, 48,
54, 60

2. 14

14, 28, 42, 56,
70, 84, 98, 112,
126, 140

3. 20

20, 40, 60, 80,
100, 120, 140,
160, 180, 200

4. 50

50, 100, 150, 200,
250, 300, 350, 400,
450, 500

5. 3

3, 6, 9, 12,
15, 18, 21, 24,
27, 30

6. 7

7, 14, 21, 28,
35, 42, 49, 56,
63, 70

7. 13

13, 26, 39, 52,
65, 78, 91, 104,
117, 130

8. 17

17, 34, 51, 68,
85, 102, 119, 136,
153, 170

9. 10

10, 20, 30, 40,
50, 60, 70, 80,
90, 100

10. 4

4, 8, 12, 16,
20, 24, 28, 32,
36, 40

11. 9

9, 18, 27, 36,
45, 54, 63, 72,
81, 90

12. 11

11, 22, 33, 44,
55, 66, 77, 88,
99, 110

13. Determine whether 26 is divisible by 7.   No

14. Determine whether 29 is divisible by 9.   No

15. Determine whether 1880 is divisible by 8.   Yes

16. Determine whether 4227 is divisible by 3.   Yes

17. Determine whether 106 is divisible by 4.   No

18. Determine whether 196 is divisible by 16.   No

19. Determine whether 4227 is divisible by 9.   No

20. Determine whether 200 is divisible by 25.   Yes

21. Determine whether 8650 is divisible by 16.   No

22. Determine whether 4143 is divisible by 7.   No

b To answer Exercises 23–28, consider the following numbers. Use the tests for divisibility.

46	300	85	256
224	36	711	8064
19	45,270	13,251	1867
555	4444	254,765	21,568

23. Which of the above are divisible by 2?

46, 224, 300, 36, 45,270, 4444, 256, 8064, 21,568

24. Which of the above are divisible by 3?

555, 300, 36, 45,270, 711, 13,251, 8064

25. Which of the above are divisible by 10?

300, 45,270

26. Which of the above are divisible by 5?

555, 300, 45,270, 85, 254,765

27. Which of the above are divisible by 6?

300, 36, 45,270, 8064

28. Which of the above are divisible by 9?

36, 45, 270, 711, 8064

To answer Exercises 29–34, consider the following numbers.

56	200	75	35
324	42	812	402
784	501	2345	111,111
55,555	3009	2001	1005

29. Which of the above are divisible by 3?

324, 42, 501, 3009, 75, 2001, 402, 111,111, 1005

30. Which of the above are divisible by 2?

56, 324, 784, 200, 42, 812, 402

31. Which of the above are divisible by 5?

55,555, 200, 75, 2345, 35, 1005

32. Which of the above are divisible by 10?

200

33. Which of the above are divisible by 9?

324

34. Which of the above are divisible by 6?

324, 42, 402

Skill Maintenance

Solve.

35. $16 \cdot t = 848$ [1.7b], [2.8b]   53

36. $m + 9 = 14$ [1.7b], [2.8a]   5

37. $23 + x = 15$ [1.7b], [2.8a] -8

38. $24 \cdot m = -576$ [1.7b], [2.8b] -24

39. Find the total cost of 12 shirts at $37 each and 4 pairs of pants at $59 each.   [1.8a] $680

40. Add: $-34 + 76$.   [2.2a]   42

Synthesis

41. ◆ Describe a test that could be used to determine whether a number is divisible by 25.

42. ◆ Is every counting number a multiple of 1? Why or why not?

43. ◆ Describe a manner in which Exercises 23, 24, and 26 can be used to answer Exercises 25 and 27.

44. ◆ Describe a test for determining whether a number is divisible by 30.

45. ▦ Find the largest five-digit number that is divisible by 47.   99,969

46. ▦ Find the largest six-digit number that is divisible by 53.   999,951

Find the smallest number that is simultaneously a multiple of the given numbers.

47. 2, 3, and 5   30

48. 3, 5, and 7   105

49. 4, 6, and 10   60

50. 6, 10, and 14   210

51. A passenger in a taxicab asks for the driver's company number. The driver says abruptly, "Sure–it's the smallest multiple of 11 that, when divided by 2, 3, 4, 5, or 6, has a remainder of 1." What is the number?   121

52. ◆ To help see why the tests for division by 3 and 9 work, note that any four-digit number $abcd$ can be rewritten as $1000 \cdot a + 100 \cdot b + 10 \cdot c + d$, or $999a + 99b + 9c + a + b + c + d$.

a) Explain why $999a + 99b + 9c$ is divisible by both 9 and 3 for all choices of a, b, c, and d.

b) Explain why the four-digit number $abcd$ is divisible by 9 if $a + b + c + d$ is divisible by 9 and is divisible by 3 if $a + b + c + d$ is divisible by 3.

Collaborative
Learning Manual

Use the divisibility rules and properties of numbers to discover an unknown number.

3.2 Factorizations

In Section 3.1, we saw that both 28 and 35 are multiples of 7. Another way of saying this is to state that 7 is a *factor* of both 28 and 35. When a number is expressed as a product of two or more factors, we say that we have *factored* the original number. Thus the word "factor" can be used as either a noun or a verb. Being able to factor is an important skill for our study of fractions.

a | Factoring Numbers

Looking at the equation $3 \cdot 4 = 12$, we see that 3 and 4 are *factors* of 12. Since $12 = 12 \cdot 1$, we know that 12 and 1 are also factors of 12.

> A number c is a **factor** of the number a if a is divisible by c.
>
> A **factorization** of a number expresses that number as a product of natural numbers.

For example, each of the following gives a factorization of 12.

$12 = 4 \cdot 3$ ⟵ This factorization shows that 4 and 3 are factors of 12.

$12 = 12 \cdot 1$ ⟵ This factorization shows that 12 and 1 are factors of 12.

$12 = 6 \cdot 2$ ⟵ This factorization shows that 6 and 2 are factors of 12.

$12 = 2 \cdot 3 \cdot 2$ ⟵ This factorization shows that 2 and 3 are factors of 12.

This shows that 1, 2, 3, 4, 6, and 12 are all factors of 12. Note that since $n = n \cdot 1$, every number has a factorization, and every number has at least itself and 1 as factors.

Example 1 Find all the factors of 24.

To help us get started, we can use some of the tests for divisibility. For example, since 24 is even, we know that 2 is a factor. Since the sum of the digits in 24 is 6 and 6 is divisible by 3, we know that 3 is a factor. We can use trial and error to determine that 4 is also a factor, but that 5 is not. A list of factorizations can then be used to make a complete list of factors.

Factorizations: $1 \cdot 24$; $2 \cdot 12$; $3 \cdot 8$; $4 \cdot 6$;

Factors: 1, 2, 3, 4, 6, 8, 12, 24

Note that, apart from the number itself, no factor can be more than half the size of the number of which it is a factor.

Do Exercises 1–4.

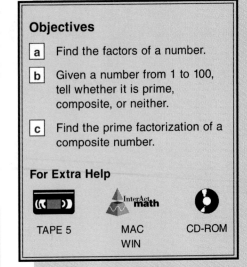

Objectives

a Find the factors of a number.

b Given a number from 1 to 100, tell whether it is prime, composite, or neither.

c Find the prime factorization of a composite number.

For Extra Help

TAPE 5   MAC WIN   CD-ROM

Find all the factors of each number listed. (*Hint*: Find some factorizations of the number.)

1. 6   1, 2, 3, 6

2. 8   1, 2, 4, 8

3. 10   1, 2, 5, 10

4. 32   1, 2, 4, 8, 16, 32

Answers on page A-7

5. Tell whether each number is prime, composite, or neither.

1, 4, 6, 8, 13, 19, 41

13, 19, 41 are prime; 4, 6, 8 are composite; 1 is neither

b | Prime and Composite Numbers

> A natural number that has exactly two different factors, itself and 1, is called a **prime number**.

Example 2 Tell whether the numbers 2, 3, 5, 7, and 11 are prime.

The number 2 is prime. It has only the factors 1 and 2.

The number 5 is prime. It has only the factors 1 and 5.

The numbers 3, 7, and 11 are also prime.

Example 3 Tell whether the numbers 4, 6, 8, 10, 63, and 1 are prime.

The number 4 is not prime. It has the factors 1, 2, and 4.

The numbers 6, 8, 10, and 63 are not prime. Each has factors other than itself and 1. For instance, 2 is a factor of 6, 8, and 10, and 7 is a factor of 63.

The number 1 is not prime. It does not have two *different* factors.

> A natural number, other than 1, that is not prime is called a **composite number**.

In other words, if a number has at least one factor other than itself and 1, it is composite. Thus, from Examples 2 and 3, we see that

2, 3, 5, 7, and 11 are prime;

4, 6, 8, 10, and 63 are composite;

and   1 is neither prime nor composite.

Do Exercise 5.

Below is a list of the prime numbers 2 to 157. The ability to recognize primes will save you time as you progress through this text.

A LIST OF PRIMES (FROM 2 TO 157)

2, 3, 5, 7, 11, 13, 17, 19, 23, 29, 31, 37, 41, 43, 47, 53, 59, 61, 67, 71, 73, 79, 83, 89, 97, 101, 103, 107, 109, 113, 127, 131, 137, 139, 149, 151, 157

Mathematicians continue to search for bigger and bigger primes. Prime numbers can be very useful when encoding messages and programming computers.

Answer on page A-7

It can be useful to note that when two different prime numbers are factors of a number, the product of those primes will also be a factor. For instance, in Example 1, since 2 and 3 are both prime factors of 24, their product, 6, is also a factor.

c Prime Factorizations

To express a composite number as a product of primes is to find a **prime factorization** of the number. To do this, we consider the primes

2, 3, 5, 7, 11, 13, 17, 19, 23, and so on,

and determine whether a given number is divisible by any of them.

Example 4 Find the prime factorization of 39.

a) We check for divisibility by the first prime, 2. Since 39 is not even, 2 is not a factor of 39.

b) Since the sum of the digits in 39 is 12 and 12 is divisible by 3, we know that 39 is divisible by 3. We then perform the division.

$$\begin{array}{r} 13 \\ 3\overline{)39} \end{array}$$ R = 0   A remainder of 0 confirms that 3 is a factor of 39.

Because 13 is a prime, we are finished. The prime factorization is

$$39 = 3 \cdot 13.$$

Example 5 Find the prime factorization of 76.

a) Since 76 is even, it must have the first prime, 2, as a factor.

$$\begin{array}{r} 38 \\ 2\overline{)76} \end{array}$$ We can write 76 = 2 · 38.

b) Because 38 is also even, we see that 76 contains a second factor of 2.

$$\begin{array}{r} 19 \\ 2\overline{)38} \end{array}$$ Note that 38 = 2 · 19, so 76 = 2 · 2 · 19.

Because 19 is prime, the complete factorization is

$$76 = 2 \cdot 2 \cdot 19.$$ All factors are prime.

We abbreviate our procedure as follows.

$$\begin{array}{r} 19 \\ 2\overline{)38} \\ 2\overline{)76} \end{array}$$ ←—— We begin here.

$$76 = 2 \cdot 2 \cdot 19$$

A factorization like $2 \cdot 2 \cdot 19$ can be written as $2^2 \cdot 19$ or $2 \cdot 19 \cdot 2$ or $19 \cdot 2 \cdot 2$ or $19 \cdot 2^2$. In any case, the prime factors are the same. For this reason, we agree that any of these may be considered "the" prime factorization of 76.

> Each composite number has just one (unique) prime factorization.

Find the prime factorization of
each number.

6. 6   2 · 3

7. 12   2 · 2 · 3

8. 45   3 · 3 · 5

9. 98   2 · 7 · 7

10. 126   2 · 3 · 3 · 7

11. 144   2 · 2 · 2 · 2 · 3 · 3

Answers on page A-7

Example 6   Find the prime factorization of 72.

$$
\begin{array}{r}
3 \\
3)\overline{9} \\
2)\overline{18} \\
2)\overline{36} \\
2)\overline{72} \leftarrow \text{ Begin here.}
\end{array}
$$

$$72 = 2 \cdot 2 \cdot 2 \cdot 3 \cdot 3$$

Another way to find a prime factorization is by using a **factor tree** as
follows:

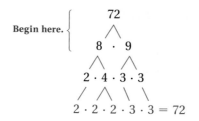

Had we begun with 2 · 36, 3 · 24,
4 · 18, or 6 · 12, the same prime
factorization would result.

Example 7   Find the prime factorization of 189.

We can use a string of successive divisions.

$$
\begin{array}{r}
7 \\
3)\overline{\ 21} \\
3)\overline{\ 63} \\
3)\overline{189}
\end{array}
$$
Since 189 is odd, 2 will not be a factor. We begin with 3.

$$189 = 3 \cdot 3 \cdot 3 \cdot 7$$

We can also use a factor tree.

$$
\begin{array}{c}
189 \\
\wedge \\
3 \cdot 63 \\
/ \quad \wedge \\
3 \cdot 7 \cdot 9 \\
/ \ / \quad \wedge \\
3 \cdot 7 \cdot 3 \cdot 3 = 189
\end{array}
$$

Example 8   Find the prime factorization of 65.

We can use a string of successive divisions.

$$
\begin{array}{r}
13 \\
5)\overline{65}
\end{array}
$$
65 is not divisible by 2 or 3 but *is* divisible by 5.

$$65 = 5 \cdot 13$$

We can also use a factor tree.

$$
\begin{array}{c}
65 \\
\wedge \\
5 \cdot 13 = 65
\end{array}
$$

Do Exercises 6–11.

Exercise Set 3.2

a Find all the factors of each number.

1. 18
1, 2, 3, 6, 9, 18

2. 16
1, 2, 4, 8, 16

3. 54
1, 2, 3, 6, 9, 18, 27, 54

4. 48
1, 2, 3, 4, 6, 8, 12, 16, 24, 48

5. 4
1, 2, 4

6. 9
1, 3, 9

7. 7
1, 7

8. 11
1, 11

9. 1
1

10. 3
1, 3

11. 98
1, 2, 7, 14, 49, 98

12. 100
1, 2, 4, 5, 10, 20, 25, 50, 100

13. 42
1, 2, 3, 6, 7, 14, 21, 42

14. 105
1, 3, 5, 7, 15, 21, 35, 105

15. 385
1, 5, 7, 11, 35, 55, 77, 385

16. 110
1, 2, 5, 10, 11, 22, 55, 110

17. 36
1, 2, 3, 4, 6, 9, 12, 18, 36

18. 196
1, 2, 4, 7, 14, 28, 49, 98, 196

19. 225
1, 3, 5, 9, 15, 25, 45, 75, 225

20. 441
1, 3, 7, 9, 21, 49, 63, 147, 441

b State whether each number is prime, composite, or neither.

21. 17   Prime

22. 24   Composite

23. 22   Composite

24. 31   Prime

25. 48   Composite

26. 43   Prime

27. 31   Prime

28. 54   Composite

29. 1   Neither

30. 2   Prime

31. 9   Composite

32. 19   Prime

33. 47   Prime

34. 27   Composite

35. 29   Prime

36. 49   Composite

c Find the prime factorization of each number.

37. 16 $2 \cdot 2 \cdot 2 \cdot 2$

38. 8 $2 \cdot 2 \cdot 2$

39. 14 $2 \cdot 7$

40. 15 $3 \cdot 5$

41. 22 $2 \cdot 11$

42. 32 $2 \cdot 2 \cdot 2 \cdot 2 \cdot 2$

43. 25 $5 \cdot 5$

44. 40 $2 \cdot 2 \cdot 2 \cdot 5$

45. 62 $2 \cdot 31$

46. 169 $13 \cdot 13$

47. 140 $2 \cdot 2 \cdot 5 \cdot 7$

48. 50 $2 \cdot 5 \cdot 5$

49. 100 $2 \cdot 2 \cdot 5 \cdot 5$ **50.** 110 $2 \cdot 5 \cdot 11$ **51.** 35 $5 \cdot 7$ **52.** 70 $2 \cdot 5 \cdot 7$

53. 78 $2 \cdot 3 \cdot 13$ **54.** 86 $2 \cdot 43$ **55.** 77 $7 \cdot 11$ **56.** 99 $3 \cdot 3 \cdot 11$

57. 112 $2 \cdot 2 \cdot 2 \cdot 2 \cdot 7$ **58.** 142 $2 \cdot 71$ **59.** 300 $2 \cdot 2 \cdot 3 \cdot 5 \cdot 5$ **60.** 175 $5 \cdot 5 \cdot 7$

76. A rectangular array of 6 rows of 9 objects each, or 9 rows of 6 objects each
77. Answers may vary. One arrangement is a three-dimensional rectangular array consisting of 2 tiers of 12 objects each, where each tier consists of a rectangular array of 4 rows with 3 objects each.

Skill Maintenance

Multiply.

61. $-2 \cdot 13$ [2.4a] -26

62. $(-8)(-32)$ [2.4a]   256

Add.

63. $-17 + 25$ [2.2a]   8

64. $-9 + (-14)$ [2.2a] -23

Divide.

65. $0 \div 22$ [2.5a]   0

66. $22 \div 22$ [1.6c]   1

Synthesis

67. ◈ Explain a method for constructing a composite number that contains exactly two factors other than itself and 1.

68. ◈ Are the divisibility tests of Section 3.1 useful for finding prime factorizations? Why or why not?

69. ◈ If a and b are both factors of c, does it follow that $a \cdot b$ is also a factor of c? Why or why not?

Find the prime factorization of each number.

70. 🖩 473,073,361 $23 \cdot 31 \cdot 61 \cdot 73 \cdot 149$ **71.** 🖩 28,502,923 $53 \cdot 53 \cdot 73 \cdot 139$ **72.** 7800 $2 \cdot 2 \cdot 2 \cdot 3 \cdot 5 \cdot 5 \cdot 13$

73. 2520 $2 \cdot 2 \cdot 2 \cdot 3 \cdot 3 \cdot 5 \cdot 7$ **74.** 2772 $2 \cdot 2 \cdot 3 \cdot 3 \cdot 7 \cdot 11$ **75.** 1998 $2 \cdot 3 \cdot 3 \cdot 3 \cdot 37$

76. Describe an arrangement of 54 objects that corresponds to the factorization $54 = 6 \times 9$.

77. Describe an arrangement of 24 objects that corresponds to the factorization $24 = 2 \cdot 3 \cdot 4$.

78. Two numbers are **relatively prime** if there is no prime number that is a factor of both numbers. For example, 10 and 21 are relatively prime but 15 and 18 are not. List five pairs of composite numbers that are relatively prime.
Answers may vary

Collaborative
Learning Manual

Find all the prime numbers less than 100, using the Sieve of Eratosthenes.

3.3 Fractions

The study of arithmetic begins with the set of whole numbers

0, 1, 2, 3, 4, 5, 6, 7, 8, 9, 10, 11, and so on.

The need soon arises for fractional parts of numbers such as halves, thirds, fourths, and so on. Here are some examples:

$\frac{1}{25}$ of the parking spaces in a commercial area in Indiana must be marked for the handicapped.

For $\frac{9}{10}$ of the people in the United States, English is the primary language.

$\frac{1}{11}$ of all women develop breast cancer at some point in their life.

$\frac{43}{200}$ of the world's population is in China.

a | Identifying Numerators and Denominators

The following are some additional examples of fractions:

$$\frac{1}{2}, \quad \frac{13}{41}, \quad \frac{-8}{5}, \quad \frac{x}{y}, \quad -\frac{4}{25}, \quad \frac{2a}{7b}.$$

This way of writing number names is called **fractional notation.** The top number is called the **numerator** and the bottom number is called the **denominator**.

Example 1 Identify the numerator and the denominator.

$$\frac{7}{8} \begin{array}{l} \leftarrow \textbf{Numerator} \\ \leftarrow \textbf{Denominator} \end{array}$$

Do Exercises 1–3.

b | Fractions and the Real World

Example 2 What part is shaded?

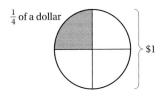

$\frac{1}{4}$ of a dollar

$1

When an object is divided into 4 parts of the same size, each of these parts is $\frac{1}{4}$ of the object. Thus, $\frac{1}{4}$ (*one-fourth* or *one-quarter*) of a dollar is shaded.

Do Exercises 4–7.

Objectives

| a | Identify the numerator and the denominator of a fraction. |

| b | Write fractional notation for part of an object or part of a set of objects. |

| c | Simplify fractional notation like n/n to 1, $0/n$ to 0, and $n/1$ to n. |

For Extra Help

| TAPE 5 | MAC WIN | CD-ROM |

Identify the numerator and the denominator of each fraction.

1. $\frac{5}{7}$ 2. $\frac{5a}{7b}$ 3. $\frac{-22}{3}$

5, numerator; 7, denominator   5a, numerator; 7b, denominator   −22, numerator; 3; denominator

What part is shaded?

4.

$1

$\$\frac{1}{2}$

5.   1 mile

$\frac{1}{3}$ mi

6.

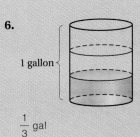

1 gallon

$\frac{1}{3}$ gal

7.

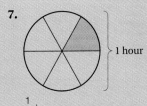

1 hour

$\frac{1}{6}$ hr

Answers on page A-7

What amount is shaded?

8.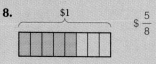

$\frac{5}{8}$

9.

1 mile

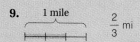

$\frac{2}{3}$ mi

10.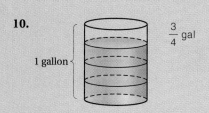

1 gallon

$\frac{3}{4}$ gal

11.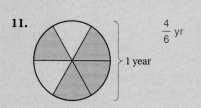

1 year

$\frac{4}{6}$ yr

What amount is shaded?

12. 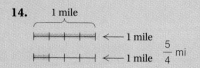 ← 1 mile

← 1 mile

$\frac{4}{3}$ mi

13.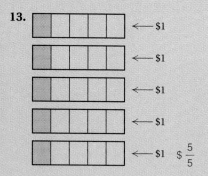

← $1

← $1

← $1

← $1

← $1 $\frac{5}{5}$

14.

1 mile

← 1 mile

← 1 mile

$\frac{5}{4}$ mi

Answers on page A-7

Chapter 3   Fractions:
Multiplication & Division

160

The diagram on the preceding page is an example of a *circle graph,* or *pie chart.* Circle graphs are often used to illustrate the relationships of fractional parts of a whole. The following graph shows color preferences of bicycles as determined by the Bicycle Market Research Institute.

Bicycle Color Preferences

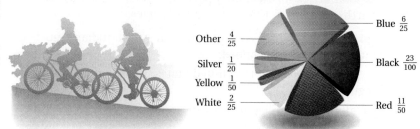

Other $\frac{4}{25}$

Silver $\frac{1}{20}$

Yellow $\frac{1}{50}$

White $\frac{2}{25}$

Blue $\frac{6}{25}$

Black $\frac{23}{100}$

Red $\frac{11}{50}$

Source: Bicycle Market Research Institute

Example 3   What amount is shaded?

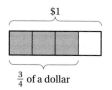

$1

$\frac{3}{4}$ of a dollar

The object is divided into 4 parts of the same size, and 3 of them are shaded. This is $3 \cdot \frac{1}{4}$, or $\frac{3}{4}$. Thus, $\frac{3}{4}$ (*three-fourths* or *three-quarters*) of a dollar is shaded.

Do Exercises 8–11.

The fraction $\frac{3}{4}$ corresponds to another situation. We take 3 objects, divide them into fourths, and take $\frac{1}{4}$ of the entire amount (which appears now as $\frac{12}{4}$). This is $\frac{1}{4} \cdot 3$, or $\frac{3}{4}$, or $3 \div 4$.

Example 4   What amount is shaded?

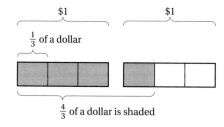

$1 $1

$\frac{1}{3}$ of a dollar

$\frac{4}{3}$ of a dollar is shaded

The objects are divided into 3 equally sized parts each, and 4 of these parts are shaded. We have more than one whole object. In this case, it is $4 \cdot \frac{1}{3}$, or $\frac{4}{3}$ of a dollar.

Do Exercises 12–15 on this page and the next.

Fractional notation also corresponds to situations involving part of a set.

Example 5 What part of this set, or collection, of workers is women?

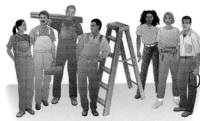

4 carpenters   3 electricians

There are 7 workers, and 3 are women. We say that three-sevenths, or $\frac{3}{7}$, of the workers are women.

Do Exercises 16–18.

c | Some Fractional Notation for Integers

Fractional Notation for 1

The number 1 corresponds to situations like the following.

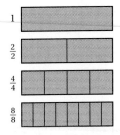

If we divide an object into n parts and take n of them, we get all of the object (1 whole object). Since a negative divided by a negative is a positive, the following is stated for *all* nonzero integers.

> $\frac{n}{n} = 1$,   for any integer n that is not 0.

Example 6 Simplify: a) $\frac{5}{5}$; b) $\frac{-9}{-9}$; c) $\frac{17x}{17x}$ (assume $x \neq 0$).

a) $\frac{5}{5} = 1$ b) $\frac{-9}{-9} = 1$ c) $\frac{17x}{17x} = 1$

Do Exercises 19–24.

15.

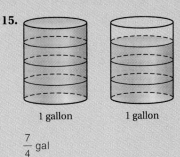

1 gallon   1 gallon

$\frac{7}{4}$ gal

16. Referring to Example 5, what part of the set of workers has dark hair?

$\frac{4}{7}$

17. What part of this set of shapes is shaded?

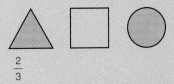

$\frac{2}{3}$

18. What part of this set were elected United States president? are recording stars?

Abraham Lincoln
Whitney Houston
Garth Brooks $\frac{2}{6}, \frac{4}{6}$
Bill Clinton
Sheryl Crow
Gloria Estefan

Simplify. Assume that $a \neq 0$.

19. $\frac{7}{7}$ 1   20. $\frac{a}{a}$ 1

21. $\frac{-34}{-34}$ 1   22. $\frac{1}{1}$ 1

23. $\frac{-2347}{-2347}$ 1   24. $\frac{54a}{54a}$ 1

Answers on page A-7

Simplify, if possible. Assume that $x \neq 0$.

25. $\dfrac{0}{2}$ 0   **26.** $\dfrac{0}{-8}$ 0

27. $\dfrac{0}{7x}$ 0   **28.** $\dfrac{4-4}{236}$ 0

29. $\dfrac{7}{0}$ **30.** $\dfrac{-4}{0}$

Undefined   Undefined

Simplify.

31. $\dfrac{8}{1}$ 8   **32.** $\dfrac{-10}{1}$ -10

33. $\dfrac{-346}{1}$ -346 **34.** $\dfrac{24-1}{23}$ 1

Answers on page A-7

Fractional Notation for 0

Consider $\frac{0}{4}$. This corresponds to dividing an object into 4 parts and taking none of them. We get 0. This result also extends to all nonzero integers.

> $\dfrac{0}{n} = 0,$ for any integer n that is not 0.

Example 7   Simplify: **a)** $\dfrac{0}{9}$;   **b)** $\dfrac{0}{1}$;   **c)** $\dfrac{0}{5a}$ (assume $a \neq 0$);   **d)** $\dfrac{0}{-23}$.

a) $\dfrac{0}{9} = 0$ **b)** $\dfrac{0}{1} = 0$

c) $\dfrac{0}{5a} = 0$ **d)** $\dfrac{0}{-23} = 0$

Fractional notation with a denominator of 0, such as $n/0$, is meaningless because we cannot speak of an object as divided into *zero* parts. (If it is not divided at all, then we say that it is undivided and remains in one part.)

> $\dfrac{n}{0}$ is not defined.
>
> $\left(\text{When asked to simplify } \dfrac{n}{0}, \text{ we write } \textit{undefined.}\right)$

Do Exercises 25–30.

Other Integers

Consider $\frac{4}{1}$. This corresponds to taking 4 objects and dividing each into 1 part. (We do not divide them.) We have 4 objects.

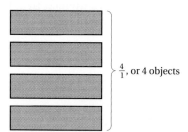

$\frac{4}{1}$, or 4 objects

> Any integer divided by 1 is the original integer. That is,
>
> $\dfrac{n}{1} = n,$ for any integer n.

Example 8   Simplify: **a)** $\dfrac{2}{1}$;   **b)** $\dfrac{-9}{1}$;   **c)** $\dfrac{3x}{1}$.

a) $\dfrac{2}{1} = 2$ **b)** $\dfrac{-9}{1} = -9$ **c)** $\dfrac{3x}{1} = 3x$

Do Exercises 31–34.

Exercise Set 3.3

a Identify the numerator and the denominator of each fraction.

1. $\dfrac{3}{4}$

3, numerator;
4, denominator

2. $\dfrac{-9}{10}$

−9, numerator;
10, denominator

3. $\dfrac{7}{-9}$

7, numerator;
−9, denominator

4. $\dfrac{15}{8}$

15, numerator;
8, denominator

5. $\dfrac{2x}{3z}$

2x, numerator;
3z, denominator

6. $\dfrac{9a}{2b}$

9a, numerator;
2b, denominator

b For each figure, what amount is shaded?

7. $1

$\$\dfrac{3}{4}$

8. $1

$\$\dfrac{1}{5}$

9. 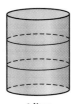 1 mile
1 mile

$\dfrac{2}{8}$ mi

10. 1 candy bar
1 candy bar
1 candy bar

$\dfrac{3}{8}$ candy bar

11. 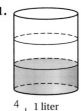 1 liter   1 liter

$\dfrac{4}{3}$ L

12. 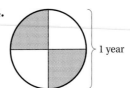 1 gold bar
1 gold bar

$\dfrac{11}{8}$ gold bar

13.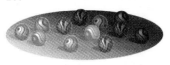

$\dfrac{3}{4}$ acre

1 acre

14.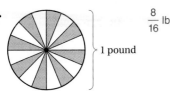

$\dfrac{2}{4}$ yr

1 year

15.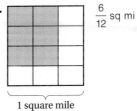

$\dfrac{8}{16}$ lb

1 pound

16.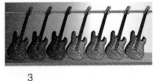

$\dfrac{6}{12}$ sq mi

1 square mile

What fractional part of each set is shaded?

17.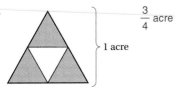

$\dfrac{5}{12}$

18.

$\dfrac{7}{10}$

19.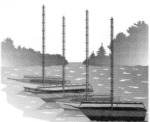

$\dfrac{1}{4}$

20.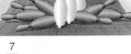

$\dfrac{3}{7}$

| c | Simplify, if possible. Assume that all variables are nonzero. |

21. $\dfrac{0}{17}$ 0

22. $\dfrac{19}{19}$ 1

23. $\dfrac{15}{1}$ 15

24. $\dfrac{10}{1}$ 10

25. $\dfrac{20}{20}$ 1

26. $\dfrac{-20}{1}$ -20

27. $\dfrac{-14}{-14}$ 1

28. $\dfrac{4a}{1}$ $4a$

29. $\dfrac{0}{-234}$ 0

30. $\dfrac{37a}{37a}$ 1

31. $\dfrac{3n}{3n}$ 1

32. $\dfrac{0}{-1}$ 0

33. $\dfrac{9x}{9x}$ 1

34. $\dfrac{-12a}{1}$ $-12a$

35. $\dfrac{-63}{1}$ -63

36. $\dfrac{-3x}{-3x}$ 1

37. $\dfrac{0}{2a}$ 0

38. $\dfrac{0}{8}$ 0

39. $\dfrac{52}{0}$ Undefined

40. $\dfrac{8-8}{1247}$ 0

41. $\dfrac{7n}{1}$ $7n$

42. $\dfrac{247}{0}$ Undefined

43. $\dfrac{6}{7-7}$ Undefined

44. $\dfrac{15}{9-9}$ Undefined

Skill Maintenance

Multiply.

45. $-7(30)$ [2.4a] -210

46. $23 \cdot (-14)$ [2.4a] -322

47. $(-71)(-12)0$ [2.4b] 0

48. $32(-29)0$ [2.4b] 0

49. Recently, the average annual income of people living in Connecticut was $30,303 per person. In Mississippi, the average annual income was $16,531. How much more do people in Connecticut make, on average, than those living in Mississippi? [1.8a]

$13,772

50. Sandy can type 62 words per minute. How long will it take Sandy to type 12,462 words? [1.8a] 201 min

---

Synthesis

51. ◆ Explain in your own words why $n/1 = n$, for any integer n.

52. ◆ Explain in your own words why $0/n = 0$, for any nonzero integer n.

53. ◆ Explain in your own words why $n/n = 1$, for any nonzero integer n.

54. The surface of Earth is 3 parts water and 1 part land. What fractional part of Earth is water? land?

55. The year 1999 began on a Friday. What fractional part of 1999 were Mondays? $\dfrac{52}{365}$

56. Rayona earned $2700 one summer. During the following semester, she spent $1200 for tuition, $540 for rent, and $360 for food. The rest went for miscellaneous expenses. What part of the income went for tuition? rent? food? miscellaneous expenses? $\dfrac{1200}{2700}, \dfrac{540}{2700}, \dfrac{360}{2700}, \dfrac{600}{2700}$

57. A couple had 3 sons, each of whom had 3 daughters. If each daughter gave birth to 3 sons, what fractional part of the couple's descendants is female? $\dfrac{9}{39}$

54. $\dfrac{3}{4}, \dfrac{1}{4}$

3.4 Multiplication

a Multiplication by an Integer

We can find $3 \cdot \frac{1}{4}$ by thinking of repeated addition. We add three $\frac{1}{4}$'s.

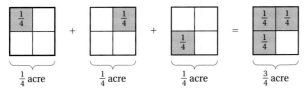

$$\frac{1}{4} \text{ acre} \qquad \frac{1}{4} \text{ acre} \qquad \frac{1}{4} \text{ acre} \qquad \frac{3}{4} \text{ acre}$$

We see that $3 \cdot \frac{1}{4} = \frac{1}{4} + \frac{1}{4} + \frac{1}{4} = \frac{3}{4}$.

Do Exercises 1 and 2.

To multiply a fraction by an integer,

a) multiply the top number (the numerator) by the integer and

$$6 \cdot \frac{4}{5} = \frac{6 \cdot 4}{5} = \frac{24}{5}$$

b) keep the same denominator.

Examples Multiply.

1. $5 \times \frac{3}{8} = \frac{5 \times 3}{8} = \frac{15}{8}$

> Skip this step when you feel comfortable doing so.

2. $\frac{2}{5} \cdot 13 = \frac{2 \cdot 13}{5} = \frac{26}{5}$

3. $-10 \cdot \frac{1}{3} = \frac{-10}{3}$, or $-\frac{10}{3}$ Recall that $\frac{-a}{b} = -\frac{a}{b}$.

4. $a \cdot \frac{4}{7} = \frac{4a}{7}$ Recall that $a \cdot 4 = 4 \cdot a$.

Do Exercises 3–6.

b Multiplication Using Fractional Notation

We find a product such as $\frac{9}{7} \cdot \frac{3}{4}$ as follows. An explanation appears on the next page.

To multiply a fraction by a fraction,

a) multiply the numerators and

$$\frac{9}{7} \cdot \frac{3}{4} = \frac{9 \cdot 3}{7 \cdot 4} = \frac{27}{28}$$

b) multiply the denominators.

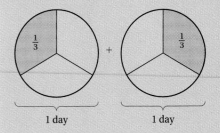
1. Find $2 \cdot \frac{1}{3}$. $\frac{2}{3}$

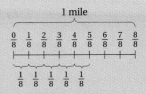

$$\frac{1}{3} \qquad + \qquad \frac{1}{3}$$

1 day   1 day

2. Find $5 \cdot \frac{1}{8}$. $\frac{5}{8}$

1 mile

$$\frac{0}{8} \quad \frac{1}{8} \quad \frac{2}{8} \quad \frac{3}{8} \quad \frac{4}{8} \quad \frac{5}{8} \quad \frac{6}{8} \quad \frac{7}{8} \quad \frac{8}{8}$$

$$\frac{1}{8} \quad \frac{1}{8} \quad \frac{1}{8} \quad \frac{1}{8} \quad \frac{1}{8}$$

Multiply.

3. $5 \times \frac{2}{3}$ $\frac{10}{3}$

4. $(-11) \times \frac{3}{8}$ $-\frac{33}{8}$ or $\frac{-33}{8}$

5. $23 \cdot \frac{2}{5}$ $\frac{46}{5}$

6. $x \cdot \frac{4}{9}$ $\frac{4x}{9}$

Answers on page A-7

Multiply.

7. $\dfrac{3}{8} \cdot \dfrac{5}{7}$ $\dfrac{15}{56}$

8. $\dfrac{4}{3} \times \dfrac{8}{5}$ $\dfrac{32}{15}$

9. $\left(-\dfrac{3}{10}\right)\left(-\dfrac{1}{10}\right)$ $\dfrac{3}{100}$

10. $(-7)\dfrac{a}{b}$ $-\dfrac{7a}{b}$ or $\dfrac{-7a}{b}$

11. Draw diagrams like those in the text to show how the multiplication $\frac{4}{5} \cdot \frac{1}{3}$ corresponds to a real-world situation.

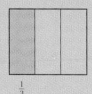

$\frac{1}{3}$

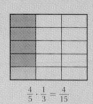

$\frac{4}{5} \cdot \frac{1}{3} = \frac{4}{15}$

Answers on page A-7

Examples Multiply.

5. $\dfrac{5}{6} \times \dfrac{7}{4} = \underbrace{\dfrac{5 \times 7}{6 \times 4}}_{} = \dfrac{35}{24}$

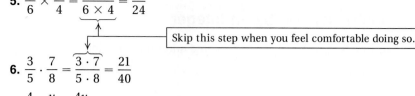

Skip this step when you feel comfortable doing so.

6. $\dfrac{3}{5} \cdot \dfrac{7}{8} = \overbrace{\dfrac{3 \cdot 7}{5 \cdot 8}} = \dfrac{21}{40}$

7. $\dfrac{4}{x} \cdot \dfrac{y}{9} = \dfrac{4y}{9x}$

8. $(-6)\left(-\dfrac{4}{5}\right) = \dfrac{-6}{1} \cdot \dfrac{-4}{5} = \dfrac{24}{5}$ Recall that $\dfrac{n}{1} = n$.

Do Exercises 7–10.

Unless one of the factors is a whole number, multiplication of fractions is hard to imagine as repeated addition. To see how multiplication of fractions corresponds to situations in the real world, consider the expressions

$$\dfrac{2}{5} \cdot \dfrac{3}{4} \quad \text{and} \quad \dfrac{2}{3} \ of \ \dfrac{3}{4}.$$

Imagine some object and take $\frac{3}{4}$ of it. We divide it into 4 parts and take 3 of them. That is shown in the shading below.

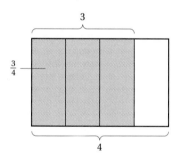

Next, we take $\frac{2}{5}$ of the result. We divide the shaded part into 5 parts and take 2 of them. That is shown below as the heavily shaded region.

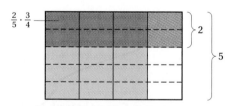

The entire object has been divided into 20 parts, of which 6 have been shaded heavily:

$$\dfrac{2}{5} \cdot \dfrac{3}{4} = \dfrac{2 \cdot 3}{5 \cdot 4} = \dfrac{6}{20}.$$

The figure above shows a rectangular array inside a rectangular array. The number of pieces in the entire array is $5 \cdot 4$ (the product of the denominators). The number of pieces shaded heavily is $2 \cdot 3$ (the product of the numerators). For the answer, we take 6 pieces out of a set of 20 to get $\frac{6}{20}$. We have shown that $\frac{2}{5} \ of \ \frac{3}{4}$ corresponds to the multiplication $\frac{2}{5} \cdot \frac{3}{4}$.

Do Exercise 11.

c | Applications and Problem Solving

Most problems that can be solved by multiplying fractions can be thought of in terms of rectangular arrays.

Example 9 A rancher owns a square mile of land. He gives $\frac{4}{5}$ of it to his daughter and she gives $\frac{2}{3}$ of her share to her son. How much land goes to the daughter's son?

1. **Familiarize.** We first make a drawing to help solve the problem. The land may not be square. It could be in a shape like A or B below, or it could even be in more than one piece. But to think about the problem, we can visualize a square, as shown by shape C.

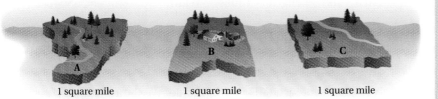

A   B   C

1 square mile   1 square mile   1 square mile

The daughter gets $\frac{4}{5}$ of the land. We shade $\frac{4}{5}$.

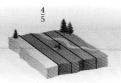

Her son gets $\frac{2}{3}$ of her part. We "raise" that.

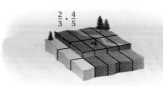

2. **Translate.** We let $n =$ the part of the land that goes to the daughter's son. We are taking "two-thirds of four-fifths." The word "of" corresponds to multiplication. Thus the following multiplication sentence corresponds to the situation:

$$\frac{2}{3} \cdot \frac{4}{5} = n.$$

3. **Solve.** The number sentence tells us what to do. We have

$$\frac{2}{3} \cdot \frac{4}{5} = n, \quad \text{or} \quad \frac{8}{15} = n.$$

4. **Check.** We can check this in the figure above, where we see that 8 of 15 equally sized parts will go to the daughter's son.

5. **State.** The daughter's son gets $\frac{8}{15}$ of a square mile of land.

Do Exercise 12.

12. A seaside hotel uses $\frac{3}{4}$ of its extra land for recreational purposes. Of that, $\frac{1}{2}$ is used for swimming pools. What part of the extra land is used for swimming pools?

$\frac{3}{8}$

Answer on page A-7

13. The length of a button on a fax machine is $\frac{9}{10}$ cm. The width is $\frac{7}{10}$ cm. What is the area?

$\frac{63}{100}$ cm²

14. Of the students at Overton Community College, $\frac{1}{8}$ participate in sports and $\frac{3}{5}$ of these play soccer. What fractional part of the student body plays soccer?

$\frac{3}{40}$

We have seen that the area of a rectangular region is found by multiplying length by width. That is true whether length and width are whole numbers or not. Remember, the area of a rectangular region is given by the formula

$$A = l \cdot w \qquad (Area = length \cdot width).$$

Example 10   The length of a rectangular key on a calculator is $\frac{7}{10}$ cm. The width is $\frac{3}{10}$ cm. What is the area?

1. **Familiarize.** Recall that area is length times width. We make a drawing, letting $A =$ the area of the calculator key.

2. **Translate.** Next, we translate.

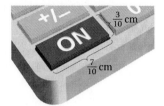

$\frac{3}{10}$ cm

$\frac{7}{10}$ cm

Area	is	Length	times	Width
A	$=$	$\frac{7}{10}$	$\times$	$\frac{3}{10}$

3. **Solve.** The sentence tells us what to do. We multiply:

$$\frac{7}{10} \cdot \frac{3}{10} = \frac{7 \cdot 3}{10 \cdot 10} = \frac{21}{100}.$$

4. **Check.** To check, we can repeat the calculation or draw a grid, as in Example 9. This is left to the student.

5. **State.** The area of the key is $\frac{21}{100}$ cm².

Do Exercise 13.

Example 11   A cornbread recipe calls for $\frac{3}{4}$ cup of cornmeal. A chef is making $\frac{1}{2}$ of the recipe. How much cornmeal will the chef need?

1. **Familiarize.** We make a drawing or at least visualize the situation. We let $n =$ the number of cups of cornmeal the chef will need.

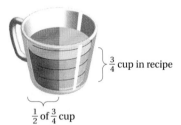

$\frac{3}{4}$ cup in recipe

$\frac{1}{2}$ of $\frac{3}{4}$ cup

2. **Translate.** The multiplication sentence $\frac{1}{2} \cdot \frac{3}{4} = n$ corresponds to the situation.

3. **Solve.** We carry out the multiplication:

$$\frac{1}{2} \cdot \frac{3}{4} = \frac{1 \cdot 3}{2 \cdot 4} = \frac{3}{8}.$$

4. **Check.** To check, we can determine what fractional part of the drawing has been heavily shaded. This is left to the student.

5. **State.** The chef will need $\frac{3}{8}$ cup of cornmeal.

Do Exercise 14.

Exercise Set 3.4

a Multiply.

1. $3 \cdot \dfrac{1}{7}$ $\dfrac{3}{7}$

2. $2 \cdot \dfrac{1}{5}$ $\dfrac{2}{5}$

3. $(-5) \times \dfrac{1}{6}$

    $\dfrac{-5}{6}$ or $-\dfrac{5}{6}$

4. $(-4) \times \dfrac{1}{7}$

    $\dfrac{-4}{7}$ or $-\dfrac{4}{7}$

5. $\dfrac{2}{3} \cdot 7$ $\dfrac{14}{3}$

6. $\dfrac{2}{5} \cdot 6$ $\dfrac{12}{5}$

7. $(-1)\dfrac{7}{9}$

    $-\dfrac{7}{9}$ or $\dfrac{-7}{9}$

8. $(-1)\dfrac{4}{11}$

    $\dfrac{-4}{11}$ or $-\dfrac{4}{11}$

9. $\dfrac{2}{5} \cdot x$ $\dfrac{2x}{5}$

10. $\dfrac{3}{8} \cdot y$ $\dfrac{3y}{8}$

11. $\dfrac{2}{5}(-3)$ $\dfrac{-6}{5}$

12. $\dfrac{3}{5}(-4)$

    $\dfrac{-12}{5}$ or $-\dfrac{12}{5}$

13. $a \cdot \dfrac{3}{4}$ $\dfrac{3a}{4}$

14. $b \cdot \dfrac{2}{5}$ $\dfrac{2b}{5}$

15. $17 \times \dfrac{m}{6}$ $\dfrac{17m}{6}$

16. $\dfrac{n}{7} \cdot 40$ $\dfrac{40n}{7}$

17. $-3 \cdot \dfrac{-2}{5}$ $\dfrac{6}{5}$

18. $-4 \cdot \dfrac{-5}{7}$ $\dfrac{20}{7}$

19. $-\dfrac{2}{7}(-x)$ $\dfrac{2x}{7}$

20. $-\dfrac{3}{4}(-a)$ $\dfrac{3a}{4}$

b Multiply.

21. $\dfrac{1}{2} \cdot \dfrac{1}{5}$

    $\dfrac{1}{10}$

22. $\dfrac{1}{4} \cdot \dfrac{1}{3}$

    $\dfrac{1}{12}$

23. $\left(-\dfrac{1}{4}\right) \times \dfrac{1}{10}$

    $\dfrac{-1}{40}$ or $-\dfrac{1}{40}$

24. $\left(-\dfrac{1}{3}\right) \times \dfrac{1}{10}$

    $\dfrac{-1}{30}$ or $-\dfrac{1}{30}$

25. $\dfrac{2}{3} \times \dfrac{1}{5}$

    $\dfrac{2}{15}$

26. $\dfrac{3}{5} \times \dfrac{1}{5}$

    $\dfrac{3}{25}$

27. $\dfrac{2}{y} \cdot \dfrac{x}{5}$

    $\dfrac{2x}{5y}$

28. $\left(-\dfrac{3}{4}\right)\left(-\dfrac{3}{5}\right)$

    $\dfrac{9}{20}$

29. $\left(-\dfrac{3}{4}\right)\left(-\dfrac{3}{4}\right)$

    $\dfrac{9}{16}$

30. $\dfrac{3}{b} \cdot \dfrac{a}{7}$

    $\dfrac{3a}{7b}$

31. $\dfrac{2}{3} \cdot \dfrac{7}{13}$

    $\dfrac{14}{39}$

32. $\dfrac{3}{11} \cdot \dfrac{4}{5}$

    $\dfrac{12}{55}$

33. $\dfrac{1}{10}\left(\dfrac{-3}{5}\right)$

    $\dfrac{-3}{50}$ or $-\dfrac{3}{50}$

34. $\dfrac{3}{10}\left(\dfrac{-7}{5}\right)$

    $\dfrac{-21}{50}$ or $-\dfrac{21}{50}$

35. $\dfrac{7}{8} \cdot \dfrac{a}{8}$

    $\dfrac{7a}{64}$

36. $\dfrac{4}{5} \cdot \dfrac{4}{b}$

    $\dfrac{16}{5b}$

37. $\dfrac{1}{y} \cdot \dfrac{1}{100}$

    $\dfrac{1}{100y}$

38. $\dfrac{x}{10} \cdot \dfrac{7}{100}$

    $\dfrac{7x}{1000}$

39. $\dfrac{-14}{15} \cdot \dfrac{13}{19}$

    $\dfrac{-182}{285}$ or $-\dfrac{182}{285}$

40. $\dfrac{-12}{13} \cdot \dfrac{12}{13}$

    $\dfrac{-144}{169}$ or $-\dfrac{144}{169}$

41. A rectangular table top measures $\frac{4}{5}$ m long by $\frac{3}{5}$ m wide. What is its area?

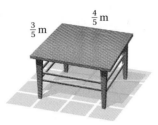

$\frac{4}{5}$ m

$\frac{3}{5}$ m

$\frac{12}{25}$ m^2

42. If each slice of pie is $\frac{1}{6}$ of a pie, how much of the pie is $\frac{1}{2}$ of a slice?

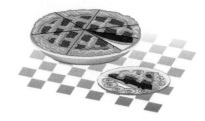

$\frac{1}{12}$

43. *Forestry.* A chain saw holds $\frac{1}{5}$ gal of fuel. Chain-saw fuel is $\frac{1}{16}$ two-cycle oil and $\frac{15}{16}$ unleaded gasoline. How much two-cycle oil is in a freshly filled chain saw? $\frac{1}{80}$ gal

44. *Football.* One of 39 high school football players plays college football. One of 39 college players plays professional football. What fraction of the number of high school players plays professional football? $\frac{1}{1521}$

45. *Cooking.* A recipe for a batch of granola calls for $\frac{2}{3}$ cup of molasses. How much molasses is needed to make $\frac{3}{4}$ of a batch? $\frac{6}{12}$ cup

46. *Sewing.* It takes $\frac{2}{3}$ yd of ribbon to make a decorative bow. How much ribbon is needed for 4 bows? $\frac{8}{3}$ yd

47. *Municipal Waste.* Of every 3 tons of municipal waste, 2 tons is dumped in landfills. Of the municipal waste that goes into landfills, $\frac{1}{10}$ is yard trimmings. What fractional part of municipal waste is trimmings that are landfilled?

$\frac{2}{30}$

48. *Muncipal Waste.* Of every 3 tons of municipal waste, 1 ton is paper and paperboard. If $\frac{2}{3}$ of all municipal waste is landfilled, what fractional part of municipal waste is paper and paperboard that is landfilled?

$\frac{2}{9}$

Skill Maintenance

Simplify.

49. $5 - 3^2$ [2.5b] -4

50. $(5 - 3)^2$ [1.9c] 4

51. $8 \cdot 12 - (7 + 13)$ [1.9c] 76

52. $8 \cdot 12 - 7 + 13$ [1.9c] 102

53. What does the digit 6 mean in 4,678,952? [1.1e]

6 hundred thousands

54. What does the digit 4 mean in 4,678,952? [1.1e]

4 millions

Synthesis

55. ◈ Following Example 8, we explained, using words and pictures, why $\frac{2}{5} \cdot \frac{3}{4}$ equals $\frac{6}{20}$. Present a similar explanation of why $\frac{2}{3} \cdot \frac{4}{7}$ equals $\frac{8}{21}$.

56. ◈ Write a problem for a classmate to solve. Design the problem so that the solution is "About $\frac{1}{30}$ of the students are lefthanded women."

57. ◈ Is mulitplication of fractions commutative? Why or why not?

Multiply. Write each answer using fractional notation.

58. ▦ $\frac{341}{517} \cdot \frac{209}{349}$ $\frac{71,269}{180,433}$

59. ▦ $\left(-\frac{57}{61}\right)^3$ $-\frac{185,193}{226,981}$ or $\frac{-185,193}{226,981}$

60. $\left(\frac{2}{5}\right)^3\left(-\frac{7}{9}\right)$ $-\frac{56}{1125}$ or $\frac{-56}{1125}$

61. $\left(-\frac{1}{2}\right)^5\left(\frac{3}{5}\right)$ $-\frac{3}{160}$ or $\frac{-3}{160}$

62. $\left(-\frac{3}{4}\right)^2\left(-\frac{5}{7}\right)^2$ $\frac{225}{784}$

63. Evaluate $-\frac{2}{3}xy$ for $x = \frac{2}{5}$ and $y = -\frac{1}{7}$. $\frac{4}{105}$

64. Evaluate $-\frac{3}{4}ab$ for $a = \frac{2}{5}$ and $b = \frac{7}{5}$. $-\frac{42}{100}$ or $\frac{-42}{100}$

3.5 Simplifying

a Multiplying by 1

Recall the following:

$$1 = \frac{1}{1} = \frac{2}{2} = \frac{3}{3} = \frac{4}{4} = \frac{-13}{-13} = \frac{45}{45} = \frac{100}{100} = \frac{n}{n}.$$

Any nonzero number divided by itself is 1.

> When we multiply a number by 1, we get the same number.
>
> $$\frac{3}{5} = \frac{3}{5} \cdot 1 = \frac{3}{5} \cdot \frac{4}{4} = \frac{12}{20}$$

Since $\frac{3}{5} \cdot 1 = \frac{12}{20}$, we know that $\frac{3}{5}$ and $\frac{12}{20}$ are two names for the same number. This means that $\frac{3}{5}$ and $\frac{12}{20}$ are *equivalent* (see Section 2.7).

Do Exercises 1–4.

Suppose we want to rename $\frac{2}{3}$, using a denominator of 15. We can multiply by 1 to find a number equivalent to $\frac{2}{3}$:

$$\frac{2}{3} = \frac{2}{3} \cdot \frac{5}{5} = \frac{2 \cdot 5}{3 \cdot 5} = \frac{10}{15}.$$

We chose $\frac{5}{5}$ for 1 because $15 \div 3$ is 5.

Example 1 Find a number equivalent to $\frac{1}{4}$ with a denominator of 24.

Since $24 \div 4 = 6$, we multiply by 1, using $\frac{6}{6}$:

$$\frac{1}{4} = \frac{1}{4} \cdot \frac{6}{6} = \frac{1 \cdot 6}{4 \cdot 6} = \frac{6}{24}.$$

Example 2 Find a number equivalent to $\frac{2}{5}$ with a denominator of -35.

Since $-35 \div 5 = -7$, we multiply by 1, using $\frac{-7}{-7}$:

$$\frac{2}{5} = \frac{2}{5}\left(\frac{-7}{-7}\right) = \frac{2(-7)}{5(-7)} = \frac{-14}{-35}.$$

Example 3 Find an expression equivalent to $\frac{9}{8}$ with a denominator of $8a$.

Since $8a \div 8 = a$, we multiply by 1, using $\frac{a}{a}$:

$$\frac{9}{8} \cdot \frac{a}{a} = \frac{9a}{8a}.$$

Do Exercises 5–9.

Objectives

a Multiply by 1 to find an equivalent expression using a different denominator.

b Simplify fractional notation.

For Extra Help

TAPE 6

MAC
WIN

CD-ROM

Multiply.

1. $\frac{1}{2} \cdot \frac{8}{8}$
    $\frac{8}{16}$

2. $\frac{3}{5} \cdot \frac{x}{x}$
    $\frac{3x}{5x}$

3. $-\frac{13}{25} \cdot \frac{4}{4}$
    $-\frac{52}{100}$

4. $\frac{8}{3}\left(\frac{-2}{-2}\right)$
    $\frac{-16}{-6}$

Find an equivalent expression for each number, but with the denominator indicated. Use multiplication by 1.

5. $\frac{4}{3} = \frac{?}{9}$
    $\frac{12}{9}$

6. $\frac{3}{4} = \frac{?}{-24}$
    $\frac{-18}{-24}$

7. $\frac{9}{10} = \frac{?}{10x}$
    $\frac{9x}{10x}$

8. $\frac{3}{15} = \frac{?}{45}$
    $\frac{9}{45}$

9. $\frac{-8}{7} = \frac{?}{49}$
    $\frac{-56}{49}$

Answers on page A-8

Simplify.

10. $\dfrac{6}{14}$ $\dfrac{3}{7}$

11. $\dfrac{-10}{12}$ $\dfrac{-5}{6}$

12. $\dfrac{40}{8}$ 5

13. $\dfrac{4a}{3a}$ $\dfrac{4}{3}$

14. $-\dfrac{50}{30}$ $-\dfrac{5}{3}$

Answers on page A-8

b   Simplifying

All of the following are names for three-fourths:

$$\frac{3}{4}, \quad \frac{-6}{-8}, \quad \frac{9}{12}, \quad \frac{12}{16}, \quad \frac{-15}{-20}.$$

We say that $\frac{3}{4}$ is **simplest** because it has the smallest positive denominator. Note that 3 and 4 have no factor in common other than 1.

To simplify, we reverse the process of multiplying by 1. This is accomplished by removing any factors other than 1 and -1 that the numerator and the denominator have in common.

$$\frac{12}{18} = \frac{2 \cdot 6}{3 \cdot 6} \quad \begin{array}{l}\longleftarrow \text{ Factoring the numerator} \\ \longleftarrow \text{ Factoring the denominator}\end{array}$$

$$= \frac{2}{3} \cdot \frac{6}{6} \qquad \text{Factoring the fraction}$$

$$= \frac{2}{3} \cdot 1 \qquad \frac{6}{6} = 1$$

$$= \frac{2}{3} \qquad \text{Removing the factor 1: } \frac{2}{3} \cdot 1 = \frac{2}{3}$$

Examples   Simplify.

4. $\dfrac{-8}{20} = \dfrac{-2 \cdot 4}{5 \cdot 4} = \dfrac{-2}{5} \cdot \dfrac{4}{4} = \dfrac{-2}{5}$ Removing a factor equal to 1: $\frac{4}{4} = 1$

5. $\dfrac{2}{6} = \dfrac{1 \cdot 2}{3 \cdot 2} = \dfrac{1}{3} \cdot \dfrac{2}{2} = \dfrac{1}{3}$ Writing 1 allows for pairing of factors in the numerator and the denominator.

6. $\dfrac{30}{6} = \dfrac{5 \cdot 6}{1 \cdot 6} = \dfrac{5}{1} \cdot \dfrac{6}{6} = \dfrac{5}{1} = 5$ $\longleftarrow$ We could also simplify $\frac{30}{6}$ by doing the division $30 \div 6$. That is, $\frac{30}{6} = 30 \div 6 = 5$.

7. $-\dfrac{15}{10} = -\dfrac{3 \cdot 5}{2 \cdot 5}$

$$= -\dfrac{3}{2} \cdot \dfrac{5}{5} \left.\begin{array}{l} \\ \\ \end{array}\right\} \text{Removing a factor equal to 1: } \frac{5}{5} = 1$$

$$= -\dfrac{3}{2}$$

8. $\dfrac{4x}{15x} = \dfrac{4 \cdot x}{15 \cdot x}$ (Assume that $x \neq 0$.)

$$= \dfrac{4}{15} \cdot \dfrac{x}{x} \left.\begin{array}{l} \\ \\ \end{array}\right\} \text{Removing a factor equal to 1: } \frac{x}{x} = 1$$

$$= \dfrac{4}{15}$$

Note that $\frac{4}{15}$ is considered simplified—the numbers 4 and 15 have no factors in common.

Do Exercises 10–14.

The tests for divisibility are also helpful when simplifying.

Example 9   Simplify: $\dfrac{105}{135}$.

Since both 105 and 135 end in 5, we know that 5 is a factor of both the numerator and the denominator:

$$\frac{105}{135} = \frac{21 \cdot 5}{27 \cdot 5} = \frac{21}{27} \cdot \frac{5}{5} = \frac{21}{27}.$$

A fraction is not "simplified" if common factors of the numerator and the denominator remain. Because 21 and 27 are both divisible by 3, we must simplify further:

$$\frac{105}{135} = \frac{21}{27} = \frac{7 \cdot 3}{9 \cdot 3} = \frac{7}{9} \cdot \frac{3}{3} = \frac{7}{9}.$$

Example 10   Simplify: $\dfrac{90}{84}$.

Since 90 and 84 are both even, we know that 2 is a common factor:

$$\frac{90}{84} = \frac{2 \cdot 45}{2 \cdot 42}$$

$$= \frac{2}{2} \cdot \frac{45}{42} = \frac{45}{42}. \qquad \text{Removing a factor equal to 1: } \frac{2}{2} = 1$$

Before stating that $\frac{45}{42}$ represents simplified form, we must check to see whether 45 and 42 share a common factor. Since the sum of the digits in 45 is 9 and 9 is divisible by 3, we know that 45 is divisible by 3. Similarly, it can be shown that 42 is divisible by 3. Thus, 3 is a common factor and we can simplify further:

$$\frac{45}{42} = \frac{3 \cdot 15}{3 \cdot 14}$$

$$= \frac{3}{3} \cdot \frac{15}{14} = \frac{15}{14}. \qquad \text{Removing a factor equal to 1: } \frac{3}{3} = 1$$

Thus $\frac{90}{84}$ simplifies to $\frac{15}{14}$.

Do Exercises 15–18.

Simplify.

15. $\dfrac{35}{40}$ $\dfrac{7}{8}$

16. $\dfrac{801}{702}$ $\dfrac{89}{78}$

17. $\dfrac{-24}{21}$ $\dfrac{-8}{7}$

18. Simplify each fraction in this circle graph.

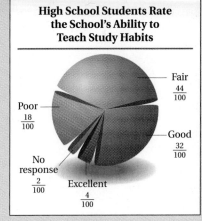

High School Students Rate the School's Ability to Teach Study Habits

Fair $\dfrac{44}{100}$

Poor $\dfrac{18}{100}$

Good $\dfrac{32}{100}$

No response $\dfrac{2}{100}$

Excellent $\dfrac{4}{100}$

$\dfrac{2}{100} = \dfrac{1}{50}, \dfrac{4}{100} = \dfrac{1}{25}, \dfrac{32}{100} = \dfrac{8}{25},$
$\dfrac{44}{100} = \dfrac{11}{25}, \dfrac{18}{100} = \dfrac{9}{50}$

Answers on page A-8

CANCELING   Canceling is a shortcut that you may have used for removing a factor that equals 1 when working with fractional notation. With *great* concern, we mention it as a possibility for speeding up your work. Canceling may be done only when removing common factors in numerators and denominators. Each common factor allows us to remove a factor equal to 1 in a product.

Our concern is that canceling be done with care and understanding. In effect, slashes are used to indicate factors equal to 1 that have been removed. For instance, Example 10 might have been done faster as follows:

$$\frac{90}{84} = \frac{2 \cdot 45}{2 \cdot 42} \qquad \text{Factoring the numerator and the denominator}$$

$$= \frac{\cancel{2} \cdot 45}{\cancel{2} \cdot 42} \qquad \begin{array}{l}\text{When a factor equal to 1 is noted,}\\ \text{it is "canceled" as shown: } \frac{2}{2} = 1.\end{array}$$

$$= \frac{45}{42} = \frac{\cancel{3} \cdot 15}{\cancel{3} \cdot 14} = \frac{15}{14}.$$

CAUTION!   The difficulty with canceling is that it is often applied incorrectly in situations like the following:

$$\frac{\cancel{2} + 3}{\cancel{2}} = 3; \qquad \frac{\cancel{4} + 1}{\cancel{4} + 2} = \frac{1}{2}; \qquad \frac{1\cancel{5}}{\cancel{5}4} = \frac{1}{4}.$$

Wrong!   Wrong!   Wrong!

The correct answers are

$$\frac{2 + 3}{2} = \frac{5}{2}; \qquad \frac{4 + 1}{4 + 2} = \frac{5}{6}; \qquad \frac{15}{54} = \frac{\cancel{3} \cdot 5}{\cancel{3} \cdot 18} = \frac{5}{18}.$$

In each of the incorrect cancellations, the numbers canceled did not form a factor equal to 1. Factors are parts of products. For example, in $2 \cdot 3$, the numbers 2 and 3 are factors, but in $2 + 3$, the numbers 2 and 3 are terms, not factors.

> • If you cannot factor, do not cancel! If in doubt, do not cancel!
>
> • Only factors can be canceled and factors are never separated by $+$ or $-$ signs.

Answers on page A-8

Exercise Set 3.5

a Find an equivalent expression for the given number, with the denominator indicated. Use multiplication by 1.

1. $\dfrac{1}{2} = \dfrac{?}{10}$ $\dfrac{5}{10}$

2. $\dfrac{1}{6} = \dfrac{?}{12}$ $\dfrac{2}{12}$

3. $\dfrac{3}{4} = \dfrac{?}{-48}$ $\dfrac{-36}{-48}$

4. $\dfrac{2}{9} = \dfrac{?}{-18}$ $\dfrac{-4}{-18}$

5. $\dfrac{9}{10} = \dfrac{?}{30}$ $\dfrac{27}{30}$

6. $\dfrac{3}{8} = \dfrac{?}{48}$ $\dfrac{18}{48}$

7. $\dfrac{11}{5} = \dfrac{?}{5t}$ $\dfrac{11t}{5t}$

8. $\dfrac{5}{3} = \dfrac{?}{3a}$ $\dfrac{5a}{3a}$

9. $\dfrac{5}{12} = \dfrac{?}{48}$ $\dfrac{20}{48}$

10. $\dfrac{7}{8} = \dfrac{?}{56}$ $\dfrac{49}{56}$

11. $-\dfrac{17}{18} = -\dfrac{?}{54}$ $-\dfrac{51}{54}$

12. $-\dfrac{11}{16} = -\dfrac{?}{256}$ $-\dfrac{176}{256}$

13. $\dfrac{2}{-5} = \dfrac{?}{-25}$ $\dfrac{10}{-25}$

14. $\dfrac{7}{-8} = \dfrac{?}{-32}$ $\dfrac{28}{-32}$

15. $\dfrac{-7}{22} = \dfrac{?}{132}$ $\dfrac{-42}{132}$

16. $\dfrac{-10}{21} = \dfrac{?}{126}$ $\dfrac{-60}{126}$

17. $\dfrac{5}{8} = \dfrac{?}{8x}$ $\dfrac{5x}{8x}$

18. $\dfrac{2}{7} = \dfrac{?}{7a}$ $\dfrac{2a}{7a}$

19. $\dfrac{7}{11} = \dfrac{?}{11m}$ $\dfrac{7m}{11m}$

20. $\dfrac{4}{3} = \dfrac{?}{3n}$ $\dfrac{4n}{3n}$

21. $\dfrac{4}{9} = \dfrac{?}{9ab}$ $\dfrac{4ab}{9ab}$

22. $\dfrac{8}{11} = \dfrac{?}{11xy}$ $\dfrac{8xy}{11xy}$

23. $\dfrac{4}{9} = \dfrac{?}{27b}$ $\dfrac{12b}{27b}$

24. $\dfrac{8}{11} = \dfrac{?}{55y}$ $\dfrac{40y}{55y}$

b Simplify.

25. $\dfrac{2}{4}$ $\dfrac{1}{2}$

26. $\dfrac{3}{6}$ $\dfrac{1}{2}$

27. $-\dfrac{6}{9}$ $-\dfrac{2}{3}$

28. $\dfrac{-9}{12}$ $\dfrac{-3}{4}$

29. $\dfrac{10}{25}$ $\dfrac{2}{5}$

30. $\dfrac{8}{10}$ $\dfrac{4}{5}$

31. $\dfrac{24}{-8}$ -3

32. $\dfrac{36}{-4}$ -9

33. $\dfrac{27}{36}$ $\dfrac{3}{4}$

34. $\dfrac{30}{40}$ $\dfrac{3}{4}$

35. $-\dfrac{24}{14}$ $-\dfrac{12}{7}$

36. $-\dfrac{16}{10}$ $-\dfrac{8}{5}$

37. $\dfrac{16n}{48n}$ $\dfrac{1}{3}$

38. $\dfrac{150a}{25a}$ 6

39. $\dfrac{-17}{51}$ $\dfrac{-1}{3}$

40. $\dfrac{-425}{525}$ $\dfrac{-17}{21}$

41. $\dfrac{420}{480}$ $\dfrac{7}{8}$

42. $\dfrac{180}{240}$ $\dfrac{3}{4}$

43. $\dfrac{136}{153}$ $\dfrac{8}{9}$

44. $\dfrac{117}{91}$ $\dfrac{9}{7}$

45. $\dfrac{3ab}{8ab}$ $\dfrac{3}{8}$

46. $\dfrac{6xy}{7xy}$ $\dfrac{6}{7}$

47. $\dfrac{9xy}{6x}$ $\dfrac{3y}{2}$

48. $\dfrac{10ab}{15a}$ $\dfrac{2b}{3}$

Skill Maintenance

49. A soccer field is 90 yd long and 40 yd wide. What is its area? [1.8a] 3600 yd²

50. Yardbird Landscaping buys 13 maple saplings and 17 oak saplings for a project. A maple costs $23 and an oak costs $37. How much is spent altogether for the saplings? [1.8a] $928

Subtract.

51. $34 - 39$ [2.3a] -5

52. $50 - 68$ [2.3a] -18

53. $803 - 617$ [1.3d] 186

54. $8344 - 5607$ [1.3d]

2737

Solve.

55. $30 \cdot x = -150$ [1.7b], [2.5a], [2.8b] -5

56. $5280 = 1760 + t$ [1.7b], [2.8a] 3520

Synthesis

57. ◆ Explain in your own words when it *is* possible to "cancel" and when it *is not* possible to "cancel."

58. ◆ Can fractional notation be simplified if the numerator and the denominator are two different prime numbers? Why or why not?

59. ◆ Why is multiplication of fractions (Section 3.4) discussed before simplification of fractions (Section 3.5)?

Simplify. Use the list of prime numbers on p. 154.

60. $\dfrac{221}{247}$ $\dfrac{17}{19}$

61. $\dfrac{209ab}{247ac}$ $\dfrac{11b}{13c}$

62. $-\dfrac{253x}{143y}$ $-\dfrac{23x}{13y}$

63. $-\dfrac{187a}{289b}$ $-\dfrac{11a}{17b}$

64. 🖩 $\dfrac{2603}{2831}$ $\dfrac{137}{149}$

65. 🖩 $\dfrac{3473}{3197}$ $\dfrac{151}{139}$

66. Sociologists have found that 4 of 10 people are shy. Write fractional notation for the part of the population that is shy; the part that is not shy. Simplify. $\dfrac{4}{10} = \dfrac{2}{5}$; $\dfrac{6}{10} = \dfrac{3}{5}$

67. Sociologists estimate that 3 of 20 people are left-handed. In a crowd of 460 people, how many would you expect to be left-handed? 69

68. The circle graph below shows how long shoppers stay when visiting a mall. What portion of shoppers stay for 0–2 hr?

$\dfrac{43}{50}$

69. A new Chevrolet Prizm costs $14,400. Pam will pay $\frac{1}{2}$ of the cost, Sam will pay $\frac{1}{4}$ of the cost, Jan will pay $\frac{1}{6}$ the cost, and Nan will pay the rest.

a) How much will Nan pay? $1200

b) What fractional part will Nan pay? $\dfrac{1}{12}$

Collaborative Learning Manual

Use fraction bars to represent equivalent fractions.

3.6 Multiplying, Simplifying, and More with Area

a Simplifying When Multiplying

We usually want a simplified answer when we multiply. To make such simplifying easier, it is generally best not to calculate the products in the numerator and the denominator until we have first factored and simplified. Consider

$$\frac{5}{6} \cdot \frac{14}{15}.$$

We proceed as follows:

$$\frac{5}{6} \cdot \frac{14}{15} = \frac{5 \cdot 14}{6 \cdot 15}$$ We do not yet carry out the multiplication. Note that 2 is a factor of 6 and 14. Also, note that 5 is a factor of 5 and 15.

$$= \frac{5 \cdot 2 \cdot 7}{2 \cdot 3 \cdot 5 \cdot 3}$$ **Factoring and identifying common factors**

$$= \frac{5 \cdot 2}{5 \cdot 2} \cdot \frac{7}{3 \cdot 3}$$ **Factoring the fraction**

$$= 1 \cdot \frac{7}{3 \cdot 3}$$

$$= \frac{7}{3 \cdot 3}$$ Removing a factor equal to 1: $\frac{5 \cdot 2}{5 \cdot 2} = 1$

$$= \frac{7}{9}.$$

> To multiply and simplify:
>
> **a)** Write the products in the numerator and the denominator, but do not calculate the products.
>
> **b)** Identify any common factors of the numerator and the denominator.
>
> **c)** Factor the fraction to remove any factors that equal 1.
>
> **d)** Calculate the remaining products.

Examples   Multiply and simplify.

1. $\dfrac{2}{3} \cdot \dfrac{5}{4} = \dfrac{2 \cdot 5}{3 \cdot 4}$ Note that 2 is a common factor of 2 and 4.

$$= \frac{2 \cdot 5}{3 \cdot 2 \cdot 2}$$ **Try to go directly to this step.**

$$= \frac{2}{2} \cdot \frac{5}{3 \cdot 2}$$

$$= 1 \cdot \frac{5}{3 \cdot 2} = \frac{5}{6}$$ Removing a factor equal to 1: $\frac{2}{2} = 1$

2. $\dfrac{6}{7} \cdot \dfrac{-5}{3} = \dfrac{3 \cdot 2 \cdot (-5)}{7 \cdot 3}$ Note that 3 is a common factor of 6 and 3.

$$= \frac{3}{3} \cdot \frac{2(-5)}{7} = \frac{-10}{7}, \text{ or } -\frac{10}{7}$$ Removing a factor equal to 1: $\frac{3}{3} = 1$

Objectives

a Multiply and simplify using fractional notation.

b Solve applied problems involving multiplication.

For Extra Help

TAPE 6   InterAct math   CD-ROM
                MAC
                WIN

Multiply and simplify.

1. $\dfrac{2}{3} \cdot \dfrac{7}{8}$ $\dfrac{7}{12}$

2. $\dfrac{4}{5} \cdot \dfrac{-5}{12}$ $-\dfrac{1}{3}$

3. $16 \cdot \dfrac{3}{8}$ 6

4. $\dfrac{5}{2x} \cdot 6$ $\dfrac{15}{x}$

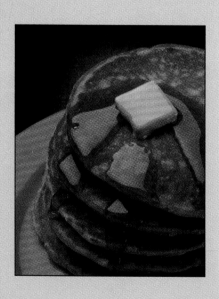

Answers on page A-8

---

3. $\dfrac{10}{21} \cdot \dfrac{14a}{15} = \dfrac{5 \cdot 2 \cdot 7 \cdot 2a}{7 \cdot 3 \cdot 5 \cdot 3}$ Note that 5 is a common factor of 10 and 15.
Note that 7 is a common factor of 21 and 14*a*.

$= \dfrac{5 \cdot 7}{5 \cdot 7} \cdot \dfrac{2 \cdot 2a}{3 \cdot 3}$

$= \dfrac{4a}{9}$ Removing a factor equal to 1: $\dfrac{5 \cdot 7}{5 \cdot 7} = 1$

4. $40 \cdot \dfrac{7}{8} = \dfrac{8 \cdot 5 \cdot 7}{8 \cdot 1}$ Note that 8 is a common factor of 40 and 8.

$= \dfrac{8}{8} \cdot \dfrac{5 \cdot 7}{1} = 35$ Removing a factor equal to 1: $\dfrac{8}{8} = 1$

CAUTION!   Canceling can be used as follows for these examples.

1. $\dfrac{2}{3} \cdot \dfrac{5}{4} = \dfrac{\cancel{2} \cdot 5}{3 \cdot \cancel{2} \cdot 2} = \dfrac{5}{6}$ Removing a factor equal to 1: $\dfrac{2}{2} = 1$

2. $\dfrac{6}{7} \cdot \dfrac{-5}{3} = \dfrac{\cancel{3} \cdot 2(-5)}{7 \cdot \cancel{3}} = \dfrac{-10}{7}$ Removing a factor equal to 1: $\dfrac{3}{3} = 1$

3. $\dfrac{10}{21} \cdot \dfrac{14a}{15} = \dfrac{\cancel{5} \cdot 2 \cdot \cancel{7} \cdot 2a}{\cancel{7} \cdot 3 \cdot \cancel{5} \cdot 3} = \dfrac{4a}{9}$ Removing a factor equal to 1: $\dfrac{5 \cdot 7}{5 \cdot 7} = 1$

4. $40 \cdot \dfrac{7}{8} = \dfrac{\cancel{8} \cdot 5 \cdot 7}{\cancel{8} \cdot 1} = 35$ Removing a factor equal to 1: $\dfrac{8}{8} = 1$

Remember, if you can't factor, you can't cancel!

Do Exercises 1–4.

b   Solving Problems

Example 5   For their annual pancake breakfast, the Colchester Boy Scouts need $\frac{2}{3}$ cup of Bisquick® per person. If at most 135 guests are expected, how much Bisquick do the scouts need?

1. **Familiarize.**   We first make a drawing or at least visualize the situation. Repeated addition will work here.

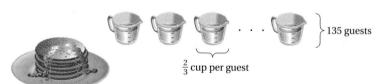

135 guests

$\frac{2}{3}$ cup per guest

We let *n* = the number of cups of Bisquick needed.

2. **Translate.**   The problem translates to the following equation:

$n = 135 \cdot \dfrac{2}{3}.$

3. Solve. To solve the equation, we carry out the multiplication:

$$n = 135 \cdot \frac{2}{3} = \frac{135 \cdot 2}{3} \qquad \text{Multiplying}$$

$$= \frac{3 \cdot 45 \cdot 2}{3 \cdot 1} \qquad \text{Note that 135 is divisible by 3.}$$

$$= \frac{3}{3} \cdot \frac{45 \cdot 2}{1} \qquad \text{Removing the factor } \frac{3}{3}$$

$$= 90. \qquad \text{Simplifying}$$

4. Check. We could repeat the calculation but this check is left to the student. We can also think about the reasonableness of the answer. Since each guest requires less than 1 cup, it makes sense that 135 guests requires fewer than 135 cups. This provides a partial check of the answer.

5. State. The scouts will need 90 cups of Bisquick.

Do Exercise 5.

Area

Multiplication of fractions can arise in geometry problems involving the area of a triangle. Consider a triangle with a base of length b and a height of h, as shown.

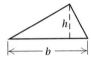

A rectangle can be formed by splitting and inverting a copy of this triangle:

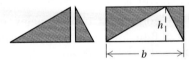

The rectangle's area, $b \cdot h$, is exactly twice the area of the triangle. We have the following result.

> The **area A of a triangle** is half the length of the base b times the height h:
>
> $$A = \frac{1}{2} \cdot b \cdot h.$$

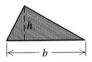

Example 6 Find the area of this triangle.

$$A = \frac{1}{2} \cdot b \cdot h$$

$$= \frac{1}{2} \cdot 9 \text{ yd} \cdot 6 \text{ yd}$$

$$= \frac{9 \cdot 6}{2} \text{ yd}^2$$

$$= 27 \text{ yd}^2$$

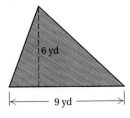

5. Yardbird Landscaping uses $\frac{2}{5}$ lb of peat moss for a rosebush. How much will be needed for 25 rosebushes?

10 lb

Answers on page A-8

Find the area.

6.

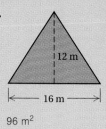

12 m

←——— 16 m ———→

96 m²

7.

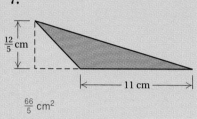

$\frac{12}{5}$ cm

←——— 11 cm ———→

$\frac{66}{5}$ cm²

8. Find the area.

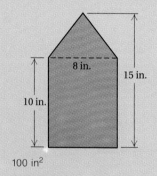

8 in.

15 in.

10 in.

100 in²

Answers on page A-8

Example 7   Find the area of this triangle.

$$A = \frac{1}{2} \cdot b \cdot h$$

$$= \frac{1}{2} \cdot \frac{10}{3} \text{ cm} \cdot 4 \text{ cm}$$

$$= \frac{1 \cdot 10 \cdot 4}{2 \cdot 3} \text{ cm}^2$$

$$= \frac{1 \cdot \cancel{2} \cdot 5 \cdot 4}{\cancel{2} \cdot 3} \text{ cm}^2 \qquad \text{Removing a factor equal to 1: } \frac{2}{2} = 1$$

$$= \frac{20}{3} \text{ cm}^2$$

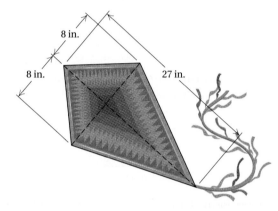

4 cm

←— $\frac{10}{3}$ cm —→

Do Exercises 6 and 7.

Example 8   Find the area of this kite.

8 in.

8 in.   27 in.

1. **Familiarize.**   We look for figures with areas we can calculate using area formulas that we already know. We let K = the kite's area.

2. **Translate.**   The kite consists of two triangles, each with a base of 27 in. and a height of 8 in. We can apply the formula $A = \frac{1}{2} \cdot b \cdot h$ for the area of a triangle and then multiply by 2.

Kite's area	is	twice	Area of long triangle
↓	↓	↓	
K	=	2	$\cdot \quad \frac{1}{2}(27 \text{ in.}) \cdot (8 \text{ in.})$

3. **Solve.**   We have

$$K = 2 \cdot \frac{1}{2} \cdot (27 \text{ in.}) \cdot (8 \text{ in.})$$

$$= 1 \cdot 27 \text{ in} \cdot 8 \text{ in.} = 216 \text{ in}^2.$$

4. **Check.**   We can check by repeating the calculations.
5. **State.**   The area of the kite is 216 in².

Do Exercise 8.

Exercise Set 3.6

a Multiply. Don't forget to simplify.

1. $\dfrac{3}{8} \cdot \dfrac{5}{3}$ $\dfrac{5}{8}$

2. $\dfrac{4}{5} \cdot \dfrac{1}{4}$ $\dfrac{1}{5}$

3. $\dfrac{7}{8} \cdot \dfrac{-1}{7}$ $-\dfrac{1}{8}$

4. $\dfrac{5}{6} \cdot \dfrac{-1}{5}$ $-\dfrac{1}{6}$

5. $\dfrac{1}{8} \cdot \dfrac{6}{5}$ $\dfrac{3}{20}$

6. $\dfrac{2}{5} \cdot \dfrac{1}{12}$ $\dfrac{1}{30}$

7. $\dfrac{1}{6} \cdot \dfrac{4}{3}$ $\dfrac{2}{9}$

8. $\dfrac{3}{6} \cdot \dfrac{1}{6}$ $\dfrac{1}{12}$

9. $\dfrac{12}{-5} \cdot \dfrac{9}{8}$ $-\dfrac{27}{10}$

10. $\dfrac{16}{-15} \cdot \dfrac{5}{4}$ $-\dfrac{4}{3}$

11. $\dfrac{5x}{9} \cdot \dfrac{7}{5}$ $\dfrac{7x}{9}$

12. $\dfrac{25}{4a} \cdot \dfrac{4}{3}$ $\dfrac{25}{3a}$

13. $\dfrac{1}{4} \cdot 8$ 2

14. $\dfrac{1}{6} \cdot 12$ 2

15. $15 \cdot \dfrac{1}{3}$ 5

16. $14 \cdot \dfrac{1}{2}$ 7

17. $-12 \cdot \dfrac{3}{4}$ -9

18. $-18 \cdot \dfrac{5}{6}$ -15

19. $\dfrac{3}{8} \cdot 8a$ $3a$

20. $\dfrac{2}{9} \cdot 9x$ $2x$

21. $\left(-\dfrac{3}{7}\right)\left(-\dfrac{7}{3}\right)$ 1

22. $\left(-\dfrac{2}{9}\right)\left(-\dfrac{9}{2}\right)$ 1

23. $\dfrac{a}{b} \cdot \dfrac{b}{a}$ 1

24. $\dfrac{n}{m} \cdot \dfrac{m}{n}$ 1

25. $\dfrac{1}{27} \cdot 360a$ $\dfrac{40a}{3}$

26. $\dfrac{1}{28} \cdot 105n$ $\dfrac{15n}{4}$

27. $176\left(\dfrac{1}{-6}\right)$ $-\dfrac{88}{3}$

28. $135\left(\dfrac{1}{-10}\right)$ $-\dfrac{27}{2}$

29. $7x \cdot \dfrac{1}{7x}$ 1

30. $5a \cdot \dfrac{1}{5a}$ 1

31. $\dfrac{2x}{9} \cdot \dfrac{27}{2x}$ 3

32. $\dfrac{10a}{3} \cdot \dfrac{3}{5a}$ 2

33. $\dfrac{7}{10} \cdot \dfrac{34}{150}$ $\dfrac{119}{750}$

34. $\dfrac{8}{10} \cdot \dfrac{45}{100}$ $\dfrac{9}{25}$

35. $\dfrac{36}{85} \cdot \dfrac{25}{-99}$ $-\dfrac{20}{187}$

36. $\dfrac{-70}{45} \cdot \dfrac{50}{49}$ $-\dfrac{100}{63}$

37. $\dfrac{-98}{99} \cdot \dfrac{27a}{175a}$ $-\dfrac{42}{275}$

38. $\dfrac{70}{-49} \cdot \dfrac{63}{300x}$ $-\dfrac{3}{10x}$

39. $\dfrac{110}{33} \cdot \dfrac{-24}{25}$ $-\dfrac{16}{5}$

40. $\dfrac{-19}{130} \cdot \dfrac{65}{38x}$ $-\dfrac{1}{4x}$

41. $\left(-\dfrac{11}{24}\right)\dfrac{3}{5}$ $-\dfrac{11}{40}$

42. $\left(-\dfrac{15}{22}\right)\dfrac{4}{7}$ $-\dfrac{30}{77}$

43. $\dfrac{10a}{21} \cdot \dfrac{3}{4a}$ $\dfrac{5}{14}$

44. $\dfrac{17}{18x} \cdot \dfrac{3x}{5}$ $\dfrac{17}{30}$

45. Anna receives $56 for working a full day doing inventory at a hardware store. How much will she receive for working $\frac{3}{4}$ of the day? $42

46. After Jack completes 60 hr of teacher training in college, he can earn $88 for working a full day as a substitute teacher. How much will he receive for working $\frac{3}{4}$ of a day? $66

47. *Food Preparation.* How much salmon is needed to serve 30 people if each person gets $\frac{2}{5}$ lb?   12 lb

48. *Mailing Lists.* Business people have determined that $\frac{1}{4}$ of the addresses on a mailing list will change in one year. A business has a mailing list of 2500 people. After one year, how many addresses on that list will be incorrect?   625

49. *Sociology.* Sociologists have determined that $\frac{2}{5}$ of the people in the world are shy. A sales manager is interviewing 650 people for a new sales position. How many of these people might be shy?

260

50. *Food Preparation.* Francesca's Sandwich Shop sells subs by the foot. If one serving is $\frac{2}{3}$ ft long, how many feet are needed to serve 30 people?   20 ft

51. A recipe for pie crust calls for $\frac{2}{3}$ cup of flour. A chef is making $\frac{1}{2}$ of the recipe. How much flour should the chef use? $\frac{1}{3}$ cup

52. Of the students in the entering class, $\frac{2}{5}$ have cameras; $\frac{1}{4}$ of these students also join the college photography club. What fraction of the students in the entering class join the photography club? $\frac{1}{10}$

53. A house worth $124,000 was assessed at $\frac{3}{4}$ of its value. What is the assessed value of the house?

$93,000

54. Roxanne's tuition was $2800. A loan was obtained for $\frac{3}{4}$ of the tuition. How much was the loan?

$2100

55. *Map Scaling.* On a map, 1 in. represents 240 mi. How much does $\frac{2}{3}$ in. represent?

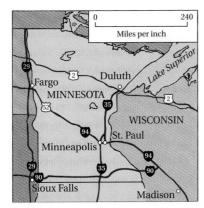

160 mi

56. *Map Scaling.* On a map, 1 in. represents 120 mi. How much does $\frac{3}{4}$ in. represent?

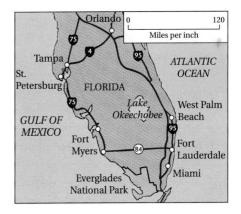

90 mi

57. *Household Budgets.* Vic has an annual income of $27,000. Of this, $\frac{1}{4}$ is spent for food, $\frac{1}{5}$ for housing, $\frac{1}{10}$ for clothing, $\frac{1}{9}$ for savings, $\frac{1}{4}$ for taxes, and the rest for other expenses. How much is spent for each?

58. *Household Budgets.* Heidi has an annual income of $25,200. Of this, $\frac{1}{4}$ is spent for food, $\frac{1}{5}$ for housing, $\frac{1}{10}$ for clothing, $\frac{1}{9}$ for savings, $\frac{1}{4}$ for taxes, and the rest for other expenses. How much is spent for each?

Household Income

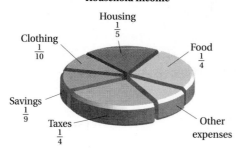

$6750 for food; $5400 for housing; $2700 for clothing; $3000 for savings; $6750 for taxes; $2400 for other expenses

$6300 for food; $5040 for housing; $2520 for clothing; $2800 for savings; $6300 for taxes; $2240 for other expenses

Find the area.

59.

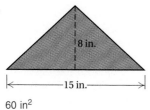

8 in.

15 in.

60 in²

60.

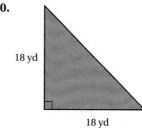

18 yd

18 yd

162 yd²

61.

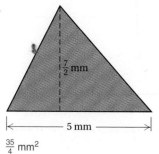

$\frac{7}{2}$ mm

5 mm

$\frac{35}{4}$ mm²

62.

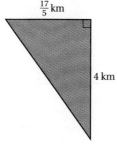

$\frac{17}{5}$ km

4 km

$\frac{34}{5}$ km²

63.

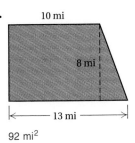

$\frac{63}{8}$ m^2

64.

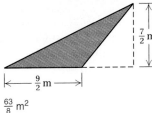

$\frac{7}{3}$ yd^2

65.

10 mi

8 mi

13 mi

92 mi^2

66.

15 cm

30 cm

30 cm

675 cm^2

67. *Construction.* Find the total area of the sides and ends of the building.   6800 ft^2

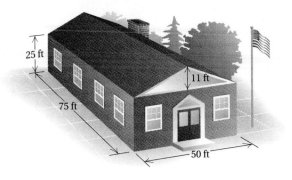

25 ft

11 ft

75 ft

50 ft

68. *Sailing* A rectangular piece of sailcloth is 36 ft by 24 ft. A triangular sail with a height of 28 ft and a base of 16 ft is cut from the sailcloth. How much area is left over?   640 ft^2

Skill Maintenance

Solve.

69. $48 \cdot t = 1680$ [1.7b], [2.8b]   35

70. $456 + x = 9002$ [1.7b], [2.8a]   8546

71. $747 = x + 270$ [1.7b], [2.8a]   477

72. $280 = 4 \cdot t$ [1.7b], [2.8b]   70

Add.

73. $(-39) + (-72)$ [2.2a] -111

74. $-59 + 37$ [2.2a] -22

75. ◈ When multiplying using fractional notation, we form products in the numerator and the denominator, but do not automatically calculate the products. Why?

76. ◈ If a fraction's numerator and denominator have no factors (other than 1) in common, can the fraction be simplified? Why or why not?

77. ◈ Is the product of two fractions always a fraction? Why or why not?

Simplify. Use the list of prime numbers on p. 154.

78. ▦ $\dfrac{201}{535} \cdot \dfrac{4601}{6499} \cdot \dfrac{129}{485}$

79. ▦ $\dfrac{5767}{3763} \cdot \dfrac{159}{395} \cdot \dfrac{219}{355}$

80. ▦ $\dfrac{667}{899} \cdot \dfrac{558}{621} \cdot \dfrac{2}{3}$

81. ▦ *Painting.* A painter needs to determine the surface area of an octagonal steeple. Find the total area, if the dimensions are as shown below. 432 ft²

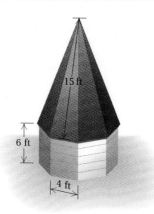

82. ▦ *Manufacturing.* A specially shaped candy box is triangular at each end, as shown below. Find the surface area of the box. 13,380 mm²

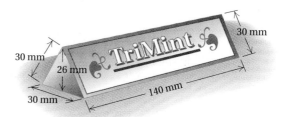

83. Of the students entering a college, $\frac{7}{8}$ have completed high school and $\frac{2}{3}$ are older than 20. If $\frac{1}{7}$ of all students are left-handed, what fraction of students entering the college are left-handed high school graduates over the age of 20? $\frac{1}{12}$

84. Refer to the information in Exercise 83. If 480 students are entering the college, how many of them are left-handed high school graduates 20 years old or younger? 20

85. Refer to Exercise 83. What fraction of students entering the college did not graduate high school, are 20 years old or younger, and are left-handed? $\frac{1}{168}$

3.7 Reciprocals and Division

a Reciprocals

Look at these products:

$$8 \cdot \frac{1}{8} = \frac{8}{8} = 1; \qquad \frac{-2}{3} \cdot \frac{3}{-2} = \frac{-6}{-6} = 1.$$

> If the product of two numbers is 1, we say that they are **reciprocals** of each other. To find a number's reciprocal, interchange the numerator and the denominator.
>
> The numbers $\frac{3}{4}$ and $\frac{4}{3}$ are reciprocals of each other.

Examples Find the reciprocal.

1. The reciprocal of $\frac{4}{5}$ is $\frac{5}{4}$.   Note that $\frac{4}{5} \cdot \frac{5}{4} = \frac{20}{20} = 1.$

2. The reciprocal of $\frac{a}{b}$ is $\frac{b}{a}$.   Note that $\frac{a}{b} \cdot \frac{b}{a} = \frac{ab}{ba} = 1.$

3. The reciprocal of 8 is $\frac{1}{8}$.   Think of 8 as $\frac{8}{1}$: $\frac{8}{1} \cdot \frac{1}{8} = \frac{8}{8} = 1.$

4. The reciprocal of $\frac{1}{3}$ is 3.   Note that $\frac{1}{3} \cdot 3 = \frac{3}{3} = 1.$

5. The reciprocal of $-\frac{5}{9}$ is $-\frac{9}{5}$.   **Negative numbers have negative reprocals:** $\left(-\frac{5}{9}\right)\left(-\frac{9}{5}\right) = \frac{45}{45} = 1.$

Do Exercises 1–5.

    Does 0 have a reciprocal? If it did, it would have to be a number x such that

$$0 \cdot x = 1.$$

But 0 times any number is 0. Thus, 0 has no reciprocal.

b Division

Recall that $a \div b$ is the number that when multiplied by b gives a. Consider the division $\frac{3}{4} \div \frac{1}{8}$. This asks how many $\frac{1}{8}$'s are in $\frac{3}{4}$. We can answer this by looking at the figure below.

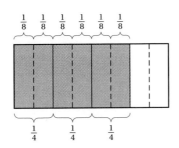

Objectives

a Find the reciprocal of a number.

b Divide and simplify using fractional notation.

c Solve problems involving division.

For Extra Help

TAPE 6   MAC   CD-ROM
        WIN

Find the reciprocal.

1. $\frac{2}{5}$ $\frac{5}{2}$

2. $\frac{-6}{x}$ $\frac{x}{-6}$

3. 9 $\frac{1}{9}$

4. $\frac{1}{5}$ 5

5. $-\frac{3}{10}$ $-\frac{10}{3}$

Answers on page A-8

We see that there are six $\frac{1}{8}$'s in $\frac{3}{4}$. Thus,

$$\frac{3}{4} \div \frac{1}{8} = 6.$$

We can check this by multiplying:

$$6 \cdot \frac{1}{8} = \frac{6}{8} = \frac{3}{4}.$$

Here is a faster way to divide. An explanation of why it works appears on the next page.

To divide a fraction, multiply by its reciprocal:

Multiply by the reciprocal of the divisor.

$$\frac{a}{b} \div \frac{c}{d} = \frac{a}{b} \cdot \frac{d}{c}.$$

Recall that when two numbers with unlike signs are multiplied or divided, the result is negative. When both numbers have the same sign, the result is positive.

Examples Divide and simplify.

6. $\dfrac{5}{6} \div \dfrac{2}{3} = \dfrac{5}{6} \cdot \dfrac{3}{2}$ Multiplying by the reciprocal of the divisor

$\qquad = \dfrac{5 \cdot 3}{3 \cdot 2 \cdot 2}$ Factoring and identifying a common factor

$\qquad = \dfrac{3}{3} \cdot \dfrac{5}{2 \cdot 2}$ Removing a factor equal to 1: $\dfrac{3}{3} = 1$

$\qquad = \dfrac{5}{4}$

7. $\dfrac{-3}{5} \div \dfrac{1}{2} = \dfrac{-3}{5} \cdot 2$ The reciprocal of $\dfrac{1}{2}$ is 2.

$\qquad = \dfrac{-3 \cdot 2}{5} = \dfrac{-6}{5}$

8. $\dfrac{2a}{5} \div 7 = \dfrac{2a}{5} \cdot \dfrac{1}{7}$ The reciprocal of 7 is $\dfrac{1}{7}$.

$\qquad = \dfrac{2a \cdot 1}{5 \cdot 7} = \dfrac{2a}{35}$

9. $\dfrac{7}{10} \div \left(-\dfrac{14}{15}\right) = \dfrac{7}{10} \cdot \left(-\dfrac{15}{14}\right)$ Multiplying by the reciprocal of the divisor

$\qquad = \dfrac{7 \cdot 5(-3)}{2 \cdot 5 \cdot 7 \cdot 2}$ Factoring and identifying common factors

$\qquad = \dfrac{7 \cdot 5}{7 \cdot 5} \cdot \dfrac{-3}{4}$ Removing a factor equal to 1: $\dfrac{7 \cdot 5}{7 \cdot 5} = 1$

$\qquad = -\dfrac{3}{4}$

CAUTION! Canceling can be used as follows for Examples 6 and 9.

6. $\dfrac{5}{6} \div \dfrac{2}{3} = \dfrac{5}{6} \cdot \dfrac{3}{2} = \dfrac{5 \cdot 3}{6 \cdot 2} = \dfrac{5 \cdot \cancel{3}}{\cancel{3} \cdot 2 \cdot 2} = \dfrac{5}{2 \cdot 2} = \dfrac{5}{4}$ Removing a factor equal to 1: $\frac{3}{3} = 1$

9. $\dfrac{7}{10} \div \left(-\dfrac{14}{15}\right) = \dfrac{7}{10} \cdot \left(-\dfrac{15}{14}\right) = \dfrac{\cancel{7} \cdot \cancel{5}(-3)}{2 \cdot \cancel{5} \cdot \cancel{7} \cdot 2} = \dfrac{-3}{4}$, or $-\dfrac{3}{4}$ Removing a factor equal to 1: $\frac{7 \cdot 5}{7 \cdot 5} = 1$

Remember, if you can't factor, you can't cancel!

Do Exercises 6–10.

Why do we multiply by a reciprocal when dividing? To see this, let's consider $\frac{2}{3} \div \frac{7}{5}$. We will multiply by 1. The name for 1 that we will use is $(5/7)/(5/7)$; it comes from the reciprocal of $\frac{7}{5}$.

$\dfrac{2}{3} \div \dfrac{7}{5} = \dfrac{\dfrac{2}{3}}{\dfrac{7}{5}}$ Writing fractional notation for the division

$= \dfrac{\dfrac{2}{3}}{\dfrac{7}{5}} \cdot 1$ Multiplying by 1

$= \dfrac{\dfrac{2}{3}}{\dfrac{7}{5}} \cdot \dfrac{\dfrac{5}{7}}{\dfrac{5}{7}}$ Multiplying by 1; $\frac{5}{7}$ is the reciprocal of $\frac{7}{5}$ and $\frac{\frac{5}{7}}{\frac{5}{7}} = 1$

$= \dfrac{\dfrac{2}{3} \cdot \dfrac{5}{7}}{\dfrac{7}{5} \cdot \dfrac{5}{7}}$ Multiplying the numerators and the denominators

$= \dfrac{\dfrac{2}{3} \cdot \dfrac{5}{7}}{1} = \dfrac{2}{3} \cdot \dfrac{5}{7} = \dfrac{10}{21}$ After we multiplied, we got 1 for the denominator. The numerator (in color) shows the multiplication by the reciprocal.

Do Exercise 11.

Answers on page A-8

Divide and simplify.

6. $\dfrac{6}{7} \div \dfrac{3}{4}$ $\dfrac{8}{7}$

7. $\left(-\dfrac{2}{3}\right) \div \dfrac{1}{4}$ $-\dfrac{8}{3}$

8. $\dfrac{4}{5} \div 8$ $\dfrac{1}{10}$

9. $60 \div \dfrac{3a}{5}$ $\dfrac{100}{a}$

10. $\dfrac{3}{5} \div \dfrac{-3}{5}$ -1

11. Divide by multiplying by 1:

$\dfrac{\dfrac{4}{5}}{\dfrac{6}{7}} \cdot \dfrac{14}{15}$

12. Each loop in a spring uses $\frac{3}{8}$ in. of wire. How many loops can be made from 120 in. of wire?

320

13. For a party, Jana made an 8-foot submarine sandwich. If one serving is $\frac{2}{3}$ ft, how many servings does Jana's sub contain?   12

Answers on page A-8

---

c   **Solving Problems**

Example 10   *Chemistry.* In a chemistry experiment, Lita needs to fill as many test tubes as possible with $\frac{3}{5}$ g of salt each. If she begins with 51 g of salt, how many test tubes can she fill?

1. Familiarize. We first make a drawing or at least visualize the situation. Repeated subtraction, or division, will work here.

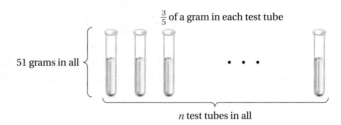

$\frac{3}{5}$ of a gram in each test tube

51 grams in all

n test tubes in all

We let $n =$ the number of test tubes that can be filled.

2. Translate. The problem can be translated to the following equation:

$$n = 51 \div \frac{3}{5}.$$

3. Solve. To solve the equation, we carry out the division:

$$n = 51 \div \frac{3}{5}$$

$$= 51 \cdot \frac{5}{3} \qquad \text{Multiplying by the reciprocal}$$

$$= \frac{51 \cdot 5}{1 \cdot 3}$$

$$= \frac{3 \cdot 17 \cdot 5}{1 \cdot 3}$$

$$= \frac{3}{3} \cdot \frac{17 \cdot 5}{1} \qquad \text{Identifying a factor equal to 1}$$

$$= 85. \qquad \text{Simplifying}$$

4. Check. If each of 85 test tubes contains $\frac{3}{5}$ g of salt, a total of

$$85 \cdot \frac{3}{5} = \frac{85 \cdot 3}{5} = \frac{\cancel{5} \cdot 17 \cdot 3}{\cancel{5}} = 17 \cdot 3,$$

or 51 g of salt is used. Since the problem states that Lita begins with 51 g, our answer checks.

5. State. Lita can fill 85 test tubes with salt.

Do Exercises 12 and 13.

Exercise Set 3.7

a Find the reciprocal.

1. $\dfrac{7}{3}$ $\dfrac{3}{7}$

2. $\dfrac{6}{5}$ $\dfrac{5}{6}$

3. 4 $\dfrac{1}{4}$

4. 7 $\dfrac{1}{7}$

5. $\dfrac{1}{6}$ 6

6. $\dfrac{1}{4}$ 4

7. $-\dfrac{10}{3}$ $-\dfrac{3}{10}$

8. $-\dfrac{12}{5}$ $-\dfrac{5}{12}$

9. $\dfrac{2}{21}$ $\dfrac{21}{2}$

10. $\dfrac{3}{28}$ $\dfrac{28}{3}$

11. $\dfrac{-3n}{m}$ $\dfrac{m}{-3n}$

12. $\dfrac{8t}{-7r}$ $\dfrac{-7r}{8t}$

13. $\dfrac{7}{-15}$ $\dfrac{-15}{7}$

14. $\dfrac{-6}{25}$ $\dfrac{25}{-6}$

15. $7m$ $\dfrac{1}{7m}$

16. $5n$ $\dfrac{1}{5n}$

b Divide. Don't forget to simplify when possible.

17. $\dfrac{3}{5} \div \dfrac{3}{4}$ $\dfrac{4}{5}$

18. $\dfrac{2}{3} \div \dfrac{3}{4}$ $\dfrac{8}{9}$

19. $\dfrac{7}{6} \div \dfrac{5}{-3}$ $-\dfrac{7}{10}$

20. $\dfrac{5}{3} \div \dfrac{4}{-9}$ $-\dfrac{15}{4}$

21. $\dfrac{4}{3} \div \dfrac{1}{3}$ 4

22. $\dfrac{10}{9} \div \dfrac{1}{2}$ $\dfrac{20}{9}$

23. $\left(-\dfrac{1}{3}\right) \div \dfrac{1}{6}$ -2

24. $\left(-\dfrac{1}{4}\right) \div \dfrac{1}{5}$ $-\dfrac{5}{4}$

25. $\dfrac{3}{8} \div 24$ $\dfrac{1}{64}$

26. $\dfrac{5}{6} \div 45$ $\dfrac{1}{54}$

27. $\dfrac{12}{7} \div (4x)$ $\dfrac{3}{7x}$

28. $\dfrac{18}{5} \div (2y)$ $\dfrac{9}{5y}$

29. $(-12) \div \dfrac{3}{2}$ -8

30. $(-24) \div \dfrac{3}{8}$ -64

31. $28 \div \dfrac{4}{5a}$ $35a$

32. $40 \div \dfrac{2}{3m}$ $60m$

33. $\left(-\dfrac{5}{8}\right) \div \left(-\dfrac{5}{8}\right)$ 1

34. $\left(-\dfrac{2}{5}\right) \div \left(-\dfrac{2}{5}\right)$ 1

35. $\dfrac{-8}{15} \div \dfrac{4}{5}$ $-\dfrac{2}{3}$

36. $\dfrac{6}{-13} \div \dfrac{3}{26}$ -4

37. $\dfrac{77}{64} \div \dfrac{49}{18}$ $\dfrac{99}{224}$

38. $\dfrac{81}{42} \div \dfrac{33}{56}$ $\dfrac{36}{11}$

39. $120a \div \dfrac{45}{14}$ $\dfrac{112a}{3}$

40. $360n \div \dfrac{27n}{8}$ $\dfrac{320}{3}$

Solve.

41. Benny uses $\frac{5}{4}$ g of toothpaste each time he brushes his teeth. How many times will Benny be able to brush his teeth with a 110-g tube of toothpaste?

88

42. Joy uses $\frac{1}{2}$ yd of dental floss each day. How long will a 45-yd container of dental floss last for Joy?

90 days

43. *Town Planning.* The Milton road crew repaves $\frac{1}{12}$ mi of road each day. How long will it take the crew to repave a $\frac{3}{4}$-mi stretch of road?   9 days

44. *Expenditures.* An airguard unit has \$9 million to spend on new helicopters. Each helicopter costs \$$\frac{3}{4}$ million. How many helicopters can be bought?

12

45. *Packaging.* Tina's Market prepackages Swiss cheese in $\frac{3}{4}$-lb packages. How many packages can be made from a 15-lb slab of cheese?   20

46. *Meal Planning.* Ian purchased 6 lb of cold cuts for a luncheon. If Ian is to allow $\frac{3}{8}$ lb per person, how many people can attend the luncheon?   16

47. *Gardening.* The Bingham community garden is to be split into 16 equally sized plots. If the garden occupies $\frac{3}{4}$ acre of land, how large will each plot be?

$\frac{3}{64}$ acre

48. *Art Supplies.* The Ferristown School District purchased $\frac{3}{4}$ T (ton) of clay. The clay is to be shared equally among the district's 6 art departments. How much will each art department receive? $\frac{1}{8}$ T

49. A piece of coaxial cable $\frac{3}{5}$ m long is to be cut into 6 pieces of the same length. What will be the length of each piece? $\frac{1}{10}$ m

50. A piece of speaker wire $\frac{4}{5}$ m long is to be cut into eight pieces of the same length. What will be the length of each piece? $\frac{1}{10}$ m

51. *Sewing.* A pair of basketball shorts requires $\frac{3}{4}$ yd of nylon. How many pairs of shorts can be made from 24 yd of the fabric?   32

52. *Sewing.* A child's shirt requires $\frac{5}{6}$ yd of cotton fabric. How many shirts can be made from 25 yd of the fabric?   30

53. *Knitting.* Brianna is knitting a sweater in which each stitch is $\frac{3}{8}$ in. long. How many stitches will Brianna need for a row that is 12 in. long?   32

54. *Knitting.* Gene is knitting a pair of socks in which each stitch is $\frac{5}{32}$ in. long. How many stitches will Gene need for a row that is 10 in. long?   64

Skill Maintenance

Multiply.

55. $(-17)(-30)$ [2.4a]   510

56. $(73)(-4)$ [2.4a] -292

Evaluate each of the following.

57. x^3, for $x = 3$ and $x = -3$ [2.6a]   27; -27

58. $5x^2$, for $x = 4$ and $x = -4$ [2.6a]   80; 80

59. $3x^2$, for $x = 7$ and $x = -7$ [2.6a]   147; 147

60. x^3, for $x = 7$ and $x = -7$ [2.6a]   343; -343

Synthesis

61. ◆ A student incorrectly insists that $\frac{2}{5} \div \frac{3}{4}$ is $\frac{15}{8}$. What mistake is the student probably making?

62. ◆ Write a problem for a classmate to solve. Devise the problem so that the solution requires the classmate to divide by a fraction. Arrange for the solution to be "The contents of the barrel will fill 40 bags with $\frac{3}{4}$ lb in each bag."

63. ◈ Without performing the division, explain why $5 \div \frac{1}{7}$ is a bigger number than $5 \div \frac{2}{3}$.

Simplify.

64. $\left(\dfrac{9}{10} \div \dfrac{2}{5} \div \dfrac{3}{8} \right)^2$ 36

65. $\dfrac{\left(-\dfrac{3}{7} \right)^2 \div \dfrac{12}{5}}{\left(\dfrac{-2}{9} \right)\left(\dfrac{9}{2} \right)}$ $-\dfrac{15}{196}$

66. $\left(\dfrac{14}{15} \div \dfrac{49}{65} \cdot \dfrac{77}{260} \right)^2$ $\dfrac{121}{900}$

67. $\left(\dfrac{10}{9} \right)^2 \div \dfrac{35}{27} \cdot \dfrac{49}{44}$ $\dfrac{35}{33}$

Simplify. Use the list of prime numbers on p. 154.

68. ▦ $\dfrac{711}{1957} \div \dfrac{10,033}{13,081}$ $\dfrac{9}{19}$

69. ▦ $\dfrac{8633}{7387} \div \dfrac{485}{581}$ $\dfrac{7}{5}$

3.8 Solving Equations: The Multiplication Principle

In Sections 1.7 and 2.8, we learned to solve an equation involving multiplication by dividing on both sides. With fractional notation, we can solve the same type of equation by using multiplication.

a   The Multiplication Principle

We have seen that to divide by a fraction, we multiply by the reciprocal of that fraction. This suggests that we restate the division principle in its more common form—the multiplication principle.

> **THE MULTIPLICATION PRINCIPLE**
>
> For any numbers a, b, and c, with $c \neq 0$,
> $$a = b \quad \text{is equivalent to} \quad a \cdot c = b \cdot c.$$

Example 1   Solve: $\frac{3}{4}x = 15$.

We can multiply by any nonzero number on both sides to produce an equivalent equation. Since we are looking for an equation of the form $1x = \blacksquare$, we multiply by the reciprocal of $\frac{3}{4}$ on both sides.

$$\frac{3}{4}x = 15$$

$$\frac{4}{3} \cdot \frac{3}{4}x = \frac{4}{3} \cdot 15 \qquad \text{Using the multiplication principle; note that } \tfrac{4}{3} \text{ is the reciprocal of } \tfrac{3}{4}.$$

$$\left(\frac{4}{3} \cdot \frac{3}{4}\right)x = \frac{4 \cdot 15}{3} \qquad \text{Using an associative law; try to do this mentally.}$$

$$1x = 20 \qquad \text{Multiplying; note that } \frac{4 \cdot 15}{3} = \frac{4 \cdot \cancel{3} \cdot 5}{\cancel{3}}.$$

$$x = 20 \qquad \text{Remember that } 1x \text{ is } x.$$

To confirm that 20 is the solution, we perform a check.

CHECK:
$$\frac{3}{4}x = 15$$
$$\frac{3}{4} \cdot 20 \;?\; 15$$
$$\frac{3 \cdot \cancel{4} \cdot 5}{\cancel{4}} \qquad \text{Removing a factor equal to 1: } \frac{4}{4} = 1$$
$$3 \cdot 5 \;\bigg|\; 15 \quad \text{TRUE}$$

The solution is 20.

Note that using the multiplication principle to multiply by $\frac{4}{3}$ on both sides is the same as using the division principle to divide by $\frac{3}{4}$ on both sides.

Do Exercises 1 and 2.

Objectives

a Use the multiplication principle to solve equations.

For Extra Help

TAPE 6   InterAct math   CD-ROM
            MAC
            WIN

Solve.

1. $\frac{2}{3}x = 10$ 15

2. $\frac{2}{7}a = -8$ -28

Answers on page A-8

Solve.

3. $-\dfrac{9}{8} = 4x$ $-\dfrac{9}{32}$

4. $-\dfrac{6}{7}a = \dfrac{9}{14}$ $-\dfrac{3}{4}$

In an expression like $\frac{3}{4}x$, the constant factor—in this case, $\frac{3}{4}$—is called the **coefficient**. In Example 1, we multiplied on both sides by $\frac{4}{3}$, the reciprocal of the coefficient of x.

Example 2   Solve: $5a = -\dfrac{7}{3}$.

We have

$$5a = -\frac{7}{3}$$

$$\frac{1}{5} \cdot 5a = \frac{1}{5} \cdot \left(-\frac{7}{3}\right) \qquad \text{Multiplying by } \tfrac{1}{5}, \text{ the reciprocal of 5, on both sides}$$

$$1a = -\frac{1 \cdot 7}{5 \cdot 3}$$

$$a = -\frac{7}{15}.$$

CHECK:
$$5a = -\frac{7}{3}$$

$$5\left(-\frac{7}{15}\right) \; \overset{?}{\vert} \; -\frac{7}{3}$$

$$-\frac{\cancel{5} \cdot 7}{\cancel{5} \cdot 3}$$

$$-\frac{7}{3} \; \bigg\vert \; -\frac{7}{3} \qquad \text{TRUE}$$

The solution is $-\dfrac{7}{15}$.

Example 3   Solve: $\dfrac{10}{3} = -\dfrac{4}{9}x$.

We have

$$\frac{10}{3} = -\frac{4}{9}x$$

$$-\frac{9}{4} \cdot \frac{10}{3} = -\frac{9}{4} \cdot \left(-\frac{4}{9}\right)x \qquad \text{The reciprocal of } -\tfrac{4}{9} \text{ is } -\tfrac{9}{4}.$$

$$-\frac{3 \cdot 3 \cdot 2 \cdot 5}{2 \cdot 2 \cdot 3} = x$$

$$-\frac{15}{2} = x. \qquad \text{Removing a factor equal to 1: } \frac{3 \cdot 2}{2 \cdot 3} = 1$$

We leave the check to the student. The solution is $-\dfrac{15}{2}$.

Do Exercises 3 and 4.

Exercise Set 3.8

a Use the multiplication principle to solve each equation. Don't forget to check!

1. $\dfrac{8}{5}x = 16$ 10

2. $\dfrac{4}{3}x = 20$ 15

3. $\dfrac{7}{3}a = 21$ 9

4. $\dfrac{4}{5}a = 24$ 30

5. $\dfrac{3}{7}x = -18$ -42

6. $\dfrac{3}{8}x = -21$ -56

7. $6a = \dfrac{12}{17}$ $\dfrac{2}{17}$

8. $3a = \dfrac{15}{14}$ $\dfrac{5}{14}$

9. $\dfrac{3}{5}x = \dfrac{2}{7}$ $\dfrac{10}{21}$

10. $\dfrac{3}{7}x = \dfrac{1}{4}$ $\dfrac{7}{12}$

11. $\dfrac{3}{2}t = -\dfrac{8}{7}$ $-\dfrac{16}{21}$

12. $\dfrac{4}{3}t = -\dfrac{5}{2}$ $-\dfrac{15}{8}$

13. $\dfrac{4}{5} = -10a$ $-\dfrac{2}{25}$

14. $\dfrac{6}{5} = -12a$ $-\dfrac{1}{10}$

15. $\dfrac{9}{5}x = \dfrac{3}{10}$ $\dfrac{1}{6}$

16. $\dfrac{10}{3}x = \dfrac{8}{15}$ $\dfrac{4}{25}$

17. $-\dfrac{3}{10}x = 8$ $-\dfrac{80}{3}$

18. $-\dfrac{2}{11}x = 5$ $-\dfrac{55}{2}$

19. $a \cdot \dfrac{9}{7} = -\dfrac{3}{14}$ $-\dfrac{1}{6}$

20. $a \cdot \dfrac{9}{4} = -\dfrac{3}{10}$ $-\dfrac{2}{15}$

21. $-x = \dfrac{9}{13}$ $-\dfrac{9}{13}$

22. $-x = \dfrac{7}{11}$ $-\dfrac{7}{11}$

23. $-x = -\dfrac{27}{31}$ $\dfrac{27}{31}$

24. $-x = -\dfrac{35}{39}$ $\dfrac{35}{39}$

25. $7t = 5$ $\dfrac{5}{7}$

26. $-6t = 1$ $-\dfrac{1}{6}$

27. $-24 = -10a$ $\dfrac{12}{5}$

28. $-18 = -20a$ $\dfrac{9}{10}$

29. $-\dfrac{15}{7} = \dfrac{3}{2}t$ $-\dfrac{10}{7}$

30. $-\dfrac{14}{9} = \dfrac{10}{3}t$ $-\dfrac{7}{15}$

31. $x \cdot \dfrac{5}{16} = \dfrac{15}{14}$ $\dfrac{24}{7}$

32. $x \cdot \dfrac{4}{15} = \dfrac{12}{25}$ $\dfrac{9}{5}$

33. $-\dfrac{3}{20}x = -\dfrac{21}{10}$ 14

34. $-\dfrac{7}{25}x = -\dfrac{21}{10}$ $\dfrac{15}{2}$

35. $-\dfrac{25}{17} = -\dfrac{35}{34}a$ $\dfrac{10}{7}$

36. $-\dfrac{49}{45} = -\dfrac{28}{27}a$ $\dfrac{21}{20}$

Skill Maintenance

Simplify.

37. $36 \div (-3)^2 \times (7 - 2)$ [2.5b]   20

38. $(-37 - 12 + 1) \div (-2)^3$ [2.5b]   6

Form an equivalent expression by combining like terms.

39. $13x + 4x$ [2.7b] $17x$

40. $9a - 5a$ [2.7b] $4a$

41. $2a + 3 + 5a$ [2.7b] $7a + 3$

42. $3x - 7 + x$ [2.7b] $4x - 7$

Synthesis

43. ◈ Does the multiplication principle enable us to solve any equations that could not have been solved with the division principle? Why or why not?

44. ◈ Example 1 was solved by multiplying by $\frac{4}{3}$ on both sides of the equation. Could we have divided by $\frac{3}{4}$ on both sides instead? Why or why not?

45. ◈ Can the multiplication principle be used to solve equations like $7x = 63$? Why or why not?

Solve.

46. $2x - 7x = -\dfrac{10}{9}$ $\dfrac{2}{9}$

47. $\left(-\dfrac{4}{7}\right)^2 = \left(\dfrac{2^3 - 9}{3}\right)^3 x$ $-\dfrac{432}{49}$

Solve using the five-step problem-solving approach.

48. After driving 180 km, $\frac{5}{8}$ of a trip is completed. How long is the total trip? How many kilometers are left to drive?   288 km; 108 km

49. After driving 240 km, $\frac{3}{5}$ of a trip is completed. How long is the total trip? How many kilometers are left to drive?   400 km; 160 km

50. A package of coffee beans weighed $\frac{21}{32}$ lb when it was $\frac{3}{4}$ full. How much could the package hold when completely filled? $\dfrac{7}{8}$ lb

51. After swimming $\frac{2}{7}$ mi, Katie had swum $\frac{3}{4}$ of the race. How long a race was Katie competing in? $\dfrac{8}{21}$ mi

52. A brick of Swiss cheese is 14 in. long. How many slices will it yield if half of the brick is cut by a slicer set for $\frac{3}{32}$-in. slices and half is cut by a slicer set for $\frac{3}{64}$-in. slices?   225

Summary and Review: Chapter 3

Important Properties and Formulas

$\dfrac{0}{n} = 0$, *for* $n \neq 0$; $\dfrac{n}{0}$ *is undefined*; $\dfrac{n}{1} = n$; $\dfrac{n}{n} = 1$, *for* $n \neq 1$

Area of a Rectangle: $A = l \cdot w$

Area of a Triangle: $A = \dfrac{1}{2} \cdot b \cdot h$

The Multiplication Principle: For $c \neq 0$, $a = b$ is equivalent to $a \cdot c = b \cdot c$.

Review Exercises

1. Determine whether 4232 is divisible by 6. Do not use long division.   [3.1b]

2. Determine whether 784 is divisible by 5. Do not use long division.   [3.1b]

3. Determine whether 4347 is divisible by 9. Do not use long division.   [3.1b]

Find the prime factorization of each number.   [3.2c]

4. 70   5. 72   6. 150

7. Determine whether 37 is prime, composite, or neither.   [3.2b]

8. Identify the numerator and the denominator of $\dfrac{9}{7}$.   [3.3a]

What part is shaded?   [3.3b]

9. 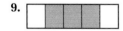   10.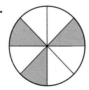

Simplify, if possible. Assume that all variables are nonzero.

11. $\dfrac{0}{4}$ [3.3c]   12. $\dfrac{23}{23}$ [3.3c]

13. $\dfrac{48}{1}$ [3.3c]   14. $\dfrac{7x}{7x}$ [3.3c]

15. $-\dfrac{10}{15}$ [3.5b]   16. $\dfrac{7}{28}$ [3.5b]

17. $\dfrac{-21}{21}$ [3.5b]   18. $\dfrac{9m}{12m}$ [3.5b]

19. $\dfrac{12}{30}$ [3.5b]   20. $\dfrac{-27}{0}$ [3.3c]

21. $\dfrac{9n}{1}$ [3.3c]   22. $\dfrac{-9}{-27}$ [3.5b]

Find an equivalent expression for the given number, but with the denominator indicated. Use multiplication by 1.   [3.5a]

23. $\dfrac{5}{7} = \dfrac{?}{21}$ 24. $\dfrac{-6}{11} = \dfrac{?}{55}$

Find the reciprocal of each number.   [3.7a]

25. $\dfrac{5}{9}$ 26. -7

27. $\dfrac{1}{8}$ 28. $\dfrac{3x}{5y}$

Perform the indicated operation and, if possible, simplify.

29. $\dfrac{2}{7} \cdot \dfrac{3}{5}$ [3.4b]

30. $\dfrac{4}{x} \cdot \dfrac{y}{9}$ [3.4b]

31. $\dfrac{3}{4} \cdot \dfrac{8}{9}$ [3.6a]

32. $-\dfrac{5}{7} \cdot \dfrac{1}{10}$ [3.6a]

33. $\dfrac{3a}{10} \cdot \dfrac{2}{15a}$ [3.6a]

34. $\dfrac{4a}{7} \cdot \dfrac{7}{4a}$ [3.6a]

35. $6 \div \dfrac{5}{3}$ [3.7b]

36. $\dfrac{3}{14} \div \dfrac{6}{7}$ [3.7b]

37. $180 \div \dfrac{3}{5}$ [3.7b]

38. $-\dfrac{5}{36} \div \left(-\dfrac{25}{12}\right)$ [3.7b]

39. $14 \div \dfrac{7}{2a}$ [3.7b]

40. $-\dfrac{23}{25} \div \dfrac{23}{25}$ [3.7b]

Solve.

41. The Mulligans have driven $\frac{4}{5}$ of a 275-mi trip. How far have they driven?   [3.6b]

42. A recipe calls for $\frac{3}{4}$ cup of sugar. In making $\frac{1}{2}$ of this recipe, how much sugar should be used?   [3.6b]

43. The Winchester swim team has 4 swimmers in a $\frac{2}{3}$-mi relay race. How far will each person swim?   [3.7c]

44. How many $\frac{2}{3}$-cup cereal bowls can be filled from 12 cups of cornflakes?   [3.7c]

Find the area.   [3.6b]

45.

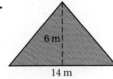

6 m

14 m

46.

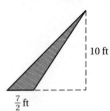

10 ft

$\frac{7}{2}$ ft

Solve.   [3.8a]

47. $\dfrac{2}{3}x = 160$

48. $\dfrac{3}{8} = -\dfrac{5}{4}t$

Skill Maintenance

49. Solve: $17 \cdot x = 408$.   [1.7b], [2.8b]

50. Simplify: $20 \div 2 \cdot 2 - 3^2$.   [1.9c]

51. Add: $(-798) + 812$.   [2.2a]

52. Multiply: $-3 \cdot (-9)$.   [2.4a]

Synthesis

53. ◈ Write in your own words a series of steps that can be used when simplifying fractional notation. [3.5b]

54. ◈ A student claims that $\frac{20}{80}$ simplifies to $\frac{2}{8}$. Is the student correct? Why or why not?   [3.5b]

55. ▦ Use a calculator and the list of prime numbers on p. 154 to find simplified fractional notation for the solution of   [3.8a]

$$\dfrac{1751}{267}x = \dfrac{3193}{2759}.$$

56. Simplify: $\dfrac{15x}{14z} \cdot \dfrac{17yz}{35xy} \div \left(-\dfrac{3}{7}\right)^2$.   [3.6a], [3.7b]

57. What digit(s) could be inserted in the ones place to make 574__ divisible by 6?   [3.1b]

Test: Chapter 3

1. Determine whether 4782 is divisible by 3. Do not use long division.

2. Determine whether 5478 is divisible by 5. Do not use long division.

Find the prime factorization of each number.

3. 36

4. 60

5. Determine whether 49 is prime, composite, or neither.

6. Identify the numerator and the denominator of $\frac{4}{9}$.

7. What part is shaded?

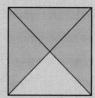

Simplify, if possible. Assume that all variables are nonzero.

8. $\frac{26}{1}$

9. $\frac{-12}{-12}$

10. $\frac{0}{16}$

11. $\frac{-8}{24}$

12. $\frac{5x}{45x}$

13. $\frac{2}{28}$

14. Find an equivalent expression for $\frac{3}{8}$ with a denominator of 40.

Find the reciprocal.

15. $\frac{x}{27}$

16. -9

Perform the indicated operation. Simplify, if possible.

17. $\frac{5}{9} \cdot \frac{7}{2}$

18. $\frac{7}{11} \div \frac{3}{4}$

19. $3 \cdot \frac{x}{8}$

20. $[3.7b]$ $-\frac{98}{3}$

21. $[3.6a]$ $\frac{6}{65}$

22. $[3.7c]$ $\frac{3}{20}$ lb

23. $[3.6b]$ 125 lb

24. $[3.8a]$ 64

25. $[3.8a]$ $-\frac{7}{4}$

26. $[3.6b]$ $\frac{91}{2}$ m²

27. $[1.9c]$ 41

28. $[1.7b]$, $[2.8b]$ 101

29. $[2.2a]$ -167

30. $[2.4a]$ 63

31. $[3.6b]$ $\frac{15}{8}$ tsp

32. $[3.6b]$ $\frac{7}{48}$ acre

33. $[3.6a]$, $[3.7b]$ $-\frac{7}{960}$

34. $[3.8a]$ $\frac{7}{5}$

20. $28 \div \left(-\frac{6}{7}\right)$

21. $\frac{4a}{13} \cdot \frac{9b}{30ab}$

Solve.

22. A $\frac{3}{4}$-lb slab of cheese is shared equally by 5 people. How much does each person receive?

23. Monroe weighs $\frac{5}{7}$ of his dad's weight. If his dad weighs 175 lb, how much does Monroe weigh?

24. $\frac{7}{8} \cdot x = 56$

25. $\frac{7}{10} = \frac{-2}{5} \cdot t$

26. Find the area.

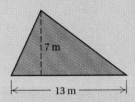

Skill Maintenance

27. Simplify: $3^2 + 2(1 + 3)^2$.

28. Solve: $47 \cdot t = 4747$.

29. Add: $(-93) + (-74)$.

30. Simplify: $(-9)(-7)$.

Synthesis

31. A recipe for a batch of buttermilk pancakes calls for $\frac{3}{4}$ teaspoon (tsp) of salt. Jacqueline plans to cut the amount of salt in half for each of 5 batches of pancakes. How much salt will she need altogether?

32. Grandma Phyllis left $\frac{2}{3}$ of her $\frac{7}{8}$-acre tree farm to Karl. Karl gave $\frac{1}{4}$ of his share to his oldest daughter, Irene. How much land did Irene receive?

33. Simplify: $\left(-\frac{3}{8}\right)^2 \div \frac{6}{7} \cdot \frac{2}{9} \div (-5)$.

34. Solve: $\frac{33}{38} \cdot \frac{34}{55} = \frac{17}{35} \cdot \frac{15}{19}x$.

Cumulative Review: Chapters 1–3

1. Write a word name: 2,056,783.

Add.

2. $\begin{array}{r} 2{,}7\ 3\ 9 \\ +\ 8{,}2\ 4\ 3 \\ \hline \end{array}$

3. $-29 + (-14)$

4. $-45 + 12$

Subtract.

5. $\begin{array}{r} 4{,}3\ 2\ 4 \\ -\ 2{,}1\ 9\ 5 \\ \hline \end{array}$

6. $17 - 40$

7. $-12 - (-4)$

Multiply and simplify.

8. $\begin{array}{r} 7\ 3\ 5 \\ \times\quad 2\ 3 \\ \hline \end{array}$

9. $-52 \cdot 6$

10. $\dfrac{6}{7} \cdot (-35x)$

11. $\dfrac{2}{9} \cdot \dfrac{21}{10}$

Divide and simplify.

12. $1\ 3\ \overline{)\ 3\ 0\ 5\ 8}$

13. $-85 \div 5$

14. $-16 \div \dfrac{4}{7}$

15. $\dfrac{3}{7} \div \dfrac{9}{14}$

16. Round 4514 to the nearest ten.

17. Estimate the product by rounding to the nearest hundred. Show your work.

$\begin{array}{r} 9\ 2\ 1 \\ \times\ 4\ 5\ 3 \\ \hline \end{array}$

18. Find the absolute value: $|879|$.

19. Simplify: $10^2 \div 5(-2) - 8(2 - 8)$.

20. Determine whether 98 is prime, composite, or neither.

21. Evaluate $a - b^2$ for $a = -5$ and $b = 4$.

Solve.

22. $a + 24 = 49$

23. $7x = 63$

24. $\dfrac{2}{9} \cdot a = -10$

25. A 1996 van that gets 25 miles per gallon is traded in toward a 1999 truck that gets 17 miles per gallon. How many more miles per gallon did the older vehicle get?

26. A 64-oz soda is poured into 8 glasses. How much will each glass hold if the soda is poured out evenly?

Combine like terms.

27. $9 - 5x - 13 + 7x$

28. $-12x + 7y + 15x$

Simplify, if possible.

29. $\dfrac{97}{97}$

30. $\dfrac{59}{1}$

31. $\dfrac{0}{72}$

32. $\dfrac{-10}{54}$

Find the reciprocal.

33. $\dfrac{2}{5}$

34. 17

35. Find an equivalent expression for $\frac{3}{10}$ with a denominator of 70. Use multiplying by 1.

36. A babysitter earns \$60 for working a full day. How much is earned for working $\frac{3}{5}$ of a day?

37. How many $\frac{3}{4}$-lb servings can be made from a 9-lb roast?

38. Tony has jogged $\frac{2}{3}$ of a course that is $\frac{9}{10}$ of a mile long. How far has Tony gone?

Synthesis

39. Evaluate $\dfrac{ab}{c}$ for $a = -\dfrac{2}{5}$, $b = \dfrac{10}{13}$, and $c = \dfrac{26}{27}$.

40. Evaluate $-|xy|^2$ for $x = -\dfrac{3}{5}$ and $y = \dfrac{1}{2}$.

41. Wayne and Patty each earn \$85 a day, while Janet earns \$90 a day. They decide to pool their earnings from three days and spend $\frac{2}{5}$ of that on entertainment and save the rest. How much will Wayne, Patty, and Janet end up saving?

4

Fractional Notation: Addition and Subtraction

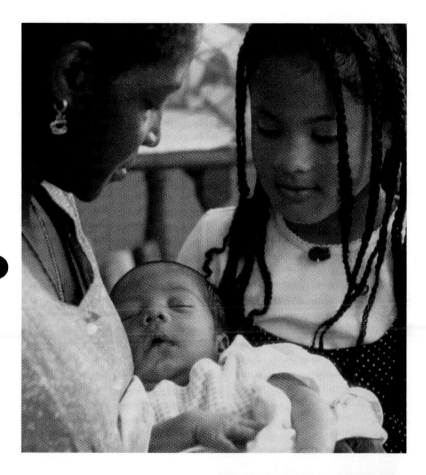

An Application

Melody has had three children. Their birth weights were $7\frac{1}{2}$ lb, $7\frac{3}{4}$ lb, and $6\frac{3}{4}$ lb. What was the average weight of her babies?

This problem appears as Example 12 in Section 4.7.

The Mathematics

We let w = the average weight, in pounds, of the babies. The problem then translates to

$$w = \frac{7\frac{1}{2} + 7\frac{3}{4} + 6\frac{3}{4}}{3}.$$

Operations using mixed numerals occur often in problem solving.

Introduction

In this chapter, we consider addition and subtraction using fractional notation. We then examine addition, subtraction, multiplication, and division using mixed numerals. These operations are then applied to the solution of equations and problems.

World Wide Web   For more information, visit us at www.mathmax.com

Pretest: Chapter 4

1. Find the least common multiple of 25 and 15.

2. Use < or > for ▊ to write a true sentence.

$$\frac{7}{9} \ \blacksquare\ \frac{4}{5}.$$

Perform the indicated operation and, if possible, simplify.

3. $\dfrac{-5}{8} + \dfrac{3}{8}$

4. $\dfrac{5}{6} + \dfrac{-7}{9} + \dfrac{1}{15}$

5. $\dfrac{2}{5} - \dfrac{1}{7}$

6. Convert to fractional notation: $5\dfrac{3}{8}$.

7. Convert to a mixed numeral: $\dfrac{13}{4}$.

8. Divide. Write a mixed numeral for the answer.

$$1\,2\,\overline{)\,4\,7\,8\,9}$$

9. Subtract. Write a mixed numeral for the answer.

$$\begin{array}{r} 14\dfrac{1}{5} \\[2mm] -\ 7\dfrac{5}{6} \\ \hline \end{array}$$

Solve.

10. $\dfrac{2}{3} + x = \dfrac{8}{9}$

11. $14 = \dfrac{2}{3}x + 20$

Perform the indicated operations. Write a mixed numeral for each answer.

12. $(-5)\left(-3\dfrac{8}{11}\right)$

13. $6\dfrac{1}{3} \cdot 5\dfrac{3}{4}$

14. $45 \div \left(-5\dfrac{5}{6}\right)$

15. $4\dfrac{5}{12} \div 3\dfrac{1}{4}$

16. Evaluate $xy \div z$ for $x = 3\dfrac{2}{5}$, $y = 6$, and $z = 2\dfrac{1}{3}$.

Solve.

17. The Colburn Inn bought 60 lb of onions and used $21\dfrac{3}{4}$ lb. How many pounds were left?

18. Water weighs $62\dfrac{1}{2}$ lb per cubic foot. How many cubic feet does $265\dfrac{5}{8}$ lb of water occupy?

19. On a trip, Janet averaged $315\dfrac{1}{2}$ miles per day for 5 days. How far did she travel altogether in those 5 days?

20. Uri is baking a birthday cake that requires $3\dfrac{3}{4}$ cups of flour and a batch of biscotti that requires $2\dfrac{1}{2}$ cups. How much flour is required altogether?

4.1 Least Common Multiples

In this chapter, we study addition and subtraction using fractional notation. Suppose we want to add $\frac{2}{3}$ and $\frac{1}{2}$. To do so, we use the least common multiple of the denominators: $\frac{2}{3} + \frac{1}{2} = \frac{4}{6} + \frac{3}{6}$. Then we add the numerators and keep the common denominator, 6. Before we do this, though, we study finding the **least common denominator (LCD),** or **least common multiple (LCM),** of the denominators.

a | Finding Least Common Multiples

> The **least common multiple,** or LCM, of two natural numbers is the smallest number that is a multiple of both.

Example 1 Find the LCM of 20 and 30.

a) First list some multiples of 20 by multiplying 20 by 1, 2, 3, and so on:

   20, 40, 60, 80, 100, 120, 140, 160, 180, 200, 220, 240, ...

b) Then list some multiples of 30 by multiplying 30 by 1, 2, 3, and so on:

   30, 60, 90, 120, 150, 180, 210, 240, ...

c) Now list the numbers *common* to both lists, the common multiples:

   60, 120, 180, 240, ...

d) These are the common multiples of 20 and 30. The *least* of these common multiples is 60. Thus the LCM of 20 and 30 is 60.

Do Exercises 1 and 2.

Next we develop two methods that are more efficient for finding LCMs. You may choose to learn either method (consult with your instructor), or both, but if you are going on to study algebra, you should definitely learn Method 2.

Method 1: Finding LCMs Using One List of Multiples

> *Method 1.* To find the LCM of a set of numbers (say, 9 and 12), determine whether the largest number is a multiple of the other(s):
>
> **1.** If it is, it is the LCM.
>
>   (Since 12 is not a multiple of 9, the LCM is not 12.)
>
> **2.** If the largest number *is not* a multiple of the other(s), check consecutive multiples of the largest number until you find one that *is a* multiple of the other number(s). That number is the LCM.
>
>   ($2 \cdot 12 = 24$, but 24 is not a multiple of 9.)
>
>   ($3 \cdot 12 = 36$, and 36 *is* a multiple of 9, so the LCM of 9 and 12 is 36.)

Objective

a Find the LCM of two or more numbers from a list of multiples or by using prime factorizations.

For Extra Help

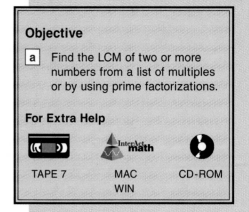

TAPE 7   MAC   CD-ROM
               WIN

1. By examining lists of multiples, find the LCM of 9 and 15. 45

2. By examining lists of multiples, find the LCM of 8 and 10. 40

Answer on page A-9

3. 6, 9   18

Example 2   Find the LCM of 12 and 15.

  1. 15 is the larger number, but it is not a multiple of 12.

  2. Check multiples of 15:

$$2 \cdot 15 = 30, \qquad \text{Not a multiple of 12}$$
$$3 \cdot 15 = 45, \qquad \text{Not a multiple of 12}$$
$$4 \cdot 15 = 60. \qquad \text{A multiple of 12}$$

The LCM = 60.

Example 3   Find the LCM of 4 and 14.

  1. 14 is the larger number, but it is not a multiple of 4.

  2. Check multiples of 14:

$$2 \cdot 14 = 28. \qquad \text{A multiple of 4}$$

The LCM = 28.

4. 6, 8   24

Do Exercises 3 and 4.

Example 4   Find the LCM of 8 and 32.

  1. 32 is the larger number and 32 is a multiple of 8, so it is the LCM.

The LCM = 32.

Example 5   Find the LCM of 10, 100, and 250.

  1. 250 is the largest number, but it is not a multiple of 100.

  2. Check multiples of 250:

$$2 \cdot 250 = 500. \qquad \text{A multiple of 10 and 100}$$

The LCM = 500.

Find the LCM.

5. 5, 10   10

Do Exercises 5 and 6.

Method 2: Finding LCMs Using Factorizations

A second method for finding LCMs uses prime factorizations. Consider again 20 and 30. Their prime factorizations are

$$20 = 2 \cdot 2 \cdot 5 \quad \text{and} \quad 30 = 2 \cdot 3 \cdot 5.$$

The least common multiple must include the factors of each number, so it must include each prime factor the greatest number of times that it appears in either of the factorizations. To find the LCM for 20 and 30, we select one factorization, say,

$$2 \cdot 2 \cdot 5,$$

and note that because it lacks the factor 3, it does not contain the entire factorization of 30. If we multiply $2 \cdot 2 \cdot 5$ by 3, every prime factor occurs just often enough to contain both 20 and 30 as factors.

6. 20, 40, 50   200

$$\text{LCM} = 2 \cdot 2 \cdot 5 \cdot 3$$

20 is a factor of the LCM.

30 is a factor of the LCM.

Note that each prime factor is used the greatest number of times that it occurs in either of the individual factorizations.

Answers on page A-9

Method 2. To find the LCM of a set of numbers (say, 9 and 12):

1. Write the prime factorization of each number.

$(9 = 3 \cdot 3; 12 = 2 \cdot 2 \cdot 3)$

2. Select one of the factorizations and see whether it contains the other(s).

$(2 \cdot 2 \cdot 3$ does not contain $3 \cdot 3.)$

a) If it does, it represents the LCM.

b) If it does not, multiply that factorization by those prime factors of the other number(s) that it lacks. The final product is the LCM.

$(2 \cdot 2 \cdot 3 \cdot 3$ is the LCM.)

3. As a check, make sure that the LCM includes each factor the greatest number of times that it occurs in any one factorization.

Example 6   Find the LCM of 18 and 21.

1. We begin by writing the prime factorization of each number:

$18 = 2 \cdot 3 \cdot 3$ and $21 = 3 \cdot 7.$

2. a) We inspect the factorization $2 \cdot 3 \cdot 3$ and note that it does not contain the other factorization, $3 \cdot 7$.

b) To find the LCM of 18 and 21, we multiply $2 \cdot 3 \cdot 3$ by the factor of 21 that it lacks, 7:

$$\text{LCM} = 2 \cdot 3 \cdot 3 \cdot 7.$$

18 is a factor.

21 is a factor.

3. The greatest number of times that 2 occurs as a factor of 18 or 21 is **one** time; the greatest number of times that 3 occurs as a factor of 18 or 21 is **two** times; and the greatest number of times that 7 occurs as a factor of 18 or 21 is **one** time. To check, note that the LCM has exactly **one** 2, **two** 3's, and **one** 7. The LCM is $2 \cdot 3 \cdot 3 \cdot 7$, or 126.

Example 7   Find the LCM of 24 and 36.

1. We begin by writing the prime factorization of each number:

$24 = 2 \cdot 2 \cdot 2 \cdot 3$ and $36 = 2 \cdot 2 \cdot 3 \cdot 3.$

2. a) The factorization $2 \cdot 2 \cdot 2 \cdot 3$ does not contain the factorization $2 \cdot 2 \cdot 3 \cdot 3$. Nor does $2 \cdot 2 \cdot 3 \cdot 3$ contain $2 \cdot 2 \cdot 2 \cdot 3$.

b) To find the LCM of 24 and 36, we multiply the factorization of 24, $2 \cdot 2 \cdot 2 \cdot 3$, by any prime factors of 36 that are lacking. In this case, a second factor of 3 is needed. We have

$$\text{LCM} = 2 \cdot 2 \cdot 2 \cdot 3 \cdot 3.$$

24 is a factor.

36 is a factor.

3. To check, note that 2 and 3 appear in the LCM the greatest number of times that each appears as a factor of 24 or 36. The LCM is

$2 \cdot 2 \cdot 2 \cdot 3 \cdot 3$,   or   72.

Do Exercises 7 and 8.

Answers on page A-9

Find the LCM.

9. 3, 18   18

10. 12, 24   24

11. 24, 35, 45   2520

Find the LCM.

12. xy, yz xyz

13. $5a^2$, a^3b $5a^3b$

Answers on page A-9

Example 8 Find the LCM of 7 and 21.

1. Because 7 is prime, we think of $7 = 7$ as a "factorization" in order to carry out our procedure:

$$7 = 7 \quad \text{and} \quad 21 = 3 \cdot 7.$$

2. One factorization, $3 \cdot 7$, contains the other. Thus the LCM is $3 \cdot 7$, or 21.

Example 9 Find the LCM of 27, 90, and 84.

1. We first find the prime factorization of each number:

$$27 = 3 \cdot 3 \cdot 3, \qquad 90 = 2 \cdot 3 \cdot 3 \cdot 5, \quad \text{and} \quad 84 = 2 \cdot 2 \cdot 3 \cdot 7.$$

2. a) No one factorization contains the other two.

b) We begin with the factorization of 90, $2 \cdot 3 \cdot 3 \cdot 5$ (we could have used any factorization listed). Since 27 contains a third factor of 3, we multiply by another factor of 3:

$$2 \cdot 3 \cdot 3 \cdot 5 \cdot 3.$$

— 90 is a factor.
— 27 is a factor.

Next, we multiply $2 \cdot 3 \cdot 3 \cdot 5 \cdot 3$ by the factors of 84 still missing, $2 \cdot 7$:

$$2 \cdot 3 \cdot 3 \cdot 5 \cdot 3 \cdot 2 \cdot 7.$$

— 90 and 27 are factors.
— 84 is a factor.

The LCM is $2 \cdot 3 \cdot 3 \cdot 5 \cdot 3 \cdot 2 \cdot 7$, or 3780.

3. The check is left to the student.

Do Exercises 9–11.

Exponential notation is often helpful when writing least common multiples. Let's reconsider Example 7:

$$24 = 2 \cdot 2 \cdot 2 \cdot 3 = 2^3 \cdot 3^1;$$
$$36 = 2 \cdot 2 \cdot 3 \cdot 3 = 2^2 \cdot 3^2;$$
$$\text{LCM} = 2 \cdot 2 \cdot 2 \cdot 3 \cdot 3 = 2^3 \cdot 3^2, \text{ or } 72.$$

Note that in the factorizations of 24 and 36, the largest power of 2 is 2^3 and the largest power of 3 is 3^2. These powers are used to create the LCM, $2^3 \cdot 3^2$, or 72.

Example 10 Find the LCM of $7a^2b$ and ab^2.

1. We have the following factorizations:

$$7a^2b = 7 \cdot a \cdot a \cdot b \quad \text{and} \quad ab^2 = a \cdot b \cdot b.$$

2. a) No one factorization contains the other.

b) Consider the factorization of $7a^2b$, $7 \cdot a \cdot a \cdot b$. Since ab^2 contains a second factor of b, we multiply by another factor of b:

$$7 \cdot a \cdot a \cdot b \cdot b.$$

— $7a^2b$ is a factor.
— ab^2 is a factor.

The LCM is $7 \cdot a \cdot a \cdot b \cdot b$, or $7a^2b^2$.

3. The check is left to the student.

Do Exercises 12 and 13.

Exercise Set 4.1

a Find the LCM of each set of numbers.

1. 2, 4
4

2. 3, 15
15

3. 10, 25
50

4. 10, 15
30

5. 20, 40
40

6. 8, 12
24

7. 18, 27
54

8. 9, 11
99

9. 30, 50
150

10. 8, 36
72

11. 30, 40
120

12. 21, 27
189

13. 18, 24
72

14. 12, 18
36

15. 60, 70
420

16. 35, 45
315

17. 16, 36
144

18. 18, 20
180

19. 32, 36
288

20. 36, 48
144

21. 2, 3, 5
30

22. 5, 18, 3
90

23. 3, 5, 7
105

24. 6, 12, 18
36

25. 24, 36, 12
72

26. 8, 16, 22
176

27. 5, 12, 15
60

28. 12, 18, 40
360

29. 9, 12, 6
36

30. 8, 16, 12
48

31. 180, 100, 450
900

32. 18, 30, 50, 48
3600

33. 75, 100
300

34. 81, 90
810

35. ab, bc
abc

36. $7x$, xy
$7xy$

37. $3x$, $9x^2$
$9x^2$

38. $10x^4$, $5x^3$
$10x^4$

39. $4x^3$, x^2y
$4x^3y$

40. $6ab^2$, a^3b
$6a^3b^2$

Applications of LCMs: Planet Orbits. Earth, Jupiter, Saturn, and Uranus all revolve around the sun. Earth takes 1 yr, Jupiter 12 yr, Saturn 30 yr, and Uranus 84 yr to make a complete revolution. On a certain night, you look at those three distant planets and wonder how many years it will take before they have the same position again. To determine this, you find the LCM of 12, 30, and 84. It will be that number of years.

41. How often will Jupiter and Saturn appear in the same direction in the night sky as seen from Earth? Once every 60 yr

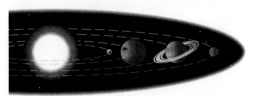

42. How often will Jupiter, Saturn, and Uranus appear in the same direction in the night sky as seen from Earth? Once every 420 yr

---

Skill Maintenance

Perform the indicated operation and, if possible, simplify.

43. $-38 + 52$ [2.2a] 14

44. $-18 \div \left(\dfrac{2}{3}\right)$ [3.7b] -27

45. $23 \cdot 345$ [1.5b] 7935

46. $\dfrac{4}{5} \cdot \dfrac{10}{12}$ [3.6a] $\dfrac{2}{3}$

47. $\dfrac{4}{5} \div \left(-\dfrac{7}{10}\right)$ [3.7b] $-\dfrac{8}{7}$

48. $382 - 549$ [2.3a] -167

Synthesis

49. ◆ Under what conditions is the LCM of two composite numbers simply the product of the two numbers?

50. ◆ Is the LCM of two prime numbers always their product? Why or why not?

51. ◆ Is the LCM of two numbers always at least twice as large as the larger of the two numbers? Why or why not?

🔲 Use a calculator and the multiples method to find the LCM of each pair of numbers.

52. 288, 324 2592

53. 2700, 7800 70,200

54. Use Example 9 to help find the LCM of 27, 90, 84, 210, 108, and 50. 18,900

55. Use Examples 6 and 7 to help find the LCM of 18, 21, 24, 36, 63, 56, and 20. 2520

56. The exhibits at a flea market are either 6 ft long or 8 ft long. How long is the shortest aisle that can accommodate exhibits of either length with no space left over? (*Note*: each aisle will be filled with either all 6-ft exhibits or all 8-ft exhibits.) 24 ft

57. Consider 8 and 12. Determine whether each of the following is the LCM of 8 and 12. Tell why or why not.

a) $2 \cdot 2 \cdot 3 \cdot 3$
b) $2 \cdot 2 \cdot 3$
c) $2 \cdot 3 \cdot 3$
d) $2 \cdot 2 \cdot 2 \cdot 3$

a) Not the LCM because 8 is not a factor of $2 \cdot 2 \cdot 3 \cdot 3$;
b) Not the LCM because 8 is not a factor of $2 \cdot 2 \cdot 3$; **c)** Not the LCM because neither 8 nor 12 is a factor of $2 \cdot 3 \cdot 3$;
d) The LCM because both 8 and 12 are factors of $2 \cdot 2 \cdot 2 \cdot 3$ and it is the smallest such number

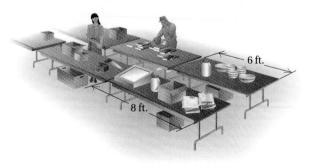

58. Find three different pairs of numbers for which 56 is the LCM. Do not use 56 itself in any one of the pairs. 8 and 7; 8 and 28; 8 and 14

59. Find three different pairs of numbers for which 54 is the LCM. Do not use 54 itself in any one of the pairs. 27 and 2; 27 and 6; 27 and 18

Find the least common multiple of two or more numbers using shaped markers.

Collaborative Learning Manual

4.2 Addition and Order

a | Like Denominators

Addition using fractional notation corresponds to combining or putting like things together, just as when we combined like terms in Section 2.7. For example,

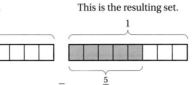

We combine two sets, each of which consists of fractional parts of one object that are the same size.

This is the resulting set.

$$\frac{2}{8} + \frac{3}{8} = \frac{5}{8}$$

2 eighths + 3 eighths = 5 eighths,

or $\quad 2 \cdot \frac{1}{8} + 3 \cdot \frac{1}{8} = 5 \cdot \frac{1}{8},$

or $\quad \frac{2}{8} + \frac{3}{8} = \frac{5}{8}.$

Do Exercise 1.

To add when denominators are the same,

a) add the numerators,

b) keep the denominator, and

$$\frac{2}{6} + \frac{5}{6} = \frac{2 + 5}{6} = \frac{7}{6}$$

c) simplify, if possible.

Examples Add and, if possible, simplify.

1. $\dfrac{2}{4} + \dfrac{1}{4} = \dfrac{2 + 1}{4} = \dfrac{3}{4}$ No simplifying is possible.

2. $\dfrac{3}{12} + \dfrac{5}{12} = \dfrac{3 + 5}{12} = \dfrac{8}{12}$ Adding numerators; the denominator remains unchanged.

$\qquad = \dfrac{4}{4} \cdot \dfrac{2}{3} = \dfrac{2}{3}$ Simplifying by removing a factor equal to 1: $\frac{4}{4} = 1$

3. $\dfrac{-11}{6} + \dfrac{3}{6} = \dfrac{-11 + 3}{6} = \dfrac{-8}{6}$

$\qquad = \dfrac{2}{2} \cdot \dfrac{-4}{3} = \dfrac{-4}{3}, \text{ or } -\dfrac{4}{3}$ Removing a factor equal to 1: $\frac{2}{2} = 1$

4. $-\dfrac{2}{a} + \left(-\dfrac{3}{a}\right) = \dfrac{-2}{a} + \dfrac{-3}{a}$ Recall that $-\dfrac{m}{n} = \dfrac{-m}{n}$. We generally try to avoid negative signs in the denominator.

$\qquad = \dfrac{-2 + (-3)}{a} = \dfrac{-5}{a}, \text{ or } -\dfrac{5}{a}$

Do Exercises 2–5.

Objectives

a | Add using fractional notation when denominators are the same.

b | Add using fractional notation when denominators are different.

c | Use < or > to form a true statement using fractional notation.

d | Solve problems involving addition with fractional notation.

For Extra Help

TAPE 7   MAC WIN   CD-ROM

1. Find $\dfrac{1}{5} + \dfrac{3}{5}$. $\dfrac{4}{5}$

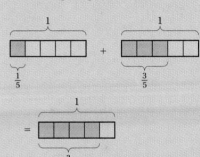

Add and, if possible, simplify.

2. $\dfrac{1}{3} + \dfrac{2}{3}$ 1

3. $\dfrac{5}{12} + \dfrac{1}{12}$ $\dfrac{1}{2}$

4. $\dfrac{-9}{16} + \dfrac{3}{16}$ $-\dfrac{3}{8}$

5. $\dfrac{3}{x} + \dfrac{-7}{x}$ $-\dfrac{4}{x}$

Answers on page A-9

4.2 **Addition and Order**

213

Simplify by combining like terms.

6. $\dfrac{3}{10}a + \dfrac{1}{10}a$ $\frac{2}{5}a$

7. $\dfrac{2}{19} + \dfrac{3}{19}x + \dfrac{5}{19} + \dfrac{7}{19}x$

$\dfrac{7}{19} + \dfrac{10}{19}x$

In some cases, we need to add fractions when combining like terms.

Example 5   Simplify by combining like terms: $\dfrac{2}{7}x + \dfrac{3}{7}x$.

$$\frac{2}{7}x + \frac{3}{7}x = \left(\frac{2}{7} + \frac{3}{7}\right)x \qquad \textbf{Try to do this step mentally.}$$
$$= \frac{5}{7}x.$$

Do Exercises 6 and 7.

b | Addition Using the Least Common Denominator

At the beginning of this section, we visualized the addition $\frac{2}{8} + \frac{3}{8}$. Consider now the addition $\frac{1}{2} + \frac{1}{3}$.

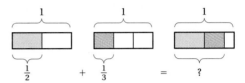

By rewriting $\frac{1}{2}$ as $\frac{1}{2} \cdot \frac{3}{3} = \frac{3}{6}$ and $\frac{1}{3}$ as $\frac{1}{3} \cdot \frac{2}{2} = \frac{2}{6}$, we can determine the sum.

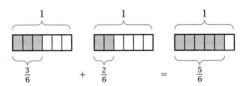

Thus, when denominators differ, before adding we must multiply by 1 to get a common denominator. There is always more than one common denominator that can be used. Consider the addition $\frac{3}{4} + \frac{1}{6}$:

A.
$$\frac{3}{4} + \frac{1}{6} = \frac{3}{4} \cdot 1 + \frac{1}{6} \cdot 1$$
$$= \frac{3}{4} \cdot \frac{6}{6} + \frac{1}{6} \cdot \frac{4}{4} \qquad \textbf{Here 24 is the common denominator.}$$
$$= \frac{18}{24} + \frac{4}{24}$$
$$= \frac{22}{24} = \frac{11}{12};$$

B.
$$\frac{3}{4} + \frac{1}{6} = \frac{3}{4} \cdot 1 + \frac{1}{6} \cdot 1$$
$$= \frac{3}{4} \cdot \frac{3}{3} + \frac{1}{6} \cdot \frac{2}{2} \qquad \textbf{Here 12 is the common denominator.}$$
$$= \frac{9}{12} + \frac{2}{12}$$
$$= \frac{11}{12}$$

We had to simplify at the end of (A), but not in (B). In (B), we used the *least* common multiple of the denominators, 12. That number is called the **least common denominator,** or **LCD**.

To add when denominators are different:

a) Find the least common multiple of the denominators. That number is the least common denominator, LCD.

b) Multiply by 1, writing 1 in the form of n/n, to find an equivalent sum in which the LCD appears.

c) Add and, if possible, simplify.

Answers on page A-9

Example 6 Add: $\frac{1}{8} + \frac{3}{4}$.

a) Since 4 is a factor of 8, the LCM of 4 and 8 is 8. Thus the LCD is 8.

b) We need to find a fraction equivalent to $\frac{3}{4}$ with a denominator of 8:

$$\frac{1}{8} + \frac{3}{4} = \frac{1}{8} + \frac{3}{4} \cdot \frac{2}{2}.$$

Think: $4 \times \blacksquare = 8$. The answer is 2, so we multiply by 1, using $\frac{2}{2}$.

c) We add: $\quad \frac{1}{8} + \frac{6}{8} = \frac{7}{8}.$ $\quad \frac{7}{8}$ cannot be simplified.

Do Exercise 8.

In Examples 7–10, we follow the same steps without spelling them out.

Example 7 Add: $\frac{5}{6} + \frac{1}{9}$.

The LCD is 18. $\quad$ $6 = 2 \cdot 3$ and $9 = 3 \cdot 3$, so the LCM of 6 and 9 is $2 \cdot 3 \cdot 3$, or 18.

$$\frac{5}{6} + \frac{1}{9} = \frac{5}{6} \cdot 1 + \frac{1}{9} \cdot 1$$

$$= \frac{5}{6} \cdot \frac{3}{3} + \frac{1}{9} \cdot \frac{2}{2}$$

Think: $9 \times \blacksquare = 18$. The answer is 2, so we multiply by 1, using $\frac{2}{2}$.

Think: $6 \times \blacksquare = 18$. The answer is 3, so we multiply by 1, using $\frac{3}{3}$.

$$= \frac{15}{18} + \frac{2}{18}$$

$$= \frac{17}{18}$$

Do Exercise 9.

Example 8 Add: $\frac{3}{-5} + \frac{11}{10}$.

$$\frac{3}{-5} + \frac{11}{10} = \frac{-3}{5} + \frac{11}{10}$$

Recall that $\frac{m}{-n} = \frac{-m}{n}$. The LCD is 10.

$$= \frac{-3}{5} \cdot \frac{2}{2} + \frac{11}{10}$$

$$= \frac{-6}{10} + \frac{11}{10}$$

$$= \frac{5}{10}$$

$$= \frac{1}{2}$$

We may still have to simplify, but simplifying is almost always easier if the LCD has been used.

---

8. Add using the least common denominator.

$$\frac{2}{3} + \frac{1}{6} \quad \frac{5}{6}$$

9. Add: $\frac{3}{8} + \frac{5}{6}$. $\frac{29}{24}$

Answers on page A-9

Add.

10. $\dfrac{1}{-6} + \dfrac{7}{18}$ $\dfrac{2}{9}$

11. $7 + \dfrac{3}{5}$ $\dfrac{38}{5}$

Add.

12. $\dfrac{4}{10} + \dfrac{1}{100} + \dfrac{3}{1000}$ $\dfrac{413}{1000}$

13. $\dfrac{7}{10} + \dfrac{-2}{21} + \dfrac{1}{7}$ $\dfrac{157}{210}$

Use < or > for ▓ to form a true sentence.

14. $\dfrac{3}{8}$ ▓ $\dfrac{5}{8}$ $<$

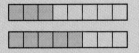

15. $\dfrac{7}{10}$ ▓ $\dfrac{6}{10}$ $>$

16. $\dfrac{-2}{9}$ ▓ $\dfrac{-5}{9}$ $>$

Answers on page A-9

Example 9   Add: $\dfrac{5}{8} + 2$.

$$\dfrac{5}{8} + 2 = \dfrac{5}{8} + \dfrac{2}{1} \qquad \text{Rewriting 2 in fractional notation}$$

$$= \dfrac{5}{8} + \dfrac{2}{1} \cdot \dfrac{8}{8} \qquad \text{The LCD is 8.}$$

$$= \dfrac{5}{8} + \dfrac{16}{8}$$

$$= \dfrac{21}{8}$$

Do Exercises 10 and 11.

Example 10   Add: $\dfrac{9}{70} + \dfrac{11}{21} + \dfrac{-6}{15}$.

We need to determine the LCM of 70, 21, and 15:

$$\left.\begin{array}{l} 70 = 2 \cdot 5 \cdot 7, \\ 21 = 3 \cdot 7, \\ 15 = 3 \cdot 5 \end{array}\right\} \quad \text{The LCM is } 2 \cdot 3 \cdot 5 \cdot 7, \text{ or } 210.$$

$$\dfrac{9}{70} + \dfrac{11}{21} + \dfrac{-6}{15} = \dfrac{9}{70} \cdot \dfrac{3}{3} + \dfrac{11}{21} \cdot \dfrac{2 \cdot 5}{2 \cdot 5} + \dfrac{-6}{15} \cdot \dfrac{7 \cdot 2}{7 \cdot 2}$$

$$= \dfrac{9 \cdot 3}{70 \cdot 3} + \dfrac{11 \cdot 10}{21 \cdot 10} + \dfrac{-6 \cdot 14}{15 \cdot 14}$$

$$= \dfrac{27}{210} + \dfrac{110}{210} + \dfrac{-84}{210}$$

$$= \dfrac{137 + (-84)}{210}$$

$$= \dfrac{53}{210}. \qquad \begin{array}{l}\text{Since 53 is prime and not a factor} \\ \text{of 210, we cannot simplify.}\end{array}$$

In each case, we multiply by 1 to obtain the LCD. To form 1, look at the prime factorization of the LCD and use the factor(s) missing from each denominator.

Do Exercises 12 and 13.

c | Order

Common denominators are also important for determining the larger of two fractions. When two fractions share a common denominator, the larger number can be found by comparing numerators. For example, 4 is greater than 3, so $\frac{4}{5}$ is greater than $\frac{3}{5}$.

$$\dfrac{4}{5} > \dfrac{3}{5}$$

Similarly, because −6 is less than −2, we have

$$\dfrac{-6}{7} < \dfrac{-2}{7}, \quad \text{or} \quad -\dfrac{6}{7} < -\dfrac{2}{7}.$$

Do Exercises 14–16.

Example 11 Use < or > for ▦ to form a true sentence:

$$\frac{5}{8} \; ▦ \; \frac{2}{3}.$$

You can confirm that the LCD is 24. We multiply by 1 to make the denominators the same:

$$\frac{5}{8} \cdot \frac{3}{3} = \frac{15}{24}; \qquad \frac{2}{3} \cdot \frac{8}{8} = \frac{16}{24}.$$

Since $15 < 16$, it follows that $\frac{15}{24} < \frac{16}{24}$. Thus,

$$\frac{5}{8} < \frac{2}{3}.$$

Example 12 Use < or > for ▦ to form a true sentence:

$$-\frac{89}{100} \; ▦ \; -\frac{9}{10}.$$

The LCD is 100.

$$\frac{-9}{10} \cdot \frac{10}{10} = \frac{-90}{100} \qquad \text{We multiply by } \frac{10}{10} \text{ to get the LCD.}$$

Since $-89 > -90$, it follows that $-\frac{89}{100} > -\frac{90}{100}$, so

$$-\frac{89}{100} > -\frac{9}{10}.$$

Do Exercises 17–19.

d Solving Problems

Example 13 *Baking.* A recipe for fudge brownies calls for $\frac{1}{4}$ cup of oil and $\frac{2}{3}$ cup of milk. How many cups of liquid ingredients are in the recipe?

1. **Familiarize.** We first make a drawing and let $n =$ the total number of cups of liquid ingredients.

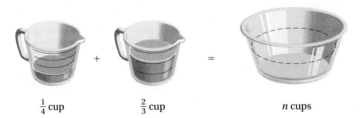

$\frac{1}{4}$ cup $+$ $\frac{2}{3}$ cup $=$ n cups

2. **Translate.** The problem can be translated to an equation as follows:

Amount of oil	plus	Amount of milk	is	Amount of liquid
↓	↓	↓	↓	↓
$\frac{1}{4}$	$+$	$\frac{2}{3}$	$=$	n

Use < or > for ▦ to form a true sentence.

17. $\frac{2}{3} \; ▦ \; \frac{3}{4}$ <

18. $\frac{-3}{4} \; ▦ \; \frac{-8}{12}$ <

19. $\frac{5}{6} \; ▦ \; \frac{7}{8}$ <

Answers on page A-9

20. Maureen bought $\frac{1}{2}$ lb of peanuts and $\frac{3}{5}$ lb of cashews. How many pounds of nuts were bought altogether? $\frac{11}{10}$ lb

3. Solve. To solve the equation, we carry out the addition:

$$\frac{1}{4} + \frac{2}{3} = n \qquad \text{The LCD is 12.}$$

$$\frac{1}{4} \cdot \frac{3}{3} + \frac{2}{3} \cdot \frac{4}{4} = n \qquad \text{Multiplying by 1}$$

$$\frac{3}{12} + \frac{8}{12} = n$$

$$\frac{11}{12} = n.$$

4. Check. As a partial check, we note that the sum is larger than either of the individual amounts, as expected. We can also check by repeating the calculations.

5. State. The recipe calls for $\frac{11}{12}$ cup of liquid ingredients.

Do Exercise 20.

Calculator Spotlight

Many calculators are equipped with a key, often labeled $\boxed{a^b\!/_c}$, that allows for computations with fractional notation. To calculate

$$\frac{2}{3} + \frac{4}{5}$$

with such a calculator, the following keystrokes can be used (note that the key $\boxed{a^b\!/_c}$ usually doubles as the $\boxed{d/c}$ key):

$$\boxed{2}\ \boxed{a^b\!/_c}\ \boxed{3}\ \boxed{+}\ \boxed{4}\ \boxed{a^b\!/_c}\ \boxed{5}\ \boxed{=}\ \boxed{\text{Shift}}\ \boxed{d/c}.$$

The display that appears,

$$\boxed{\qquad 22\ \lrcorner\ 15\quad},$$

represents the fraction $\frac{22}{15}$.

Note that we used the keystrokes $\boxed{\text{Shift}}$ $\boxed{d/c}$ to convert from a mixed numeral (see Section 4.5) to fractional notation.

Graphing calculators can also perform computations with fractional notation. To do the above addition on a graphing calculator, we use the $\boxed{\text{MATH}}$ key as follows:

$$\boxed{2}\ \boxed{\div}\ \boxed{3}\ \boxed{+}\ \boxed{4}\ \boxed{\div}\ \boxed{5}\ \boxed{\text{MATH}}\ \boxed{1}\ \boxed{\text{ENTER}}.$$

> **CAUTION!** Although it is possible to add on a calculator using fractional notation, it is still very important for you to understand how such addition is performed longhand. For this reason, your instructor may disallow the use of calculators on this chapter's test.

Exercises

Calculate.

1. $\dfrac{3}{8} + \dfrac{1}{4}$ $\dfrac{5}{8}$

2. $\dfrac{5}{12} + \dfrac{7}{10}$ $\dfrac{67}{60}$

3. $\dfrac{15}{7} + \dfrac{1}{3}$ $\dfrac{52}{21}$

4. $\dfrac{19}{20} + \dfrac{17}{35}$ $\dfrac{201}{140}$

5. $\dfrac{29}{30} + \dfrac{18}{25}$ $\dfrac{253}{150}$

6. $\dfrac{17}{23} + \dfrac{13}{29}$ $\dfrac{792}{667}$

Answers on page A-9

Exercise Set 4.2

a, **b** Add and, if possible, simplify.

1. $\dfrac{4}{9} + \dfrac{5}{9}$ 1

2. $\dfrac{1}{4} + \dfrac{1}{4}$ $\dfrac{1}{2}$

3. $\dfrac{1}{8} + \dfrac{5}{8}$ $\dfrac{3}{4}$

4. $\dfrac{7}{8} + \dfrac{1}{8}$ 1

5. $\dfrac{7}{10} + \dfrac{3}{-10}$ $\dfrac{2}{5}$

6. $\dfrac{1}{-6} + \dfrac{5}{6}$ $\dfrac{2}{3}$

7. $\dfrac{9}{a} + \dfrac{4}{a}$ $\dfrac{13}{a}$

8. $\dfrac{4}{t} + \dfrac{3}{t}$ $\dfrac{7}{t}$

9. $\dfrac{-5}{11} + \dfrac{3}{11}$ $-\dfrac{2}{11}$

10. $\dfrac{7}{12} + \dfrac{-5}{12}$ $\dfrac{1}{6}$

11. $\dfrac{2}{9}x + \dfrac{5}{9}x$ $\dfrac{7}{9}x$

12. $\dfrac{3}{11}a + \dfrac{2}{11}a$ $\dfrac{5}{11}a$

13. $\dfrac{5}{32} + \dfrac{3}{32}t + \dfrac{7}{32} + \dfrac{13}{32}t$
$\dfrac{3}{8} + \dfrac{1}{2}t$

14. $\dfrac{3}{25}x + \dfrac{7}{25} + \dfrac{12}{25}x + \dfrac{-2}{25}$
$\dfrac{3}{5}x + \dfrac{1}{5}$

15. $-\dfrac{3}{x} + \left(-\dfrac{7}{x}\right)$ $-\dfrac{10}{x}$

16. $-\dfrac{9}{a} + \dfrac{5}{a}$ $-\dfrac{4}{a}$

17. $\dfrac{1}{8} + \dfrac{1}{6}$ $\dfrac{7}{24}$

18. $\dfrac{1}{9} + \dfrac{1}{6}$ $\dfrac{5}{18}$

19. $\dfrac{-4}{5} + \dfrac{7}{10}$ $-\dfrac{1}{10}$

20. $\dfrac{-3}{4} + \dfrac{1}{12}$ $-\dfrac{2}{3}$

21. $\dfrac{5}{12} + \dfrac{3}{8}$ $\dfrac{19}{24}$

22. $\dfrac{7}{8} + \dfrac{1}{16}$ $\dfrac{15}{16}$

23. $\dfrac{3}{20} + 4$ $\dfrac{83}{20}$

24. $\dfrac{2}{15} + 3$ $\dfrac{47}{15}$

25. $\dfrac{5}{-8} + \dfrac{5}{6}$ $\quad\dfrac{5}{24}$

26. $\dfrac{5}{-6} + \dfrac{7}{9}$ $\quad -\dfrac{1}{18}$

27. $\dfrac{3}{10}x + \dfrac{7}{100}x$ $\quad\dfrac{37}{100}x$

28. $\dfrac{9}{20}a + \dfrac{3}{40}a$ $\quad\dfrac{21}{40}a$

29. $\dfrac{5}{12} + \dfrac{4}{15}$ $\quad\dfrac{41}{60}$

30. $\dfrac{3}{16} + \dfrac{1}{12}$ $\quad\dfrac{13}{48}$

31. $\dfrac{9}{10} + \dfrac{-99}{100}$ $\quad -\dfrac{9}{100}$

32. $\dfrac{3}{10} + \dfrac{-27}{100}$ $\quad\dfrac{3}{100}$

33. $5 + \dfrac{7}{12}$ $\quad\dfrac{67}{12}$

34. $7 + \dfrac{3}{8}$ $\quad\dfrac{59}{8}$

35. $-5t + \dfrac{2}{7}t$ $\quad -\dfrac{33}{7}t$

36. $-4x + \dfrac{3}{5}x$ $\quad -\dfrac{17}{5}x$

37. $-\dfrac{5}{12} + \dfrac{7}{-24}$ $\quad -\dfrac{17}{24}$

38. $-\dfrac{1}{18} + \dfrac{5}{-12}$ $\quad -\dfrac{17}{36}$

39. $\dfrac{4}{10} + \dfrac{3}{100} + \dfrac{7}{1000}$ $\quad\dfrac{437}{1000}$

40. $\dfrac{7}{10} + \dfrac{2}{100} + \dfrac{9}{1000}$ $\quad\dfrac{729}{1000}$

41. $\dfrac{3}{10} + \dfrac{5}{12} + \dfrac{8}{15}$ $\quad\dfrac{5}{4}$

42. $\dfrac{1}{2} + \dfrac{3}{8} + \dfrac{1}{4}$ $\quad\dfrac{9}{8}$

43. $\dfrac{5}{6} + \dfrac{25}{52} + \dfrac{7}{4}$ $\quad\dfrac{239}{78}$

44. $\dfrac{15}{24} + \dfrac{7}{36} + \dfrac{91}{48}$ $\quad\dfrac{391}{144}$

45. $\dfrac{2}{9} + \dfrac{7}{10} + \dfrac{-4}{15}$ $\quad\dfrac{59}{90}$

46. $\dfrac{5}{12} + \dfrac{-3}{8} + \dfrac{1}{10}$ $\quad\dfrac{17}{120}$

c Use < or > for ▇ to form a true sentence.

47. $\dfrac{5}{8}$ ▇ $\dfrac{6}{8}$ <

48. $\dfrac{7}{9}$ ▇ $\dfrac{5}{9}$ >

49. $\dfrac{2}{3}$ ▇ $\dfrac{5}{6}$ <

50. $\dfrac{11}{18}$ ▇ $\dfrac{5}{9}$ >

51. $\dfrac{-2}{3}$ ▇ $\dfrac{-5}{7}$ >

52. $\dfrac{-3}{5}$ ▇ $\dfrac{-4}{7}$ <

53. $\dfrac{11}{15}$ ▇ $\dfrac{7}{10}$ >

54. $\dfrac{5}{14}$ ▇ $\dfrac{8}{21}$ <

55. $\dfrac{3}{4}$ ▇ $-\dfrac{1}{5}$ >

56. $\dfrac{3}{8}$ ▇ $-\dfrac{13}{16}$ >

57. $\dfrac{-7}{20}$ ▇ $\dfrac{-6}{15}$ >

58. $\dfrac{-7}{12}$ ▇ $\dfrac{-9}{16}$ <

Arrange each grouping of fractions from smallest to largest.

59. $\dfrac{3}{10}, \dfrac{5}{12}, \dfrac{4}{15}$ $\dfrac{4}{15}, \dfrac{3}{10}, \dfrac{5}{12}$

60. $\dfrac{5}{6}, \dfrac{19}{21}, \dfrac{11}{14}$ $\dfrac{11}{14}, \dfrac{5}{6}, \dfrac{19}{21}$

d Solve.

61. Rose bought $\frac{1}{3}$ lb of orange pekoe tea and $\frac{1}{2}$ lb of English cinnamon tea. How many pounds of tea were bought altogether? $\frac{5}{6}$ lb

62. Mitch bought $\frac{1}{4}$ lb of gumdrops and $\frac{1}{2}$ lb of caramels. How many pounds of candy were bought altogether?

$\frac{3}{4}$ lb

63. Ruwanda walked $\frac{3}{8}$ mi to Juan's dormitory, and then $\frac{3}{4}$ mi to class. How far did Ruwanda walk? $\frac{9}{8}$ mi

64. Ola walked $\frac{7}{8}$ mi to the student union, and then $\frac{2}{5}$ mi to class. How far did Ola walk? $\frac{51}{40}$ mi

65. *Baking.* A recipe for muffins calls for $\frac{1}{2}$ qt (quart) of buttermilk, $\frac{1}{3}$ qt of skim milk, and $\frac{1}{16}$ qt of oil. How many quarts of liquid ingredients does the recipe call for? $\frac{43}{48}$ qt

66. *Baking.* A recipe for bread calls for $\frac{2}{3}$ cup of water, $\frac{1}{4}$ cup of milk, and $\frac{1}{8}$ cup of oil. How many cups of liquid ingredients does the recipe call for? $\frac{25}{24}$ cups

67. *Masonry.* A cubic meter of concrete mix contains 420 kg of cement, 150 kg of stone, and 120 kg of sand. What is the total weight of the cubic meter of concrete mix? What fractional part is cement? stone? sand? Add these amounts. What is the result?

690 kg; $\frac{14}{23}$; $\frac{5}{23}$; $\frac{4}{23}$; 1

68. *Bartending.* A recipe for cherry punch calls for $\frac{1}{5}$ L of ginger ale and $\frac{3}{5}$ L of black cherry soda. How much liquid is needed? If the recipe is doubled, how much liquid is needed? If the recipe is halved, how much liquid is needed? $\frac{4}{5}$ L; $\frac{8}{5}$ L; $\frac{2}{5}$ L

69. A park ranger hikes $\frac{3}{5}$ mi to a lookout, another $\frac{3}{10}$ mi to an osprey's nest, and finally, $\frac{3}{4}$ mi to a campsite. How far did the ranger hike? $\frac{33}{20}$ mi

70. A triathlete runs $\frac{7}{8}$ mi, canoes $\frac{1}{3}$ mi, and swims $\frac{1}{6}$ mi. How many miles does the triathlete cover? $\frac{11}{8}$ mi

71. A tile $\frac{5}{8}$ in. thick is glued to a board $\frac{7}{8}$ in. thick. The glue is $\frac{3}{32}$ in. thick. How thick is the result? $\frac{51}{32}$ in.

72. A baker used $\frac{1}{2}$ lb of flour for rolls, $\frac{1}{4}$ lb for donuts, and $\frac{1}{3}$ lb for cookies. How much flour was used? $\frac{13}{12}$ lb

---

Skill Maintenance

Subtract. [2.3a]

73. $-7 - 6$ -13

74. $-5 - (-9)$ 4

75. $9 - 17$ -8

76. $-8 - 23$ -31

Evaluate. [2.6a]

77. $\dfrac{x - y}{3}$, for $x = 7$ and $y = -3$ $\dfrac{10}{3}$

78. $3(x + y)$ and $3x + 3y$, for $x = 5$ and $y = 9$ 42; 42

Synthesis

79. ◆ Suppose that a classmate believes, incorrectly, that $\frac{2}{5} + \frac{4}{5} = \frac{6}{10}$. How could you convince the classmate that he or she is mistaken?

80. ◆ Explain how pictures could be used to convince someone that $\frac{5}{7}$ is larger than $\frac{13}{21}$.

81. ◆ To add numbers with different denominators, a student consistently uses the product of the denominators as a common denominator. Is this correct? Why or why not?

Add and, if possible, simplify.

82. $\dfrac{3}{10}t + \dfrac{2}{7} + \dfrac{2}{15}t + \dfrac{3}{5}$ $\dfrac{13}{30}t + \dfrac{31}{35}$

83. $\dfrac{2}{9} + \dfrac{4}{21}x + \dfrac{4}{15} + \dfrac{3}{14}x$ $\dfrac{22}{45} + \dfrac{17}{42}x$

84. $5t^2 + \dfrac{6}{a}t + 2t^2 + \dfrac{3}{a}t$ $7t^2 + \dfrac{9}{a}t$

Use <, >, or = for ▓ to form a true sentence.

85. ▦ $\dfrac{12}{97} + \dfrac{67}{137}$ ▓ $\dfrac{8144}{13,289}$ <

86. ▦ $\dfrac{37}{157} + \dfrac{19}{107}$ ▓ $\dfrac{6941}{16,799}$ >

87. A guitarist's band is booked for Friday and Saturday night at a local club. The guitarist is part of a trio on Friday and part of a quintet on Saturday. Thus the guitarist is paid one-third of one-half the weekend's pay for Friday and one-fifth of one-half the weekend's pay for Saturday. What fractional part of the band's pay did the guitarist receive for the weekend's work? If the band was paid $1200, how much did the guitarist receive? $\frac{4}{15}$; $320

Collaborative Learning Manual

Arrange sockets and drill bits in fractional sizes from smallest to largest.

4.3 Subtraction, Equations, and Applications

a | Subtraction

Like Denominators

We can consider the difference $\frac{4}{8} - \frac{3}{8}$ as we did before, as either "take away" or "how much more." Let's consider "take away."

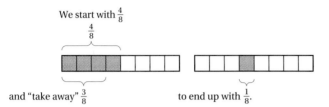

We start with $\frac{4}{8}$

$\frac{4}{8}$

and "take away" $\frac{3}{8}$ to end up with $\frac{1}{8}$.

We start with 4 eighths and take away 3 eighths:

$$4 \text{ eighths} - 3 \text{ eighths} = 1 \text{ eighth},$$

or $\quad 4 \cdot \frac{1}{8} - 3 \cdot \frac{1}{8} = \frac{1}{8}, \quad$ or $\quad \frac{4}{8} - \frac{3}{8} = \frac{1}{8}.$

To subtract when denominators are the same,

a) subtract the numerators,

b) keep the denominator, and

c) simplify, if possible.

$$\frac{7}{10} - \frac{4}{10} = \frac{7 - 4}{10} = \frac{3}{10}$$

Examples   Subtract and simplify.

1. $\dfrac{8}{13} - \dfrac{3}{13} = \dfrac{8 - 3}{13} = \dfrac{5}{13}$

2. $\dfrac{3}{35} - \dfrac{13}{35} = \dfrac{3 - 13}{35} = \dfrac{-10}{35} = \dfrac{5}{5} \cdot \dfrac{-2}{7} = \dfrac{-2}{7}$, or $-\dfrac{2}{7}$ **Removing a factor equal to 1: $\frac{5}{5} = 1$**

3. $\dfrac{13}{2a} - \dfrac{5}{2a} = \dfrac{13 - 5}{2a} = \dfrac{8}{2a} = \dfrac{2}{2} \cdot \dfrac{4}{a} = \dfrac{4}{a}$ **Removing a factor equal to 1: $\frac{2}{2} = 1$**

Do Exercises 1–3.

Different Denominators

To subtract when denominators are different:

a) Find the least common multiple of the denominators. That number is the least common denominator, LCD.

b) Multiply by 1, writing 1 in the form of n/n, to find an equivalent subtraction in which the LCD appears.

c) Subtract and, if possible, simplify.

Subtract and simplify.

1. $\dfrac{7}{8} - \dfrac{3}{8}$ $\dfrac{1}{2}$

2. $\dfrac{9}{5a} - \dfrac{6}{5a}$ $\dfrac{3}{5a}$

3. $\dfrac{8}{10} - \dfrac{13}{10}$ $-\dfrac{1}{2}$

Answers on page A-10

4. Subtract: $\dfrac{3}{4} - \dfrac{2}{3}$. $\dfrac{1}{12}$

Subtract.

5. $\dfrac{5}{6} - \dfrac{2}{3}$ $\dfrac{1}{6}$

6. $\dfrac{2}{5} - \dfrac{7}{10}$ $-\dfrac{3}{10}$

7. $\dfrac{2}{3} - \dfrac{5}{6}$ $-\dfrac{1}{6}$

8. $\dfrac{11}{28} - \dfrac{5}{16}$ $\dfrac{9}{112}$

9. Simplify: $\dfrac{9}{10}x - \dfrac{3}{5}x$. $\dfrac{3}{10}x$

Answers on page A-10

Example 4   Subtract: $\dfrac{2}{5} - \dfrac{3}{8}$.

a) The LCM of 5 and 8 is 40, so the LCD is 40.

b) We need to find numbers equivalent to $\frac{2}{5}$ and $\frac{3}{8}$ with denominators of 40:

$$\dfrac{2}{5} - \dfrac{3}{8} = \dfrac{2}{5} \cdot \dfrac{8}{8} - \dfrac{3}{8} \cdot \dfrac{5}{5}$$

Think: $8 \times \blacksquare = 40$. The answer is 5, so we multiply by 1, using $\frac{5}{5}$.

Think: $5 \times \blacksquare = 40$. The answer is 8, so we multiply by 1, using $\frac{8}{8}$.

c) We subtract: $\dfrac{16}{40} - \dfrac{15}{40} = \dfrac{16 - 15}{40} = \dfrac{1}{40}$.

Do Exercise 4.

Example 5   Subtract: $\dfrac{7}{12} - \dfrac{5}{6}$.

Since 6 is a factor of 12, the LCM of 6 and 12 is 12. The LCD is 12.

$$\dfrac{7}{12} - \dfrac{5}{6} = \dfrac{7}{12} - \dfrac{5}{6} \cdot \dfrac{2}{2}$$

Think: $6 \times \blacksquare = 12$. The answer is 2, so we multiply by 1, using $\frac{2}{2}$.

$$= \dfrac{7}{12} - \dfrac{10}{12}$$

$$= \dfrac{7 - 10}{12} = \dfrac{-3}{12}$$

If we prefer, we can add the opposite: $7 + (-10)$.

$$= \dfrac{3}{3} \cdot \dfrac{-1}{4} = \dfrac{-1}{4}, \text{ or } -\dfrac{1}{4}$$

Simplifying by removing a factor equal to 1: $\frac{3}{3} = 1$

Example 6   Subtract: $\dfrac{17}{24} - \dfrac{4}{15}$.

We need to find the LCM of 24 and 15:

$$\left. \begin{array}{l} 24 = 2 \cdot 2 \cdot 2 \cdot 3, \\ 15 = 3 \cdot 5 \end{array} \right\} \quad \text{The LCM is } 2 \cdot 2 \cdot 2 \cdot 3 \cdot 5, \text{ or } 120.$$

$$\dfrac{17}{24} - \dfrac{4}{15} = \dfrac{17}{24} \cdot \dfrac{5}{5} - \dfrac{4}{15} \cdot \dfrac{8}{8}$$

Multiplying by 1 to obtain the LCD. To form 1, look at the prime factorization of the LCM and use the factors that each denominator lacks.

$$= \dfrac{85}{120} - \dfrac{32}{120} = \dfrac{85 - 32}{120} = \dfrac{53}{120}.$$

Do Exercises 5–8.

Example 7   Simplify by combining like terms: $\dfrac{7}{8}x - \dfrac{3}{4}x$.

$$\dfrac{7}{8}x - \dfrac{3}{4}x = \left(\dfrac{7}{8} - \dfrac{3}{4} \right)x$$

Try to do this step mentally.

$$= \left(\dfrac{7}{8} - \dfrac{6}{8} \right)x = \dfrac{1}{8}x$$

Multiplying $\frac{3}{4}$ by $\frac{2}{2}$ and subtracting

Do Exercise 9.

b | Solving Equations

In Section 2.8, we introduced the addition principle as one way to form equivalent equations. We can use that principle here to solve equations containing fractions.

Example 8 Solve: $x - \dfrac{1}{3} = \dfrac{6}{7}$.

$$x - \frac{1}{3} = \frac{6}{7}$$

$$x - \frac{1}{3} + \frac{1}{3} = \frac{6}{7} + \frac{1}{3} \qquad \text{Using the addition principle: adding } \tfrac{1}{3} \text{ on both sides}$$

$$x + 0 = \frac{6}{7} + \frac{1}{3} \qquad \text{Adding } \tfrac{1}{3} \text{ "undoes" the subtraction of } \tfrac{1}{3}.$$

$$x = \frac{6}{7} \cdot \frac{3}{3} + \frac{1}{3} \cdot \frac{7}{7} \qquad \text{Multiplying by 1 to obtain the LCD, 21}$$

$$x = \frac{18}{21} + \frac{7}{21} = \frac{25}{21}$$

CHECK:

$$\frac{x - \dfrac{1}{3} = \dfrac{6}{7}}{\begin{array}{c|c} \dfrac{25}{21} - \dfrac{1}{3} \ ? \ \dfrac{6}{7} \\[2mm] \dfrac{25}{21} - \dfrac{1}{3} \cdot \dfrac{7}{7} \\[2mm] \dfrac{25}{21} - \dfrac{7}{21} \\[2mm] \dfrac{18}{21} \\[2mm] \dfrac{6 \cdot \cancel{3}}{7 \cdot \cancel{3}} \ \Big| \ \dfrac{6}{7} \quad \text{TRUE} \end{array}}$$

Recall that since subtraction can be regarded as adding the opposite of the number being subtracted, the addition principle allows us to subtract the same number on both sides of an equation.

Example 9 Solve: $x + \dfrac{1}{4} = \dfrac{3}{5}$.

$$x + \frac{1}{4} - \frac{1}{4} = \frac{3}{5} - \frac{1}{4} \qquad \text{Using the addition principle to add } -\tfrac{1}{4} \text{ or to subtract } \tfrac{1}{4} \text{ on both sides}$$

$$x + 0 = \frac{3}{5} \cdot \frac{4}{4} - \frac{1}{4} \cdot \frac{5}{5} \qquad \text{The LCD is 20. We multiply by 1 to get the LCD.}$$

$$x = \frac{12}{20} - \frac{5}{20} = \frac{7}{20}$$

The solution is $\frac{7}{20}$. We leave the check to the student.

Do Exercises 10-12.

Solve.

10. Solve: $x - \dfrac{2}{5} = \dfrac{1}{5}$. $\dfrac{3}{5}$

11. $x + \dfrac{2}{3} = \dfrac{5}{6}$ $\dfrac{1}{6}$

12. $\dfrac{3}{5} + t = -\dfrac{7}{8}$ $-\dfrac{59}{40}$

Answers on page A-10

13. A $\frac{4}{5}$-cup bottle of salad dressing consists of olive oil and vinegar. The bottle contains $\frac{2}{3}$ cup of oil. How much vinegar is in the bottle?

$\frac{2}{15}$ cup

---

c | ## Solving Problems

Example 10 *Woodworking.* Celeste is replacing a $\frac{3}{4}$-in. thick shelf in her bookcase. If her replacement board is $\frac{15}{16}$ in. thick, how much should it be planed down before the repair can be completed?

1. **Familiarize.** We first make a drawing or at least visualize the situation.

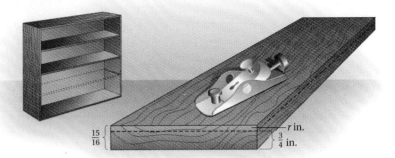

If necessary, we consult a reference book to learn that to plane a piece of wood is to use a tool for removing thin amounts of wood while producing a smooth surface. We let r = the amount of wood, in inches, that needs to be removed.

2. **Translate.** The problem translates to a "take-away" situation.

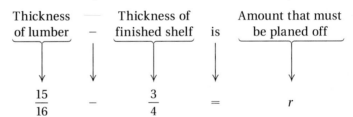

Thickness of lumber	−	Thickness of finished shelf	is	Amount that must be planed off
$\frac{15}{16}$	−	$\frac{3}{4}$	=	r

3. **Solve.** To solve the equation, we carry out the subtraction:

$$\frac{15}{16} - \frac{3}{4} = r \qquad \text{The LCD is 16.}$$

$$\frac{15}{16} - \frac{3}{4} \cdot \frac{4}{4} = r \qquad \text{Multiplying by 1}$$

$$\frac{15}{16} - \frac{12}{16} = r$$

$$\frac{3}{16} = r.$$

4. **Check.** We can check by adding $\frac{3}{16}$ to $\frac{3}{4}$:

$$\frac{3}{16} + \frac{3}{4} = \frac{3}{16} + \frac{12}{16} = \frac{15}{16}.$$

Since $\frac{15}{16}$ in. is the board's original thickness, our answer checks.

5. **State.** Celeste should plane $\frac{3}{16}$ in. from the replacement board.

Do Exercise 13.

Answer on page A-10

Exercise Set 4.3

a Subtract and, if possible, simplify.

1. $\dfrac{5}{6} - \dfrac{1}{6}$ $\dfrac{2}{3}$

2. $\dfrac{7}{5} - \dfrac{2}{5}$ 1

3. $\dfrac{11}{16} - \dfrac{15}{16}$ $-\dfrac{1}{4}$

4. $\dfrac{5}{12} - \dfrac{7}{12}$ $-\dfrac{1}{6}$

5. $\dfrac{7}{a} - \dfrac{3}{a}$ $\dfrac{4}{a}$

6. $\dfrac{4}{t} - \dfrac{9}{t}$ $-\dfrac{5}{t}$

7. $\dfrac{10}{3t} - \dfrac{4}{3t}$ $\dfrac{2}{t}$

8. $\dfrac{9}{2a} - \dfrac{5}{2a}$ $\dfrac{2}{a}$

9. $\dfrac{3}{5a} - \dfrac{7}{5a}$ $-\dfrac{4}{5a}$

10. $\dfrac{3}{7t} - \dfrac{9}{7t}$ $-\dfrac{6}{7t}$

11. $\dfrac{7}{8} - \dfrac{1}{16}$ $\dfrac{13}{16}$

12. $\dfrac{4}{3} - \dfrac{5}{6}$ $\dfrac{1}{2}$

13. $\dfrac{7}{15} - \dfrac{4}{5}$ $-\dfrac{1}{3}$

14. $\dfrac{3}{4} - \dfrac{3}{28}$ $\dfrac{9}{14}$

15. $\dfrac{3}{4} - \dfrac{1}{20}$ $\dfrac{7}{10}$

16. $\dfrac{3}{4} - \dfrac{4}{16}$ $\dfrac{1}{2}$

17. $\dfrac{2}{15} - \dfrac{5}{12}$ $-\dfrac{17}{60}$

18. $\dfrac{11}{16} - \dfrac{9}{10}$ $-\dfrac{17}{80}$

19. $\dfrac{6}{10} - \dfrac{7}{100}$ $\dfrac{53}{100}$

20. $\dfrac{9}{10} - \dfrac{3}{100}$ $\dfrac{87}{100}$

21. $\dfrac{7}{15} - \dfrac{3}{25}$ $\dfrac{26}{75}$

22. $\dfrac{18}{25} - \dfrac{4}{35}$ $\dfrac{106}{175}$

23. $\dfrac{69}{100} - \dfrac{9}{10}$ $-\dfrac{21}{100}$

24. $\dfrac{42}{100} - \dfrac{11}{20}$ $-\dfrac{13}{100}$

www.mathmax.com   World Wide Web   Exercise Set 4.3

227

25. $\dfrac{2}{3} - \dfrac{1}{8}$ $\dfrac{13}{24}$

26. $\dfrac{3}{4} - \dfrac{1}{2}$ $\dfrac{1}{4}$

27. $\dfrac{3}{5} - \dfrac{1}{2}$ $\dfrac{1}{10}$

28. $\dfrac{5}{6} - \dfrac{2}{3}$ $\dfrac{1}{6}$

29. $\dfrac{11}{18} - \dfrac{7}{24}$ $\dfrac{23}{72}$

30. $\dfrac{-7}{25} - \dfrac{2}{15}$ $-\dfrac{31}{75}$

31. $\dfrac{13}{90} - \dfrac{17}{120}$ $\dfrac{1}{360}$

32. $\dfrac{8}{25} - \dfrac{29}{150}$ $\dfrac{19}{150}$

33. $\dfrac{2}{3}x - \dfrac{4}{9}x$ $\dfrac{2}{9}x$

34. $\dfrac{7}{4}x - \dfrac{5}{12}x$ $\dfrac{4}{3}x$

35. $\dfrac{3}{5}a - \dfrac{3}{4}a$ $-\dfrac{3}{20}a$

36. $\dfrac{4}{7}a - \dfrac{1}{3}a$ $\dfrac{5}{21}a$

b Solve.

37. $x - \dfrac{5}{9} = \dfrac{2}{9}$ $\dfrac{7}{9}$

38. $x - \dfrac{3}{11} = \dfrac{7}{11}$ $\dfrac{10}{11}$

39. $a + \dfrac{2}{11} = \dfrac{8}{11}$ $\dfrac{6}{11}$

40. $a + \dfrac{4}{15} = \dfrac{13}{15}$ $\dfrac{3}{5}$

41. $x + \dfrac{2}{3} = \dfrac{7}{9}$ $\dfrac{1}{9}$

42. $x + \dfrac{1}{2} = \dfrac{7}{8}$ $\dfrac{3}{8}$

43. $a - \dfrac{3}{8} = \dfrac{3}{4}$ $\dfrac{9}{8}$

44. $x - \dfrac{3}{10} = \dfrac{2}{5}$ $\dfrac{7}{10}$

45. $\frac{2}{3} + x = \frac{4}{5}$ $\frac{2}{15}$

46. $\frac{4}{5} + x = \frac{6}{7}$ $\frac{2}{35}$

47. $\frac{3}{8} + a = \frac{1}{12}$ $-\frac{7}{24}$

48. $\frac{5}{6} + a = \frac{2}{9}$ $-\frac{11}{18}$

49. $n - \frac{1}{10} = -\frac{1}{30}$ $\frac{1}{15}$

50. $n - \frac{3}{4} = -\frac{5}{12}$ $\frac{1}{3}$

51. $x + \frac{3}{4} = -\frac{1}{2}$ $-\frac{5}{4}$

52. $x + \frac{5}{6} = -\frac{11}{12}$ $-\frac{7}{4}$

c | Solve.

53. Monica spent $\frac{3}{4}$ hr listening to tapes of Beethoven and Brahms. She spent $\frac{1}{3}$ hr listening to Beethoven. How many hours were spent listening to Brahms?

$\frac{5}{12}$ hr

54. From a $\frac{4}{5}$-lb wheel of cheese, a $\frac{1}{4}$-lb piece was served. How much cheese remained on the wheel?

$\frac{11}{20}$ lb

55. *Exercise.* As part of an exercise program, Hugo is to walk $\frac{7}{8}$ mi each day. He has already walked $\frac{1}{3}$ mi. How much farther should Hugo walk? $\frac{13}{24}$ mi

56. *Fitness.* As part of a fitness program, Deb swims $\frac{1}{2}$ mi every day. She has already swum $\frac{1}{5}$ mi. How much farther should Deb swim? $\frac{3}{10}$ mi

57. *Tire Tread.* A new long-life tire has a tread depth of $\frac{3}{8}$ in. instead of the more typical $\frac{11}{32}$ in. (***Source**: Popular Science*). How much deeper is the new tread depth? $\frac{1}{32}$ in.

58. *Furniture Cleaner.* A $\frac{3}{4}$-cup mixture of lemon juice and olive oil makes an excellent cleaner for wood furniture. If the mixture contains $\frac{1}{3}$ cup of lemon juice, how much olive oil is in the cleaner? $\frac{5}{12}$ cup

Skill Maintenance

Divide and simplify. [3.7b]

59. $\dfrac{9}{10} \div \dfrac{3}{5}$ $\dfrac{3}{2}$

60. $\dfrac{3}{7} \div \dfrac{9}{4}$ $\dfrac{4}{21}$

61. $(-7) \div \dfrac{1}{3}$ -21

62. $8 \div \left(-\dfrac{1}{4}\right)$ -32

63. A small box of cornflakes weighs $\frac{3}{4}$ lb. How much do 8 small boxes of cornflakes weigh? [3.6b]

6 lb

64. A batch of fudge requires $\frac{3}{4}$ cup of sugar. How much sugar is needed to make 12 batches? [3.6b]   9 cups

Synthesis

65. ◈ If a negative fraction is subtracted from another negative fraction, is the result always negative? Why or why not?

66. ◈ Victor incorrectly writes $\frac{8}{5} - \frac{8}{2} = \frac{8}{3}$. How could you convince Victor that his subtraction is incorrect?

67. ◈ Without performing the actual computation, explain how you can tell that $\frac{3}{7} - \frac{5}{9}$ is negative.

Solve.

68. ▦ $x + \dfrac{16}{323} = \dfrac{10}{187}$ $\dfrac{14}{3553}$

69. ▦ $x + \dfrac{7}{253} = \dfrac{12}{299}$ $\dfrac{41}{3289}$

70. A mountain climber, beginning at sea level, climbs $\frac{3}{5}$ km, descends $\frac{1}{4}$ km, climbs $\frac{1}{3}$ km, and then descends $\frac{1}{7}$ km. At what elevation does the climber finish? $\dfrac{227}{420}$ km

Simplify.

71. $\dfrac{2}{5} - \dfrac{1}{6}(-3)^2$ $-\dfrac{11}{10}$

72. $\dfrac{7}{8} - \dfrac{1}{10}\left(-\dfrac{5}{6}\right)^2$ $\dfrac{29}{36}$

73. $-4 \times \dfrac{3}{7} - \dfrac{1}{7} \times \dfrac{4}{5}$ $-\dfrac{64}{35}$

74. $\left(\dfrac{5}{6}\right)^2 + \left(\dfrac{3}{4}\right)^2$ $\dfrac{181}{144}$

75. Mazzi's meat slicer cut 8 slices of turkey and 3 slices of Vermont cheddar. If each turkey slice was $\frac{1}{16}$-in. thick and each cheddar slice was $\frac{5}{32}$-in. thick, how tall was the pile of cold cuts? $\dfrac{31}{32}$ in.

76. As part of a rehabilitation program, an athlete must swim and then walk a total of $\frac{9}{10}$ km each day. If one lap in the swimming pool is $\frac{3}{80}$ km, how far must the athlete walk after swimming 10 laps?

$\dfrac{21}{40}$ km

77. The Fullerton estate was left to four children. One received $\frac{1}{4}$ of the estate, one received $\frac{3}{8}$, and the twins split the rest. What fractional piece did each twin receive? $\dfrac{3}{16}$

78. Mark Romano owns $\frac{7}{12}$ of Romano-Chrenka Chevrolet and Lisa Romano owns $\frac{1}{6}$. If Paul and Ella Chrenka own the remaining share of the dealership equally, what fractional piece does Paul own? $\dfrac{1}{8}$

4.4 Solving Equations: Using the Principles Together

The equations that we solved in Sections 2.8, 3.8, and 4.3 required the use of either the addition principle or the multiplication principle. In this section, we will learn to solve equations that require the use of *both* principles. As review, let's restate both principles.

> **THE ADDITION PRINCIPLE**
>
> For any numbers a, b, and c,
>
> $$a = b \text{ is equivalent to } a + c = b + c.$$

> **THE MULTIPLICATION PRINCIPLE**
>
> For any numbers a, b, and c, with $c \neq 0$,
>
> $$a = b \text{ is equivalent to } a \cdot c = b \cdot c.$$

a   Using the Principles Together

Suppose we want to determine whether 6 is the solution of $5x - 8 = 27$. To check, we replace x with 6 and simplify.

CHECK:

$$
\begin{array}{c}
5x - 8 = 27 \\
\hline
5 \cdot 6 - 8 \; ? \; 27 \\
30 - 8 \\
22 \; \mid \; 27 \quad \text{FALSE}
\end{array}
$$

This shows that 6 is *not* the solution.

Do Exercises 1 and 2.

In the check above, note that the rules for order of operations dictate that we multiply (or divide) before we subtract (or add).

When solving an equation, we find an equivalent equation in which the variable is isolated on one side. Until now, this has been accomplished by "undoing" the operation present:

To solve $x - 7 = -2$, we added 7 on both sides.

To solve $9x = 63$, we divided by 9 on both sides.

To solve an equation like $5x - 8 = 27$, we need to "undo" both subtraction *and* multiplication in order to isolate x. Because the subtraction is performed *after* the multiplication in $5x - 8$, we will use addition *before* division when solving.

Objectives

a Solve equations that require use of both the addition principle and the multiplication principle.

For Extra Help

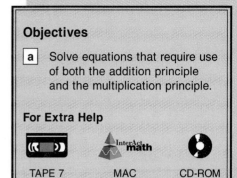

TAPE 7   MAC   CD-ROM
                WIN

1. Determine whether -9 is the solution of $7x + 8 = -55$.

   Yes

2. Determine whether -6 is the solution of $4x + 3 = -25$.

   No

Answers on page A-10

3. Solve: $2x - 9 = 43$ 26

4. Solve: $-3x + 2 = 47$ −15

Example 1   Solve: $5x - 8 = 27$.

We first isolate $5x$ by adding 8 on both sides:

$$5x - 8 = 27$$
$$5x - 8 + 8 = 27 + 8 \qquad \text{Using the addition principle}$$
$$5x + 0 = 35 \qquad \text{Try to do this step mentally.}$$
$$5x = 35.$$

Next, we isolate x by dividing by 5 $\left(\text{or multiplying by } \frac{1}{5}\right)$ on both sides:

$$5x = 35$$
$$\frac{5x}{5} = \frac{35}{5} \qquad \text{Using the division principle or the multiplication}$$
$$\qquad\qquad \text{principle (multiplying by } \tfrac{1}{5} \text{ on both sides)}$$
$$1x = 7 \qquad \text{Try to do this step mentally.}$$
$$x = 7.$$

CHECK:
$$\frac{5x - 8 = 27}{5 \cdot 7 - 8 \;?\; 27}$$
$$35 - 8$$
$$27 \mid 27 \quad \text{TRUE}$$

The solution is 7.

Note that we subtracted *last* in the check and used the addition principle *first* when solving.

Do Exercise 3.

Example 2   Solve: $38 = 9x + 2$.

We first isolate $9x$ by subtracting 2 on both sides:

$$38 = 9x + 2$$
$$38 - 2 = 9x + 2 - 2 \qquad \text{Subtracting 2 (or adding −2) on both sides}$$
$$36 = 9x + 0 \qquad \text{Try to do this step mentally.}$$
$$36 = 9x.$$

Now that we have isolated $9x$ on one side of the equation, we can divide by 9 to isolate x:

$$36 = 9x$$
$$\frac{36}{9} = \frac{9x}{9} \qquad \text{Dividing by 9} \left(\text{or multiplying by } \tfrac{1}{9} \text{ on both sides}\right)$$
$$4 = x. \qquad \text{Simplifying}$$

CHECK:
$$\frac{38 = 9x + 2}{38 \;?\; 9 \cdot 4 + 2}$$
$$\mid 36 + 2$$
$$38 \mid 38 \qquad \text{TRUE}$$

The solution is 4.

Do Exercise 4.

Example 3 Solve: $20 = 6 - \dfrac{2}{3}x$.

Our plan is to first use the addition principle to isolate $-\frac{2}{3}x$ and to then use the multiplication principle to isolate x.

$$20 = 6 - \frac{2}{3}x$$

$$20 - 6 = 6 - \frac{2}{3}x - 6 \qquad \text{Subtracting 6 (or adding } -6\text{) on both sides}$$

$$14 = -\frac{2}{3}x$$

$$\left(-\frac{3}{2}\right)14 = \left(-\frac{3}{2}\right)\left(-\frac{2}{3}x\right) \qquad \text{Multiplying by } -\tfrac{3}{2} \left(\text{or dividing by } -\tfrac{2}{3}\right) \\ \text{on both sides}$$

$$-\frac{3 \cdot 14}{2} = 1x$$

$$-\frac{3 \cdot 7 \cdot \cancel{2}}{\cancel{2}} = 1x \qquad \text{Removing a factor equal to 1: } \tfrac{2}{2} = 1$$

$$-21 = x.$$

CHECK:
$$20 = 6 - \frac{2}{3}x$$
$$\begin{array}{c|l} \hline 20 & 6 - \dfrac{2}{3}(-21) \\[2mm] & 6 + \dfrac{42}{3} \\[2mm] 20 & 6 + 14 \qquad \text{TRUE} \end{array}$$

The solution is -21.

Do Exercise 5.

The same steps are used to solve the next example on page 234.

5. Solve: $9 - \dfrac{3}{4}x = 21$. -16

Answer on page A-10

6. Solve: $3 + \dfrac{14}{5}t = -\dfrac{21}{5}$. $-\dfrac{18}{7}$

Example 4   Solve: $5 + \dfrac{9}{2}t = -\dfrac{7}{2}$.

$$5 + \frac{9}{2}t = -\frac{7}{2}$$

$$5 + \frac{9}{2}t - 5 = -\frac{7}{2} - 5 \qquad \text{Subtracting 5 on both sides}$$

$$\frac{9}{2}t = -\frac{7}{2} - \frac{10}{2} \qquad \text{Writing 5 as } \frac{10}{2} \text{ to use the LCD}$$

$$\frac{9}{2}t = -\frac{17}{2}$$

$$\frac{2}{9} \cdot \frac{9}{2}t = \frac{2}{9}\left(-\frac{17}{2}\right) \qquad \text{Multiplying by } \frac{2}{9} \text{ on both sides}$$

$$1t = -\frac{\cancel{2} \cdot 17}{9 \cdot \cancel{2}} \qquad \text{Removing a factor equal to 1: } \frac{2}{2} = 1$$

$$t = -\frac{17}{9}$$

CHECK:

$$5 + \frac{9}{2}t = -\frac{7}{2}$$

$$5 + \frac{\cancel{9}}{2}\left(-\frac{17}{\cancel{9}}\right) \overset{?}{\mid} -\frac{7}{2} \qquad \text{Removing a factor equal to 1: } \frac{9}{9} = 1$$

$$5 + \left(-\frac{17}{2}\right)$$

$$\frac{10}{2} + \left(\frac{-17}{2}\right)$$

$$\frac{10 - 17}{2}$$

$$\frac{-7}{2} \quad \Big| \quad -\frac{7}{2} \qquad \text{TRUE}$$

The solution is $-\dfrac{17}{9}$.

Do Exercise 6.

Answer on page A-10

Chapter 4   Fractions: Addition &
Subtraction

234

Exercise Set 4.4

a Solve using the addition principle and/or the multiplication principle. Don't forget to check!

1. $6x - 4 = 14$ 3

2. $7x - 6 = 22$ 4

3. $3a + 8 = 23$ 5

4. $19 = 2x - 7$ 13

5. $4a + 9 = 37$ 7

6. $2a - 9 = -7$ 1

7. $31 = 3x - 5$ 12

8. $5x + 7 = -8$ -3

9. $-5t + 4 = 39$ -7

10. $-8t + 7 = 39$ -4

11. $3x + 4 = -11$ -5

12. $3a - 7 = -1$ 2

13. $\dfrac{4}{5}x = 20$ 25

14. $\dfrac{3}{4}x = 18$ 24

15. $\dfrac{3}{2}x - 3 = 12$ 10

16. $\dfrac{7}{3}x - 1 = 6$ 3

17. $\dfrac{3}{5}t - 4 = 8$ 20

18. $6 - \dfrac{2}{9}t = -4$ 45

19. $x + \dfrac{7}{3} = \dfrac{19}{6}$ $\dfrac{5}{6}$

20. $-\dfrac{41}{10} + x = \dfrac{7}{2}$ $\dfrac{38}{5}$

21. $7 = a + \dfrac{14}{5}$ $\dfrac{21}{5}$

22. $9 = a + \dfrac{47}{10}$ $\dfrac{43}{10}$

23. $\dfrac{2}{5}t - 1 = \dfrac{7}{5}$ 6

24. $-\dfrac{53}{4} = \dfrac{3}{2}a + 2$ $-\dfrac{61}{6}$

25. $\dfrac{39}{8} = \dfrac{11}{4} + \dfrac{1}{2}x$ $\dfrac{17}{4}$

26. $\dfrac{17}{2} = \dfrac{2}{7}t - \dfrac{3}{2}$ 35

27. $\dfrac{13}{3}s + \dfrac{11}{2} = \dfrac{35}{4}$ $\dfrac{3}{4}$

28. $\dfrac{11}{5}t + \dfrac{36}{5} = \dfrac{7}{2}$ $-\dfrac{37}{22}$

Solve.   [2.3b]

29. Jeremy withdraws $200 from an ATM (automated teller machine), makes a $90 deposit, and then withdraws another $40. How much has Jeremy's account balance changed?

The balance has decreased $150.

30. Animal Instinct, a pet supply store, makes a profit of $850 on Friday, and $375 on Saturday, but suffers a loss of $45 on Sunday. Find the total profit or loss for the three days. $1180 profit

Divide and simplify.   [3.7b]

31. $\dfrac{10}{7} \div 2m$ $\dfrac{5}{7m}$

32. $45n \div \dfrac{9}{4}$ $20n$

Multiply.   [2.7a]

33. $3(a + b)$ $3a + 3b$

34. $7(m - 3)$ $7m - 21$

Synthesis

35. ◆ Describe a procedure that a classmate could use to solve the equation $ax + b = c$ for x.

36. ◆ Nathan begins solving the equation $-\dfrac{2}{3}x + 7 = -9$ by adding 9 on both sides. Is this a wise thing to do? Why or why not?

37. ◆ Lorin begins solving the equation $\dfrac{2}{3}x + 1 = \dfrac{5}{6}$ by multiplying on both sides by 12. Is this a wise thing to do? Why or why not?

Solve.

38. ▦ $\dfrac{1081}{3599}x - \dfrac{17}{61} = \dfrac{19}{59}$ 2

39. ▦ $\dfrac{553}{2451}a - \dfrac{13}{57} = \dfrac{29}{43}$ 4

40. $-\dfrac{a}{5} + \dfrac{31}{4} = \dfrac{16}{3}$ $\dfrac{145}{12}$

41. $\dfrac{47}{5} - \dfrac{a}{4} = \dfrac{44}{7}$ $\dfrac{436}{35}$

42. $\dfrac{49}{8} + \dfrac{2x}{9} = 4$ $-\dfrac{153}{16}$

43. The perimeter of the figure shown is 15 cm. Solve for x.   2 cm

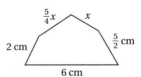

4.5 Mixed Numerals

a | What Is a Mixed Numeral?

A symbol like $2\frac{3}{4}$ is called a **mixed numeral.**

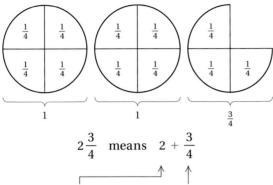

1   1 $\frac{3}{4}$

$$2\frac{3}{4} \quad \text{means} \quad 2 + \frac{3}{4}$$

This is a whole number.   This is a fraction less than 1.

Examples Convert to a mixed numeral.

1. $7 + \frac{2}{5} = 7\frac{2}{5}$ **2.** $4 + \frac{3}{10} = 4\frac{3}{10}$

Do Exercises 1–3.

The notation $2\frac{3}{4}$ has a plus sign left out. To aid in understanding, we sometimes write the missing plus sign. Similarly, the notation $-5\frac{2}{3}$ has a minus sign left out since $-5\frac{2}{3} = -\left(5 + \frac{2}{3}\right) = -5 - \frac{2}{3}$.

Mixed numbers can be displayed easily on a number line, as shown here.

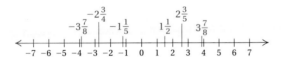

Examples Convert to fractional notation.

3. $2\frac{3}{4} = 2 + \frac{3}{4}$ Inserting the missing plus sign

$= \frac{2}{1} + \frac{3}{4}$ $2 = \frac{2}{1}$

$= \frac{2}{1} \cdot \frac{4}{4} + \frac{3}{4}$ Finding a common denominator

$= \frac{8}{4} + \frac{3}{4}$

$= \frac{11}{4}$ Adding

4. $4\frac{3}{10} = 4 + \frac{3}{10} = \frac{4}{1} + \frac{3}{10} = \frac{4}{1} \cdot \frac{10}{10} + \frac{3}{10} = \frac{40}{10} + \frac{3}{10} = \frac{43}{10}$

Do Exercises 4 and 5.

1. $1 + \frac{2}{3} =$ Convert to a mixed numeral.

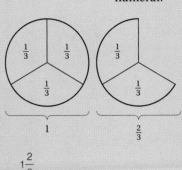

1       $\frac{2}{3}$

$1\frac{2}{3}$

Convert to a mixed numeral.

2. $8 + \frac{3}{4}$ **3.** $12 + \frac{2}{3}$

$8\frac{3}{4}$ $12\frac{2}{3}$

Convert to fractional notation.

4. $4\frac{2}{5}$ **5.** $6\frac{1}{10}$

$\frac{22}{5}$ $\frac{61}{10}$

Answers on page A-10

Convert to fractional notation.
Use the faster method.

6. $4\frac{5}{6}$ $\frac{29}{6}$

7. $9\frac{1}{4}$ $\frac{37}{4}$

8. $20\frac{2}{3}$ $\frac{62}{3}$

Convert to fractional notation.

9. $-6\frac{2}{5}$ $-\frac{32}{5}$

10. $-8\frac{3}{7}$ $-\frac{59}{7}$

Answers on page A-10

Using Example 4, we can develop a faster way to convert.

To convert from a mixed numeral like $4\frac{3}{10}$ to fractional notation:

ⓐ Multiply: $4 \cdot 10 = 40$.

ⓑ Add: $40 + 3 = 43$.

ⓒ Keep the denominator.

$$\overset{ⓑ}{\nearrow} \underset{ⓐ}{\nwarrow} 4\frac{3}{10} = \frac{43}{10} \swarrow$$

Examples   Convert to fractional notation.

5. $6\frac{2}{3} = \frac{20}{3}$ $6 \cdot 3 = 18, \ 18 + 2 = 20$; keep the denominator

6. $8\frac{2}{9} = \frac{74}{9}$ $9 \cdot 8 = 72; \ 72 + 2 = 74$; keep the denominator

7. $10\frac{7}{8} = \frac{87}{8}$ $8 \cdot 10 = 80; \ 80 + 7 = 87$; keep the denominator

Do Exercises 6–8.

To find the opposite of the number in Example 5, we can write either $-6\frac{2}{3}$ or $-\frac{20}{3}$. Thus, to convert a negative mixed numeral to fractional notation, we remove the negative sign for purposes of computation and then include it in the answer.

Examples   Convert to fractional notation.

8. $-5\frac{1}{3} = -\frac{16}{3}$ $3 \cdot 5 = 15; \ 15 + 1 = 16$; include the negative sign

9. $-7\frac{5}{6} = -\frac{47}{6}$ $6 \cdot 7 = 42; \ 42 + 5 = 47$

Do Exercises 9 and 10.

b **Writing Mixed Numerals**

We can find a mixed numeral for $\frac{5}{3}$ as follows:

$$\frac{5}{3} = \frac{3}{3} + \frac{2}{3} = 1 + \frac{2}{3} = 1\frac{2}{3}.$$

Fractional symbols like $\frac{5}{3}$ also indicate division:

$$\begin{array}{r} 1\frac{2}{3} \leftarrow \\ 3\overline{)5} \\ \underline{3} \\ 2 \end{array} \leftarrow \text{Now divide 2 by 3: } 2 \div 3 = \frac{2}{3}$$

Thus, $\frac{5}{3} = 1\frac{2}{3}$.

We can also visualize $\frac{5}{3}$ as one-third of 5 objects, as shown below.

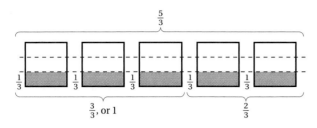

$\frac{5}{3}$

$\frac{1}{3}$ $\frac{1}{3}$ $\frac{1}{3}$ $\frac{1}{3}$ $\frac{1}{3}$

$\frac{3}{3}$, or 1 $\frac{2}{3}$

To convert from fractional notation to a mixed numeral, divide.

$$\frac{13}{5};$$

$$\begin{array}{r} 2 \\ 5\overline{)13} \\ 10 \\ \hline 3 \end{array}$$ → The quotient

→ The remainder

$2\frac{3}{5};$

$$\frac{13}{5} = 2\frac{3}{5}$$

Examples   Convert to a mixed numeral.

10. $\frac{8}{5}$ $\begin{array}{r} 1 \\ 5\overline{)8} \\ 5 \\ \hline 3 \end{array}$ $\frac{8}{5} = 1\frac{3}{5}$

> A fraction larger than 1, such as $\frac{8}{5}$, is sometimes referred to as an "improper" fraction. We have intentionally avoided such terminology. The use of such notation as $\frac{8}{5}$, $\frac{69}{10}$, and so on, is quite proper and very common in algebra.

11. $\frac{69}{10}$ $\begin{array}{r} 6 \\ 10\overline{)69} \\ 60 \\ \hline 9 \end{array}$ $\frac{69}{10} = 6\frac{9}{10}$

12. $\frac{122}{8}$ $\begin{array}{r} 15 \\ 8\overline{)122} \\ 80 \\ \hline 42 \\ 40 \\ \hline 2 \end{array}$ $\frac{122}{8} = 15\frac{2}{8} = 15\frac{1}{4}$

> Whenever possible, simplify the fractional part of the numeral.

Do Exercises 11–13.

The same procedure also works with negative numbers. Of course, the result will be a negative mixed numeral.

Example 13   Convert $\frac{-9}{4}$ to a mixed numeral.

Since $\begin{array}{r} 2 \\ 4\overline{)9} \\ 8 \\ \hline 1 \end{array}$,   we have $\frac{9}{4} = 2\frac{1}{4}$.

Thus, $\frac{-9}{4} = -2\frac{1}{4}$.

Do Exercises 14 and 15.

Convert to a mixed numeral.

11. $\frac{7}{3}$ $2\frac{1}{3}$

12. $\frac{11}{10}$ $1\frac{1}{10}$

13. $\frac{110}{6}$ $18\frac{1}{3}$

Convert to a mixed numeral.

14. $\frac{-12}{5}$ $-2\frac{2}{5}$

15. $-\frac{134}{12}$ $-11\frac{1}{6}$

Answers on page A-10

16. Divide. Write a mixed numeral for the answer.

$$6 \overline{)\,4\ 8\ 4\ 6}$$

$807\frac{2}{3}$

17. Over the last 4 yr, Roland Thompson's raspberry patch has yielded 48, 35, 65, and 75 qt of berries. Find the average yield for the four years.

$55\frac{3}{4}$ qt

It is quite common when performing long division to express the quotient as a mixed numeral. As in Examples 10–13, the remainder becomes the numerator of the fractional part of the mixed numeral.

Example 14   Divide. Write a mixed numeral for the quotient.

$$7 \overline{)\,6\ 3\ 4\ 1}$$

We first divide as usual.

$$
\begin{array}{r}
9\ 0\ 5 \\
7 \overline{)\,6\ 3\ 4\ 1} \\
6\ 3\ 0\ 0 \\
\hline
4\ 1 \\
3\ 5 \\
\hline
6
\end{array}
$$

The answer is 905 R 6, or, as a mixed numeral $905\frac{6}{7}$. Using fractional notation, we write $\frac{6341}{7} = 905\frac{6}{7}$.

Do Exercise 16.

Example 15   *Charities.*   The American Institute of Philanthropy monitors how much charitable organizations spend in order to raise $100. (*Source: AIP 1996–97 Watchdog Report.* American Institute of Philanthropy, St. Louis, MO 63108). Five of the best organizations in this respect are listed below. How much did they spend, on average, to raise $100?

African–American Institute	$3
Asia Foundation	$4
International Rescue Committee	$8
Make-A-Wish Foundation	$7
National Hispanic Scholarship Fund	$4

Recall from Section 1.9 that to find the *average* of a set of values, we add the values and divide that sum by the number of values being added.

$$\text{Average spent} = \frac{3 + 4 + 8 + 7 + 4}{5} = \frac{26}{5} = 5\frac{1}{5}$$

On average, these groups spent $5\frac{1}{5}$ to raise $100.

Do Exercise 17.

Calculator Spotlight

Exercises

If your calculator has the capability of finding whole-number quotients and remainders (see Section 1.6), use it to find mixed numerals for the answers to each of the following divisions.

1. $6 \overline{)\,8\ 8\ 5\ 7}$ $1476\frac{1}{6}$ **2.** $9 \overline{)\,6\ 0\ 8\ 8}$ $676\frac{4}{9}$

3. $5\ 6 \overline{)\,4\ 4,8\ 5\ 1}$ $800\frac{51}{56}$ **4.** $1\ 8 \overline{)\,2\ 3\ 4,5\ 6\ 7}$ $13{,}031\frac{1}{2}$

5. $1\ 1 \overline{)\,5\ 6\ 7,8\ 9\ 5}$ $51{,}626\frac{9}{11}$ **6.** $3\ 2 \overline{)\,2\ 3\ 4,5\ 6\ 7}$ $7330\frac{7}{32}$

7. $4\ 5 \overline{)\,6\ 0\ 3\ 3}$ $134\frac{1}{15}$ **8.** $2\ 1\ 3 \overline{)\,5\ 6\ 7,9\ 8\ 8}$ $2666\frac{130}{213}$

9. $1\ 1\ 2 \overline{)\,4\ 0\ 0,0\ 0\ 3}$ $3571\frac{51}{112}$ **10.** $9\ 0\ 8 \overline{)\,1\ 1,2\ 3\ 4}$ $12\frac{169}{454}$

Exercise Set 4.5

a Convert to fractional notation.

1. $3\frac{2}{5}$ $\quad \frac{17}{5}$

2. $5\frac{2}{3}$ $\quad \frac{17}{3}$

3. $6\frac{1}{4}$ $\quad \frac{25}{4}$

4. $8\frac{1}{2}$ $\quad \frac{17}{2}$

5. $-20\frac{1}{8}$ $\quad -\frac{161}{8}$

6. $-10\frac{1}{3}$ $\quad -\frac{31}{3}$

7. $5\frac{1}{10}$ $\quad \frac{51}{10}$

8. $8\frac{1}{10}$ $\quad \frac{81}{10}$

9. $20\frac{3}{5}$ $\quad \frac{103}{5}$

10. $30\frac{4}{5}$ $\quad \frac{154}{5}$

11. $-9\frac{5}{6}$ $\quad -\frac{59}{6}$

12. $-8\frac{7}{8}$ $\quad -\frac{71}{8}$

13. $6\frac{9}{10}$ $\quad \frac{69}{10}$

14. $1\frac{3}{5}$ $\quad \frac{8}{5}$

15. $-12\frac{3}{4}$ $\quad -\frac{51}{4}$

16. $-15\frac{2}{3}$ $\quad -\frac{47}{3}$

17. $5\frac{7}{10}$ $\quad \frac{57}{10}$

18. $7\frac{3}{100}$ $\quad \frac{703}{100}$

19. $-5\frac{7}{100}$ $\quad -\frac{507}{100}$

20. $-6\frac{4}{15}$ $\quad -\frac{94}{15}$

b Convert to a mixed numeral.

21. $\frac{14}{3}$ $\quad 4\frac{2}{3}$

22. $\frac{19}{8}$ $\quad 2\frac{3}{8}$

23. $\frac{-27}{6}$ $\quad -4\frac{1}{2}$

24. $\frac{30}{9}$ $\quad 3\frac{1}{3}$

25. $\frac{57}{10}$ $\quad 5\frac{7}{10}$

26. $\frac{-89}{10}$ $\quad -8\frac{9}{10}$

27. $\frac{53}{7}$ $\quad 7\frac{4}{7}$

28. $\frac{65}{8}$ $\quad 8\frac{1}{8}$

29. $\frac{45}{6}$ $\quad 7\frac{1}{2}$

30. $\frac{-50}{8}$ $\quad -6\frac{1}{4}$

31. $\frac{46}{4}$ $\quad 11\frac{1}{2}$

32. $\frac{39}{9}$ $\quad 4\frac{1}{3}$

33. $\frac{-12}{8}$ $\quad -1\frac{1}{2}$

34. $\frac{757}{100}$ $\quad 7\frac{57}{100}$

35. $\frac{28}{6}$ $\quad 4\frac{2}{3}$

36. $-\frac{345}{8}$ $\quad -43\frac{1}{8}$

37. $-\frac{223}{4}$ $\quad -55\frac{3}{4}$

38. $\frac{467}{100}$ $\quad 4\frac{67}{100}$

c Divide. Write a mixed numeral for the answer.

39. $8\,)\,8\,6\,9$

$108\frac{5}{8}$

40. $3\,)\,2\,1\,2\,6$

$708\frac{2}{3}$

41. $7\,)\,6\,3\,4\,5$

$906\frac{3}{7}$

42. $9\,)\,9\,1\,1\,0$

$1012\frac{2}{9}$

43. $2\,1\,)\,8\,5\,2$

$40\frac{4}{7}$

44. $8\,5\,)\,7\,6\,7\,2$

$90\frac{22}{85}$

45. $-302 \div 15$

$-20\frac{2}{15}$

46. $-475 \div 13$

$-36\frac{7}{13}$

47. $471 \div (-21)$

$-22\frac{3}{7}$

48. $542 \div (-25)$

$-21\frac{17}{25}$

Nutrition. For Exercises 49–52, consider the list at right of the 20 least fatty fast foods. (**Source:** *The Consumer Bible* by Mark Green. New York: Workman, 1995, p. 25).

Chain	Food	Fat
Boston Market	Fruit salad side dish	0 g
Boston Market	Steamed vegetables	0 g
Hardee's	Mashed potatoes and gravy side	0 g
KFC	Garden rice side dish	1 g
KFC	Mashed potatoes with gravy side dish	1 g
KFC	Green beans side dish	1 g
Arby's	Chicken Noodle Soup	2 g
Jack-in-the-Box	Chicken Teriyaki Bowl	2 g
KFC	Baked Beans side dish	2 g
KFC	Mean Greens side dish	2 g
Boston Market	Chicken Soup	3 g
Church's	Potatoes & Gravy	3 g
Jack-in-the-Box	Beef Teriyaki Bowl	3 g
KFC	Red Beans & Rice	3 g
Popeye's	Corn on the cob	3 g
Arby's	Mixed Vegetable Soup	4 g
Boston Market	Chicken breast sandwich, no mayo or mustard	4 g
Boston Market	White meat chicken quarter, no skin or wing	4 g
Dairy Queen/Brazier	BBQ Beef Sandwich	4 g
KFC	Vegetable Medley Salad	4 g

49. What is the average number of grams (g) of fat in the foods from Boston Market? $2\frac{1}{5}$ g

50. What is the average number of grams of fat in the foods from Arby's and Jack-in-the-Box taken together? $2\frac{3}{4}$ g

51. What is the average number of grams of fat for the entire list? $2\frac{3}{10}$ g

52. What is the average number of grams of fat for the last 10 items on the list? $3\frac{1}{2}$ g

Skill Maintenance

Multiply and simplify. [3.6a]

53. $\dfrac{7}{9} \cdot \dfrac{24}{21}$ $\dfrac{8}{9}$

54. $\dfrac{6}{5} \cdot 15$ 18

55. $\dfrac{5}{12} \cdot (-6)$ $-\dfrac{5}{2}$

56. $\dfrac{7}{10} \cdot \dfrac{5}{14}$ $\dfrac{1}{4}$

Synthesis

57. ◆ Describe in your own words a method for rewriting a mixed numeral as a fraction.

58. ◆ Describe in your own words a method for rewriting a fraction as a mixed numeral.

59. ◆ Are the numbers $2\frac{1}{3}$ and $2 \cdot \frac{1}{3}$ equal? Why or why not?

Write a mixed numeral.

60. 🖩 $\dfrac{128,236}{541}$ $237\dfrac{19}{541}$

61. 🖩 $\dfrac{103,676}{349}$ $297\dfrac{23}{349}$

62. $\dfrac{56}{7} + \dfrac{2}{3}$ $8\dfrac{2}{3}$

63. $\dfrac{72}{12} + \dfrac{5}{6}$ $6\dfrac{5}{6}$

64. $\dfrac{12}{5} + \dfrac{19}{15}$ $3\dfrac{2}{3}$

65. There are $\frac{366}{7}$ weeks in a leap year. $52\frac{2}{7}$

66. There are $\frac{365}{7}$ weeks in a year. $52\frac{1}{7}$

67. *Athletics.* At a track and field meet, the hammer that is thrown has a wire length ranging from 3 ft, $10\frac{1}{4}$ in. to 3 ft, $11\frac{3}{4}$ in., a $4\frac{1}{8}$-in. grip, and a 16-lb ball with a diameter of from $4\frac{3}{8}$ in. to $5\frac{1}{8}$ in. Give specifications for the wire length and diameter of an "average" hammer.

wire length: 3 ft, 11 in. diameter: $4\frac{3}{4}$ in.

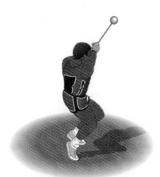

4.6 Addition and Subtraction Using Mixed Numerals; Applications

a | Addition

To find the sum $1\frac{5}{8} + 3\frac{1}{8}$, we first add the fractions. Then we add the whole numbers.

$$1 \frac{5}{8} = \qquad 1 \frac{5}{8}$$
$$+ 3 \frac{1}{8} = \qquad + 3 \frac{1}{8}$$
$$\overline{\qquad \frac{6}{8} \qquad} \qquad \overline{4 \frac{6}{8} = 4\frac{3}{4}}$$

Simplify the fractional part of the result when possible.

↑ Add the fractions. ↑ Add the whole numbers.

Do Exercise 1.

Example 1 Add: $5\frac{2}{3} + 3\frac{5}{6}$. Write a mixed numeral for the answer.

We first rewrite $\frac{2}{3}$, using the LCD, 6. Then we add.

$$5 \frac{2}{3} \cdot \frac{2}{2} = \quad 5 \frac{4}{6}$$
$$+ 3 \frac{5}{6} \qquad = + 3 \frac{5}{6}$$
$$\overline{\qquad 8 \frac{9}{6} = 8 + \frac{9}{6}}$$
$$= 8 + 1\frac{1}{2}$$
$$= 9\frac{1}{2}$$

To find a mixed numeral for $\frac{9}{6}$, we divide:

$$6)\overline{9} \qquad \frac{9}{6} = 1\frac{3}{6} = 1\frac{1}{2}$$
$$\underline{6}$$
$$3$$

$\frac{19}{2}$ is also a correct answer, but it is not a mixed numeral, which is what we are working with in Sections 4.5, 4.6, and 4.7.

Do Exercise 2.

Example 2 Add: $10\frac{5}{6} + 7\frac{3}{8}$.

The LCD is 24.

$$10 \frac{5}{6} \cdot \frac{4}{4} = \quad 10\frac{20}{24}$$
$$+ 7 \frac{3}{8} \cdot \frac{3}{3} = + 7\frac{9}{24}$$
$$\overline{\qquad 17\frac{29}{24} = 18\frac{5}{24}}$$

The fractional part of a mixed numeral should always be less than 1.

Do Exercise 3.

Objectives

a Add using mixed numerals.

b Subtract and combine like terms using mixed numerals.

c Solve applied problems involving addition and subtraction with mixed numerals.

d Add and subtract using negative mixed numerals.

For Extra Help

TAPE 8 MAC WIN CD-ROM

1. Add.

$$2\frac{3}{10}$$
$$+ 5\frac{1}{10}$$
$$\overline{7\frac{2}{5}}$$

2. Add.

$$8\frac{2}{5}$$
$$+ 3\frac{7}{10}$$
$$\overline{12\frac{1}{10}}$$

3. Add.

$$9\frac{3}{4}$$
$$+ 3\frac{5}{6}$$
$$\overline{13\frac{7}{12}}$$

Answers on page A-10

Subtract.

4. $10\dfrac{7}{8}$
$-\ 9\dfrac{3}{8}$
——————
$1\dfrac{1}{2}$

5. $8\dfrac{2}{3}$
$-\ 5\dfrac{1}{2}$
——————
$3\dfrac{1}{6}$

6. Subtract.

$5\dfrac{1}{12}$
$-\ 1\dfrac{3}{4}$
——————
$3\dfrac{1}{3}$

7. Subtract.

5
$-\ 1\dfrac{1}{3}$
——————
$3\dfrac{2}{3}$

Answers on page A-10

---

b | Subtraction

Example 3   Subtract: $7\dfrac{3}{4} - 2\dfrac{1}{4}$.

$$7\,\boxed{\dfrac{3}{4}} = \qquad 7\,\dfrac{3}{4}$$
$$-\ 2\,\boxed{\dfrac{1}{4}} = \qquad -\ 2\,\dfrac{1}{4}$$
$$\overline{\qquad\boxed{\dfrac{2}{4}}\qquad} \qquad \overline{\ 5\,\boxed{\dfrac{2}{4}}} = 5\dfrac{1}{2}$$

↑   ↑   ↑
                                    Simplifying

Subtract the   Subtract the
fractions.   whole numbers.

Example 4   Subtract: $9\dfrac{4}{5} - 3\dfrac{1}{2}$.

The LCD is 10.

$$9\,\boxed{\dfrac{4}{5}\cdot\dfrac{2}{2}} = \qquad 9\,\dfrac{8}{10}$$
$$-\ 3\,\boxed{\dfrac{1}{2}\cdot\dfrac{5}{5}} = -\ 3\,\dfrac{5}{10}$$
$$\overline{\qquad\qquad\qquad\qquad\qquad 6\,\dfrac{3}{10}}$$

Do Exercises 4 and 5.

Example 5   Subtract: $7\dfrac{1}{6} - 2\dfrac{1}{4}$.

The LCD is 12.

$$7\,\boxed{\dfrac{1}{6}\cdot\dfrac{2}{2}} = \qquad 7\,\dfrac{2}{12}\;\Big\}$$
$$-\ 2\,\boxed{\dfrac{1}{4}\cdot\dfrac{3}{3}} = -\ 2\,\dfrac{3}{12}\;\Big\}$$

> To subtract $2\dfrac{3}{12}$ from $7\dfrac{2}{12}$ we borrow 1, or $\dfrac{12}{12}$, from 7: $7\dfrac{2}{12} = 6 + 1 + \dfrac{2}{12} = 6 + \dfrac{12}{12} + \dfrac{2}{12} = 6\dfrac{14}{12}$.

Once $7\dfrac{1}{6}$ has been written as $6\dfrac{14}{12}$, we can subtract as we did in Examples 3 and 4:

$$7\,\dfrac{2}{12} = \qquad 6\,\dfrac{14}{12}$$
$$-\ 2\,\dfrac{3}{12} = -\ 2\,\dfrac{3}{12}$$
$$\overline{\qquad\qquad\qquad\qquad 4\,\dfrac{11}{12}}.$$

Do Exercise 6.

Example 6   Subtract: $12 - 9\dfrac{3}{8}$.

$$12 \quad = \quad 11\,\dfrac{8}{8} \leftarrow 12 = 11 + 1 = 11 + \dfrac{8}{8} = 11\dfrac{8}{8}$$
$$-\ 9\,\dfrac{3}{8} = -\ 9\,\dfrac{3}{8}$$
$$\overline{\qquad\qquad\qquad\qquad 2\,\dfrac{5}{8}}$$

Do Exercise 7.

To combine like terms, we use the distributive law and add or subtract as above.

Example 7   Combine like terms: **(a)** $9\frac{3}{4}x - 4\frac{1}{2}x$; **(b)** $4\frac{5}{6}t + 2\frac{7}{9}t$.

a) $9\frac{3}{4}x - 4\frac{1}{2}x = \left(9\frac{3}{4} - 4\frac{1}{2}\right)x$ Using the distributive law.
                                                                   This is often done mentally.

$= \left(9\frac{3}{4} - 4\frac{2}{4}\right)x$ The LCD is 4.

$= 5\frac{1}{4}x$ Subtracting

b) $4\frac{5}{6}t + 2\frac{7}{9}t = \left(4\frac{5}{6} + 2\frac{7}{9}\right)t$ This step is often performed mentally.

$= \left(4\frac{15}{18} + 2\frac{14}{18}\right)t$ The LCD is 18.

$= 6\frac{29}{18}t = 7\frac{11}{18}t$

Do Exercises 8–10.

c | Solving Problems

Example 8   *Intel Stock.* One day, the stock of Intel Corporation opened at $100\frac{3}{8}$ and then rose $4\frac{3}{4}$. Find the price of the stock at the end of the day.

1. Familiarize.   We first make a drawing or at least visualize the situation. We let p = the price, in dollars, at the end of the day.

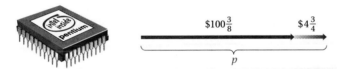

$$\$100\frac{3}{8} \qquad \$4\frac{3}{4}$$
$$p$$

Note that $100\frac{3}{8}$ is close to $100 and that $4\frac{3}{4}$ is close to $5, so we expect the answer to be close to 100 + 5, or $105.

2. Translate.   From the work above, we see that the price at the end of the day is the opening price plus the amount of the rise. Thus,

$$p = 100\frac{3}{8} + 4\frac{3}{4}.$$

3. Solve.   The equation tells us what to do. We add, using the LCD, 8:

$$100\frac{3}{8} = \quad 100\frac{3}{8} \quad = \quad 100\frac{3}{8}$$

$$+ \quad 4\frac{3}{4} = + \quad 4\frac{3}{4}\cdot\frac{2}{2} = + \quad 4\frac{6}{8}$$

$$104\frac{9}{8} = 105\frac{1}{8}.$$

Thus, $p = \$105\frac{1}{8}$.

Combine like terms.

8. $7\frac{1}{6}t + 5\frac{2}{3}t$ $12\frac{5}{6}t$

9. $7\frac{11}{12}x - 5\frac{2}{3}x$ $2\frac{1}{4}x$

10. $4\frac{3}{10}x + 9\frac{11}{15}x$ $14\frac{1}{30}x$

Answers on page A-10

11. Executive Car Care sold two pieces of synthetic leather. One piece was $3\frac{1}{4}$ yd long and the other was $3\frac{5}{6}$ yd long. What was the total length sold?

$7\frac{1}{12}$ yd

4. Check. We check by repeating the calculation or by noting that $\$105\frac{1}{8}$ is close to $\$105$, as predicted in the *Familiarize* step.

5. State. The price of the stock was $\$105\frac{1}{8}$ at the end of the day.

Do Exercise 11.

Example 9 *NCAA Football Goalposts.* Recently, in college football, the distance between goalposts was reduced from $23\frac{1}{3}$ ft to $18\frac{1}{2}$ ft. By how much was it reduced?

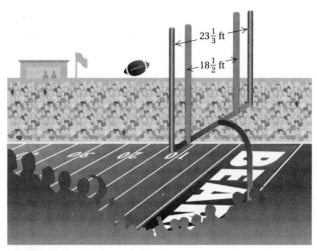

Source: NCAA

1. Familiarize. We let d = the size of the reduction in feet and make a drawing to illustrate the situation.

2. Translate. We translate as follows.

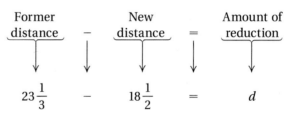

Former distance	−	New distance	=	Amount of reduction
$23\frac{1}{3}$	−	$18\frac{1}{2}$	=	d

12. *Knives.* The Damascus blade of a pearl-handled folding knife is $3\frac{3}{4}$ in. long. The same blade in an ATS-34 is $4\frac{1}{8}$ in. long (**Source:** *Blade Magazine* 23, no. 10, October 1996: 26–27). How many inches longer is the ATS-34 blade?

$\frac{3}{8}$ in.

3. Solve. To solve the equation, we carry out the subtraction. The LCD is 6.

$$23\frac{1}{3} = 23\frac{1}{3}\cdot\frac{2}{2} = 23\frac{2}{6} = 22\frac{8}{6}$$
$$-18\frac{1}{2} = -18\frac{1}{2}\cdot\frac{3}{3} = -18\frac{3}{6} = -18\frac{3}{6}$$
$$\overline{\phantom{-18\frac{1}{2} = -18\frac{1}{2}\cdot\frac{3}{3} = -18}4\frac{5}{6}}$$

Thus, $d = 4\frac{5}{6}$ ft.

4. Check. To check, we add the reduction to the new distance:

$$18\frac{1}{2} + 4\frac{5}{6} = 18\frac{3}{6} + 4\frac{5}{6} = 22\frac{8}{6} = 23\frac{2}{6} = 23\frac{1}{3}.$$

This checks.

5. State. The reduction in the goalpost distance was $4\frac{5}{6}$ ft.

Answers on page A-10

Do Exercise 12.

d | Negative Mixed Numerals

Consider the numbers $5\frac{3}{4}$ and $-5\frac{3}{4}$ on a number line.

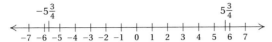

Note that just as $5\frac{3}{4}$ means $5 + \frac{3}{4}$, we can regard $-5\frac{3}{4}$ as $-5 - \frac{3}{4}$.

To subtract a larger number from a smaller number, we must modify the approach of Examples 3–6. To see why, consider the subtraction $4 - 4\frac{1}{2}$. We know that if we have \$4 and make a \$$4\frac{1}{2}$ purchase, we will owe half a dollar. Thus,

$$4 - 4\frac{1}{2} = -\frac{1}{2}.$$

The following is *not* correct:

$$
\left.
\begin{aligned}
4 \phantom{\frac{2}{2}} &= 3\frac{2}{2}\\
-4\frac{1}{2} &= -4\frac{1}{2}\\
\hline
&\ -1\frac{1}{2}
\end{aligned}
\right\}\quad \textbf{Wrong!}
$$

The correct answer, $-\frac{1}{2}$, can be obtained by rewriting the subtraction as addition (see Section 2.3):

$$4 - 4\frac{1}{2} = 4 + \left(-4\frac{1}{2}\right).$$

Because $-4\frac{1}{2}$ has the greater absolute value, the answer will be negative. The difference in absolute values is $4\frac{1}{2} - 4 = \frac{1}{2}$, so

$$4 - 4\frac{1}{2} = -\frac{1}{2}.$$

Do Exercise 13.

Example 10 Subtract: $3\frac{2}{7} - 4\frac{2}{5}$.

Since $4\frac{2}{5}$ is greater than $3\frac{2}{7}$, the answer will be negative. We can also see this by rewriting the subtraction as $3\frac{2}{7} + \left(-4\frac{2}{5}\right)$. The difference in absolute values is

$$
\begin{aligned}
4\frac{2}{5} &= 4\frac{2}{5}\cdot\frac{7}{7} = 4\frac{14}{35}\\
-3\frac{2}{7} &= -3\frac{2}{7}\cdot\frac{5}{5} = -3\frac{10}{35}\\
\hline
&1\frac{4}{35}.
\end{aligned}
$$

> Because $-4\frac{2}{5}$ has the larger absolute value, we make the answer negative.

Thus, $3\frac{2}{7} - 4\frac{2}{5} = -1\frac{4}{35}$. ◄

---

13. Subtract: $7 - 7\frac{3}{4}$.　$-\dfrac{3}{4}$

Answer on page A-10

Subtract.

14. $1\frac{3}{4} - 5\frac{1}{2}$ $-3\frac{3}{4}$

15. $-7\frac{1}{3} - \left(-5\frac{1}{2}\right)$ $-1\frac{5}{6}$

16. Subtract: $-7\frac{1}{10} - 6\frac{2}{15}$. $-13\frac{7}{30}$

Example 11   Subtract: $-6\frac{4}{5} - \left(-9\frac{3}{10}\right)$.

We rewrite the subtraction as addition:

$$-6\frac{4}{5} - \left(-9\frac{3}{10}\right) = -6\frac{4}{5} + 9\frac{3}{10}.$$ **Instead of subtracting, we add the opposite.**

Since $9\frac{3}{10}$ has the greater absolute value, the answer will be positive. The difference in absolute values is

$$
\begin{array}{llll}
9\frac{3}{10} = & 9\ \frac{3}{10} & = & 9\ \frac{3}{10} = & 8\frac{13}{10} \\
-6\frac{4}{5} = & -6\ \frac{4}{5}\cdot\frac{2}{2} & = & -6\frac{8}{10} = & -6\frac{8}{10} \\
\hline
 & & & & 2\frac{5}{10} = 2\frac{1}{2}.
\end{array}
$$

Thus, $-6\frac{4}{5} - \left(-9\frac{3}{10}\right) = 2\frac{1}{2}$.

Do Exercises 14 and 15.

In Section 2.2, we saw that to add two negative numbers we add absolute values and make the answer negative. The same approach is used with mixed numerals.

Example 12   Subtract: $-4\frac{1}{6} - 5\frac{2}{9}$.

We rewrite the subtraction as addition:

$$
\begin{aligned}
-4\frac{1}{6} - 5\frac{2}{9} &= -4\frac{1}{6} + \left(-5\frac{2}{9}\right) \\
&= -\left(4\frac{1}{6} + 5\frac{2}{9}\right) \quad \text{The LCD is 18.} \\
&= -\left(4\frac{3}{18} + 5\frac{4}{18}\right) \quad \frac{1}{6}\cdot\frac{3}{3} = \frac{3}{18}; \frac{2}{9}\cdot\frac{2}{2} = \frac{4}{18} \\
&= -9\frac{7}{18}.
\end{aligned}
$$

Thus, $-4\frac{1}{6} - 5\frac{2}{9} = -9\frac{7}{18}$.

Do Exercise 16.

Exercise Set 4.6

a Perform the indicated operation. Write a mixed numeral for each answer.

1. $5\frac{7}{8}$
   $+ 3\frac{5}{8}$

   $9\frac{1}{2}$

2. $4\frac{5}{6}$
   $+ 3\frac{5}{6}$

   $8\frac{2}{3}$

3. $1\frac{1}{4}$
   $+ 1\frac{2}{3}$

   $2\frac{11}{12}$

4. $4\frac{1}{3}$
   $+ 5\frac{2}{9}$

   $9\frac{5}{9}$

5. $7\frac{3}{4}$
   $+ 5\frac{5}{6}$

   $13\frac{7}{12}$

6. $4\frac{3}{8}$
   $+ 6\frac{5}{12}$

   $10\frac{19}{24}$

7. $3\frac{2}{5}$
   $+ 8\frac{7}{10}$

   $12\frac{1}{10}$

8. $5\frac{1}{2}$
   $+ 3\frac{7}{10}$

   $9\frac{1}{5}$

9. $6\frac{3}{8}$
   $+ 10\frac{5}{6}$

   $17\frac{5}{24}$

10. $\frac{5}{8}$
    $+ 1\frac{5}{6}$

    $2\frac{11}{24}$

11. $12\frac{4}{5}$
    $+ 8\frac{7}{10}$

    $21\frac{1}{2}$

12. $15\frac{5}{8}$
    $+ 11\frac{3}{4}$

    $27\frac{3}{8}$

13. $14\frac{5}{8}$
    $+ 13\frac{1}{4}$

    $27\frac{7}{8}$

14. $16\frac{1}{4}$
    $+ 15\frac{7}{8}$

    $32\frac{1}{8}$

15. $4\frac{1}{5}$
    $- 2\frac{3}{5}$

    $1\frac{3}{5}$

16. $5\frac{1}{8}$
    $- 2\frac{3}{8}$

    $2\frac{3}{4}$

17. $6\frac{3}{5}$
    $- 2\frac{1}{2}$

    $4\frac{1}{10}$

18. $7\frac{2}{3}$
    $- 6\frac{1}{2}$

    $1\frac{1}{6}$

19. $34\frac{1}{3}$
    $- 12\frac{5}{8}$

    $21\frac{17}{24}$

20. $23\frac{5}{16}$
    $- 16\frac{3}{4}$

    $6\frac{9}{16}$

21. 21
    $- 8\frac{3}{4}$

    $12\frac{1}{4}$

22. 42
    $- 3\frac{7}{8}$

    $38\frac{1}{8}$

23. 34
    $- 18\frac{5}{8}$

    $15\frac{3}{8}$

24. 23
    $- 19\frac{3}{4}$

    $3\frac{1}{4}$

25. $21\frac{1}{6}$
    $- 13\frac{3}{4}$

    $7\frac{5}{12}$

26. $42\frac{1}{10}$
    $- 23\frac{7}{12}$

    $18\frac{31}{60}$

27. $25\frac{1}{9}$
    $- 13\frac{5}{6}$

    $11\frac{5}{18}$

28. $23\frac{5}{16}$
    $- 14\frac{7}{12}$

    $8\frac{35}{48}$

29. $5\frac{3}{14}t + 3\frac{2}{21}t$ $8\frac{13}{42}t$

30. $9\frac{1}{2}x + 5\frac{3}{4}x$ $15\frac{1}{4}x$

31. $9\frac{1}{2}x - 7\frac{3}{8}x$ $2\frac{1}{8}x$

32. $7\frac{3}{4}x - 2\frac{3}{8}x$ $5\frac{3}{8}x$

33. $3\frac{7}{8}t + 4\frac{9}{10}t$ $8\frac{31}{40}t$

34. $5\frac{3}{8}x + 6\frac{2}{7}x$ $11\frac{37}{56}x$

35. $37\frac{5}{9}t - 25\frac{4}{5}t$ $11\frac{34}{45}t$

36. $23\frac{1}{6}t - 19\frac{2}{5}t$ $3\frac{23}{30}t$

37. $2\frac{5}{6}x + 3\frac{1}{3}x$ $6\frac{1}{6}x$

38. $7\frac{3}{20}t + 1\frac{2}{15}t$ $8\frac{17}{60}t$

39. $4\frac{3}{11}x + 5\frac{2}{3}x$ $9\frac{31}{33}x$

40. $4\frac{11}{12}t + 5\frac{7}{10}t$ $10\frac{37}{60}t$

c Solve.

41. *Fishing.* Candy caught two trout. One weighed $1\frac{1}{2}$ lb and the other weighed $2\frac{3}{4}$ lb. What was the total weight of the fish?

$4\frac{1}{4}$ lb

42. *Shopping.* Hubert purchased two packages of cheese weighing $1\frac{1}{3}$ lb and $4\frac{3}{5}$ lb. What was the total weight of the cheese?

$5\frac{14}{15}$ lb

43. *Heights.* Rocky is $187\frac{1}{10}$ cm tall and his daughter is $180\frac{3}{4}$ cm tall. How much taller is Rocky?

$6\frac{7}{20}$ cm

44. *Heights.* Aunt Louise is $168\frac{1}{4}$ cm tall and her son is $150\frac{7}{10}$ cm tall. How much taller is Aunt Louise?

$17\frac{11}{20}$ cm

45. *Plumbing.* Janet uses pipes of lengths $10\frac{5}{16}$ ft and $8\frac{3}{4}$ ft in the installation of a sink. How much pipe was used?

$19\frac{1}{16}$ ft

46. *Writing Supplies.* The standard pencil is $6\frac{7}{8}$ in. wood and $\frac{1}{2}$ in. eraser (***Source:*** Eberhard Faber American). What is the total length of the standard pencil?

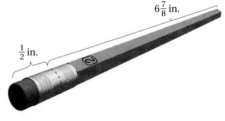

$6\frac{7}{8}$ in.

$\frac{1}{2}$ in.

$7\frac{3}{8}$ in.

47. *Writing Supplies.* A standard sheet of paper is $8\frac{1}{2}$ in. by 11 in. What is the total distance around (perimeter of) the paper?   39 in.

48. *Book Size.* One standard book size is $8\frac{1}{2}$ in. by $9\frac{3}{4}$ in. What is the total distance around (perimeter of) the front cover of such a book?

$36\frac{1}{2}$ in.

49. *Toys "R" Us Stock.* During a recent year, the price of one share of stock in Toys "R" Us varied between a low of $20\frac{1}{2}$ and a high of $37\frac{5}{8}$ (***Source:*** Toys "R" Us annual report). What was the difference between the high and the low?

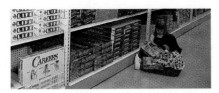

$17\frac{1}{8}$

50. *Coca-Cola Stock.* On a recent day, the stock of Coca-Cola opened at $86\frac{1}{8}$ and closed at $84\frac{9}{16}$. How much did the price of the stock drop that day?

$1\frac{9}{16}$

51. *Carpentry.* When cutting wood with a saw, a carpenter must take into account the thickness of the saw blade. Suppose that from a piece of wood 36 in. long, a carpenter cuts a $15\frac{3}{4}$-in. length with a saw blade that is $\frac{1}{8}$ in. in thickness. How long is the piece that remains?

$20\frac{1}{8}$ in.

52. *Painting.* When redecorating, a painter used $1\frac{3}{4}$ gal of paint for the living room and $1\frac{1}{3}$ gal for the family room. How much paint was used in all?

$3\frac{1}{12}$ gal

53. Sue, an interior designer, worked $10\frac{1}{2}$ hr over a three-day period. If Sue worked $2\frac{1}{2}$ hr on the first day and $4\frac{1}{5}$ hr on the second, how many hours did Sue work on the third day?

$3\frac{4}{5}$ hr

54. A DC-10 flew 640 mi on a nonstop flight. On the return flight, it landed after having flown $320\frac{3}{10}$ mi. How far was the plane from its original point of departure?

$319\frac{7}{10}$ mi

Find the perimeter of (distance around) each figure.

55.

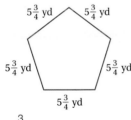

$5\frac{3}{4}$ yd $\quad$ $5\frac{3}{4}$ yd

$5\frac{3}{4}$ yd $\quad$ $5\frac{3}{4}$ yd

$5\frac{3}{4}$ yd

$28\frac{3}{4}$ yd

56.

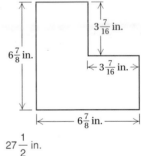

$3\frac{7}{16}$ in.

$6\frac{7}{8}$ in.

$3\frac{7}{16}$ in.

$6\frac{7}{8}$ in.

$27\frac{1}{2}$ in.

Find the length *d* in each figure.

57.

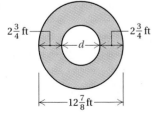

$2\frac{3}{4}$ ft $\qquad$ $2\frac{3}{4}$ ft

d

$12\frac{7}{8}$ ft

$7\frac{3}{8}$ ft

58.

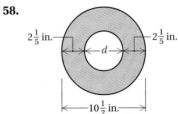

$2\frac{1}{5}$ in. $\qquad$ $2\frac{1}{5}$ in.

d

$10\frac{1}{2}$ in.

$6\frac{1}{10}$ in.

59. Find the smallest length of a bolt that will pass through a piece of tubing with an outside diameter of $\frac{1}{2}$ in., a washer $\frac{1}{16}$ in. thick, a piece of tubing with a $\frac{3}{4}$-in. outside diameter, another washer $\frac{1}{16}$ in. thick, and a nut $\frac{3}{16}$ in. thick.

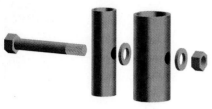

$1\frac{9}{16}$ in.

60. The front of the stage at the Lagrange Town Hall is $6\frac{1}{2}$ yd long. If renovation work succeeds in adding $2\frac{3}{4}$ yd in length, how long is the renovated stage?

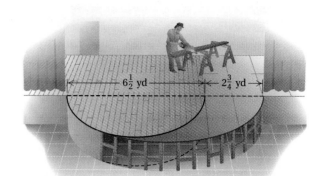

$9\frac{1}{4}$ yd

| d | Subtract.

61. $8\frac{3}{5} - 9\frac{2}{5}$ $-\frac{4}{5}$

62. $4\frac{5}{7} - 8\frac{3}{7}$ $-3\frac{5}{7}$

63. $3\frac{1}{2} - 6\frac{3}{4}$ $-3\frac{1}{4}$

64. $5\frac{1}{2} - 7\frac{3}{4}$ $-2\frac{1}{4}$

65. $3\frac{4}{5} - 7\frac{2}{3}$ $-3\frac{13}{15}$

66. $2\frac{3}{7} - 5\frac{1}{2}$ $-3\frac{1}{14}$

67. $-3\frac{1}{5} - 4\frac{2}{5}$ $-7\frac{3}{5}$

68. $-5\frac{3}{8} - 4\frac{1}{8}$ $-9\frac{1}{2}$

69. $-4\frac{2}{5} - 6\frac{3}{7}$ $-10\frac{29}{35}$

70. $-2\frac{3}{4} - 3\frac{3}{8}$ $-6\frac{1}{8}$

71. $-6\frac{1}{9} - \left(-4\frac{2}{9}\right)$ $-1\frac{8}{9}$

72. $-2\frac{3}{5} - \left(-1\frac{1}{5}\right)$ $-1\frac{2}{5}$

Skill Maintenance

Perform the indicated operation and, if possible, simplify.

73. $\frac{12}{25} \div \frac{24}{5}$ [3.7b] $\frac{1}{10}$

74. $\left(-\frac{15}{9}\right)\left(\frac{18}{39}\right)$ [3.6a] $-\frac{10}{13}$

75. $\left(-\frac{3}{4}\right)\left(-\frac{32}{33}\right)$ [3.6a] $\frac{8}{11}$

76. $-\frac{49}{54} \div \frac{7}{6}$ [3.7b] $-\frac{7}{9}$

Synthesis

77. ◆ Explain how "borrowing" is used in this section.

78. ◆ Is the sum of two mixed numerals always a mixed numeral? Why or why not?

79. ◆ Write a problem for a classmate to solve. Design the problem so the solution is "The larger package holds $4\frac{1}{2}$ oz more than the smaller package."

Calculate each of the following. Write the result as a mixed numeral.

80. ▦ $3289\frac{1047}{1189} + 5278\frac{32}{41}$ $8568\frac{786}{1189}$

81. ▦ $5798\frac{17}{53} - 3909\frac{1957}{2279}$ $1888\frac{1053}{2279}$

82. ▦ $4230\frac{19}{73} - 5848\frac{17}{29}$ $-1618\frac{690}{2117}$

83. A post for a pier is 29 ft long. Half of the post extends above the water's surface and $8\frac{3}{4}$ ft of the post is buried in mud. How deep is the water at that location? $5\frac{3}{4}$ ft

Solve.

84. $35\frac{2}{3} + n = 46\frac{1}{4}$ $10\frac{7}{12}$

85. $42\frac{7}{9} = x - 13\frac{2}{5}$ $56\frac{8}{45}$

86. $-15\frac{7}{8} = 12\frac{1}{2} + t$ $-28\frac{3}{8}$

Collaborative Learning Manual

Add and subtract mixed numerals using fraction strips.

4.7 Multiplication and Division Using Mixed Numerals; Applications

Whereas addition and subtraction of mixed numerals are usually performed by leaving the numbers as mixed numerals, multiplication and division are usually performed by first converting the numbers to fractional notation.

a Multiplication

> To multiply using mixed numerals, first convert to fractional notation. Then multiply with fractional notation and, if appropriate, rewrite the answer as a mixed numeral.

Example 1 Multiply: $6 \cdot 2\frac{1}{2}$.

$$6 \cdot 2\frac{1}{2} = \frac{6}{1} \cdot \frac{5}{2} = \frac{6 \cdot 5}{1 \cdot 2} = \frac{\cancel{2} \cdot 3 \cdot 5}{\cancel{2} \cdot 1} = 15$$

Removing a factor equal to 1: $\frac{2}{2} = 1$

↑   ↑

Here we write fractional notation.

Do Exercise 1.

Example 2 Multiply: $3\frac{1}{2} \cdot \frac{3}{4}$.

$$3\frac{1}{2} \cdot \frac{3}{4} = \frac{7}{2} \cdot \frac{3}{4} = \frac{21}{8} = 2\frac{5}{8}$$

Although fractional notation is needed, *common denominators are not required.*

Do Exercise 2.

Example 3 Multiply: $-8 \cdot 4\frac{2}{3}$.

$$-8 \cdot 4\frac{2}{3} = -\frac{8}{1} \cdot \frac{14}{3} = -\frac{112}{3} = -37\frac{1}{3}$$

Do Exercise 3.

Example 4 Multiply: $2\frac{1}{4} \cdot 3\frac{2}{5}$.

$$2\frac{1}{4} \cdot 3\frac{2}{5} = \frac{9}{4} \cdot \frac{17}{5} = \frac{153}{20} = 7\frac{13}{20}$$

CAUTION! $2\frac{1}{4} \cdot 3\frac{2}{5} \neq 6\frac{2}{20}$. A common error is to multiply the whole numbers and then the fractions. The correct answer, $7\frac{13}{20}$, is found after converting first to fractional notation.

Do Exercise 4.

1. Multiply: $6 \cdot 3\frac{1}{3}$. 20

2. Multiply: $2\frac{1}{2} \cdot \frac{3}{4}$. $1\frac{7}{8}$

3. Multiply: $-2 \cdot 6\frac{2}{5}$. $-12\frac{4}{5}$

4. Multiply: $3\frac{1}{3} \cdot 2\frac{1}{2}$. $8\frac{1}{3}$

Answers on page A-10

5. Divide: $84 \div 5\frac{1}{4}$.   16

Divide.

6. $2\frac{1}{4} \div 1\frac{1}{5}$ $1\frac{7}{8}$

7. $1\frac{3}{4} \div \left(-2\frac{1}{2}\right)$ $-\frac{7}{10}$

Answers on page A-10

---

b   Division

The division $1\frac{1}{2} \div \frac{1}{6}$ is shown here.

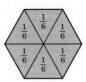 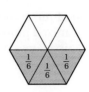

We see that $\frac{1}{6}$ goes into $1\frac{1}{2}$ nine times.

$$1\frac{1}{2} \div \frac{1}{6} = \frac{3}{2} \div \frac{1}{6}$$

$$= \frac{3}{2} \cdot 6 = \frac{3 \cdot 6}{2} = \frac{3 \cdot 3 \cdot 2}{2 \cdot 1} = \frac{3 \cdot 3}{1} \cdot \frac{2}{2} = \frac{3 \cdot 3}{1} \cdot 1 = 9$$

To divide using mixed numerals, first write fractional notation. Then divide (multiply by the reciprocal of the divisor) and, if appropriate, rewrite the answer as a mixed numeral.

Example 5   Divide: $32 \div 3\frac{1}{5}$.

$$32 \div 3\frac{1}{5} = \frac{32}{1} \div \frac{16}{5} \qquad \text{Converting to fractional notation}$$

$$= \frac{32}{1} \cdot \frac{5}{16} = \frac{32 \cdot 5}{1 \cdot 16} = \frac{2 \cdot 16 \cdot 5}{1 \cdot 16} = 10 \qquad \text{Removing a factor equal to 1: } \frac{16}{16} = 1$$

      Remember to multiply by the reciprocal of the divisor.

CAUTION!   The reciprocal of $3\frac{1}{5}$ is neither $5\frac{1}{3}$ nor $3\frac{5}{1}$!

Do Exercise 5.

Example 6   Divide: $2\frac{1}{3} \div 1\frac{3}{4}$.

$$2\frac{1}{3} \div 1\frac{3}{4} = \frac{7}{3} \div \frac{7}{4} = \frac{7}{3} \cdot \frac{4}{7} = \frac{7 \cdot 4}{7 \cdot 3} = \frac{4}{3} = 1\frac{1}{3} \qquad \text{Removing a factor equal to 1: } \frac{7}{7} = 1$$

Example 7   Divide: $-1\frac{3}{5} \div \left(-3\frac{1}{3}\right)$.

$$-1\frac{3}{5} \div \left(-3\frac{1}{3}\right) = -\frac{8}{5} \div \left(-\frac{10}{3}\right) = \frac{8}{5} \cdot \frac{3}{10} \qquad \text{The product or quotient of two negatives is positive.}$$

$$= \frac{2 \cdot 4 \cdot 3}{5 \cdot 2 \cdot 5} = \frac{12}{25} \qquad \text{Removing a factor equal to 1: } \frac{2}{2} = 1$$

Do Exercises 6 and 7.

c | Evaluating Expressions

Mixed numerals can appear in algebraic expressions just as the integers of Section 2.6 did.

Example 8 A train traveling r miles per hour for t hours travels a total of rt miles. (*Remember*: Distance = Rate · Time.)

a) Find the distance traveled by a 60-mph train in $2\frac{3}{4}$ hr.

b) Find the distance traveled if the speed of the train is $26\frac{1}{2}$ mph and the time is $2\frac{2}{3}$ hr.

a) We evaluate rt for $r = 60$ and $t = 2\frac{3}{4}$:

$$rt = 60 \cdot 2\frac{3}{4}$$

$$= \frac{60}{1} \cdot \frac{11}{4}$$

$$= \frac{15 \cdot \cancel{4} \cdot 11}{1 \cdot \cancel{4}} = 165. \qquad \text{Removing a factor equal to 1: } \frac{4}{4} = 1$$

In $2\frac{3}{4}$ hr, a 60-mph train travels 165 mi.

b) We evaluate rt for $r = 26\frac{1}{2}$ and $t = 2\frac{2}{3}$:

$$rt = 26\frac{1}{2} \cdot 2\frac{2}{3}$$

$$= \frac{53}{2} \cdot \frac{8}{3} = \frac{53 \cdot \cancel{2} \cdot 4}{\cancel{2} \cdot 3} \qquad \text{Removing a factor equal to 1: } \frac{2}{2} = 1$$

$$= \frac{212}{3} = 70\frac{2}{3}.$$

In $2\frac{2}{3}$ hr, a $26\frac{1}{2}$-mph train travels $70\frac{2}{3}$ mi.

Example 9 Evaluate $x + yz$ for $x = 7\frac{1}{3}$, $y = \frac{1}{3}$, and $z = 5$.

We substitute and follow the rules for order of operations:

$$x + yz = 7\frac{1}{3} + \frac{1}{3} \cdot 5 \qquad \text{The dot indicates the multiplication, } yz.$$

$$= 7\frac{1}{3} + \frac{1}{3} \cdot \frac{5}{1} \qquad \text{Multiply first; then add.}$$

$$= 7\frac{1}{3} + \frac{5}{3}$$

$$= 7\frac{1}{3} + 1\frac{2}{3} \qquad\Big\}$$

$$= 8\frac{3}{3} = 9. \qquad\Big\} \text{Adding mixed numerals}$$

Do Exercises 8–10.

Evaluate.

8. rt, for $r = 78$ and $t = 2\frac{1}{4}$ $\quad 175\frac{1}{2}$

9. $7xy$, for $x = 9\frac{2}{5}$ and $y = 2\frac{3}{7}$

$\quad 159\frac{4}{5}$

10. $x - y \div z$, for $x = 5\frac{7}{8}$, $y = \frac{1}{4}$, and $z = 2$ $\quad 5\frac{3}{4}$

Answers on page A-10

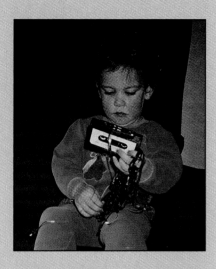

11. Kyle's pickup truck travels on an interstate highway at 65 mph for $3\frac{1}{2}$ hr. How far does it travel?

$227\frac{1}{2}$ mi

12. Holly's minivan travels 302 mi on $15\frac{1}{10}$ gal of gas. How many miles per gallon did it get?

20 mpg

d Applications and Problem Solving

Example 10 *Cassette Tape Music.* The tape in an audio cassette is played at a rate of $1\frac{7}{8}$ in. per second. A recording has 30 in. of damaged tape. How many seconds of music have been lost?

1. Familiarize. We can make a drawing.

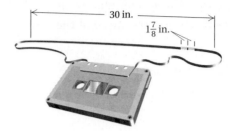

Since each $1\frac{7}{8}$ in. of tape represents 1 sec of lost music, the question can be regarded as asking how many times 30 can be divided by $1\frac{7}{8}$. We let $t =$ the number of seconds of music lost.

2. Translate. The situation corresponds to a division sentence:

$$t = 30 \div 1\frac{7}{8}.$$

3. Solve. To solve the equation, we perform the division:

$$t = 30 \div 1\frac{7}{8}$$

$$= \frac{30}{1} \div \frac{15}{8} \qquad \text{Rewriting in fractional notation}$$

$$= \frac{30}{1} \cdot \frac{8}{15}$$

$$= \frac{15 \cdot 2 \cdot 8}{1 \cdot 15} \qquad \text{Removing a factor equal to 1: } \frac{15}{15} = 1$$

$$= 16.$$

4. Check. We check by multiplying. If 16 sec of music were lost, then

$$16 \cdot 1\frac{7}{8} = \frac{16}{1} \cdot \frac{15}{8}$$

$$= \frac{8 \cdot 2 \cdot 15}{1 \cdot 8} = 30 \text{ in.} \qquad \text{Removing a factor equal to 1: } \frac{8}{8} = 1$$

of tape were destroyed. Our answer checks. A quick, partial, check uses approximations:

$$16 \cdot 1\frac{7}{8} \approx 16 \cdot 2 = 32 \approx 30. \qquad \text{The symbol } \approx \text{ means "approximately equal to."}$$

5. State. The cassette has lost 16 sec of music.

Do Exercises 11 and 12.

Example 11 *Home Furnishings.* An L-shaped room consists of a rectangle that is $8\frac{1}{2}$ ft by 11 ft adjacent to one that is $6\frac{1}{2}$ by $7\frac{1}{2}$ ft. What is the total area of a carpet that covers the floor?

1. **Familiarize.** We make a drawing of the situation. We let a = the total floor area.

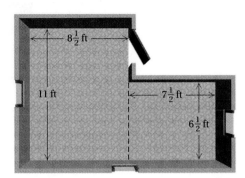

2. **Translate.** The total area is the sum of the areas of the two rectangles. This gives us the following equation:

$$a = 8\frac{1}{2} \cdot 11 + 7\frac{1}{2} \cdot 6\frac{1}{2}.$$

3. **Solve.** This is a multistep problem. We perform each multiplication and then add. This follows the rules for order of operations:

$$a = 8\frac{1}{2} \cdot 11 + 7\frac{1}{2} \cdot 6\frac{1}{2}$$

$$= \frac{17}{2} \cdot \frac{11}{1} + \frac{15}{2} \cdot \frac{13}{2} \qquad \text{Rewriting in fractional notation}$$

$$= \frac{17 \cdot 11}{2 \cdot 1} + \frac{15 \cdot 13}{2 \cdot 2}$$

$$= \frac{187}{2} + \frac{195}{4}$$

$$= 93\frac{1}{2} + 48\frac{3}{4}$$

$$= 93\frac{2}{4} + 48\frac{3}{4} \qquad \text{For addition, a common denominator is needed.}$$

$$= 141\frac{5}{4}$$

$$= 142\frac{1}{4}.$$

4. **Check.** We perform a partial check by estimating the total area as $11 \cdot 9 + 7 \cdot 7 = 99 + 49 = 148$ ft². Our answer, $142\frac{1}{4}$ ft², seems reasonable.

5. **State.** The total area of the carpet is $142\frac{1}{4}$ ft².

Do Exercise 13.

13. A room is $22\frac{1}{2}$ ft by $15\frac{1}{2}$ ft. A 9-ft by 12-ft Oriental rug is placed in the center of the room. How much area is not covered by the rug?

$240\frac{3}{4}$ ft²

Answer on page A-10

14. After two weeks, Kurt's tomato seedlings measure $9\frac{1}{2}$ in., $10\frac{3}{4}$ in., $10\frac{1}{4}$ in., and 9 in. tall. Find their average height. $9\frac{7}{8}$ in.

Example 12   Melody has had three children. Their birth weights were $7\frac{1}{2}$ lb, $7\frac{3}{4}$ lb, and $6\frac{3}{4}$ lb. What was the average weight of her babies?

1. **Familiarize.**   Recall that to compute an *average*, we add the values and then divide the sum by the number of values. We let $w =$ the average weight, in pounds.

2. **Translate.**   We have

$$w = \frac{7\frac{1}{2} + 7\frac{3}{4} + 6\frac{3}{4}}{3}.$$

3. **Solve.**   We first add:

$$7\frac{1}{2} + 7\frac{3}{4} + 6\frac{3}{4} = 7\frac{2}{4} + 7\frac{3}{4} + 6\frac{3}{4}$$

$$= 20\frac{8}{4} = 22. \qquad 20\frac{8}{4} = 20 + \frac{8}{4} = 20 + 2$$

Then we divide:

$$w = \frac{7\frac{1}{2} + 7\frac{3}{4} + 6\frac{3}{4}}{3} = \frac{22}{3} = 7\frac{1}{3}. \qquad \text{Dividing by 3.}$$

4. **Check.**   As a partial check, we note that the average is smaller than the largest individual value and larger than the smallest individual value. We could also repeat our calculations.

5. **State.**   The average weight of the three babies is $7\frac{1}{3}$ lb.

Answers on page A-10

Do Exercise 14.

Calculator Spotlight

Calculators equipped with a key, often labeled $\boxed{a^b/c}$, allow for computations with fractional notation and mixed numerals. To calculate

$$\frac{2}{3} + \frac{4}{5}$$

with such a calculator, press:

$\boxed{2}\ \boxed{a^b/c}\ \boxed{3}\ \boxed{+}\ \boxed{4}\ \boxed{a^b/c}\ \boxed{5}\ \boxed{=}$.

The display that appears,

$\boxed{1\ \lrcorner\ 7\ \lrcorner\ 15}$,

represents the mixed numeral $1\frac{7}{15}$.

To express the answer in fractional notation, we press $\boxed{\text{Shift}}\ \boxed{d/c}$ and 22 ⌐ 15 appears, representing $\frac{22}{15}$.

To enter a mixed numeral like $3\frac{2}{5}$ on a fraction calculator equipped with an $\boxed{a^b/c}$ key, we press

$\boxed{3}\ \boxed{a^b/c}\ \boxed{2}\ \boxed{a^b/c}\ \boxed{5}$.

The calculator's display is in the form

$\boxed{3\ \lrcorner\ 2\ \lrcorner\ 5}$.

Some calculators are capable of displaying mixed numerals in the way in which we write them, as shown below.

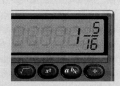

Exercises

Calculate using a fraction calculator. Write the answers in fractional notation.

1. $\dfrac{3}{8} + \dfrac{1}{4}$ **2.** $\dfrac{5}{12} + \dfrac{7}{10} - \dfrac{5}{12}$ **3.** $\dfrac{15}{7} \cdot \dfrac{1}{3}$

4. $\dfrac{19}{20} \div \dfrac{17}{35}$ **5.** $\dfrac{29}{30} - \dfrac{18}{25} \cdot \dfrac{2}{3}$ **6.** $\dfrac{1}{2} + \dfrac{13}{29} \cdot \dfrac{3}{4}$

Calculate using a fraction calculator. Write the answers as mixed numerals.

7. $4\frac{1}{2} \cdot 5\frac{3}{7}$ $24\frac{3}{7}$ **8.** $7\frac{2}{3} \div 9\frac{4}{5}$ $\frac{115}{147}$

9. $8\frac{3}{7} + 5\frac{2}{9}$ $13\frac{41}{63}$ **10.** $13\frac{4}{9} - 7\frac{5}{8}$ $5\frac{59}{72}$

11. $13\frac{1}{4} - 2\frac{1}{5} \cdot 4\frac{3}{8}$ $3\frac{5}{8}$ **12.** $2\frac{5}{6} + 5\frac{1}{6} \cdot 3\frac{1}{4}$ $19\frac{5}{8}$

1. $\frac{5}{8}$ **2.** $\frac{7}{10}$ **3.** $\frac{5}{7}$ **4.** $\frac{133}{68}$ **5.** $\frac{73}{150}$ **6.** $\frac{97}{116}$

Exercise Set 4.7

a Multiply. Write a mixed numeral for each answer.

1. $10 \cdot 2\frac{5}{6}$

$28\frac{1}{3}$

2. $5 \cdot 3\frac{3}{4}$

$18\frac{3}{4}$

3. $6\frac{2}{3} \cdot \frac{1}{4}$

$1\frac{2}{3}$

4. $-9 \cdot 2\frac{3}{5}$

$-23\frac{2}{5}$

5. $-10 \cdot 7\frac{1}{3}$

$-73\frac{1}{3}$

6. $7\frac{3}{8} \cdot 4\frac{1}{3}$

$31\frac{23}{24}$

7. $3\frac{1}{2} \cdot 4\frac{2}{3}$

$16\frac{1}{3}$

8. $4\frac{1}{5} \cdot 5\frac{1}{4}$

$22\frac{1}{20}$

9. $-2\frac{3}{10} \cdot 4\frac{2}{5}$

$-10\frac{3}{25}$

10. $4\frac{7}{10} \cdot 5\frac{3}{10}$

$24\frac{91}{100}$

11. $6\frac{3}{10} \cdot 5\frac{7}{10}$

$35\frac{91}{100}$

12. $-20\frac{1}{2} \cdot \left(-10\frac{1}{5}\right)$

$209\frac{1}{10}$

b Divide. Write a mixed numeral for each answer whenever possible.

13. $20 \div 2\frac{3}{5}$

$7\frac{9}{13}$

14. $18 \div 2\frac{1}{4}$

8

15. $8\frac{2}{5} \div 7$

$1\frac{1}{5}$

16. $3\frac{3}{8} \div 3$

$1\frac{1}{8}$

17. $4\frac{3}{4} \div 1\frac{1}{3}$

$3\frac{9}{16}$

18. $5\frac{4}{5} \div 2\frac{1}{2}$

$2\frac{8}{25}$

19. $-1\frac{7}{8} \div 1\frac{2}{3}$

$-1\frac{1}{8}$

20. $-4\frac{3}{8} \div 2\frac{5}{6}$

$-1\frac{37}{68}$

21. $5\frac{1}{10} \div 4\frac{3}{10}$

$1\frac{8}{43}$

22. $4\frac{1}{10} \div 2\frac{1}{10}$

$1\frac{20}{21}$

23. $20\frac{1}{4} \div (-90)$

$-\frac{9}{40}$

24. $12\frac{1}{2} \div (-50)$

$-\frac{1}{4}$

c Evaluate.

25. lw, for $l = 2\frac{3}{5}$ and $w = 9$ $\quad 23\frac{2}{5}$

26. mv, for $m = 7$ and $v = 3\frac{2}{5}$ $\quad 23\frac{4}{5}$

27. rs, for $r = 5$ and $s = 3\frac{1}{7}$ $\quad 15\frac{5}{7}$

28. rt, for $r = 5\frac{2}{3}$ and $t = -2\frac{3}{8}$ $\quad -13\frac{11}{24}$

29. mt, for $m = 6\frac{2}{9}$ and $t = -4\frac{3}{5}$ $\quad -28\frac{28}{45}$

30. $M \div NP$, for $M = 2\frac{1}{4}$, $N = -5$, and $P = 2\frac{1}{3}$ $\quad -1\frac{1}{20}$

31. $R \cdot S \div T$, for $R = 4\frac{2}{3}$, $S = 1\frac{3}{7}$, and $T = -5$ $\quad -1\frac{1}{3}$

32. $a - bc$, for $a = 18$, $b = 2\frac{1}{5}$, and $c = 3\frac{3}{4}$ $\quad 9\frac{3}{4}$

33. $r + ps$, for $r = 5\frac{1}{2}$, $p = 3$, and $s = 2\frac{1}{4}$ $\quad 12\frac{1}{4}$

34. $s + rt$, for $s = 3\frac{1}{2}$, $r = 5\frac{1}{2}$, and $t = 7\frac{1}{2}$ $\quad 44\frac{3}{4}$

35. $m + n \div p$, for $m = 7\frac{2}{5}$, $n = 4\frac{1}{2}$, and $p = 6$ $\quad 8\frac{3}{20}$

36. $x - y \div z$, for $x = 9$, $y = 2\frac{1}{2}$, and $z = 3\frac{3}{4}$ $\quad 8\frac{1}{3}$

d Solve.

37. *Home Furnishings.* Each shelf in June's entertainment center is 27 in. long. A videocassette is $1\frac{1}{8}$ in. thick. How many cassettes can she place on each shelf? 24

38. *Exercise.* At one point during a spinning class at Ray's health club, his bicycle wheel was completing $76\frac{2}{3}$ revolutions per minute. How many revolutions did the wheel complete in 6 min? 460

39. *Sodium Consumption.* The average American woman consumes $1\frac{1}{3}$ tsp of sodium each day (**Source**: *Nutrition Action Health Letter*, March 1994, p. 6. 1875 Connecticut Ave., N.W., Washington, DC 20009-5728). How much sodium do 10 average American women consume in one day? $13\frac{1}{3}$ tsp

40. *Aeronautics.* Most space shuttles orbit the earth once every $1\frac{1}{2}$ hr. How many orbits are made every 24 hr? 16

41. A serving of filleted fish is generally considered to be about $\frac{1}{3}$ lb. How many servings can be prepared from $5\frac{1}{2}$ lb of flounder fillet? $16\frac{1}{2}$

42. A serving of fish steak (cross section) is generally $\frac{1}{2}$ lb. How many servings can be prepared from a cleaned $18\frac{3}{4}$-lb tuna? $37\frac{1}{2}$

43. The weight of water is $62\frac{1}{2}$ lb per cubic foot. What is the weight of $5\frac{1}{2}$ cubic feet of water? $343\frac{3}{4}$ lb

44. The weight of water is $62\frac{1}{2}$ lb per cubic foot. What is the weight of $2\frac{1}{4}$ cubic feet of water? $140\frac{5}{8}$ lb

45. *Video Recording.* The tape in a VCR operating in the short-play mode travels at a rate of $1\frac{3}{8}$ in. per second. How many inches of tape are used to record for 60 sec in the short-play mode? $82\frac{1}{2}$ in.

46. *Audio Recording.* The tape in an audio cassette is played at the rate of $1\frac{7}{8}$ in. per second. How many inches of tape are used when a cassette is played for $5\frac{1}{2}$ sec? $10\frac{5}{16}$ in.

47. *Temperatures.* Fahrenheit temperature can be obtained from Celsius (centigrade) temperature by multiplying by $1\frac{4}{5}$ and adding 32°. What Fahrenheit temperature corresponds to a Celsius temperature of 20°?   68°

48. *Temperature.* Fahrenheit temperature can be obtained from Celsius (centigrade) temperature by multiplying by $1\frac{4}{5}$ and adding 32°. What Fahrenheit temperature corresponds to the Celsius temperature of boiling water, which is 100°?   212°

49. *Weightlifting.* In 1997, weightlifter Gao Shihong of China snatched $103\frac{1}{2}$ kg (**Source:** *The Guinness Book of Records,* 1998). This amount was about $1\frac{1}{2}$ times her body weight. How much did Shihong weigh?

69 kg

50. *Weightlifting.* In 1983, weightlifter Stefan Topurov of Bulgaria hoisted $396\frac{3}{4}$ lb over his head (**Source:** *The Guinness Book of Records,* 1998). This amount was about three times his body weight. How much did Topurov weigh? $132\frac{1}{4}$ lb

51. *Birth Weights.* The Piper quadruplets of Great Britain weighed $2\frac{9}{16}$ lb, $2\frac{9}{32}$ lb, $2\frac{1}{8}$ lb, and $2\frac{5}{16}$ lb at birth. (*Source:* *The Guinness Book of Records,* 1998). Find their average birth weight. $2\frac{41}{128}$ lb

52. *Vertical Leaps.* Eight-year-old Zachary registered vertical leaps of $12\frac{3}{4}$ in., $13\frac{3}{4}$ in., $13\frac{1}{2}$ in., and 14 in. Find his average vertical leap. $13\frac{1}{2}$ in.

53. *Manufacturing.* A test of five light bulbs showed that they burned for the lengths of time given on the graph below. For how many days, on average, did the bulbs burn? $18\frac{3}{5}$ days

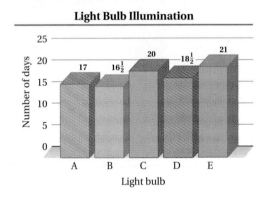

54. *Packaging.* A sample of four bags of beef jerky showed the weights given on the graph below. What was the average weight? $4\frac{5}{32}$ oz

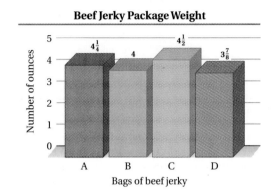

Find the area of each shaded region.

55.

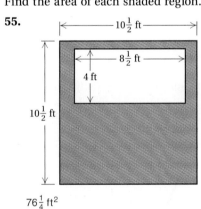

$76\frac{1}{4}$ ft^2

56.

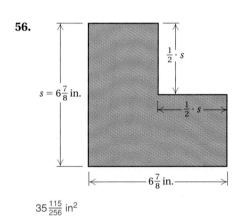

$35\frac{115}{256}$ in^2

57. *Word Processing.* Kelly wants to create a table using Microsoft® Word software for word processing. She needs to have two columns, each $1\frac{1}{2}$ in. wide, and five columns, each $\frac{3}{4}$ in. wide. Will this table fit on a piece of standard paper that is $8\frac{1}{2}$ in. wide? If so, how wide will each margin be if her margins on each side are to be of equal width?   Yes; $\frac{7}{8}$ in.

58. *Construction.* A rectangular lot has dimensions of $302\frac{1}{2}$ ft by $205\frac{1}{4}$ ft. A building with dimensions of 100 ft by $25\frac{1}{2}$ ft is built on the lot. How much area is left over? $59,538\frac{1}{8}$ ft^2

59. Multiply: $-8(x - 3)$ [2.7a] $-8x + 24$

60. On a winter night, the temperature dropped from 7°F to −12°F. How many degrees did it drop?   [2.3b]

19°F

61. Solve: $-9x = 189$.   [2.8b] -21

62. Solve: $-9 + x = 189$.   [2.8a]   198

63. Divide: $-198 \div (-6)$.   [2.5a]   33

64. Multiply: $(-7)(185)(0)$.   [2.4a]   0

Synthesis

65. ◈ If Kate and Jessie are both less than 5 ft, $6\frac{1}{2}$ in. tall, but Dot is over 5 ft, $6\frac{1}{2}$ in. tall, is it possible that the average height of the three exceeds 5 ft, $6\frac{1}{2}$ in.? Why or why not?

66. ◈ Write a problem for a classmate to solve. Design the problem so that its solution is found by performing the multiplication $4\frac{1}{2} \cdot 33\frac{1}{3}$.

67. ◈ Under what circumstances is a pair of mixed numerals more easily added than multiplied?

Simplify. Write each answer as a mixed numeral whenever possible.

68. ▦ $15\frac{2}{11} \cdot 23\frac{31}{43}$ $360\frac{60}{473}$

69. ▦ $17\frac{23}{31} \cdot 19\frac{13}{15}$ $352\frac{44}{93}$

70. $-8 \div \frac{1}{2} + \frac{3}{4} + \left(-5 - \frac{5}{8}\right)^2$ $16\frac{25}{64}$

71. $\left(\frac{5}{9} - \frac{1}{4}\right)(-12) + \left(-4 - \frac{3}{4}\right)^2$ $18\frac{43}{48}$

72. $\frac{1}{3} \div \left(\frac{1}{2} - \frac{1}{5}\right) \times \frac{1}{4} + \frac{1}{6}$ $\frac{4}{9}$

73. $\frac{7}{8} - 1\frac{1}{8} \times \frac{2}{3} + \frac{9}{10} \div \frac{3}{5}$ $1\frac{5}{8}$

Evaluate.

74. $ab + ac$ and $a(b + c)$, for $a = 3\frac{1}{4}$, $b = 5\frac{1}{3}$, and $c = 4\frac{5}{8}$ $32\frac{35}{96}$; $32\frac{35}{96}$

75. $a^3 + a^2$ and $a^2(a + 1)$, for $a = -3\frac{1}{2}$ $-30\frac{5}{8}$; $-30\frac{5}{8}$

76. 🖩 Use a calculator to determine what whole number a must be in order for the following to be true:

$$\frac{a}{17} + \frac{10 + a}{23} = \frac{330}{391}.\quad 4$$

77. *Heights.* Find the average height of the following NBA stars:

Shawn Kemp	6 ft, 10 in.
Grant Hill	6 ft, 7 in.
Damon Stoudamire	5 ft, 10 in.
Kobe Bryant	6 ft, 6 in.
Shaquille O'Neal	7 ft, 1 in.

6 ft, $6\frac{4}{5}$ in.

Recipes. The following heart-healthy recipes serve four. How much of each ingredient would you use to serve ten?

78.

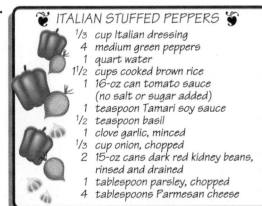

🍂 *ITALIAN STUFFED PEPPERS* 🍂

- ⅓ cup Italian dressing
- 4 medium green peppers
- 1 quart water
- 1½ cups cooked brown rice
- 1 16-oz can tomato sauce (no salt or sugar added)
- 1 teaspoon Tamari soy sauce
- ½ teaspoon basil
- 1 clove garlic, minced
- ⅓ cup onion, chopped
- 2 15-oz cans dark red kidney beans, rinsed and drained
- 1 tablespoon parsley, chopped
- 4 tablespoons Parmesan cheese

$\frac{5}{6}$ cup Italian dressing; 10 medium green peppers; $2\frac{1}{2}$ qt water; $3\frac{3}{4}$ cup cooked brown rice; $2\frac{1}{2}$ 16-oz cans tomato sauce; $2\frac{1}{2}$ tsp Tamari soy sauce; $1\frac{1}{4}$ tsp basil; $2\frac{1}{2}$ cloves garlic, minced; $\frac{5}{6}$ cup onion, chopped; 5 15-oz cans dark red kidney beans, rinsed and drained; $2\frac{1}{2}$ tbsp parsley, chopped; 10 tbsp Parmesan cheese

79.

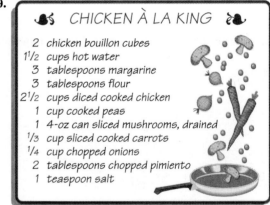

🍄 *CHICKEN À LA KING* 🍄

- 2 chicken bouillon cubes
- 1½ cups hot water
- 3 tablespoons margarine
- 3 tablespoons flour
- 2½ cups diced cooked chicken
- 1 cup cooked peas
- 1 4-oz can sliced mushrooms, drained
- ⅓ cup sliced cooked carrots
- ¼ cup chopped onions
- 2 tablespoons chopped pimiento
- 1 teaspoon salt

5 chicken bouillon cubes; $3\frac{3}{4}$ cups hot water; $7\frac{1}{2}$ tbsp margarine; $7\frac{1}{2}$ tbsp flour; $6\frac{1}{4}$ cups diced cooked chicken; $2\frac{1}{2}$ cups cooked peas, $2\frac{1}{2}$ 4-oz cans sliced mushrooms, drained; $\frac{5}{6}$ cup sliced cooked carrots; $\frac{5}{8}$ cup chopped onions; 5 tbsp chopped pimiento; $2\frac{1}{2}$ tsp salt

Analyze stock market prices.

Summary and Review: Chapter 4

Important Properties and Formulas

The Addition Principle: $a = b$ is equivalent to $a + c = b + c$.
The Multiplication Principle: For $c \neq 0$, $a = b$ is equivalent to $c \cdot a = c \cdot b$.

Review Exercises

Find the LCM. [4.1a]

1. 12 and 18 **2.** 18 and 45 **3.** 3, 6, and 30

Perform the indicated operation and, if possible, simplify. [4.2a, b], [4.3a]

4. $\frac{2}{9} + \frac{5}{9}$

5. $\frac{3}{a} + \frac{4}{a}$

6. $-\frac{6}{5} + \frac{11}{15}$

7. $\frac{5}{16} + \frac{3}{24}$

8. $\frac{5}{9} - \frac{2}{9}$

9. $\frac{3}{4} - \frac{7}{8}$

10. $\frac{11}{27} - \frac{2}{9}$

11. $\frac{5}{6} - \frac{2}{9}$

Use < or > for ▢ to form a true sentence. [4.2c]

12. $\frac{4}{7}$ ▢ $\frac{5}{9}$

13. $-\frac{8}{9}$ ▢ $-\frac{11}{13}$

Solve. [4.3b], [4.4a]

14. $x + \frac{2}{5} = \frac{7}{8}$

15. $7a - 2 = 26$

16. $5 + \frac{16}{3}x = \frac{5}{9}$

17. $\frac{22}{5} = \frac{16}{5} + \frac{5}{2}x$

Convert to fractional notation. [4.5a]

18. $7\frac{1}{2}$

19. $8\frac{3}{8}$

20. $-4\frac{1}{3}$

21. $10\frac{5}{7}$

Convert to a mixed numeral. [4.5b]

22. $\dfrac{7}{3}$

23. $\dfrac{-27}{4}$

24. $\dfrac{63}{5}$

25. $\dfrac{7}{2}$

26. Divide. Write a mixed numeral for the answer. [4.5c]

$7896 \div (-9)$

27. Gina's golf scores were 79, 81, and 84. What was her average score? [4.5c]

Perform the indicated operation. Write a mixed numeral for each answer. [4.6a, b, d]

28. $\begin{aligned} 5\dfrac{3}{5} \\ + 4\dfrac{4}{5} \\ \hline \end{aligned}$

29. $\begin{aligned} 8\dfrac{1}{3} \\ + 3\dfrac{2}{5} \\ \hline \end{aligned}$

30. $-5\dfrac{5}{6} + \left(-3\dfrac{1}{6}\right)$

31. $-2\dfrac{3}{4} + 4\dfrac{1}{2}$

32. $\begin{aligned} 12 \\ - \ 4\dfrac{2}{9} \\ \hline \end{aligned}$

33. $\begin{aligned} 9\dfrac{3}{5} \\ - 4\dfrac{13}{15} \\ \hline \end{aligned}$

34. $4\dfrac{5}{8} - 9\dfrac{3}{4}$

35. $-7\dfrac{1}{2} - 6\dfrac{3}{4}$

Combine like terms. [4.2a], [4.6b]

36. $\dfrac{4}{9}x + \dfrac{1}{3}x$

37. $5\dfrac{3}{10}a - 2\dfrac{1}{8}a$

Perform the indicated operation. Write a mixed numeral or integer for each answer. [4.7a, b]

38. $6 \cdot 2\dfrac{2}{3}$

39. $-5\dfrac{1}{4} \cdot \dfrac{2}{3}$

40. $2\dfrac{1}{5} \cdot 1\dfrac{1}{10}$

41. $2\dfrac{2}{5} \cdot 2\dfrac{1}{2}$

42. $27 \div 2\frac{1}{4}$

43. $2\frac{2}{5} \div \left(-1\frac{7}{10}\right)$

44. $3\frac{1}{4} \div 26$

45. $4\frac{1}{5} \div 4\frac{2}{3}$

Evaluate. [4.7c]

46. $5x - y$, for $x = 3\frac{1}{5}$ and $y = 2\frac{2}{7}$

47. $2a \div b$, for $a = 5\frac{2}{11}$ and $b = 3\frac{4}{5}$

Solve.

48. A curtain requires $2\frac{3}{5}$ m of material. How many curtains can be made from 39 m of material? [4.7d]

49. On the first day of trading on the stock market, stock in Alcoa opened at $\$67\frac{3}{4}$ and rose by $\$2\frac{5}{8}$ at the close of trading. What was the stock's closing price? [4.6c]

50. Mica pedals up a $\frac{1}{10}$-mi hill and then coasts for $\frac{1}{2}$ mi down the other side. How far has she traveled? [4.2d]

51. A wedding-cake recipe requires 12 cups of shortening. Being calorie-conscious, the wedding couple decides to reduce the shortening by $3\frac{5}{8}$ cups and replace it with prune purée. How many cups of shortening are used in their new recipe? [4.6c]

52. What is the sum of the areas in the figure below? [4.6c], [4.7d]

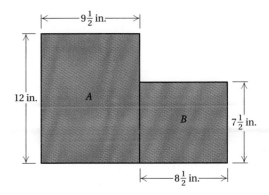

53. In the figure in Exercise 52, how much larger is the area of rectangle A than the area of rectangle B? [4.6c], [4.7d]

54. Multiply and simplify: $\dfrac{9}{10} \cdot \left(-\dfrac{4}{3} \right)$. [3.6a]

55. Divide and simplify: $\dfrac{5}{4} \div \left(-\dfrac{5}{6} \right)$. [3.7b]

56. Bright Sunshine Landscaping made $230 Monday but lost $150 on Tuesday and $110 on Wednesday. Find the total profit or loss. [2.3b]

57. Multiply: $5(a - 9)$. [2.7a]

Synthesis

58. ◈ Rachel insists that $3\frac{2}{5} \cdot 1\frac{3}{7} = 3\frac{6}{35}$. What mistake is she probably making and how should she have proceeded instead? [4.7a]

59. ◈ Do least common multiples play any role in the addition or subtraction of mixed numerals? Why or why not? [4.6a, b]

60. ▦ Find the LCM of 141, 2419, and 1357. [4.1a]

61. Find r if
$$\frac{1}{r} = \frac{1}{100} + \frac{1}{150} + \frac{1}{200}. \quad [4.2b]$$

62. Find the smallest integer for which each fraction is greater than $\frac{1}{2}$. [4.2c]

a) $\dfrac{\blacksquare}{11}$ b) $\dfrac{\blacksquare}{8}$

c) $\dfrac{\blacksquare}{23}$ d) $\dfrac{\blacksquare}{35}$

e) $\dfrac{-51}{\blacksquare}$ f) $\dfrac{-78}{\blacksquare}$

g) $\dfrac{-2}{\blacksquare}$ h) $\dfrac{-1}{\blacksquare}$

63. Find the largest integer for which each fraction is greater than 1. [4.2c]

a) $\dfrac{7}{\blacksquare}$ b) $\dfrac{11}{\blacksquare}$

c) $\dfrac{47}{\blacksquare}$ d) $\dfrac{\frac{9}{8}}{\blacksquare}$

e) $\dfrac{\blacksquare}{-13}$ f) $\dfrac{\blacksquare}{-27}$

g) $\dfrac{\blacksquare}{-1}$ h) $\dfrac{\blacksquare}{-\frac{1}{2}}$

Test: Chapter 4

1. Find the LCM of 12 and 16.

Perform the indicated operation and, if possible, simplify.

2. $\dfrac{1}{2} + \dfrac{5}{2}$　　3. $-\dfrac{7}{8} + \dfrac{2}{3}$　　4. $\dfrac{5}{t} - \dfrac{3}{t}$　　5. $\dfrac{5}{6} - \dfrac{3}{4}$　　6. $\dfrac{5}{8} - \dfrac{17}{24}$

7. Use < or > for ▮ to form a true sentence.

$$\dfrac{6}{7} \ ▮ \ \dfrac{21}{25}$$

Solve.

8. $x + \dfrac{2}{3} = \dfrac{11}{12}$　　　9. $-5x - 2 = 10$　　　10. $32 = 2 + \dfrac{5}{3}x$

Convert to fractional notation.

11. $3\dfrac{1}{2}$　　　　　　　　　12. $-9\dfrac{7}{8}$

13. Convert to a mixed numeral:

$$-\dfrac{74}{9}.$$

14. Divide. Write a mixed numeral for the answer.

$$11\ \overline{)\ 1\,7\,8\,9}$$

Perform the indicated operation. Write a mixed numeral for each answer.

15. $\begin{array}{r} 6\frac{2}{5} \\ +\,7\frac{4}{5} \\ \hline \end{array}$　　16. $\begin{array}{r} 9\frac{1}{4} \\ +\,5\frac{1}{6} \\ \hline \end{array}$　　17. $\begin{array}{r} 10\frac{1}{6} \\ -\,5\frac{7}{8} \\ \hline \end{array}$

18. $14 + \left(-5\dfrac{3}{7}\right)$　　　19. $3\dfrac{4}{5} - 9\dfrac{1}{2}$

Combine like terms.

20. $\dfrac{3}{8}x - \dfrac{1}{2}x$　　　　　　21. $5\dfrac{2}{11}a - 3\dfrac{1}{5}a$

Answers

1. [4.1a] 48

2. [4.2a] 3

3. [4.2b] $-\frac{5}{24}$

4. [4.3a] $\frac{2}{t}$

5. [4.3a] $\frac{1}{12}$

6. [4.3a] $-\frac{1}{12}$

7. [4.2c] $>$

8. [4.3b] $\frac{1}{4}$

9. [4.4a] $-\frac{12}{5}$

10. [4.4a] 18

11. [4.5a] $\frac{7}{2}$

12. [4.5a] $-\frac{79}{8}$

13. [4.5b] $-8\frac{2}{9}$

14. [4.5c] $162\frac{7}{11}$

15. [4.6a] $14\frac{1}{5}$

16. [4.6a] $14\frac{5}{12}$

17. [4.6b] $4\frac{7}{24}$

18. [4.6d] $8\frac{4}{7}$

19. [4.6d] $-5\frac{7}{10}$

20. [4.3a] $-\frac{1}{8}x$

21. [4.6d] $1\frac{54}{55}a$

Perform the indicated operation. Write a mixed numeral for each answer.

22. $9 \cdot 4\frac{1}{3}$

23. $6\frac{3}{4} \cdot \left(-2\frac{2}{3}\right)$

24. $33 \div 5\frac{1}{2}$

25. $2\frac{1}{3} \div 1\frac{1}{6}$

Evaluate.

26. $\frac{2}{3}ab$, for $a = 7$ and $b = 4\frac{1}{5}$

27. $4 + mn$, for $m = 7\frac{2}{5}$ and $n = 3\frac{1}{4}$

Solve.

28. One batch of low-cholesterol turkey chili calls for $1\frac{1}{2}$ lb of roasted turkey breast. How much turkey is needed for 5 batches?

29. An order of books for a math course weighs 220 lb. Each book weighs $2\frac{3}{4}$ lb. How many books are in the order?

30. Marilyn weighs 123 lb. Her twin brother Mike weighs 174 lb. What is the average of their weights?

31. A standard piece of paper is $\frac{43}{200}$ m by $\frac{7}{25}$ m. By how much does the length exceed the width?

Skill Maintenance

32. Multiply: $9(x - 6)$.

33. Divide and simplify:

$$\left(-\frac{4}{3}\right) \div \left(-\frac{5}{6}\right).$$

34. Multiply and simplify: $\frac{4}{3} \cdot \frac{5}{6}$.

35. A rock climber descended from an altitude of 720 ft to a depth of 470 ft below sea level. How many feet did the climber descend?

Synthesis

36. Yuri and Olga are orangutans who perform in a circus by riding bicycles around a circular track. It takes Yuri $\frac{6}{25}$ min and Olga $\frac{8}{25}$ min to complete one lap. They start their act together at one point and complete their act when they are next together at that point. How long does the act last?

37. Dolores runs 17 laps at her health club. Terence runs 17 laps at his health club. If the track at Dolores's health club is $\frac{1}{7}$ mi long, and the track at Terence's is $\frac{1}{8}$ mi long, who runs farther? How much farther?

38. The students in a math class can be organized into study groups of 8 each such that no students are left out. The same class of students can also be organized into groups of 6 such that no students are left out.

a) Find some class sizes for which this will work.

b) Find the smallest such class size.

39. Simplify each of the following, using fractional notation. Try to answer part (e) by recognizing a pattern in parts (a) through (d).

a) $\frac{1}{1 \cdot 2}$

b) $\frac{1}{1 \cdot 2} + \frac{1}{2 \cdot 3}$

c) $\frac{1}{1 \cdot 2} + \frac{1}{2 \cdot 3} + \frac{1}{3 \cdot 4}$

d) $\frac{1}{1 \cdot 2} + \frac{1}{2 \cdot 3} + \frac{1}{3 \cdot 4} + \frac{1}{4 \cdot 5}$

e) $\frac{1}{1 \cdot 2} + \frac{1}{2 \cdot 3} + \frac{1}{3 \cdot 4} + \frac{1}{4 \cdot 5} + \frac{1}{5 \cdot 6}$

$+ \frac{1}{6 \cdot 7} + \frac{1}{7 \cdot 8} + \frac{1}{8 \cdot 9} + \frac{1}{9 \cdot 10}$

Cumulative Review: Chapters 1–4

1. In the number 2753, what digit names tens?

2. Write expanded notation for 6075.

3. Write a word name for the number in the following sentence: The diameter of Uranus is 29,500 miles.

Add and, if possible, simplify.

4.
$$\begin{array}{r} 3\ 7\ 5 \\ +\ 2\ 4\ 8 \\ \hline \end{array}$$

5. $29 + (-37)$

6. $\dfrac{3}{8} + \dfrac{1}{24}$

7.
$$\begin{array}{r} 2\dfrac{3}{4} \\ +\ 5\dfrac{1}{2} \\ \hline \end{array}$$

Subtract and, if possible, simplify.

8.
$$\begin{array}{r} 7\ 4\ 6\ 9 \\ -\ 2\ 3\ 4\ 5 \\ \hline \end{array}$$

9. $-9 - (-25)$

10. $\dfrac{1}{3} - \dfrac{3}{4}$

11.
$$\begin{array}{r} 2\dfrac{1}{3} \\ -\ 1\dfrac{1}{6} \\ \hline \end{array}$$

Multiply and, if possible, simplify.

12.
$$\begin{array}{r} 2\ 7\ 8 \\ \times\ \ \ 1\ 8 \\ \hline \end{array}$$

13. $29(-5)$

14. $\dfrac{9}{10} \cdot \dfrac{5}{3}$

15. $18\left(-\dfrac{5}{6}\right)$

16. $2\dfrac{1}{3} \cdot 3\dfrac{1}{7}$

Divide. Write the answer with the remainder in the form 34 R 7.

17. $731 \div 15$

18. $4\ 5 \overline{)\ 2\ 5\ 3\ 1}$

19. In Question 18, write a mixed numeral for the answer.

Divide and, if possible, simplify.

20. $\dfrac{2}{5} \div \left(-\dfrac{7}{10}\right)$

21. $2\dfrac{1}{5} \div \dfrac{3}{10}$

22. Round 38,478 to the nearest hundred.

23. Find the LCM of 24 and 36.

24. Without performing the division, determine whether 4296 is divisible by 6.

25. Find all factors of 16.

26. What part is shaded?

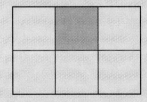

Use $<$, $>$, or $=$ for ▩ to form a true sentence.

27. $\dfrac{4}{5}$ ▩ $\dfrac{4}{6}$

28. $-\dfrac{3}{7}$ ▩ $-\dfrac{5}{12}$

Simplify.

29. $\dfrac{36}{45}$

30. $-\dfrac{420}{30}$

31. Convert to fractional notation: $4\dfrac{5}{8}$.

32. Convert to a mixed numeral: $-\dfrac{17}{3}$.

Solve.

33. $x + 24 = 117$

34. $x + \dfrac{7}{9} = \dfrac{4}{3}$

35. $\dfrac{7}{9} \cdot t = -\dfrac{4}{3}$

36. $\dfrac{5}{7} = \dfrac{1}{3} + 4a$

37. Evaluate $\dfrac{t + p}{3}$ for $t = -4$ and $p = 16$.

38. Multiply: $7(b - 5)$.

39. Multiply: $-3(x - 2 + z)$.

40. Combine like terms: $x - 5 - 7x - 4$.

Solve.

41. A jacket costs $87 and a coat costs $148. How much does it cost to buy both?

42. The emergency soup kitchen fund contains $978. From this fund, $148 and $167 are withdrawn for expenses. How much is left in the fund?

43. A rectangular lot measures 27 ft by 11 ft. What is its area?

44. How many people can get equal $16 shares from a total of $496?

45. A recipe calls for $\dfrac{4}{5}$ tsp of salt. How much salt should be used in $\dfrac{1}{2}$ recipe?

46. A book weighs $2\dfrac{3}{5}$ lb. How much do 15 books weigh?

47. How many pieces, each $2\dfrac{3}{8}$ cm long, can be cut from a piece of wire 38 cm long?

48. How long is the shortest bolt that will pass through a $\dfrac{1}{16}$-in. thick washer, a $\dfrac{3}{4}$-in. thick backboard, and a $\dfrac{3}{8}$-in thick nut? Disregard the head of the bolt.

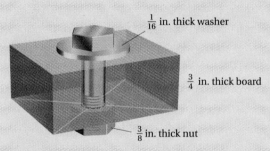

$\dfrac{1}{16}$ in. thick washer

$\dfrac{3}{4}$ in. thick board

$\dfrac{3}{8}$ in. thick nut

Synthesis

49. Solve: $7x - \dfrac{2}{3}(x - 6) = 6\dfrac{5}{7}$.

50. Each floor of a seven-story office building is 25 m by $22\dfrac{1}{2}$ m, with a 5-m by $4\dfrac{1}{2}$-m elevator/stairwell. How many square meters of office space are in the building?

5

Decimal Notation

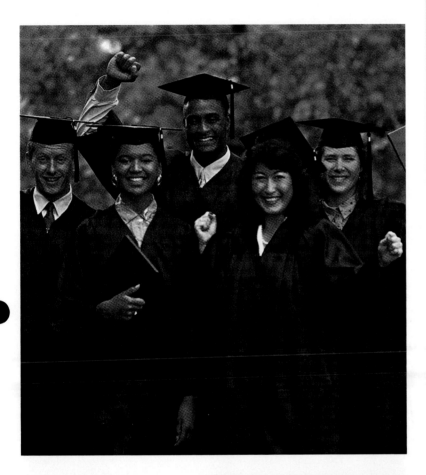

An Application

The Mathematics

Upon graduation from college, Jannette will be faced with repaying a Stafford loan that totals $23,334. The loan is to be paid back over 10 yr in equal payments. Find the amount of each payment.

This problem appears as Example 3 in Section 5.8.

This is a multistep problem. First, we determine the number of payments (10 · 12, or 120), and then we divide:

Monthly payment size	is	Total owed	Divided by	Number of payments
m	=	23,334	÷	120.

Division like this is most easily performed using *decimal notation*.

For more information, visit us at www.mathmax.com

Pretest: Chapter 5

1. Write a word name for 17.369.

2. Write $625.27 in words, as on a check.

Write fractional notation. Do not simplify.

3. 0.21

4. 5.408

Write decimal notation.

5. $\dfrac{379}{100}$

6. $-\dfrac{79}{10,000}$

7. Round 21.0448 to the nearest tenth.

Perform the indicated operation.

8.
$$\begin{array}{r} 6\ 0\ 1.3 \\ 5.8\ 1 \\ +\quad 0.1\ 0\ 9 \\ \hline \end{array}$$

9.
$$\begin{array}{r} 9\ 4.0\ 6\ 1 \\ -\quad 2.3\ 2\ 9 \\ \hline \end{array}$$

10.
$$\begin{array}{r} 7.3\ 2\ 5 \\ \times\quad 0.6\ 4 \\ \hline \end{array}$$

11. $91.6851 - 344.6788$

12. $-6.6\,)\,\overline{2\ 0\ 0.6\ 4}$

13. Combine like terms: $8.3a + 4.6a$.

14. Combine like terms: $-2.7x + 5.1 - 4.2x + 1.7$.

15. Simplify: $(2 - 1.7)^2 - 4.1 \times 3.1$.

16. Estimate the sum $3.649 + 4.038$ to the nearest tenth.

17. Multiply by 1 to find decimal notation for $\frac{7}{5}$.

18. Use division to find decimal notation for $\frac{29}{7}$.

19. Calculate: $\frac{3}{4} \times 2.378$.

20. Find the area of a triangular sail that is 2.8 m wide at the base and 3.1 m tall.

Solve.

21. $x + 3.91 = 7.26$

22. $-9.6y = 808.896$

23. $4.2x - 3.8 = 18.88$

24. $4.7a - 1.9 = 3.2a + 7.1$

25. $2.3(t + 4) - 0.5t = 5.8t - 9$

Solve.

26. A checking account contained $434.19. After a $148.24 check was drawn, how much was left in the account?

27. On a three-day trip, Doris drove the following distances: 432.6 mi, 179.2 mi, and 469.8 mi. What was the total number of miles driven?

28. What is the cost of 6 compact discs at $14.95 each?

29. Costas Construction paid $47,567.89 for 14 acres of land. How much did 1 acre of land cost? Round to the nearest cent.

30. Jorge filled the gas tank of his Ford Explorer and noted that the odometer read 52,091.7. At the next fillup, when the odometer read 52,214.9, it took 8 gal to fill the tank. How many miles per gallon did Jorge's Explorer get?

5.1 Decimal Notation

The set of **rational numbers** consists of the **integers**

$$\dots, -3, -2, -1, 0, 1, 2, 3, \dots,$$

and fractions like

$$\frac{1}{2}, \frac{2}{3}, \frac{-7}{8}, \frac{17}{-10}, \text{ and so on.}$$

We used fractional notation for rational numbers in Chapters 3 and 4. In Chapter 5, we will use *decimal notation.* We will still consider the same set of numbers, but now with a different notation. For example, instead of using fractional notation for $\frac{7}{8}$, we use decimal notation, 0.875.

a Decimal Notation and Word Names

Decimal notation for the women's shotput record is 74.249 ft. To understand what 74.249 means, we use a **place-value chart.** The value of each place is $\frac{1}{10}$ as large as the one to its left. To the right of the decimal point, each place value ends with *ths.*

PLACE-VALUE CHART							
Hundreds	Tens	Ones	Ten*ths*	Hundred*ths*	Thousand*ths*	Ten-Thousand*ths*	Hundred-Thousand*ths*
100	10	1	$\frac{1}{10}$	$\frac{1}{100}$	$\frac{1}{1000}$	$\frac{1}{10,000}$	$\frac{1}{100,000}$
7	4 .	2	4	9			

The decimal notation 74.249 means

$$7 \text{ tens} + 4 \text{ ones} + 2 \text{ tenths} + 4 \text{ hundredths} + 9 \text{ thousandths},$$

or

$$74 + \frac{2}{10} + \frac{4}{100} + \frac{9}{1000}$$

or

$$74 + \frac{200}{1000} + \frac{40}{1000} + \frac{9}{1000}, \text{ or } 74\frac{249}{1000}.$$

A mixed numeral for 74.249 is $74\frac{249}{1000}$. We read 74.249 as "seventy-four and two hundred forty-nine thousandths." When we come to the decimal point (that is, the dot in front of the 2), we read "and." We can also read 74.249 as "seventy-four *point* two four nine."

To write a word name from decimal notation,

a) write the name of the integer that appears to the left of the decimal point,

    397.685
    ⎣⟶ Three hundred ninety-seven

b) write the word "and" for the decimal point, and

    397.685
    Three hundred ninety-seven and

c) write the name of the integer that appears to the right of the decimal point, followed by the place value of the last digit.

    397.685
    Three hundred ninety-seven and six hundred eighty-five *thousandths*

Write a word name for each number.

1. Each person in this country consumes an average of 20.5 gallons of coffee per year (*Source*: Department of Agriculture).

Twenty and five tenths

2. The racehorse *Swale* won the Belmont Stakes in a time of 2.4533 minutes.

Two and four thousand five hundred thirty-three ten-thousandths

3. −453.27

Negative four hundred fifty-three and twenty-seven hundredths

4. 51,739.082

Fifty-one thousand, seven hundred thirty-nine and eighty-two thousandths

Write in words, as on a check.

5. $4217.56

Four thousand, two hundred seventeen and $\frac{56}{100}$ dollars

6. $13.98

Thirteen and $\frac{98}{100}$ dollars

Answers on pages A-11

Example 1 Write a word name for the number in this sentence: Each person consumes an average of 41.2 gallons of water per year.

Forty-one and two tenths

Example 2 Write a word name for −413.07.

Negative four hundred thirteen and seven hundredths

Example 3 Write a word name for the number in this sentence: The world record in the men's marathon is 2.1008 hours.

Two and one thousand eight ten-thousandths

Example 4 Write a word name for the number in this sentence: The fastest time in the women's marathon is 2.341 hours.

Two and three hundred forty-one thousandths

Do Exercises 1–4.

Decimal notation is also used with money. It is common on a check to write "and ninety-five cents" as "and $\frac{95}{100}$ dollars."

Example 5 Write $5876.95 in words, as on a check.

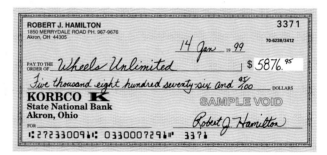

Five thousand, eight hundred seventy-six and $\frac{95}{100}$ dollars

Do Exercises 5 and 6.

b | Converting from Decimal Notation to Fractional Notation

We can find fractional notation as follows:

$$9.875 = 9 + \frac{875}{1000}$$

$$= \frac{9000}{1000} + \frac{875}{1000} = \frac{9875}{1000}$$

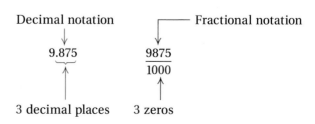

To convert from decimal to fractional notation,

a) count the number of decimal places,   4.98
          2 places

b) move the decimal point that many   4.98.   Move
    places to the right, and   2 places.

c) write the answer over a denominator $\dfrac{498}{100}$ 2 zeros
    with a 1 followed by that number of zeros.

Example 6   Write fractional notation for 0.876. Do not simplify.

$$0.876 \qquad 0.876. \qquad 0.876 = \frac{876}{1000}$$

3 places   3 zeros

For a number like 0.876, we generally write a 0 before the decimal point to avoid forgetting or overlooking the decimal point.

Example 7   Write fractional notation for 56.23. Do not simplify.

$$56.23 \qquad 56.23. \qquad 56.23 = \frac{5623}{100}$$

2 places   2 zeros

Negative numbers written in decimal notation can also be converted.

Example 8   Write fractional notation for −1.5018. Do not simplify.

$$-1.5018 \qquad -1.5018. \qquad -1.5018 = -\frac{15{,}018}{10{,}000}, \quad \text{or} \quad \frac{15{,}018}{-10{,}000}$$

4 places   4 zeros

Do Exercises 7–10.

c   Converting from Fractional Notation and Mixed Numerals to Decimal Notation

Suppose we wish to write $\frac{5328}{10}$ in decimal notation. In Section 4.5, we learned that division can be used to find an equivalent mixed numeral:

$$\frac{5328}{10} = 532\frac{8}{10}.$$

Note that

$$532\frac{8}{10} = 532 + \frac{8}{10}$$

$$= 532.8.$$

$$\begin{array}{r} 5\ 3\ 2 \\ 1\ 0\ \overline{)\ 5\ 3\ 2\ 8} \\ \underline{5\ 0} \\ 3\ 2 \\ \underline{3\ 0} \\ 2\ 8 \\ \underline{2\ 0} \\ 8 \end{array}$$

This procedure can be generalized. It is the reverse of the procedure used in Examples 6–8.

Write fractional notation. Do not simplify.

7. 0.896

$$\frac{896}{1000}$$

8. −39.08

$$\frac{3908}{100}$$

9. 5.6789

$$\frac{56{,}789}{10{,}000}$$

10. −3.7

$$\frac{37}{10}$$

Answers on page A-11

Write decimal notation.

11. $\dfrac{743}{100}$ 7.43

12. $\dfrac{48}{1000}$ 0.048

13. $\dfrac{67{,}089}{10{,}000}$ 6.7089

14. $-\dfrac{9}{10}$ −0.9

Write decimal notation.

15. $-7\dfrac{3}{100}$ −7.03

16. $23\dfrac{47}{1000}$ 23.047

Answers on page A-11

To convert from fractional notation to decimal notation when the denominator is 10, 100, 1000, and so on,

a) count the number of zeros, and

$$\dfrac{8679}{1000}$$

3 zeros

b) move the decimal point that number of places to the left. Leave off the denominator.

8.679.   Move 3 places.

$$\dfrac{8679}{1000} = 8.679$$

Example 9   Write decimal notation for $\dfrac{47}{10}$.

$$\dfrac{47}{10}$$

1 zero

4.7. $\dfrac{47}{10} = 4.7$ **The decimal point is moved 1 place.**

Example 10   Write decimal notation for $\dfrac{123{,}067}{10{,}000}$.

$$\dfrac{123{,}067}{10{,}000}$$

4 zeros

12.3067. $\dfrac{123{,}067}{10{,}000} = 12.3067$ **The decimal point is moved 4 places.**

Example 11   Write decimal notation for $-\dfrac{9}{100}$.

$$-\dfrac{9}{100}$$

2 zeros

−0.09. $-\dfrac{9}{100} = -0.09$ **The decimal point is moved 2 places.**

Do Exercises 11–14.

For denominators other than 10, 100, and so on, we will usually perform long division. This is examined in Section 5.5.

If a mixed numeral has a fractional part with a denominator that is a power of ten, such as 10, 100, or 1000, and so on, we first write the mixed numeral as a sum of a whole number and a fraction. Then we convert to decimal notation.

Example 12   Write decimal notation for $23\dfrac{59}{100}$.

$$23\dfrac{59}{100} = 23 + \dfrac{59}{100} = 23 \text{ and } \dfrac{59}{100} = 23.59$$

Do Exercises 15 and 16.

d | Order

To compare numbers in decimal notation, consider 0.85 and 0.9. First note that $0.9 = 0.90$ because $\frac{9}{10} = \frac{90}{100}$. Since $0.85 = \frac{85}{100}$, it follows that $\frac{85}{100} < \frac{90}{100}$ and $0.85 < 0.9$. This leads us to a quick way to compare two numbers in decimal notation.

> ▶ To compare two positive numbers in decimal notation, start at the left and compare corresponding digits. When two digits differ, the number with the larger digit is the larger of the two numbers. To ease the comparison, extra zeros can be written to the right of the last decimal place.

Example 13 Which is larger: 2.109 or 2.1?

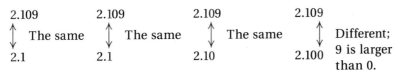

Thus, 2.109 is larger. In symbols, $2.109 > 2.1$.

Example 14 Which is larger: 0.09 or 0.108?

0.09		0.09	Different;
↕	The same	↕	1 is larger than 0.
0.108		0.108	

Thus, 0.108 is larger. In symbols, $0.108 > 0.09$.

As before, we can use a number line to visualize order. We illustrate Examples 13 and 14 below. Larger numbers are always to the right.

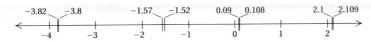

Note from the number line that $-2 < -1$. Similarly, $-1.57 < -1.52$.

> To compare two negative numbers in decimal notation, start at the left and compare corresponding digits. When two digits differ, the number with the smaller digit is the larger of the two numbers.

Example 15 Which is larger: -3.8 or -3.82?

-3.8		-3.80	
↕	The same	↕	Different; 0 is smaller than 2.
-3.82		-3.82	

Thus, -3.8 is larger. In symbols, $-3.8 > -3.82$. (See the graph above.)

Do Exercises 17–24.

Which number is larger?

17. 2.04, 2.039 2.04

18. 0.06, 0.008 0.06

19. 0.5, 0.58 0.58

20. 1, 0.9999 1

21. 0.8989, 0.09898 0.8989

22. 21.006, 21.05 21.05

23. −34.01, −34.008 −34.008

24. −9.12s, −8.98 −8.98

Answers on page A-11

Round to the nearest tenth.

25. 2.76

　　2.8

26. 13.85

　　13.9

27. −234.448

　　−234.4

28. 7.009

　　7.0

Round to the nearest hundredth.

29. 0.636

　　0.64

30. −7.834

　　−7.83

31. 34.695

　　34.70

32. −0.025

　　−0.03

Round to the nearest thousandth.

33. 0.9434

　　0.943

34. −8.0038

　　−8.004

35. −43.1119

　　−43.112

36. 37.4005

　　37.401

Round 7459.3598 to the nearest:

37. Thousandth.

　　7459.360

38. Hundredth.

　　7459.36

39. Tenth.

　　7459.4

40. One.

　　7459

41. Ten. (*Caution*: "Tens" are not "tenths.")

　　7460

42. Hundred.

　　7500

43. Thousand.

　　7000

Answers on pages A-11 and A-12

e | Rounding

Rounding is done as for whole numbers. To see how, we use a number line.

Example 16 Round 0.37 to the nearest tenth.

Here is part of a number line, magnified.

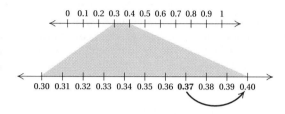

We see that 0.37 is closer to 0.40 than to 0.30. Thus, when 0.37 is rounded to the nearest tenth, we round *up* to 0.4.

To round to a certain place:

a) Locate the digit in that place.

b) Consider the next digit to the right.

c) If the digit to the right is 5 or greater, round up; if the digit to the right is 4 or less, round down.

Example 17 Round 72.3846 to the nearest hundredth.

a) Locate the digit in the hundredths place.

　　7 2.3 8 4 6
　　　　↑

b) Consider the next digit to the right.

　　7 2.3 8 4 6
　　　　└↑

CAUTION! 72.39 is not a correct answer to Example 17. It is incorrect to round sequentially from right to left as follows:

72.3846,　72.385,　72.39.

c) Since that digit, 4, is less than 5, we round *down* from 72.3846 to 72.38.

Example 18 Round −0.06 to the nearest tenth.

a) Locate the digit in the tenths place.

b) Consider the next digit to the right.

−0.0 6
　　↑

−0.0 6
　　└↑

c) Since that digit, 6, is greater than 5, round from −0.06 to −0.1.

The answer is −0.1. Since −0.1 < −0.06, we actually rounded *down*.

Do Exercises 25–43.

Exercise Set 5.1

a   Write a word name for the number in each sentence.

1. The largest pumpkin ever grown weighed 481.27 kilograms (**Source:** *Guinness Book of Records,* 1998).

Four hundred eighty-one and twenty-seven hundredths

2. The average loss of daylight in October in Anchorage, Alaska, is 5.63 min per day.

Five and sixty-three hundredths

3. Recently, one British pound was worth about $1.5599 in U.S. currency.

One and five thousand five hundred ninety-nine ten-thousandths

4. The cost of a fast modem for a computer was $289.95.

Two hundred eighty-nine and ninety-five hundredths

Write a word name.

5. 34.891

Thirty-four and eight hundred ninety-one thousandths

6. 27.1245

Twenty-seven and one thousand two hundred forty-five ten-thousandths

Write in words, as on a check.

7. $326.48   See answer below.

8. $125.99   See answer below.

9. $36.72   Thirty-six and $\frac{72}{100}$ dollars

10. $0.67   Zero and $\frac{67}{100}$ dollars

b   Write fractional notation. Do not simplify.

11. 8.3 $\frac{83}{10}$ **12.** 0.17 $\frac{17}{100}$ **13.** 203.6 $\frac{2036}{10}$ **14.** -57.32 $-\frac{5732}{100}$ **15.** -2.703 $-\frac{2703}{1000}$

16. 0.00013 $\frac{13}{100,000}$ **17.** 0.0109 $\frac{109}{10,000}$ **18.** 1.0008 $\frac{10,008}{10,000}$ **19.** -6.004 $-\frac{6004}{1000}$ **20.** -9.012 $-\frac{9012}{1000}$

c   Write decimal notation.

21. $\frac{8}{10}$ 0.8   **22.** $\frac{51}{10}$ 5.1   **23.** $-\frac{59}{100}$ -0.59 **24.** $-\frac{67}{100}$ -0.67 **25.** $\frac{3798}{1000}$ 3.798

26. $\frac{780}{1000}$ 0.780   **27.** $\frac{78}{10,000}$ 0.0078   **28.** $\frac{56,788}{100,000}$ 0.56788   **29.** $\frac{-18}{100,000}$ -0.00018 **30.** $\frac{-2347}{100}$ -23.47

31. $\frac{376,193}{1,000,000}$ 0.376193   **32.** $\frac{8,953,074}{1,000,000}$ 8.953074   **33.** $99\frac{44}{100}$ 99.44   **34.** $4\frac{909}{1000}$ 4.909   **35.** $-8\frac{431}{1000}$ -8.431

36. $-49\frac{32}{1000}$ -49.032 **37.** $2\frac{1739}{10,000}$ 2.1739   **38.** $9243\frac{1}{10}$ 9243.1   **39.** $8\frac{953,073}{1,000,000}$ 8.953073   **40.** $2256\frac{3059}{10,000}$ 2256.3059

d   Which number is larger?

41. 0.06,   0.58   0.58   **42.** 0.008,   0.8   0.8   **43.** 0.905,   0.91   0.91   **44.** 42.06,   42.1   42.1

45. -5.046, -5.043 -5.043 **46.** -324.19, -325.19 -324.19 **47.** 234.07,   235.07   235.07   **48.** 0.99999,   1   1

49. 0.004, $\frac{4}{100}$ $\frac{4}{100}$ **50.** $\frac{73}{10}$,   0.73 $\frac{73}{10}$ **51.** -0.872, -0.873 -0.872 **52.** -0.8437, -0.84384 -0.8437

e   Round to the nearest tenth.

53. 0.11   0.1   **54.** 0.85   0.9   **55.** -0.37 -0.4 **56.** -0.26 -0.3

57. 2.951   3.0   **58.** 4.98   5.0   **59.** -327.2347 -327.2 **60.** -8.749 -8.7

Round to the nearest hundredth.

61. 0.893   0.89   **62.** 0.675   0.68   **63.** -0.6666 -0.67 **64.** -7.525 -7.53

65. 0.995   1.00   **66.** 207.9976   208.00   **67.** -0.0348 -0.03 **68.** -9.2748 -9.27

---

7. Three hundred twenty-six and $\frac{48}{100}$ dollars   **8.** One hundred twenty-five and $\frac{99}{100}$ dollars

Round to the nearest thousandth.

69. 0.3246   0.325

70. 0.6666   0.667

71. 17.0015   17.002

72. 123.4562   123.456

73. −20.20202   −20.202

74. −0.10346   −0.103

75. 9.9848   9.985

76. 67.100602   67.101

Round 809.4732 to the nearest:

77. Tenth.   809.5

78. Thousandth.   809.473

79. Hundredth.   809.47

80. One.   809

Skill Maintenance

81. Simplify: $\dfrac{0}{-19}$.   [3.3c]   0

82. Add: $\dfrac{2}{15} + \dfrac{5}{9}$.   [4.2b] $\dfrac{31}{45}$

83. Subtract: $\dfrac{4}{9} - \dfrac{2}{3}$.   [4.3a] $-\dfrac{2}{9}$

84. Solve: $7x + 5 = 3$.   [4.4a] $-\dfrac{2}{7}$

85. Solve: $3x - 8 = 21$.   [4.4a] $\dfrac{29}{3}$

86. Subtract: $\dfrac{3}{14} - \dfrac{2}{7}$.   [4.3a] $-\dfrac{1}{14}$

Synthesis

87. ◆ Brian rounds 536.447 to the nearest one and, incorrectly, gets 537. How might he have made this mistake?

88. ◆ Explain why −73.69 is smaller than −73.67.

89. ◆ Describe in your own words a procedure for converting from decimal notation to fractional notation.

Global Warming. The graph below is based on the average global temperatures from January through May of 1880 through 1998. Each bar indicates, in Fahrenheit degrees, how much above or below average the temperature was for the year.

90. For what year(s) was the yearly temperature more than 0.4 degree above average?
1983, 1988, 1990, 1991, 1992, 1995, 1997, 1998

91. What was the last year in which the yearly temperature was more than 0.6 degree below average?   1979

92. What was the last year in which the yearly temperature was below average?   1985

93. For what year(s) was the yearly temperature more than 1.0 degree above average?   1998

A Warming Trend

Degrees above or below the average global temperature between 1880 and 1998 for January through May. In degrees Fahrenheit.

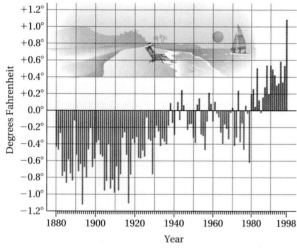

Source: *Council on Environmental Quality*, The New York Times.

There are other methods of rounding decimal notation. A computer often uses a method called **truncating**. To round using truncating, simply drop all decimal places past the rounding place, which is the same as changing all digits to the right to zeros. For example, truncating 6.78163 to the third decimal place gives 6.781. Use truncating to round each of the following to the fifth decimal place.

94. 6.78346123   6.78346

95. 0.07070707   0.07070

5.2 Addition and Subtraction with Decimals

Objectives

a Add using decimal notation.

b Subtract using decimal notation.

c Add and subtract negative decimals.

d Combine like terms with decimal coefficients.

For Extra Help

TAPE 9   MAC   CD-ROM
           WIN

a   Addition

Adding with decimal notation is similar to adding whole numbers. First we line up the decimal points so that we can add corresponding place-value digits. Then we add digits from the right. For example, we add the thousandths, then the hundredths, and so on, carrying if necessary. If desired, we can write extra zeros to the right of the last decimal place so that the number of places is the same.

Example 1   Add: 56.314 + 17.78.

```
    5 6 . 3 1 4      Lining up the decimal points in order to add
  + 1 7 . 7 8 0      Writing an extra zero to the right
                     of the last decimal place

    5 6 . 3 1 4      Adding thousandths
  + 1 7 . 7 8 0
              4

    5 6 . 3 1 4      Adding hundredths
  + 1 7 . 7 8 0
            9 4

      1
    5 6 . 3 1 4      Adding tenths
  + 1 7 . 7 8 0      Write a decimal point in the answer.
        . 0 9 4      We get 10 tenths = 1 one + 0 tenths,
                     so we carry the 1 to the ones column.

    1 1
    5 6 . 3 1 4      Adding ones
  + 1 7 . 7 8 0
      4 . 0 9 4      We get 14 ones = 1 ten + 4 ones,
                     so we carry the 1 to the tens column.

    1 1
    5 6 . 3 1 4      Adding tens
  + 1 7 . 7 8 0
    7 4 . 0 9 4
```

Do Exercises 1 and 2.

Remember, we can write extra zeros to the right of the last decimal place to get the same number of decimal places.

Example 2   Add: 3.42 + 0.237 + 14.1.

```
      3.4 2 0     Lining up the decimal points
      0.2 3 7     and writing extra zeros
  + 1 4.1 0 0
    1 7.7 5 7     Adding
```

Do Exercises 3–5.

Add.

1.
```
      0.8 4 7
  + 1 0.0 7
```
10.917

2.
```
      2.1
      0.7 3 9
  + 3 1.3 6 8 9
```
34.2079

Add.

3. 0.02 + 4.3 + 0.649

4.969

4. 0.12 + 3.006 + 0.4357

3.5617

5. 0.4591 + 0.2374 + 8.70894

9.40544

Answers on page A-12

Add.

6. 789 + 123.67

912.67

7. 45.78 + 2467 + 1.993

2514.773

Subtract.

8. 37.428 − 26.674

10.754

9.   0.3 4 7
     − 0.0 0 8

0.339

Answers on page A-12

Consider the addition 3456 + 19.347. Keep in mind that an integer, such as 3456, has an "unwritten" decimal point at the right, with 0 fractional parts. When adding, we can always write in that decimal point and extra zeros if desired.

Example 3   Add: 3456 + 19.347.

```
          1
    3 4 5 6.0 0 0     Writing in the decimal point and extra zeros
  +      1 9.3 4 7    Lining up the decimal points
    3 4 7 5.3 4 7     Adding
```

Do Exercises 6 and 7.

b | Subtraction

Subtracting with decimal notation is similar to subtracting integers. First we line up the decimal points so that we can subtract corresponding place-value digits. Then we subtract digits from the right. For example, we subtract the thousandths, then the hundredths, the tenths, and so on, borrowing if necessary.

Example 4   Subtract: 56.314 − 17.78.

```
    5 6.3 1 4     Lining up the decimal points in order to subtract
  − 1 7.7 8 0     Writing an extra 0
```

```
    5 6.3 1 4     Subtracting thousandths
  − 1 7.7 8 0
              4
```

```
        2 11
    5 6.3 1 4     Borrowing a tenth to subtract hundredths
  − 1 7.7 8 0
            3 4
```

```
         12
       5 2 11
    5 6.3 1 4     Borrowing a one to subtract tenths
  − 1 7.7 8 0
          .5 3 4  Writing a decimal point
```

```
      15 12
     4 5 2 11
    5 6.3 1 4     Borrowing a ten to subtract ones
  − 1 7.7 8 0
      8.5 3 4
```

```
      15 12
     4 5 2 11
    5 6.3 1 4     Subtracting tens
  − 1 7.7 8 0
    3 8.5 3 4
```

```
              1  1  1
CHECK:      3 8.5 3 4
          + 1 7.7 8 0
            5 6.3 1 4
```

Do Exercises 8 and 9.

Example 5 Subtract: 23.08 − 5.0053.

$$\begin{array}{r} \overset{1\ 13\ \ \ 7\ 9\ 10}{2\,\cancel{3}.0\ \cancel{8}\ \cancel{0}\ \cancel{0}} \\ -\quad 5.0\ 0\ 5\ 3 \\ \hline 1\ 8.0\ 7\ 4\ 7 \end{array}$$ Writing two extra zeros

Subtracting

Do Exercises 10–12.

As with addition, when subtraction involves an integer, there is an "unwritten" decimal point that can be written in. Extra zeros can then be written in to the right of the decimal point.

Example 6 Subtract: 456 − 2.467.

$$\begin{array}{r} \overset{5\ 9\ 9\ 10}{4\ 5\ 6.\cancel{0}\ \cancel{0}\ \cancel{0}} \\ -\quad 2.4\ 6\ 7 \\ \hline 4\ 5\ 3.5\ 3\ 3 \end{array}$$ Writing in the decimal point and extra zeros

Subtracting

Do Exercises 13 and 14.

c | Adding and Subtracting with Negatives

Negative numbers in decimal notation are added or subtracted just like integers.

To add a negative number and a positive number:

a) Determine which number has the greater absolute value.

b) Subtract the smaller absolute value from the larger one.

c) The answer is the difference from part (b) with the sign from part (a).

Example 7 Add: −13.82 + 4.69.

a) Note that |−13.82| = 13.82, and |4.69| = 4.69. Since |−13.82| > |4.69|, the answer is negative.

b)
$$\begin{array}{r} \overset{7\ 12}{1\ 3.\cancel{8}\ \cancel{2}} \\ -\quad 4.6\ 9 \\ \hline 9.1\ 3 \end{array}$$ Finding the difference of the absolute values

Next, use the result of part (a).

c) −13.82 + 4.69 = −9.13

Do Exercises 15 and 16.

To add two negative numbers:

a) Add the absolute values.

b) Make the answer negative.

Example 8 Add: −2.306 + (−3.125).

a)
$$\left.\begin{array}{r} 2.3\ 0\ 6 \\ +\ 3.1\ 2\ 5 \end{array}\right\}$$ Note that |−2.306| = 2.306 and |−3.125| = 3.125.

$$5.4\ 3\ 1$$ Adding the absolute values

b) −2.306 + (−3.125) = −5.431   The sum of two negatives is negative.

Do Exercise 17.

Subtract.

10. 1.7 − 0.23   1.47

11. 0.43 − 0.18762   0.24238

12. 7.37 − 0.00008   7.36992

Subtract.

13. 1277 − 82.78   1194.22

14. 5 − 0.0089   4.9911

Add.

15. 7.42 + (−9.38)   −1.96

16. −4.201 + 7.36   3.159

17. Add: −4.95 + (−3.6).   −8.55

Answers on page A-12

Subtract.

18. $9.25 - 13.41$ -4.16

19. $-4.26 - 3.18$ -7.44

20. $9.8 - (-2.6)$ 12.4

21. $-5.9 - (-3.2)$ -2.7

Combine like terms.

22. $7.9x - 3.2x$ $4.7x$

23. $-5.9a + 7.6a$ $1.7a$

24. $-4.8y + 7.5 + 2.1y - 2.1$

$-2.7y + 5.4$

Answers on page A-12

To subtract, we add the opposite of the number being subtracted.

Example 9   Subtract: $-3.1 - 4.8$.

$$-3.1 - 4.8 = -3.1 + (-4.8) \qquad \text{Adding the opposite of 4.8}$$
$$= -7.9 \qquad \text{The sum of two negatives is negative.}$$

Example 10   Subtract: $-7.9 - (-8.5)$.

$$-7.9 - (-8.5) = -7.9 + 8.5 \qquad \text{Adding the opposite of } -8.5$$
$$= 0.6 \qquad \text{Subtracting absolute values. The answer is positive since 8.5 has the larger absolute value.}$$

Do Exercises 18–21.

d | Combining Like Terms

Recall that like, or similar, terms have exactly the same variable factors. When we combine like terms, we add or subtract coefficients to form an equivalent expression.

Example 11   Combine like terms: $3.2x + 4.6x$.

These are the coefficients.

$$3.2x + 4.6x = (3.2 + 4.6)x \qquad \text{Using the distributive law \\ Try to do this step mentally}$$
$$= 7.8x \qquad \text{Adding}$$

A similar procedure is used when subtracting like terms.

Example 12   Combine like terms: $4.13a - 7.56a$.

$$4.13a - 7.56a = (4.13 - 7.56)a \qquad \text{Using the distributive law}$$
$$= (4.13 + (-7.56))a \qquad \text{Adding the opposite of 7.56}$$
$$= -3.43a \qquad \text{Subtracting absolute values. The coefficient is negative since } |-7.56| > |4.13|.$$

When more than one pair of like terms is present, we can rearrange the terms and then simplify.

Example 13   Combine like terms: $5.7x - 3.9y - 2.4x + 4.5y$.

$$5.7x - 3.9y - 2.4x + 4.5y$$
$$= 5.7x + (-3.9y) + (-2.4x) + 4.5y \qquad \text{Rewriting as addition}$$
$$= 5.7x + (-2.4x) + 4.5y + (-3.9y) \qquad \text{Using the commutative law to rearrange}$$
$$= 3.3x + 0.6y \qquad \text{Combining like terms}$$

With practice, you will be able to perform many of the above steps mentally.

Do Exercises 22–24.

Exercise Set 5.2

a Add.

1. 3 1 6.2 5
   +   1 8.1 2
   334.37

2.   4 1.8 2 3
   + 6 1 4.9 1 5
   656.738

3.   6 5 9.4 0 3
   + 9 1 6.8 1 2
   1576.215

4.   3.2 5
   + 1 1 2 3.3 9
   1126.64

5.   9.1 0 4
   + 1 2 3.4 5 6
   132.56

6.   4.1 5 2 3
   + 3.2 7 7 8
   7.4301

7.   6 1.0 0 6
   +   3.4 0 7
   64.413

8. 0.8096 + 0.7856   1.5952

9. 20.0124 + 30.0124   50.0248

10. 0.263 + 0.8   1.063

11. 0.83 + 0.005   0.835

12. 0.347 + 10.04   10.387

13. 0.34 + 3.5 + 0.127 + 768
   771.967

14. 2.3 + 0.729 + 23
   26.029

15. 17 + 3.24 + 0.256 + 0.3689
   20.8649

16.   4 7.8
   2 1 9.8 5 2
   4 3.5 9
   + 6 6 6.7 1 3
   977.955

17.   2.7 0 3
   7 8.3 3
   2 8.0 0 0 9
   + 1 1 8.4 3 4 1
   227.468

18.   1 3.7 2
   9.1 1 2
   6 5 4 2.7 9 0 8
   +   2 3.9 0 1
   6589.5238

b Subtract.

19.   5.2
   − 3.1
   2.1

20. 1 1.3 4 5
   −   2.1 0 5
   9.24

21.   5 1.3 1
   −   2.2 9
   49.02

22.   3 7.4 5
   −   6.3 2
   31.13

23.
```
    2.5
 - 0.0 0 2 5
```
2.4975

24.
```
   2 8.0
 -    0.2 8
```
27.72

25.
```
   9 2.3 4 1
 -    6.4 2
```
85.921

26.
```
   0.3 4 6
 - 0.0 3 4 6
```
0.3114

27.
```
   3.0 0 7 4
 - 1.3 4 0 8
```
1.6666

28.
```
   3 2.7 9 7 8
 -     0.0 5 9 2
```
32.7386

29.
```
   6.0 7
 - 2.0 0 7 8
```
4.0622

30.
```
   1.0
 - 0.9 9 9 9
```
0.0001

31. 28.2 − 19.35

8.85

32. 100.12 − 0.112

100.008

33. 34.07 − 30.7

3.37

34. 36.2 − 16.28

19.92

35. 8.45 − 7.405

1.045

36. 3.801 − 2.81

0.991

37. 6.003 − 2.3

3.703

38. 1 − 0.0098

0.9902

39. 2 − 1.0908

0.9092

40. 100 − 0.34

99.66

41. 624 − 18.79

605.21

42. 7.48 − 2.6

4.88

43. 3 − 2.006

0.994

44. 25.008 − 12.4

12.608

45. 263.7 − 102.08

161.62

46. 19 − 1.198

17.802

47. 45 − 0.999

44.001

48. 10.056 − 0.392

9.664

c Add or subtract, as indicated.

49. −8.02 + 9.73

1.71

50. −4.31 + 7.66

3.35

51. 12.9 − 15.4

−2.5

52. 27.2 − 31.9

−4.7

53. −2.9 + (−4.3)

−7.2

54. −5.7 + (−1.9)

−7.6

55. −4.301 + 7.68

3.379

56. −5.952 + 7.98

2.028

57. $-13.4 - 9.2$
-22.6

58. $-8.7 - 12.4$
-21.1

59. $-2.1 - (-4.6)$
2.5

60. $-4.3 - (-2.5)$
-1.8

61. $14.301 + (-17.82)$
-3.519

62. $13.45 + (-18.701)$
-5.251

63. $7.201 - (-2.4)$
9.601

64. $2.901 - (-5.7)$
8.601

65. $23.9 + (-9.4)$
14.5

66. $43.2 + (-10.9)$
32.3

67. $-8.9 - (-12.7)$
3.8

68. $-4.5 - (-7.3)$
2.8

69. $-4.9 - 5.392$
-10.292

70. $89.3 - 92.1$
-2.8

71. $14.7 - 23.5$
-8.8

72. $-7.201 - 1.9$
-9.101

$\boxed{\text{d}}$ Combine like terms.

73. $5.1x + 3.6x$
$8.7x$

74. $7.9x + 1.8x$
$9.7x$

75. $17.59a - 12.73a$
$4.86a$

76. $23.28a - 15.79a$
$7.49a$

77. $15.2t + 7.9 + 5.9t$
$21.1t + 7.9$

78. $29.5t - 4.8 + 7.6t$
$37.1t - 4.8$

79. $9.208t - 14.519t$
$-5.311t$

80. $6.317t - 9.429t$
$-3.112t$

81. $4.906y - 7.1 + 3.2y$
$8.106y - 7.1$

82. $9.108y + 4.2 + 3.7y$
$12.808y + 4.2$

83. $4.8x + 1.9y - 5.7x + 1.2y$
$-0.9x + 3.1y$

84. $3.2r - 4.1t + 5.6t + 1.9r$
$5.1r + 1.5t$

85. $4.9 - 3.9t + 2.3 - 4.5t$
$7.2 - 8.4t$

86. $5.8 + 9.7x - 7.2 - 12.8x$
$-1.4 - 3.1x$

87. Simplify: $\dfrac{0}{-92}$. [3.3c]   0

88. Add: $\dfrac{-2}{7} + \dfrac{5}{21}$. [4.2b] $-\dfrac{1}{21}$

89. Subtract: $\dfrac{3}{5} - \dfrac{7}{10}$. [4.3a] $-\dfrac{1}{10}$

90. Solve: $9x - 16 = 5$. [4.4a] $\dfrac{7}{3}$

91. Solve: $7x + 19 = 40$. [4.4a]   3

92. Subtract: $\dfrac{2}{9} - \dfrac{2}{3}$. [4.3a] $-\dfrac{4}{9}$

Synthesis

93. ◈ Explain the error in the following:

Subtract.

$$
\begin{array}{r}
7\,3.0\,8\,9 \\
-\ 5.0\,0\,6\,1 \\
\hline
2.3\,0\,2\,8
\end{array}
$$

94. ◈ A student claims to be able to add negative numbers but not subtract them. What advice would you give this student?

95. ◈ Although the step in which it is used may not always be written out, the commutative law is often used when combining like terms. Under what circumstances would the commutative law *not* be needed for combining like terms?

Combine like terms.

96. ▦ $-3.928 - 4.39a + 7.4b - 8.073 + 2.0001a - 9.931b - 9.8799a + 12.897b$ $-12.001 - 12.2698a + 10.366b$

97. ▦ $79.02x + 0.0093y - 53.14z - 0.02001y - 37.987z - 97.203x - 0.00987y$ $-18.183x - 0.02058y - 91.127z$

98. ▦ $39.123a - 42.458b - 72.457a + 31.462b - 59.491 + 37.927a$ $4.593a - 10.996b - 59.491$

99. Fred presses the wrong key when using a calculator and adds 235.7 instead of subtracting it. The incorrect answer is 817.2. What is the correct answer?   345.8

100. Millie presses the wrong key when using a calculator and subtracts 349.2 instead of adding it. The incorrect answer is −836.9. What is the correct answer?   −138.5

101. ▦ Find the errors, if any, in the balances in this checkbook.

19 ___	BE SURE TO DEDUCT ANY PER ITEN CHARGES, SEVICE CHARGES, OR FEES THAT MAY APPLY IN 'OTHER' COLUMN						BALANCE FORWARD
DATE	CHECK NUMBER	TRANSACTION DESCRIPTION	✓ T	AMOUNT OF PAYMENT OR DEBIT	(+ OR −) OTHER	(+) AMOUNT OF CREDIT	8767 73
8/16	432	Burch Laundry		23 56			8744 16
8/19	433	Rogers TV		20 49			8764 65
8/20		Deposit				85 00	8848 65
8/21	434	Galaxy Records		48 60			8801 05
8/22	435	Electric Works		267 95			8533 09

101. $8744.16 should be $8744.17; $8764.65 should be $8723.68; $8848.65 should be $8808.68; $8801.05 should be $8760.08; $8533.09 should be $8492.13

5.3 Multiplication with Decimals

a Multiplication

To develop an understanding of how decimals are multiplied, consider

$$2.3 \times 1.12.$$

One way to find this product is to first convert each factor to fractional notation:

$$2.3 \times 1.12 = \frac{23}{10} \times \frac{112}{100}.$$

Next, we multiply the fractions and then return to decimal notation:

$$\frac{23}{10} \times \frac{112}{100} = \frac{2576}{1000} = 2.576.$$

Note that the number of decimal places in the product is the sum of the number of decimal places in the factors.

```
    1.1 2     (2 decimal places)
 ×    2.3     (1 decimal place)
   2.5 7 6    (3 decimal places)
```

Now consider 0.02×3.412:

$$0.02 \times 3.412 = \frac{2}{100} \times \frac{3412}{1000}$$

$$= \frac{6824}{100{,}000} = 0.06824.$$

Again, note the number of decimal places in the product is the sum of the number of decimal places in the factors.

```
      3.4 1 2     (3 decimal places)
 ×      0.0 2     (2 decimal places)
   0.0 6 8 2 4    (5 decimal places)
         ↑
```
It is important to write in this zero.

We have the following rule for multiplying decimals.

To multiply using decimals:	0.8×0.43
a) Ignore the decimal points, for the moment, and multiply as though both factors were integers.	$\begin{array}{r} 2 \\ 0.4\ 3 \\ \times\quad 0.8 \\ \hline 3\ 4\ 4 \end{array}$ Ignore the decimal points for now.
b) Then place the decimal point in the result. The number of decimal places in the product is the sum of the number of places in the factors (count places from the right).	$\begin{array}{r} 0.4\ 3 \\ \times\quad 0.8 \\ \hline 0.3\ 4\ 4 \end{array}$ (2 decimal places) (1 decimal place) (3 decimal places)

Objectives

a Multiply using decimal notation.

b Convert from dollars to cents and cents to dollars, and from notation like 45.7 million to standard notation.

c Evaluate algebraic expressions using decimal notation.

For Extra Help

TAPE 9   MAC   CD-ROM
                WIN

1. Multiply.

$$\begin{array}{r} 7\ 6.3 \\ \times\ \ \ \ 8.2 \\ \hline \end{array}$$

625.66

Multiply.

2.
$$\begin{array}{r} 4\ 2\ 1\ 3 \\ \times\ 0.0\ 0\ 5\ 1 \\ \hline \end{array}$$

21.4863

3. 2.3×0.0041 0.00943

4. $5.2014 \times (-2.41)$ -12.535374

Example 1   Multiply: 8.3×74.6.

a) Ignore the decimal points and multiply as if both factors were integers:

$$\begin{array}{r} {\scriptstyle 3\ 4} \\ {\scriptstyle 1\ 1} \\ 7\ 4.6 \\ \times\ \ \ \ \ 8.3 \\ \hline 2\ 2\ 3\ 8 \\ 5\ 9\ 6\ 8\ 0 \\ \hline 6\ 1\ 9\ 1\ 8 \end{array}$$ **We are not yet finished.**

b) Place the decimal point in the result. The number of decimal places in the product is the sum, $1 + 1$, of the number of decimal places in the factors.

$$\begin{array}{r} 7\ 4.6 \\ \times\ \ \ \ \ 8.3 \\ \hline 2\ 2\ 3\ 8 \\ 5\ 9\ 6\ 8\ 0 \\ \hline 6\ 1\ 9.1\ 8 \end{array}$$ (1 decimal place)
(1 decimal place)

(2 decimal places)

Do Exercise 1.

As we catch on to the skill, we can combine the two steps.

Example 2   Multiply: 0.0032×2148.

$$\begin{array}{r} 2\ 1\ 4\ 8 \\ \times\ 0.0\ 0\ 3\ 2 \\ \hline 4\ 2\ 9\ 6 \\ 6\ 4\ 4\ 4\ 0 \\ \hline 6.8\ 7\ 3\ 6 \end{array}$$ (0 decimal places)
(4 decimal places)

(4 decimal places)

Example 3   Multiply: -0.14×0.867.

Multiplying the absolute values, we have

$$\begin{array}{r} 0.8\ 6\ 7 \\ \times\ \ \ \ \ 0.1\ 4 \\ \hline 3\ 4\ 6\ 8 \\ 8\ 6\ 7\ 0 \\ \hline 0.1\ 2\ 1\ 3\ 8 \end{array}$$ (3 decimal places)
(2 decimal places)

(5 decimal places)

Since the product of a negative and a positive is negative, the answer is -0.12138.

Do Exercises 2–4.

Suppose that a product involves multiplication by a tenth, hundredth, thousandth, and so on. From the following products, a pattern emerges.

$$\begin{array}{r} 4\ 5.6 \\ \times\ \ \ 0.1 \\ \hline 4.5\ 6 \end{array} \quad \begin{array}{r} 4\ 5.6 \\ \times 0.0\ 1 \\ \hline 0.4\ 5\ 6 \end{array} \quad \begin{array}{r} 4\ 5.6 \\ \times 0.0\ 0\ 1 \\ \hline 0.0\ 4\ 5\ 6 \end{array} \quad \begin{array}{r} 4\ 5.6 \\ \times 0.0\ 0\ 0\ 1 \\ \hline 0.0\ 0\ 4\ 5\ 6 \end{array}$$

Note the location of the decimal point in each product. In each case, the product is *smaller* than 45.6 and contains the digits 456.

To multiply any number by a tenth, hundredth, or thousandth, and so on,

a) count the number of decimal places in the tenth, hundredth, or thousandth, and

$$0.001 \times 34.45678$$

⟶ 3 places

b) move the decimal point that many places to the left. Use zeros as placeholders if necessary.

$$0.001 \times 34.45678 = 0.034.45678$$

Move 3 places to the left.

$$0.001 \times 34.45678 = 0.03445678$$

Examples Multiply.

5. 0.1×359 35.9

4. $0.1 \times 45 = 4.5$ — Moving the decimal point one place to the left

5. $0.01 \times 243.7 = 2.437$ — Moving the decimal point two places to the left

6. $0.001 \times (-8.2) = -0.0082$ — Moving the decimal point three places to the left. This requires writing two extra zeros.

7. $0.0001 \times 536.9 = 0.05369$ — Moving the decimal point four places to the left. This requires writing one extra zero.

6. 0.001×732.4 0.7324

Do Exercises 5–8.

Next we consider multiplication of a decimal by a power of ten such as 10, 100, 1000, and so on. From the following products, a pattern emerges.

```
    5.2 3 7          5.2 3 7               5.2 3 7
  ×     1 0       ×     1 0 0           ×     1 0 0 0
    0 0 0 0          0 0 0 0               0 0 0 0
  5 2 3 7          0 0 0 0               0 0 0 0
  5 2.3 7 0      5 2 3 7                 0 0 0 0
                 5 2 3.7 0 0           5 2 3 7
                                       5 2 3 7.0 0 0
```

7. $(-0.01) \times 5.8$ −0.058

Note the location of the decimal point in each product. In each case, the product is *larger* than 5.237 and contains the digits 5237.

To multiply any number by a power of ten, such as 10, 100, 1000, and so on,

a) count the number of zeros, and

$$1000 \times 34.45678$$

⟶ 3 zeros

b) move the decimal point that many places to the right. Use zeros as placeholders if necessary.

$$1000 \times 34.45678 = 34.456.78$$

Move 3 places to the right.

$$1000 \times 34.45678 = 34{,}456.78$$

8. 0.0001×723.6 0.07236

Answers on page A-12

Multiply.

9. 10×53.917 539.17

10. $100 \times (-62.417)$ -6241.7

11. 1000×64.7 64,700

12. $10,000 \times 43.01$ 430,100

Answers on page A-12

Examples   Multiply.

8. $10 \times 32.98 = 329.8$ Moving the decimal point one place to the right

9. $100 \times 4.7 = 470$ Moving the decimal point two places to the right. The 0 in 470 is a placeholder.

10. $1000 \times (-2.4167) = -2416.7$ Moving the decimal point three places to the right

11. $10,000 \times 7.52 = 75,200$ Moving the decimal point four places to the right and using two zeros as placeholders

Do Exercises 9–12.

b | Applications Using Multiplication with Decimal Notation

Naming Large Numbers

We often see notation like the following in newspapers, magazines and on television.

> O'Hare International Airport handles 67.3 million passengers per year.
>
> In 1995, the Internal Revenue Service collected \$1.39 trillion.
>
> The population of the world is 6.6 billion.

To understand such notation, it helps to consider the following table.

1 hundred = 100 = 10^2
→ 2 zeros

1 thousand = 1000 = 10^3
→ 3 zeros

1 million = 1,000,000 = 10^6
→ 6 zeros

1 billion = 1,000,000,000 = 10^9
→ 9 zeros

1 trillion = 1,000,000,000,000 = 10^{12}
→ 12 zeros

To convert to standard notation, we proceed as follows.

Example 12 Convert the number in this sentence to standard notation: O'Hare International Airport handles 67.3 million passengers per year.

$$67.3 \text{ million} = 67.3 \times 1 \text{ million}$$
$$= 67.3 \times 1{,}000{,}000$$
$$= 67{,}300{,}000$$

Do Exercises 13 and 14.

Money Conversion

Converting from dollars to cents is like multiplying by 100. To see why, consider $19.43.

$\$19.43 = 19.43 \times \$1$	We think of $19.43 as 19.43 × 1 dollar, or 19.43 × $1.
$= 19.43 \times 100¢$	Substituting 100¢ for $1: $1 = 100¢
$= 1943¢$	Multiplying

> To convert from dollars to cents, move the decimal point two places to the right and change from the $ sign in front to the ¢ sign at the end.

Examples Convert from dollars to cents.

13. $\$189.64 = 18{,}964¢$

14. $\$0.75 = 75¢$

Do Exercises 15 and 16.

Converting from cents to dollars is like multiplying by 0.01. To see why, consider 65¢.

$65¢ = 65 \times 1¢$	We think of 65¢ as 65 × 1 cent, or 65 × 1¢.
$= 65 \times \$0.01$	Substituting $0.01 for 1¢: 1¢ = $0.01
$= \$0.65$	Multiplying

> To convert from cents to dollars, move the decimal point two places to the left and change from the ¢ sign at the end to the $ sign in front.

Examples Convert from cents to dollars.

15. $395¢ = \$3.95$

16. $8503¢ = \$85.03$

Do Exercises 17 and 18.

Convert the number in each sentence to standard notation.

13. In a recent year, there were more than 4.3 million skateboarders in the United States (*Source: Statistical Abstract of the United States, 1997*).

4,300,000

14. In a recent year, the U.S. trade deficit with Japan was $44.1 billion.

$44,100,000,000

Convert from dollars to cents.

15. $15.69

1569¢

16. $0.17

17¢

Convert from cents to dollars.

17. 35¢

$0.35

18. 577¢

$5.77

Answers on page A-12

19. Evaluate lwh for $l = 3.2$, $w = 2.6$, and $h = 0.8$. (This is the formula for the volume of a rectangular box.)

6.656

20. Find the area of the stamp in Example 18.   8.125 sq cm

21. Evaluate $6.28rh + 3.14r^2$ for $r = 1.5$ and $h = 5.1$. (This is the formula for the area of an open can.)

55.107

Answers on page A-12

---

c Evaluating

Algebraic expressions are often evaluated using numbers written in decimal notation.

Example 17   Evaluate Prt for $P = 80$, $r = 0.12$, and $t = 0.5$.

We will see in Chapter 8 that this product could be used to determine the interest earned on $80, invested at 12 percent simple interest, for half a year. We substitute as follows:

$$Prt = 80 \cdot 0.12 \cdot 0.5 = 80 \cdot 0.06 = 4.8.$$

Do Exercise 19.

Example 18   Find the perimeter of a stamp that is 3.25 cm long and 2.5 cm wide.

Recall that the perimeter, P, of a rectangle of length l and width w is given by the formula

$$P = 2l + 2w.$$

Thus we evaluate $2l + 2w$ for $l = 3.25$ and $w = 2.5$:

$$2l + 2w = 2 \cdot 3.25 + 2 \cdot 2.5$$
$$= 6.5 + 5.0 \qquad \text{Remember the rules for order of operations.}$$
$$= 11.5.$$

The perimeter is 11.5 cm.

Example 19   Evaluate $4.9t^2$ for $t = 5.1$.

This formula is used in physics to find the distance, in meters, traveled by a falling body. We substitute as follows:

$$4.9t^2 = 4.9 \cdot 5.1^2$$
$$= 4.9 \cdot (5.1)(5.1) \qquad \text{Square first, then multiply.}$$
$$= 4.9 \cdot 26.01 = 127.449.$$

Do Exercises 20 and 21.

Calculator Spotlight

Most scientific and graphing calculators are equipped with a key labeled $\boxed{x^2}$. On a scientific calculator, pressing $\boxed{x^2}$ usually squares whatever number was last displayed. For instance, to compute 7^2, we press

$$\boxed{7} \; \boxed{x^2} .$$

To compute 7^2 on most graphing calculators, we press

$$\boxed{7} \; \boxed{x^2} \; \boxed{\text{ENTER}} .$$

Exercises

1. Use a scientific or graphing calculator to check Example 19.

2. Use a scientific or graphing calculator to evaluate Pm^2 for each of the following.

   a) $P = 7536$ and $m = 1.046$ 8245.258176

   b) $P = 927.45$ and $m = 1.057$ 1036.192585

   c) $P = 10,475$ and $m = 1.062$ 11,814.1659

Exercise Set 5.3

a Multiply.

1. 6.8
  × 7
  47.6

2. 5.7
  × 0.9
  5.13

3. 0.8 4
  × 8
  6.72

4. 7.3
  × 0.6
  4.38

5. 6.3
  × 0.0 4
  0.252

6. 7.8
  × 0.0 9
  0.702

7. 1 7.2
  × 0.0 0 6
  0.1032

8. 8.7
  × 0.0 6
  0.522

9. 10×42.63
  426.3

10. 100×2.8793
  287.93

11. -1000×783.686852
  $-783,686.852$

12. -0.34×1000
  -340

13. -7.8×100
  -780

14. $0.00238 \times (-10)$
  -0.0238

15. 0.1×79.18
  7.918

16. 0.01×789.235
  7.89235

17. 0.001×97.68
  0.09768

18. 8976.23×0.001
  8.97623

19. $28.7 \times (-0.01)$
  -0.287

20. $0.0325 \times (-0.1)$
  -0.00325

21. 2.7 3
  × 1 6
  43.68

22. 8.2 7
  × 5.4
  44.658

23. 0.9 8 4
  × 3.3
  3.2472

24. 7.4 8 9
  × 8.2
  61.4098

25. $(-37.4)(-2.4)$
  89.76

26. $569(-1.05)$
  -597.45

27. $749(-0.43)$
  -322.07

28. $(-876)(-20.4)$
  17,870.4

29. 0.8 7
  × 6 4
  55.68

30. 7.2 5
  × 6 0
  435

31. 4 6.5 0
  × 7 5
  3487.5

32. 8.2 4
  × 7 0 3
  5792.72

33. $(-0.231)(-0.5)$
  0.1155

34. $(-12.3)(-1.08)$
  13.284

35. $9.42 \times (-1000)$
  -9420

36. $-7.6 \times (-1000)$
  7600

37. $-95.3 \times (-0.0001)$
  0.00953

38. $-4.23 \times (-0.001)$
  0.00423

b Convert from dollars to cents.

39. $28.88
  2888¢

40. $67.43
  6743¢

41. $0.66
  66¢

42. $1.78
  178¢

Convert from cents to dollars.

43. 34¢
  $0.34

44. 95¢
  $0.95

45. 3445¢
  $34.45

46. 933¢
  $9.33

Convert the number in each sentence to standard notation.

47. AMTRAK operating revenues for 1995 were $32.279 billion. $32,279,000,000

48. AMTRAK operating expenses for 1995 were $27.897 billion. $27,897,000,000

49. In a recent year, the daily circulation of the *Los Angeles Times* was 1.03 million.   1,030,000

50. The total surface area of Earth is 196.8 million square miles.   196,800,000

c Evaluate.

51. $P + Prt$, for $P = 10{,}000$, $r = 0.04$, and $t = 2.5$
(*A formula for adding interest*)   11,000

52. $6.28r(h + r)$, for $r = 10$ and $h = 17.2$
(*Surface area of a cylinder*)   1708.16

53. $vt + 0.5at^2$, for $v = 10$, $t = 1.5$, and $a = 9.8$
(*A physics formula*)   26.025

54. $4lh + 2h^2$, for $l = 3.5$ and $h = 1.2$
(*Surface area of a rectangular prism*)   19.68

Find **(a)** the perimeter and **(b)** the area of a rectangular room with the given dimensions.

55. 12.5 ft long, 9.5 ft wide   **(a)** 44 ft; **(b)** 118.75 sq ft

56. 10.25 ft long, 8 ft wide   **(a)** 36.5 ft; **(b)** 82 sq ft

Skill Maintenance

57. Simplify: $\dfrac{-109}{-109}$.   [3.3c]   1

58. Add: $\dfrac{-2}{10} + \dfrac{4}{15}$.   [4.2b] $\dfrac{1}{15}$

59. Subtract: $\dfrac{2}{9} - \dfrac{5}{18}$.   [4.3a] $-\dfrac{1}{18}$

60. Solve: $7x - 4 = -2$.   [4.4a] $\dfrac{2}{7}$

61. Add: $-\dfrac{3}{20} + \dfrac{3}{4}$.   [4.2b] $\dfrac{3}{5}$

62. Simplify: $\dfrac{0}{-19}$.   [3.3c]   0

Synthesis

63. ◆ Is it easier to multiply numbers written in decimal notation or fractional notation? Why?

64. ◆ If two rectangles have the same perimeter, will they also have the same area? Why?

65. ◆ A student insists that 346.708×0.1 is 3467.08. How can you convince the student that a mistake has been made?

▦ Evaluate using a calculator.

66. $d + vt + at^2$, for $d = 79.2$, $v = 3.029$, $t = 7.355$, and $a = 4.9$ (*A physics formula*)   366.5488175

67. $3.14r^2 + 6.28rh$, for $r = 5.756$ and $h = 9.047$
(*Surface area of a silo*)   431.061084

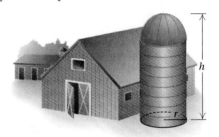

Express as a power of 10.

68. (1 trillion) · (1 billion) 10^{21}

69. (1 million) · (1 billion) 10^{15}

Electric Bills. Recently, electric bills from the Central Vermont Public Service Corporation consisted of a "customer charge" of $0.35 per day plus an "energy charge" of $0.10470 per kilowatt-hour (kWh) for the first 250 kWh used and $0.09079 per kilowatt-hour for each kilowatt-hour in excess of 250 (***Source:*** 1999 CVPS monthly statement).

70. From April 20 to May 20, the Coy-Bergers used 480 kWh of electricity. What was their bill for the period? $57.56

71. From June 20 to July 20, the D'Amicos used 430 kWh of electricity. What was their bill for the period? $53.02

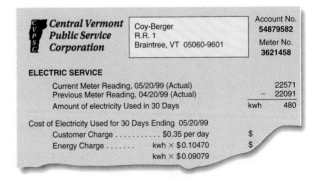

5.4 Division with Decimals

a Division

Whole-Number Divisors

Now that we have studied multiplication of decimals, we can develop a procedure for division. The following divisions are justified by the multiplication in each *check*:

This is the dividend. ⟶ $\dfrac{651}{7} = 93$ *Check:* 7 · 93 = 651.
This is the divisor. ⟶

This is the quotient.

$\dfrac{65.1}{7} = 9.3$ *Check:* 7 · 9.3 = 65.1.

$\dfrac{6.51}{7} = 0.93$ *Check:* 7 · 0.93 = 6.51.

$\dfrac{0.651}{7} = 0.093$ *Check:* 7 · 0.093 = 0.651.

Note that the number of decimal places in each quotient is the same as the number of decimal places in the dividend.

To divide by a whole number,

a) place the decimal point directly above the decimal point in the dividend, and

b) divide as though dividing whole numbers.

```
          0.8 4  ⟵ Quotient
      7 ) 5.8 8  ⟵ Dividend
     ↑    5 6 0
 Divisor  ─────
            2 8
            2 8
          ─────
              0  ⟵ Remainder
```

Example 1 Divide: 82.08 ÷ 24.

We have

```
                Place the decimal point.
            3.4 2
     2 4 ) 8 2.0 8
           7 2 0 0
           ───────
           1 0 0 8    Divide as though dividing whole numbers.
             9 6 0
           ───────
             4 8
             4 8
           ───────
               0
```

Estimation can be used as a partial check: 24 ≈ 25 and 82.08 ≈ 75; since 75 ÷ 25 = 3 and 3 ≈ 3.42, we have at least a partial check.

Do Exercises 1–3.

Sometimes it helps to write some extra zeros to the right of the dividend's decimal point. They don't change the number.

Objectives

a Divide using decimal notation.

b Simplify expressions using the rules for order of operations.

For Extra Help

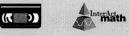

TAPE 9   MAC   CD-ROM
                WIN

Divide.

1. 9) 5.4   0.6

2. 1 5) 2 5.5   1.7

3. 8 2) 3 8.5 4   0.47

Answers on page A-12

Example 2 Divide: $30 \div 8$.

```
       3.
   8 ) 3 0.
       2 4
         6
```
Place the decimal point and divide to find how many ones.

```
       3.
   8 ) 3 0.0
       2 4 ↓
         6 0
```
Write an extra zero. This does not change the number.

```
       3.7
   8 ) 3 0.0
       2 4
         6 0
         5 6
           4
```
Divide to find how many tenths.

```
       3.7
   8 ) 3 0.0 0
       2 4
         6 0
         5 6 ↓
           4 0
```
Write an extra zero.

```
       3.7 5
   8 ) 3 0.0 0
       2 4
         6 0
         5 6 ↓
           4 0
           4 0
             0
```
Repeat the procedure: Divide to find how many hundredths are in the quotient.

Since the remainder is 0, we are finished.

Calculator Spotlight

It is possible to use a calculator to find whole-number remainders when doing division. To see how one method works, consider the quotient $17 \div 8$. We know that

$$17 \div 8 = 2.125.$$

To check, we can multiply:

$$8 \times 2.125 = 17,$$

or

$$8 \times (2 + 0.125) = 8 \times 2 + 8 \times 0.125$$
$$= 16 + 1 = 17.$$

Note that $17 \div 8 = 2$ R 1. Thus we can find a whole-number remainder by multiplying the decimal portion of a quotient by the divisor.

To find the quotient and the whole-number remainder for $567 \div 13$, we can use a calculator to find that

$$567 \div 13 \approx 43.61538462. \leftarrow \text{To isolate the decimal part, we can subtract 43.}$$

When the decimal part of the quotient is multiplied by the divisor, we have

$$0.61538462 \times 13 = 8.00000006.$$

The rounding error in the result may vary, depending on the calculator used. We see that $567 \div 13 = 43$ R 8.

Exercises Find the quotient and the whole-number remainder for each of the following.

1. $478 \div 17$ 28 R 2   **2.** $815 \div 7$ 116 R 3

3. $824 \div 11$ 74 R 10   **4.** $7888 \div 19$ 415 R 3

Example 3 Divide: $-4 \div 25$.

We first consider $4 \div 25$:

$$
\begin{array}{r}
0.1\,6 \\
2\,5 \overline{)\,4.0\,0} \leftarrow \text{We can write as many extra zeros as needed.} \\
\underline{2\,5} \\
1\,5\,0 \\
\underline{1\,5\,0} \\
0 \leftarrow \text{Since the remainder is 0, we are finished.}
\end{array}
$$

Since a negative number divided by a positive numer is negative, the answer is -0.16.

Do Exercises 4–6.

Divisors That Are Not Whole Numbers

Consider the division

$$0.2\,4 \overline{)\,8.2\,0\,8}$$

We write the division as $\dfrac{8.208}{0.24}$. Multiplying by a form of 1, we can find an equivalent division with a whole-number divisor, as in Examples 1–3:

$$\frac{8.208}{0.24} = \frac{8.208}{0.24} \times \frac{100}{100} = \frac{820.8}{24}.$$ We chose to use 100 in order to move the decimal point in 0.24 two places.

Since the divisor is now a whole number, we have effectively traded a "new" problem for an equivalent problem that is more familiar:

$$0.2\,4 \overline{)\,8.2\,0\,8}$$

is equivalent to

$$2\,4 \overline{)\,8\,2\,0.8}$$

To divide when the divisor is not a whole number,	
a) move the decimal point (multiply by 10, 100, and so on) to make the divisor a whole number;	$0.2\,4 \overline{)\,8.2\,0\,8}$ Move 2 places to the right.
b) move the decimal point the same number of places (multiply the same way) in the dividend; and	$0.2\,4 \overline{)\,8.2\,0\,8}$ Move 2 places to the right.
c) place the decimal point for the answer directly above the new decimal point in the dividend and divide as though dividing whole numbers.	$$\begin{array}{r} 3\,4.2 \\ 0.2\,4 \overline{)\,8.2\,0_{\wedge}8} \\ 7\,2\,0\,0 \\ 1\,0\,0\,8 \\ \underline{9\,6\,0} \\ 4\,8 \\ \underline{4\,8} \\ 0 \end{array}$$ (The new decimal point in the dividend is indicated by a caret.)

Divide.

4. $2\,5 \overline{)\,8}$ 0.32

5. $-23 \div 4$ -5.75

6. $8\,6 \overline{)\,2\,1.5}$ 0.25

Answers on page A-12

7. a) Complete.

$$\frac{3.75}{0.25} = \frac{3.75}{0.25} \times \frac{100}{100}$$

$$= \frac{(\quad)}{25}$$

375

b) Divide.

$$0.2\,5\,\overline{\smash{\big)}\,3.7\,5}$$

15

Divide.

8. $0.8\,3\,\overline{\smash{\big)}\,4.0\,6\,7}$

4.9

9. $-44.8 \div (-3.5)$

12.8

10. Divide.

$$1.6\,\overline{\smash{\big)}\,2\,5}$$

15.625

Answer on page A-12

Example 4   Divide: $5.848 \div 8.6$.

$$8.6\,\overline{\smash{\big)}\,5.8\,4\,8}$$

Multiply the divisor by 10 (move the decimal point 1 place). Multiply the same way in the dividend (move 1 place).

$$
\begin{array}{r}
0.6\,8 \\
8.6\,\overline{\smash{\big)}\,5.8\,4\,8} \\
5\,1\,6\,0 \\
\hline
6\,8\,8 \\
6\,8\,8 \\
\hline
0
\end{array}
$$

Then divide.

Note: $\dfrac{5.848}{8.6} = \dfrac{5.848}{8.6} \cdot \dfrac{10}{10} = \dfrac{58.48}{86}$.

Do Exercises 7–9.

Example 5   Divide: $12 \div 0.64$.

$$0.6\,4\,\overline{\smash{\big)}\,1\,2.}$$

Put a decimal point at the end of the whole number.

$$0.6\,4\,\overline{\smash{\big)}\,1\,2.0\,0}$$

Multiply the divisor by 100 (move the decimal point 2 places). Multiply the same way in the dividend (move 2 places).

$$
\begin{array}{r}
1\,8.7\,5 \\
0.6\,4\,\overline{\smash{\big)}\,1\,2.0\,0\,0\,0} \\
6\,4\,0 \\
\hline
5\,6\,0 \\
5\,1\,2 \\
\hline
4\,8\,0 \\
4\,4\,8 \\
\hline
3\,2\,0 \\
3\,2\,0 \\
\hline
0
\end{array}
$$

Then divide.

Since the remainder is 0, we are finished.

Do Exercise 10.

To divide quickly by a thousandth, hundredth, tenth, ten, hundred, and so on, consider

$$\frac{43.9}{100} \quad \text{and} \quad \frac{43.9}{0.001}.$$

$$
\begin{array}{r}
.4\,3\,9 \\
1\,0\,0\,\overline{\smash{\big)}\,4\,3.9\,0\,0} \\
4\,0\,0 \\
\hline
3\,9\,0 \\
3\,0\,0 \\
\hline
9\,0\,0 \\
9\,0\,0 \\
\hline
0
\end{array}
\qquad
\begin{array}{r}
4\,3\,9\,0\,0. \\
0.0\,0\,1\,\overline{\smash{\big)}\,4\,3.9\,0\,0}
\end{array}
$$

Division of 43.9 by a number greater than 1 results in a quotient *smaller* than 43.9, whereas division by a positive number less than 1 results in a quotient that is *larger* than 43.9.

To divide by a power of ten, such as 10, 100, or 1000, and so on,

a) count the number of zeros in the divisor, and

$$\frac{713.495}{100}$$

↳ 2 zeros

b) move the decimal point that number of places to the left.

$$\frac{713.495}{100}, \quad 7.13495 \quad \frac{713.495}{100} = \frac{7.13495}{1.00} = 7.13495$$

2 places to the left

To divide by a tenth, hundredth, or thousandth, and so on,

a) count the number of decimal places in the divisor, and

$$\frac{89.12}{0.001}$$

↳ 3 places

b) move the decimal point that number of places to the right.

$$\frac{89.12}{0.001}, \quad 89.120. \quad \frac{89.12}{0.001} = \frac{89120}{1.0} = 89{,}120$$

3 places to the right

Example 6 Divide: $\dfrac{0.0732}{10}$.

$$\frac{0.0732}{10}, \quad 0.0.0732, \quad \frac{0.0732}{10} = 0.00732$$

1 zero   1 place to the left to change 10 to 1

Example 7 Divide: $\dfrac{23.738}{0.001}$.

$$\frac{23.738}{0.001}, \quad 23.738. \quad \frac{23.738}{0.001} = 23{,}738$$

3 places   3 places to the right to change 0.001 to 1

Do Exercises 11–14.

b | Order of Operations: Decimal Notation

The same rules for order of operations used with integers apply when we are simplifying expressions involving decimal notation.

RULES FOR ORDER OF OPERATIONS
1. Do all calculations within parentheses before operations outside.
2. Evaluate all exponential expressions.
3. Do all multiplications and divisions in order from left to right.
4. Do all additions and subtractions in order from left to right.

Divide.

11. $\dfrac{0.1278}{0.01}$ 12.78

12. $\dfrac{0.1278}{100}$ 0.001278

13. $\dfrac{98.47}{1000}$ 0.09847

14. $\dfrac{6.7832}{-0.1}$ −67.832

Answers on page A-12

Simplify.

15. $0.25 \cdot (1 + 0.08) - 0.0274$

0.2426

16. $[(19.7 - 17.2)^2 + 3] \div (-1.25)$

-7.4

17. *Movie Attendance.* The number of tickets sold at the movies, in billions, in each of the four years from 1993 to 1996 is shown in the bar graph below. Find the average number of tickets sold.

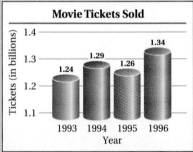

Movie Tickets Sold

Source: Motion Picture Association of America

1.2825 billion

Example 8   Simplify: $(5 - 0.06) \div 2 + 3.42 \times 0.1$.

$(5 - 0.06) \div 2 + 3.42 \times 0.1 = 4.94 \div 2 + 3.42 \times 0.1$ Carrying out operations inside parentheses

$= 2.47 + 0.342$ Doing all multiplications and divisions in order from left to right

$= 2.812$

Example 9   Simplify: $13 - [5.4(1.3^2 + 0.21) \div 0.6]$.

$13 - [5.4(1.3^2 + 0.21) \div 0.6]$

$= 13 - [5.4(1.69 + 0.21) \div 0.6]$ Working in the innermost parentheses first

$= 13 - [5.4 \times 1.9 \div 0.6]$

$= 13 - [10.26 \div 0.6]$ Multiplying

$= 13 - 17.1$ Dividing

$= -4.1$

Do Exercises 15 and 16.

Example 10   *Movie Revenue.* The bar graph shows movie box-office revenue (money taken in), in billions of dollars, in each of the four years from 1993 to 1996. Find the average revenue.

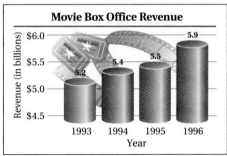

Source: Motion Picture Association of America

To find the average of a set of numbers, we add them. Then we divide by the number of addends. In this case, we are finding the average of 5.2, 5.4, 5.5, and 5.9. The average is given by

$(5.2 + 5.4 + 5.5 + 5.9) \div 4$.

Thus,

$(5.2 + 5.4 + 5.5 + 5.9) \div 4 = 22 \div 4 = 5.5$.

The average box-office revenue was $5.5 billion.

Do Exercise 17.

Exercise Set 5.4

a Divide.

1. $5\overline{)8\,2}$

16.4

2. $5\overline{)1\,8}$

3.6

3. $4\overline{)9\,5.1\,2}$

23.78

4. $8\overline{)2\,5.9\,2}$

3.24

5. $1\,2\overline{)8\,9.7\,6}$

7.48

6. $2\,3\overline{)2\,5.0\,7}$

1.09

7. $3\,3\overline{)2\,3\,7.6}$

7.2

8. $12.4 \div (-4)$

-3.1

9. $9.144 \div (-8)$

-1.143

10. $3.6 \div 4$

0.9

11. $-5.4 \div 6$

-0.9

12. $0.0\,4\overline{)1.6\,8}$

42

13. $0.1\,2\overline{)8.4}$

70

14. $3.2\overline{)1\,2\,8}$

40

15. $2.6\overline{)1\,0\,4}$

40

16. $6 \div (-15)$

-0.4

17. $1.8 \div (-12)$

-0.15

18. $3\,6\overline{)1\,4.7\,6}$

0.41

19. $2.7\overline{)1\,2\,9.6}$

48

20. $6.2\overline{)4\,6.5}$

7.5

21. $8.5\overline{)2\,7.2}$

3.2

22. $39.06 \div (-4.2)$

-9.3

23. $-5 \div (-8)$

0.625

24. $-7 \div (-8)$

0.875

25. $0.4\,7\overline{)0.1\,2\,2\,2}$

0.26

26. $0.5\,4\overline{)0.2\,7}$

0.5

27. $0.0\,3\,2\overline{)0.0\,7\,4\,8\,8}$

2.34

28. $0.0\,1\,7\overline{)1.5\,8\,1}$

93

29. $-24.969 \div 82$

-0.3045

30. $-25.221 \div 42$

-0.6005

31. $\dfrac{-213.4567}{100}$

-2.134567

32. $\dfrac{-213.4567}{10}$

-21.34567

33. $\dfrac{1.0237}{0.001}$

1023.7

34. $\dfrac{1.0237}{-0.01}$

-102.37

35. $\dfrac{56.78}{-0.001}$

$-56,780$

36. $\dfrac{0.5678}{1000}$

0.0005678

37. $\dfrac{0.97}{0.1}$ 9.7

38. $\dfrac{0.97}{0.001}$ 970

39. $\dfrac{75.3}{-0.001}$ −75,300

40. $\dfrac{-75.3}{1000}$ −0.0753

41. $\dfrac{23,001}{100}$ 230.01

42. $\dfrac{23,001}{0.01}$ 2,300,100

| b | Simplify.

43. $14 \times (82.6 + 67.9)$
2107

44. $(26.2 - 14.8) \times 12$
136.8

45. $0.003 + 3.03 \div (-0.01)$
−302.997

46. $42 \times (10.6 + 0.024)$
446.208

47. $(4.9 - 18.6) \times 13$
−178.1

48. $4.2 \times 5.7 + 0.7 \div 3.5$
24.14

49. $123.3 - 4.24 \times 1.01$
119.0176

50. $-9.0072 + 0.04 \div 0.1^2$
−5.0072

51. $12 \div (-0.03) - 12 \times 0.03^2$
−400.0108

52. $(5 - 0.04)^2 \div 4 + 8.7 \times 0.4$
9.6304

53. $(4 - 2.5)^2 \div 100 + 0.1 \times 6.5$
0.6725

54. $4 \div 0.4 - 0.1 \times 5 + 0.1^2$
9.51

55. $6 \times 0.9 - 0.1 \div 4 + 0.2^3$

5.383

56. $5.5^2 \times [(6 - 7.8) \div 0.06 + 0.12]$

-903.87

57. $12^2 \div (12 + 2.4) - [(2 - 2.4) \div 0.8]$

10.5

58. $0.01 \times \{[(4 - 0.25) \div 2.5] - (4.5 - 4.025)\}$

0.01025

59. *World Population.* Using the information in the following bar graph, determine the average population of the world for the years 1950 through 2000.   4.229 billion

60. *Manufacturing.* Using the information in the following bar graph, determine the average amount of aluminum in a particular automobile during four recent years.   113.25 lb

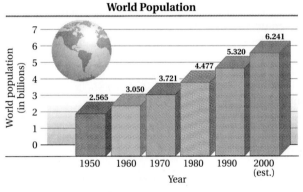

World Population

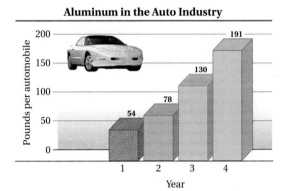

Aluminum in the Auto Industry

Source: Francis Urban and Philip Rose. *World Population by Country and Region*, 1950–86, and *Projections to 2050*, U.S. Dept. of Agriculture.

The following table lists the global average temperature for the years 1987 through 1998. Use the table for Exercises 61 and 62.

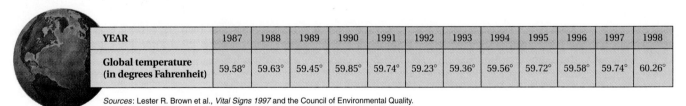

YEAR	1987	1988	1989	1990	1991	1992	1993	1994	1995	1996	1997	1998
Global temperature (in degrees Fahrenheit)	59.58°	59.63°	59.45°	59.85°	59.74°	59.23°	59.36°	59.56°	59.72°	59.58°	59.74°	60.26°

Sources: Lester R. Brown et al., *Vital Signs 1997* and the Council of Environmental Quality.

61. Find the average temperature for the years 1992 through 1996.   59.49°

62. Find the average temperature for the years 1987 through 1991.   59.65°

63. Add: $-4\dfrac{1}{3} + 7\dfrac{5}{6}$.   [4.6a] $3\dfrac{1}{2}$

64. Subtract: $7 - 8\dfrac{1}{3}$.   [4.6b] $-1\dfrac{1}{3}$

Solve.   [4.4a]

65. $-3x + 7 = 31$. -8

66. $38 = 9 - 2x$ $-\dfrac{29}{2}$, or $-14\dfrac{1}{2}$

67. $-28 = 5 - 3x$ 11

68. $9 = \dfrac{2}{3}x - 1$ 15

Synthesis

69. ◈ Which is easier and why: Dividing a decimal by a decimal or dividing a fraction by a fraction?

70. ◈ Maurice insists that $0.247 \div 0.1$ is 0.0247. How could you convince him that a mistake has been made?

71. ◈ Ellie insists that $0.247 \div 10$ is 2.47. How could you convince her that a mistake has been made?

Simplify.

72. 🖩 $9.0534 - 2.041^2 \times 0.731 \div 1.043^2$ 6.254194585

73. 🖩 $23.042(7 - 4.037 \times 1.46 - 0.932^2)$ 5.469156952

In Exercises 74–76, find the missing value.

74. $439.57 \times 0.01 \div 1000 \times \blacksquare = 4.3957$ 1000

75. $5.2738 \div 0.01 \times 1000 \div \blacksquare = 52.738$ 10,000

76. $0.0329 \div 0.001 \times 10^4 \div \blacksquare = 3290$ 100

77. *Television Ratings.* A television rating point represents 980,000 households. The 1998 NBA finals was viewed in approximately 18.5 million households, which was a record for the NBA (***Source:*** *Burlington Free Press,* 6/16/98). How many rating points did the finals receive? Round to the nearest tenth.   18.9

Electric Bills. Recently, electric bills from the Central Vermont Public Service Corporation consisted of a "customer charge" of $0.35 per day plus an "energy charge" of $0.10470 per kilowatt-hour (kWh) for the first 250 kWh used and $0.09079 per kWh for each kWh in excess of 250.

78. From August 20 to September 20, the Kaufmans' bill was $54.28. How many kilowatt-hours of electricity did they use?   440

79. From July 20 to August 20, the McGuires' bill was $67.89. How many kilowatt-hours of electricity did they use?   590

5.5 More with Fractional Notation and Decimal Notation

Now that we know how to divide using decimal notation, we can express *any* fraction as a decimal.

a | Using Division to Find Decimal Notation

Recall that the expression $\frac{a}{b}$ means $a \div b$. This gives us one way of converting fractional notation to decimal notation.

Example 1 Find decimal notation for $\frac{3}{20}$.

We have

$$\frac{3}{20} = 3 \div 20 \qquad \begin{array}{r} 0.1\,5 \\ 20 \overline{)\ 3.0\,0} \\ 2\,0 \\ \hline 1\,0\,0 \\ 1\,0\,0 \\ \hline 0 \end{array} \qquad \frac{3}{20} = 0.15$$

We are finished when the remainder is 0. $\longrightarrow 0$

Example 2 Find decimal notation for $\frac{7}{8}$.

We have

$$\frac{7}{8} = 7 \div 8 \qquad \begin{array}{r} 0.8\,7\,5 \\ 8 \overline{)\ 7.0\,0\,0} \\ 6\,4 \\ \hline 6\,0 \\ 5\,6 \\ \hline 4\,0 \\ 4\,0 \\ \hline 0 \end{array} \qquad \frac{7}{8} = 0.875$$

Do Exercises 1 and 2.

Note that the fractional notation in Examples 1 and 2 had already been simplified as much as possible. Furthermore, note that because each denominator contained only 2's and/or 5's as prime factors, each division eventually led to a remainder of 0. When the division ends, or *terminates*, with a remainder of 0, we have what is called a **terminating decimal.**

Often the denominator of a number written in simplified fractional form contains a prime factor other than 2 or 5. In such cases we can still divide to get decimal notation, but answers will be *repeating* decimals. For example, $\frac{5}{6}$ can be converted to decimal notation, but since 6 contains 3 as a prime factor, the answer will be a repeating decimal, as follows.

Objectives

a Use division to convert fractional notation to decimal notation.

b Round numbers named by repeating decimals.

c Convert certain fractions to decimal notation by using equivalent fractions.

d Simplify expressions that contain both fractional and decimal notation.

For Extra Help

TAPE 10   MAC WIN   CD-ROM

Find decimal notation.

1. $\frac{2}{5}$ 0.4

2. $\frac{3}{8}$ 0.375

Answers on page A-12

Find decimal notation.

3. $\dfrac{1}{6}$ $0.1\overline{6}$

4. $\dfrac{2}{3}$ $0.\overline{6}$

Find decimal notation.

5. $\dfrac{5}{11}$ $0.\overline{45}$

6. $-\dfrac{12}{11}$ $-1.\overline{09}$

Answers on page A-12

Example 3   Find decimal notation for $\dfrac{5}{6}$.

We have

$$\dfrac{5}{6} = 5 \div 6 \qquad \begin{array}{r} 0.8\,3\,3 \\ 6\,)\overline{5.0\,0\,0} \\ \underline{4\,8} \\ 2\,0 \\ \underline{1\,8} \\ 2\,0 \\ \underline{1\,8} \\ 2 \end{array}$$

Since 2 keeps reappearing as a remainder, the digits repeat and will continue to do so; therefore,

$$\dfrac{5}{6} = 0.83333\ldots.$$

The dots indicate an endless sequence of digits in the quotient. When there is a repeating pattern, the dots are often replaced by a bar to indicate the repeating part—in this case, only the 3:

$$\dfrac{5}{6} = 0.8\overline{3}.$$

Do Exercises 3 and 4.

Example 4   Find decimal notation for $-\dfrac{4}{11}$.

First consider $\dfrac{4}{11}$. Because 11 is not a product of 2's and/or 5's, we expect a repeating decimal:

$$\dfrac{4}{11} = 4 \div 11 \qquad \begin{array}{r} 0.3\,6\,3\,6 \\ 1\,1\,)\overline{4.0\,0\,0\,0} \\ \underline{3\,3} \\ 7\,0 \\ \underline{6\,6} \\ 4\,0 \\ \underline{3\,3} \\ 7\,0 \\ \underline{6\,6} \\ 4 \end{array}$$

Since 7 and 4 keep reappearing as remainders, the sequence of digits "36" repeats in the quotient, and

$$\dfrac{4}{11} = 0.363636\ldots, \quad \text{or} \quad 0.\overline{36}.$$

Thus, $-\dfrac{4}{11} = -0.\overline{36}$.

Do Exercises 5 and 6.

Example 5 Find decimal notation for $\frac{3}{7}$.

Because 7 is not a product of 2's and/or 5's, we again expect a repeating decimal:

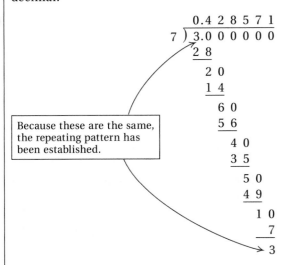

```
        0.4 2 8 5 7 1
   7 ) 3.0 0 0 0 0 0
        2 8
          2 0
          1 4
            6 0
            5 6
              4 0
              3 5
                5 0
                4 9
                  1 0
                     7
                     3
```

Because these are the same, the repeating pattern has been established.

Since we have already divided 7 into 3, the sequence of digits "428571" repeats in the quotient, and

$$\frac{3}{7} = 0.428571428571\ldots, \quad \text{or} \quad 0.\overline{428571}.$$

It is possible for the repeating part of a repeating decimal to be so long that it will not fit on a calculator. For example, when $\frac{5}{97}$ is written in decimal form, its repeating part is 96 digits long! Most calculators round off repeating decimals to 9 or 10 decimal places.

Do Exercise 7.

b Rounding Repeating Decimals

In applied problems, repeating decimals are generally rounded to a predetermined degree of accuracy.

Example 6 Round $4.\overline{27}$ to the nearest thousandth.

We first rewrite the decimal without the bar. The repeating part is rewritten until we have passed the thousandths place:

$$4.\overline{27} = 4.2727\ldots.$$

Now we round as in Section 5.1.

a) Locate the digit in the thousandths place.   4.2 7 2 7...

b) Consider the next digit to the right.   4.2 7 2 7...

c) Since that digit, 7, is greater than or equal to 5, round up.

  4.273   **This is the answer.**

---

7. Find decimal notation for $\frac{5}{7}$.

0.$\overline{714285}$

Answer on page A-12

Round each to the nearest tenth, hundredth, and thousandth.

8. $0.\overline{6}$

0.7; 0.67; 0.667

9. $0.6\overline{08}$

0.6; 0.61; 0.608

10. $-7.3\overline{49}$

-7.3; -7.35; -7.349

11. $2.6\overline{891}$

2.7; 2.69; 2.689

Find decimal notation. Use multiplying by 1.

12. $\dfrac{4}{5}$ 0.8

13. $-\dfrac{9}{20}$ -0.45

14. $\dfrac{7}{200}$ 0.035

15. $\dfrac{33}{25}$ 1.32

Answers on page A-12

Examples Round each to the nearest tenth, hundredth, and thousandth.

	Nearest tenth	*Nearest hundredth*	*Nearest thousandth*
7. $0.8\overline{3} = 0.83333\ldots$	0.8	0.83	0.833
8. $3.\overline{09} = 3.090909\ldots$	3.1	3.09	3.091
9. $-4.1\overline{763} = -4.1763763\ldots$	-4.2	-4.18	-4.176

Do Exercises 8–11.

c | More with Conversions

Recall that fractional notation like $\frac{3}{10}$ or $-\frac{71}{1000}$ can be converted quickly to decimal notation, without performing long division. When a denominator is a factor of 10, 100, and so on, we can convert to decimal notation by finding (perhaps mentally) an equivalent fraction in which the denominator is a power of 10.

Example 10   Find decimal notation for $\frac{3}{20}$.

Note that 20 is a factor of 100 ($20 \cdot 5 = 100$). Thus, by using $\frac{5}{5}$ as an expression for 1, we can easily find an equivalent fraction with a denominator that is a power of 10:

$$\frac{3}{20} = \frac{3}{20} \cdot \frac{5}{5} = \frac{15}{100} = 0.15.$$

To perform this mentally, you might say to yourself "20 goes into 100 five times; 5 times 3 is 15; $\frac{15}{100}$ is 0.15."

Example 11   Find decimal notation for $-\frac{7}{500}$.

Since $500 \cdot 2 = 1000$, a power of 10, we use $\frac{2}{2}$ as an expression for 1:

$$-\frac{7}{500} = -\frac{7}{500} \cdot \frac{2}{2} = -\frac{14}{1000} = -0.014.$$

Example 12   Find decimal notation for $\frac{9}{25}$.

$$\frac{9}{25} = \frac{9}{25} \cdot \frac{4}{4} = \frac{36}{100} = 0.36 \qquad \text{Using } \tfrac{4}{4} \text{ for 1 to get a denominator of 100}$$

As a check, we can divide:

```
        0.3 6
  2 5 ) 9.0 0
        7 5          Note that multiplication by 1 is much faster.
        1 5 0
        1 5 0
            0
```

Example 13   Find decimal notation for $\frac{7}{4}$.

$$\frac{7}{4} = \frac{7}{4} \cdot \frac{25}{25} = \frac{175}{100} = 1.75 \qquad \begin{array}{l}\text{Using } \tfrac{25}{25} \text{ for 1 to get a denominator of 100.} \\ \text{You might also note that 7 quarters is \$1.75.}\end{array}$$

Do Exercises 12–15.

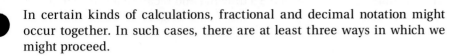

d | Calculations with Fractional and Decimal Notation Together

In certain kinds of calculations, fractional and decimal notation might occur together. In such cases, there are at least three ways in which we might proceed.

Example 14   Calculate: $\frac{2}{3} \times 0.576$.

METHOD 1.   Perhaps the quickest method is to treat 0.576 as $\frac{0.576}{1}$. Then we multiply 0.576 by 2, and divide the result by 3.

$$\frac{2}{3} \times 0.576 = \frac{2}{3} \times \frac{0.576}{1}$$

$$= \frac{2 \times 0.576}{3} = \frac{1.152}{3}$$

$$= 0.384$$

$$\begin{array}{r} 0.3\ 8\ 4 \\ 3\overline{)\ 1.1\ 5\ 2} \\ \underline{9} \\ 2\ 5 \\ \underline{2\ 4} \\ 1\ 2 \\ \underline{1\ 2} \\ 0 \end{array}$$

METHOD 2.   A second way to do this calculation is to convert the fractional notation to decimal notation so that both numbers are in decimal notation. Since $\frac{2}{3}$ converts to repeating decimal notation, it is first rounded to some chosen decimal place. We choose three decimal places. Then, using decimal notation, we multiply. Note that the answer is not as accurate as that found by Method 1, due to the rounding.

$$\frac{2}{3} \times 0.576 = 0.\overline{6} \times 0.576$$

$$\approx 0.667 \times 0.576 = 0.384192$$

METHOD 3.   Another way to do this calculation is to convert the decimal notation to fractional notation so that both numbers are in fractional notation. The answer can be left in fractional notation and simplified, or we can convert back to decimal notation and, if appropriate, round.

$$\frac{2}{3} \times 0.576 = \frac{2}{3} \cdot \frac{576}{1000} = \frac{2 \cdot 576}{3 \cdot 1000}$$

$$= \frac{2 \cdot 2 \cdot 2 \cdot 2 \cdot 2 \cdot 2 \cdot 2 \cdot 3 \cdot 3}{2 \cdot 2 \cdot 2 \cdot 3 \cdot 5 \cdot 5 \cdot 5} \qquad \text{Factoring}$$

$$= \frac{2 \cdot 2 \cdot 2 \cdot 3}{2 \cdot 2 \cdot 2 \cdot 3} \cdot \frac{2 \cdot 2 \cdot 2 \cdot 2 \cdot 3}{5 \cdot 5 \cdot 5} \qquad \begin{array}{l}\text{Removing a factor equal to 1:} \\ \dfrac{2 \cdot 2 \cdot 2 \cdot 3}{2 \cdot 2 \cdot 2 \cdot 3} = 1\end{array}$$

$$= \frac{2 \cdot 2 \cdot 2 \cdot 2 \cdot 3}{5 \cdot 5 \cdot 5} = \frac{48}{125}, \text{ or } 0.384$$

Do Exercises 16 and 17.

Calculate.

16. Calculate: $\dfrac{5}{6} \times 0.864$ 0.72

17. $\dfrac{1}{3} \times 0.384 + \dfrac{5}{8} \times 0.6784$

0.552

Answers on page A-12

18. Find the area of a triangular window that is 3.25 ft wide and 2.6 ft tall. 4.225 ft²

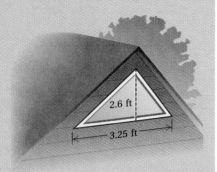

2.6 ft
3.25 ft

Example 15 *Boating.* A triangular sail from a single-sail day cruiser is 3.4 m wide and 4.2 m tall. Find the area of the sail.

1. **Familiarize.** We first make a drawing and recall that the formula for the area, A, of a triangle with base b and height h is $A = \frac{1}{2}bh$.

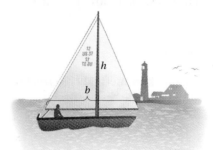

2. **Translate.** We substitute 3.4 for b and 4.2 for h:

$$A = \frac{1}{2}bh = \frac{1}{2}(3.4)(4.2). \qquad \text{Evaluating}$$

3. **Solve.** We simplify as follows:

$$A = \frac{1}{2}(3.4)(4.2)$$

$$= \frac{3.4}{2}(4.2) \qquad \text{Multiplying } \frac{1}{2} \text{ and } \frac{3.4}{1}$$

$$= 1.7(4.2) \qquad \text{Dividing}$$

$$= 7.14. \qquad \text{Multiplying}$$

4. **Check.** To check, we repeat the calculations, using the commutative law to multiply in a different order. We also rewrite $\frac{1}{2}$ as 0.5:

$$\frac{1}{2}(4.2)(3.4) = 0.5(4.2)(3.4)$$

$$= (2.1)(3.4) = 7.14.$$

Our answer checks.

5. **State.** The area of the sail is 7.14 m² (square meters).

Do Exercise 18.

Calculator Spotlight

Many geometric applications of decimal notation involve the number π (see Exercises 86–89 of this section).

Most calculators are now equipped with a key that provides an approximation of π to at least six decimal places. Often a key labeled `SHIFT` or `2nd` must be pressed first.

To calculate the value of an expression like $2\pi(7.5)$, on most calculators we simply press

`2` `×` `2nd` `π` `×` `7` `.` `5`

and then `=` or `ENTER`.

Exercises

1. Calculate $4\pi(9.8)$. 123.150432

2. Evaluate $2\pi r$ for $r = 8.37$. 52.59026102

Answer on page A-12

Exercise Set 5.5

a , c Find decimal notation.

1. $\dfrac{5}{16}$ 0.3125

2. $\dfrac{9}{20}$ 0.45

3. $\dfrac{19}{40}$ 0.475

4. $\dfrac{1}{16}$ 0.0625

5. $-\dfrac{1}{5}$ −0.2

6. $-\dfrac{3}{20}$ −0.15

7. $\dfrac{13}{20}$ 0.65

8. $\dfrac{3}{40}$ 0.075

9. $\dfrac{17}{40}$ 0.425

10. $-\dfrac{39}{40}$ −0.975

11. $\dfrac{49}{40}$ 1.225

12. $\dfrac{13}{40}$ 0.325

13. $-\dfrac{13}{25}$ −0.52

14. $-\dfrac{21}{125}$ −0.168

15. $\dfrac{2502}{125}$ 20.016

16. $\dfrac{121}{200}$ 0.605

17. $\dfrac{-1}{4}$ −0.25

18. $\dfrac{-1}{2}$ −0.5

19. $\dfrac{23}{40}$ 0.575

20. $\dfrac{11}{20}$ 0.55

21. $-\dfrac{5}{8}$ −0.625

22. $-\dfrac{19}{16}$ −1.1875

23. $\dfrac{37}{25}$ 1.48

24. $\dfrac{18}{25}$ 0.72

25. $\dfrac{8}{15}$ $0.5\overline{3}$

26. $\dfrac{7}{9}$ $0.\overline{7}$

27. $\dfrac{1}{3}$ $0.\overline{3}$

28. $\dfrac{1}{9}$ $0.\overline{1}$

29. $\dfrac{-4}{3}$ $-1.\overline{3}$

30. $\dfrac{-8}{9}$ $-0.\overline{8}$

31. $\dfrac{7}{6}$ $1.1\overline{6}$

32. $\dfrac{7}{11}$ $0.\overline{63}$

33. $\dfrac{4}{7}$ $0.\overline{571428}$

34. $\dfrac{14}{11}$ $1.\overline{27}$

35. $-\dfrac{11}{12}$ $-0.91\overline{6}$

36. $-\dfrac{5}{12}$ $-0.41\overline{6}$

b

37.–47. Round each answer of the odd-numbered
(odd) Exercises 25–35 to the nearest tenth,
hundredth, and thousandth.

37. 0.5; 0.53; 0.533 **39.** 0.3; 0.33; 0.333
41. −1.3; −1.33; −1.333 **43.** 1.2; 1.17; 1.167
45. 0.6; 0.57; 0.571 **47.** −0.9; −0.92; −0.917

38.–48. Round each answer of the even-numbered
(even) Exercises 26–36 to the nearest tenth,
hundredth, and thousandth.

38. 0.8; 0.78; 0.778 **40.** 0.1; 0.11; 0.111
42. −0.9; −0.89; −0.889 **44.** 0.6; 0.64; 0.636
46. 1.3; 1.27; 1.273 **48.** −0.4; −0.42; −0.417

Round each of the following to the nearest tenth, hundredth, and thousandth.

49. $0.\overline{74}$

50. $0.\overline{38}$

51. $-7.9\overline{6}$

52. $-3.09\overline{7}$

0.7; 0.75; 0.747

0.4; 0.38; 0.384

−8.0; −7.97; −7.967

−3.1; −3.10; −3.098

Calculate.

53. $\dfrac{7}{8}(10.84)$ 9.485

54. $\dfrac{4}{5}(264.8)$ 211.84

55. $\dfrac{47}{9}(-79.95)$ $-417.51\overline{6}$

56. $\dfrac{7}{11}(-2.7873)$ $-1.7737\overline{36}$

57. $\left(\dfrac{1}{6}\right)0.0765 + \left(\dfrac{3}{4}\right)0.1124$ 0.09705

58. $\left(\dfrac{2}{5}\right)6384.1 - \left(\dfrac{5}{8}\right)156.56$

2455.79

59. $\dfrac{3}{4} \times 2.56 - \dfrac{7}{8} \times 3.94$ -1.5275

60. $\dfrac{2}{5} \times 3.91 - \dfrac{7}{10} \times 4.15$ -1.341

61. $5.2 \times 1\dfrac{7}{8} \div 0.4$ 24.375

62. $4\dfrac{3}{4} \times 0.5 \div 0.1$ 23.75

Solve.

63. Find the area of a triangular shawl that is 1.8 m long and 1.2 m wide.   1.08 m²

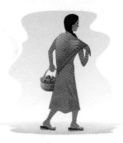

64. Find the area of a triangular sign that is 1.5 m wide and 1.5 m tall.   1.125 m²

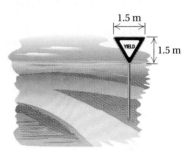

65. Find the area of a triangular stamp that is 3.4 cm wide and 3.4 cm tall.   5.78 cm²

66. Find the area of a triangular reflector that is 7.4 cm wide and 9.1 cm tall.   33.67 cm²

Exercise Set 5.5

317

67. Subtract: $20 - 16\frac{3}{5}$.   [4.6b] $3\frac{2}{5}$

68. Add: $14\frac{3}{5} + 16\frac{1}{10}$.   [4.6a] $30\frac{7}{10}$

69. Simplify: $\dfrac{95}{-1}$.   [3.3c] -95

70. Solve: $5x - 9 = 7x + 11$.   [4.4a] -10

71. Simplify: $9 - 4 + 2 \div (-1) \cdot 6$.   [2.6b] -7

72. Simplify: $\dfrac{-9}{-9}$.   [3.3c] 1

Synthesis

73. ◈ When is long division *not* the fastest way of converting a fraction to decimal notation?

74. ◈ Examine Example 14 of this section. How could the problem be changed so that method 2 would give a result that is completely accurate?

75. ◈ Are the numbers $6.2\overline{35}$ and $6.23\overline{535}$ equal? Why or why not?

▦ Find decimal notation. Save the answers for Exercise 81.

76. $\dfrac{1}{7}$ $0.\overline{142857}$

77. $\dfrac{2}{7}$ $0.\overline{285714}$

78. $\dfrac{3}{7}$ $0.\overline{428571}$

79. $\dfrac{4}{7}$ $0.\overline{571428}$

80. $\dfrac{5}{7}$ $0.\overline{714285}$

81. ▦ From the pattern of Exercises 76–80, predict the decimal notation for $\frac{6}{7}$. Check your answer on a calculator.
$0.\overline{857142}$

Find decimal notation. Save the answers for Exercise 85.

82. $\dfrac{1}{9}$ $0.\overline{1}$

83. $\dfrac{1}{99}$ $0.\overline{01}$

84. $\dfrac{1}{999}$ $0.\overline{001}$

85. ▦ From the pattern of Exercises 82–84, predict the decimal notation for $\frac{1}{9999}$. Check your answer on a calculator.
$0.\overline{0001}$

The formula $A = \pi r^2$ is used to find the area, A, of a circle with radius r. For Exercises 86 and 87, find the area of a circle with the given radius, using $\frac{22}{7}$ for π. For Exercises 88 and 89, use 3.14 for π or a calculator with a π key.

86. $r = 2.1$ cm

13.86 cm^2

87. $r = 1.4$ cm

6.16 cm^2

88. $r = \dfrac{3}{4}$ ft

1.76625 ft^2 or
1.767145868 ft^2

89. $r = 4\dfrac{1}{2}$ yd

63.585 yd^2, or
63.61725124 yd^2

90. ◈ ▦ A scientific calculator indicates that

$$\frac{5}{6} = 0.833333333 \quad \text{and} \quad \frac{4{,}999{,}999{,}998}{6{,}000{,}000{,}000} = 0.833333333.$$

a) Is it true that $\frac{5}{6} = \frac{4{,}999{,}999{,}998}{6{,}000{,}000{,}000}$? Why or why not?

b) Should decimal notation for $\frac{4{,}999{,}999{,}998}{6{,}000{,}000{,}000}$ repeat? Why or why not?

5.6 Estimating

a Estimating Sums, Differences, Products and Quotients

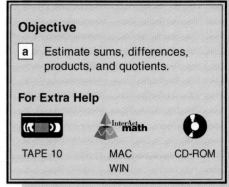
Estimating has many uses. It can be done before a problem is even attempted in order to get an idea of the answer. It can be done afterward as a check, even when we are using a calculator. In many situations, an estimate is all we need. We usually estimate by rounding the numbers so that there are one or two nonzero digits. Consider the following advertisements for Examples 1–4.

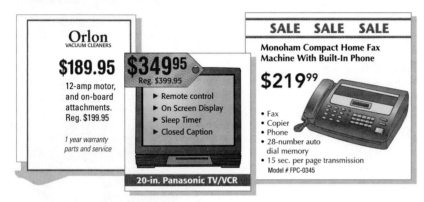

1. Estimate to the nearest ten the total cost of one TV/VCR and one vacuum cleaner. $540

Example 1   Estimate to the nearest ten the total cost of one fax machine and one TV/VCR.

We are estimating the sum

$219.99 + $349.95 = Total cost.

The estimate to the nearest ten is

$220 + $350 = $570.   (Estimated total cost)

We rounded $219.99 to the nearest ten and $349.95 to the nearest ten. The estimated sum is $570.

Do Exercise 1.

2. About how much more does the TV/VCR cost than the vacuum cleaner? $160

Example 2   About how much more does the TV/VCR cost than the fax machine? Estimate to the nearest ten.

We are estimating the difference

$349.95 − $219.99 = Price difference.

The estimate to the nearest ten is

$350 − $220 = $130.   (Estimated price difference)

Do Exercise 2.

Answers on page A-13

3. Estimate the total cost of 6 fax machines. $1320

4. About how many vacuum cleaners can be bought for $830?   4

Estimate each product. Do not find the actual product.

5. 2.1 × 8.02   16

6. 36 × 0.54   18

7. 0.93 × 472   470

8. 0.72 × 0.1   0.07

9. 0.12 × 180.3   18

10. 24.359 × 5.2   125

Answers on page A-13

Example 3   Estimate the total cost of 4 vacuum cleaners. (See p. 319.)

We are estimating the product

4 × $189.95 = Total cost.

The estimate is found by rounding $189.95 to the nearest ten:

4 × $190 = $760.

Do Exercise 3.

Example 4   About how many fax machines can be bought for $1480? (See p. 319.)

To estimate 1480 ÷ 219.99, we mentally search for a number near 1480 that is a multiple of a number near 219.99. Rounding $219.99 to the nearest hundred, we get $200. Since $1480 is close to $1400, which is a multiple of 200, we have

1480 ÷ 219.99 ≈ 1400 ÷ 200 = 7,

so the answer is 7.

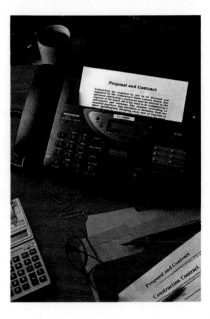

Do Exercise 4.

Example 5   Estimate: 4.8 × 52. Do not find the actual product.

We round 4.8 to the nearest one and 52 to the nearest ten. This gives us two easy numbers with which to work, 5 and 50. Since

4.8 × 52 ≈ 5 × 50

and

5 × 50 = 250,

the estimated product is 250.

Compare these estimates for the product 4.94 × 38:

5 × 40 = 200,   5 × 38 = 190,   4.9 × 40 = 196,   4.9 × 38 = 186.2.

The first estimate was the easiest. You could probably do it mentally. The others had more nonzero digits and were more accurate but required more work.

When making estimates, we usually look for numbers that are easy to work with mentally. For example, if multiplying, we might round 0.43 to 0.5 and 8.9 to 10, because 0.5 and 10 are such convenient numbers by which to multiply.

Do Exercises 5–10.

Example 6 Which of the following is the best estimate of 82.08 ÷ 24?

a) 400   **b)** 16   **c)** 40   **d)** 4

This is about 80 ÷ 20, so the answer is about 4. We could also estimate the division as 75 ÷ 25, or 3. In any case, of the choices listed, (d) is the most appropriate.

Example 7 Which of the following is the best estimate of 94.18 ÷ 3.2?

a) 30   **b)** 300   **c)** 3   **d)** 60

This is about 90 ÷ 3, so the answer is about 30. Thus the most appropriate choice is (a).

Example 8 Which of the following is the best estimate of 0.0156 ÷ 1.3?

a) 0.2   **b)** 0.002   **c)** 0.02   **d)** 20

This is about 0.02 ÷ 1, so the answer is about 0.02. Thus the most appropriate choice is (c).

Do Exercises 11–13.

In some cases, it is easier to estimate a quotient by checking products than by rounding the divisor and the dividend.

Example 9 Which of the following is the best estimate of 0.0074 ÷ 0.23?

a) 0.3   **b)** 0.03   **c)** 300   **d)** 3

Note that 0.23 is close to 0.25 and that 0.25 is easier to multiply by than divide by. Thus we use 0.25 to check some products.

We first try 3:

$0.23 \times 3 \approx 0.25 \times 3 = 0.75.$ **This is too large.**

We try a smaller estimate, 0.3:

$0.23 \times 0.3 \approx 0.25 \times 0.3 = 0.075.$ **This is also too large.**

We make the estimate smaller still, 0.03:

$0.23 \times 0.03 \approx 0.25 \times 0.03 = 0.0075.$

This is close to 0.0074, so the quotient is close to 0.03. Thus the most appropriate choice is (b).

Do Exercise 14.

Select the most appropriate estimate for each quotient.

11. 59.78 ÷ 29.1

     a) 200   **b)** 20

     c) 2   **d)** 0.2

     (c)

12. 82.08 ÷ 2.4

     a) 40   **b)** 4.0

     c) 400   **d)** 0.4

     (a)

13. 0.1768 ÷ 0.08

     a) 8   **b)** 10

     c) 2   **d)** 20

     (c)

14. Which of the following is an appropriate estimate of 0.0069 ÷ 0.15?

     a) 0.5   **b)** 50

     c) 0.05   **d)** 23.4

     (c)

Answers on page A-13

Improving Your Math Study Skills

Other study tips appear on pages 50, 90, 100, 150, 368, and 596.

Study Tips for Trouble Spots

By now you have probably encountered certain topics that gave you more difficulty than others. It is important to know that this happens to every person who studies mathematics. Unfortunately, frustration is often part of the learning process and it is important not to give up when difficulty arises.

One source of frustration for many students is not being able to set aside sufficient time for studying. Family commitments, work schedules, and athletics are just a few of the time demands that many students face. Couple these demands with a math lesson that seems to require a greater than usual amount of study time, and it is no wonder that many students often feel frustrated. Below are some study tips that might be useful if and when troubles arise.

- **Realize that everyone—even your instructor—has been stymied at times when studying math.** You are not the first person, nor will you be the last, to encounter a "roadblock."

- **Whether working alone or with a classmate, try to allow enough study time so that you won't need to constantly glance at a clock.** Difficult material is best mastered when your mind is completely focused on the subject matter. Thus, if you are tired, it is usually best to study early the next morning or to take a ten-minute "power-nap" in order to make the most productive use of your time.

- **Talk about your trouble spot with a classmate.** It is possible that she or he is also having difficulty with the same material. If that is the case, perhaps the majority of your class is confused and your instructor's coverage of the topic is not yet finished. If your classmate *does* understand the topic that is troubling you, patiently allow him or her to explain it to you. By verbalizing the math in question, your classmate may help clarify the material for both of you. Perhaps you will be able to return the favor for your classmate when he or she is struggling with a topic that you understand.

- **Try to study in a "controlled" environment.** What we mean by this is that you can often put yourself in a setting that will enable you to maximize your powers of concentration. For example, whereas some students may succeed in studying at home or in a dorm room, for many these settings are filled with distractions. Consider a trip to a library, classroom building, or perhaps the attic or basement if such a setting is more conducive to studying. If you plan on working with a classmate, try to find a location in which conversation will not be bothersome to others.

- **When working on difficult material, it is often helpful to first "back up" and review the most recent material that *did* make sense.** This can build your confidence and create a momentum that can often carry you through the roadblock. Sometimes a small piece of information that appeared in a previous section is all that is needed for your problem spot to disappear. When the difficult material is finally mastered, try to make use of what is fresh in your mind by taking a "sneak preview" of what your next topic for study will be.

- Consider keeping a mathematical journal and/or toolbox. In a mathematical journal, you write study tips and observations that have been gleaned from the most recent lesson. In a mathematical toolbox, you use a designated notebook or portion of a notebook to list important formulas and concepts as they are encountered throughout the course.

  Maintaining your journal or toolbox can often help you to clarify your understanding of course material.

Exercise Set 5.6

a Consider the following advertisements for Exercises 1–8. Estimate the sums, differences, products, or quotients involved in these problems.

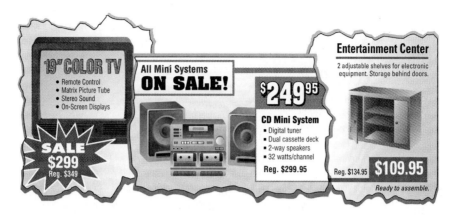

1. Estimate the total cost of one entertainment center and one mini system. $360

2. Estimate the total cost of one entertainment center and one TV. $410

3. About how much more does the TV cost than the mini system? $50

4. About how much more does the TV cost than the entertainment center? $190

5. Estimate the total cost of 9 TVs. $2700

6. Estimate the total cost of 16 mini systems. $4000

7. About how many TVs can be bought for $1700? 5

8. About how many mini systems can be bought for $1300? 5

Estimate by rounding as directed.

9. 0.02 + 1.31 + 0.34; nearest tenth

1.6

10. 0.88 + 2.07 + 1.54; nearest one

5

11. 6.03 + 0.007 + 0.214; nearest one

6

12. 1.11 + 8.888 + 99.94; nearest one

110

13. 52.367 + 1.307 + 7.324 nearest one

60

14. 12.9882 + 1.0115; nearest tenth

14.0

15. 2.678 − 0.445; nearest tenth

2.3

16. 12.9882 − 1.0115; nearest one

12

17. 198.67432 − 24.5007; nearest ten

180

Estimate. Choose a rounding digit that gives one or two nonzero digits. Indicate which of the choices is an appropriate estimate.

18. $234.12321 - 200.3223$ (d)

    a) 600   **b)** 60
    c) 300   **d)** 30

19. 49×7.89 (a)

    a) 400   **b)** 40
    c) 4   **d)** 0.4

20. 7.4×8.9 (b)

    a) 95   **b)** 63
    c) 124   **d)** 6

21. 98.4×0.083 (c)

    a) 80   **b)** 14
    c) 8   **d)** 0.8

22. 78×5.3 (a)

    a) 400   **b)** 800
    c) 40   **d)** 8

23. $3.6 \div 4$ (b)

    a) 10   **b)** 1
    c) 0.1   **d)** 0.01

24. $0.0713 \div 1.94$ (c)

    a) 4   **b)** 0.4
    c) 0.04   **d)** 40

25. $74.68 \div 24.7$ (b)

    a) 9   **b)** 3
    c) 12   **d)** 120

26. $914 \div 0.921$ (c)

    a) 9   **b)** 90
    c) 900   **d)** 0.9

27. *Movie Revenue.* Total summer box-office revenue (money taken in) for the movie *Eraser* was $53.6 million (**Source:** *Hollywood Reporter Magazine*). Each theater showing the movie averaged $6716 in revenue. Estimate how many screens were showing this movie.   8000

28. *Nintendo and the Sears Tower.* The Nintendo Game Boy portable video game is 4.5 in. (0.375 ft) tall (**Source:** Nintendo of America). Estimate how many game units it would take to reach the top of the Sears Tower, which is 1454 ft tall. Round to the nearest one.   4000

Skill Maintenance

Find the prime factorization.   [3.2c]

29. 108 $2 \cdot 2 \cdot 3 \cdot 3 \cdot 3$

30. 400 $2 \cdot 2 \cdot 2 \cdot 2 \cdot 5 \cdot 5$

31. 325 $5 \cdot 5 \cdot 13$

32. 666 $2 \cdot 3 \cdot 3 \cdot 37$

Simplify.   [2.5a]

33. $\dfrac{125}{400}$ $\dfrac{5}{16}$

34. $\dfrac{3225}{6275}$ $\dfrac{129}{251}$

35. $\dfrac{72}{81}$ $\dfrac{8}{9}$

36. $\dfrac{325}{625}$ $\dfrac{13}{25}$

Synthesis

37. ◆ Under what circumstance(s) would you round down from 5.8 to 5.0 when rounding to the nearest one?

38. ◆ A roll of fiberglass insulation costs $21.95. Describe two situations involving estimating and the cost of fiberglass insulation. Devise one situation so that $21.95 is rounded to $22. Devise the other situation so that $21.95 is rounded to $20.

39. ◆ Describe a situation in which an estimation is made by rounding to the nearest 10,000 and then multiplying.

The following were done on a calculator. Estimate to see if the decimal point was placed correctly.

40. $178.9462 \times 61.78 = 11,055.29624$ Yes

41. $14,973.35 \div 298.75 = 501.2$ No

42. $19.7236 - 1.4738 \times 4.1097 = 1.366672414$ No

43. $28.46901 \div 4.9187 - 2.5081 = 3.279813473$ Yes

Estimate the food cost for catering a party.

Collaborative Learning Manual

5.7 Solving Equations

In Section 4.4, we saw how the addition and multiplication principles can be used to solve equations like $5x + 7 = -3$. We now use those same properties to solve similar equations involving decimals.

a Equations with One Variable Term

Recall that to solve equations like $3x = 12$, we can use the multiplication principle to multiply by $\frac{1}{3}$ on both sides. This is the same as dividing by 3 on both sides. The same procedure works with decimals.

Example 1 Solve: $3.4x = 6.97$.

We have

$$3.4x = 6.97$$

$$\frac{3.4x}{3.4} = \frac{6.97}{3.4} \quad \textbf{Dividing by 3.4} \left(\textbf{or multiplying by } \tfrac{1}{3.4}\right) \textbf{ on both sides}$$

$$x = 2.05.$$

$$
\begin{array}{r}
2.0\,5 \\
3.4_{\curvearrowleft}\overline{)\,6.9_{\wedge}7\,0} \\
6\,8\,0\,0 \\
\hline
1\,7\,0 \\
1\,7\,0 \\
\hline
0
\end{array}
$$

To check, we can approximate: Note that $3.4 \approx 3.5$ and $2.05 \approx 2$. Since $3.5 \cdot 2 = 7.0 \approx 6.97$, we have a partial check. The solution is 2.05.

Do Exercises 1 and 2.

To solve equations like $x + 7 = -3$, we use the addition principle to add -7 on both sides or, equivalently, to subtract 7 on both sides. The same approach is used with decimals.

Example 2 Solve: $x + 7.4 = -3.1$.

We have

$$x + 7.4 = -3.1$$

$$x + 7.4 + (-7.4) = -3.1 + (-7.4) \quad \textbf{Adding } -7.4 \textbf{ on both sides}$$

$$x = -10.5.$$

To check, note that $-10.5 + 7.4 = -3.1$. The solution is -10.5.

In Examples 1 and 2, we used the addition and multiplication principles to produce equivalent equations from which we could easily read the solution. A similar approach, involving more steps, will be used in the examples that follow.

Do Exercises 3 and 4.

Solve.

1. $23x = 96.6$ 4.2

2. $1.25t = 7.125$ 5.7

Solve.

3. $x + 9.8 = 12.4$ 2.6

4. $6.5 + t = -4.3$ −10.8

Answers on page A-13

Solve.

5. $7.4t + 1.25 = 27.89$ 3.6

As we saw in Section 4.4, when an equation requires both multiplication *and* addition, we generally "undo" the addition before we "undo" the multiplication. This reverses the order of operations in which we multiply first and then add.

Example 3   Solve: $4.2x + 3.7 = -26.12$.

$$4.2x + 3.7 = -26.12$$

$$4.2x + 3.7 - 3.7 = -26.12 - 3.7$$ Subtracting 3.7 or adding -3.7 on both sides

$$4.2x = -29.82$$ Simplifying

$$\frac{4.2x}{4.2} = \frac{-29.82}{4.2}$$ Multiplying by $\frac{1}{4.2}$ or dividing by 4.2 on both sides

$$x = -7.1$$ Simplifying

CHECK:

$$4.2x + 3.7 = -26.12$$

$$4.2(-7.1) + 3.7 \;?\; -26.12$$
$$-29.82 + 3.7$$
$$-26.12 \quad | \quad -26.12 \quad \text{TRUE}$$

The solution is -7.1.

Do Exercises 5 and 6.

6. $-2.7 + 4.8x = -11.82$ -1.9

Answers on page A-13

b | Equations with Two or More Variable Terms

Some equations have variable terms on both sides. To solve such an equation, we use the addition principle to get all variable terms on one side of the equation and all constant terms on the other side.

Example 4   Solve: $10x - 7 = 2x + 13$.

We begin by subtracting $2x$ (or adding $-2x$) on both sides. This will group all variable terms on one side of the equation:

$$10x - 7 - 2x = 2x + 13 - 2x \qquad \text{Adding } -2x \text{ on both sides}$$
$$8x - 7 = 13. \qquad \text{Combining like terms}$$

This last equation is similar to Example 3. As in that example, we use the addition principle to isolate all constant terms on one side:

$$8x - 7 = 13$$
$$8x - 7 + 7 = 13 + 7 \qquad \text{Adding 7 on both sides}$$
$$8x = 20 \qquad \text{Simplifying (combining like terms)}$$
$$\frac{8x}{8} = \frac{20}{8} \qquad \text{Dividing on both sides, as in Example 1}$$
$$x = 2.5.$$

CHECK:

$$\begin{array}{c|c} \multicolumn{2}{c}{10x - 7 = 2x + 13} \\ \hline 10(2.5) - 7 \ ? \ 2(2.5) + 13 \\ 25 - 7 \ \big| \ 5 + 13 \\ 18 \ \big| \ 18 \qquad \text{TRUE} \end{array}$$

The solution is 2.5.

Sometimes it may be easier to combine all variable terms on the right side and all constant terms on the left side.

Example 5   Solve: $11 - 3t = 7t + 8$.

We can combine all variable terms on the right side by adding $3t$ on both sides:

$$11 - 3t = 7t + 8$$
$$11 - 3t + 3t = 7t + 8 + 3t \qquad \text{Using the addition principle}$$
$$11 = 10t + 8 \qquad \text{Combining like terms}$$
$$11 - 8 = 10t + 8 - 8 \qquad \text{Adding } -8 \text{ on both sides}$$
$$3 = 10t$$
$$\frac{3}{10} = \frac{10t}{10} \qquad \text{Dividing by 10 on both sides}$$
$$0.3 = t.$$

CHECK:

$$\begin{array}{c|c} \multicolumn{2}{c}{11 - 3t = 7t + 8} \\ \hline 11 - 3(0.3) \ ? \ 7(0.3) + 8 \\ 11 - 0.9 \ \big| \ 2.1 + 8 \\ 10.1 \ \big| \ 10.1 \qquad \text{TRUE} \end{array}$$

The solution is 0.3.

Solve.

7. $10t - 3 = 4t + 18$ 3.5

8. $8 + 4x = 9x - 3$ 2.2

9. $2.1x - 45.3 = 17.3x + 23.1$

  −4.5

10. Solve:

  $3(x + 4) = 17 - x.$ 1.25

Answers on page A-13

Because equations are reversible, it does not matter whether the variable is isolated on the right or left side. What is important is that you have a clear direction to your work as you proceed from step to step.

Do Exercises 7–9.

Note that after we had combined all variable terms on one side of the equation, Examples 4 and 5 were similar to Example 3.

PROBLEM-SOLVING TIP

When faced with a new type of problem, see if you can change the problem into an equivalent problem that you find easier to solve.

Example 6   Solve: $5(x + 1) = 3x + 12$.

By using the distributive law, we can find an equivalent equation:

$$5(x + 1) = 3x + 12$$
$$5 \cdot x + 5 \cdot 1 = 3x + 12 \qquad \text{Using the distributive law to remove parentheses}$$
$$5x + 5 = 3x + 12. \qquad \text{Simplifying}$$

We now solve as we did in Examples 4 and 5:

$$5x + 5 - 3x = 3x + 12 - 3x \qquad \text{Subtracting } 3x \text{ on both sides}$$
$$2x + 5 = 12 \qquad \text{Simplifying}$$
$$2x + 5 - 5 = 12 - 5 \qquad \text{Subtracting } 5 \text{ on both sides}$$
$$2x = 7$$
$$\frac{2x}{2} = \frac{7}{2} \qquad \text{Dividing by } 2 \text{ on both sides}$$
$$x = 3.5.$$

CHECK:

$$5(x + 1) = 3x + 12$$

$5(3.5 + 1)$? $3(3.5) + 12$
$5(4.5)$ ∣ $10.5 + 12$
22.5 ∣ 22.5 TRUE

The solution is 3.5.

Do Exercise 10.

Exercise Set 5.7

a Solve. Remember to check.

1. $5x = 27$ 5.4

2. $36 \cdot y = 14.76$ 0.41

3. $100t = 52.39$ 0.5239

4. $789.23 = 0.25 \cdot q$ 3156.92

5. $-23.4 = 5.2a$ −4.5

6. $-40.74 = 4.2x$ −9.7

7. $-9.2x = -94.76$ 10.3

8. $-7.6a = -29.64$ 3.9

9. $t - 19.27 = 24.51$ 43.78

10. $t - 3.012 = 10.478$ 13.49

11. $4.1 = -3.6 + n$ 7.7

12. $2.7 = -5.31 + m$ 8.01

13. $x + 13.9 = 4.2$ −9.7

14. $x + 15.7 = 3.1$ −12.6

15. $4x - 7 = 13$ 5

16. $5x - 8 = 22$ 6

17. $7.1x - 9.3 = 8.45$ 2.5

18. $6.9x - 8.4 = 4.02$ 1.8

19. $12.4 + 3.7t = 2.04$ −2.8

20. $21.6 + 4.1t = 6.43$ −3.7

21. $-26.05 = 7.5x + 9.2$ -4.7

22. $-43.42 = 8.7x + 5.3$ -5.6

23. $-4.2x + 3.04 = -4.1$ 1.7

24. $-2.9x - 2.24 = -17.9$ 5.4

b Solve. Remember to check.

25. $9x - 6 = 5x + 30$ 9

26. $8x - 5 = 6x + 9$ 7

27. $3x + 15 = 11x + 5$ 1.25

28. $2x + 18 = 7x + 2$ 3.2

29. $6y - 5 = 8 + 10y$ -3.25

30. $5y - 3 = 4 + 9y$ -1.75

31. $5.9x + 67 = 7.6x + 16$ 30

32. $2.1x + 42 = 5.2x - 20$ 20

33. $7.8a + 2 = 2.4a + 19.28$ 3.2

34. $7.5a - 5.16 = 3.1a + 12$ 3.9

35. $5(x + 2) = 3x + 18$ 4

36. $6(x + 2) = 4x + 30$ 9

37. $2(x + 3) = 4x - 11$ 8.5

38. $5(x + 3) = 15x - 6$ 2.1

39. $2a + 17 = 12(a - 1)$ 2.9

40. $7a + 6 = 15(a - 2)$ 4.5

41. $2(x + 7.3) = 6x - 0.83$ 3.8575

42. $2.9(x + 8.1) = 7.8x - 3.95$ 5.6

43. $-7.37 - 3.2t = 4.9(t + 6.1)$ −4.6

44. $-6.21 - 4.3t = 9.8(t + 2.1)$ −1.9

45. $9(x - 4) + 8 = 4x + 7$ 7

46. $4(x - 2) - 9 = 2x + 9$ 13

47. $34(5 - 3.5x) = 12(3x - 8) + 653.5$ −2.5

48. $43(7 - 2x) + 34 = 50(x - 4.1) + 744$ −1.5

49. Simplify: $\dfrac{-43}{-43}$. [3.3a] 1

50. Add: $\dfrac{4}{9} + \dfrac{5}{6}$. [4.2b] $\dfrac{23}{18}$

51. Subtract: $\dfrac{3}{25} - \dfrac{7}{10}$. [4.3a] $-\dfrac{29}{50}$

52. Simplify: $\dfrac{0}{-18}$. [3.3a] 0

53. Add: $-17 + 24 + (-9)$. [2.2a] -2

54. Solve: $3x - 10 = 14$. [4.4a] 8

Synthesis

55. ◆ When solving linear equations, can the multiplication principle be used before the addition principle? Why or why not?

56. ◆ Is it possible for an equation like $x + 3 = x + 5$ to have a solution? Why or why not?

57. ◆ Describe a method for constructing an equation similar in form to Exercise 17, but with 8.3 as the solution.

Solve.

58. ▦ $7.035(4.91x - 8.21) + 17.401 = 23.902x - 7.372815$ 3.1

59. ▦ $8.701(3.4 - 5.1x) - 89.321 = 5.401x + 74.65787$ -2.7

60. $5(x - 4.2) + 3[2x - 5(x + 7)] = 39 + 2(7.5 - 6x) + 3x$ 36

61. $14(2.5x - 3) + 9x + 5 = 4(3.25 - x) + 2[5x - 3(x + 1)]$ 1

Create and solve equations as a group.

Collaborative Learning Manual

5.8 Applications and Problem Solving

a Solving applied problems with decimals is like solving applied problems with integers. We translate first to an equation that corresponds to the situation. Then we solve the equation.

Example 1 *Dining Out.* More and more Americans are eating meals outside the home. The following graph compares the average check for meals of various types for the years 1997 and 1998. How much more is the average check for fast food in 1998 than in 1997?

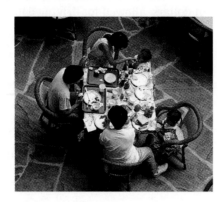

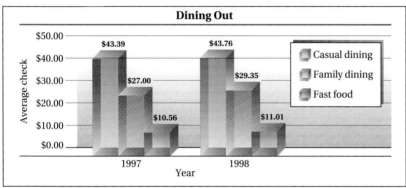

Source: Sandelman and Associates, Brea, California

1. **Familiarize.** We use the bar graph to visualize the situation and to obtain the appropriate data. We let c = the additional amount spent on fast food in 1998.

2. **Translate.** This is a "how-much-more" situation. We translate as follows, using the data from the bar graph.

Average check in 1997	plus	Additional amount	is	Average check in 1998
↓	↓	↓	↓	↓
$10.56	+	c	=	$11.01

3. **Solve.** We solve the equation by subtracting 10.56 from both sides:

$$10.56 + c - 10.56 = 11.01 - 10.56$$
$$c = 0.45.$$

$$\begin{array}{r} {}^{0\ \ 9\ \ 11} \\ 1\ \cancel{1}.\cancel{0}\ \cancel{1} \\ -\ 1\ 0.5\ 6 \\ \hline 0.4\ 5 \end{array}$$

4. **Check.** We can check by adding 0.45 to 10.56 to get 11.01.

5. **State.** The average check for fast food in 1998 was 45¢ more than in 1997.

Do Exercise 1.

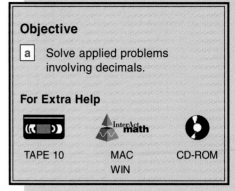

1. *Body Temperature.* Normal body temperature is 98.6°F. When fevered, most people will die if their bodies reach 107°F. This is a rise of how many degrees?

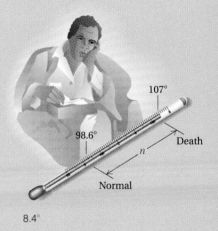

8.4°

Answer on page A-13

2. At Copylot Printing, the cost of copying is 8 cents per page. How much, in dollars, would it cost to make 466 copies?

$37.28

Example 2 *IRS Driving Allowance.* In 1997, the Internal Revenue Service (IRS) allowed a tax deduction of 31.5¢ per mile for mileage driven for business purposes. What deduction, in dollars, could Jill take for driving 640 work-related miles?

1. **Familiarize.** We first make a drawing or at least visualize the situation. Repeated addition fits this situation. We let d = the deduction, in dollars, allowed for driving 640 mi. Note that 31.5¢ is $0.315.

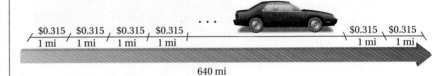

$640 mi

2. **Translate.** We translate as follows.

Deduction for each mile	times	Number of miles driven	is	Total deduction
$0.315	×	640	=	d

3. **Solve.** To solve the equation, we carry out the multiplication.

$$\begin{array}{r} 0.3\ 1\ 5 \\ \times \quad\ \ 6\ 4\ 0 \\ \hline 0\ 0\ 0 \\ 1\ 2\ 6\ 0 \\ 1\ 8\ 9\ 0 \\ \hline 2\ 0\ 1.6\ 0\ 0 \end{array}$$

Thus, $d = 201.60$.

4. **Check.** We can obtain a partial check by rounding and estimating:

$$0.315 \times 640 \approx 0.3 \times 650$$
$$= 195 \approx 201.6.$$

5. **State.** Jill could take a tax deduction of $201.60.

Do Exercise 2.

Multistep Problems

Example 3 *Student Loans.* Upon graduation from college, Jannette will be faced with repaying a Stafford loan that totals $23,334. The loan is to be paid back over 10 yr in equal payments. Find the amount of each payment.

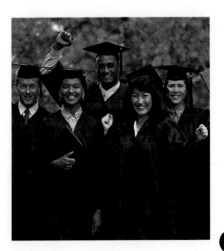

Answer on page A-13

1. **Familiarize.** We imagine the situation as one in which money that was borrowed is then repaid in monthly checks that are always the same amount. Since we are not told how many checks there will be, one part of solving this problem is to determine how many months are in 10 yr. We let $m =$ the size of each monthly payment.

2. **Translate.** To find the amount of the monthly payment, we note that the amount owed is split up, or *divided,* into payments of equal size. The size of each payment will depend on how many payments there are. To find the number of payments, we first determine that in 10 yr there are

$10 \cdot 12 = 120$ months.   **There are 12 months in a year.**

We have

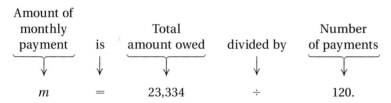

Amount of monthly payment	is	Total amount owed	divided by	Number of payments
m	$=$	$23{,}334$	$\div$	$120.$

3. **Solve.** To solve, we carry out the division.

$$
\begin{array}{r}
1\ 9\ 4.4\ 5 \\
1\ 2\ 0\ \overline{)\ 2\ 3{,}3\ 3\ 4.0\ 0} \\
\underline{1\ 2\ 0} \\
1\ 1\ 3\ 3 \\
\underline{1\ 0\ 8\ 0} \\
5\ 3\ 4 \\
\underline{4\ 8\ 0} \\
5\ 4\ 0 \\
\underline{4\ 8\ 0} \\
6\ 0\ 0 \\
\underline{6\ 0\ 0} \\
0
\end{array}
$$

$m = 194.45$

4. **Check.** To check, we first verify that there are 120 months in 10 yr. We can do this with division:

120 months $\div$ 12 months per year $=$ 10 years.

To check that the amount of the monthly payment is correct, we can estimate the product:

$194.45 \cdot 120 \approx 200 \cdot 120 = 24{,}000 \approx 23{,}334.$

5. **State.** Jannette's monthly payments will be $194.45.

Do Exercise 3.

3. *Car Payments.* Kevin's car loan totals $11,370 and is to be paid over 5 yr in monthly payments of equal size. Find the amount of each payment? $189.50

Answer on page A-13

4. *Gas Mileage.* Ivan filled his Dodge Stratus and noted that the odometer read 38,320.8. After the next filling, the odometer read 38,735.5. It took 14.5 gal to fill the tank. How many miles per gallon (mpg) did Ivan's Dodge get?

28.6 mpg

Example 4 *Gas Mileage.* Emma filled her Ford Contour with gas and noted that the odometer read 67,507.8. After the next filling, the odometer read 67,890.3. It took 12.5 gal to fill the tank. How many miles per gallon did Emma's Ford get?

1. Familiarize. We make a drawing.

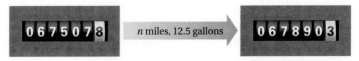

This is a two-step problem. First, we find the number of miles driven between fillups. We let n = the number of miles driven.

2., 3. Translate and **Solve.** To find the number of miles driven, we translate and solve as follows.

Second odometer reading	minus	First odometer reading	is	Number of miles driven
67,890.3	−	67,507.8	=	n

To solve the equation, we simplify on the left side:

$$67,890.3 - 67,507.8 = n$$
$$382.5 = n.$$

$$\begin{array}{r} 6\,7,8\,9\,0.3 \\ -\ 6\,7,5\,0\,7.8 \\ \hline 3\,8\,2.5 \end{array}$$

Next, we divide the number of miles driven by the number of gallons used. This gives us m = the number of miles per gallon—that is, the mileage. The division that corresponds to the situation is

$$382.5 \div 12.5 = m.$$

To find the number m, we divide.

$$\begin{array}{r} 3\,0.6 \\ 1\,2.5.\ \overline{)\,3\,8\,2\,5._\wedge 0} \\ \underline{3\,7\,5\,0} \\ 7\,5\,0 \\ \underline{7\,5\,0} \\ 0 \end{array}$$

Thus, m = 30.6.

4. Check. To check, we first multiply the number of miles per gallon times the number of gallons:

$$12.5 \times 30.6 = 382.5. \qquad \textbf{12.5 gal would take Emma 382.5 mi.}$$

Then we add 382.5 to 67,507.8:

$$67,507.8 + 382.5 = 67,890.3.$$

The mileage 30.6 checks.

5. State. Emma's Ford Contour got 30.6 miles per gallon.

Do Exercise 4.

Answer on page A-13

Some problems may require us to recall important formulas. Example 5 involves a formula from geometry that is worth remembering.

5. Suppose that an 8-in.–wide disc is punched out of an 8-in. by 8-in. sheet of metal. How much material is left over?

13.76 in^2

> In any circle, a **diameter** is a segment that passes through the center of the circle with endpoints on the circle. A **radius** is a segment with one endpoint on the center and the other endpoint on the circle. The area, A, of a circle with radius of length r is given by
>
> $$A = \pi \cdot r^2,$$
>
> where $\pi \approx 3.14$.

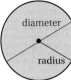

Example 5 The Northfield Tap and Die Company stamps 6-cm–wide discs out of metal squares that are 6 cm by 6 cm. How much metal remains after the disc has been punched out?

1. **Familiarize.** We make, and label, a drawing. The question deals with discs, squares, and leftover material, so we list the relevant area formulas.

   For a square with sides of length s,

   $$Area = s^2.$$

   For a circle with radius of length r,

   $$Area = \pi \cdot r^2,$$

   where $\pi \approx 3.14$.

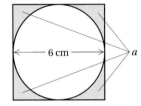

2. **Translate.** To find the amount left over, we subtract the area of the disc from the area of the square. Note that a circle's radius is half of its diameter, or width.

Area of square	minus	Area of disc	is	Area left over
6^2	$-$	$3.14 \times \left(\dfrac{6}{2}\right)^2$	$=$	a

3. **Solve.** We simplify as follows:

   $$6^2 - 3.14\left(\frac{6}{2}\right)^2 = a$$
   $$36 - 3.14(3)^2 = a$$
   $$36 - 3.14 \cdot 9 = a$$
   $$36 - 28.26 = a$$
   $$7.74 = a.$$

4. **Check.** We can repeat our calculation as a check. Note that 7.74 is less than the area of the disc, which in turn is less than the area of the square. This agrees with the impression given by our drawing.

5. **State.** The amount of material left over is 7.74 cm^2.

Do Exercise 5.

Answer on page A-13

6. Yardbird Landscaping charges customers $25 plus $20 per hour to rototill a garden. For how many hours can Emily hire Yardbird if she has budgeted $50 for rototilling?

1.25 hr

Example 6 *Truck Rentals.* Yardbird Landscaping has rented a 22-ft truck at a daily rate of $49.95 plus 35 cents a mile. They have budgeted $125 for renting a truck to deliver trees to customers around the county. How many miles can a one-day rental truck be driven without exceeding the budget?

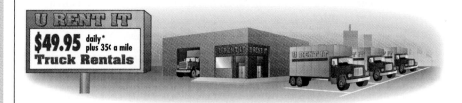

1. Familiarize. Suppose the landscapers drive 100 mi. Then the cost would be

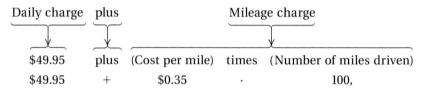

$$\underbrace{\$49.95}_{\text{Daily charge}} \quad \underbrace{\text{plus}}_{\text{plus}} \quad \underbrace{\text{(Cost per mile)} \quad \text{times} \quad \text{(Number of miles driven)}}_{\text{Mileage charge}}$$

$$\$49.95 \quad + \quad \$0.35 \quad \cdot \quad 100,$$

which is $49.95 + $35, or $84.95. This familiarizes us with the way in which a calculation is made. Note that we convert 35 cents to $0.35 so that only one unit, dollars, is used. Note also that the landscapers can exceed 100 mi and still be within budget. To see just how many miles the budget allows for, we could make and check more guesses, but this would be very time-consuming. Instead we let m = the number of miles that can be driven within a $125 budget.

2. Translate. The problem can be rephrased and translated as follows.

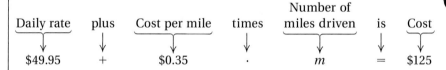

$$\underbrace{\$49.95}_{\text{Daily rate}} \;\; \underbrace{+}_{\text{plus}} \;\; \underbrace{\$0.35}_{\text{Cost per mile}} \;\; \underbrace{\cdot}_{\text{times}} \;\; \underbrace{m}_{\substack{\text{Number of} \\ \text{miles driven}}} \;\; \underbrace{=}_{\text{is}} \;\; \underbrace{\$125}_{\text{Cost}}$$

3. Solve. We solve the equation:

$$49.95 + 0.35m = 125$$

$$0.35m = 75.05 \qquad \text{Subtracting 49.95 on both sides}$$

$$m = \frac{75.05}{0.35} \qquad \text{Dividing by 0.35 on both sides}$$

$$m \approx 214.4. \qquad \text{Rounding to the nearest tenth}$$

4. Check. We check in the original problem. We multiply 214.4 by $0.35, getting $75.04. Then we add $75.04 to $49.95 and get $124.99, which is just about the $125 allotted. Our answer is not exact because we rounded.

5. State. Yardbird Landscaping can drive the truck about 214.4 mi without exceeding the budget.

Do Exercise 6.

Answer on page A-13

Exercise Set 5.8

a Solve.

1. What is the cost of 7 shirts at $32.98 each? $230.86

2. What is the cost of 8 pairs of socks at $4.95 each?
$39.60

3. What is the cost, in dollars, of 20.4 gal of gasoline at 129.9 cents per gallon? (129.9 cents = $1.299) Round the answer to the nearest cent. $26.50

4. What is the cost, in dollars, of 17.7 gal of gasoline at 119.9 cents per gallon? (119.9 cents = $1.199) Round the answer to the nearest cent. $21.22

5. Madeleine buys a book for $44.68 and pays with a $50 bill. How much change does she receive?

$5.32

6. Roberto bought a CD for $16.99 and paid with a $20 bill. How much change was there?

$3.01

7. *Nursing.* A nurse draws 17.85 mg of blood and uses 9.68 mg in a blood test. How much is left?   8.17 mg

8. *Medicine.* Normal body temperature is 98.6°F. During an illness, a patient's temperature rose 4.2°. What was the new temperature?   102.8°F

9. *Finance.* A car loan totaling $4425 is to be paid off in 12 monthly payments of equal size. How much is each payment? $368.75

10. *Culinary Arts.* One pound of crabmeat makes three servings at the Key West Seafood Restaurant. If the crabmeat costs $16.95 per pound, what is the cost per serving? $5.65

11. *Medicine.* After being tested for allergies, Mike was given allergy shots of 0.25 mg, 0.4 mg, 0.5 mg, and 0.5 mg over a 2-month period. What was the total amount of the injections?   1.65 mg

12. *Beverage Consumption.* Each year, the average American drinks about 49.0 gal of soft drinks, 41.2 gal of water, 25.3 gal of milk, 24.8 gal of coffee, and 7.8 gal of fruit juice. What is the total amount that the average American drinks?   148.1 gal

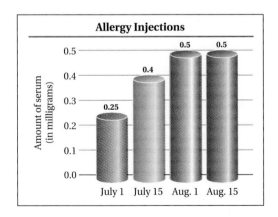

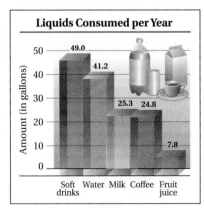

Source: U.S. Department of Agriculture

13. *Lotteries.* In Texas, one of the state lotteries is called "Cash 5." In a recent weekly game, the lottery prize of $127,315 was shared equally by 6 winners. How much was each winner's share? Round to the nearest cent. $21,219.17

14. A group of 4 students pays $40.76 for lunch. What is each person's share? $10.19

15. A rectangular poster measures 73.2 cm by 61.8 cm. What is its area?   4523.76 cm²

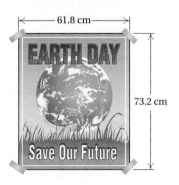

16. A rectangular fenced yard measures 40.3 yd by 65.7 yd. What is its area?   2647.71 yd²

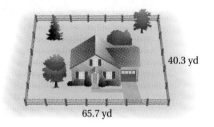

17. The length of the Panama Canal is 81.6 kilometers (km). The length of the Suez Canal is 175.5 km. How much longer is the Suez Canal?   93.9 km

18. In 1970, the median age of a first-time bride was 20.8 yr. In 1992, the median age was 24.4 yr. How much greater was the median age of a bride in 1992 than in 1970?   3.6 yr

19. *Taxes.* The Colavitos own a house with an assessed value of $124,500. For every $1000 of assessed value, they pay $7.68 in taxes. How much in taxes do they pay? $956.16

20. *Chemistry.* The water in a filled tank weighs 748.45 lb. One cubic foot of water weighs 62.5 lb. How many cubic feet of water does the tank hold?   11.9752 cu ft

Find the distance around (perimeter of) each figure.

21.
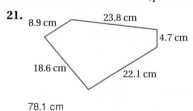

8.9 cm   23.8 cm   4.7 cm   18.6 cm   22.1 cm   78.1 cm

22.
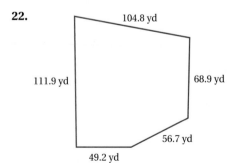

104.8 yd   111.9 yd   68.9 yd   56.7 yd   49.2 yd

391.5 yd

23. 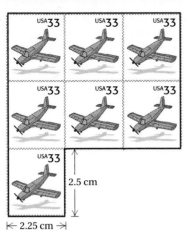 28.5 cm

2.5 cm

2.25 cm

24. 2.5 cm 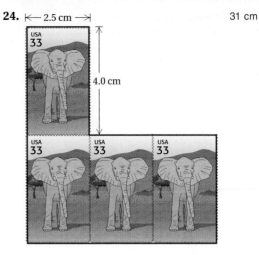 31 cm

4.0 cm

Find the length *d* in each figure.

25.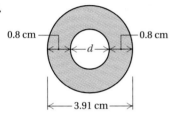

0.8 cm   0.8 cm

d

3.91 cm

2.31 cm

26.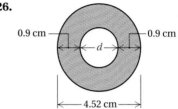

0.9 cm   0.9 cm

d

4.52 cm

2.72 cm

27. *Mileage.* Peggy filled her van's gas tank and noted that the odometer read 26,342.8. After the next filling, the odometer read 26,736.7. It took 19.5 gal to fill the tank. How many miles per gallon (mpg) did the van get?   20.2 mpg

28. *Mileage.* Peter filled his Honda's gas tank and noted that the odometer read 18,943.2. After the next filling, the odometer read 19,306.2. It took 13.2 gal to fill the tank. How many miles per gallon did the car get?   27.5 mpg

29. Roberto bought 3 CDs at $12.99 (tax included). He paid with a $50 bill. How much change did he receive? $11.03

30. Natalie Clad had $185.00 to spend for fall clothes: She spent $44.95 for shoes, $71.95 for a jacket, and $55.35 for pants. How much was left? $12.75

31. *Carpentry.* A round, 6-ft–wide, hot tub is being built into a 12-ft by 30-ft rectangular deck. How much decking is needed for the surface of the deck?

331.74 ft^2

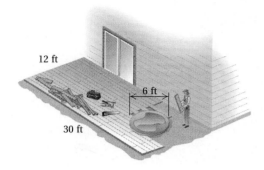

32. *Landscaping.* A rectangular yard is 20 ft by 15 ft. The yard is covered with grass except for a circular flower garden with an 8-ft diameter. How much grass is in the yard?   249.76 ft^2

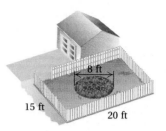

33. A 4-ft by 6-ft table top is cut from a round table top that is 9 ft wide. How much wood will be left over?

39.585 ft^2

34. A 4-ft by 4-ft tablecloth is cut from a round tablecloth that is 6 ft wide. How much cloth will be left over?   12.26 ft^2

35. Zachary worked 53 hr during a week one summer. He earned $8.50 per hour for the first 40 hr and $12.75 per hour for overtime. How much did Zachary earn during the week? $505.75

36. It costs $24.95 a day plus 27 cents per mile to rent a compact car at Shuttles Rent-A-Car. How much, in dollars, would it cost to drive the car 120 mi in 1 day? $57.35

37. *Car Rentals.* Badger Rent-A-Car rents a midsize car at a daily rate of $34.95 plus 10 cents per mile. A businessperson is allotted $80 for car rental. How many miles can the businessperson travel on the $80 budget?   450.5 mi

38. *Car Rentals.* Badger also rents a full-size car at $43.95 plus 10 cents per mile. A businessperson has a car rental allotment of $90. How many miles can the businessperson travel on the $90 budget?

460.5 mi

39. *Bike Rentals.* Mike's Bikes rents mountain bikes. The shop charges $5.50 insurance for each rental plus $2.40 per hour. For how many hours can a person rent a bike with $25.00? 8.125 hr

40. *Phone Bills.* Auritech Communication charges 50¢ for the first minute and 32¢ for each additional minute for a certain phone call. For how long could two parties speak if the bill for the call cannot exceed $5.30? 16 min

41. *Service Calls.* JoJo's Service Center charges $30 for a house call plus $37.50 for each hour the job takes. For how long has a repairperson worked on a house call if the bill comes to $123.75? 2.5 hr

42. *Electric Rates.* Southeast Electric charges 9¢ per kilowatt-hour for the first 200 kWh. The company charges 11¢ per kilowatt-hour for all electrical usage in excess of 200 kWh. How many kilowatt-hours were used if a monthly electric bill was $57.60? 560 kWh

43. *Field Dimensions.* The dimensions of a World Cup soccer field are 114.9 yd by 74.4 yd. The dimensions of a standard football field are 120 yd by 53.3 yd. How much greater is the area of a World Cup soccer field? 2152.56 yd^2

44. *Overtime Pay.* A construction worker earned $17 per hour for the first 40 hr of work and $25.50 per hour for work in excess of 40 hr. One week she earned $896.75. How much overtime did she work? 8.5 hr

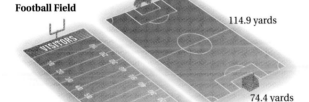

World Cup Soccer Field

Football Field

114.9 yards

74.4 yards

120 yards

53.3 yards

45. Frank has been sent to the store with $40 to purchase 6 lb of cheese at $4.79 a pound and as many bottles of seltzer, at $0.64 a bottle, as possible. How many bottles of seltzer should Frank buy? 17

46. Janice has been sent to the store with $30 to purchase 5 pt of salsa at $2.49 a pint and as many bags of chips, at $1.39 a bag, as possible. How many bags of chips should Janice buy? 12

47. Simplify: $\dfrac{0}{-13}$. [3.3a] 0

48. Add: $-\dfrac{4}{5} + \dfrac{7}{10}$. [4.2b] $-\dfrac{1}{10}$

49. Subtract: $\dfrac{8}{11} - \dfrac{4}{3}$. [4.3a] $-\dfrac{20}{33}$

50. Solve: $4x - 7 = 9x + 13$. [5.7b] -4

51. Add: $4\dfrac{1}{3} + 2\dfrac{1}{2}$. [4.6a] $6\dfrac{5}{6}$

52. Simplify: $\dfrac{-72}{-72}$. [3.3a] 1

Synthesis

53. ◆ Write a problem for a classmate to solve. Design the problem so that the solution is "The larger field is 200 m² bigger."

54. ◆ Write a problem for a classmate to solve. Design the problem so that the solution is "Mona's Buick got 23.5 mpg."

55. ◆ 🖩 Which is a better deal and why: a 14-in. pizza that costs $9.95 or a 16-in. pizza that costs $11.95?

56. You can drive from home to work using either of two routes:

Route A: Via interstate highway, 7.6 mi, with a speed limit of 65 mph.
Route B: Via a country road, 5.6 mi, with a speed limit of 50 mph.

Assuming you drive at the posted speed limit, how much time can you save by taking the faster route?

$\dfrac{96}{325}$ min

57. 🖩 A 25-ft by 30-ft yard contains an 8-ft–wide, round fountain. How many 1-lb bags of grass seed should be purchased to seed the lawn if 1 lb of seed covers 300 ft²? 3

58. If the daily rental for a car is $18.90 plus a certain price per mile and Lindsey must drive 190 mi and still stay within a $55.00 budget, what is the highest price per mile that Lindsey can afford?

$0.19

59. Find the shaded area. What assumptions must you make?

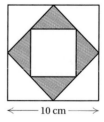

←— 10 cm —→

25 cm². We assume that the figures are nested squares formed by connecting the midpoints of consecutive sides of the next larger square.

60. *Fast-Food Meals.* In 1995, the average fast-food meal cost $9.42; in 1996, it was $10.06; in 1997, it was $10.56; and in 1998, it was $11.01 (**Source:** Sandelman and Associates, Brea, California). Determine the average yearly increase in the cost of a fast-food meal. $0.53

61. *Family Dining.* In 1995, the average cost of a family's dinner outside the home was $25.39; in 1996, it was $27.40; in 1997, it was $27.00; and in 1998, it was $29.35 (**Source:** Sandelman and Associates, Brea, California). Determine the average yearly increase in what it costs a family to eat out.

$1.32

Copyright © 2000 Addison Wesley Longman

Prepare a budget for redecorating the classroom.

Collaborative Learning Manual

Summary and Review Exercises: Chapter 5

1. Write a word name for 3.47. [5.1a]

2. Write $597.25 in words, as on a check. [5.1a]

Write fractional notation. [5.1b]

3. 0.09

4. −3.0227

Write decimal notation. [5.1c]

5. $-\dfrac{34}{1000}$

6. $\dfrac{2791}{100}$

Which number is larger? [5.1d]

7. 0.034, 0.0185

8. −0.67, −0.19

Round 39.4287 to the nearest: [5.1e]

9. Tenth.

10. Hundredth.

Perform the indicated operation.

11.
```
  2 3 6.2 3 1
    2 6 3.4
+     0.1 9 8   [5.2a]
```

12.
```
  3 7.6 4 5
−    8.4 9 7   [5.2b]
```

13. 219.3 + 2.8 + 7
   [5.2a]

14. 745.0109 − 59.959
   [5.2b]

15. −37.8 + (−19.5)
   [5.2c]

16. −7.52 − (−9.89)
   [5.2c]

17.
```
    4 8
× 0.2 7   [5.3a]
```

18. −3.7(0.29) [5.3a]

19.
```
  2 4.6 8
× 1 0 0 0   [5.3a]
```

20. $2\,5\,\overline{)\,8\,0}$ [5.4a]

21. 11.52 ÷ (−7.2) [5.4a]

22. $\dfrac{276.3}{1000}$ [5.4a]

Combine like terms. [5.2d]

23. $3.7x - 5.2y - 1.5x - 3.9y$

24. $7.94 - 3.89a + 4.63 + 1.05a$

25. Evaluate $P - Prt$ for $P = 1000$, $r = 0.05$, and $t = 1.5$. (*A formula for depreciation*) [5.3c]

26. Simplify: $9 - 3.2(-1.5) + 5.2^2$. [5.4b]

27. Estimate the sum 7.298 + 3.961 to the nearest tenth. [5.6a]

28. About how many videotapes, at $2.45 each, can be purchased with $49.95? [5.6a]

29. Which of the following is an appropriate estimate of 7.9 × 4.8?   [5.6a]

a) 240   b) 24
c) 40   d) 4

30. Convert 1549 cents to dollars.   [5.3b]

31. Round 248.$\overline{27}$ to the nearest hundredth.   [5.5b]

Find decimal notation. Use multiplying by 1.   [5.5c]

32. $\dfrac{13}{5}$ **33.** $\dfrac{32}{25}$

Find decimal notation. Use division.   [5.5a]

34. $\dfrac{13}{4}$ **35.** $-\dfrac{7}{6}$

36. Calculate: $\dfrac{4}{15} \times 79.05$.   [5.5d]

Solve. Remember to check.

37. $t - 4.3 = -7.5$ **38.** $4.1x + 5.6 = -6.7$
   [5.7a]   [5.7a]

39. $6x - 11 = 8x + 4$ **40.** $3(x + 2) = 5x - 7$
   [5.7b]   [5.7b]

Solve.   [5.8a]

41. In the United States, there are 51.81 telephone poles for every 100 people. In Canada, there are 40.65. How many more telephone poles for every 100 people are there in the United States?

42. Zack's times in the quarter-mile run were 89.3 sec, 88.9 sec, and 90.0 sec. What was his average time?

43. The McCoys have 4 corn fields. One year the harvest in each field was 1419.3 bushels, 1761.8 bushels, 1095.2 bushels, and 2088.8 bushels. What was the year's total harvest?

44. A florist sold 13 potted palms for a total of $423.65. What was the cost for each palm? Round to the nearest cent.

45. Worldwide, the average person drinks 3.48 cups of tea per day. How many cups of tea does the average person drink in a week? in a month (30 days)?

46. A taxi driver charges $7.25 plus 95 cents a mile for out-of-town fares. How far can an out-of-towner travel on $15.23?

Skill Maintenance

47. Simplify: $\dfrac{-29}{-29}$.   [3.3c]

48. Add and simplify: $-\dfrac{1}{9} + \dfrac{1}{6}$.   [4.2b]

49. Subtract and simplify: $\dfrac{4}{5} - \dfrac{1}{2}$.   [4.3a]

50. Simplify: $\dfrac{1}{2}x + \dfrac{3}{4}y - \dfrac{3}{4}x - y$.   [4.3a]

Synthesis

51. ◆ Explain how fractional notation can be used when explaining why we add decimal places when multiplying with decimal notation.   [5.3a]

52. ◆ Explain what mistake is made in the following calculation.   [5.2a]

$$\begin{array}{r} 1\,3.0\,7 \\ +\ 9.2\,0\,5 \\ \hline 1\,0.5\,1\,2 \end{array}$$

53. ▦ Arrange from smallest to largest: [5.1d], [5.5a]

$$-\dfrac{2}{3},\ -\dfrac{15}{19},\ -\dfrac{11}{13},\ \dfrac{-5}{7},\ \dfrac{-13}{15},\ \dfrac{-17}{20}.$$

54. The Fit Fiddle health club generally charges a $79 membership fee and $42.50 a month. Alayn has a coupon that will allow her to join the club for $299 for six months. How much will Alayn save if she uses the coupon?   [5.8a]

Test: Chapter 5

1. Write a word name for 6.0401.

   [5.1a] Six and four hundred one ten-thousandths

2. Write $1234.78 in words, as on a check.

   [5.1a] One thousand two hundred thirty-four and $\frac{78}{100}$ dollars

Write fractional notation. Do not simplify.

3. −0.2

4. 7.308

Write decimal notation.

5. $\dfrac{49}{10,000}$

6. $-\dfrac{528}{100}$

Which number is larger?

7. 0.07, 0.162

8. −0.173, −0.25

Round 9.4523 to the nearest:

9. Tenth.

10. Thousandth.

Perform the indicated operation.

11.
```
   4 0 2.3
     2.8 1
+    0.1 0 9
```

12.
```
   0.1 2 5
×    0.2 4
```

13.
```
   2 1 3.4 5
×     0.0 0 1
```

14.
```
   5 2.0 9 1
−    7.3 4 5
```

15. 342.9 + 8.1 + 5.37

16. −9.5 + 7.3

17. 2 − 0.0054

18. $2\,5\,)\overline{1\,1}$

19. $3.3\,)\overline{1\,0\,0.3\,2}$

20. $\dfrac{-346.82}{1000}$

21. Convert $179.82 to cents.

22. Combine like terms:

    4.1x + 5.2 − 3.9y + 5.7x − 9.8.

23. Evaluate 2l + 4w + 2h for l = 2.4, w = 1.3, and h = 0.8.
    (*The total girth of a postal package*)

24. Simplify: 20 ÷ 5(−2)² − 8.4.

25. About how many gallons of gasoline, at $1.269 per gallon, can be bought with $10? Round to the nearest gallon.

26. Round 48.$\overline{74}$ to the nearest tenth.

Find decimal notation. Use multiplying by 1.

27. $\dfrac{8}{5}$

28. $\dfrac{21}{4}$

Answers

1.

2.

3. [5.1b] $-\frac{2}{10}$

4. [5.1b] $\frac{7308}{1000}$

5. [5.1c] 0.0049

6. [5.1c] −5.28

7. [5.1d] 0.162

8. [5.1d] −0.173

9. [5.1e] 9.5

10. [5.1e] 9.452

11. [5.2a] 405.219

12. [5.3a] 0.03

13. [5.3a] 0.21345

14. [5.2b] 44.746

15. [5.2a] 356.37

16. [5.2c] −2.2

17. [5.2b] 1.9946

18. [5.4a] 0.44

19. [5.4a] 30.4

20. [5.4a] −0.34682

21. [5.3b] 17,982¢

22. [5.2d] 9.8x − 3.9y − 4.6

23. [5.3c] 11.6

24. [5.4b] 7.6

25. [5.6a] 8 gal

26. [5.5b] 48.7

27. [5.5c] 1.6

28. [5.5c] 5.25

Find decimal notation. Use division.

29. $-\dfrac{7}{16}$

30. $\dfrac{11}{9}$

31. Calculate: $\dfrac{3}{8} \times 45.6 - \dfrac{1}{5} \times 36.9$.

Solve. Remember to check.

32. $17y - 3.12 = -58.2$

33. $9t - 4 = 6t + 26$

34. $4 + 2(x - 3) = 7x - 9$

Solve.

35. Raul wrote checks of $123.89, $56.78, and $3446.98. What was the average amount of the checks? Round to the nearest cent.

36. In 1896, Alfred Hajos set the world record in the 100-m freestyle swim with a time of 82.2 sec. A hundred years later, Aleksandr Popov set a new record of 48.74 sec. How much better was Popov's time?

37. Alexia bought 6 books at $19.95 each. How much was spent?

38. The three Szmansky sisters commute 3 mi, 5.2 mi, and 16.4 mi to their jobs each day. How far do they commute on average?

39. Air-Tight Heating Service charges $35 for a house call plus $32.50 an hour for labor. A family's bill is $83.75 for repairs to their furnace. How long did the repairs take?

Skill Maintenance

40. Simplify: $\dfrac{0}{57}$.

41. Add and simplify: $\dfrac{2}{7} + \dfrac{3}{21}$.

42. Subtract and simplify: $\dfrac{2}{3} - \dfrac{7}{10}$.

43. Simplify: $\dfrac{4}{5}x + \dfrac{2}{3}y - \dfrac{1}{10}x - \dfrac{3}{5}y$.

Synthesis

44. Use one of the words *sometimes, never,* or *always* to complete each of the following.

a) The product of two numbers greater than 0 and less than 1 is _____ less than 1.

b) The product of two numbers greater than 1 is _____ less than 1.

c) The product of a number greater than 1 and a number less than 1 is _____ equal to 1.

d) The product of a number greater than 1 and a number less than 1 is _____ equal to 0.

Copyright © 2000 Addison Wesley Longman

Cumulative Review: Chapters 1–5

1. Write expanded notation: 12,758.

2. Write $802.53 in words, as on a check.

3. Write fractional notation: 10.09.

4. Convert to fractional notation: $3\frac{3}{8}$.

5. Write decimal notation: $\dfrac{-35}{1000}$.

6. List all the factors of 66.

7. Find the prime factorization of 66.

8. Find the LCM of 28 and 35.

9. Round 6962.4721 to the nearest hundred.

10. Round 6962.4721 to the nearest hundredth.

Add and, if possible, simplify.

11.
$$3\frac{2}{3}$$
$$+\,2\frac{5}{9}$$

12.
```
  1 1 0.8 6 3
      0.7 3
  1 2 1.9
+     1.9 0 4
```

13.
```
  5 2 4 9
    2 1 5
+     3 1
```

14. $-\dfrac{4}{15}+\dfrac{7}{30}$

Subtract.

15. $29-(-17)$

16. $9010-563.47$

17. $\dfrac{8}{9}-\dfrac{7}{8}$

18. $7\dfrac{1}{5}-3\dfrac{4}{5}$

Multiply and simplify.

19.
```
  2 3.9
×   0.2
```

20. $-\dfrac{3}{5}\times\dfrac{10}{21}$

21. $3\dfrac{2}{11}\cdot 4\dfrac{2}{7}$

22. $5\cdot\dfrac{3}{10}$

Divide and simplify.

23. $2\dfrac{4}{5}\div 1\dfrac{13}{15}$

24. $\dfrac{6}{5}\div\dfrac{7}{8}$

25. $-43.795\div 0.001$

26. $2.1\,\overline{)\,4\,3.2\,6}$

Use $<$, $>$, or $=$ for ▓ to write a true sentence.

27. $\dfrac{5}{7}$ ▓ $\dfrac{2}{3}$

28. -3 ▓ -5

29. Evaluate $\dfrac{x}{3} - y$ for $x = 15$ and $y = 7$.

30. Multiply: $4(x - y + 3)$.

Combine like terms.

31. $-4p + 28 + 11p - 33$

32. $x - 9 + 13x - 2$

Solve. Remember to check.

33. $8.32 + x = 9.1$

34. $-75 \cdot x = 2100$

35. $y \cdot 9.47 = 81.6314$

36. $1062 - y = -368{,}313$

37. $t + \dfrac{5}{6} = \dfrac{8}{9}$

38. $\dfrac{7}{8} \cdot t = \dfrac{7}{16}$

39. $2.4x - 7.1 = 2.05$

40. $9 = -\dfrac{2}{3}x - 1$

Solve.

41. In 1996, there were 2344 heart transplants, 12,080 kidney transplants, 4064 liver transplants, and 811 lung transplants.* How many transplants of these four organs were performed?

42. After making a $150 down payment on a motorcycle, $\dfrac{3}{10}$ of the total cost was paid. How much did the motorcycle cost?

43. There are 60 seconds in a minute and 60 minutes in an hour. How many seconds are in a day?

44. Claude's college tuition was $4200. A loan was obtained for $\dfrac{2}{3}$ of the tuition. For how much was the loan?

45. The balance in a checking account is $314.79. After a check is written for $56.02, what is the balance in the account?

46. A clerk in a deli sold $1\dfrac{1}{2}$ lb of ham, $2\dfrac{3}{4}$ lb of turkey, and $2\dfrac{1}{4}$ lb of roast beef. How many pounds of meat were sold altogether?

47. A triangular sail has a height of 16 ft and a base of 11 ft. Find its area.

48. A rectangular billboard measures 19.8 ft by 23.6 ft. Find its area.

Synthesis

49. A box of Jello®-mix packages weighs $15\dfrac{3}{4}$ lb. Each package weighs $1\dfrac{3}{4}$ oz. How many packages are in the box?

50. In the Newton Market, Brenda used a manufacturer's coupon to buy juice. With the coupon, if 5 cartons of juice were purchased, the sixth carton was free. The price of each carton was $1.89. What was the cost per carton with the coupon? Round to the nearest cent.

———————

*United Network for Organ Sharing, cited in *The Statistical Abstract of the United States, 1998*.

6

Introduction to Graphing and Statistics

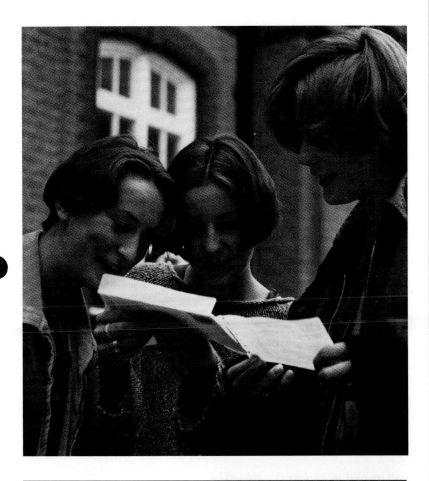

Introduction

There are many ways in which data can be represented and analyzed. One way is to use graphs. In this chapter, we examine several kinds of graphs: pictographs, bar graphs, line graphs, and graphs drawn from equations in two variables. Another way to analyze data is to study certain numbers, or *statistics*, that are related to the data. We will consider three statistics in this chapter: the *mean*, the *median*, and the *mode*.

An Application	The Mathematics
Meg earned grades of B, A, A, C, and D in courses that carried credit values of 3, 4, 3, 4, and 1, respectively. Find Meg's grade point average if an A corresponds to 4.0, a B corresponds to 3.0, a C corresponds to 2.0, and a D corresponds to 1.0.	We first multiply each grade point value by the number of credit hours in the course. Then we add and divide by the total number of credits to find the grade point average (GPA). This problem appears as Example 3 in Section 6.5.

World Wide Web For more information, visit us at www.mathmax.com

Pretest: Chapter 6

1. The table at right shows the comparison of the cost of a $100,000 life insurance policy for female smokers and nonsmokers at certain ages.

   a) How much does it cost a female smoker, age 32, for insurance?

   b) How much does it cost a female nonsmoker, age 32, for insurance?

   c) How much more does it cost a female smoker, age 35, than a nonsmoker of the same age?

LIFE INSURANCE: FEMALE		
Age	Cost (Smoker)	Cost (Nonsmoker)
31	$294	$170
32	298	172
33	302	176
34	310	178
35	316	182

2. Using the data in Question 1, draw a vertical bar graph showing the cost of insurance for a female smoker, ages 31–35. Use age on the horizontal scale and cost on the vertical scale.

3. Using the data in Question 1, draw a line graph showing the cost of insurance for a female smoker, ages 31–35. Use age on the horizontal scale and cost on the vertical scale.

The line graph at right shows the relationship between blood cholesterol level and risk of coronary heart disease.

4. Which of the cholesterol levels listed has the highest risk?

5. About how much higher is the risk at 260 than at 200?

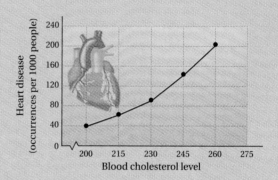

6. Plot these points:

   (−2, 4), (5, −3), (0, 6), (3, 0), (−4, −1), (2, 4).

7. In which quadrant is the point (−5, 7) located?

8. Determine whether the ordered pair (−2, 4) is a solution of the equation $2x − y = 0$.

Graph on a plane.

9. $y = −x$

10. $x + 2y = 9$

11. $y = \frac{2}{3}x − 1$

In Questions 12–14, find (a) the mean, (b) the median, and (c) any modes that exist.

12. 46, 50, 53, 55

13. 5, 5, 3, 1, 1

14. 4, 17, 4, 18, 4, 17, 18, 20

15. Wynton drove 660 mi in 12 hr. What was his average rate of travel?

16. To get a B in chemistry, Delia must average 80 on four tests. Scores on the first three tests were 78, 81, and 75. What is the lowest score that she can receive on the last test and still get a B?

17. Use the graph from Question 4 to estimate the frequency of occurrence of heart disease among people whose blood cholesterol level is 207.

18. A die is about to be rolled. Find the probability that a 2 will be rolled.

6.1 Tables and Pictographs

a | Reading and Interpreting Tables

A **table** is often used to present data in rows and columns.

Example 1 *Cereal Data.* Let's assume that you generally have a 2-cup bowl of cereal each morning. The following table lists nutritional information for five name-brand cereals. (It does not consider the use of milk, sugar, or sweetener.) The data have been determined by doubling the information given for a 1-cup serving that is found in the Nutrition Facts panel on a box of cereal.

Cereal	Calories	Fat	Total Carbohydrate	Sodium
Ralston Rice Chex	240	0 g	54 g	460 mg
Kellogg's Complete Bran Flakes	240	1.3 g	64 g	613.3 mg
Kellogg's Special K	220	0 g	44 g	500 mg
Honey Nut Cheerios	240	3 g	48 g	540 mg
Wheaties	220	2 g	48 g	440 mg

a) Which cereal has the least amount of sodium per serving?

b) Which cereal has the greatest amount of fat?

c) Which cereal has the least amount of fat?

d) Find the average total carbohydrate in the cereals.

Careful examination of the table will give the answers.

a) To determine which cereal has the least amount of sodium, look down the column headed "Sodium" until you find the smallest number. That number is 440 mg. Then look across that row to find the brand of cereal, Wheaties.

b) To determine which cereal has the greatest amount of fat, look down the column headed "Fat" until you find the largest number. That number is 3 g. Then look across that row to find the cereal, Honey Nut Cheerios.

c) To determine which cereal has the least amount of fat, look down the column headed "Fat" until you find the smallest number. There are two listings of 0 g. Then look across those rows to find the cereals, Ralston Rice Chex and Kellogg's Special K.

d) Find the average of all the numbers in the column labeled "Total Carbohydrate":

$$\frac{54 + 64 + 44 + 48 + 48}{5} = 51.6.$$

The average total carbohydrate content is 51.6 g.

Do Exercises 1–5.

Objectives

a | Extract and interpret data from tables.

b | Extract and interpret data from pictographs.

c | Draw simple pictographs.

For Extra Help

TAPE 11   InterAct math   CD-ROM
            MAC
            WIN

Use the table in Example 1 to answer each of the following.

1. Which cereal has the most total carbohydrate?

   Kellogg's Complete Bran Flakes

2. Which cereal has the least total carbohydrate?

   Kellogg's Special K

3. Which cereal has the least number of calories?

   Kellogg's Special K, Wheaties

4. Which cereal has the greatest number of calories?

   Ralston Rice Chex, Kellogg's Complete Bran Flakes, Honey Nut Cheerios

5. Find the average amount of sodium in the cereals.

   510.66 mg

Answers on page A-14

Use the table in Example 2 to answer each of the following.

6. Which plan has the highest off-peak rate? AT&T, LCI

7. Which plan has a peak rate of 14¢/min. GTE

8. Using an off-peak rate of 8¢/min for MCI, find the average off-peak rate for the seven companies. 11.7¢/min

9. What is the average of the three most expensive off-peak rates? Round to the nearest tenth of a cent. 14.7¢/min

Example 2 *Phone Rates.* The following table shows the rates for several popular long-distance calling plans during a recent year.

Company	Plan	Peak Rate	Off-Peak Rate	Info Number
AT&T	One rate ☐1	15¢/min	15¢/min	800 222-0300
GTE	One Price	14	14	800 483-3737
Sprint	Sprint Sense	25	10	800 366-1044
LCI	One rate ☐2	15	15	800 860-2255
Matrix	SmartWorld	19.9	9.9	800 282-0242
MCI	MCI One	25	5–10	800 444-3333
WorldCom	Home Adv.	25	10	800 275-0100

☐1 With Plus plan, U.S. calls cost 10¢/min anytime, with a $4.95 monthly fee.

☐2 This plan costs an additional $1.00 per month.

a) Of the plans listed, which has the least expensive peak rate?

b) Of the plans listed, which has the least expensive off-peak rate?

c) Shannon has the Sprint Sense plan. She spoke for 50 min at the peak rate and for 75 min at the off-peak rate. What was the total cost for these calls?

d) For the plans listed, what is the average peak rate?

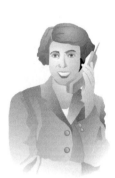

Careful examination of the table will give the answers.

a) To determine the least expensive peak rate, we look down the column labeled "Peak Rate" for the lowest rate listed. When we find that rate (14¢/min), we read across to the left and find that this rate is for the GTE One Price plan.

b) To determine which plan has the least expensive off-peak rate, we look down the column labeled "Off-Peak Rate" for the lowest rate listed. We note there that the lowest rate is part of a range, from 5¢ to 10¢ per minute. Next, we read across that line, to the left, and find that the MCI One plan has the lowest off-peak rate, 5¢/min.

c) Under the Sprint Sense plan, if Shannon spoke for 50 min at the peak rate, her bill for those minutes would be (50 min)(25¢/min), or $12.50. If she spoke for 75 min at the off-peak rate of 10¢/min, her bill for those minutes would be (75 min)(10¢/min), or $7.50. Altogether, 50 min at the peak rate and 75 min at the off-peak rate would cost $12.50 + $7.50, or $20.

d) To find the average peak rate of all the plans, we add the peak rates for the seven companies and then divide by 7:

$$\text{Average peak rate} = \frac{15¢ + 14¢ + 25¢ + 15¢ + 19.9¢ + 25¢ + 25¢}{7}$$

$$\approx 19.8¢/\text{min}. \quad \text{Rounding to the nearest tenth}$$

Do Exercises 6–9.

b Reading and Interpreting Pictographs

Pictographs (or *picture graphs*) are another way to show information. Instead of actually listing the amounts to be considered, a **pictograph** uses symbols to represent the amounts. In addition, a *key* is given telling what each symbol represents.

Example 3 *Coffee Consumption.* For selected countries, the following pictograph shows approximately how many cups of coffee each person (per capita) drinks annually. A key indicates that each symbol ☕ represents 100 cups.

Coffee Consumption (per Capita)

Source: Beverage Marketing Corporation and *The Statistical Abstract of the United States, 1997*

a) Determine the approximate annual coffee consumption per capita of Germany.

b) Which two countries have the greatest difference in coffee consumption? Estimate that difference.

We use the data from the pictograph as follows.

a) Germany's consumption is represented by 11 whole symbols (1100 cups) and, though it is visually debatable, about $\frac{1}{8}$ of another symbol (about 13 cups), for a total of 1113 cups.

b) Visually, we see that, of the countries listed, Switzerland has the most consumption and the United States the least. Switzerland's annual coffee consumption per capita is represented by 12 whole symbols (1200 cups) and about $\frac{1}{5}$ of another symbol (20 cups), for a total of 1220 cups. U.S. consumption is represented by 4 whole symbols (400 cups) and about $\frac{1}{3}$ of another symbol (33 cups), for a total of 433 cups. The difference between these amounts is $1220 - 433$, or 787 cups.

One advantage of pictographs is that the appropriate choice of a symbol will tell you, at a glance, the kind of measurement being made. Another advantage is that the comparison of amounts represented in the graph can be expressed more easily by just counting symbols. For instance, in Example 3, we can tell at a glance that the annual coffee consumption per capita in Germany is more than twice that of the United States.

One disadvantage of pictographs is that, in order to make a pictograph easy to read, we must generally round amounts to the unit that a symbol represents. Another disadvantage is that it is difficult to determine how much a partial symbol represents. A third disadvantage is that we must usually multiply to compute the amount represented, since the total amounts are rarely listed.

Do Exercises 10–12.

Use the pictograph in Example 3 to answer each of the following.

10. Approximate the annual coffee consumption per capita in France.

795 cups; answers may vary

11. Approximate the annual coffee consumption per capita in Italy. 750 cups; answers may vary

12. The approximate annual coffee consumption in Finland is about the same as the combined coffee consumption in Switzerland and the United States. What is the approximate coffee consumption in Finland?

1650 cups; answers may vary

Answers on page A-14

13. *Concert Revenue.* The following is a list of three other groups active during the same time and their total gross revenues. Draw a pictograph to represent the data.

Boyz II Men $43.2 million   (1995)
REM $38.7 million   (1995)
Kiss $43.6 million   (1996)

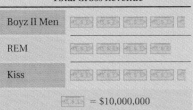

c   Drawing Pictographs

Example 4   *North American Concert Revenue.* The following is a list of the gross revenue (money taken in) during one year by five of the top concert acts for the years 1992–1998 (**Source:** *The World Almanac*). Draw a pictograph to represent the data. Let the symbol [🖼] represent $10,000,000.

The Rolling Stones	$121.2 million	(1994)
Pink Floyd	$103.5 million	(1994)
The Eagles	$79.4 million	(1994)
U2	$67.0 million	(1992)
The Grateful Dead	$52.4 million	(1994)

Some computation is necessary before we can draw the pictograph.

The Rolling Stones: Note that $121.2 \div 10 = 12.12$. Thus we need 12 whole symbols and 0.12 of another symbol. Now 0.12 is hard to draw, but we estimate it to be about $\frac{1}{10}$ of a symbol.

Pink Floyd: Note that $103.5 \div 10 = 10.35$. Thus we need 10 whole symbols and 0.35, or about $\frac{1}{3}$ of another symbol.

The Eagles: Note that $79.4 \div 10 = 7.94$. Thus we need 7 whole symbols and 0.94, or about $\frac{9}{10}$ of another symbol.

U2: Note that $67 \div 10 = 6.7$. Thus we need 6 whole symbols and $\frac{7}{10}$ of another symbol.

The Grateful Dead: Note that $52.4 \div 10 = 5.24$. Thus we need 5 whole symbols and 0.24, or about $\frac{1}{4}$ of another symbol.

The pictograph can now be drawn as follows. We list the concert act in one column, draw the monetary amounts using symbols, and title the overall graph "Total Gross Revenue."

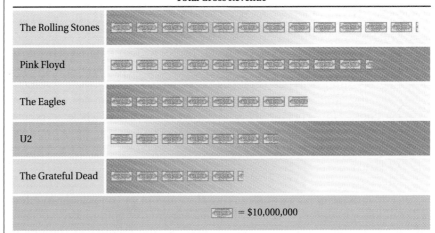

Do Exercise 13.

Answer on page A-14

Exercise Set 6.1

a *Astronomy.* Use the following table, which lists information about the planets, for Exercises 1–10.

Planet	Average Distance from Sun (in miles)	Diameter (in miles)	Length of Planet's Day in Earth Time (in days)	Time of Revolution in Earth Time (in years)
Mercury	35,983,000	3,031	58.82	0.24
Venus	67,237,700	7,520	224.59	0.62
Earth	92,955,900	7,926	1.00	1.00
Mars	141,634,800	4,221	1.03	1.88
Jupiter	483,612,200	88,846	0.41	11.86
Saturn	888,184,000	74,898	0.43	29.46
Uranus	1,782,000,000	31,763	0.45	84.01
Neptune	2,794,000,000	31,329	0.66	164.78
Pluto	3,666,000,000	1,423	6.41	248.53

Source: Handy Science Answer Book, Gale Research, Inc.

1. Find the average distance from the sun to Jupiter.

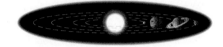

483,612,200 mi

2. How long is a day on Venus?   224.59 days

3. Which planet has a time of revolution of 164.78 yr?   Neptune

4. Which planet has a diameter of 4221 mi?   Mars

5. Which planets have an average distance from the sun that is greater than 1,000,000 mi?   All

6. Which planets have a diameter that is less than 100,000 mi?   All

7. About how many earth diameters would it take to equal the diameter of Jupiter?   11

8. How much longer is the longest time of revolution than the shortest?   248.29 yr

9. What is the average diameter of a planet?
27,884.$\overline{1}$ mi

10. What is the average distance from the sun to a planet?   1,105,734,178 mi

Global Warming. Ecologists are increasingly concerned about global warming, that is, the trend of average global temperatures to rise over recent years. One possible effect is the melting of the polar icecaps. Use the following table for Exercises 11–18.

Year	Average Global Temperature (°F)
1986	59.29°
1987	59.58°
1988	59.63°
1989	59.45°
1990	59.85°
1991	59.74°
1992	59.23°
1993	59.36°
1994	59.56°
1995	59.72°
1996	59.58°

Source: Vital Signs, 1997

11. In what year was the average global temperature the lowest?   1992

12. In what year was the average global temperature the highest?   1990

13. Find the average global temperatures for 1986 and 1987.   59.29°, 59.58°

14. Find the average global temperatures for 1992 and 1993.   59.23°, 59.36°

15. Find the average of the average global temperatures for the years 1986 through 1988. Find the eight-year average global temperature for the years 1989 through 1996. By how many degrees does the latter average exceed the former?

59.50°; 59.56125°; 0.06125°

16. Find the average of the average global temperatures for the years 1994 to 1996. Find the ten-year average global temperature for the years 1987 to 1996. By how many degrees does the former average exceed the latter?   59.62°; 59.57°; 0.05°

17. Between which two years did the average global temperature increase the most?   1989 and 1990

18. Between which two years did the average global temperature decrease the most?   1991 and 1992

b *World Population Growth.* The following pictograph shows world population in various years. Use the pictograph for Exercises 19–26.

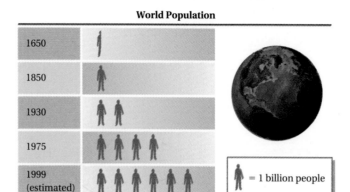

World Population

1650	
1850	
1930	
1975	
1999 (estimated)	

= 1 billion people

19. What was the world population in 1850?   1.0 billion

20. What was the world population in 1975?   4.0 billion

21. In which year is the population the greatest?
1999

22. In which year was the population the least?   1650

23. Between which two years was the amount of growth the least?   1650 and 1850

24. Between which two years was the amount of growth the greatest?   1930 and 1975, or 1975 and 1999

25. How much greater will the world population in 1999 be than in 1975?

2.0 billion

26. How much greater will the world population be in 1999 than in 1930?

4.0 billion

TV News Magazine Programs. The number of network news magazine programs has increased dramatically since the early 1980s when there were just two—ABC's "20/20" and CBS's "60 Minutes." In the pictograph below, each symbol represents a 1-hr prime-time news magazine in the network's weekly fall schedule. Use the pictograph for Exercises 27–34.

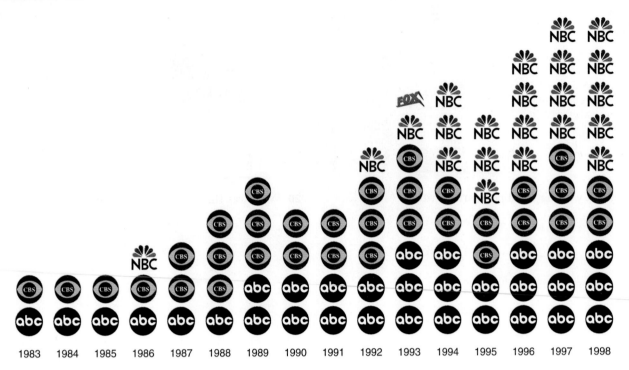

Sources: "Total Television," by Alex McNeil. Penguin Books; The Hollywood Reporter; Fox Broadcasting.
The New York Times, June 8, 1998

27. In which year was there exactly 7 hr of prime-time news magazine programming per week?   1995

28. In which year was there exactly 5 hr of prime-time news magazine programming per week?   1989

29. How many hours per week of prime-time news magazine programming were there in 1994?   8 hr

30. How many hours per week of prime-time news magazine programming were there in 1997?   10 hr

31. How much did prime-time news magazine programming increase from 1991 through 1993?

4 hr/wk

32. How much did prime-time news magazine programming increase from 1991 through 1997?

6 hr/wk

33. Between which two years did weekly prime-time news magazine programming increase the most?

1991 and 1992, or 1992 and 1993, or 1995 and 1996

34. Between which two years did weekly news magazine programming first decrease?

1989 and 1990

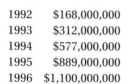

35. *Lettuce Sales.* The sales of lettuce have experienced a tremendous increase in recent years due to the convenience of prepackaged, prewashed, and prechopped lettuce. Sales for recent years are listed below (***Source:*** International Fresh-Cut Produce Association). Draw a pictograph to represent lettuce sales for these years. Use the symbol to represent $100,000,000.

1992	$168,000,000
1993	$312,000,000
1994	$577,000,000
1995	$889,000,000
1996	$1,100,000,000

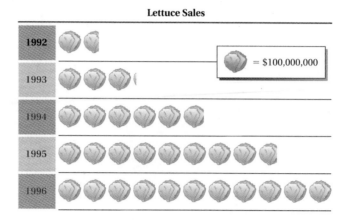

Skill Maintenance

Solve.

36. $9x - 5 = -23$ [4.4a] -2

37. $3x - 2 = 7x + 10$ [5.7b] -3

38. $-4x = 3x - 7$ [5.7b] 1

Convert to decimal notation.   [5.5a]

39. $\dfrac{3}{8}$ 0.375

40. $\dfrac{3}{50}$ 0.06

41. $\dfrac{29}{25}$ 1.16

42. $\dfrac{5}{6}$ $0.8\overline{3}$

43. ◈ Loreena is drawing a pictograph in which dollar bills are used as symbols to represent the tuition at various private colleges. Should each dollar bill represent $10,000, $5000, or $500? Why?

44. ◈ Suppose you are drawing a pictograph in which stopwatches are used as symbols to represent the number of minutes each of three professors spends on the phone each month. Should each stopwatch represent 1 min, 10 min, or 100 min? Why?

45. ◈ What advantage(s) does a table have over a pictograph?

46. Redraw the pictograph appearing in Example 3 as one in which each symbol represents 150 cups of coffee.

Coffee Consumption

47. Use the pictograph from Exercises 27–34 to determine the average yearly increase in prime-time news magazine programming for the years 1983 to 1998. (For example, the yearly increase between 1991 and 1992 was 2 hr.) $0.5\overline{3}$ hr

48. Refer to the table in Example 2. Bridget spoke the same number of minutes at the peak rate as she did at the off-peak rate. If her Sprint Sense bill was for $42, how many minutes did she speak for at each rate?   120 min

6.2 Bar Graphs and Line Graphs

Beginning in Chapter 1, we have used *bar graphs* to convey information (see pages 3, 61, 262, 282, 304, and 333). In this section, we make further use of bar graphs and also introduce *line graphs*.

a Reading and Interpreting Bar Graphs

Example 1 *Fat Content in Fast Foods.* Wendy's Hamburgers is a national chain of fast-food restaurants. The following bar graph shows the fat content of various sandwiches sold by Wendy's.

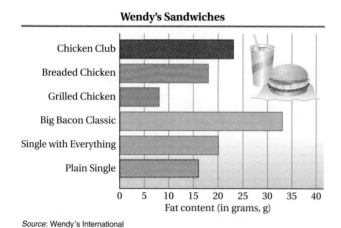

Wendy's Sandwiches

Source: Wendy's International

a) About how much fat is in a Chicken Club sandwich?

b) Which sandwich contains the least amount of fat?

c) Which sandwich contains about 20 g of fat?

We look at the graph to answer the questions.

a) We move to the right along the bar representing Chicken Club sandwiches. We can read, fairly accurately, that there is approximately 23 g of fat in the Chicken Club sandwich.

b) The shortest bar is for the Grilled Chicken sandwich. Thus that sandwich contains the least amount of fat.

c) We locate the line representing 20 g and then go up until we reach a bar that ends at approximately 20 g. We then go across to the left and read the name of the sandwich, which is the Single with Everything.

Do Exercises 1–3.

Use the bar graph in Example 1 to answer each of the following.

1. About how much fat is in the plain single sandwich?

16 g

2. Which sandwich contains the greatest amount of fat?

Big Bacon Classic

3. Which sandwiches contain 20 g or more of fat?

Chicken Club, Big Bacon Classic, Single with Everything

Answers on page A-15

Use the bar graph in Example 2 to answer each of the following.

4. Approximately how many women, per 100,000, develop breast cancer between the ages of 35 and 39?

60

5. In what age group is the mortality rate the highest?

85+

6. In what age group do about 350 out of every 100,000 women develop breast cancer?

60–64

7. Does the breast-cancer mortality rate seem to increase from the youngest to the oldest age group?

Yes

Answers on page A-15

Bar graphs are often drawn vertically and sometimes a double bar graph is used to make comparisons.

Example 2 *Breast Cancer.* The following graph indicates the incidence and mortality rates of breast cancer for women of various age groups.

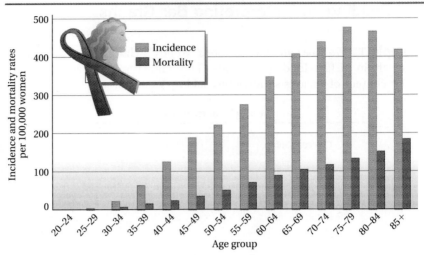

When Breast Cancer Strikes

Source: National Cancer Institute

a) Approximately how many women, per 100,000, develop breast cancer between the ages of 40 and 44?

b) In what age range is the mortality rate for breast cancer approximately 100 for every 100,000 women?

c) In what age range is the incidence of breast cancer the highest?

d) Does the incidence of breast cancer always increase from the younger to older age groups?

We look at the graph to answer the questions.

a) We go to the right, across the bottom, to the green bar above the age group 40–44. Next, we go up to the top of that bar and, from there, back to the left to read approximately 130 on the vertical scale. About 130 out of every 100,000 women develop breast cancer between the ages of 40 and 44.

b) We read up the vertical scale to the number 100. From there we move to the right until we come to the top of a red bar. Moving down that bar, we find that in the 65–69 age group, about 100 out of every 100,000 women die of breast cancer.

c) We look for the tallest green bar and read the age range below it. The incidence of breast cancer is highest for women in the 75–79 age group.

d) Looking at the heights of the bars, we see that the incidence of breast cancer actually *decreases* after ages 75–79. Thus the incidence of breast cancer does not always increase from the younger to older age groups.

Do Exercises 4–7.

b | Drawing Bar Graphs

Example 3 *Centenarians.* The number of centenarians—that is, people 100 yr or older—is growing rapidly. Projections from the U.S. Bureau of the Census and the National Center for Health Statistics are shown below. Use the projections to form a bar graph.

Year	Projected Number of Centenarians
2000	72,000
2010	131,000
2020	214,000
2030	324,000
2040	447,000
2050	834,000

Source: The New York Times, 6/22/98, p. A14

First, we draw a horizontal scale with six equally spaced intervals and the different years listed. We title that scale "Year." (See the figure on the left below.) Next, we label the vertical scale "Projected Number (in thousands)." Note that the largest number (in thousands) is 834 and the smallest is 72. If we count by 100s, we can range from 0 to 900 with just nine marks. Finally, we draw vertical bars to represent the number of centenarians projected for each year and title the graph. (See the figure on the right below.)

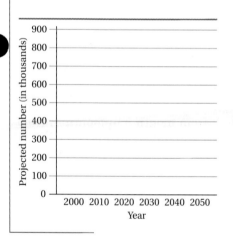

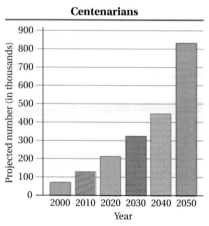

Do Exercise 8.

8. *Planetary Moons.* Make a horizontal bar graph to show the number of moons orbiting the various planets.

Planet	Number of Moons
Earth	1
Mars	2
Jupiter	16
Saturn	18
Uranus	15
Neptune	8
Pluto	1

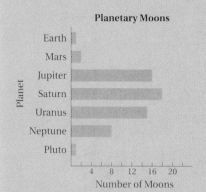

Answer on page A-15

Use the line graph in Example 4 to answer each of the following.

9. For which month were new home sales lowest?

Month 7

10. Between which months did new home sales decrease?

Months 1 and 2, 4 and 5, 6 and 7, 11 and 12

11. For which months were new home sales below 700 thousand?

Months 2, 5, 6, 7, 8, 9, 12

Answers on page A-15

c | Reading and Interpreting Line Graphs

Line graphs are often used to show a change over time as well as to indicate patterns or trends.

Example 4 *New Home Sales.* The following line graph shows the number of new home sales, in thousands, over a recent twelve-month period. The jagged line at the base of the vertical scale indicates an unnecessary portion of the scale. Note that the vertical scale differs from the horizontal scale so that the data can be easily shown.

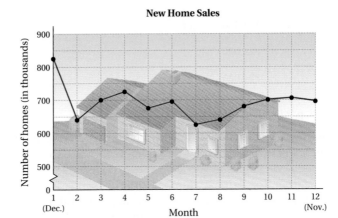

New Home Sales

Source: U.S. Department of Commerce

a) For which month were new home sales the greatest?

b) Between which months did new home sales increase?

c) For which months were new home sales about 700 thousand?

We look at the graph to answer the questions.

a) The greatest number of new home sales was about 825 thousand in month 1.

b) Reading the graph from left to right, we see that new home sales increased from month 2 to month 3, from month 3 to month 4, from month 5 to month 6, from month 7 to month 8, from month 8 to month 9, from month 9 to month 10, and from month 10 to month 11.

c) We look from left to right along the line at 700.

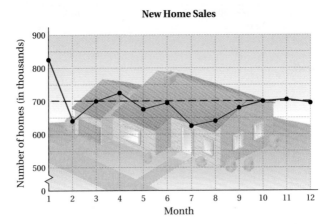

New Home Sales

We see that points are closest to 700 thousand at months 3, 6, 10, 11, and 12.

Do Exercises 9–11.

d | Drawing Line Graphs

Example 5 *Movie Releases.* Draw a line graph to show how the number of movies released each year has changed over a period of 6 yr. Use the following data (**Source**: Motion Picture Association of America).

1991:	164 movies
1992:	150 movies
1993:	161 movies
1994:	184 movies
1995:	234 movies
1996:	260 movies

First, we indicate on the horizontal scale the different years and title it "Year." (See the graph below.) Then we mark the vertical scale appropriately by 50s to show the number of movies released and title it "Number per Year." We also give the overall title "Movies Released" to the graph.

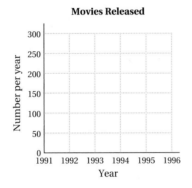

Next, we mark at the appropriate level above each year the points that indicate the number of movies released. Then we draw line segments connecting the points. The change over time can now be observed easily from the graph.

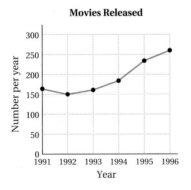

Do Exercise 12.

---

12. *SAT Scores.* Draw a line graph to show how the average combined verbal–math SAT score has changed over a period of 6 yr. Use the following data (**Source**: The College Board).

1991:	999
1992:	1001
1993:	1003
1994:	1003
1995:	1010
1996:	1013
1997:	1016

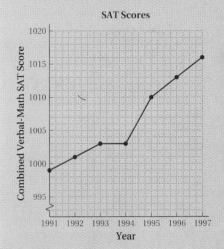

Answer on page A-15

Improving Your Math Study Skills

How Many Women Have Won the Ultimate Math Contest?

Although this Study Skill feature does not contain specific tips on studying mathematics, we hope that you will find this 1997 article both challenging and encouraging.

Every year on college campuses across the United States and Canada, the most brilliant math students face the ultimate challenge. For six hours, they struggle with problems from the merely intractable to the seemingly impossible.

Every spring, five are chosen winners of the William Lowell Putnam Mathematical Competition, the Olympics of college mathematics. Every year for 56 years, all have been men.

Until this year.

This spring, Ioana Dumitriu (pronounced yo-AHN-na doo-mee-TREE-oo), 20, a New York University sophomore from Romania, became the first woman to win the award.

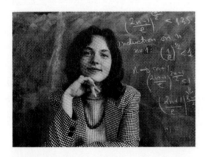

Ms. Dumitriu, the daughter of two electrical engineering professors in Romania, who as a girl solved math puzzles for fun, was identified as a math talent early in her schooling in Bucharest. At 11, Ms. Dumitriu was steered into years of math training camps as preparation for the Romanian entry in the International Mathematics Olympiad.

It was this training, and a handsome young coach, that led her to New York City. He was several years older. They fell in love. He chose N.Y.U. for its graduate school in mathematics, and at 19 she joined him in New York.

The test Ms. Dumitriu won is dauntingly difficult, even for math majors. About half of the 2,407 test-takers scored 2 or less of a possible 120, and a third scored 0. Some students simply walk out after staring at the questions for a while.

Ms. Dumitriu said that in the six hours allotted, she had time to do 8 of the 12 problems, each worth a maximum of 10 points. The last one she did in 10 minutes. This year, Ms. Dumitriu and her five co-winners (there was a tie for fifth place) scored between 76 and 98. She does not know her exact score or rank because the organizers do not announce them.

"I didn't ever tell myself that I was unlikely to win, that no woman before had ever won and therefore I couldn't," she said. "It is not that I forget that I'm a woman. It's just that I don't see it as an obstacle or a ——."

Her English is near-perfect, but she paused because she could not find the right word. "The mathematics community is made up of persons, and that is what I am primarily."

Prof. Joel Spencer, who was a Putnam winner himself, said her work for his class in problem solving last year was remarkable. "What really got me was her fearlessness," he said. "To be good at math, you have to go right at it and start playing around with it, and she had that from the start."

In the graduate lounge in the Courant Institute of Mathematical Sciences at N.Y.U., Ms. Dumitriu, a tall, striking redhead, stands out. Instead of jeans and T-shirts, she wears gray pin-striped slacks and a rust-colored turtleneck and vest.

"There is a social perception of women and math, a stereotype," Ms. Dumitriu said during an interview. "What's happening right now is that the stereotype is defied. It starts breaking."

Still, even as women began to flock to sciences, math has remained largely a male bastion.

"Math remains the bottom line of sex differences for many," said Sheila Tobias, author of "Overcoming Math Anxiety" (W.W. Norton & Company, 1994). "It's one thing for women to write books, negotiate bills through Congress, litigate, fire missiles; quite another for them to do math."

Besides collecting the $1,000 awarded to each Putnam fellow, Ms. Dumitriu also won the $500 Elizabeth Lowell Putnam prize for the top woman finisher for the second year in a row, a prize created five years ago to encourage women to take the test. This year 414 did.

In her view, there are never too many problems, never too much practice.

Besides, each new problem holds its own allure: "When you have all the pieces and you put them together and you see the puzzle, that moment always amazes me."

Exercise Set 6.2

a *Chocolate Sweets.* The following horizontal bar graph shows the average caloric content of various kinds of chocolate foods or beverages. Use the bar graph for Exercises 1–12.

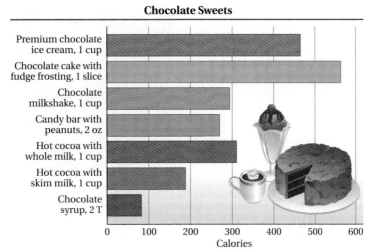

Chocolate Sweets

Source: *Better Homes and Gardens*, December 1996

1. Estimate how many calories there are in 1 cup of hot cocoa with skim milk.   190

2. Estimate how many calories there are in 1 cup of premium chocolate ice cream.   460

3. Which food or beverage has the highest caloric content?

   1 slice of chocolate cake with fudge frosting

4. Which food or beverage has the lowest caloric content?

   2 T of chocolate syrup

5. Which food or beverage contains about 460 calories?

   1 cup of premium chocolate ice cream

6. Which foods or beverages contain about 300 calories?

   1 cup of chocolate milkshake, 1 cup of hot cocoa made with whole milk

7. How many more calories are there in 1 cup of hot cocoa made with whole milk than in 1 cup of hot cocoa made with skim milk?   120 calories

8. Fred generally drinks a 4-cup chocolate milkshake. How many calories does he consume?   1160 calories

9. Kristin likes to eat 2 cups of premium chocolate ice cream in the course of a weekend. How many calories does she consume?   920 calories

10. Barney likes to eat a 6-oz chocolate bar with peanuts for lunch. How many calories does he consume?   810 calories

11. Paul adds a 2-oz chocolate bar with peanuts to his diet each day for 1 yr (365 days) and makes no other changes in his eating or exercise habits. Consumption of 3500 extra calories will add about 1 lb to his body weight. How many pounds will he gain? 28 lb

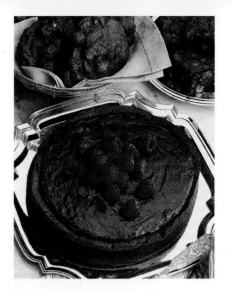

12. Tricia adds one slice of chocolate cake with fudge frosting to her diet each day for 1 yr (365 days) and makes no other changes in her eating or exercise habits. Consumption of 3500 extra calories will add about 1 lb to her body weight. How many pounds will she gain? 58 lb

Deforestation. The world is gradually losing its tropical forests. The following triple bar graph shows the amount of forested land of three tropical regions in the years 1980 and 1990. Use the bar graph for Exercises 13–20.

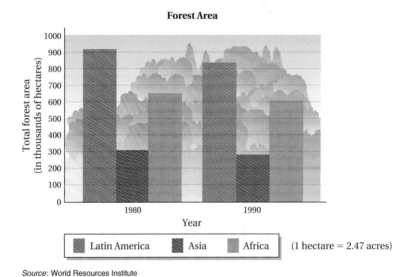

Forest Area

(1 hectare = 2.47 acres)

Legend: Latin America, Asia, Africa

Source: World Resources Institute

13. What was the forest area of Latin America in 1980?
920,000 hectares

14. What was the forest area of Africa in 1990?
600,000 hectares

15. Which region experienced the greatest loss of forest area from 1980 to 1990? Latin America

16. Which region experienced the smallest loss of forest area from 1980 to 1990? Asia

17. Which region had a forest area of about 600 thousand hectares in 1990? Africa

18. Which region had a forest area of about 300 thousand hectares in 1980? Asia

19. What was the average forest area in Latin America for the two years? 880,000 hectares

20. What was the average forest area in Asia for the two years? 290,000 hectares

b

21. *Commuting Time.* The following table lists the average commuting time in several metropolitan areas with more than 1 million people. Make a vertical bar graph to illustrate the data.

City	Commuting Time (in minutes)
New York	30.6
Los Angeles	26.4
Phoenix	23.0
Dallas	24.1
Indianapolis	21.9
Orlando	22.9

Source: Census Bureau

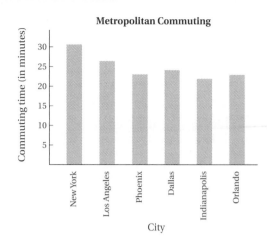

Use the data and the bar graph in Exercise 21 for Exercises 22–25.

22. Which city has the greatest commuting time?

New York

23. Which city has the least commuting time?

Indianapolis

24. What is the average commuting time for all six cities? Round to the nearest tenth.   24.8 min

25. What is the average commuting time for New York and Los Angeles?   28.5 min

26. *Calorie Expenditure.* Use the following information to make a horizontal bar graph showing the number of calories burned during each activity by a person weighing 152 lb.

Tennis: 420 calories per hour

Jogging: 650 calories per hour

Hiking: 590 calories per hour

Office work: 180 calories per hour

Sleeping: 70 calories per hour

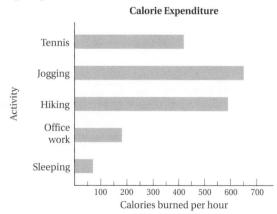

Use the data and the bar graph in Exercise 26 for Exercises 27–30.

27. What is the difference in the number of calories burned per hour between sleeping and jogging?

580 calories

28. Suppose you were trying to lose weight by exercising and had to choose one of these exercises. If your doctor told you not to jog, what would be the most beneficial exercise?   Hiking

29. Ryan works at the office for 8 hr and then sleeps for 7 hr. How many calories does Ryan burn doing this?   1930 calories

30. Nancy hiked for 6 hr and then slept for 8 hr. How many calories did she burn doing this?   4100 calories

c *Average Salary of Major-League Baseball Players.* The following graph shows the average salary of major-league baseball players over a recent 8-yr period. Use the graph for Exercises 31–36.

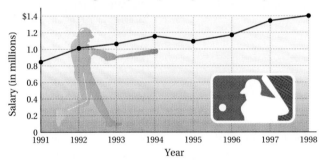

Average Salary of Major League Baseball Players

31. In which year was the average salary the highest?

1998

32. In which year was the average salary the lowest?

1991

33. What was the difference in salary between the highest and lowest salaries?   About $0.55 million

34. Between which two years was the increase in salary the greatest?   1996 and 1997

35. Between which two years did the salary decrease?

1994 and 1995

36. In what year was the average salary about $1.2 million?   1996

37. *Ozone Layer.* Make a line graph of the data, listing years on the horizontal scale.

Year	Ozone Level (in parts per billion)
1991	2981
1992	3133
1993	3148
1994	3138
1995	3124

Source: National Oceanic and Atmospheric Administration

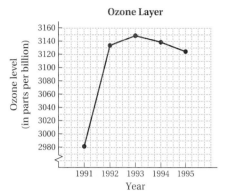

Use the data and the line graph in Exercise 37 for Exercises 38–41.

38. Between which two years was the increase in the ozone level the greatest?   1991 and 1992

39. Between which two years was the decrease in the ozone level the greatest?   1994 and 1995

40. What was the average ozone level over the 5-yr period?   3104.8 parts per billion

41. What was the average ozone level from 1992 through 1995?   3135.75 parts per billion

42. *Motion Picture Expense.* Make a line graph of the data, listing years on the horizontal scale.

Year	Average Expense per Picture (in millions)
1991	$38.2
1992	42.4
1993	44.0
1994	50.4
1995	54.1
1996	61.0

Source: Motion Picture Association of America

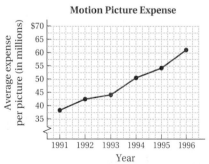

Use the data and the line graph in Exercise 42 for Exercises 43–46.

43. Between which two years was the increase in motion-picture expense the greatest? 1995 and 1996

44. Between which two years was the increase in motion-picture expense the least? 1992 and 1993

45. What was the average motion-picture expense over the 6-yr period? $48.35 million

46. What was the average motion-picture expense from 1994 through 1996? Round to the nearest tenth of a million dollars. $55.2 million

---

Skill Maintenance

47. How many 12-oz bottles can be filled from a vat containing 408 oz of catsup? [1.8a] 34

48. It is known to operators of pizza restaurants that if 50 pizzas are ordered in an evening, people will request extra cheese on 9 of them. What fraction of the pizzas sold are ordered with extra cheese? [3.3b] $\frac{9}{50}$

49. A can of Coca-Cola contains 12 fluid ounces. How many fluid ounces are in a six-pack? [1.8a] 72 fl oz

50. 24 is $\frac{3}{4}$ of what number? [3.4c] 32

51. $\frac{2}{3}$ of 75 is what number? [3.4c] 50

52. $\frac{3}{5}$ of 30 is what number? [3.4c] 18

Synthesis

53. ◆ Can bar graphs always, sometimes, or never be converted to line graphs? Why?

54. ◆ Consider the graph in Example 4. Sam states that the initial drop shows that sales were nearly cut in half over the first month of the year. What mistake is Sam making?

55. ◆ Using the data in Exercise 42, how could someone make a reasonable estimate of the average expense per motion picture in 1998?

56. ▦ Bonnie eats a 700-Cal breakfast, jogs for 45 min, works in her office for $2\frac{1}{2}$ hr, and eats a 615-Cal lunch. She then works for another $5\frac{1}{2}$ hr before eating a 235-Cal snack and playing tennis for 40 min. If Bonnie weighs 152 lb (see Exercise 26), how many calories has she lost or gained in the course of the day? Lost 657.5 calories

57. ▦ Use the information in Example 2 to approximate the average rate of incidence of breast cancer for all women above the age of 24. 268 per 100,000

Analyze class grades using line graphs and bar graphs.

6.3 Ordered Pairs and Equations in Two Variables

Bar graphs and line graphs are used to illustrate relationships between the items or quantities listed along the bottom and the side of the graph. The horizontal and vertical sides of a bar graph or line graph are often called the **axes** (pronounced ăk´ sēź; singular: **axis**). By using two perpendicular number lines as axes, we can use points to represent solutions of certain equations. First, however, we must learn to graph points.

a | Points and Ordered Pairs

When two number lines are used as axes, a grid can be formed. The grid provides a helpful way of locating any point on the plane. Just as a location in a city might be given as the intersection of an avenue and a side street, a point on a plane can be regarded as the intersection of a vertical line and a horizontal line. In the figure below, these lines pass through 3 on the horizontal axis and 4 on the vertical axis. Thus the **first coordinate** of this point is 3 and the **second coordinate** is 4. **Ordered pair** notation, (3, 4), provides a quick way of listing these coordinates.

> **CAUTION!** When writing an ordered pair, you should always list the coordinate from the horizontal axis first.

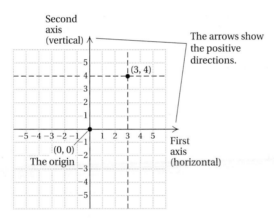

The point (0, 0), where the axes cross each other, is called the **origin**. To graph, or *plot*, the point (3, 4), we can begin at the origin and move horizontally (along the first axis) to the number 3. From there, we move up 4 units vertically and make a "dot."

It is important to always make sure that the first coordinate matches the number that would be below (or above) the point on the horizontal axis. Similarly, the second coordinate should always match the number that would be to the left (or right) of the point on the vertical axis.

Do Exercises 1 and 2.

Objectives

a Plot a point, given its coordinates. Find coordinates, given a point.

b Determine the quadrant in which a point lies.

c Determine whether an ordered pair is a solution of an equation with two variables.

For Extra Help

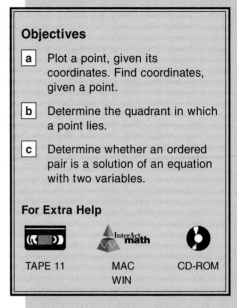

TAPE 11   MAC WIN   CD-ROM

Plot these points on the graph below.

1.

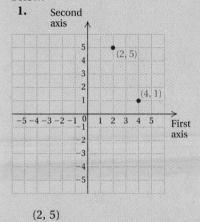

(2, 5)

2. (4, 1)

Answers on page A-15

Plot these points on the graph below.

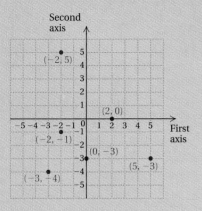

3. (−2, 5)

4. (−3, −4)

5. (5, −3)

6. (−2, −1)

7. (0, −3)

8. (2, 0)

9. Find the coordinates of points *A, B, C, D, E, F,* and *G* on the graph below.

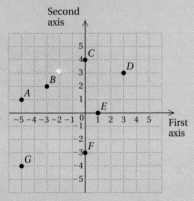

A: (−5, 1); *B*: (−3, 2); *C*: (0, 4); *D*: (3, 3); *E*: (1, 0); *F*: (0, −3); *G*: (−5, −4)

Answers on page A-16

Example 1 Plot the points (−5, 2) and (2, −5).

To plot (−5, 2), we locate −5 on the first, or horizontal, axis. Then we go up 2 units and make a dot.

To plot (2, −5), we locate 2 on the first, or horizontal, axis. Then we go down 5 units and make a dot. Note that the order of the numbers within a pair is important: (2, −5) ≠ (−5, 2).

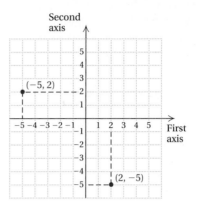

Do Exercises 3–8.

To find the coordinates of a given point, we first look above (or below) the point and list the point's horizontal coordinate. Then we look to the left (or right) of the point and list the vertical coordinate.

Example 2 Find the coordinates of points *A, B, C, D, E, F,* and *G.*

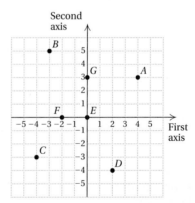

We look below point *A* to see that its first coordinate is 4. Looking to the left of point *A*, we find that its second coordinate is 3. Thus the coordinates of point *A* are (4, 3). The coordinates of the other points are given below.

B: (−3, 5);   *C*: (−4, −3);   *D*: (2, −4);

E: (0, 0);   *F*: (−2, 0);   *G*: (0, 3).

Do Exercise 9.

b | Quadrants

The axes divide the plane into four regions, or **quadrants**. In region I (the *first quadrant*), both coordinates of any point are positive. In region II (the *second quadrant*), the first coordinate is negative and the second coordinate is positive. In region III (the *third quadrant*), both coordinates are negative. In region IV (the *fourth quadrant*), the first coordinate is positive and the second coordinate is negative.

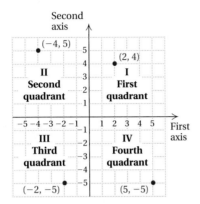

As the figure above illustrates, the point (2, 4) is in the first quadrant, (−4, 5) is in the second quadrant, (−2, −5) is in the third quadrant, and (5, −5) is in the fourth quadrant.

Do Exercises 10–15.

c | Solutions of Equations

The coordinate system we have just introduced is called the **Cartesian** coordinate system, in honor of the great mathematician and philosopher René Descartes (1596–1650). Descartes devised this coordinate system in part as a method of presenting solutions of equations containing two variables. Equations like $3x + 2y = 8$ have ordered pairs as solutions. In Section 6.4, we will find solutions and graph them. Here we simply practice checking to see if an ordered pair is a solution.

To determine whether an ordered pair is a solution of an equation, we substitute the first coordinate for the letter that comes first alphabetically and the second coordinate for the letter that is last alphabetically. The letters x and y are used most often.

Example 3 Determine whether the ordered pair (2, 1) is a solution of the equation $3x + 2y = 8$.

We substitute:

$$\frac{3x + 2y = 8}{}$$

$$3 \cdot 2 + 2 \cdot 1 \ ? \ 8 \qquad \text{Substituting 2 for } x \text{ and 1 for } y$$
$$6 + 2 \qquad \qquad \text{(alphabetical order of variables)}$$
$$8 \ \big| \ 8 \qquad \text{TRUE}$$

Since the equation becomes true, (2, 1) is a solution.

In a similar manner, we can show that (0, 4) and (4, −2) are also solutions of $3x + 2y = 8$. In fact, there is an infinite number of solutions of $3x + 2y = 8$.

---

10. What can you say about the coordinates of a point in the third quadrant?

Both are negative numbers.

11. What can you say about the coordinates of a point in the fourth quadrant?

The first, or horizontal, coordinate is positive; the second, or vertical, coordinate is negative.

In which quadrant is the point located?

12. (5, 3)   I

13. (−6, −4)   III

14. (10, −14)   IV

15. (−13, 9)   II

Answers on page A-16

16. Determine whether (5, 1) is a solution of $y = 2x + 3$.   No

17. Determine whether (4, −1) is a solution of $3x + 2y = 10$.   Yes

Answers on page A-16

Example 4   Determine whether the ordered pair (−2, 3) is a solution of the equation $2t = 4s − 8$.

We substitute:

$$
\begin{array}{c|c}
\multicolumn{2}{c}{2t = 4s - 8} \\
\hline
2 \cdot 3 \;\; ? & 4(-2) - 8 \\
6 & -8 - 8 \\
6 & -16 \quad \text{FALSE}
\end{array}
$$

Substituting −2 for s and 3 for t

Since the equation becomes false, (−2, 3) is not a solution.

Do Exercises 16 and 17.

Calculator Spotlight

Solutions of equations in two variables can be easily checked on a calculator. For instance, to show that (5.1, −3.65) is a solution of $3x + 2y = 8$, on many calculators we press

[3] [×] [5] [.] [1] [+] [2] [×] [3] [.] [6] [5] [+/−] [=] .

The result, 8, shows that (5.1, −3.65) is a solution.

Most calculators now have memory keys. These keys enable us to store and recall a number as needed. Any number being displayed can be stored by pressing a particular key. On many calculators, this key is labeled [STO], [M], or [Min]. Once a number has been stored, we can retrieve the number by pressing a key labeled [RCL] or [MR].

To show that (7.35, 10.7) is a solution of $2t = 4s − 8$, we can first evaluate the right side of the equation:

[4] [×] [7] [.] [3] [5] [−] [8] [=] [STO] .

The result, 21.4, has been stored in the calculator's memory, so we need not worry about writing it down. To complete the check, we clear the calculator and evaluate the left side of the equation:

[2] [×] [1] [0] [.] [7] [=] .

To show that this result matches the earlier number that was stored, we do not clear the display, but instead press

[−] [RCL] [=] .

The result, 0, indicates that 2 × 10.7 and 4 × 7.35 − 8 are equal. A result other than 0 would indicate that the ordered pair in question does not check.

Exercises

Determine whether each point is a solution of the given equation.

1. (7.9, 3.2); $5x + 4y = 52.3$ Yes
2. (1.9, 2.3); $7x − 8y = 5.1$ No
3. (4.3, 4.75); $5y = 6x − 7$ No
4. (3.8, −4.3); $9a = 17 − 4b$
5. (9.4, −3.9); $3a − 15 = 29 + 4b$
6. (5.6, 8.8); $4y + 23 = 7x + 19$
7. (−2.4, 8.5625); $3.5x + 17.4 = 3.2y − 18.4$
8. (1.8, 2.6); $9.2x − 15.3 = 4.8y − 13.7$

4. Yes   5. No   6. Yes   7. Yes   8. No

Exercise Set 6.3

a Plot each group of points on the given graph below.

1. (2, 5)   (−1, 3)   (3, −2)   (−2, −4)
(0, 4)   (0, −5)   (5, 0)   (−5, 0)

2. (4, 4)   (−2, 4)   (5, −3)   (−5, −5)
(0, 4)   (0, −4)   (3, 0)   (−4, 0)

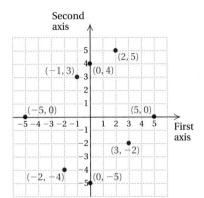

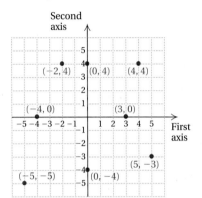

3. (−3, −1)   (5, 1)   (−1, −5)   (0, 0)
(0, 1)   (−4, 0) $\left(2, 3\frac{1}{2}\right)$ $\left(4\frac{1}{2}, -2\right)$

4. (−2, −4)   (5, −4) $\left(0, 3\frac{1}{2}\right)$ $\left(4, 3\frac{1}{2}\right)$
(−1, −3)   (−1, 5)   (4, −1)   (−2, 0)

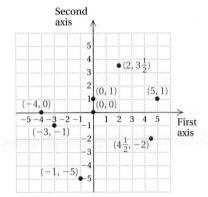

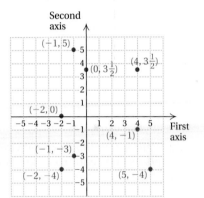

Find the coordinates of points *A, B, C, D, E,* and *F*.

5.

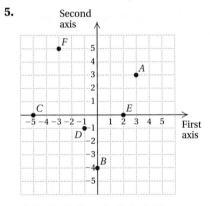

A: (3, 3); *B*: (0, −4); *C*: (−5, 0);
D: (−1, −1); *E*: (2, 0); *F*: (−3, 5)

6.

A: (4, 1); *B*: (0, −5); *C*: (−4, 0);
D: (−3, −2); *E*: (3, 0); *F*: (1, 5)

7.

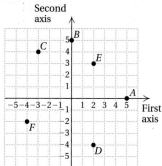

A: (5, 0); B: (0, 5); C: (−3, 4);
D: (2, −4); E: (2, 3); F: (−4, −2)

8.

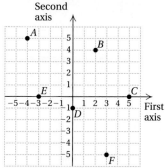

A: (−4, 5); B: (2, 4); C: (5, 0);
D: (0, −1); E: (−3, 0); F: (3, −5)

b In which quadrant is each point located?

9. (−5, 3)   II

10. (−12, 1)   II

11. (100, −1)   IV

12. $\left(35\frac{1}{2}, -2\frac{1}{2}\right)$ IV

13. (−6.5, −1.9)   III

14. (−3.4, −5.9)   III

15. $\left(3\frac{7}{10}, 9\frac{1}{11}\right)$ I

16. (1895, 1492)   I

Complete each sentence using the words *positive* or *negative* or the numerals I, II, III, or IV.

17. In quadrant IV, first coordinates are always _____ and second coordinates are always _____.   Positive; negative

18. In quadrant III, first coordinates are always _____ and second coordinates are always _____.   Negative; negative

19. In quadrant _____, both coordinates are always negative.   III

20. In quadrant _____, both coordinates are always positive.   I

21. In quadrants I and _____, the first coordinate is always _____.   IV; positive

22. In quadrants II and _____, the second coordinate is always _____.   I; positive

$\boxed{\text{c}}$ Determine whether each ordered pair is a solution of the given equation.

23. $(2, 7)$; $\quad y = 3x + 1$ Yes

24. $(1, 7)$; $\quad y = 2x + 5$ Yes

25. $(2, -3)$; $\quad 3x - y = 4$ No

26. $(-1, 4)$; $\quad 2x + y = 6$ No

27. $(-2, -1)$; $\quad 2c + 3d = -7$ Yes

28. $(0, -4)$; $\quad 4p + 2q = -9$ No

29. $(5, -4)$; $\quad 3x + y = 19$ No

30. $(-1, 7)$; $\quad x - y = -8$ Yes

31. $\left(2\frac{1}{3}, 5\right)$; $\quad 2q - 3p = 3$ Yes

32. $\left(3, 1\frac{1}{4}\right)$; $\quad 2p - 4q = 1$ Yes

33. $(2.4, 0.7)$; $\quad y = 5x - 6.3$ No

34. $(1.8, 7.4)$; $\quad y = 3x + 2$ Yes

Skill Maintenance

Solve.

35. $3x - 4 = 17$ [4.4a]   7

36. $7 + 2x = 25$ [4.4a]   9

37. $5(x - 2) = 3x - 4$ [5.7b]   3

38. Simplify: $\frac{90}{51}$.   [3.5b] $\frac{30}{17}$

39. Combine like terms: [4.6b]

$$7\frac{2}{11}a - 5\frac{1}{3}a. \quad \frac{61}{33}a$$

40. Simplify: [2.7b]

$$3(x - 5) + 4x - 9. \quad 7x - 24$$

Synthesis

41. ◈ Under what conditions will the points (a, b) and (b, a) be in the same quadrant?

42. ◈ Describe in your own words how to plot the point (a, b).

43. ◈ In which quadrant, if any, is the point $(5, 0)$? Why?

Determine whether each ordered pair is a solution of the given equation.

44. ▦ $(-2.37, 1.23)$; $5.2x + 6.1y = -4.821$ Yes

45. ▦ $(4.16, -9.35)$; $6.5x - 7.2y = -94.36$ No

In Exercises 46–49, tell in which quadrant(s) the point could be located.

46. The first coordinate is positive.   I, IV

47. The second coordinate is negative.   III, IV

48. The first and second coordinates are equal.   I, III

49. The first coordinate is the opposite of the second coordinate.   II, IV

50. The points $(-1, 1)$, $(4, 1)$, and $(4, -5)$ are three vertices of a rectangle. Find the coordinates of the fourth vertex. $(-1, -5)$

51. A parallelogram is a four-sided polygon with two pairs of parallel sides. Three parallelograms share the vertices $(-2, -3)$, $(-1, 2)$, and $(4, -3)$. Find the fourth vertex of each parallelogram.

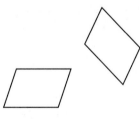

$(5, 2)$; $(-7, 2)$; $(3, -8)$

52. Graph eight points such that the sum of the coordinates in each pair is 6.   Answers may vary.

53. Graph eight points such that for each point the first coordinate minus the second coordinate is 1.

Answers may vary.

54. Find the perimeter of a rectangle with vertices at $(5, 3)$, $(5, -2)$, $(-3, -2)$, and $(-3, 3)$.   26

55. Find the area of a rectangle with vertices at $(0, 9)$, $(0, -4)$, $(5, -4)$, and $(5, 9)$.   65

Chapter 6   Introduction to Graphing and Statistics

Collaborative Learning Manual

Practice finding and plotting ordered pairs by playing a variation of the game Battleship.

6.4 Graphing Linear Equations

In Section 6.3, we saw how to determine whether an ordered pair is a solution of an equation in two variables. We now develop a way of finding such solutions on our own. Once we are able to find a few ordered pairs that solve an equation, we will be able to graph the equation.

a | Finding Solutions

To solve an equation with one variable, like $3x + 2 = 8$, we isolate the variable, x, on one side of the equation. To solve an equation with two variables, we will first replace one variable with some number choice and then solve the resulting equation.

Example 1   Find a solution of $x + y = 7$. Let $x = 5$.

If x is 5, then $x + y = 7$ can be rewritten as

$$5 + y = 7.$$

We solve as follows:

$$5 + y = 7$$
$$5 + y - 5 = 7 - 5 \qquad \text{Subtracting 5 or adding } -5 \text{ on both sides}$$
$$y = 2.$$

The ordered pair $(5, 2)$ is a solution of $x + y = 7$.

Do Exercise 1.

Example 2   Complete these solutions of $2x + 3y = 8$: (, 2); $(-2,$).

To complete the pair (, 2), we replace y with 2 and solve for x:

$$2x + 3y = 8$$
$$2x + 3 \cdot 2 = 8 \qquad \text{Substituting 2 for } y$$
$$2x + 6 = 8$$
$$2x + 6 - 6 = 8 - 6 \qquad \text{Subtracting 6 on both sides}$$
$$2x = 2$$
$$\tfrac{1}{2} \cdot 2x = \tfrac{1}{2} \cdot 2 \qquad \text{Multiplying by } \tfrac{1}{2} \text{ on both sides}$$
$$x = 1.$$

Thus, $(1, 2)$ is a solution of $2x + 3y = 8$.

To complete the pair $(-2,$), we replace x with -2 and solve for y:

$$2x + 3y = 8$$
$$2(-2) + 3y = 8 \qquad \text{Substituting } -2 \text{ for } x$$
$$-4 + 3y = 8$$
$$3y = 12 \qquad \text{Adding 4 on both sides}$$
$$y = 4. \qquad \text{Dividing by 3 on both sides}$$

Thus, $(-2, 4)$ is also a solution of $2x + 3y = 8$.

Do Exercise 2.

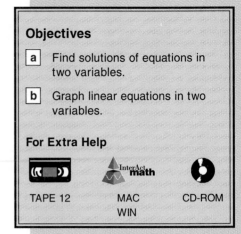

Objectives

a   Find solutions of equations in two variables.

b   Graph linear equations in two variables.

For Extra Help

TAPE 12   MAC   CD-ROM
                 WIN

1. Find a solution of $x - y = 3$. Let $y = 5$.   (8, 5)

2. Complete these solutions of $5x + y = 10$: $(1,$); ($, -5)$.

   (1, 5); (3, −5)

Answers on page A-16

3. Find three solutions of $x + 2y = 7$. Answers may vary.

(1, 3), (7, 0), (5, 1)

Example 3 Find three solutions of $2x - y = 5$.

We are free to choose *any* number as a replacement for x or y. To find one solution, we choose to replace x with 1. We then solve for y:

$$2x - y = 5$$
$$2 \cdot 1 - y = 5 \qquad \text{Substituting 1 for } x. \text{ Other choices are possible.}$$
$$2 - y = 5$$
$$-y = 3 \qquad \text{Subtracting 2 on both sides}$$
$$-1y = 3 \qquad \text{Recall that } -a = -1 \cdot a.$$
$$y = -3. \qquad \text{Dividing by } -1 \text{ on both sides}$$

Thus, $(1, -3)$ is one solution of $2x - y = 5$.

To find a second solution, we choose to replace y with 3 and solve for x:

$$2x - y = 5$$
$$2x - 3 = 5 \qquad \text{Substituting 3 for } y. \text{ Other choices are possible.}$$
$$2x = 8 \qquad \text{Adding 3 on both sides}$$
$$x = 4. \qquad \text{Dividing by 2 on both sides}$$

Thus, $(4, 3)$ is a second solution of $2x - y = 5$.

To find a third solution, we can replace x with 0 and solve for y:

$$2x - y = 5$$
$$2 \cdot 0 - y = 5 \qquad \text{Substituting 0 for } x. \text{ Other choices are possible.}$$
$$0 - y = 5$$
$$-y = 5$$
$$-1y = 5 \qquad \text{Try to do this step mentally.}$$
$$y = -5. \qquad \text{Dividing by } -1 \text{ on both sides}$$

The pair $(0, -5)$ is a third solution of $2x - y = 5$.

Note that three different choices for x or y would have given three different solutions. There is an infinite number of ordered pairs that are solutions, so it is unlikely for two students to have solutions that match entirely.

4. Find three solutions of $y = -2x + 7$. Answers may vary.

(0, 7), (2, 3), (−2, 11)

Do Exercises 3 and 4.

b Graphing Equations

Equations like those considered in Examples 1–3 are in the form $Ax + By = C$. All equations that can be written this way are said to be **linear** because the solutions of each equation, when graphed, form a straight line. When the appropriate line is drawn, we say that we have *graphed* the equation.

Example 4 Graph: $2x - y = 5$.

In Example 3, we found that $(1, -3)$, $(4, 3)$, and $(0, -5)$ are solutions of $2x - y = 5$. Had we not known that, before graphing we would need to calculate two or three solutions, much as we did in Example 3.

Answer on page A-16

Next, we plot the points and look for a pattern. As expected, the points describe a straight line. We draw the line, as shown on the right below.

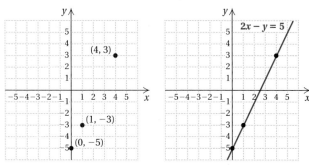

Note that two points are enough to determine a line, but if either point is calculated incorrectly, the wrong line will be drawn. For this reason, we generally calculate at least three ordered pairs before drawing a line. If when we plot these pairs we note that they do not all line up, we know that a mistake has been made.

Do Exercise 5.

Equations like $y = 2x$ or $y = x + 2$ are also linear. To find pairs that solve such equations, it is usually easiest to substitute for x and then find y.

Example 5   Graph: $y = 2x$.

First, we find some ordered pairs that are solutions. Suppose we choose 3 for x. Then

$$y = 2x = 2 \cdot 3 = 6,$$

so (3, 6) is one solution.
 To find a second solution, we can replace x with -2:

$$y = 2x = 2(-2) = -4.$$

Thus, $(-2, -4)$ is a solution.
 To find a third solution, we can replace x with 0:

$$y = 2x = 2 \cdot 0 = 0.$$

Thus, (0, 0) is a solution.
 We can compute additional pairs if we wish and form a table.

x	y $y = 2x$	(x, y)
3	6	(3, 6)
-2	-4	(-2, -4)
0	0	(0, 0)
1	2	(1, 2)

(1) Choose x.
(2) Compute y.
(3) Form the pair (x, y).
(4) Plot the points.
(5) Draw and label the graph.

Next, we plot these points. We draw the line, or graph, with a ruler and label it $y = 2x$.

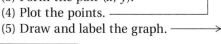

5. Graph $x + 2y = 7$. Use the results from Margin Exercise 3.

Graph.

6. $y = 3x$

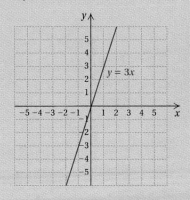

7. $y = \frac{1}{2}x$

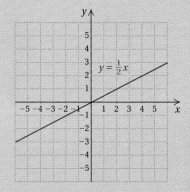

Answers on page A-16

Graph.

8. $y = -x$ (or $y = -1 \cdot x$)

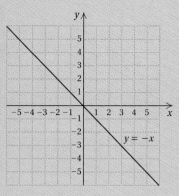

9. $y = -2x$

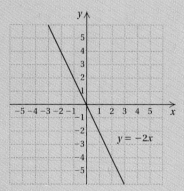

Do Exercises 6 and 7 on the preceding page.

Example 6 Graph: $y = -3x$.

We make a table of solutions. Then we plot the points, draw the line with a ruler, and label the line $y = -3x$.

If x is 0, then $y = -3 \cdot 0 = 0$.
If x is 1, then $y = -3 \cdot 1 = -3$.
If x is -2, then $y = -3(-2) = 6$.
If x is 2, then $y = -3 \cdot 2 = -6$.

x	y $y = -3x$	(x, y)
0	0	$(0, 0)$
1	-3	$(1, -3)$
-2	6	$(-2, 6)$
2	-6	$(2, -6)$

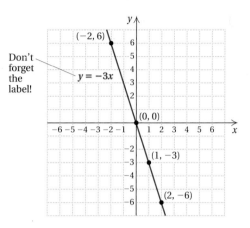

Do Exercises 8 and 9.

Example 7 Graph: $y = x + 2$.

We make a table of solutions. Then we plot the points, draw the line with a ruler, and label it.

If x is 0, then $y = 0 + 2 = 2$.
If x is 1, then $y = 1 + 2 = 3$.
If x is -1, then $y = -1 + 2 = 1$.
If x is 3, then $y = 3 + 2 = 5$.

x	y $y = x + 2$	(x, y)
0	2	$(0, 2)$
1	3	$(1, 3)$
-1	1	$(-1, 1)$
3	5	$(3, 5)$

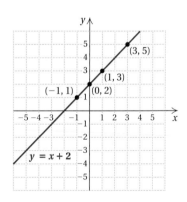

Example 8 Graph: $y = \frac{2}{3}x$.

We make a table of solutions, plot the points, and draw and label the line. It is important to note that by selecting multiples of 3 as x-values, we avoid fractional values for y.

If x is 6, then $y = \frac{2}{3} \cdot 6 = 4$.

If x is 3, then $y = \frac{2}{3} \cdot 3 = 2$.

If x is 0, then $y = \frac{2}{3} \cdot 0 = 0$.

If x is -3, then $y = \frac{2}{3}(-3) = -2$.

x	$y = \frac{2}{3}x$	(x, y)
6	4	(6, 4)
3	2	(3, 2)
0	0	(0, 0)
-3	-2	$(-3, -2)$

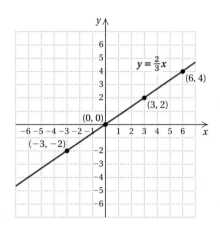

Do Exercises 10–12.

As is the case with many skills, your ability to graph linear equations will grow with practice. By carefully plotting at least three points for each equation, you can check your work for errors before any line is drawn. It is extremely unlikely for three points to line up if one of them was calculated incorrectly.

Graph.

10. $y = x + 1$

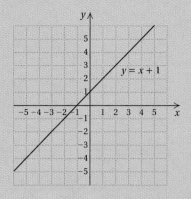

11. $y = -2x + 1$

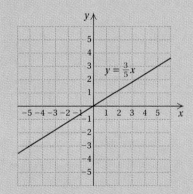

12. $y = \frac{3}{5}x$

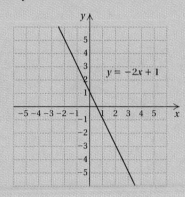

Answers on pages A-16 and A-17

6.4   Graphing Linear Equations

Calculator Spotlight

Calculators or computers with graphing capability have become increasingly common. This technology is generally used for graphing equations that are more complicated than $y = x + 2$ and $y = \frac{2}{3}x$ (Examples 7 and 8) and *in no way decreases the importance of understanding how such equations are graphed by hand.* The purpose of the following discussion is to show how graphing technology can be used to check some of your work and how it might enable you to handle more challenging problems.

All graphing technology utilizes a *window,* the rectangular portion of the screen in which a graph appears. For our purposes, a window extending from −10 to 10 on the *x*- and *y*-axes will suffice. Such settings may be standard or can be easily adjusted with keystrokes that vary depending on the technology in use (consult a user's manual or an instructor for the exact procedure).

To graph the equation $y = x + 2$, we press a key (often labeled $\boxed{Y=}$) and then

$$\boxed{X, T, \theta}\ \boxed{+}\ \boxed{2}\ \boxed{GRAPH}$$

(keystrokes will vary with the technology used). A graph similar to that shown on the left below should appear. To view some of the ordered pairs that are solutions, a TRACE key can be used to move a cursor along the line. Near the bottom of the window the cursor's coordinates appear (see the graph on the right below).

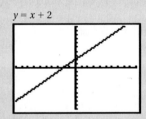

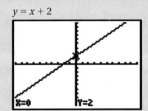

Exercises

Use graphing technology to graph each of the following.

1. $y = \frac{2}{3}x$
(Example 8)

2. $y = x + 1$
(Margin Exercise 10)

3. $y = -2x + 1$
(Margin Exercise 11)

4. $y = \frac{3}{5}x$
(Margin Exercise 12)

1. $y = \frac{2}{3}x$

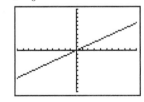

2. $y = x + 1$

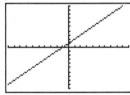

3. $y = -2x + 1$

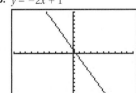

4. $y = \frac{3}{5}x$

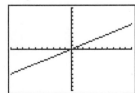

Exercise Set 6.4

a For each equation, use the indicated value to find an ordered pair that is a solution. See Example 1.

1. $x - y = 3$; let $x = 8$

(8, 5)

2. $x + y = 5$; let $x = 4$

(4, 1)

3. $2x + y = 7$; let $x = 3$

(3, 1)

4. $x + 2y = 9$; let $y = 4$

(1, 4)

5. $y = 3x - 1$; let $x = 5$

(5, 14)

6. $y = 2x + 7$; let $x = 3$

(3, 13)

7. $x + 3y = 1$; let $x = 7$

(7, −2)

8. $5x + y = 7$; let $y = 2$

(1, 2)

9. $2x + 5y = 17$; let $x = 1$

(1, 3)

10. $5x + 2y = 19$; let $x = 1$

(1, 7)

11. $3x - 2y = 8$; let $y = -1$

(2, −1)

12. $2x - 5y = 12$; let $y = -2$

(1, −2)

For each equation, complete the given ordered pairs. See Example 2.

13. $x + y = 7$; (, 8); (4,   )

(−1, 8); (4, 3)

14. $x - y = 6$; (, 2); (9,   )

(8, 2); (9, 3)

15. $x - y = 4$; (, 3); (10,   )

(7, 3); (10, 6)

16. $x + y = 10$; (, 8); (3,   )

(2, 8); (3, 7)

17. $2x + 3y = 15$; (3,   ); (, 1)

(3, 3); (6, 1)

18. $3x + 2y = 16$; (4,   ); (, −1)

(4, 2); (6, −1)

19. $5x + 2y = 11$; $(3, \blacksquare)$; $(\blacksquare, 3)$
$(3, -2)$; $(1, 3)$

20. $4x + 3y = 11$; $(5, \blacksquare)$; $(\blacksquare, 2)$
$(5, -3)$; $\left(\frac{5}{4}, 2\right)$

21. $y = 4x$; $(\blacksquare, 4)$; $(-2, \blacksquare)$
$(1, 4)$; $(-2, -8)$

22. $y = 6x$; $(\blacksquare, 6)$; $(-2, \blacksquare)$
$(1, 6)$; $(-2, -12)$

23. $2x + 5y = 3$; $(0, \blacksquare)$; $(\blacksquare, 0)$
$\left(0, \frac{3}{5}\right)$; $\left(\frac{3}{2}, 0\right)$

24. $5x + 7y = 9$; $(0, \blacksquare)$; $(\blacksquare, 0)$
$\left(0, \frac{9}{7}\right)$; $\left(\frac{9}{5}, 0\right)$

For each equation, find three solutions. Answers may vary.

25. $x + y = 12$
$(0, 12)$, $(5, 7)$, $(14, -2)$

26. $x + y = 19$
$(19, 0)$, $(20, -1)$, $(10, 9)$

27. $y = 4x$
$(0, 0)$, $(1, 4)$, $(2, 8)$

28. $y = 5x$
$(0, 0)$, $(1, 5)$, $(2, 10)$

29. $3x + y = 13$
$(0, 13)$, $(1, 10)$, $(2, 7)$

30. $x + 5y = 12$
$(12, 0)$, $(7, 1)$, $(22, -2)$

31. $y = 3x - 1$
$(0, -1)$, $(2, 5)$, $(-1, -4)$

32. $y = 2x + 5$
$(0, 5)$, $(1, 7)$, $(-2, 1)$

33. $y = -5x$
$(0, 0)$, $(1, -5)$, $(-1, 5)$

34. $y = -3x$
$(0, 0)$, $(1, -3)$, $(-2, 6)$

35. $4 + y = x$
$(0, -4)$, $(4, 0)$, $(1, -3)$

36. $3 + y = x$
$(0, -3)$, $(3, 0)$, $(1, -2)$

37. $3x + 2y = 12$
$(0, 6)$, $(4, 0)$, $\left(1, \frac{9}{2}\right)$

38. $2x + 3y = 18$
$(0, 6)$, $(9, 0)$, $\left(1, \frac{16}{3}\right)$

39. $y = \frac{1}{3}x + 2$
$(0, 2)$, $(3, 3)$, $(-3, 1)$

40. $y = \frac{1}{2}x + 5$
$(0, 5)$, $(2, 6)$, $(-2, 4)$

b Use your own graph paper. Draw and label x- and y-axes. Then graph each equation.

41. $x + y = 4$

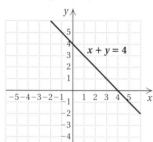

42. $x + y = 6$

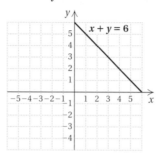

43. $x - 1 = y$

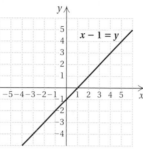

44. $x - 2 = y$

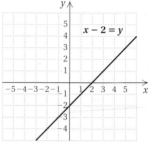

45. $y = x - 3$

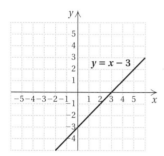

46. $y = x - 5$

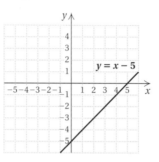

47. $y = \frac{1}{3}x$

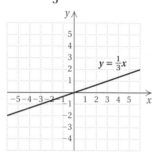

48. $y = -\frac{1}{3}x$

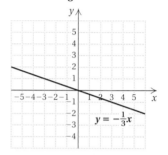

49. $y = x$

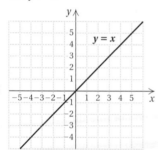

50. $y = x - 7$

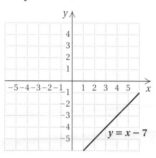

51. $y = 2x - 1$

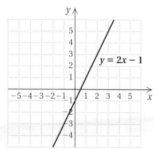

52. $y = 2x - 3$

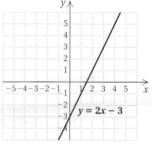

53. $y = 2x - 7$

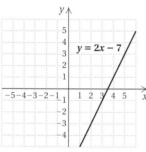

54. $y = 3x - 7$

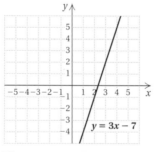

55. $y = \frac{2}{5}x$

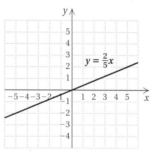

56. $y = \frac{3}{4}x$

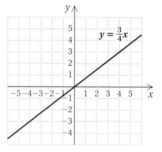

57. $y = -x + 4$

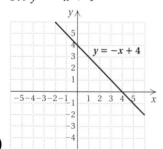

58. $y = -x + 5$

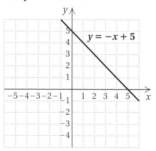

68.

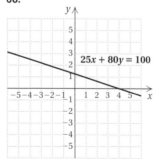

69.

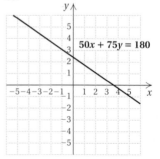

59. A recipe for a batch of chili calls for $\frac{3}{4}$ cup of red wine vinegar. How much vinegar is needed to make $2\frac{1}{2}$ batches of chili? [4.7d] $1\frac{7}{8}$ cup

Simplify.

60. $-\dfrac{49}{77}$ [3.5b] $-\dfrac{7}{11}$

61. $-8 - 5^2 \cdot 2(3 - 4)$ [2.5b] 42

62. $\dfrac{3}{10}\left(-\dfrac{25}{12}\right)$ [3.4b] $-\dfrac{5}{8}$

73.

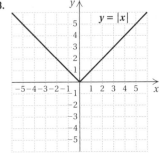

Solve.

63. $4.8 - 1.5x = 0.9$ [5.7a] 2.6

64. $3x - 8 = 5x - 12$ [5.7b] 2

Synthesis

65. ◈ What is the greatest number of quadrants that a line can pass through? Why?

66. ◈ In Example 8, we found that by choosing multiples of 3 for x, we could avoid fractions. What is the advantage of avoiding fractions? Would it have been incorrect to substitute values for x that are *not* multiples of 3? Why or why not?

67. ◈ To graph a linear equation, a student plots three points and discovers that the points do not line up with each other. What should the student do next?

Find three solutions of each equation. Then graph the equation.

68. ▦ $25x + 80y = 100$

(0, 1.25), (4, 0), (0.8, 1); answers may vary.
See figure on page 391.

69. ▦ $50x + 75y = 180$

(−3, 4.4), (−3.9, 5), (3, 0.4) See figure on page 391.

70. Use the graph in Example 4 to find three solutions of $2x - y = 5$. Do not use the ordered pairs already listed.

(2, −1), (3, 1), (5, 5); answers may vary

71. Use the graph in Example 7 to find three solutions of $y = x + 2$. Do not use the ordered pairs already listed.

(2, 4), (−3, −1), (−5, −3); answers may vary

72. Find all the whole-number solutions of $x + y = 6$.

(0, 6), (1, 5), (2, 4), (3, 3), (4, 2), (5, 1), (6, 0)

73. Graph three solutions of $y = |x|$ in the second quadrant and another three solutions in the first quadrant.

Answers may vary, but all should appear on this graph.

6.5 Means, Medians, and Modes

We have seen that pictographs, bar graphs, and line graphs provide three ways of representing a collection of data *visually*. Sometimes it is useful to describe a set of data *numerically*, using *statistics*. A **statistic** is simply a number that is derived from a set of data. There are three statistics that are considered *center point*, that is, numbers that serve to represent the entire data set. Let's examine all three.

a | Means

The most commonly used center point is the *average* of the set of numbers. We have already computed an average several times in this book (see pages 76, 240, 258, and 304). Although the word "average" is often used in everyday speech, in math we more often use the word *mean* instead.

> To find the **mean** of a set of numbers, add the numbers and then divide by the number of items of data.

Example 1 *Golfing.* In 1997, Tiger Woods set the record for the lowest total score in a golf tournament consisting of four rounds. His scores were 70, 66, 65, and 69. Find his mean score per round.

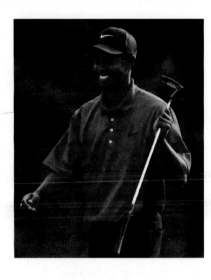

To find the mean, we add the scores together and then divide by the number of scores, 4:

$$\frac{70 + 66 + 65 + 69}{4} = \frac{270}{4} = 67.5.$$

Tiger Woods' mean score was 67.5.

Do Exercises 1–4.

Example 2 *Food Waste.* Courtney is a typical American consumer. In the course of 1 yr, she discards 100 lb of food waste. What is the average number of pounds of food waste discarded each week? Round to the nearest tenth.

We already know the total amount of food waste for the year. Since there are 52 weeks in a year, we divide by 52 and round:

$$\frac{100}{52} \approx 1.9.$$

On average, Courtney discards 1.9 lb of food waste per week.

Do Exercise 5.

Find the mean.

1. 14, 175, 36   75

2. 75, 36.8, 95.7, 12.1   54.9

3. Wendy scored the following on five tests: 96, 85, 82, 74, 68. What was her mean score?

   81

4. In the first five games, a basketball player scored points as follows: 26, 21, 13, 14, 23. Find the mean number of points scored per game.   19.4

5. *Food Waste.* Courtney also composts (converts to dirt) 5 lb of food waste each year. How much, on average, does Courtney compost per month? Round to the nearest tenth.

   0.4 lb

Answers on page A-18

6. *GPA.* Alex earned the following grades one semester.

Grade	Number of Credit Hours in Course
B	3
C	4
C	4
A	2

What was Alex's grade point average? Assume that the grade point values are 4.0 for an A, 3.0 for a B, and so on. Round to the nearest tenth.

2.5

Example 3 *GPA.* In most colleges, students are assigned grade point values for grades obtained. The **grade point average,** or **GPA,** is the average of the grade point values for each credit hour taken. At most colleges, grade point values are assigned as follows:

A: 4.0
B: 3.0
C: 2.0
D: 1.0
F: 0.0

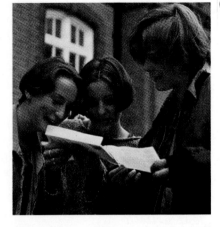

Meg earned the following grades for one semester. What was her grade point average?

Course	Grade	Number of Credit Hours in Course
Colonial History	B	3
Basic Mathematics	A	4
English Literature	A	3
French	C	4
Physical Education	D	1

To find the GPA, we first multiply the grade point value (in color below) by the number of credit hours in the course and then add, as follows:

Colonial History	$3.0 \cdot 3 =$	9
Basic Mathematics	$4.0 \cdot 4 =$	16
English Literature	$4.0 \cdot 3 =$	12
French	$2.0 \cdot 4 =$	8
Physical Education	$1.0 \cdot 1 =$	1
		46 (Total)

The total number of credit hours taken is $3 + 4 + 3 + 4 + 1$, or 15. We divide 46 by 15 and round to the nearest tenth:

$$\text{GPA} = \frac{46}{15} \approx 3.1.$$

Meg's grade point average was 3.1.

Do Exercise 6.

Answers on page A-18

Example 4 To get a B in math, Geraldo must have a mean test score of at least 80. On the first four tests, his scores were 79, 88, 64, and 78. What is the lowest score that Geraldo can get on the last test and still get a B?

We can find the total of the five scores needed as follows:

$$80 + 80 + 80 + 80 + 80 = 5 \cdot 80, \quad \text{or} \quad 400.$$

The total of the scores on the first four tests is

$$79 + 88 + 64 + 78 = 309.$$

Thus Geraldo needs to get at least

$$400 - 309, \quad \text{or} \quad 91$$

in order to get a B. We can check this as follows:

$$\frac{79 + 88 + 64 + 78 + 91}{5} = \frac{400}{5}, \quad \text{or} \quad 80.$$

Do Exercise 7.

b Medians

Another type of center-point statistic is the *median*. Medians are useful when we wish to de-emphasize unusually extreme scores. For example, suppose a small class scored as follows on an exam.

Phil:	78	Pat:	56
Jill:	81	Olga:	84
Matt:	82		

Let's first list the scores in order from smallest to largest:

$$56, \quad 78, \quad \underset{\uparrow}{81}, \quad 82, \quad 84.$$
$$\text{Middle score}$$

The middle score—in this case, 81—is called the **median.** Note that because of the extremely low score of 56, the average of the scores is 76.2. In this example, the median may be more indicative of how the class as a whole performed.

Example 5 What is the median of this set of numbers?

$$99, \quad 870, \quad 91, \quad 98, \quad 106, \quad 90, \quad 98$$

We first rearrange the numbers in order from smallest to largest. Then we locate the middle number, 98.

$$90, \quad 91, \quad 98, \quad \underset{\uparrow}{98}, \quad 99, \quad 106, \quad 870$$
$$\text{Middle number}$$

The median is 98.

Do Exercises 8–10.

> Once a set of data is listed in order, from smallest to largest, the **median** is the middle number if there is an odd number of data items. If there is an even number of items, the median is the number that is the average of the two middle numbers.

7. To get an A in math, Rosa must have a mean test grade of at least 90. On the first three tests, her scores were 80, 100, and 86. What is the lowest score that Rosa can get on the last test and still get an A?   94

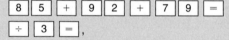
Find the median.

8. 17, 13, 18, 14, 19   17

9. 20, 14, 13, 19, 16, 18, 17   17

10. 78, 81, 83, 91, 103, 102, 122, 119, 88   91

Answers on page A-18

Find the median.

11. $1300, $2000, $3900, $1600, $1800, $1400 $1700

12. 68, 34, 67, 69, 58, 70   67.5

Find the modes.

13. 23, 45, 45, 45, 78   45

14. 34, 34, 67, 67, 68, 70   34, 67

15. 13, 24, 27, 28, 67, 89

No mode exists.

16. In a lab, Gina determined the mass, in grams, of each of five eggs:

15 g, 19 g, 19 g, 14 g, 18 g.

a) What is the mean?   17 g

b) What is the median?   18 g

c) What is the mode?   19 g

Answers on page A-18

Example 6   What is the median of this set of yearly salaries?

$35,000, $500,000, $28,000, $34,000, $27,000, $42,000

We rearrange the numbers in order from smallest to largest. The two middle numbers are $34,000 and $35,000. Thus the median is halfway between $34,000 and $35,000 (the average of $34,000 and $35,000):

$27000, $28,000, $34,000, $35,000, $42,000, $500,000

$$\text{Median} = \frac{\$34,000 + \$35,000}{2} = \frac{\$69,000}{2} = \$34,500.$$

Do Exercises 11 and 12.

c | Modes

The final type of center-point statistic is the **mode**.

> The **mode** of a set of data is the number or numbers that occur most often. If each number occurs the same number of times, there is *no* mode.

Example 7   Find the mode of these data.

13,   14,   17,   17,   18,   19

The number that occurs most often is 17. Thus the mode is 17.

A set of data has just one mean and just one median, but it can have more than one mode. It is also possible for a set of data to have no mode — when all numbers are equally represented. For example, the set of data 5, 7, 11, 13, 19 has no mode.

Example 8   Find the modes of these data.

33,   34,   34,   34,   35,   36,   37,   37,   37,   38,   39,   40

There are two numbers that occur most often, 34 and 37. Thus the modes are 34 and 37.

Do Exercises 13–16.

Which statistic is best for a particular situation? If someone is bowling, the *average* from several games is a good indicator of that person's ability. If someone is applying for a job, the *median* salary at that business is often most indicative of what people are earning there. Finally, if someone is reordering for a clothing store, the *mode* of the waist sizes sold is probably the most important statistic.

Exercise Set 6.5

a, **b**, **c** For each set of numbers, find the mean, the median, and any modes that exist.

1. 16, 18, 29, 14, 29, 19, 15

Mean: 20; median: 18; mode: 29

2. 72, 83, 85, 88, 92

Mean: 84; median: 85; no mode exists

3. 5, 30, 20, 20, 35, 5, 25

Mean: 20; median: 20; modes: 5, 20

4. 13, 32, 25, 27, 13

Mean: 22; median: 25; mode: 13

5. 1.2, 4.3, 5.7, 7.4, 7.4

Mean: 5.2; median: 5.7; mode: 7.4

6. 12.6, 13.4, 12.6, 43.7

Mean: 20.575; median: 13.0; mode: 12.6

7. 134, 128, 128, 129, 128, 178

Mean: 137.5; median: 128.5; mode: 128

8. $29.95, $28.79, $30.95, $29.95

Mean: $29.91; median: $29.95; mode: $29.95

9. *Basketball.* Lisa Leslie of the Los Angeles Spark once scored 23, 21, 19, 23, and 20 points in consecutive games. What was the mean for the five games? the median? the mode?

Mean: 21.2; median: 21; mode: 23

10. The following temperatures were recorded for seven days in Hartford:

43°, 40°, 23°, 38°, 54°, 35°, 47°.

What was the mean temperature? the median? the mode?   Mean: 40°; median: 40°; no mode exists

11. *Gas Mileage.* According to recent EPA estimates, an Achieva can be expected to travel 297 mi (highway) on 9 gal of gasoline (**Source:** *Motor Trend Magazine*). What is the mean number of miles expected per gallon?   33 mpg

12. *Gas Mileage.* According to recent EPA estimates an Aurora can be expected to travel 192 mi (highway) on 8 gal of gasoline (**Source:** *Motor Trend Magazine*). What is the mean number of miles expected per gallon?   24 mpg

GPA. In Exercises 13 and 14 are the grades of a student for one semester. In each case, find the grade point average. Assume that the grade point values are 4.0 for an A, 3.0 for a B, and so on. Round to the nearest tenth.

13.   2.9

Grades	Number of Credit Hours in Course
B	4
A	3
B	3
C	4

14.   3.1

Grades	Number of Credit Hours in Course
A	4
B	4
B	3
C	3

15. *Fish Prices.* The following prices per pound of Atlantic salmon were found at five fish markets:

$7.99, $9.49, $9.99, $7.99, $10.49.

What was the mean price per pound? the median price? the mode?

Mean: $9.19; median: $9.49; mode: $7.99

16. *Cheese Prices.* The following prices per pound of Vermont cheddar cheese were found at five supermarkets:

$4.99, $5.79, $4.99, $5.99, $5.79.

What was the mean price per pound? the median price? the mode?

Mean: $5.51; median: $5.79; modes: $4.99, $5.79

17. *Grading.* To get a B in math, Rich must average at least 80 on five tests. Scores on the first four tests were 80, 74, 81, and 75. What is the lowest score that Rich can get on the last test and still receive a B? 90

18. *Grading.* To get an A in math, Cybil must average at least 90 on five tests. Scores on the first four tests were 90, 91, 81, and 92. What is the lowest score that Cybil can get on the last test and still receive an A? 96

19. *Length of Pregnancy.* Marta was pregnant 270 days, 259 days, and 272 days for her first three pregnancies. In order for Marta's mean pregnancy to equal the worldwide average of 266 days, how long must her fourth pregnancy last? (***Source:*** David Crystal (ed.), *The Cambridge Factfinder.* Cambridge CB2 1RP: Cambridge University Press, 1997, p. 84.) 263 days

20. *Male Height.* Jason's brothers are 174 cm, 180 cm, 179 cm, and 172 cm tall. The average male is 176.5 cm tall. How tall is Jason if he and his brothers have a mean height of 176.5 cm? 177.5 cm

---

Skill Maintenance

Multiply.

21. $14 \cdot 14$ [1.5b] 196

22. $-144 \div (-9)$ [2.5a] 16

23. 1.4×1.4 [5.3a] 1.96

24. $-\dfrac{4}{9} \cdot \dfrac{15}{22}$ [3.4b]

$-\dfrac{10}{33}$

Solve. [5.8a]

25. A disc jockey charges a $40 setup fee and $50 an hour. How long can the disc jockey work for $165?

2.5 hr

26. To rent a floor sander costs $15 an hour plus a $10 supply fee. For how long can the machine be rented if $100 has been budgeted for the sander? 6 hr

---

Synthesis

27. ◆ Why might a firm's median salary be more indicative of what employees earn than the average, or mean, salary would be? (*Hint:* See Example 6.)

28. ◆ The following is a list of the number of children in each family in a certain Glen View neighborhood: 0, 2, 3, 0, 5, 2, 2, 0, 0, 2, 0, 0. Explain why the mode might be the most indicative statistic for the number of children in a family.

29. ◆ Is it possible for a driver to average 20 mph on a 30-mi trip and still receive a ticket for driving 75 mph? Why or why not?

Bowling Averages. Bowling averages are always computed by rounding down to the nearest integer. For example, suppose a bowler gets a total of 599 for 3 games. To find the average, we divide 599 by 3 and drop the amount to the right of the decimal point:

$$\dfrac{599}{3} \approx 199.67. \qquad \text{The bowler's average is 199.}$$

30. ▦ If Frances bowls 4176 in 23 games, what is her average? 181

31. ▦ If Eric bowls 4621 in 27 games, what is his average? 171

32. The ordered set of data 18, 21, 24, *a*, 36, 37, *b* has a median of 30 and an mean of 32. Find *a* and *b*.

$a = 30$; $b = 58$

33. *Hank Aaron.* Hank Aaron averaged $34\frac{7}{22}$ home runs per year over a 22-yr career. After 21 yr, Aaron had averaged $35\frac{10}{21}$ home runs per year. How many home runs did Aaron hit in his final year? 10

34. Because of a poor grade on the fifth and final test, Chris's mean test grade fell from 90.5 to 84.0. What did Chris score on the fifth test? Assume that all tests are equally important. 58

35. *Price Negotiations.* Amy offers $3200 for a used Ford Taurus advertised at $4000. The first offer from Jim, the car's owner, is to "split the diffence" and sell the car for $(3200 + 4000) \div 2$, or $3600. Amy's second offer is to split the difference between Jim's offer and her first offer. Jim's second offer is to split the difference between Amy's second offer and his first offer. If this pattern continues and Amy accepts Jim's third (and final) offer, how much will she pay for the car? $3475

Use averages to negotiate the price of a car.

Collaborative Learning Manual

6.6 Predictions and Probability

a | Making Predictions

Sometimes we use data to make predictions or estimates of missing data points. One process for doing so is called **interpolation**. Interpolation enables us to estimate missing "in-between values" on the basis of known information.

Example 1 *Monthly Mortgage Payments.* When money is borrowed and then repaid in monthly installments, the size of the payments increases as the length of the loan, in years, decreases. The table below lists the size of a monthly payment when $110,000 is borrowed (at 9% interest) for various lengths of time. Use interpolation to estimate the monthly payment on a 35-yr loan.

Year	Monthly Payment
5	$2283.42
10	1393.43
15	1115.69
20	989.70
25	923.12
30	885.08
35	?
40	848.50

To use interpolation, we first plot the points and look for a trend. It seems reasonable to draw a line between the points corresponding to 30 and 40. We can "zoom-in" to better visualize the situation. To estimate the second coordinate that is paired with 35, we trace a vertical line up from 35 to the graph and then left to the vertical axis. Thus we estimate the value to be 867. We can also estimate this value by averaging $885.08 and $848.50:

$$\frac{\$885.08 + \$848.50}{2} = \$866.79.$$

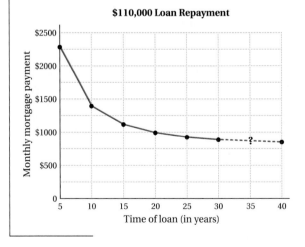

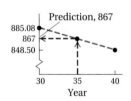

Objectives

a Make predictions from a set of data using interpolation or extrapolation.

b Calculate the probability of an event occurring.

For Extra Help

TAPE 12   InterAct math   CD-ROM
             MAC
             WIN

1. *World Bicycle Production.* Use interpolation to estimate world bicycle production in 1994 from the information in the following table.   111 million

Year	World Bicycle Production (in millions)
1989	95
1990	90
1991	96
1992	103
1993	108
1994	?
1995	114

Source: United Nations Interbike Directory

2. *Study Time and Test Scores.* A professor gathered the following data comparing study time and test scores. Use extrapolation to estimate the test score received when studying for 23 hr.   94%

Study Time (in hours)	Test Grade (in percent)
19	83
20	85
21	88
22	91
23	?

When we estimate in this way to find an in-between value, we are *interpolating*. Real-world information about the data might tell us that an estimate found in this way is unreliable. For example, data from the stock market might be too erratic for interpolation.

Do Exercise 1.

We often analyze data with the view of going "beyond" the data. One process for doing so is called **extrapolation**.

Example 2   *Movies Released.* The data in the following table and graphs show the number of movie releases over a period of years. Use extrapolation to estimate the number of movies released in 1997.

Year	Movies Released
1991	164
1992	150
1993	161
1994	184
1995	234
1996	260
1997	?

Source: Motion Picture Association of America

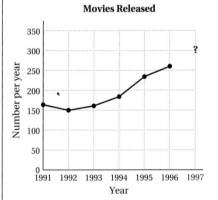

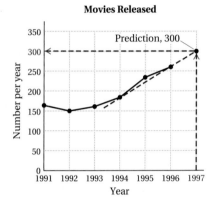

First, we analyze the data and note that they tend to follow a straight line past 1994. Keeping this trend in mind, we draw a "representative" line through the data and beyond. To estimate a value for 1997, we draw a vertical line up from 1997 until it hits the representative line. We go to the left and read off a value—about 300. When we estimate in this way to find a "go-beyond value," we are *extrapolating*. Answers found with this method can vary greatly depending on the points chosen to determine the "representative" line.

Do Exercise 2.

Answer on page A-18

b   Probability

The predictions made in Examples 1 and 2 have a good chance of being reasonably accurate. A branch of mathematics known as *probability* is used to attach a numerical value to the likelihood that a specific event will occur.

Suppose we were to flip a coin. Because the coin is just as likely to land heads as it is to land tails, we say that the *probability* of it landing heads is $\frac{1}{2}$. Similarly, if we roll a die (plural: dice), we are as likely to roll a ⚄ as we are to roll a ⚀, ⚁, ⚂, ⚃, or ⚅. Because of this, we say that the probability of rolling a ⚄ is $\frac{1}{6}$.

Example 3   A die is about to be rolled. Find the probability that a number greater than 4 will be rolled.

Since rolling a ⚀, ⚁, ⚂, ⚃, ⚄, or ⚅ are all equally likely to occur, and since two of these possibilities involve numbers greater than 4, we have

$$\begin{matrix} \text{The probability of rolling} \\ \text{a number greater than 4} \end{matrix} = \frac{2}{6} \quad \begin{matrix} \longleftarrow \text{Number of ways to roll a 5 or 6} \\ \longleftarrow \text{Number of (equally likely) possible outcomes} \end{matrix}$$

$$= \frac{1}{3}.$$

The reasoning shown in Example 3 can be used in a variety of applications.

Example 4   A cloth bag contains 20 equally sized marbles: 5 are red, 7 are blue, and 8 are yellow. A marble is randomly selected. Find the probability that **(a)** a red marble is selected; **(b)** a blue marble is selected; **(c)** a yellow marble is selected.

a) Since all 20 marbles are equally likely to be selected we have

$$\begin{matrix} \text{The probability of} \\ \text{selecting a red marble} \end{matrix} = \frac{\text{Number of ways to select a red marble}}{\text{Number of ways to select any marble}}$$

$$= \frac{5}{20} = \frac{1}{4}, \text{ or } 0.25.$$

b) $$\begin{matrix} \text{The probability of} \\ \text{selecting a blue marble} \end{matrix} = \frac{\text{Number of ways to select a blue marble}}{\text{Number of ways to select any marble}}$$

$$= \frac{7}{20}, \text{ or } 0.35.$$

c) $$\begin{matrix} \text{The probability} \\ \text{of selecting a} \\ \text{yellow marble} \end{matrix} = \frac{\text{Number of ways to select a yellow marble}}{\text{Number of ways to select any marble}}$$

$$= \frac{8}{20} = \frac{2}{5}, \text{ or } 0.4.$$

Do Exercise 3.

3. A presentation of *The Lion King* is attended by 250 people: 40 children, 60 seniors, and 150 (nonsenior) adults. After everyone has been seated, one audience member is selected at random. Find the probability of each of the following.

a) A child is selected.

b) A senior is selected.

c) A (nonsenior) adult is selected.

(a) $\frac{4}{25}$, or 0.16   (b) $\frac{6}{25}$, or 0.24
(c) $\frac{3}{5}$, or 0.6

Answers on page A-18

4. A card is randomly selected from a well-shuffled deck of cards. Find the probability of each of the following.

a) The card is a diamond.

b) The card is a king or queen.

(a) $\frac{1}{4}$, or 0.25   (b) $\frac{2}{13}$

Many probability problems involve a standard deck of 52 playing cards. Such a deck is made up as shown below.

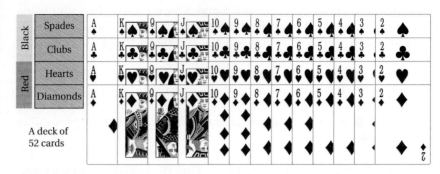

A deck of 52 cards

Example 5   A card is randomly selected from a well-shuffled (mixed) deck of cards. Find the probability that **(a)** the card is a jack; **(b)** the card is a club.

a) The probability of selecting a jack $= \dfrac{\text{Number of ways to select a jack}}{\text{Number of ways to select any card}}$

$$= \frac{4}{52} = \frac{1}{13}$$

b) The probability of selecting a club $= \dfrac{\text{Number of ways to select a club}}{\text{Number of ways to select any card}}$

$$= \frac{13}{52} = \frac{1}{4}$$

Do Exercise 4.

In Examples 3–5, several "events" were discussed: rolling a number greater than 4, selecting a marble of a certain color, and selecting a certain type of playing card. The likelihood of each event occurring was determined by considering the total number of possible outcomes, using the principle formally stated below.

> **THE PRIMARY PRINCIPLE OF PROBABILITY**
>
> If an event E can occur m ways out of n possible equally likely outcomes, then
>
> $$\text{The probability of } E \text{ occurring} = \frac{m}{n}.$$

Answers on page A-18

Exercise Set 6.6

a Use interpolation or extrapolation to find the missing data values.

1. *Study Time and Grades.* A math instructor asked her students to keep track of how much time each spent studying the chapter on decimal notation in her basic mathematics course. They collected the information together with test scores from that chapter's test. The data are given in the following table. Estimate the missing data value. 83

Study Time (in hours)	Test Grade
9	75
11	93
13	80
15	85
16	85
17	80
19	?
21	86
23	91

2. *Maximum Heart Rate.* A person's maximum heart rate depends on his or her gender, age, and resting heart rate. The following table relates resting heart rate and maximum heart rate for a 20-yr-old man. Estimate the missing data value. 169

Resting Heart Rate (in beats per minute)	Maximum Heart Rate (in beats per minute)
50	166
60	168
65	?
70	170
80	172

Source: American Heart Association

Estimate the missing data value in each of the following tables.

3. *Ozone Layer.* About 3112 parts per billion

Year	Ozone Level (in parts per billion)
1991	2981
1992	3133
1993	3148
1994	3138
1995	3124
1996	?

Source: National Oceanic and Atmospheric Administration

4. *Motion Picture Expense.* About $66.5 million

Year	Average Expense per Picture (in millions)
1991	$38.2
1992	42.4
1993	44.0
1994	50.4
1995	54.1
1996	61.0
1997	?

Source: Motion Picture Association of America

5. *Credit-Card Spending.* About $148.8 billion

Year	Credit-Card Spending from Thanksgiving to Christmas (in billions)
1991	$ 59.8
1992	66.8
1993	79.1
1994	96.9
1995	116.3
1996	131.4
1997	?

Source: RAM Research Group, National Credit Counseling Services

6. *U.S. Book-Buying Growth.* About $27 billion

Year	Book Sales (in billions)
1992	$21
1993	23
1994	24
1995	25
1996	26
1997	?

Source: Book Industry Trends 1995

7. *FedEx Priority Rates.* $27.30

FedEx Letter	FedEx Priority Overnight®
up to 8 oz.	$ 13.25

Weight in lbs.	
1 lb.	$ 18.30
2 lbs.	19.20
3	21.00
4	22.80
5	24.90
6	?
7	29.70
8	31.80
9	34.20
10	36.80
11	37.80

Delivery by 10:00 a.m. next business day

Source: Federal Express Corporation

8. *FedEx Standard Rates.* $23.50

FedEx Letter	FedEx Standard Overnight®
up to 8 oz.	$ 11.50

Weight in lbs.	
1 lb.	$ 16.00
2 lbs.	17.00
3	18.00
4	19.00
5	20.00
6	21.75
7	?
8	25.25
9	27.00
10	28.75
11	30.75

Delivery by 3:00 p.m. next business day

Source: Federal Express Corporation

b Find each of the following probabilities.

Rolling a die. In Exercises 9–12, assume that a die is about to be rolled.

9. Find the probability that a ⚁ is rolled.

$\frac{1}{6}$, or $0.1\overline{6}$

10. Find the probability that a ⚄ is rolled.

$\frac{1}{6}$, or $0.1\overline{6}$

11. Find the probability that an odd number is rolled.

$\frac{1}{2}$, or 0.5

12. Find the probability that a number greater than 2 is rolled. $\frac{2}{3}$, or $0.\overline{6}$

Copyright © 2000 Addison Wesley Longman

Playing Cards. In Exercises 13–18, assume that one card is randomly selected from a well-shuffled deck.

13. Find the probability that the card is the ace of spades. $\frac{1}{52}$

14. Find the probability that the card is a picture card (jack, queen, or king). $\frac{3}{13}$

15. Find the probability that an 8 or a 6 is selected. $\frac{2}{13}$

16. Find the probability that a red 2 is selected. $\frac{1}{26}$

17. Find the probability that a black picture card (jack, queen, or king) is selected. $\frac{3}{26}$

18. Find the probability that a 10 is selected. $\frac{1}{13}$

Candy Colors. Made by the Tootsie Industries of Chicago, Illinois, Mason Dots® is a gumdrop candy. A box was opened by the authors and found to contain the following number of gumdrops:

Strawberry	7
Lemon	8
Orange	9
Cherry	4
Lime	5
Grape	6

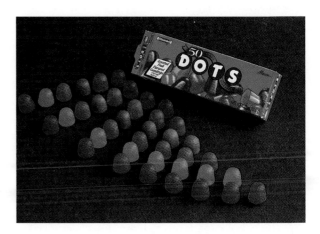

In Exercises 19–22, assume that one gumdrop is randomly choosen from the box.

19. Find the probability that a cherry gumdrop is selected. $\frac{4}{39}$

20. Find the probability that an orange gumdrop is selected. $\frac{9}{39}$

21. Find the probability that a gumdrop is *not* lime. $\frac{34}{39}$

22. Find the probability that the gumdrop is *not* lemon. $\frac{31}{39}$

Solve. [5.7b]

23. $-3x + 8 = 2x - 7$ 3

24. $3(x - 4) = 7x - 2$ $-\frac{5}{2}$

25. $-7 + 3x - 5 = 8x - 1$ $-\frac{11}{5}$

Convert to decimal notation. [5.5a]

26. $\frac{4}{9}$ $0.\overline{4}$

27. $\frac{17}{15}$ $1.1\overline{3}$

28. $-\frac{5}{8}$ -0.625

Synthesis

29. ◆ Would a company considering expansion be more interested in interpolation or extrapolation? Why?

30. ◆ Would a bookkeeper who is lacking records from a firm's third year of operation be more interested in interpolation or extrapolation? Why?

31. ◆ Is it possible for the probability of an event occurring to exceed 1? Why or why not?

32. A coin is flipped twice. What is the probability that two heads will occur? $\frac{1}{4}$, or 0.25

33. A coin is flipped twice. What is the probability that one head and one tail will occur? $\frac{1}{2}$, or 0.5

34. A die is rolled twice. What is the probability that a ■ is rolled twice? $\frac{1}{36}$

35. A day is chosen randomly during a leap year. What is the probability that the day is in July? $\frac{31}{366}$

Summary and Review Exercises: Chapter 6

For Exercises 1–5, use the following tables, which list the ideal body weights for men and women over age 25.

DESIRABLE WEIGHT OF MEN			
Height	Small Frame (in pounds)	Medium Frame (in pounds)	Large Frame (in pounds)
5 ft, 7 in.	138	152	166
5 ft, 9 in.	146	160	174
5 ft, 11 in.	154	169	184
6 ft, 1 in.	163	179	194
6 ft, 3 in.	172	188	204

DESIRABLE WEIGHT OF WOMEN			
Height	Small Frame (in pounds)	Medium Frame (in pounds)	Large Frame (in pounds)
5 ft, 1 in.	105	113	122
5 ft, 3 in.	111	120	130
5 ft, 5 in.	118	128	139
5 ft, 7 in.	126	137	147
5 ft, 9 in.	134	144	155

1. What is the ideal weight for a 6 ft, 1 in. man with a medium frame? [6.1a]

2. What is the ideal weight for a 5 ft, 5 in. woman with a small frame? [6.1a]

3. What size woman has an ideal weight of 120 lb? [6.1a]

4. What size man has an ideal weight of 169 lb? [6.1a]

5. Use the information provided to draw a line graph showing the ideal body weight for a large-framed woman. Use height on the horizontal axis and weight, in pounds, on the vertical axis. [6.2d]

This pictograph shows the number of officers in the largest U.S. police forces. Use the pictorgraph for Exercises 6–9.

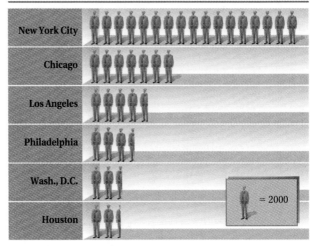

America's Largest Police Forces

= 2000

Source: International Association of Chiefs of Police

6. About how many officers are in the Chicago police force? [6.1b]

7. Which city has about 9000 officers on its force? [6.1b]

8. Of the cities listed, which has the smallest police force? [6.1b]

9. Estimate the average size of these six police forces. [6.1b], [6.5a]

The following bar graph shows the number of U.S. households that owned different types of pets in a recent year. Use the graph for Exercises 10–15.   [6.2a]

American Pet Ownership
(Millions of U.S. households)

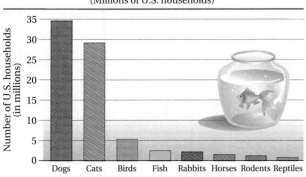

Source: American Veterinary Medical Association

10. About how many U.S. households have pet fish?

11. What type of pet is owned by about 5 million U.S. households?

12. Of the pets listed, which type is owned by the smallest number of U.S. households?

13. About how many more dog owners are there than cat owners?

14. True or false? There are more cat owners than bird, fish, rabbit, horse, rodent, and reptile owners combined.

15. True of false? There are more dog owners than all other pet owners combined.

The following line graph shows the number of accidents per 100 drivers, by age. Use the graph for Exercises 16–21.   [6.2c]

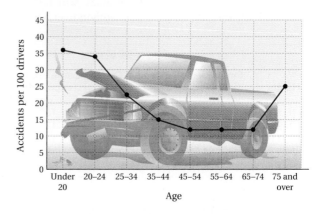

16. Which age group has the most accidents per 100 drivers?

17. What is the fewest number of accidents per 100 in any age group?

18. How many more accidents do people over 75 yr of age have than those in the age range of 65–74?

19. Between what ages does the number of accidents stay basically the same?

20. How many fewer accidents do people 25–34 yr of age have than those 20–24 yr of age?

21. Which age group has accidents more than three times as often as people 55–64 yr of age?

Find the coordinates for each point. [6.3a]

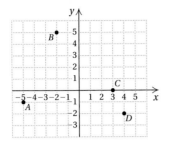

22. *A*   **23.** *B*

24. *C*   **25.** *D*

Plot these points using graph paper. [6.3a]

26. (2, 5)   **27.** (0, −3)   **28.** (−4, −2)

In which quadrant is the point located? [6.3b]

29. (3, −8)   **30.** (−20, −14)   **31.** $\left(4\frac{9}{10}, 1\frac{3}{10}\right)$

Determine whether the given point is a solution of the equation $2y − x = 10$. [6.3c]

32. (2, −6)   **33.** (0, 5)

Graph on a plane. [6.4b]

34. $y = 2x − 5$ **35.** $y = -\frac{3}{4}x$

36. $x + y = 4$ **37.** $y = 3 − 4x$

In Exercises 38–43, find **(a)** the mean, **(b)** the median, and **(c)** any modes that exist. [6.5a, b, c]

38. 26, 51, 34, 26, 43   **39.** 11, 14, 17, 17, 21, 7, 11

40. 500, 25, 470, 190, 470, 280

41. 700, 700, 1900, 2700, 3000

42. $2, $14, $17, $17, $26, $29

43. $30,000, $75,000, $20,000, $25,000

44. One summer, a student earned the following amounts over a four-week period: $302, $312, $330, and $298. What was the mean of his weekly earnings? the median?   [6.5a, b]

45. The following temperatures were recorded in St. Louis every 4 hr on a certain day in June: 63°, 58°, 66°, 72°, 71°, 67°. What was the mean temperature for that day?   [6.5a]

46. To get an A in math, Sasha must average at least 90 on four tests. Scores on her first three tests were 94, 78, and 92. What is the lowest score that she can receive on the last test and still get an A?   [6.5a]

47. Use interpolation and the graph in Exercises 16–21 to estimate the number of accidents per 100 drivers that are 22.5 to 27.5 yr old.   [6.6a]

A deck of 52 playing cards is thoroughly shuffled and a car is randomly selected.   [6.6b]

48. Find the probability that the five of clubs was selected.

49. Find the probability that a red card was selected.

50. Divide: $-405 \div 3$.   [2.5a]

51. A cutting board measures $\frac{2}{3}$ m by $\frac{1}{2}$ m. What is its area?   [3.4c]

52. Simplify: $-\frac{32}{4}$.   [3.5b]

53. Solve: $3.1 + 4x = -2.7$.   [5.7a]

Synthesis

54. ◆ Is it possible for the graph of a linear equation to pass through all four quadrants? Why or why not?   [6.4b]

55. ◆ Write a statistics problem for which the solution is

$$\frac{21,500 + 23,800 + 24,400 + 27,000}{4} = 24,175.$$

[6.5a]

56. ▦ Find three solutions and then graph $34x + 47y = 100$.   [6.4a, b]

57. ▦ A typing pool consists of four senior typists who earn $12.35 per hour and nine other typists who earn $11.15 per hour. Find the mean hourly wage.   [6.5a]

For Exercises 58–61, refer to the table and graph in Exercises 1–5 and 10–15.

58. If the average dog-owning household has 1.2 dogs, how many pet dogs are there in the United States?   [6.2a]

59. If the average fish-owning household has 14.3 fish, how many pet fish are there in the United States?   [6.2a]

60. Is it possible for a woman's ideal body weight to exceed the ideal body weight for a man of the same height?   [6.1a]

61. Is it possible for a woman's ideal body weight to exceed the ideal body weight of a taller man?   [6.1a]

Graph on a plane.   [6.4b]

62. $1\frac{2}{3}x + \frac{3}{4}y = 2$ **63.** $\frac{3}{4}x - 2\frac{1}{2}y = 3$

Test: Chapter 6

This table lists the number of calories burned during various walking activities. Use it for Questions 1 and 2.

Walking Activity	Calories Burned in 30 Min		
	110 lb	132 lb	154 lb
Walking			
Fitness (5 mph)	183	213	246
Mildly energetic (3.5 mph)	111	132	159
Strolling (2 mph)	69	84	99
Hiking			
3 mph with 20-lb load	210	249	285
3 mph with 10-lb load	195	228	264
3 mph with no load	183	213	246

1. Which activity provides the greatest benefit in burned calories for a person who weighs 132 lb?

2. What is the least strenuous activity you must perform if you weigh 154 lb and you want to burn at least 250 calories every 30 min?

3. Draw a vertical bar graph using an appropriate scale, showing the recent starting salary of college graduates in various fields. Be sure to label the axes properly.

Accounting: $28,500

Marketing: $26,500

Humanities: $24,000

Computer science: $34,000

Mathematics: $31,000

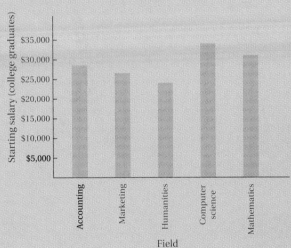

The following pictograph shows the number of hits in 1998 for several major-league baseball players. Use the graph for Questions 4–7.

Number of Hits in 1998 for 5 Professional Players

Tony Gwynn	
Bernie Williams	
Aaron Boone	
Alex Rodriguez	
Tony Fernandez	

= 25 hits

4. How many hits did Bernie Williams have?

5. Who had the most hits?

6. Who had the fewest hits?

7. Who had 150 hits?

The following line graph shows the revenues of Nike, Inc. Use the graph for Questions 8–13.

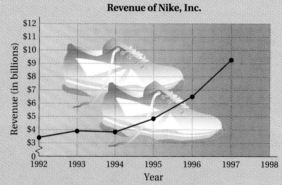

Revenue of Nike, Inc.

Source: Nike, Inc., annual report and The World Almanac 1999.

8. How much revenue was earned in 1996?

9. What was the mean revenue for the six years?

10. How much more revenue was earned in 1997 than in 1992?

11. In which year did revenue increase the most?

12. What was the median revenue for the six years?

13. Use extrapolation to estimate the revenue in 1998.

In which quadrant is each point located?

14. $\left(-\frac{1}{2}, 7\right)$

15. $(-5, -6)$

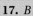

Find the coordinates of each point.

16. A

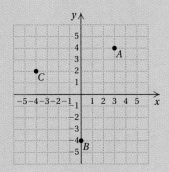

17. B

18. C

19. Determine whether $(2, -4)$ is a solution of the equation $y - 3x = -10$.

Graph.

20. $y = 2x - 1$

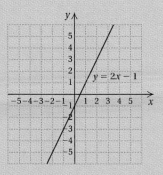

21. $y = -\dfrac{3}{2}x$

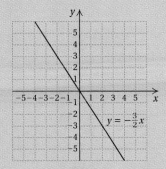

22. $x + 2y = 8$

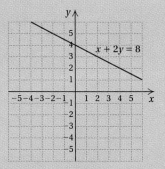

14. [6.3b] II

15. [6.3b] III

16. [6.3a] (3, 4)

17. [6.3a] (0, −4)

18. [6.3a] (−4, 2)

19. [6.3c] Yes

20. [6.4b] See graph.

21. [6.4b] See graph.

22. [6.4b] See graph.

Find the mean.

23. 45, 49, 52, 54   **24.** 1, 2, 3, 4, 5   **25.** 3, 17, 17, 18, 18, 20

Find the median and any modes that exist.

26. 45, 47, 54, 54   **27.** 1, 2, 3, 4, 5   **28.** 20, 17, 17, 18, 3, 18

29. Bill drove 754 km in 13 hr. What was the average number of kilometers per hour?

30. To get a C in chemistry, Ernie must score an average of 70 on four tests. Scores on his first three tests were 68, 71, and 65. What is the lowest score that Ernie can receive on the last test and still get a C?

31. A month of the year is randomly selected for a company's party. What is the probability that a month whose name begins with J is chosen?

36. 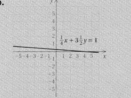   **37.**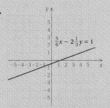

Skill Maintenance

32. Divide: $\dfrac{-700}{35}$.   **33.** Simplify: $\dfrac{75}{45}$.

34. A recipe for nachos calls for $\frac{3}{4}$ lb of shredded cheese. How much cheese should be used to make $\frac{1}{3}$ of a recipe?   **35.** Solve: $-9.8 = 5x - 1.7$.

Synthesis

Graph.

36. $\dfrac{1}{4}x + 3\dfrac{1}{2}y = 1$ **37.** $\dfrac{5}{6}x - 2\dfrac{1}{3}y = 1$

38. Find the area of a rectangle whose vertices are $(-3, 1)$, $(5, 1)$, $(5, 8)$, and $(-3, 8)$.

Cumulative Review: Chapters 1–6

1. Write expanded notation for 3671.

2. Jonathan pedals 23 mi on each of 5 days. How many miles are bicycled in all?

3. Write standard notation for the number in this sentence: Experts predict the global population to surpass 8 billion by the year 2030.

4. Find the perimeter and the area of the rectangle.

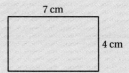

5. Kati poured 129 g of carbon and then 87 g of sodium chloride into a beaker. How many grams of chemicals were poured into the beaker altogether?

6. Write exponential notation: $7 \cdot 7 \cdot 7 \cdot 7$.

7. Tell which integers correspond to this situation: Monique lost 9 lb and Jacques gained 4 lb.

Use either < or > for ▒ to form a true statement.

8. $1 \ \blacksquare \ -7$

9. $\dfrac{4}{9} \ \blacksquare \ \dfrac{3}{7}$

10. $-4.8 \ \blacksquare \ -4.09$

11. Find $-x$ when $x = -5$.

12. Find $-(-x)$ when $x = 17$.

13. Evaluate $2x - y$ for $x = 3$ and $y = 8$.

14. Combine like terms: $6x + 4y - 8x - 3y$.

15. Find all the factors of 36.

16. Determine whether 732 is divisible by 6.

17. Write two different expressions for $\dfrac{-7}{x}$ with negative signs in different places.

18. Multiply: $5(2a - 3b + 1)$.

19. What part is shaded?

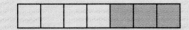

20. Find another name for the given number but with the denominator indicated.

$$\frac{2}{7} = \frac{?}{35}$$

Simplify, if possible. Assume that all variables are nonzero.

21. $427 - 398$

22. $17 \cdot 28$

23. $63 \div (-7)$

24. $-32 + (-83)$

25. $\dfrac{3}{7} + \dfrac{2}{7}$

26. $\dfrac{3}{7} \div \dfrac{9}{5}$

27. $\dfrac{5}{6} - \dfrac{1}{9}$

28. $\dfrac{-2}{15} + \dfrac{3}{10}$

29. $\dfrac{8}{11} \cdot \dfrac{11}{8}$

30. $3\dfrac{1}{4} + 5\dfrac{7}{8}$

31. $7\dfrac{2}{3}x - 5\dfrac{1}{4}x$

32. $4\dfrac{1}{5} \cdot 3\dfrac{1}{7}$

33. $39.72 + 43.56$

34. $1334.183 \div 21.4$

35. $17.4(-2.43)$

36. $\dfrac{9a}{9a}$

37. $\dfrac{4x}{1}$

38. $\dfrac{0}{7x}$

Solve.

39. $x + \dfrac{2}{3} = -\dfrac{2}{5}$

40. $\dfrac{3}{8}x + 2 = 14$

41. $3(x - 5) = 7x + 2$

42. In which quadrant is the point $(-4, 9)$ located?

43. Graph: $y = \dfrac{1}{2}x - 4$.

44. Find the mean:

    19, 39, 34, 52.

45. Find the median:

    7, 9, 12, 35.

46. Find the mode:

    43, 56, 56, 43, 49, 49, 49.

47. A marathoner ran 59 km in 3 hr. What was the average number of kilometers per hour?

Synthesis

48. Simplify:

$$\left(\dfrac{3}{4}\right)^2 - \dfrac{1}{8} \cdot \left(3 - 1\dfrac{1}{2}\right)^2.$$

49. Add and write the answer as a mixed numeral:

$$-5\dfrac{42}{100} + \dfrac{355}{100} + \dfrac{89}{10} + \dfrac{17}{1000}.$$

50. A square with sides parallel to the axes has the point $(2, 3)$ at its center. Find the coordinates of the square's vertices if each side is 8 units long.

Ratio and Proportion

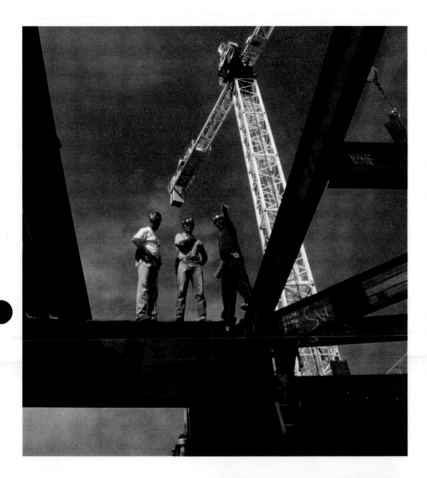

Introduction

The equation shown below is an example of a *proportion*. Fractional expressions appearing in a proportion are examples of *ratios*. In this chapter, we will study ratios and proportions and then use them for problem solving. A topic of interest to consumers, unit pricing, is also examined.

An Application	**The Mathematics**

A scale model of an addition to an athletic facility is 12 cm wide at the base and rises to a height of 15 cm. If the actual base is to be 116 ft, what will be the actual height of the addition?

This problem appears as Example 5 in Section 7.5.

We let $h =$ the height of the addition, in feet. Then we translate to a proportion and solve.

Each of these is a ratio.

$$\text{Width} \longrightarrow \frac{12}{15} = \frac{116}{h} \longleftarrow \text{Width}$$
$$\text{Height} \longrightarrow \qquad\qquad \longleftarrow \text{Height}$$

This is a proportion.

World Wide Web   For more information, visit us at www.mathmax.com

1. Write fractional notation for the ratio 31 to 54.

2. In this rectangle, find the ratio of width to length and simplify.

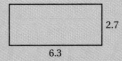

3. Craig's Ford Windstar can travel 336 mi on 14 gal of gasoline. What is the rate in miles per gallon?

4. A 16-oz bottle of Snapple iced tea costs $1.05. Find the unit cost in dollars per ounce. Round to the nearest hundredth of a cent.

5. Which has the lower unit price?

MINERAL WATER
Sparkle: 93¢ for 12 oz
Cleary's: $1.07 for 16 oz

6. Determine whether the pairs 3, 5 and 21, 35 are proportional.

Solve.

7. $\dfrac{6}{5} = \dfrac{27}{x}$

8. $\dfrac{y}{0.25} = \dfrac{0.3}{0.1}$

9. The clock on Sharon's stove loses 5 min in 10 hr. At this rate, how many minutes will it lose in 24 hr?

10. On a California state map, 4 in. represents 225 mi. If two cities are 7 in. apart on the map, how far apart are they in reality?

11. The figures below represent two similar polygons. Find the missing lengths.

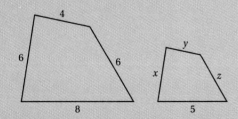

12. How high is a steeple that casts a 97.5-ft shadow at the same time that an 8-ft road sign casts a 13-ft shadow?

7.1 Introduction to Ratios

a Ratio

> A **ratio** is the quotient of two quantities.

For every 26 lb of waste produced in the United States, about 7 lb are recycled. The *ratio* of the amount of waste recycled to the amount of waste produced is shown by the fractional notation

$$\frac{7}{26}, \quad \text{or by the notation} \quad 7:26.$$

We can read such notation as "the ratio of 7 to 26," listing the numerator first and the denominator second. Note that a ratio indicates how important, or sizable, one quantity is in comparison to a second quantity.

> The ratio of a to b is written $\frac{a}{b}$, or $a:b$.

For most of our work, we will use fractional notation for ratios.

Example 1 Write fractional notation for the ratio of 7 to 8.

The ratio is $\frac{7}{8}$.

Example 2 Write fractional notation for the ratio of 31.4 to 100.

The ratio is $\frac{31.4}{100}$.

Example 3 Write fractional notation for the ratio of $4\frac{2}{3}$ to $5\frac{7}{8}$.

The ratio is $\dfrac{4\frac{2}{3}}{5\frac{7}{8}}$.

Do Exercises 1–3.

Example 4 *Drive-Through Fast Food.* For every 6 Americans who use a fast-food restaurant's drive-through window, 4 others order indoors. What is the ratio of drive-through orders to indoor orders?

The ratio is $\frac{6}{4}$.

Example 5 *Car Expenses.* A family earning $42,800 per year allots about $6420 for car expenses. What is the ratio of car expenses to yearly income?

The ratio is $\frac{6420}{42,800}$.

Objectives

a Find fractional notation for ratios.

b Simplify ratios.

For Extra Help

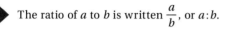

TAPE 13   MAC   CD-ROM
               WIN

1. Write fractional notation for the ratio of 5 to 11.

$\frac{5}{11}$

2. Write fractional notation for the ratio of 57.3 to 86.1.

$\frac{57.3}{86.1}$

3. Write fractional notation for the ratio of $6\frac{3}{4}$ to $7\frac{2}{5}$.

$\dfrac{6\frac{3}{4}}{7\frac{2}{5}}$

4. *Household Economics.* A family earning $28,500 per year will spend abut $7410 for food. What is the ratio of food expenses to yearly income?

$\frac{7410}{28,500}$

5. *Beverage Consumption.* The average American drinks 182.5 gal of liquid each year. Of this, 21.1 gal is milk. Find the ratio of milk consumed to total amount of liquid consumed.

$\frac{21.1}{182.5}$

Answers on page A-20

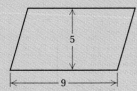

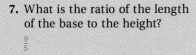

In the parallelogram above:

6. What is the ratio of the height to the length of the base?

$\frac{5}{9}$

7. What is the ratio of the length of the base to the height?

$\frac{9}{5}$

8. *Commuting by Car.* According to an Eno Transportation Foundation study, 73 of every 100 American workers drive to work alone. Find the ratio of single drivers to those who do not drive to work alone.

$\frac{73}{27}$

9. In Example 8, what is the ratio of the length of the shortest side of the television screen to the length of the longest side?

$\frac{3}{4}$

Write the ratio of the two given numbers. Then simplify each to find two other numbers in the same ratio.

10. 18 to 27

18 is to 27 as 2 is to 3.

11. 3.6 to 12

3.6 is to 12 as 3 is to 10.

12. 1.2 to 1.5

1.2 is to 1.5 as 4 is to 5.

Answers on page A-20

Example 6   In the triangle at right:

a) What is the ratio of the length of the longest side to the length of the shortest side?

The ratio is $\frac{5}{3}$.

b) What is the ratio of the length of the shortest side to the length of the longest side?

The ratio is $\frac{3}{5}$.

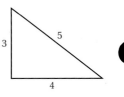

Do Exercises 4–7. (Exercises 4 and 5 are on the preceding page.)

Example 7   *Packaging.* For every dollar spent on food, about 13 cents goes to pay for the package. What is the ratio of the cost of the package to the cost of the package's contents?

If 13 cents of each dollar pays for packaging, then $100 - 13 = 87$ cents of each dollar pays for the package's contents. Thus the ratio of the cost of the package to the cost of the contents is

$$\frac{13}{87}.$$

Do Exercise 8.

b | Simplifying Notation for Ratios

Sometimes a ratio can be simplified. This provides a means of finding other numbers with the same ratio.

Example 8   Most television screens have the same ratio of length to width. Emilio's television has a screen that is 20 in. long and 15 in. wide. What is the ratio of length to width?

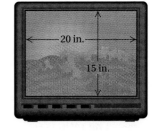

We write the ratio in fractional notation and then simplify:

$$\frac{20}{15} = \frac{5 \cdot 4}{5 \cdot 3} = \frac{5}{5} \cdot \frac{4}{3} = \frac{4}{3}.$$

Thus we can say that the ratio of length to width is 4 to 3.

Example 9   Write the ratio of 2.4 to 9.2. Then simplify and find two other numbers in the same ratio.

We first write the ratio. Next, we multiply by $\frac{10}{10}$, or 1, to clear the decimals from the numerator and the denominator. Then we simplify:

$$\frac{2.4}{9.2} = \frac{2.4}{9.2} \cdot \frac{10}{10} = \frac{24}{92} = \frac{4 \cdot 6}{4 \cdot 23} = \frac{4}{4} \cdot \frac{6}{23} = \frac{6}{23}.$$

We can say that 2.4 is to 9.2 as 6 is to 23.

Do Exercises 9–12.

Exercise Set 7.1

a Write fractional notation for each ratio. You need not simplify.

1. 4 to 5

$\frac{4}{5}$

2. 3 to 2

$\frac{3}{2}$

3. 178 to 572

$\frac{178}{572}$

4. 329 to 967

$\frac{329}{967}$

5. 0.4 to 12

$\frac{0.4}{12}$

6. 2.3 to 22

$\frac{2.3}{22}$

7. 3.8 to 7.4

$\frac{3.8}{7.4}$

8. 0.6 to 0.7

$\frac{0.6}{0.7}$

9. 56.78 to 98.35

$\frac{56.78}{98.35}$

10. 456.2 to 333.1

$\frac{456.2}{333.1}$

11. $8\frac{3}{4}$ to $9\frac{5}{6}$

$\frac{8\frac{3}{4}}{9\frac{5}{6}}$

12. $10\frac{1}{2}$ to $43\frac{1}{4}$

$\frac{10\frac{1}{2}}{43\frac{1}{4}}$

13. One person in four plays a musical instrument. In a typical group of people, what is the ratio of those who play an instrument to the total number of people? What is the ratio of those who do not play an instrument to those who do?

$\frac{1}{4}$; $\frac{3}{1}$

14. Of the 365 days in each year, it takes 107 days of work for the average person to pay his or her taxes. What is the ratio of days worked for taxes to total number of days in a year?

$\frac{107}{365}$

15. *Corvette Accidents.* Of every 5 fatal accidents involving a Corvette, 4 do not involve another vehicle (**Source:** *Harper's Magazine*). Find the ratio of fatal accidents involving just a Corvette to those involving a Corvette and at least one other vehicle.

$\frac{4}{1}$

16. *New York Commuters.* Of every 5 people who commute to work in New York City, 2 spend more than 90 min a day commuting (**Source:** *The Amicus Journal*). Find the ratio of people whose daily commute to New York exceeds 90 min a day to those whose commute is 90 min or less.

$\frac{2}{3}$

17. In this rectangle, find the ratios of length to width and of width to length.

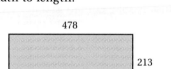

478

213

$\frac{478}{213}$; $\frac{213}{478}$

18. In this right triangle, find the ratios of shortest length to longest length and of longest length to shortest length.

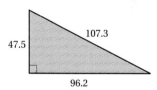

107.3

47.5

96.2

$\frac{47.5}{107.3}$; $\frac{107.3}{47.5}$

b Simplify each ratio.

19. 4 to 6

$\frac{2}{3}$

20. 6 to 10

$\frac{3}{5}$

21. 18 to 24

$\frac{3}{4}$

22. 28 to 36

$\frac{7}{9}$

23. 4.8 to 10

$\frac{12}{25}$

24. 5.6 to 10

$\frac{14}{25}$

25. 2.8 to 3.6

$\frac{7}{9}$

26. 4.8 to 6.4

$\frac{3}{4}$

27. 20 to 30

$\frac{2}{3}$

28. 40 to 60

$\frac{2}{3}$

29. 56 to 100

$\frac{14}{25}$

30. 42 to 100

$\frac{21}{50}$

31. 128 to 256

$\frac{1}{2}$

32. 232 to 116

$\frac{2}{1}$

33. 0.48 to 0.64

$\frac{3}{4}$

34. 0.32 to 0.96

$\frac{1}{3}$

35. The ratio of females to males worldwide is 51 to 49. Write this ratio in simplified fractional form.

$\frac{51}{49}$

36. The ratio of Americans aged 18–24 living with their parents to all Americans aged 18–24 is 54 to 100. Write this ratio in simplified fractional form.

$\frac{27}{50}$

37. In this right triangle, find the ratio of shortest length to longest length and simplify.

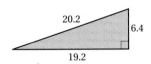

$\frac{32}{101}$

38. In this rectangle, find the ratio of width to length and simplify.

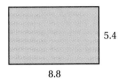

$\frac{27}{44}$

Skill Maintenance

Use < or > for ▨ to write a true sentence. [4.2c]

39. $-\dfrac{5}{6}$ ▨ $-\dfrac{3}{4}$ <

40. $\dfrac{12}{8}$ ▨ $\dfrac{7}{4}$ <

41. $\dfrac{5}{9}$ ▨ $\dfrac{6}{11}$ >

42. $-\dfrac{3}{4}$ ▨ $-\dfrac{2}{3}$ <

Solve. [4.6c]

43. Rocky is $187\frac{1}{10}$ cm tall and his daughter is $180\frac{3}{4}$ cm tall. How much taller is Rocky?

$6\frac{7}{20}$ cm

44. Aunt Louise is $168\frac{1}{4}$ cm tall and her son is $150\frac{7}{10}$ cm tall. How much taller is Aunt Louise?

$17\frac{11}{20}$ cm

Synthesis

45. ◆ Is it possible for the ratio of the lengths of the two legs of a right triangle to be 1:5? Why or why not?

46. ◆ Can every ratio be written as the ratio of some number to 1? Why or why not?

47. ◆ What can be concluded about the width of a rectangle if the ratio of length to perimeter is 1 to 3? Make some sketches and explain your reasoning.

48. ▦ In 1996, the total payroll of major league baseball teams was $937,905,284. The New York Yankees won the World Series that year. Their payroll was the highest at $61,511,870. Find the ratio in decimal notation of the Yankees payroll to the overall payroll. 0.065584309 to 1

49. ▦ See Exercise 48. In 1995, the total payroll of major league baseball teams was $927,334,416. Find the ratio of the payroll in 1996 to the payroll in 1995. 1.011399197 to 1

50. Write simplified fractional form for the ratio of $3\frac{3}{4}$ to $5\frac{7}{8}$. $\frac{30}{47}$

Exercises 51 and 52 refer to a common fertilizer known as "5, 10, 15." This mixture contains 5 parts of potassium for every 10 parts of phosphorus and 15 parts of nitrogen (this is often denoted 5:10:15).

51. Find the ratio of potassium to nitrogen and of nitrogen to phosphorus. $\frac{1}{3}$; $\frac{3}{2}$

52. Simplify the ratio 5:10:15. 1:2:3

Analyze the ratios of different colored M&M candies.

Collaborative Learning Manual

7.2 Rates and Unit Prices

a Rates

When a ratio is used to compare two different kinds of measure, we call it a **rate.** Suppose that a car is driven 200 km in 4 hr. The ratio

$$\frac{200 \text{ km}}{4 \text{ hr}}, \quad \text{or } 50\frac{\text{km}}{\text{hr}}, \quad \text{or } 50 \text{ kilometers per hour}, \quad \text{or } 50 \text{ km/h}$$

> Recall that "per" means "division," or "for each."

is the rate of travel in kilometers per hour, which is the division of the number of kilometers by the number of hours. A ratio of distance traveled to time is also called **speed.**

Example 1 Pierre's moped travels 145 km on 2.5 L of gas. What is the rate in kilometers per liter?

$$\text{The rate is } \frac{145 \text{ km}}{2.5 \text{ L}}, \quad \text{or } \quad 58\frac{\text{km}}{\text{L}}.$$

Example 2 It takes 60 oz of grass seed to seed 3000 sq ft of lawn. What is the rate in ounces per square foot?

$$\text{The rate is } \frac{60 \text{ oz}}{3000 \text{ sq ft}} = \frac{1}{50}\frac{\text{oz}}{\text{sq ft}}, \quad \text{or } \quad 0.02\frac{\text{oz}}{\text{sq ft}}.$$

Example 3 A cook buys 10 lb of potatoes for \$3.69. What is the rate in cents per pound?

$$\text{The rate is } \frac{\$3.69}{10 \text{ lb}} = \frac{369 \text{ cents}}{10 \text{ lb}}, \quad \text{or } \quad 36.9\frac{\text{cents}}{\text{lb}}.$$

Example 4 A student nurse working in a health center earned \$3690 for working 3 months one summer. What was the rate of pay per month?

  The rate of pay is the ratio of money earned per length of time worked, or

$$\frac{\$3690}{3 \text{ mo}} = 1230\frac{\text{dollars}}{\text{month}}, \quad \text{or } \quad \$1230 \text{ per month.}$$

Example 5 *At-Bats to Home-Run Ratio.* At one point during the 1998 baseball season, slugger Mark McGwire had hit 50 home runs in 390 at-bats (times at bat). Find his at-bats per home-run rate.*

$$\text{His rate was } \frac{390 \text{ at-bats}}{50 \text{ home runs}} = 7.8\frac{\text{at-bats}}{\text{home runs}}.$$

Do Exercises 1–8.

---

*See also Exercise 53 on p. 428.

*See also Exercise 53 on p. 428.

Objectives

a Give the ratio of two different kinds of measure as a rate.

b Find unit prices and use them to determine which of two possible purchases has the lower unit price.

For Extra Help

TAPE 13   MAC   CD-ROM
            WIN

What is the rate, or speed, in miles per hour?

1. 45 mi, 9 hr   5 mi/hr

2. 120 mi, 10 hr   12 mi/hr

3. 3 mi, 10 hr   0.3 mi/hr

What is the rate, or speed, in feet per second?

4. 2200 ft, 2 sec   1100 ft/sec

5. 52 ft, 13 sec   4 ft/sec

6. 232 ft, 16 sec   14.5 ft/sec

7. A well-hit golf ball can travel 500 ft in 2 sec. What is the rate, or speed, of the golf ball in feet per second?

250 ft/sec

8. A leaky faucet can lose 14 gal of water in a week. What is the rate in gallons per day?

2 gal/day

Answers on page A-20

9. Kate bought a 14-oz package of cereal for $2.89. What is the unit price in cents per ounce? Round to the nearest hundredth of a cent.

20.64 ¢/oz

10. Which has the lower unit price? [*Note*: 1 qt = 32 fl oz (fluid ounces).]

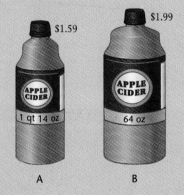

A   B

Container B

Answers on page A-20

b Unit Pricing

> A **unit price** or **unit rate** is the ratio of price to the number of units.

By carrying out the division indicated by the ratio, we can find the price per unit.

Example 6   Ruby bought a 40-lb bag of Nutro™ dog food for $34. What is the unit price in dollars per pound?

The unit price is the price in dollars for each pound.

$$\text{Unit price} = \frac{\text{Price}}{\text{Number of units}}$$

$$= \frac{\$34}{40 \text{ lb}} = \frac{34}{40} \cdot \frac{\$}{\text{lb}}$$

$$= 0.85 \text{ dollar per pound}$$

Do Exercise 9.

For comparison shopping, it helps to find unit prices. Make sure that the same units are being used in all items being compared.

Example 7   Which has the lower unit price?

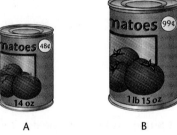

A   B

To find out, we compare the unit prices—in this case, the price per ounce.

For can A: $\dfrac{48 \text{ cents}}{14 \text{ oz}} \approx 3.429 \dfrac{\text{cents}}{\text{oz}}$.

For can B: We need to find the total number of ounces:

1 lb, 15 oz = 16 oz + 15 oz = 31 oz.

Then

$\dfrac{99 \text{ cents}}{31 \text{ oz}} \approx 3.194 \dfrac{\text{cents}}{\text{oz}}$.

Thus can B has the lower unit price.

In supermarkets, unit prices are usually listed below the items on the shelves.

Do Exercise 10.

Exercise Set 7.2

a In Exercises 1–6, find the rate as a ratio of distance to time. Use the units given.

1. 120 km, 3 hr

40 km/h

2. 18 mi, 9 hr

2 mi/hr

3. 440 m, 40 sec

11 m/sec

4. 200 mi, 25 sec

8 mi/sec

5. 342 yd, 2.25 days

152 yd/day

6. 492 m, 60 sec

8.2 m/sec

7. A delivery van is driven 500 mi in 20 hr. What is the rate in miles per hour? in hours per mile?

25 mi/hr; 0.04 hr/mi

8. Franny eats 3 hamburgers in 15 min. What is the rate in hamburgers per minute? in minutes per hamburger?

0.2 hamburger/min; 5 min/hamburger

9. A long-distance telephone call between two cities costs $5.75 for 10 min. What is the rate in cents per minute?

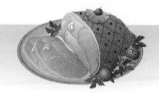

57.5 ¢/min

10. An 8-lb boneless ham contains 36 servings of meat. What is the ratio in servings per pound?

4.5 servings/lb

11. A thoroughly watered lawn requires 623 gal of water for every 1000 ft^2. What is the rate in gallons per square foot?

0.623 gal/ft^2

12. A limousine is driven 200 km on 40 L of gasoline. What is the rate in kilometers per liter?

5 km/L

13. Sound travels 66,000 ft in 1 min. What is its rate, or speed, in feet per second?

1100 ft/sec

14. Light travels 11,160,000 mi in 1 min. What is its rate, or speed, in miles per second?

186,000 mi/sec

15. Impulses in nerve fibers can travel 310 km in 2.5 hr. What is the rate, or speed, in kilometers per hour?

124 km/h

16. A black racer snake can travel 4.6 km in 2 hr. What is its rate, or speed, in kilometers per hour?

2.3 km/h

17. A jet flew 2660 mi in 4.75 hr. What was its speed?

560 mi/hr

18. A turtle traveled 0.42 mi in 2.5 hr. What was its speed?

0.168 mi/hr

b

19. The fabric for a wedding gown costs $165.75 for 8.5 yd. Find the unit price.

$19.50/yd

20. An 8-oz tube of toothpaste costs $2.59. Find the unit price.

$0.32375/oz, or 32.375 ¢/oz

21. A 2-lb can of coffee costs $6.59. What is the unit price in cents per ounce? Round to the nearest hundredth of a cent.

20.59 ¢/oz

22. A 24-can package of 12-oz cans of soda is on sale for $6.99. What is the unit price in cents per ounce? Round to the nearest hundredth of a cent.

2.43 ¢/oz

23. A $\frac{2}{3}$-lb package of Monterey Jack cheese costs $2.89. Find the unit price in dollars per pound. Round to the nearest hundredth of a dollar.

$4.34/lb

24. A $1\frac{1}{4}$-lb container of cottage cheese costs $1.62. Find the unit price in dollars per pound. Round to the nearest hundredth of a dollar.

$1.30/lb

Which has the lower unit price?

25.

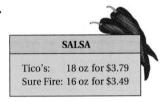

SALSA	
Tico's:	18 oz for $3.79
Sure Fire:	16 oz for $3.49

Tico's

26.

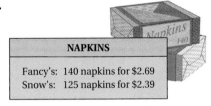

NAPKINS	
Fancy's:	140 napkins for $2.69
Snow's:	125 napkins for $2.39

Snow's

27.

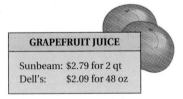

GRAPEFRUIT JUICE	
Sunbeam:	$2.79 for 2 qt
Dell's:	$2.09 for 48 oz

Dell's

28.

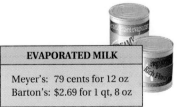

EVAPORATED MILK	
Meyer's:	79 cents for 12 oz
Barton's:	$2.69 for 1 qt, 8 oz

Meyer's

29.

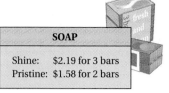

SOAP	
Shine:	$2.19 for 3 bars
Pristine:	$1.58 for 2 bars

Shine

30.

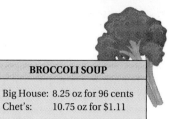

BROCCOLI SOUP	
Big House:	8.25 oz for 96 cents
Chet's:	10.75 oz for $1.11

Chet's

31.

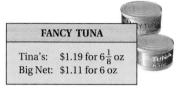

FANCY TUNA	
Tina's:	$1.19 for $6\frac{1}{8}$ oz
Big Net:	$1.11 for 6 oz

Big Net

32.

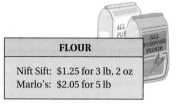

FLOUR	
Nift Sift:	$1.25 for 3 lb, 2 oz
Marlo's:	$2.05 for 5 lb

Nift Sift

33.

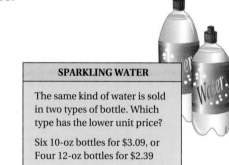

SPARKLING WATER

The same kind of water is sold in two types of bottle. Which type has the lower unit price?

Six 10-oz bottles for $3.09, or
Four 12-oz bottles for $2.39

Four 12-oz bottles

34.

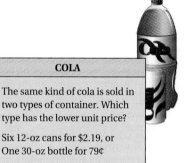

COLA

The same kind of cola is sold in two types of container. Which type has the lower unit price?

Six 12-oz cans for $2.19, or
One 30-oz bottle for 79¢

30-oz bottle

35.

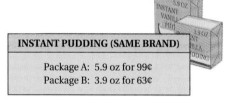

INSTANT PUDDING (SAME BRAND)

Package A: 5.9 oz for 99¢
Package B: 3.9 oz for 63¢

B

36.

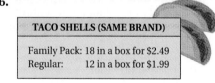

TACO SHELLS (SAME BRAND)

Family Pack: 18 in a box for $2.49
Regular: 12 in a box for $1.99

Family Pack

37.

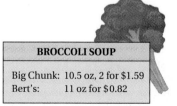

BROCCOLI SOUP	
Big Chunk:	10.5 oz, 2 for $1.59
Bert's:	11 oz for $0.82

Bert's

38.

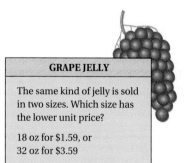

GRAPE JELLY

The same kind of jelly is sold in two sizes. Which size has the lower unit price?

18 oz for $1.59, or
32 oz for $3.59

18 oz

Skill Maintenance

Solve.

39. There are 20.6 million people in this country who play the piano and 18.9 million who play the guitar. How many more play the piano than the guitar? [5.8a] 1.7 million

40. A serving of fish steak (cross section) is generally $\frac{1}{2}$ lb. How many servings can be prepared from a cleaned $12\frac{3}{4}$-lb salmon? [4.7d] $25\frac{1}{2}$

Multiply. [5.3a]

41. 4 5.6 7
      $\times$ 2.4
      ───────
      109.608

42. 6 7 8.1 9
      $\times$ 1 0 0
      ───────
      67,819

In which quadrant is each point located? [6.3b]

43. (3, −8) IV

44. (−5, 4.1) II

Synthesis

45. ◆ The unit price of an item generally drops when larger packages of that item are purchased. Why?

46. ◆ Suppose that the same type of juice is available in two sizes and that the larger bottle has the lower unit price. If the larger bottle costs $3.79 and contains twice as much juice, what can you conclude about the price of the smaller bottle? Why?

47. ◆ Manufacturers of laundry detergent sometimes charge a higher unit price for their larger packages. Why do you think they do so?

48. Recently, certain manufacturers have been changing the size of their containers in such a way that the consumer thinks the price of a product has been lowered when, in reality, a higher unit price is being charged.

a) Some aluminum juice cans are now concave (curved in) on the bottom. Suppose the volume of the can in the figure has been reduced from a fluid capacity of 6 oz to 5.5 oz, and the price of each can has been reduced from 65¢ to 60¢. Find the unit price of each container in cents per ounce. 10.83¢/oz; 10.91¢/oz

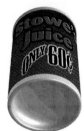

b) Suppose that at one time the cost of a certain kind of paper towel was $0.89 for a roll containing 78 ft^2 of absorbent surface. Later the surface area was changed to 65 ft^2 and the price was decreased to $0.79. Find the unit price of each product in cents per square foot. 1.14¢/ft^2; 1.22¢/ft^2

49. In 1994, Coca-Cola introduced a 20-oz soda bottle. At first it was sold for 64¢ a bottle, the same price as their 16-oz bottle. After about a month, the price of a 20-oz bottle rose to 80¢. How did the unit price change for a consumer who made the switch from the 16-oz to the 20-oz bottle? See below.

50. Suppose that a pasta manufacturer shrinks the size of a box from 1 lb to 14 oz, but keeps the price at 85 cents a box. How does the unit price change?

The unit price increases by 0.76 ¢/oz.

51. ▦ Use the formula for the area of a circle, $A = \pi r^2$, to determine which is a better deal: a 14-in. pizza for $10.50 or a 16-in. pizza for $11.95. Use 3.14 for π.

16-in pizza

52. ▦ Suppose that, 25 mi from where you're standing, a bolt of lightning splits a tree. How long will it take for you to hear the accompanying crack of thunder? How long will it take for you to see the flash of light? (*Hint*: Use the information in Exercises 13 and 14.) 2 min; 0.0000022 min

53. ▦ In 1998, Mark McGwire set a major-league record, hitting 70 home runs in 509 at-bats. Find his at-bats per home run rate. About 7.27 at-bats per home run

49. For about a month, the unit price decreased by 0.8¢/oz. Then it changed to the same unit cost as the 16-oz bottle.

7.3 Proportions

a | Proportion

When two pairs of numbers (such as 3, 2 and 6, 4) have the same ratio, we say that they are **proportional**. The equation

$$\frac{3}{2} = \frac{6}{4}$$

states that the pairs 3, 2 and 6, 4 are proportional. Such an equation is called a **proportion**. We sometimes read $\frac{3}{2} = \frac{6}{4}$ as "3 is to 2 as 6 is to 4." Because proportions arise frequently and in many fields of study, being able to solve them is an extremely useful skill. Several important applications of proportions are considered in Section 7.4.

Checking to see whether two pairs of numbers are proportional is the same as checking to see whether two fractions are equal. To develop a quick way of doing this, consider a/b and c/d and assume that neither b nor d is 0.

Note that if

$$\frac{a}{b} = \frac{c}{d}$$

is true, then (using the multiplication principle)

$$bd \cdot \frac{a}{b} = bd \cdot \frac{c}{d} \qquad \textbf{Multiplying by } \textit{bd} \textbf{ on both sides}$$

is also true. Simplifying, we have

$$da = bc.$$

If neither b nor d is 0, the above equations are equivalent. Thus any time that $da = bc$ (with $d \neq 0$ and $b \neq 0$), it follows that

$$\frac{a}{b} = \frac{c}{d}.$$

> **A Test for Equality**
>
> We multiply these two numbers: $3 \cdot 4$.
>
> We multiply these two numbers: $2 \cdot 6$.
>
> $$\frac{3}{2} \overset{?}{=} \frac{6}{4}$$
>
> Since $3 \cdot 4 = 2 \cdot 6$, we know that
>
> $$\frac{3}{2} = \frac{6}{4}.$$
>
> We call $3 \cdot 4$ and $2 \cdot 6$ *cross products*.

Example 1 Determine whether 1, 2 and 3, 6 are proportional.

We can use cross products to check an equivalent equation:

$$1 \cdot 6 = 6 \qquad \frac{1}{2} \overset{?}{=} \frac{3}{6} \qquad 2 \cdot 3 = 6$$

$$1 \cdot 6 \overset{?}{=} 2 \cdot 3$$

$$6 = 6.$$

Since this last equation is true, we know that the first equation is also true and the numbers 1, 2 and 3, 6 are proportional.

Objectives

a | Determine whether two pairs of numbers are proportional.

b | Solve proportions.

For Extra Help

TAPE 13

MAC
WIN

CD-ROM

Determine whether the two pairs of numbers are proportional.

4. $4\frac{2}{3}$, $5\frac{1}{2}$ and 14, $16\frac{1}{2}$.

Yes

5. 7.4, 6.8 and 4.2, 3.6

No

Answers on page A-20

Example 2   Determine whether 2, 5 and 4, 7 are proportional.

We can check an equivalent equation using cross products:

$2 \cdot 7 = 14$ $\dfrac{2}{5} \overset{?}{=} \dfrac{4}{7}$ $5 \cdot 4 = 20$

$$2 \cdot 7 \overset{?}{=} 5 \cdot 4$$

$$14 \neq 20.$$

Since $14 \neq 20$, we know that $\frac{2}{5} \neq \frac{4}{7}$, so 2, 5 and 4, 7 are not proportional.

Do Exercises 1–3.

Example 3   Determine whether $1\frac{1}{4}$, $\frac{1}{2}$ and 1, $\frac{2}{5}$ are proportional.

We can use cross products:

$1\frac{1}{4} \cdot \dfrac{2}{5} = \dfrac{5}{4} \cdot \dfrac{2}{5}$ $\dfrac{1\frac{1}{4}}{\frac{1}{2}} \overset{?}{=} \dfrac{1}{\frac{2}{5}}$ $\dfrac{1}{2} \cdot 1 = \dfrac{1}{2}$

$$\dfrac{5}{4} \cdot \dfrac{2}{5} \overset{?}{=} \dfrac{1}{2}$$

$$\dfrac{10}{20} = \dfrac{1}{2}.$$

Since $\frac{10}{20} = \frac{1}{2}$, we know that

$$\dfrac{1\frac{1}{4}}{\frac{1}{2}} = \dfrac{1}{\frac{2}{5}}.$$

The numbers $1\frac{1}{4}$, $\frac{1}{2}$ and 1, $\frac{2}{5}$ are proportional.

Do Exercises 4 and 5.

b   Solving Proportions

Often one of the four numbers in a proportion is unknown. Cross products can be used to find the missing number and "solve" the proportion.

Example 4   Solve: $\dfrac{x}{8} = \dfrac{3}{5}$.

We form an equivalent equation by equating cross products. Then we solve for x.

$$5 \cdot x = 8 \cdot 3 \quad \text{Equating cross products}$$

$$\dfrac{5x}{5} = \dfrac{24}{5} \quad \text{Dividing by 5 on both sides}$$

$$x = \dfrac{24}{5} \quad \text{Simplifying}$$

$$= 4.8. \quad \text{Dividing}$$

To check that 4.8 is the solution, we replace x with 4.8 and use cross products:

$4.8 \cdot 5 = 24$ $\dfrac{4.8}{8} \overset{?}{=} \dfrac{3}{5}$ $8 \cdot 3 = 24$.   The cross products are the same.

Since the cross products are the same, it follows that $\frac{4.8}{8} = \frac{3}{5}$. Thus, 4.8, 8 and 3, 5 are proportional, and 4.8 is the solution of the equation.

> To solve $\frac{a}{b} = \frac{c}{d}$ for a specific variable, equate cross products and then divide on both sides to get that variable alone. (Assume b, $d \neq 0$.)

Do Exercise 6.

Example 5 Solve: $\frac{x}{7} = \frac{5}{3}$. Write a mixed numeral for the answer.

We have

$$\frac{x}{7} = \frac{5}{3}$$

$3 \cdot x = 7 \cdot 5$ **Equating cross products**

$\frac{3x}{3} = \frac{35}{3}$ **Dividing by 3 on both sides**

$x = \frac{35}{3}$, or $11\frac{2}{3}$.

The solution is $11\frac{2}{3}$.

Do Exercise 7.

Example 6 Solve: $\frac{7.7}{15.4} = \frac{y}{2.2}$. Write decimal notation for the answer.

We have

$$\frac{7.7}{15.4} = \frac{y}{2.2}$$

$(7.7)(2.2) = 15.4y$ **Equating cross products**

$\frac{(7.7)(2.2)}{15.4} = \frac{15.4y}{15.4}$ **Dividing by 15.4 on both sides**

$\frac{16.94}{15.4} = y$ **Simplifying**

$1.1 = y.$ **Dividing:**
$$\begin{array}{r} 1.1 \\ 15.4\overline{)16.9.4} \\ \underline{1\,5\,4\,0} \\ 1\,5\,4 \\ \underline{1\,5\,4} \\ 0 \end{array}$$

The solution is 1.1.

Do Exercise 8.

6. Solve: $\frac{x}{63} = \frac{2}{9}$.   14

7. Solve: $\frac{x}{9} = \frac{5}{4}$. $11\frac{1}{4}$

8. Solve: $\frac{21}{5} = \frac{n}{2.5}$.   10.5

Answers on page A-20

9. Solve: $\dfrac{2}{3} = \dfrac{6}{x}$.　9

Example 7　Solve: $\dfrac{3}{x} = \dfrac{6}{4}$.

We have

$$\dfrac{3}{x} = \dfrac{6}{4}$$

$3 \cdot 4 = x \cdot 6$ 　　**Equating cross products**

$$\dfrac{12}{6} = \dfrac{6x}{6}$$ 　　**Dividing by 6 on both sides**

$2 = x.$ 　　**Simplifying**

The solution is 2.

Do Exercise 9.

Example 8　Solve: $\dfrac{3.4}{4.93} = \dfrac{10}{n}$.

We have

$$\dfrac{3.4}{4.93} = \dfrac{10}{n}$$

$(n)(3.4) = (4.93)(10)$ 　　**Equating cross products**

$$\dfrac{3.4n}{3.4} = \dfrac{(4.93)(10)}{3.4}$$ 　　**Dividing by 3.4 on both sides**

$$n = \dfrac{49.3}{3.4}$$ 　　**Multiplying**

10. Solve: $\dfrac{0.4}{0.9} = \dfrac{4.8}{t}$.　10.8

$= 14.5.$ 　　Dividing:
$$\begin{array}{r} 1\,4.5 \\ 3.4\,)\overline{4\,9.3\,0} \\ 3\,4\,0\,0 \\ \hline 1\,5\,3\,0 \\ 1\,3\,6\,0 \\ \hline 1\,7\,0 \\ 1\,7\,0 \\ \hline 0 \end{array}$$

The solution is 14.5.

Do Exercise 10.

Answer on page A-20

Exercise Set 7.3

a Determine whether the two pairs of numbers are proportional.

1. 5, 6 and 7, 9

No

2. 7, 5 and 6, 4

No

3. 1, 2 and 10, 20

Yes

4. 7, 3 and 21, 9

Yes

5. 2.4, 3.6 and 1.8, 2.7

Yes

6. 4.5, 3.8 and 6.7, 5.2

No

7. $5\frac{1}{3}$, $8\frac{1}{4}$ and $2\frac{1}{5}$, $9\frac{1}{2}$

No

8. $2\frac{1}{3}$, $3\frac{1}{2}$ and 14, 21

Yes

b Solve.

9. $\dfrac{18}{4} = \dfrac{x}{10}$

45

10. $\dfrac{x}{45} = \dfrac{20}{25}$

36

11. $\dfrac{x}{8} = \dfrac{9}{6}$

12

12. $\dfrac{8}{10} = \dfrac{n}{5}$

4

13. $\dfrac{t}{12} = \dfrac{5}{6}$

10

14. $\dfrac{12}{4} = \dfrac{x}{3}$

9

15. $\dfrac{2}{5} = \dfrac{8}{n}$

20

16. $\dfrac{10}{6} = \dfrac{5}{x}$

3

17. $\dfrac{n}{15} = \dfrac{10}{30}$

5

18. $\dfrac{2}{24} = \dfrac{x}{36}$

3

19. $\dfrac{16}{12} = \dfrac{24}{x}$

18

20. $\dfrac{7}{11} = \dfrac{2}{x}$

$3\frac{1}{7}$ or $\frac{22}{7}$

21. $\dfrac{6}{11} = \dfrac{12}{x}$

22

22. $\dfrac{8}{9} = \dfrac{32}{n}$

36

23. $\dfrac{20}{7} = \dfrac{80}{x}$

28

24. $\dfrac{5}{x} = \dfrac{4}{10}$

$12\frac{1}{2}$ or $\frac{25}{2}$

25. $\dfrac{12}{9} = \dfrac{x}{7}$

$9\frac{1}{3}$ or $\frac{28}{3}$

26. $\dfrac{x}{20} = \dfrac{16}{15}$

$21\frac{1}{3}$ or $\frac{64}{3}$

27. $\dfrac{x}{13} = \dfrac{2}{9}$

$2\frac{8}{9}$ or $\frac{26}{9}$

28. $\dfrac{1.2}{4} = \dfrac{x}{9}$

2.7

29. $\dfrac{t}{0.16} = \dfrac{0.15}{0.40}$

0.06

30. $\dfrac{x}{11} = \dfrac{7.1}{2}$

39.05

31. $\dfrac{100}{25} = \dfrac{20}{n}$

5

32. $\dfrac{35}{125} = \dfrac{7}{m}$

25

33. $\dfrac{7}{\frac{1}{4}} = \dfrac{28}{x}$ 1

34. $\dfrac{x}{6} = \dfrac{1}{6}$ 1

35. $\dfrac{\frac{1}{4}}{\frac{1}{2}} = \dfrac{\frac{1}{2}}{x}$ 1

36. $\dfrac{1}{7} = \dfrac{x}{4\frac{1}{2}}$ $\frac{9}{14}$

37. $\dfrac{x}{\frac{4}{5}} = \dfrac{0}{\frac{9}{11}}$ 0

38. $\dfrac{\frac{2}{7}}{\frac{3}{4}} = \dfrac{\frac{5}{6}}{y}$ $2\frac{3}{16}$, or $\frac{35}{16}$

39. $\dfrac{2\frac{1}{2}}{3\frac{1}{3}} = \dfrac{x}{4\frac{1}{4}}$ $\frac{51}{16}$, or $3\frac{3}{16}$

40. $\dfrac{5\frac{1}{5}}{6\frac{1}{6}} = \dfrac{y}{3\frac{1}{2}}$ $\frac{546}{185}$, or $2\frac{176}{185}$

41. $\dfrac{1.28}{3.76} = \dfrac{4.28}{y}$ 12.5725

42. $\dfrac{10.4}{12.4} = \dfrac{6.76}{t}$ 8.06

43. $\dfrac{10\frac{3}{8}}{12\frac{2}{3}} = \dfrac{5\frac{3}{4}}{y}$ $\frac{1748}{249}$, or $7\frac{5}{249}$

44. $\dfrac{12\frac{7}{8}}{20\frac{3}{4}} = \dfrac{5\frac{2}{3}}{y}$ $\frac{2822}{309}$, or $9\frac{41}{309}$

Skill Maintenance

In which quadrant is each point located?   [6.3b]

45. $(-3.2, -5.7)$ III

46. $\left(-7\frac{1}{2}, 13\right)$ II

47. $(9, -0.1)$ IV

48. $(19, 57)$ I

Divide. Write decimal notation for the answer.   [5.4a]

49. $260 \div (-5)$ -52

50. $395 \div (-20)$ -19.75

51. $4648 \div 16$ 290.5

52. $3427 \div 2.25$ $1523.\overline{1}$

Synthesis

53. ◆ Instead of equating cross products, a student solves $\frac{x}{7} = \frac{5}{3}$ (see Example 5) by multiplying on both sides by the least common denominator, 21. Is the student's approach a good one? Why or why not?

54. ◆ An instructor predicts that a student's test grade will be proportional to the amount of time the student spends studying. What is meant by this? Write an example of a proportion that involves the grades of two students and their study times.

55. ◆ Joaquin argues that $\frac{0}{0}$ is equal to $\frac{3}{4}$ because $0 \cdot 3 = 4 \cdot 0$. Is he correct? Why or why not?

Solve.

56. 🖩 $\dfrac{1728}{5643} = \dfrac{836.4}{x}$ Approximately 2731.4

57. 🖩 $\dfrac{328.56}{627.48} = \dfrac{y}{127.66}$ Approximately 66.85

58. $\dfrac{x}{4} = \dfrac{x-1}{6}$ -2

59. $\dfrac{x+3}{5} = \dfrac{x}{7}$ -10.5

60. Show using a sequence of steps—each of which can be justified—that for $a, b, c, d, \neq 0$,

$$\dfrac{a}{b} = \dfrac{c}{d} \quad \text{is equivalent to} \quad \dfrac{d}{b} = \dfrac{c}{a}.$$

7.4 Applications of Proportions

a Problem Solving

Proportions have applications in business, the natural and social sciences, home economics, and many areas of daily life.

Example 1 *Calories Burned.* Heather's stairmaster tells her that if she exercises for 24 min, she will burn 356 calories. How many calories will she burn if she exercises for 30 min?

We let n = the number of calories that Heather will burn in 30 min. Then we translate to a proportion in which each side is the ratio of the number of calories burned to the number of minutes spent exercising.

Calories burned in 30 min → $\dfrac{n}{30} = \dfrac{356}{24}$ ← Calories burned in 24 min
Time → — — ← Time

Each side of the equation represents the same ratio. It may help to verbalize the proportion as "the unknown number of carlories is to 30 min, as 356 calories is to 24 min."

Solve: $24 \cdot n = 30 \cdot 356$ **Equating cross products**

$\left\{\begin{array}{l}\dfrac{24n}{24} = \dfrac{30 \cdot 356}{24} \quad\text{\textbf{Dividing by 24 on both sides}}\\[2mm] n = \dfrac{6 \cdot 5 \cdot 4 \cdot 89}{6 \cdot 4} \quad\text{\textbf{Factoring}}\\[2mm] = 5 \cdot 89 \quad\text{\textbf{Removing a factor equal to 1: } } \dfrac{6 \cdot 4}{6 \cdot 4} = 1\\[2mm] = 445\end{array}\right.$

A calculator can shorten these steps

Heather will burn 445 calories in 30 min.

Do Exercise 1.

Proportion problems can be solved in more than one way. For Example 1, any one of the following equations could have been used:

$$\frac{356}{24} = \frac{n}{30}, \quad \frac{30}{n} = \frac{24}{356}, \quad \frac{30}{24} = \frac{n}{356}, \quad \frac{356}{n} = \frac{24}{30}.$$

Example 2 To control a fever, a doctor suggests that a child weighing 28 kg be given 420 mg of Tylenol™. Under similar circumstances, how much Tylenol could be recommended for a child weighing 35 kg?

We let t = the number of milligrams of Tylenol and form a proportion.

Tylenol suggested → $\dfrac{420}{28} = \dfrac{t}{35}$ ← Tylenol suggested
Child's weight → — — ← Child's weight

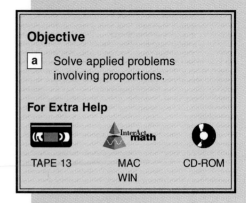

1. Brian drives his delivery van 800 mi in 5 days. At this rate, how far will he travel in 7 days?   1120 mi

Answer on page A-20

2. Campus Painting, Inc., can paint 1700 ft² of clapboard with 4 gal of paint. How much paint would be needed for a building with 6800 ft² of clapboard?　16 gal

3. *Purchasing Shirts.* If 2 shirts can be bought for $47, how many shirts can be bought with $200?　8

4. *Waist-to-Hip Ratio.* It is also recommended that a man's waist-to-hip ratio be 0.95 (or lower). Uri's hip measurement is 45 in. To meet the recommendation, what should Uri's waist measurement be?

$42\frac{3}{4}$ in. or less

Answers on page A-20

Solve: $\quad 420 \cdot 35 = 28 \cdot t$　　**Equating cross products**

$$\frac{420 \cdot 35}{28} = \frac{28t}{28}$$　　**Dividing by 28 on both sides**

$$\frac{\cancel{4} \cdot 105 \cdot 5 \cdot \cancel{7}}{\cancel{4} \cdot \cancel{7}} = t$$　　**Removing a factor equal to 1:** $\frac{4 \cdot 7}{4 \cdot 7} = 1$

$$525 = t.$$

Thus, 525 mg could be recommended for a 35-kg child.

Do Exercise 2.

Example 3　*Ticket Purchases.* Rosa bought 8 tickets to an international food festival for $52. How many tickets could she purchase with $90?

We let n = the number of tickets that can be purchased with $90. Then we translate to a proportion.

$$\begin{array}{c} \text{Cost} \rightarrow \\ \text{Tickets} \rightarrow \end{array} \frac{52}{8} = \frac{90}{n} \begin{array}{c} \leftarrow \text{Cost} \\ \leftarrow \text{Tickets} \end{array}$$

Solve: $\quad 52n = 8 \cdot 90$　　**Equating cross products**

$$n = \frac{8 \cdot 90}{52}$$　　**Dividing by 52 on both sides**

$$\approx 13.8.$$　　**Simplifying and rounding**

Because it is impossible to buy a fractional part of a ticket, we must round our answer *down* to 13. As a check, we use a different approach: We find the cost per ticket and then divide $90 by that price. Since $52 \div 8 = 6.50$ and $90 \div 6.50 \approx 13.8$, we have a check. Rosa could purchase 13 tickets with $90.

Do Exercise 3.

Example 4　*Waist-to-Hip Ratio.* For improved health, it is recommended that a woman's waist-to-hip ratio be 0.85 (or lower) (***Source:*** David Schmidt, "Lifting Weight Myths," *Nutrition Action Newsletter* 20, no. 4, October 1993). Marta's hip measurement is 40 in. To meet the recommendation, what should Marta's waist measurement be?

 Hip measurement is the largest measurement around the widest part of the buttocks.

 Waist measurement is the smallest measurement below the ribs but above the navel.

Note that $0.85 = \frac{85}{100}$. We let w = Marta's waist measurement and translate to a proportion.

$$\begin{array}{c} \text{Waist measurement} \rightarrow \\ \text{Hip measurement} \rightarrow \end{array} \frac{w}{40} = \frac{85}{100} \begin{array}{c} \searrow \text{Recommended} \\ \nearrow \text{waist-to-hip ratio} \end{array}$$

Solve: $\quad 100w = 40 \cdot 85$　　**Equating cross products**

$$w = \frac{40 \cdot 85}{100}$$　　**Dividing by 100 on both sides**

$$= 34$$

Marta's recommended waist measurement is 34 in. (or less).

Do Exercise 4.

Exercise Set 7.4

a Solve.

1. *Gasoline Mileage.* Nancy's van traveled 84 mi on 6.5 gal of gasoline. At this rate, how many gallons would be needed to travel 126 mi?   9.75 gal

2. *Bicycling.* Roy bicycled 234 mi in 14 days. At this rate, how far would Roy travel in 42 days?   702 mi

3. *Quality Control.* A quality-control inspector examined 100 lightbulbs and found 7 of them to be defective. At this rate, how many defective bulbs will there be in a lot of 2500?   175

4. *Grading.* A professor must grade 32 essays in a literature class. She can grade 5 essays in 40 min. At this rate, how long will it take her to grade all 32 essays?   256 min

5. *Painting.* Fred uses 3 gal of paint to cover 1275 ft^2 of siding. How much siding can Fred paint with 7 gal of paint?   2975 ft^2

6. *Waterproofing.* Bonnie can waterproof 450 ft^2 of decking with 2 gal of sealant. How many gallons should Bonnie buy for a 1200-ft^2 deck?   6 gal

7. *Publishing.* Every 6 pages of an author's manuscript corresponds to 5 published pages. How many published pages will a 540-page manuscript become?   450

8. *Turkey Servings.* An 8-lb turkey breast contains 36 servings of meat. How many pounds of turkey breast would be needed for 54 servings?   12 lb

9. *Lefties.* In a class of 40 students, on average, 6 will be left-handed. If a class includes 9 "lefties," how many students would you estimate are in the class?
60

10. *Sugaring.* When 38 gal of maple sap are boiled down, the result is 2 gal of maple syrup. How much sap is needed to produce 9 gal of syrup?   171 gal

11. *Mileage.* Jean bought a new car. In the first 8 months, it was driven 9000 mi. At this rate, how many miles will the car be driven in 1 yr?
13,500 mi

12. *Coffee Production.* Coffee beans from 14 trees are required to produce the 17 lb of coffee that the average person in the United States drinks each year. How many trees are required to produce 375 lb of coffee?   309

13. *Metallurgy.* In a metal alloy, the ratio of zinc to copper is 3 to 13. If there are 520 lb of copper, how many pounds of zinc are there?   120 lb

14. *Class Size.* A college advertises that its student-to-faculty ratio is 14 to 1. If 56 students register for Introductory Spanish, how many sections of the course would you expect to see offered?   4

15. *Painting.* Helen can paint 950 ft^2 with 2 gal of paint. How many 1-gal cans does she need in order to paint a 30,000-ft^2 wall?   64 cans

16. *Snow to Water.* Under typical conditions, $1\frac{1}{2}$ ft of snow will melt to 2 in. of water. To how many inches of water will $5\frac{1}{2}$ ft of snow melt? $7\frac{1}{3}$ in.

17. *Map Scaling.* On a map, $\frac{1}{4}$ in. represents 50 mi. If two cities are $3\frac{1}{4}$ in. apart on the map, how far apart are they in reality?   650 mi

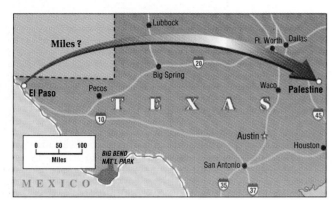

18. *Map Scaling.* On a road atlas map, 1 in. represents 16.6 mi. If two cities are 3.5 in. apart on the map, how far apart are they in reality?   58.1 mi

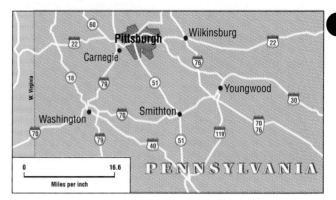

19. At the Bertocinis' church, two pews can seat 14 people. How many pews will be needed for a wedding party of 44 people?   7

20. Halo grass seed is sold in 1-lb bags. Each bag covers 800 ft^2 of lawn. How many bags must be purchased in order to cover a 4300 ft^2 lawn?   6

Skill Maintenance

21. Plot the following points. [6.3a]

$(-3, 2),\ (4, 5),\ (-4, -1),\ (0, 3)$

22. Multiply: $-19.3(4.1)$. [5.3a] -79.13

23. Divide: $-13.11 \div 5.7$. [5.4a] -2.3

24. Divide: $169.36 \div (-23.2)$. [5.4a] -7.3

25. Add: $-19.7 + 12.5$. [5.2c] -7.2

26. Subtract: $-3.7 - (-1.9)$. [5.2c] -1.8

Synthesis

27. ◈ Polly solved Example 1 by forming the proportion

$$\frac{24}{30} = \frac{356}{n},$$

whereas Rudy wrote

$$\frac{24}{n} = \frac{356}{30}.$$

Are both approaches valid? Why or why not?

28. ◈ Rob's waist and hips measure 35 in. and 33 in., respectively (see Margin Exercise 4). Suppose that Rob can either gain or lose 1 in. from one of his measurements. Where should the inch come from or go to? Why?

21.

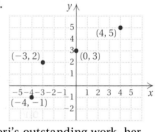

29. ◈ Can unit prices be used to solve proportions that involve money? Why or why not?

30. ▦ Carlson College is expanding from 850 to 1050 students. To avoid any rise in the student-to-faculty ratio, the faculty of 69 professors must also increase. How many new faculty positions should be created?   17

31. ▦ In recognition of Sheri's outstanding work, her salary has been increased from $26,000 to $29,380. Tim is earning $23,000 and is requesting a proportional raise. How much more should he ask for? $2990

32. *Baseball Statistics.* Cy Young, one of the greatest baseball pitchers of all time, gave up an average of 2.63 earned runs every 9 innings. Young pitched 7356 innings, more than anyone in the history of baseball. How many earned runs did he give up?

2150

33. ▦ *Real-Estate Values.* According to Coldwell Banker Real Estate Corporation, a home selling for $89,000 in Austin, Texas, would sell for $286,000 in San Francisco. How much would a $450,000 home in San Francisco sell for in Austin? Round to the nearest $1000. $140,000

34. ▦ The ratio 1:3:2 is used to estimate the relative costs of a CD player, receiver, and speakers when shopping for a stereo. That is, the receiver should cost three times the amount spent on the CD player and the speakers should cost twice as much as the amount spent on the CD player. If you had $900 to spend, how would you allocate the money, using this ratio? $150: CD player; $450: receiver; $300: speakers

Collaborative
Learning Manual

Use proportions to make predictions of your college's student population.

7.5 Geometric Applications

a Proportions and Similar Triangles

Look at the pair of triangles below. Note that they appear to have the same shape, but their sizes are different. These are examples of **similar triangles**. By using a magnifying glass, you could imagine enlarging the smaller triangle to get the larger. This process works because the corresponding sides of each triangle have the same ratio. That is, the following proportion is true.

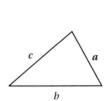
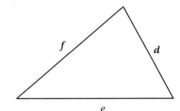

$$\frac{a}{d} = \frac{b}{e} = \frac{c}{f}$$

> **Similar triangles** have the same shape. The lengths of their corresponding sides have the same ratio—that is, they are proportional.

Example 1 The triangles at right are similar triangles. Find the missing length x.

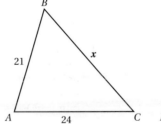

The ratio of x to 9 is the same as the ratio of 24 to 8 or 21 to 7. We get the proportions

$$\frac{x}{9} = \frac{24}{8} \quad \text{and} \quad \frac{x}{9} = \frac{21}{7}.$$

We can solve either one of these proportions as follows:

$\frac{x}{9} = 3$ **Simplifying**

$x = 3 \cdot 9$ **Multiplying by 9 on both sides**

$= 27.$ **Simplifying**

The missing length x is 27. Other proportions could also be used.

Do Exercise 1.

Similar triangles and proportions can often be used to find lengths that would ordinarily be difficult to measure. For example, we could find the height of a flagpole without climbing it or the distance across a river without crossing it.

Objectives

a Find lengths of sides of similar triangles using proportions.

b Use proportions to find lengths in pairs of figures that differ only in size.

For Extra Help

TAPE 13   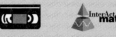 MAC WIN   CD-ROM

1. This pair of triangles is similar. Find the missing length x.

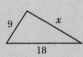
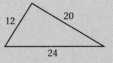

Answer on page A-20

2. How high is a flagpole that casts a 45-ft shadow at the same time that a 5.5-ft woman casts a 10-ft shadow?

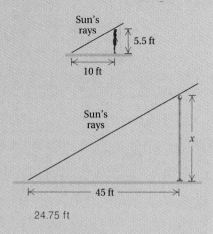

24.75 ft

3. *F-106 Blueprint.* Referring to Example 3, find the length x of the wing.

34.9 ft

Answers on page A-20

Example 2   How high is a flagpole that casts a 56-ft shadow at the same time that a 6-ft man casts a 5-ft shadow?

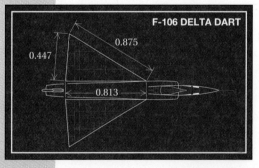

If we use the sun's rays to represent the third side of the triangle in our drawing of the situation, we see that we have similar triangles. Let p = the height of the flagpole. The ratio of 6 to p is the same as the ratio of 5 to 56. Thus we have the proportion

Height of man $\rightarrow \dfrac{6}{p} = \dfrac{5}{56}$. $\leftarrow$ Length of shadow of man
Height of pole $\rightarrow$ $\quad\quad\quad$ $\leftarrow$ Length of shadow of pole

Solve: $6 \cdot 56 = 5 \cdot p$ **Equating cross products**

$\dfrac{6 \cdot 56}{5} = p$ **Dividing by 5 on both sides**

$67.2 = p$ **Simplifying**

The height of the flagpole is 67.2 ft.

Do Exercise 2.

Example 3   *F-106 Blueprint.* A blueprint for an F-106 Delta Dart military plane is a scale drawing. Each wing of the plane has a triangular shape. The blueprint shows similar triangles. Find the length of side a of the wing.

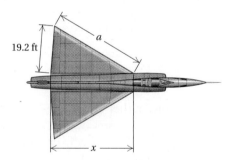

We let a = the length of the wing. Thus we have the proportion

Length on the blueprint $\rightarrow \dfrac{0.447}{19.2} = \dfrac{0.875}{a}$. $\leftarrow$ Length on the blueprint
Length of the wing $\rightarrow$ $\quad\quad\quad$ $\leftarrow$ Length of the wing

Solve: $0.447 \cdot a = 19.2 \cdot 0.875$ **Equating cross products**

$a = \dfrac{19.2 \cdot 0.875}{0.447}$ **Dividing by 0.447 on both sides**

≈ 37.6 ft

The length of side a of the wing is about 37.6 ft.

Do Exercise 3.

b Proportions and Other Geometric Shapes

When one geometric figure is a magnification of another, the figures are similar. Thus the corresponding lengths are proportional.

Example 4   The sides in the negative and photograph below are proportional. Find the width of the photograph.

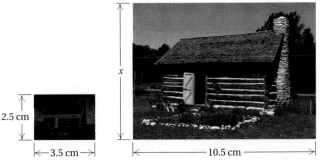

2.5 cm

3.5 cm

x

10.5 cm

We let x = the width of the photograph. Then we translate to a proportion.

Photo width $\rightarrow \dfrac{x}{2.5} = \dfrac{10.5}{3.5} \leftarrow$ Photo length
Negative width $\rightarrow \quad \quad \leftarrow$ Negative length

Solve: $\dfrac{x}{2.5} = 3$ \qquad **Simplifying**

$\quad x = 3(2.5)$ \qquad **Multiplying by 2.5 on both sides**

$\quad \ = 7.5$ \qquad **Simplifying**

Thus the width of the photograph is 7.5 cm.

Do Exercise 4.

Example 5   A scale model of an addition to an athletic facility is 12 cm wide at the base and rises to a height of 15 cm. If the actual base is to be 116 ft, what will be the actual height of the addition?

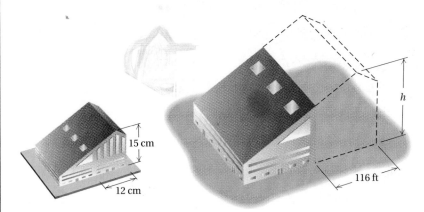

15 cm

12 cm

h

116 ft

We let h = the height of the addition. Then we translate to a proportion.

Width in model $\rightarrow \dfrac{12}{116} = \dfrac{15}{h} \leftarrow$ Height in model
Actual width $\rightarrow \quad \quad \quad \leftarrow$ Actual height

4. The sides in the photographs below are proportional. Find the width of the larger photograph.   21 cm

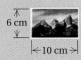

6 cm

10 cm

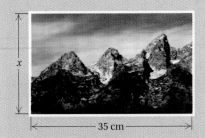

x

35 cm

Answer on page A-20

5. Refer to the figures in Example 5. If a model skylight is 3 cm wide, how wide will the actual skylight be? 29 ft

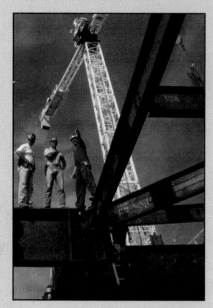

Solve:

$$12h = 116 \cdot 15 \qquad \text{Equating cross products}$$

$$h = \frac{116 \cdot 15}{12} \qquad \text{Dividing by 12 on both sides}$$

$$= \frac{\cancel{4} \cdot 29 \cdot \cancel{3} \cdot 5}{\cancel{4} \cdot \cancel{3}} \qquad \text{Removing a factor equal to 1: } \frac{4 \cdot 3}{4 \cdot 3} = 1$$

$$= 145. \qquad \text{Multiplying}$$

Thus the height of the addition will be 145 ft.

Do Exercise 5.

Calculator Spotlight

Proportions can be solved easily with the aid of a calculator. For example, earlier in this section we solved

$$\frac{0.447}{19.2} = \frac{0.875}{a}$$

by equating cross products and then dividing. The solution,

$$\frac{19.2 \cdot 0.875}{0.447},$$

uses the three numbers that were given: The numerator is a cross product that uses two of those numbers, and the denominator is the remaining number. This pattern can be used to solve *any* proportion. For instance, to solve

$$\frac{5}{8} = \frac{x}{20},$$

we can press [5] [×] [2] [0] [÷] [8] [=]. When a calculator is not available, it is usually easiest to simplify first by removing a factor equal to 1, as in Example 5.

Exercises

Solve each proportion.

1. $\dfrac{15.75}{20} = \dfrac{a}{35}$ 27.5625

2. $\dfrac{32}{x} = \dfrac{25}{20}$ 25.6

3. $\dfrac{t}{57} = \dfrac{17}{64}$ 15.140625

4. $\dfrac{16}{29} = \dfrac{23}{a}$ 41.6875

5. $\dfrac{71.2}{a} = \dfrac{42.5}{23.9}$ 40.03952941

6. $\dfrac{29.6}{3.15} = \dfrac{x}{4.23}$ 39.74857143

7. $\dfrac{0.023}{0.15} = \dfrac{0.401}{t}$ 2.615217391

8. $\dfrac{a}{3.01} = \dfrac{1.7}{0.043}$ 119

Answer on page A-20

Exercise Set 7.5

a The triangles in each exercise are similar. Find the missing lengths.

1.

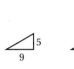
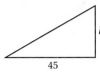

25

2.

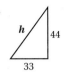
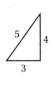

55

3.

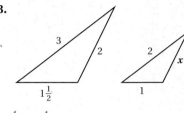

$\frac{4}{3}$, or $1\frac{1}{3}$

4.

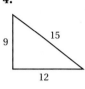
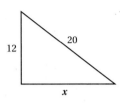

16

5.

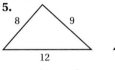

$x = \frac{27}{4}$, or $6\frac{3}{4}$; $y = 9$

6.

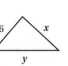
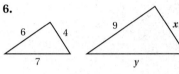

$x = 6$; $y = \frac{21}{2}$, or $10\frac{1}{2}$

7.

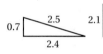
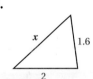

$x = 7.5$; $y = 7.2$

8.

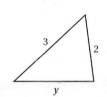

$x = 2.4$; $y = 2.5$

9. When a tree 8 m high casts a shadow 5 m long, how long a shadow is cast by a person 2 m tall?

1.25 m

10. How high is a flagpole that casts a 42-ft shadow at the same time that a $5\frac{1}{2}$-ft woman casts a 7-ft shadow?

33 ft

11. How high is a tree that casts a 27-ft shadow at the same time that a 4-ft fence post casts a 3-ft shadow?

36 ft

12. How high is a tree that casts a 32-ft shadow at the same time that an 8-ft light pole casts a 9-ft shadow?

$28\frac{4}{9}$ ft

13. Find the height *h* of the wall.   7 ft

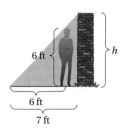

14. Find the length *L* of the lake.   2880 yd

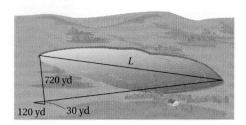

15. Find the distance across the river. Assume that the ratio of *d* to 25 ft is the same as the ratio of 40 ft to 10 ft.   100 ft

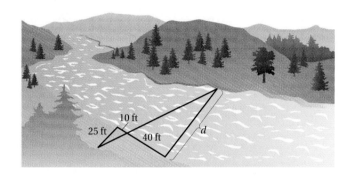

16. To measure the height of a hill, a string is drawn tight from level ground to the top of the hill. A 3-ft stick is placed under the string, touching it at point *P*, a distance of 5 ft from point *G*, where the string touches the ground. The string is then detached and found to be 120 ft long. How high is the hill?   72 ft

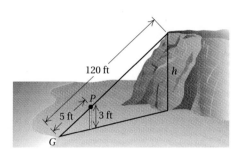

b The sides in each pair of figures are proportional. Find the missing lengths.

17.

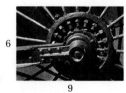

6

9   *x*

6

4

18.

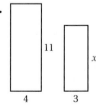

5

x

7   14

10

19.

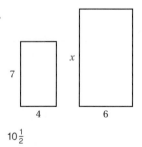

7   *x*

4   6

$10\frac{1}{2}$

20.

11   *x*

4   3

8.25

21.

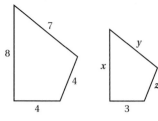

$x = 6$, $y = 5.25$, $z = 3$

22.

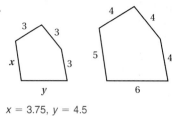

$x = 3.75$, $y = 4.5$

23.

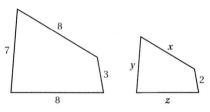

$x = 5\frac{1}{3}$, or $5.\overline{3}$; $y = 4\frac{2}{3}$, or $4.\overline{6}$; $z = 5\frac{1}{3}$, or $5.\overline{3}$

24.

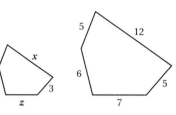

$x = 7.2$, $y = 3.6$, $z = 4.2$

25.

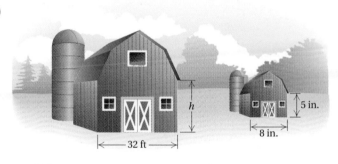

20 ft

26.

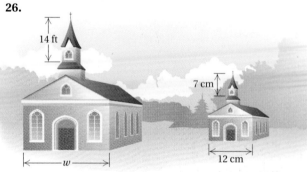

24 ft

Skill Maintenance

27. Kathy has $34.97 to spend for a book at $49.95, a CD at $14.88, and a sweatshirt at $29.95. How much more money does she need to make these purchases? [5.8a] $59.81

28. Divide: $80.892 \div 8.4$. [5.4a] 9.63

Multiply. [5.3a]

29. -8.4×80.892 -679.4928

30. 0.01×274.568 2.74568

31. 100×274.568 27,456.8

32. $-0.002(-274.568)$ 0.549136

33. ◆ Is it possible for two triangles to have two pairs of sides that are proportional without the triangles being similar? Why or why not?

34. ◆ Suppose that all the sides in one triangle are half the size of the corresponding sides in a similar triangle. Does it follow that the area of the smaller triangle is half the area of the larger triangle? Why or why not? (*Hint*: $A = \frac{1}{2}bh$ for any triangle.)

35. ◆ Design for a classmate a problem involving similar triangles for which

$$\frac{18}{128.95} = \frac{x}{789.89}.$$

Hockey Goals. An official hockey goal is 6 ft wide. To make scoring more difficult, goalies often locate themselves far in front of the goal to "cut down the angle." In Exercises 36 and 37, suppose that a slapshot from point A is attempted and that the goalie is 2.7 ft wide. Determine how far from the goal the goalie should be located if point A is the given distance from the goal. (*Hint*: First find how far the goalie should be from point A.)

36. ▦ 25 ft   13.75 ft

37. ▦ 35 ft   19.25 ft

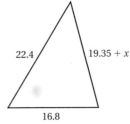

▦ The triangles in each exercise are similar triangles. Find the lengths not given.

38.

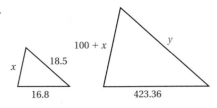

$x \approx 4.13$, $y = 466.2$

39.

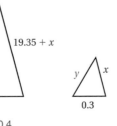

$x \approx 0.35$, $y = 0.4$

40. ▦ A miniature basketball hoop is built for the model referred to in Example 5. An actual hoop is 10 ft high. How high should the model hoop be? Round to the nearest thousandth of a centimeter.   1.034 cm

41. ▦ A miniature baseball diamond is drawn to accompany the model used in Example 5. If the actual baseball diamond is a 90-ft by 90-ft square, what will the area of the model diamond be?   86.68 cm²

Summary and Review Exercises: Chapter 7

1. Write fractional notation for the ratio 37 to 85. [7.1a]

2. In this rectangle, find the ratio of width to length and simplify. [7.1b]

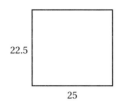

22.5

25

3. In 1996, approximately 66 million citizens were registered to vote. Of those registered, about 54 million voted. Write simplified fractional notation for the ratio of those who voted to those were registered. [7.1a, b]

4. An Olympic marathoner ran 20 km in 57 min. What is the rate in kilometers per minute? in minutes per kilometer? [7.2a]

5. A bicycle racer biked 25 mi in 1.25 hr. What was the racer's rate in minutes per mile? [7.2a]

6. A 12-oz container of Jones' Hot Pepper Jelly costs $3.24. Find the unit price in dollars per ounce. [7.2b]

7. Which has the lower unit cost? [7.2b]

CANNED PINEAPPLE JUICE
Delacorte: 12 oz for 99 cents
BiteFine: 18 oz for $1.26

8. Determine whether the pairs 7, 5 and 13, 11 are proportional. [7.3a]

Solve. [7.3b]

9. $\dfrac{8}{9} = \dfrac{x}{36}$

10. $\dfrac{120}{\frac{3}{7}} = \dfrac{7}{x}$

11. $\dfrac{6}{x} = \dfrac{48}{56}$

12. $\dfrac{4.5}{120} = \dfrac{0.9}{x}$

Solve. [7.4a]

13. If 3 dozen eggs cost $3.99, how much will 5 dozen eggs cost?

14. In a factory, it was discovered that 39 circuits in a lot of 65 were defective. At this rate, how many defective circuits can be expected in a lot of 585 circuits?

15. The ratio of children to adults at the Ever Ready Daycare Center cannot exceed 13 to 2. If there are 35 children at the center, how many adults must be present?

16. A train travels 448 km in 7 hr. At this rate, how far would it travel in 13 hr?

17. It has been estimated that, on average, 5 people produce 13 kg of garbage each day. San Antonio, Texas, has a population of 936,000 people. Estimate the quantity of garbage produced in San Antonio each day.

18. In Michigan, there are 2.3 lawyers for every 1000 people. The population of the Detroit metropolitan area is 4,307,000. Estimate the number of lawyers in Detroit.

Each pair of triangles in Exercises 19 and 20 is similar. Find the missing length(s). [7.5a]

19.

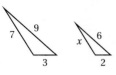

20.

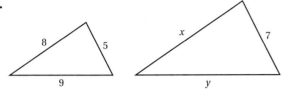

21. How high is a billboard that casts a 25-ft shadow at the same time that an 8-ft sapling casts a 5-ft shadow? [7.5a]

22. The lengths in the figures below are proportional. Find the missing lengths. [7.5b]

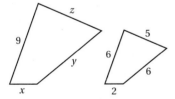

Skill Maintenance

23. A family has $2347.89 in its checking account. It writes checks for $678.95 and $38.54. How much is left in the checking account? [5.8a]

24. In which quadrant is each point located? [6.3b]

$(-4, -3)$, $(-2, 7)$, $(1, 4)$, and $(3, -2)$

25. Multiply: $456.1(-23.4)$. [5.3a]

26. Divide. Write decimal notation for the answer. [5.4a]

$$5.6 \overline{)254.8}$$

Synthesis

27. ◈ Write a proportion problem for a classmate to solve. Design the problem so that the solution is "Leslie would need 16 gal of gasoline in order to travel 368 mi." [7.4a]

28. ◈ If you were a college president, which would you prefer: a low or high faculty-to-student ratio? Why? What about the student-to-faculty ratio? [7.1a]

State Lottery Prizes. The chart below shows the prizes awarded in certain state lotteries in a recent year. (*Source: Statistical Abstract of the United States, 1998*). Use the information to do Exercises 29–32.

State	Prizes (in millions)
California	$1132
Colorado	192
*Connecticut	402
Florida	1024
Illinois	839
*Maine	84
Maryland	609
*Massachusetts	2140
Michigan	736
*New Hampshire	98
New Jersey	796
New York	1827
Ohio	1363
Pennsylvania	891
*Rhode Island	303
*Vermont	44
Washington	224

* = a New England State

29. 🖩 What is the ratio of the lottery prizes in New York to the total prizes awarded by all lotteries? [7.1a]

30. 🖩 What is the ratio of the lottery prizes in New England to the total prizes awarded by all lotteries? [7.1a]

31. 🖩 The population of California is 31,858,000. If all prize money were equally shared, how much would the average Californian receive? [7.2a]

32. 🖩 The population of New York is 18,134,000. If all prize money were equally shared, how much would the average New Yorker receive? [7.2a]

33. Shine-and-Glo Painters uses 2 gal of finishing paint for every 3 gal of primer. Each gallon of finishing paint covers 450 ft². If a surface of 4950 ft² needs both primer and finishing paint, how many gallons should be purchased altogether? [7.4a]

34. It takes Yancy Martinez 10 min to type two-thirds of a page of his term paper. At this rate, how long will it take him to type a 7-page term paper? [7.4a]

Test: Chapter 7

Write fractional notation for each ratio. Do not simplify.

1. 83 to 94

2. 0.34 to 124

3. Simplify the ratio of length to width in this rectangle.

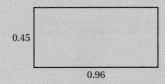

0.45

0.96

4. A diver descends 10 ft in 16 sec. What is the rate of descent in feet per second?

5. In 1 hr 20 min, a bicycle racer biked 48 km. What was the racer's rate in minutes per kilometer?

6. An 8-oz package of extra-sharp cheddar cheese costs $2.79. Find the unit price in dollars per ounce.

7. Determine whether the pairs 8, 6 and 15, 10 are proportional.

Solve.

8. $\dfrac{27}{x} = \dfrac{9}{4}$

9. $\dfrac{150}{2.5} = \dfrac{x}{6}$

10. An ocean liner traveled 432 km in 12 hr. At this rate, how far would the boat travel in 42 hr?

11. A watch loses 2 min in 10 hr. At this rate, how much will it lose in 24 hr.?

12. On a map, 3 in. represents 225 mi. If two cities are 7 in. apart on the map, how far are they apart in reality?

13. A birdhouse built on a pole that is 3 m high casts a shadow 5 m long. At the same time, the shadow of a tower is 110 m long. How high is the tower?

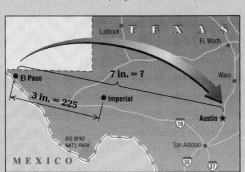

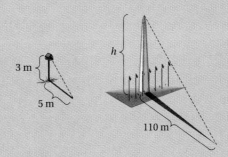

3 m

5 m

h

110 m

Answers

1. [7.1a] $\frac{83}{94}$

2. [7.1a] $\frac{0.34}{124}$

3. [7.1b] $\frac{32}{15}$

4. [7.2a] $\frac{5}{8}$ ft/sec

5. [7.2a] $1\frac{2}{3}$ min/km

6. [7.2b] $0.35/oz

7. [7.3a] No

8. [7.3b] 12

9. [7.3b] 360

10. [7.4a] 1512 km

11. [7.4a] 4.8 min

12. [7.4a] 525 mi

13. [7.5a] 66 m

The lengths in each pair of figures are proportional. Find the missing lengths.

14.

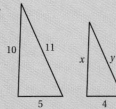

15.

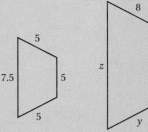

Skill Maintenance

16. In a recent year, Kellogg sold 146.2 million lb of Corn Flakes and 120.4 million lb of Frosted Flakes. How many more pounds of Corn Flakes did they sell than Frosted Flakes?

17. In which quadrant is each point located?

$(-2, 4)$, $(5, -2)$, $(7, 1)$, and $(-1, -6)$

18. Multiply: $-24.13(-7.2)$.

19. Divide: $\dfrac{-99.44}{100}$.

Synthesis

Solve.

20. $\dfrac{5}{9} = \dfrac{2x - 1}{x + 3}$

21. $\dfrac{3x + 1}{7} = \dfrac{4x - 5}{6}$

22. Nancy Morano-Smith wants to guess the number of marbles in an 8-gal jar. Knowing that there are 128 oz in a gallon, Nancy goes home and fills an 8-oz jar with 46 marbles. How many marbles should she guess are in the 8-gal jar?

23. The Johnson triplets and the Solomini twins went out to dinner and decided to split the bill of $79.85 proportionately. How much will the Johnsons pay?

24. A soccer goalie wishing to block an opponent's shot moves toward the shooter to reduce the shooter's view of the goal. If the goalie can only defend a region 10 ft wide, how far in front of the goal should the goalie be (see the following figure)?

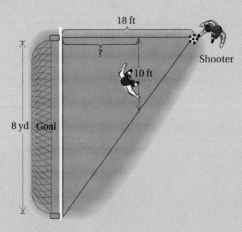

Cumulative Review: Chapters 1–7

Add and simplify.

1.
$$\begin{array}{r} 1\ 3\ 7.1\ 8\ 6 \\ 2\ 3.0\ 1\ 9 \\ +\ 4\ 8\ 3.2\ 9\ 7 \\ \hline \end{array}$$

2.
$$\begin{array}{r} 2\frac{1}{3} \\ +\ 4\frac{5}{12} \\ \hline \end{array}$$

3. $\dfrac{6}{35} + \dfrac{5}{28}$

Perform the indicated operation and simplify.

4.
$$\begin{array}{r} 6\ 0.2\ 1 \\ -\quad 9.7\ 0\ 9 \\ \hline \end{array}$$

5. $-32 - (-15)$

6. $\dfrac{4}{15} - \dfrac{3}{20}$

7.
$$\begin{array}{r} 3\ 7.6\ 4 \\ \times\qquad 5.9 \\ \hline \end{array}$$

8. $-43(15)$

9. $2\dfrac{1}{3} \cdot 1\dfrac{2}{7}$

10. $2.3\ )\overline{9\ 8.9}$

11. $-306 \div 6$

12. $\dfrac{7}{11} \div \dfrac{14}{33}$

13. Write expanded notation for 30,074.

14. Write a word name for 120.07.

Which number is larger?

15. 0.7, 0.698

16. -0.799, -0.8

17. Find the prime factorization of 144.

18. Find the LCM of 44 and 55.

19. What part is shaded?

20. Simplify: $\dfrac{90}{144}$.

Calculate.

21. $\dfrac{3}{5} \times 9.53$

22. $7.2 \div 0.4(-1.5) + (1.2)^2$

23. Find the mean: 23, 49, 52, 71.

24. Determine whether the pairs 3, 9 and 25, 75 are proportional.

25. Graph on a plane: $y = -x - 4$.

26. Evaluate $\dfrac{t-7}{w}$ for $t = -3$ and $w = -2$.

Solve.

27. $\dfrac{14}{25} = \dfrac{x}{54}$

28. $-423 = 16 \cdot t$

29. $9x - 7 = -43$

30. $2(x - 3) + 9 = 5x - 6$

31. $34.56 + n = 67.9$

32. $\dfrac{2}{3}x = \dfrac{16}{27}$

Solve.

33. A car travels 337.62 mi in 8 hr. How far does it travel in 1 hr?

34. A machine can stamp out 925 washers in 5 min. How much time would be needed to stamp out 1295 washers?

35. Elise drove 347.6 mi, 249.8 mi, and 379.5 mi on three separate trips. What was the total mileage?

36. In a recent year, 1,635,000 people camped at Yosemite National Park. In the same year, 1,221,000 people camped at Yellowstone National Park. How many more people camped at Yosemite than at Yellowstone?

37. A triangular window is 4 ft high and has a base that measures 5 ft. Find its area.

38. It takes Jose $\frac{2}{3}$ hr to hang a door. How many doors can he hang in 8 hr?

39. A 46-oz juice can contains $5\frac{3}{4}$ cups of juice. A recipe calls for $3\frac{1}{2}$ cups of juice. How many cups are left?

40. A space shuttle recently made 16 orbits a day during an 8.25-day mission. How many orbits were made during the entire mission?

Synthesis

41. A car travels 88 ft in 1 sec. What is the rate in miles per hour?

42. A 12-oz bag of shredded mozzarella cheese is on sale for $2.07. Blocks of mozzarella cheese are on sale for $2.79 per pound. Which is the better buy?

43. Hans attends a university where the academic year consists of two 16-week semesters. He budgets $1200 for incidental expenses for the academic year. After 3 weeks, Hans has spent $150 for incidental expenses. Assuming he continues to spend at the same rate, will the budget for incidental expenses be adequate? If not, when will the money be exhausted and how much more will be needed to complete the year?

44. A basic sound system consists of a CD player, a receiver, and two speakers. A standard rule of thumb on the relative investment in these components is 1:3:2. That is, the receiver should cost three times as much as the CD player and the speakers should cost twice as much as the CD player.

a) You have $1200 to spend. How should you allocate the funds if you use this rule of thumb?

b) How should you spend $3000?

8

Percent Notation

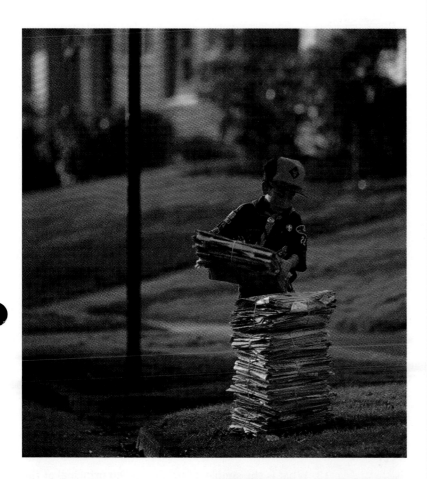

An Application	The Mathematics

Recently, the United States was generating 79.9 million tons of paper waste per year, of which 32.6 million tons were recycled (**Source**: Franklin Associates, Ltd., Prairie Village, KS). What percent of paper waste was recycled?

This problem appears as Example 1 in Section 8.4.

We let $n =$ the percent of paper waste that was recycled. The problem can be translated as follows:

$$
\underset{\substack{\downarrow \\ 32.6}}{\underbrace{32.6 \text{ million}}} \quad \underset{\downarrow}{\text{is}} \quad \underset{\substack{\downarrow \\ n \\ \uparrow}}{\underbrace{\text{what percent}}} \quad \underset{\downarrow}{\text{of}} \quad \underset{\substack{\downarrow \\ 79.9}}{79.9?}
$$

$$32.6 = n \cdot 79.9$$

Once n has been found, we will change it from decimal notation to percent notation.

 For more information, visit us at www.mathmax.com

Pretest: Chapter 8

1. Write decimal notation for 87%.

2. Write percent notation for 0.537.

3. Write percent notation for $\dfrac{3}{4}$.

4. Write fractional notation for 37%.

5. Translate to an equation. Then solve.
   What is 60% of 75?

6. Translate to a proportion. Then solve.
   What percent of 50 is 35?

Solve.

7. The weight of muscles in an adult male is 40% of total body weight. A man weighs 225 lb. What do the muscles weigh?

8. The population of Winchester increased from 3000 to 3600. Write the percent of increase in population.

9. The sales tax rate in California is 6%. How much tax is charged on a purchase of $286? What is the total price?

10. Anwar's commission rate is 28%. What is his commission from the sale of $18,400 worth of merchandise?

11. The marked price of a Panasonic camcorder is $450. This camera is on sale at Lowland Appliances for 25% off. What is the discount and what is the sale price?

12. What is the simple interest on $1200 principal at the interest rate of 8.3% for 1 year?

13. What is the simple interest on $500 at 8% for $\frac{1}{2}$ year?

14. Interest is compounded quarterly. Write the amount in an account if $6000 is invested at 8% for 6 months.

8.1 Percent Notation

a | Understanding Percent Notation

Of all wood harvested, 35% is used for paper. What does this mean? It means that, on average, of every 100 tons of wood harvested, 35 tons is made into paper. Thus, 35% is a ratio of 35 to 100, or $\frac{35}{100}$. Percent means parts of 100.

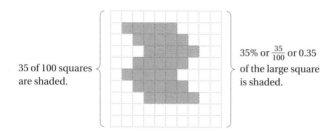

35 of 100 squares are shaded.

35% or $\frac{35}{100}$ or 0.35 of the large square is shaded.

Objectives

a Write three kinds of notation for a percent.

b Convert between percent notation and decimal notation.

c Convert between fractional notation and percent notation.

For Extra Help

TAPE 14   MAC WIN   CD-ROM

Percent notation is used extensively in our lives. Here are some examples:

Astronauts lose 1% of their bone mass for each month of weightlessness.

95% of hair spray is alcohol.

55% of all baseball merchandise sold is purchased by women.

62.4% of all aluminum cans were recycled in a recent year.

56% of all fruit juice purchased is orange juice.

45.8% of us sleep between 7 and 8 hours per night.

Percent notation is often represented by pie charts to show how the parts of a quantity are related. For example, the chart below relates the length of time couples are engaged before marrying.

Length of Engagement Before Marriage

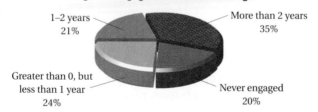

1–2 years 21%

More than 2 years 35%

Greater than 0, but less than 1 year 24%

Never engaged 20%

To draw a pie chart like the one above, think of a pie cut into 100 equally sized pieces. Then shade in a wedge equal in size to 20 of these pieces to represent 20%. Shade in a wedge equal in size to 35 of the 100 pieces to represent 35% and so on.

Do Exercise 1.

The notation *n*% arose historically meaning "*n* per hundred." This rate can be expressed as *n*/100, $n \times \frac{1}{100}$, or $n \times 0.01$.

> **Percent notation, *n*%,** is defined in three ways:
>
> ratio ➤ *n*% = the ratio of *n* to 100 = $\frac{n}{100}$;
>
> fractional notation ➤ *n*% = $n \times \frac{1}{100}$;
>
> decimal notation ➤ *n*% = $n \times 0.01$.

1. The circle below is divided into 100 sections. Use the following information on the amounts of fruit juices sold to draw and label a circle graph.

Apple:	14%
Orange:	56%
Grapefruit:	4%
Blends:	6%
Grape:	5%
Other:	15%

Source: Beverage Marketing Corporation

Fruit Juice Sales

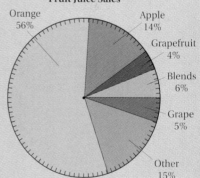

Orange 56%

Apple 14%

Grapefruit 4%

Blends 6%

Grape 5%

Other 15%

Answer on page A-21

Write three kinds of notation as in Examples 1 and 2.

2. 70%

$\frac{70}{100}$; $70 \times \frac{1}{100}$; 70×0.01

3. 23.4%

$\frac{23.4}{100}$; $23.4 \times \frac{1}{100}$; 23.4×0.01

4. 100%

$\frac{100}{100}$; $100 \times \frac{1}{100}$; 100×0.01

It is thought that the Roman Emperor Augustus began percent notation by taxing goods sold at a rate of $\frac{1}{100}$. In time, the symbol "%" evolved by interchanging the parts of the symbol "100" to "0/0" and then to "%".

Answers on page A-21

Example 1   Write three kinds of notation for 35%.

Using ratio: $\qquad 35\% = \dfrac{35}{100}$ **A ratio of 35 to 100**

Using fractional notation: $\quad 35\% = 35 \times \dfrac{1}{100}$ **Replacing % with $\times \frac{1}{100}$**

Using decimal notation: $\quad 35\% = 35 \times 0.01$ **Replacing % with $\times$ 0.01**

Example 2   Write three kinds of notation for 67.8%.

Using ratio: $\qquad 67.8\% = \dfrac{67.8}{100}$ **A ratio of 67.8 to 100**

Using fractional notation: $\quad 67.8\% = 67.8 \times \dfrac{1}{100}$ **Replacing % with $\times \frac{1}{100}$**

Using decimal notation: $\quad 67.8\% = 67.8 \times 0.01$ **Replacing % with $\times$ 0.01**

Do Exercises 2–4.

b │ Converting Between Percent Notation and Decimal Notation

To write decimal notation for a number like 78%, we can replace "%" with "$\times 0.01$" and multiply:

$$78\% = 78 \times 0.01 \qquad \text{Replacing \% with } \times \text{ 0.01}$$
$$= 0.78. \qquad \text{Multiplying}$$

Similarly,

$$4.9\% = 4.9 \times 0.01 \qquad \text{Replacing \% with } \times \text{ 0.01}$$
$$= 0.049 \qquad \text{Multiplying}$$

and

$$265\% = 265 \times 0.01 \qquad \text{Replacing \% with } \times \text{ 0.01}$$
$$= 2.65. \qquad \text{Multiplying}$$

When we multiply by 0.01, the decimal point is moved two places to the left. Thus, to quickly convert from percent notation to decimal notation, we can drop the percent symbol and move the decimal point two places to the left.

To convert from percent notation to decimal notation,	29.7%
a) replace the percent symbol % with $\times$ 0.01, and	29.7×0.01
b) multiply by 0.01, which means move the decimal point two places to the left.	0.29.7 **Move 2 places to the left.** $29.7\% = 0.297$

Example 3 Write decimal notation for 92.43%.

a) Replace the percent symbol with × 0.01.   92.43 × 0.01

b) Multiply to move the decimal point   0.92.43
   two places to the left.

Thus, 92.43% = 0.9243. With practice, you will be able to make this conversion mentally.

Sometimes it may be necessary to write zeros as placeholders.

Example 4 In 1997, the population of North America was 7.9% of the world population. Write decimal notation for 7.9%.

a) Replace the percent symbol with × 0.01.   7.9 × 0.01

b) Multiply to move the decimal point
   two places to the left.

┌─── This zero serves as
     a placeholder.

0.07.9

Thus, 7.9% = 0.079.

Do Exercises 5–8.

The procedure used in Examples 3 and 4 can be reversed to write a decimal, like 0.38, in percent notation. To see why, consider the following:

$$0.38 = 0.38 \times 100\%$$ **Multiplying by 100% or 1**
$$= 0.38 \times 100 \times 0.01$$ **Replacing 100% with 100 × 0.01**
$$= (0.38 \times 100) \times 0.01$$ **Using an associative law**
$$= 38 \times 0.01$$
$$= 38\%.$$ **Replacing × 0.01 with %**

To summarize, $0.38 = 0.38 \times 100\% = (0.38 \times 100)\% = 38\%$.

┌───┐
│ To convert from decimal notation to $0.675 = 0.675 \times 100\%$ │
│ percent notation, multiply by 100%.   │
│ That is,   │
│ a) move the decimal point two   0.67.5   Move 2 places   │
│   places to the right, and   to the right.   │
│ b) write a % symbol.   67.5%   │
│ $0.675 = 67.5\%$ │
└───┘

Example 5 Babies are born before their "due" date 0.3 of the time. Write percent notation for 0.3.

a) Multiply by 100 to move the
   decimal point two places to the
   right. Recall that 0.3 = 0.30
   since $\frac{3}{10} = \frac{30}{100}$.

┌─── This zero serves as
     a placeholder.

0.30.

b) Write a % symbol.   30%

Thus, 0.3 = 30%.

Write decimal notation.

5. 34%

0.34

6. 78.9%

0.789

7. Electricity prices in 1996 were 104.5% of the prices in 1990. (*Source*: *Statistical Abstract of the United States, 1997*). Write decimal notation for this number.

1.045

8. Soft drink sales in the United States have grown 4.2% annually over the past decade. Write decimal notation for this number.

0.042

Answers on page A-21

8.1   Percent Notation

457

Write percent notation.

9. 0.24   24%

10. 3.47   347%

11. 1   100%

12. Muscles make up 0.4 of an adult male's body. Find percent notation for 0.4.   40%

13. The average television set is on 0.25 of the time. Find percent notation for 0.25.   25%

Write percent notation.

14. $\frac{1}{4}$ 25%

15. $\frac{7}{8}$ 87.5%

Answers on page A-21

Example 6   Property values in Dorchester were multiplied by 1.23 when reassessment was performed. Find percent notation for 1.23.

a) Multiply by 100 to move the decimal point two places to the right.

1.23.

b) Write a % symbol.   123%

Thus, 1.23 = 123%.

Do Exercises 9–13.

c | Converting Between Fractional Notation and Percent Notation

To convert from fractional notation to percent notation,	$\frac{3}{5}$ Fractional notation
a) find decimal notation by division, and	$5\overline{)3.0}$ with quotient 0.6, $\;\;3\,0$, $\;\;0$
b) convert the decimal notation to percent notation.	$0.6 = 0.60 = 60\%$ Percent $\frac{3}{5} = 60\%$ notation

Example 7   Write percent notation for $\frac{3}{8}$.

a) Find decimal notation by division.

$$8\overline{)3.000}$$
with work: 0.375 quotient, $2\,4$, $6\,0$, $5\,6$, $4\,0$, $4\,0$, 0

$$\frac{3}{8} = 0.375$$

b) Convert the decimal notation to percent notation. To do so, multiply by 100 to move the decimal point two places to the right, and write a % symbol.

0.37.5

$$\frac{3}{8} = 0.375 = 37.5\%, \text{ or } 37\frac{1}{2}\%$$

Don't forget the % symbol.

Do Exercises 14 and 15.

Example 8 Of all meals, $\frac{1}{3}$ are eaten outside the home. Write percent notation for $\frac{1}{3}$.

a) Find decimal notation by division.

```
        0.3 3 3
3 ) 1.0 0 0
      9
      1 0
        9
        1 0
          9
          1
```

> Remember that to find percent notation, we will need to move the decimal point two places to the right.

We get a repeating decimal: $0.33\overline{3}$.

b) Convert the answer to percent notation.

$$0.33.\overline{3}$$

$$\frac{1}{3} = 33.\overline{3}\%, \text{ or } 33\frac{1}{3}\%$$

Do Exercises 16 and 17.

In some cases, division is not the fastest way to convert to percent notation. The following are some optional ways in which conversion might be done.

Example 9 Write percent notation for $\frac{69}{100}$.

We use the definition of percent as a ratio.

$$\frac{69}{100} = 69\%$$

Example 10 Write percent notation for $\frac{17}{20}$.

We multiply $\frac{17}{20}$ by 1 to get 100 in the denominator. We think of what we have to multiply 20 by in order to get 100. That number is 5, so we multiply by 1 using $\frac{5}{5}$.

$$\frac{17}{20} \cdot \frac{5}{5} = \frac{85}{100} = 85\%$$

Check:
```
        .8 5
2 0 ) 1 7.0 0
      1 6 0
        1 0 0
        1 0 0
            0
```

Note that this shortcut works only when the denominator is a factor of 100.

Do Exercises 18 and 19.

---

16. The human body is $\frac{2}{3}$ water. Write percent notation for $\frac{2}{3}$.

$66\frac{2}{3}\%$

17. Write percent notation: $\frac{15}{8}$.

187.5%

Write percent notation.

18. $\frac{57}{100}$ 57%

19. $\frac{19}{25}$ 76%

3. 107.69%   5. 59.62%

Answers on page A-21

Write fractional notation.

20. 180% $\frac{9}{5}$

21. 3.25% $\frac{13}{400}$

22. $66\frac{2}{3}$% $\frac{2}{3}$

23. Complete this table.

Fractional Notation	$\frac{1}{5}$	$\frac{5}{6}$	$\frac{3}{8}$
Decimal Notation	0.2	$0.8\overline{33}$	0.375
Percent Notation	20%	$83\frac{1}{3}$%	$37\frac{1}{2}$%

Answers on pages A-21 and A-22

The method used in Examples 9 and 10 is reversed when we convert from percent notation to fractional notation.

To convert from percent notation to fractional notation,

a) use the definition of percent as a ratio, and

b) simplify, if possible.

30%   Percent notation

$\frac{30}{100}$

$\frac{3}{10}$ Fractional notation

Example 11   Write fractional notation for 75%.

$$75\% = \frac{75}{100} \qquad \text{Using the definition of percent}$$

$$= \frac{3 \cdot 25}{4 \cdot 25} = \frac{3}{4} \cdot \frac{25}{25}$$

$$= \frac{3}{4} \qquad \Bigg\} \text{Simplifying}$$

Example 12   Write fractional notation for 112.5%.

$$112.5\% = \frac{112.5}{100} \qquad \text{Using the definition of percent}$$

$$= \frac{112.5}{100} \times \frac{10}{10} \qquad \text{Multiplying by 1 to eliminate the decimal point in the numerator}$$

$$= \frac{1125}{1000}$$

$$= \frac{5 \cdot 225}{5 \cdot 200} = \frac{5}{5} \cdot \frac{225}{200}$$

$$= \frac{225}{200} = \frac{25 \cdot 9}{25 \cdot 8} = \frac{9}{8} \qquad \Bigg\} \text{Simplifying}$$

Example 13   Write fractional notation for $16\frac{2}{3}$%.

$$16\frac{2}{3}\% = \frac{50}{3}\% \qquad \text{Converting from the mixed numeral to fractional notation}$$

$$= \frac{50}{3} \times \frac{1}{100} \qquad \text{Using the definition of percent}$$

$$= \frac{50 \cdot 1}{3 \cdot 50 \cdot 2} = \frac{1}{6} \cdot \frac{50}{50} = \frac{1}{6}$$

Do Exercises 20–22.

Had we noticed that $16\frac{2}{3}$% is half of $33\frac{1}{3}$%, and if we remembered that $33\frac{1}{3}\% = \frac{1}{3}$, Example 13 could have been solved as follows:

$$16\frac{2}{3}\% = \frac{1}{2} \times 33\frac{1}{3}\% = \frac{1}{2} \times \frac{1}{3} = \frac{1}{6}.$$

By memorizing the fractional, decimal, and percent equivalents that are listed on the inside back cover, you can greatly simplify some of your work.

Do Exercise 23.

Exercise Set 8.1

a Use the given information to complete a circle graph. Note that each circle is divided into 100 sections.

1. *Reasons for Drinking Coffee.*

To get going in the morning:	32%
Like the taste:	33%
Not sure:	2%
To relax:	4%
As a pick-me-up:	10%
It's a habit:	19%

Source: LMK Associates survey for Au Bon Pain Co., Inc.

2. *How Vacation Money is Spent.*

Transportation:	15%
Meals:	20%
Lodging:	32%
Recreation:	18%
Other:	15%

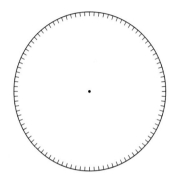

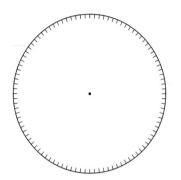

Answers to Exercises 1–2 can be found on p. A-22.

Write three kinds of notation as in Examples 1 and 2 on p. 456.

3. 90%

$\frac{90}{100}$; $90 \times \frac{1}{100}$; 90×0.01

4. 43.8%

$\frac{43.8}{100}$; $43.8 \times \frac{1}{100}$; 43.8×0.01

5. 12.5%

$\frac{12.5}{100}$; $12.5 \times \frac{1}{100}$; 12.5×0.01

6. 120%

$\frac{120}{100}$; $120 \times \frac{1}{100}$; 120×0.01

b Write decimal notation.

7. 12%

0.12

8. 42%

0.42

9. 34.7%

0.347

10. 69.7%

0.697

11. 59.01%

0.5901

12. 20.08%

0.2008

13. 10%

0.1

14. 20%

0.2

15. 1%

0.01

16. 100%

1

17. 300%

3

18. 700%

7

19. 0.6%

0.006

20. 0.2%

0.002

21. 0.23%

0.0023

22. 0.19%

0.0019

23. 105.24%

1.0524

24. 103.76%

1.0376

Write decimal notation for the percent notation in each sentence.

25. On average, about 40% of the body weight of an adult male is muscle.

0.4

26. On average, about 23% of the body weight of an adult female is muscle.

0.23

27. A person's brain is 2.5% of his or her body weight.

0.025

28. It is known that 16% of all dessert orders in restaurants is for pie.

0.16

29. It is known that 62.2% of us think Monday is the worst day of the week.

0.622

30. Of all 18-year-olds, 68.4% have a driver's license.

0.684

Write percent notation.

31. 0.47

47%

32. 0.87

87%

33. 0.03

3%

34. 0.01

1%

35. 8.7

870%

36. 4

400%

37. 0.334

33.4%

38. 0.889

88.9%

39. 0.75

75%

40. 0.99

99%

41. 0.4

40%

42. 0.5

50%

43. 0.8925

89.25%

44. 0.0258

2.58%

Write percent notation for the decimal notation in each sentence.

45. Around the fourth of July, about 0.000104 of all children aged 15 to 19 suffer injuries from fireworks.   0.0104%

46. With a relative humidity of 0.80, a temperature of 75°F feels like 88°F.   80%

47. It is known that 0.24 of us go to the movies once a month.   24%

48. It is known that 0.458 of us sleep between 7 and 8 hours.   45.8%

49. Of all money spent on sound recordings, 0.326 is spent on rock music.   32.6%

50. About 0.026 of all college football players go on to play professional football.   2.6%

c Write percent notation.

51. $\dfrac{41}{100}$ **52.** $\dfrac{36}{100}$ **53.** $\dfrac{5}{100}$ **54.** $\dfrac{1}{100}$ **55.** $\dfrac{2}{10}$ **56.** $\dfrac{7}{10}$

     41%   36%   5%   1%   20%   70%

57. $\dfrac{7}{25}$ **58.** $\dfrac{1}{20}$ **59.** $\dfrac{3}{20}$ **60.** $\dfrac{3}{4}$ **61.** $\dfrac{5}{8}$ **62.** $\dfrac{13}{50}$

     28%   5%   15%   75%   62.5%, or $62\frac{1}{2}$%   26%

63. $\dfrac{4}{5}$ **64.** $\dfrac{2}{5}$ **65.** $\dfrac{2}{3}$ **66.** $\dfrac{1}{3}$ **67.** $\dfrac{29}{50}$ **68.** $\dfrac{13}{25}$

     80%   40% $66.\overline{6}$%, or $66\frac{2}{3}$% $33.\overline{3}$%, or $33\frac{1}{3}$%   58%   52%

Write percent notation for the fractional notation in each sentence.

69. Bread is $\frac{9}{25}$ water.

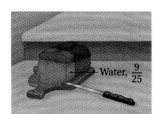
Water, $\frac{9}{25}$

     36%

70. Milk is $\frac{7}{8}$ water.

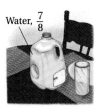
Water, $\frac{7}{8}$

     87.5%, or $87\frac{1}{2}$%

Write fractional notation. Try to remember the information in the table that appears on the inside back cover.

71. 85%   **72.** 55%   **73.** 62.5%   **74.** 12.5%

   $\frac{17}{20}$ $\frac{11}{20}$ $\frac{5}{8}$ $\frac{1}{8}$

75. $33\dfrac{1}{3}$%   **76.** $83\dfrac{1}{3}$%   **77.** $16.\overline{6}$%   **78.** $66.\overline{6}$%

   $\frac{1}{3}$ $\frac{5}{6}$ $\frac{1}{6}$ $\frac{2}{3}$

79. 7.25%   **80.** 4.85%   **81.** 0.8%   **82.** 0.2%

   $\frac{29}{400}$ $\frac{97}{2000}$ $\frac{1}{125}$ $\frac{1}{500}$

Write percent notation for the fractions in this pie chart.

Engagement Times of Married Couples

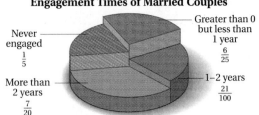

Never engaged $\frac{1}{5}$

Greater than 0 but less than 1 year $\frac{6}{25}$

More than 2 years $\frac{7}{20}$

1–2 years $\frac{21}{100}$

83. $\frac{21}{100}$ 21%

84. $\frac{1}{5}$ 20%

85. $\frac{6}{25}$ 24%

86. $\frac{7}{20}$ 35%

Use this bar graph to write fractional notation for the percentage of people who "greatly enjoy" each type of food.

Popularity of Ethnic Foods

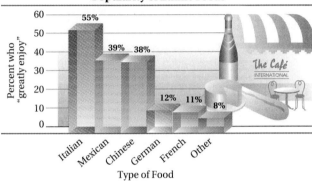

Percent who "greatly enjoy"

Italian 55%, Mexican 39%, Chinese 38%, German 12%, French 11%, Other 8%

Type of Food

Note that there can be multiple responses.

87. Italian $\frac{11}{20}$

88. Mexican $\frac{39}{100}$

89. Chinese $\frac{19}{50}$

90. German $\frac{3}{25}$

91. French $\frac{11}{100}$

92. Other $\frac{2}{25}$

93. *Energy Consumption.* The United States uses 26.4% of the world's energy (*Source:* U.S. Energy Information Administration, *International Energy Annual*). Write fractional notation for 26.4%. $\frac{33}{125}$

94. *World Population.* The United States has 4.5% of the world's population. Write fractional notation for 4.5%. $\frac{9}{200}$

95. *Election Turnouts.* In the 1996 presidential election, 45.7% of the voting-age population voted. Write fractional notation for 45.7%. $\frac{457}{1000}$

96. *Recordings Purchased.* Of the money spent on all sound recordings, 84.5% comes from people less than 45 yr old (*Source:* Recording Industry Association of America, Inc., *1997 Consumer Profile*). Write fractional notation for 84.5%. $\frac{169}{200}$

Complete the table.

97.

Fractional Notation	Decimal Notation	Percent Notation
$\frac{1}{8}$	0.125	$12\frac{1}{2}\%$, or 12.5%
$\frac{1}{6}$	$0.1\overline{6}$	$16\frac{2}{3}\%$, or $16.\overline{6}\%$
$\frac{1}{5}$	0.2	20%
$\frac{1}{4}$	0.25	25%
$\frac{1}{3}$	$0.\overline{3}$	$33\frac{1}{3}\%$, or $33.\overline{3}\%$
$\frac{3}{8}$	0.375	$37\frac{1}{2}\%$, or 37.5%
$\frac{2}{5}$	0.4	40%
$\frac{1}{2}$	0.5	50%

98.

Fractional Notation	Decimal Notation	Percent Notation
$\frac{3}{5}$	0.6	60%
$\frac{5}{8}$	0.625	$62\frac{1}{2}\%$, or 62.5%
$\frac{2}{3}$	$0.\overline{6}$	$66\frac{2}{3}\%$, or $66.\overline{6}\%$
$\frac{3}{4}$	0.75	75%
$\frac{4}{5}$	0.8	80%
$\frac{5}{6}$	$0.8\overline{3}$	$83\frac{1}{3}\%$, or $83.\overline{3}\%$
$\frac{7}{8}$	0.875	$87\frac{1}{2}\%$, or 87.5%
$\frac{1}{1}$	1	100%

99.

Fractional Notation	Decimal Notation	Percent Notation
$\frac{1}{2}$	0.5	50%
$\frac{1}{3}$	$0.\overline{3}$	$33\frac{1}{3}\%$, or $33.\overline{3}\%$
$\frac{1}{4}$	0.25	25%
$\frac{1}{6}$	$0.1\overline{6}$	$16\frac{2}{3}\%$, or $16.\overline{6}\%$
$\frac{1}{8}$	0.125	$12\frac{1}{2}\%$, or 12.5%
$\frac{3}{4}$	0.75	75%
$\frac{5}{6}$	$0.8\overline{3}$	$83\frac{1}{3}\%$, or $83.\overline{3}\%$
$\frac{3}{8}$	0.375	$37\frac{1}{2}\%$, or 37.5%

100.

Fractional Notation	Decimal Notation	Percent Notation
$\frac{2}{5}$	0.4	40%
$\frac{5}{8}$	0.625	$62\frac{1}{2}\%$, or 62.5%
$\frac{7}{8}$	0.875	$87\frac{1}{2}\%$, or 87.5%
$\frac{1}{1}$	1	100%
$\frac{3}{5}$	0.6	60%
$\frac{2}{3}$	$0.\overline{6}$	$66\frac{2}{3}\%$, or $66.\overline{6}\%$
$\frac{1}{5}$	0.2	20%
$\frac{4}{5}$	0.8	80%

Convert to a mixed numeral. [4.5b]

101. $\dfrac{100}{3}$ $33\dfrac{1}{3}$

102. $-\dfrac{75}{2}$ $-37\dfrac{1}{2}$

Solve.

103. $0.05 \times b = 20$ [5.7a]   400

104. $3 = 0.16 \times b$ [5.7a]   18.75

105. $\dfrac{24}{37} = \dfrac{15}{x}$ [7.3b]   23.125

106. $\dfrac{17}{18} = \dfrac{x}{27}$ [7.3b]   25.5

Synthesis

107. ◈ Tammy remembers that $\frac{1}{4} = 25\%$. Explain how she can use this to (a) write $\frac{1}{8}$ in percent notation and (b) write $\frac{5}{8}$ in percent notation.

108. ◈ Is it always best to convert from fractional notation to percent notation by first finding decimal notation? Why or why not?

109. ◈ Athletes sometimes speak of "giving 110%" effort. Does this make sense? Why or why not?

Write percent notation.

110. ▦ $\dfrac{41}{369}$ $11.\overline{1}\%$

111. ▦ $\dfrac{54}{999}$ $5.\overline{405}\%$

112. $2.5\overline{74631}$ $257.4\overline{6317}\%$

113. $3.2\overline{93847}$ $329.\overline{38479}\%$

Write decimal notation.

114. $\dfrac{14}{9}\%$ $0.01\overline{5}$

115. $\dfrac{19}{12}\%$ $0.0158\overline{3}$

116. $\dfrac{729}{7}\%$ $1.04\overline{142857}$

117. $\dfrac{637}{6}\%$ $1.061\overline{6}$

Collaborative Learning Manual

Use percent squares to develop a number sense for percents.

8.2 Solving Percent Problems Using Proportions*

a | Translating to Proportions

A percent is a ratio of some number to 100. For example, 75% is the ratio $\frac{75}{100}$. The numbers 3 and 4 have the same ratio as 75 and 100. Thus,

$$75\% = \frac{75}{100} = \frac{3}{4}.$$

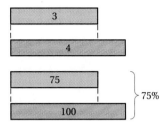

To solve a percent problem using a proportion, we translate as follows:

$$\text{Number} \rightarrow \frac{N}{100} = \frac{a}{b} \begin{matrix} \leftarrow \text{Amount} \\ \leftarrow \text{Base} \end{matrix}$$
$$100 \longrightarrow$$

> You might find it helpful to read this as "part is to whole as part is to whole."

For example,

> 60% of 25 is 15

translates to

$$\frac{60}{100} = \frac{15}{25}. \begin{matrix} \leftarrow \text{Amount} \\ \leftarrow \text{Base} \end{matrix}$$

A clue in translating is that the base, b, corresponds to 100 and usually follows the wording "percent of." Also, $N\%$ always translates to $N/100$. Another aid in translating is to make a comparison drawing. To do this, we start with the percent side and list 0% at the top and 100% near the bottom. Then we estimate where the specified percent—in this case, 60%—is located. The corresponding quantities are then filled in. The base—in this case, 25—always corresponds to 100% and the amount—in this case, 15—corresponds to the specified percent.

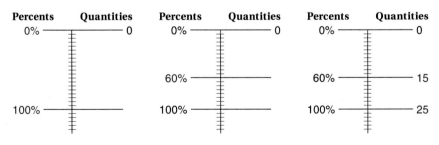

The proportion can then be read easily from the drawing.

*Note: Sections 8.2 and 8.3 present two methods for solving percent problems. You may prefer one method over the other, or your instructor may specify the method to be used. Section 8.2 is used as a check in Section 8.4, but otherwise it is not used in future sections of this book.

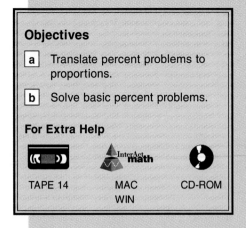

Objectives

a Translate percent problems to proportions.

b Solve basic percent problems.

For Extra Help

TAPE 14   MAC   CD-ROM
            WIN

Translate to a proportion. Do not solve.

1. 12% of 50 is what?

$$\frac{12}{100} = \frac{a}{50}$$

2. What is 40% of 60?

$$\frac{40}{100} = \frac{a}{60}$$

3. 130% of 72 is what?

$$\frac{130}{100} = \frac{a}{72}$$

Translate to a proportion. Do not solve.

4. 45 is 20% of what?

$$\frac{20}{100} = \frac{45}{b}$$

5. 120% of what is 60?

$$\frac{120}{100} = \frac{60}{b}$$

Answers on page A-22

Example 1 Translate to a proportion.

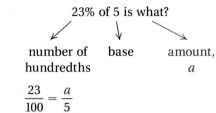

$$\frac{23}{100} = \frac{a}{5}$$

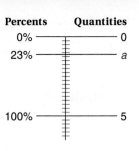

Example 2 Translate to a proportion.

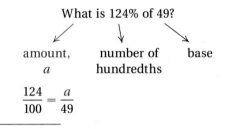

$$\frac{124}{100} = \frac{a}{49}$$

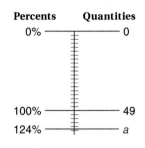

Do Exercises 1–3.

Example 3 Translate to a proportion.

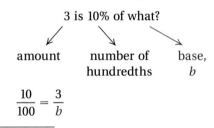

$$\frac{10}{100} = \frac{3}{b}$$

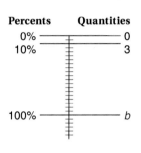

Example 4 Translate to a proportion.

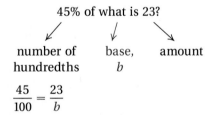

$$\frac{45}{100} = \frac{23}{b}$$

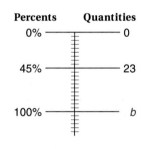

Do Exercises 4 and 5.

Example 5 Translate to a proportion.

10 is what percent of 20?

amount   number of   base
          hundredths, N

$$\frac{N}{100} = \frac{10}{20}$$

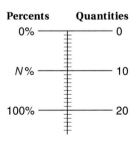

Example 6 Translate to a proportion.

What percent of 50 is 7?

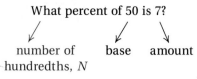

number of   base   amount
hundredths, N

$$\frac{N}{100} = \frac{7}{50}$$

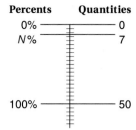

Percents	Quantities
0%	0
N%	7
100%	50

Do Exercises 6 and 7.

b Solving Percent Problems

After a percent problem has been translated to a proportion, we solve as in Section 7.3.

Example 7 5% of what is $20?

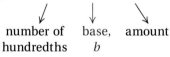

number of   base,   amount
hundredths b

Translate: $\dfrac{5}{100} = \dfrac{20}{b}$

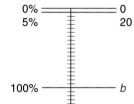

Percents	Quantities
0%	0
5%	20
100%	b

Solve: $5 \cdot b = 100 \cdot 20$ **Equating cross products**

$\dfrac{5b}{5} = \dfrac{2000}{5}$ **Dividing by 5**

$b = 400$ **Simplifying**

Thus, 5% of $400 is $20. The answer is $400.

Do Exercise 8.

Example 8 120% of 42 is what?

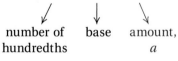

number of   base   amount,
hundredths a

Translate: $\dfrac{120}{100} = \dfrac{a}{42}$

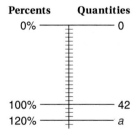

Percents	Quantities
0%	0
100%	42
120%	a

Solve: $120 \cdot 42 = 100 \cdot a$ **Equating cross products**

$\dfrac{5040}{100} = \dfrac{100a}{100}$ **Dividing by 100**

$50.4 = a$ **Simplifying**

Thus, 120% of 42 is 50.4. The answer is 50.4.

Do Exercises 9 and 10.

Translate to a proportion. Do not solve.

6. 16 is what percent of 40?

$$\frac{N}{100} = \frac{16}{40}$$

7. What percent of 84 is 10.5?

$$\frac{N}{100} = \frac{10.5}{84}$$

8. Solve:

20% of what is $45?

$225

Solve.

9. 64% of 55 is what?

35.2

10. What is 12% of 50?

6

Answers on page A-22

11. Solve:

60 is 120% of what?

50

12. Solve:

$12 is what percent of $40?

30%

13. Solve:

What percent of 84 is 10.5?

12.5%

Example 9   3 is 16% of what?

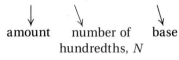

amount   number of   base,
           hundredths b

Translate: $\dfrac{3}{b} = \dfrac{16}{100}$

Solve: $3 \cdot 100 = b \cdot 16$ **Equating cross products**

$\dfrac{300}{16} = \dfrac{16b}{16}$ **Dividing by 16**

$18.75 = b$ **Simplifying**

Thus, 3 is 16% of 18.75. The answer is 18.75.

Percents	Quantities
0%	0
16%	3
100%	b

Do Exercise 11.

Example 10 $10 is what percent of $20?

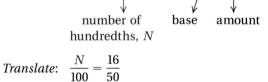

amount   number of   base
           hundredths, N

Translate: $\dfrac{10}{20} = \dfrac{N}{100}$

Solve: $10 \cdot 100 = 20 \cdot N$ **Equating cross products**

$\dfrac{1000}{20} = \dfrac{20N}{20}$ **Dividing by 20**

$50 = N$ **Simplifying**

Thus, $10 is 50% of $20. The answer is 50%.

Percents	Quantities
0%	0
N%	$10
100%	$20

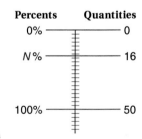

Always "look before you leap." Many students can solve this problem mentally: $10 is half, or 50%, of $20.

Do Exercise 12.

Example 11   What percent of 50 is 16?

number of   base   amount
hundredths, N

Translate: $\dfrac{N}{100} = \dfrac{16}{50}$

Solve: $50 \cdot N = 100 \cdot 16$ **Equating cross products**

$\dfrac{50 \cdot N}{50} = \dfrac{100 \cdot 16}{50}$ **Dividing by 50**

$N = \dfrac{2 \cdot 50 \cdot 16}{50}$ **Removing a factor equal to 1:** $\dfrac{50}{50} = 1$

$N = 32$ **Multiplying**

Thus, 32% of 50 is 16. The answer is 32%. A quick alternative approach is to note that, since $50 \cdot 2 = 100$, we have $\frac{16}{50} = \frac{16 \cdot 2}{50 \cdot 2} = \frac{32}{100}$, or 32%.

Percents	Quantities
0%	0
N%	16
100%	50

Do Exercise 13.

Exercise Set 8.2

a Translate to a proportion. Do not solve.

1. What is 37% of 74?

$$\frac{37}{100} = \frac{a}{74}$$

2. 66% of 74 is what?

$$\frac{66}{100} = \frac{a}{74}$$

3. 4.3 is what percent of 5.9?

$$\frac{N}{100} = \frac{4.3}{5.9}$$

4. What percent of 6.8 is 5.3?

$$\frac{N}{100} = \frac{5.3}{6.8}$$

5. 14 is 25% of what?

$$\frac{25}{100} = \frac{14}{b}$$

6. 133% of what is 40?

$$\frac{133}{100} = \frac{40}{b}$$

7. 9% of what is 37?

$$\frac{9}{100} = \frac{37}{b}$$

8. What is 132% of 75?

$$\frac{132}{100} = \frac{a}{75}$$

9. 70% of 660 is what?

$$\frac{70}{100} = \frac{a}{660}$$

10. 17 is 23% of what?

$$\frac{23}{100} = \frac{17}{b}$$

b Solve.

11. What is 4% of 1000?
40

12. What is 6% of 2000?
120

13. 4.8% of 60 is what?
2.88

14. 63.1% of 80 is what?
50.48

15. $24 is what percent of $96?
25%

16. $14 is what percent of $70?
20%

17. 102 is what percent of 100?
102%

18. 103 is what percent of 100?
103%

19. What percent of $480 is $120?
25%

20. What percent of $80 is $60?
75%

21. What percent of 160 is 150?
93.75%

22. What percent of 33 is 11?
$33.\overline{3}$%, or $33\frac{1}{3}$%

23. $18 is 25% of what?
$72

24. $75 is 20% of what?
$375

25. 60% of what is 54?
90

26. 80% of what is 96?
120

27. 65.12 is 74% of what?
88

28. 63.7 is 65% of what?
98

29. 80% of what is 16?
20

30. 80% of what is 10?
12.5

31. What is $62\frac{1}{2}$% of 40? 25

32. What is $43\frac{1}{4}$% of 2600? 1124.5

33. What is 9.4% of $8300? $780.20

34. What is 8.7% of $76,000? $6612

35. 9.48 is 120% of what? 7.9

36. 8.45 is 130% of what? 6.5

37.
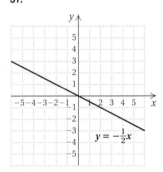

38.
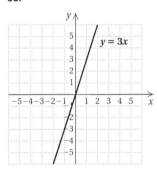

39.
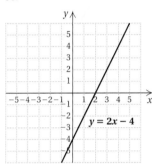

40.
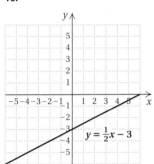

Skill Maintenance

Graph. [6.4b]

37. $y = -\dfrac{1}{2}x$

38. $y = 3x$

39. $y = 2x - 4$

40. $y = \dfrac{1}{2}x - 3$

Solve.

41. A recipe for pancakes calls for $\frac{1}{2}$ qt of buttermilk, $\frac{1}{3}$ qt of skim milk, and $\frac{1}{16}$ qt of oil. How many quarts of liquid ingredients does the recipe call for? [4.2d]

$\frac{43}{48}$ qt

42. Guilford Gardeners purchased $\frac{3}{4}$ ton (T) of top soil. If the soil is to be shared equally among 6 gardeners, how much will each gardener receive? [3.7c]

$\frac{1}{8}$ T

Synthesis

43. ◆ In your own words, list steps that a classmate could use to solve any percent problem in this section.

44. ◆ In solving Example 10, a student simplifies $\frac{10}{20}$ before solving. Is this a good idea? Why or why not?

45. ◆ Can "comparison drawings," like those used in this section, be used to solve *any* proportion? Why or why not?

Solve.

46. ▦ What is 8.85% of $12,640?
Estimate _____ $1134; can vary
Calculate _____ $1118.64

47. ▦ 78.8% of what is 9809.024?
Estimate _____ 12,500; can vary
Calculate _____ 12,448

8.3 Solving Percent Problems Using Equations

a Translating to Equations

A second method for solving percent problems is to translate a problem's wording directly to an equation. For example, "23% of 5 is what?" translates as follows.

$$
\begin{array}{ccccc}
23\% & \text{of} & 5 & \text{is} & \text{what?} \\
\downarrow & \downarrow & \downarrow & \downarrow & \downarrow \\
23\% & \cdot & 5 & = & a
\end{array}
$$

> Note how the key words are translated.

> "**Of**" translates to "$\cdot$", or "$\times$".   "**Is**" translates to "$=$".
>
> "**What**" translates to a variable.   **%** translates to "$\times \frac{1}{100}$" or "$\times 0.01$".

Example 1 Translate:

$$
\begin{array}{ccccc}
\text{What} & \text{is} & 11\% & \text{of} & 49? \\
\downarrow & \downarrow & \downarrow & \downarrow & \downarrow \\
a & = & 11\% & \cdot & 49
\end{array}
$$

Any letter can be used as a variable.

Do Exercises 1 and 2.

Example 2 Translate:

$$
\begin{array}{ccccc}
3 & \text{is} & 10\% & \text{of} & \text{what?} \\
\downarrow & \downarrow & \downarrow & \downarrow & \downarrow \\
3 & = & 10\% & \cdot & b
\end{array}
$$

Example 3 Translate:

$$
\begin{array}{ccccc}
45\% & \text{of} & \text{what} & \text{is} & 23? \\
\downarrow & \downarrow & \downarrow & \downarrow & \downarrow \\
45\% & \cdot & b & = & 23
\end{array}
$$

Do Exercises 3 and 4.

Example 4 Translate:

$$
\begin{array}{ccccc}
10 & \text{is} & \text{what percent} & \text{of} & 20? \\
\downarrow & \downarrow & \downarrow & \downarrow & \downarrow \\
10 & = & n & \cdot & 20
\end{array}
$$

Example 5 Translate:

$$
\begin{array}{ccccc}
\text{What percent} & \text{of} & 50 & \text{is} & 7? \\
\downarrow & \downarrow & \downarrow & \downarrow \\
n & \cdot & 50 & = & 7
\end{array}
$$

Do Exercises 5 and 6.

Translate to an equation. Do not solve.

1. 12% of 50 is what?

$12\% \cdot 50 = a$

2. What is 40% of 60?

$a = 40\% \cdot 60$

Translate to an equation. Do not solve.

3. 45 is 20% of what?

$45 = 20\% \cdot t$

4. 120% of what is 60?

$120\% \cdot y = 60$

Translate to an equation. Do not solve.

5. 16 is what percent of 40?

$16 = n \cdot 40$

6. What percent of 84 is 10.5?

$n \cdot 84 = 10.5$

Answers on page A-23

7. Solve:

What is 12% of 50?

6

b | Solving Percent Problems

In solving percent problems, we use the *Translate* and *Solve* steps in the problem-solving strategy used throughout this text.

Percent problems are actually of three different types. Although the method we present does *not* require that you be able to identify which type we are studying, it is helpful to know them.

We know that

15 is 25% of 60, or

$15 = 25\% \cdot 60.$

We can think of this as:

> Amount = Percent number · Base.

Each of the three types of percent problems depends on which of the three pieces of information is missing.

1. Finding the *amount* (the result of taking the percent)

Example: What is   25% of   60?

Translation: y =   25%   ·   60

2. Finding the *base* (the number you are taking the percent of)

Example: 15   is   25%   of   what number?

Translation: 15   =   25%   · y

3. Finding the *percent number* (the percent itself)

Example: 15   is   what percent   of   60?

Translation: 15   = y ·   60

Finding the Amount

Example 6   What is 11% of 49?

Translate: $a = 11\% \cdot 49.$

Solve: The variable is by itself. To solve the equation, we just convert 11% to decimal notation and multiply.

$a = 0.11(49)$

$$\begin{array}{r} 4\ 9 \\ \times\ 0.1\ 1 \\ \hline 4\ 9 \\ 4\ 9\ 0 \\ \hline 5.3\ 9 \end{array}$$

$a = 5.39$

> A way of checking answers is by estimating as follows:
>
> $11\% \times 49 \approx 10\% \cdot 50$
> $= 0.10(50) = 5.$
>
> Since 5 is close to 5.39, our answer is reasonable.

Thus, 5.39 is 11% of 49. The answer is 5.39.

Do Exercise 7.

Answer on page A-23

Example 7 120% of $42 is what?

Translate: 120% · 42 = a.

Solve: The variable is by itself. To solve the equation, we convert 120% to 1.2 and carry out the calculation.

$$1.2(42) = a$$

$$\begin{array}{r} 4\ 2 \\ \times\ 1.2 \\ \hline 8\ 4 \\ 4\ 2\ 0 \\ \hline \end{array}$$

$$50.4 = a \qquad 5\ 0.4$$

Thus, 120% of $42 is $50.40. The answer is $50.40.

Do Exercise 8.

Finding the Base

Example 8 5% of what is 20?

Translate: 5% · b = 20.

Solve: This time the variable is *not* by itself. To solve the equation, we convert 5% to 0.05 and divide by 0.05 on both sides:

$$\frac{0.05 \cdot b}{0.05} = \frac{20}{0.05} \qquad \text{Dividing by 0.05 on both sides}$$

$$b = \frac{20}{0.05}$$

$$= 400.$$

$$\begin{array}{r} 4\ 0\ 0. \\ 0.0\ 5\ )\overline{2\ 0.0\ 0}_{\wedge} \\ 2\ 0\ 0\ 0 \\ \hline 0 \end{array}$$

Thus, 5% of 400 is 20. The answer is 400.

Example 9 $3 is 16% of what?

Translate:

$$\begin{array}{ccccc} \$3 & \text{is} & 16\% & \text{of} & \text{what?} \\ \downarrow & \downarrow & \downarrow & \downarrow & \downarrow \\ 3 & = & 16\% & \cdot & b. \end{array}$$

Solve: Again, the variable is not by itself. To solve the equation, we convert 16% to 0.16 and divide by 0.16 on both sides:

$$\frac{3}{0.16} = \frac{0.16 \cdot b}{0.16} \qquad \text{Dividing by 0.16 on both sides}$$

$$\frac{3}{0.16} = b$$

$$18.75 = b.$$

$$\begin{array}{r} 1\ 8.7\ 5 \\ 0.1\ 6\ )\overline{3.0\ 0}_{\wedge}0\ 0 \\ 1\ 6 \\ \hline 1\ 4\ 0 \\ 1\ 2\ 8 \\ \hline 1\ 2\ 0 \\ 1\ 1\ 2 \\ \hline 8\ 0 \\ 8\ 0 \\ \hline 0 \end{array}$$

Thus, $3 is 16% of $18.75. The answer is $18.75.

Do Exercises 9 and 10.

8. Solve:

64% of $55 is what?

$35.20

Solve.

9. 20% of what is 45?

225

10. $60 is 120% of what?

$50

Answers on page A-23

16 is what percent of 40?

40%

Finding the Percent

In solving these problems, you *must* remember to convert to percent notation after you have solved the equation.

Example 10   17 is what percent of 20?

Translate: 17   is   what percent   of   20?

17   = n ·   20.

Solve: To solve the equation, we divide by 20 on both sides and convert the result to percent notation:

$$17 = n \cdot 20$$

$$\frac{17}{20} = \frac{n \cdot 20}{20}$$ **Dividing by 20 on both sides:**

$$0.85 = n, \text{ or } n = 85\%.$$

$$\begin{array}{r} .85 \\ 20 \overline{)\ 17.00} \\ 160 \\ \hline 100 \\ 100 \\ \hline 0 \end{array}$$

Thus, 17 is 85% of 20. The answer is 85%.

Do Exercise 11.

12. Solve:

What percent of $84 is $10.50?

12.5%

Example 11   What percent of $50 is $16?

Translate: What percent   of $50   is $16?

n ·   50   =   16.

Solve: To solve the equation, we divide by 50 on both sides and convert the answer to percent notation:

$$\frac{n \cdot 50}{50} = \frac{16}{50}$$ **Dividing by 50 on both sides**

$$n = \frac{16}{50}$$

$$= \frac{16}{50} \cdot \frac{2}{2}$$ **Multiplying by $\frac{2}{2}$, or 1, to get a denominator of 100**

$$= \frac{32}{100}$$

$$= 32\%.$$ **Converting to percent notation**

Thus, 32% of $50 is $16. The answer is 32%.

Do Exercise 12.

CAUTION!   When a question asks "what percent?", be sure to give the answer in percent notation.

Answers on page A-23

Exercise Set 8.3

a Translate to an equation. Do not solve.

1. What is 32% of 78?

$y = 32\% \cdot 78$

2. 98% of 57 is what?

$98\% \cdot 57 = p$

3. 89 is what percent of 99?

$89 = a \cdot 99$

4. What percent of 25 is 8?

$y \cdot 25 = 8$

5. 13 is 25% of what?

$13 = 25\% \cdot y$

6. 21.4% of what is 20?

$21.4\% \cdot m = 20$

b Solve.

7. What is 85% of 276?

234.6

8. What is 74% of 53?

39.22

9. 150% of 30 is what?

45

10. 100% of 13 is what?

13

11. What is 6% of $300?

$18

12. What is 4% of $45?

$1.80

13. 3.8% of 50 is what?

1.9

14. $33\frac{1}{3}\%$ of 480 is what? $\left(\textit{Hint: } 33\frac{1}{3}\% = \frac{1}{3}.\right)$

160

15. $39 is what percent of $50?

78%

16. $16 is what percent of $90?

$17.\overline{7}\%$, or $17\frac{7}{9}\%$

17. 20 is what percent of 10?

200%

18. 60 is what percent of 20?

300%

19. What percent of $300 is $150?

50%

20. What percent of $50 is $40?

80%

21. What percent of 80 is 100?

125%

22. What percent of 60 is 15?

25%

23. 20 is 50% of what?

40

24. 57 is 20% of what?

285

25. 40% of what is $16?

$40

26. 100% of what is $74?

$74

27. 56.32 is 64% of what?

88

28. 71.04 is 96% of what?

74

29. 70% of what is 14?

20

30. 70% of what is 35?

50

31. What is $62\frac{1}{2}$% of 10?

6.25

32. What is $35\frac{1}{4}$% of 1200?

423

33. What is 8.3% of $10,200?

$846.60

34. What is 9.2% of $5600?

$515.20

35. $66\frac{2}{3}$% of what is 27.4?

$\left(\textit{Hint}: 66\frac{2}{3}\% = \frac{2}{3}.\right)$ 41.1

36. $33\frac{1}{3}$% of what is 17.2?   51.6

Skill Maintenance

Write fractional notation.   [5.1b]

37. 0.623 $\frac{623}{1000}$

38. 1.9 $\frac{19}{10}$

39. 2.37 $\frac{237}{100}$

Write decimal notation.   [5.1c]

40. $\frac{9}{1000}$ 0.009

41. $\frac{39}{100}$ 0.39

42. $\frac{57}{10}$ 5.7

Synthesis

43. ◈ Write a percent problem that could be translated to the equation

$30 = n \cdot 80.$

44. ◈ Write a percent problem that could be translated to the equation

$25 = 4\% \cdot b.$

45. ◈ To calculate a 15% tip on a $24 bill, a customer adds $2.40 and half of $2.40, or $1.20, to get $3.60. Is this procedure valid? Why or why not?

Solve.

46. 🖩 What is 7.75% of $10,880?
   Estimate _____ $880; can vary
   Calculate _____ $843.20

47. 🖩 50,951.775 is what percent of 78,995?
   Estimate _____   62.5% (can vary)
   Calculate _____   64.5%

48. *Recyclables.* It is estimated that 40% to 50% of all trash is recyclable. If a community produces 270 tons of trash, how much of their trash is recyclable?

108 to 135 tons

49. 40% of $18\frac{3}{4}$% of $25,000 is what? $1875

8.4 Applications of Percent

a Applied Problems Involving Percent

Applied problems involving percent are not always stated in a manner easily translated to an equation. In such cases, it is helpful to rephrase the problem before translating. Sometimes it also helps to make a drawing.

Example 1 *Paper Recycling.* In a recent year, the United States generated 81.5 million tons of paper waste, of which about 32.6 million tons were recycled (**Source:** Environmental Protection Agency). What percent of paper waste was recycled?

1. **Familiarize.** The question asks for a percent. We know that 10% of 81.5 is approximately 8. Since 8 · 4 = 32, which is close to 32.6, we expect the answer to be close to 40%. We let n = the percent of paper waste that was recycled.

2. **Translate.** We can rephrase the question and translate as follows:

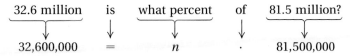

32.6 million	is	what percent	of	81.5 million?
32,600,000	=	n	·	81,500,000

3. **Solve.** We solve as we did in Section 8.3:

$$32{,}600{,}000 = n \cdot 81{,}500{,}000$$

$$\frac{32{,}600{,}000}{81{,}500{,}000} = \frac{n \cdot 81{,}500{,}000}{81{,}500{,}000} \qquad \text{Dividing by 81,500,000 on both sides}$$

$$0.4 = n$$

$$40\% = n. \qquad \text{Remember to write percent notation.}$$

4. **Check.** To check, we note that 40% is just what we predicted in the *Familiarize* step.

5. **State.** About 40% of the paper waste was recycled.

Do Exercise 1.

Example 2 *"Junk" Mail.* The U.S. Postal Service estimates that we read 78% of the junk mail we receive. Suppose that a business sends out 9500 advertising brochures. How many brochures can the business expect to be opened and read?

1. **Familiarize.** Since 78% ≈ 75% and 9500 ≈ 10,000, we can estimate that about 75% of 10,000, or 7500 brochures will be opened and read. To find a more exact answer, we let a = the number of brochures that will be opened and read.

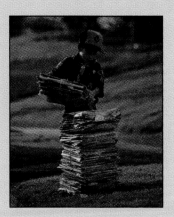
1. *Desserts.* If a restaurant sells 250 desserts in an evening, it is typical that 40 of them will be pie. What percent of the desserts sold will be pie?

16%

Answer on page A-23

---

2. *Human Anatomy.* The weight of a human brain is 2.5% of total body weight. A person weighs 200 lb. What does the brain weigh?   5 lb

Brain Weight vs. Body Weight

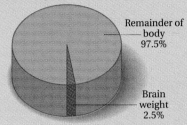

Remainder of body
97.5%

Brain weight
2.5%

2. Translate.   The question can be rephrased and translated as follows.*

What number   is   78%   of   9500?

$$a = 78\% \cdot 9500$$

3. Solve.   We convert 78% to decimal notation and multiply:

$$a = 78\% \cdot 9500 = 0.78(9500) = 7410.$$

4. Check.   To check, we note that our answer, 7410, is not far from 7500, our estimate in the *Familiarize* step. The student can also check that $7410 \div 9500$ is 0.78, or 78%.

5. State.   The business can expect 7410 of its brochures to be opened and read.

Do Exercise 2.

b   Percent of Increase or Decrease

What do we mean when we say that the price of Swiss cheese has decreased 8%? If the price was $5.00 per pound and it went down to $4.60 per pound, then the decrease is $0.40, which is 8% of the original price. We can see this in the following figure.

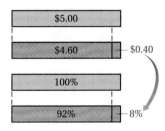

Example 3   *Energy Consumption.* With proper furnace maintenance, a family that pays a monthly fuel bill of $78.00 can reduce their bill to $70.20. What is the percent of decrease?

1. Familiarize.   We find the amount of decrease and then make a drawing.

```
  7 8.0 0     Original bill
- 7 0.2 0     New bill
  ───────
    7.8 0     Decrease
```

We let n = the percent of decrease.

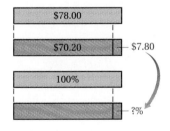

2. Translate.   We rephrase and translate as follows.*

7.80   is   what percent   of   78.00?

$$7.80 = n \cdot 78.00$$

*We can also use the proportion method of Section 8.2 to solve.

3. Solve. To solve the equation, we divide by 78 on both sides:

$$\frac{7.80}{78.00} = \frac{n \cdot 78.00}{78.00}$$ Dividing by 78 on both sides

$$0.1 = n$$ You may have noticed earlier that 7.8 is 10% of 78.

$$10\% = n.$$ Changing from decimal to percent notation

4. Check. To check, we note that, with a 10% decrease, the reduced bill should be 90% of the original bill. Since 90% of 78 = 0.9(78) = 70.20, our answer checks.

5. State. The percent of decrease of the fuel bill is 10%.

Do Exercise 3.

Example 4 *Wages.* A sixth-grade teacher earns $27,000 one year and receives a 6% raise the next. What is the new salary?

1. Familiarize. We note that the amount of the raise can be found and then added to the old salary. A drawing can help us visualize this. We let x = the new salary.

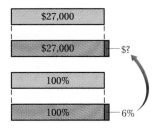

2. Translate. We rephrase the question and translate as follows.

What	is	the old salary	plus	6%	of	the old salary?
↓	↓	↓	↓	↓	↓	↓
x	=	27,000	+	6%	·	27,000

3. Solve. To solve, we convert 6% to a decimal and simplify:

$$x = 27,000 + 0.06(27,000)$$

$$= 27,000 + 1620 \quad \text{The value of the raise is \$1620.}$$

$$= 28,620.$$

4. Check. To check, we note that the new salary is 100% of the old salary plus 6% of the old salary. Thus the new salary is 106% of the old salary. Since 1.06(27,000) = 28,620, our answer checks.

5. State. The new salary is $28,620.

Do Exercise 4.

Percents provide a way to measure increases or decreases relative to the original amount. For example, the average salary of an NBA basketball player increased from $1.558 million in 1994 to $1.867 million in 1995. To find the *percent of increase* in salary, we first subtract to find out how much more the salary was in 1995: $1.867 million − $1.558 million = $0.309 million. Then we determine what percent of the original amount the increase was.

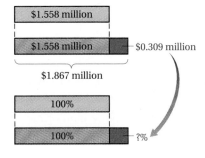

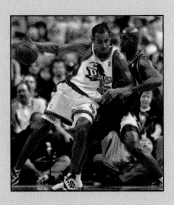

3. *Energy Consumption.* By using only cold water in the washing machine, a household with a monthly fuel bill of $78.00 can reduce their bill to $74.88. What is the percent of decrease? 4%

4. *Wages.* A daycare worker earns $17,500 one year and receives a 9% raise the next. What is the new salary? $19,075

Answers on page A-23

5. *Automobile Price.* The price of an automobile increased from $15,800 to $17,222. What was the percent of increase?   9%

Since $0.309 million = $309,000, we are asking

$309,000 is what percent of $1,558,000?

This translates to the following:

309,000 = x · 1,558,000.

This is an equation of the type studied in Sections 8.2 and 8.3. Solving the equation, we can confirm that $0.309 million, or $309,000, is about 19.8% of $1.558 million. Thus the percent of increase in salary was 19.8%.

To find a percent of increase or decrease:

a) Find the amount of increase or decrease.

b) Then determine what percent this is of the original amount.

Example 5 *Digital-Camera Screen Size.* The diagonal of the display screen of a digital camera was recently increased from 1.8 in. to 2.5 in. What was the percent of increase in the diagonal?

1. **Familiarize.** We note that the increase in the diagonal was 2.5 − 1.8, or 0.7 in. A drawing can help us to visualize the situation. We let n = the percent of increase.

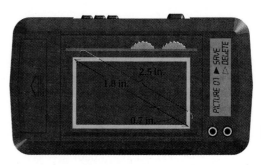

2. **Translate.** We rephrase the question and translate.

0.7 in. is what percent of 1.8 in.?

0.7 = n · 1.8

3. **Solve.** To solve the equation, we divide by 1.8 on both sides:*

$$\frac{0.7}{1.8} = \frac{n \cdot 1.8}{1.8}$$

$0.389 \approx n$ Rounded to the nearest thousandth

$38.9\% \approx n.$ Remember to write percent notation.

4. **Check.** To check, we take 38.9% of 1.8:

$38.9\% \cdot 1.8 = 0.389(1.8) = 0.7002.$

Since we rounded the percent, this approximation is close enough to 0.7 to be a good check.

5. **State.** The percent of increase of the screen diagonal is 38.9%.

Do Exercise 5.

---

*We can also use the proportion method of Section 8.2 and solve:

$$\frac{0.7}{1.8} = \frac{N}{100}.$$

Answer on page A-23

Exercise Set 8.4

a Solve.

1. *Left-handed Professional Bowlers.* It has been determined by sociologists that 17% of the population is left-handed. Each tournament conducted by the Professional Bowlers Association has 120 entrants. How many would you expect to be left-handed? not left-handed? Round to the nearest one.

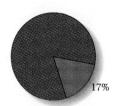

Total: 120

20; 100

2. *Advertising Budget.* A common guideline for businesses is to use 5% of their operating budget for advertising. Ariel Electronics has an operating budget of $8000 per week. How much should it spend each week for advertising? for other expenses?

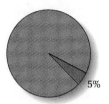

Total: $8000

$400; $7600

3. Of all moviegoers, 67% are in the 12–29 age group. A five-screen cinema complex is filled with 600 moviegoers. How many would you expect to find in the 12–29 age group?

402

4. Deming, New Mexico, claims to have the purest drinking water in the world. It is 99.9% pure. If you had 240 L of water from Deming, how much of it, in liters, would be pure? impure?

239.76 L; 0.24 L

5. A baseball player gets 13 hits in 40 at-bats. What percent are hits? not hits?

32.5%; 67.5%

6. On a test of 80 items, Erika had 76 correct. What percent were correct? incorrect?

95%; 5%

7. A lab technician has 680 mL of a solution of water and acid; 3% is acid. How many milliliters are acid? water?

20.4 mL; 659.6 mL

8. A lab technician has 540 mL of a solution of alcohol and water; 8% is alcohol. How many milliliters are alcohol? water?

43.2 mL; 496.8 mL

9. *TV Usage.* Of the 8760 hr in a year, most television sets are on for 2190 hr. What percent is this?

25%

10. *Colds from Kissing.* In a medical study, it was determined that if 800 people kiss someone who has a cold, only 56 will actually catch a cold. What percent is this?

7%

11. *Maximum Heart Rate.* Treadmill tests are often administered to diagnose heart ailments. A guideline in such a test is to try to get you to reach your *maximum heart rate,* in beats per minute. The maximum heart rate is found by subtracting your age from 220 and then multiplying by 85%. What is the maximum heart rate of someone whose age is 25? 36? 48? 55? 76? Round to the nearest one.

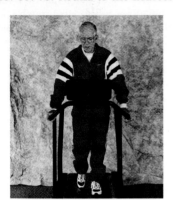

166; 156; 146; 140; 122

12. *Tampoline Injuries.* As the number of home trampolines has increased, so too has the number of trampoline-related injuries. In 1995, there were 58,400 injuries (**Source:** *The New York Times,* March 3, 1998).

a) Research shows that 93% of all trampoline-related injuries occur at home. How many occurred at home in 1995?   54,312

b) From 1990 to 1995, a total of 249,400 trampoline-related injuries occurred. What percentage of these occurred in 1995?   23.4%

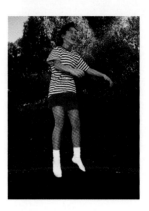

b Solve.

13. The amount in a savings account increased from $150 to $162. What was the percent of increase?

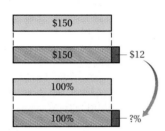

8%

14. The population of South Creek increased from 840 to 882. What was the percent of increase?

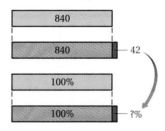

5%

15. During a sale, the price of a dress decreased from $90 to $72. What was the percent of decrease?

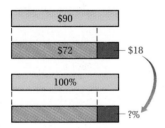

20%

16. A person on a diet goes from a weight of 125 lb to a weight of 110 lb. What is the percent of decrease?

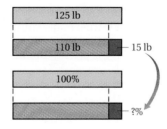

12%

17. Rachel earns $28,600 one year and receives a 5% raise in salary. What is the new salary?

$30,030

18. Derek earns $20,400 one year and receives an 8% raise in salary. What is the new salary?

$22,032

19. The value of a car typically decreases by 30% in the first year. A car is bought for $18,000. What is its value one year later? $12,600

20. One year the pilots of an airline shocked the business world by taking an 11% pay cut. The former salary was $55,000. What was the reduced salary? $48,950

21. *World Population.* World population is increasing by 1.6% each year. In 1999, it was 6.0 billion. How much will it be in 2000? 2001? 2002?

6.096 billion; 6.194 billion; 6.293 billion

22. *Cooling Costs.* By increasing the thermostat from 72° to 78°, a family can reduce its cooling bill by 50%. If the cooling bill was $106.00, what would the new bill be? By what percent has the temperature been increased?

$53.00; 8.$\overline{3}$%, or $8\frac{1}{3}$%

23. *Car Depreciation.* A car generally depreciates 30% of its original value in the first year. A car is worth $25,480 after the first year. What was its original cost? $36,400

24. *Car Depreciation.* Given normal use, an American-made car will depreciate 30% of its original cost the first year and 14% of its remaining value in the second year. What is the value of a car at the end of the second year if its original cost was $36,400? $28,400? $26,800?

$21,912.80; $17,096.80; $16,133.60

25. *Tipping.* Diners frequently add a 15% tip when charging a meal to a credit card. What is the total amount charged if the cost of the meal, without tip, is $15? $34? $49? $17.25; $39.10; $56.35

26. *Carpentry.* A cross section of a standard "two-by-four" board actually measures $1\frac{1}{2}$ in. by $3\frac{1}{2}$ in. The rough board is 2 in. by 4 in. but is planed and dried to the finished size. What percent of the wood is removed in planing and drying?   34.375%, or $34\frac{3}{8}$%

27. *Drunk Driving.* Despite efforts by groups such as MADD (Mothers Against Drunk Driving), the number of alcohol-related deaths rose in 1995 after many years of decline. The data in the table show the number of deaths from 1986 to 1995.

a) What is the percent of increase in the number of alcohol-related deaths from 1994 to 1995?   4.1%
b) What is the percent of decrease in the number of alcohol-related deaths from 1986 to 1994?   31.0%

Alcohol-Related Traffic Deaths Back on the Increase!!	
Year	Deaths
1986	24,045
1987	23,641
1988	23,626
1989	22,436
1990	22,084
1991	19,887
1992	17,859
1993	17,473
1994	16,589
1995	17,274

Source: National Highway Traffic Safety Administration

28. *Fetal Acoustic Stimulation.* Each year there are about 4 million births in the United States. Of these, about 120,000 births occur in breech position (delivery of a fetus with the buttocks or feet appearing first). A new technique, called *fetal acoustic stimulation (FAS)*, uses sound directed through a mother's abdomen in order to stimulate movement of the fetus to a safer position. In a recent study of this low-risk and low-cost procedure, FAS enabled doctors to turn the baby in 34 of 38 cases (***Source:*** Johnson and Elliott, "Fetal Acoustic Stimulation, an Adjunct to External Cephalic Versions: A Blinded, Randomized Crossover Study," *American Journal of Obstetrics & Gynecology* **173**, no. 5 (1995): 1369–1372).

a) What percent of U.S. births are breech?   3%
b) What percent (rounded to the nearest tenth) of cases showed success with FAS?   89.5%
c) About how many breech babies yearly might be turned if FAS could be implemented in all breech births in the United States?   107,400
d) Breech position is one reason for performing Caesarean section (or C-section) birth surgery. Researchers expect that FAS alone can eliminate the need for about 2000 C-sections yearly in the United States. Given this information, how many C-sections per year are due to breech position alone?   2235

29. *Strike Zone.* In baseball, the *strike zone* is normally a 17-in. by 40-in. rectangle. Some batters give the pitcher an advantage by swinging at pitches thrown out of the strike zone. By what percent is the area of the strike zone increased if a 2-in. border is added to the outside?

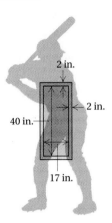

35.9%

30. *Gardening.* Tony is planting grass on a 24-ft by 36-ft area in his back yard. He installs a 6-ft by 8-ft garden. By what percent has he reduced the area he has to mow?

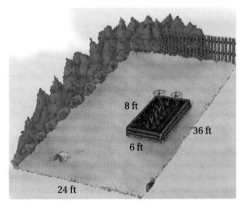

5.$\overline{5}$%

Skill Maintenance

Convert to decimal notation.   [5.1c]

31. $\dfrac{25}{11}$ 2.$\overline{27}$

32. $\dfrac{11}{25}$ 0.44

33. $\dfrac{27}{8}$ 3.375

34. $\dfrac{43}{9}$ 4.$\overline{7}$

35. $\dfrac{23}{25}$ 0.92

36. $\dfrac{20}{24}$ 0.8$\overline{3}$

37. $\dfrac{14}{32}$ 0.4375

38. $\dfrac{2317}{1000}$ 2.317

39. $\dfrac{34,809}{10,000}$ 3.4809

40. $\dfrac{27}{40}$ 0.675

Synthesis

41. ◆ Which is better for a wage earner, and why: a 10% raise followed by a 5% raise a year later, or a 5% raise followed by a 10% raise a year later?

42. ◆ Write a problem for a classmate to solve. Design the problem so that the solution is "Jackie's raise was 7$\frac{1}{2}$%."

43. ◆ The former baseball player and manager Yogi Berra once said that "ninety percent of the game is half mental." If this is true, what percent of the game is mental? Explain your reasoning.

44. ◆ ▦ A workers' union is offered either a 5% "across-the-board" raise in which all salaries would increase 5%, or a flat $1650 raise for each worker. If the total payroll for the 123 workers is $4,213,365, which offer should the union select? Why?

45. *Adult Height.* It has been determined that at the age of 10, a girl has reached 84.4% of her final adult growth. Cynthia is 4 ft, 8 in. at the age of 10. What will be her final adult height?   About 5 ft, 6 in.

46. *Adult Height.* It has been determined that at the age of 15, a boy has reached 96.1% of his final adult height. Claude is 6 ft, 4 in. at the age of 15. What will be his final adult height?   About 6 ft, 7 in.

47. If p is 120% of q, then q is what percent of p?   83$\frac{1}{3}$%

48. A coupon allows a couple to have dinner and then have $10 subtracted from the bill. Before subtracting $10, however, the restaurant adds a tip of 15%. If the couple is presented with a bill for $44.05, how much would the dinner (without tip) have cost without the coupon? $47

49. ▦ A worker receives raises of 3%, 6%, and then 9%. By what percent has the original salary increased?   19%

8.5 Consumer Applications: Sales Tax, Commission, and Discount

a Sales Tax

Sales tax computations represent a special type of percent of increase problem. The sales tax rate in Colorado is 3%. This means that the tax is 3% of the purchase price. Suppose the purchase price on a coat is $124.95. The sales tax is then

$$3\% \text{ of } \$124.95, \quad \text{or} \quad 0.03 \cdot 124.95,$$

or

$$3.7485, \quad \text{or about} \quad \$3.75.$$

The total that you pay is the price plus the sales tax:

$$\$124.95 + \$3.75, \quad \text{or} \quad \$128.70.$$

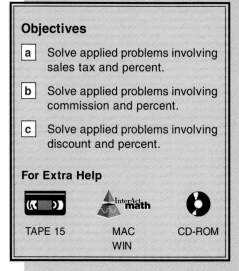

$124.95 + 3% sales tax

Bill:		
Purchase price	=	$124.95
Sales tax (3% of $124.95)	=	+ 3.75
Total price		$128.70

▶ **Sales tax** = Sales tax rate · Purchase price

Total price = Purchase price + Sales tax

Example 1 *New Jersey Sales Tax.* In 1998, the sales tax rate in New Jersey was 6%. How much tax was charged on the purchase of 3 CDs at $13.95 each? What was the total price?

a) We first find the cost of the CDs. It is

$$3 \cdot \$13.95 = \$41.85.$$

b) The sales tax on items costing $41.85 is

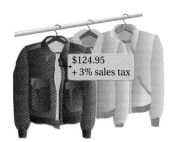

Sales tax rate · Purchase price

6% · $41.85,

or 0.06 · 41.85, or 2.511. Thus the tax is $2.51.

c) The total price is given by the purchase price plus the sales tax:

$$\$41.85 + \$2.51, \quad \text{or} \quad \$44.36.$$

To check, note that the total price is the purchase price plus 6% of the purchase price. Thus the total price is 106% of the purchase price. Since 1.06 · 41.85 = 44.361 and 44.361 rounds to 44.36, we have a check. The total price was $44.36.

Do Exercises 1 and 2.

Objectives

a Solve applied problems involving sales tax and percent.

b Solve applied problems involving commission and percent.

c Solve applied problems involving discount and percent.

For Extra Help

TAPE 15   MAC WIN   CD-ROM

1. *Connecticut Sales Tax.* In 1998, the sales tax rate in Connecticut was 6%. How much tax was charged on the purchase of a refrigerator that sold for $668.95? What was the total price?

   $40.14; $709.09

2. *Rhode Island Sales Tax.* Morris buys 5 blank audiocassettes in Rhode Island, where the sales tax rate is 7%. If each tape costs $2.95, how much tax will be charged? What is the total price?

   $1.03; $15.78

Answers on page A-23

3. The sales tax is $33 on the purchase of a $550 washer. What is the sales tax rate?

6%

4. The sales tax on a 27-inch television is $25.20 and the sales tax rate is 6%. Find the purchase price (the price before taxes are added).

$420

Answers on page A-23

Example 2   The sales tax is $32 on the purchase of an $800 sofa. What is the sales tax rate?

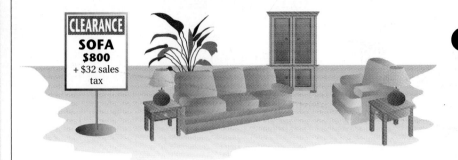

Rephrase: Sales tax   is   what percent   of   purchase price?

Translate: 32   =   r   ·   800

To solve the equation, we divide by 800 on both sides:

$$\frac{32}{800} = \frac{r \cdot 800}{800}$$

$$0.04 = r$$

$$4\% = r.$$

The sales tax rate is 4%.

Do Exercise 3.

Example 3   The sales tax on a laser printer is $31.74 and the sales tax rate is 5%. Find the purchase price (the price before taxes are added).

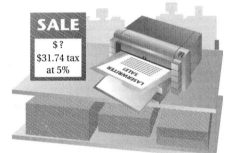

Rephrase: Sales tax   is   5%   of   what?

Translate: 31.74   =   5%   ·   b,   or   31.74 = 0.05 · b.

To solve, we divide by 0.05 on both sides:

$$\frac{31.74}{0.05} = \frac{0.05 \cdot b}{0.05}$$

$$634.8 = b.$$

```
                    6 3 4.8
        0.0 5 ) 3 1.7 4 0
                  3 0 0 0
                    1 7 4
                    1 5 0
                      2 4
                      2 0
                        4 0
                        4 0
                         0
```

The purchase price is $634.80.

Do Exercise 4.

b | Commission

When you work for a **salary**, you receive the same amount of money each week or month. When you work for a **commission**, you are paid a percentage of the total sales for which you are responsible.

> Commission = Commission rate · Sales

Example 4 *Stereo Equipment Sales.* A salesperson's commission rate is 20%. What is the commission from the sale of $25,560 worth of stereo equipment?

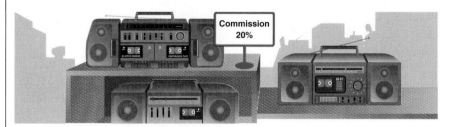

$$\begin{array}{ccccc} Commission & = & Commission\ rate & \cdot & Sales \\ C & = & 20\% & \cdot & 25{,}560 \end{array}$$

This tells us what to do. We multiply.

$$\begin{array}{r} 2\,5{,}5\,6\,0 \\ \times\qquad 0.2 \\ \hline 5\ 1\ 1\ 2.0 \end{array} \qquad \text{20\% = 0.20 = 0.2}$$

The commission is $5112.

Do Exercise 5.

Example 5 *Farm Machinery Sales.* Dawn earns a commission of $3000 selling $60,000 worth of farm machinery. What is the commission rate?

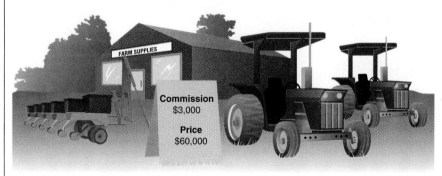

$$\begin{array}{ccccc} Commission & = & Commission\ rate & \cdot & Sales \\ 3000 & = & r & \cdot & 60{,}000 \end{array}$$

To solve this equation, we divide by 60,000 on both sides:

$$\frac{3000}{60{,}000} = \frac{r \cdot 60{,}000}{60{,}000} = r.$$

5. Raul's commission rate is 30%. What is the commission from the sale of $18,760 worth of air conditioners?

$5628

Answer on page A-23

6. Liz earns a commission of $6000 selling $24,000 worth of refrigerators. What is the commission rate?

25%

We can divide, but this time we simplify by removing a factor equal to 1:

$$r = \frac{3000}{60{,}000} = \frac{1}{20} \cdot \frac{3000}{3000} = \frac{1}{20} = 0.05 = 5\%.$$

The commission rate is 5%.

Do Exercise 6.

Example 6 *Motorcycle Sales.* Joyce's commission rate is 25%. She receives a commission of $425 on the sale of a motorcycle. How much did the motorcycle cost?

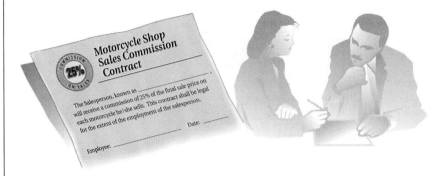

$$
\begin{array}{ccccc}
Commission & = & Commission\ rate & \cdot & Sales \\
425 & = & 25\% & \cdot & S
\end{array}
$$

To solve this equation, we divide by 0.25 on both sides:

$$\frac{425}{0.25} = \frac{0.25 \cdot S}{0.25}$$

$$1700 = S.$$

$$
\begin{array}{r}
1\ 7\ 0\ 0. \\
0.2\ 5\ )\overline{4\ 2\ 5.0\ 0_\wedge} \\
2\ 5\ 0 \\
\hline
1\ 7\ 5 \\
1\ 7\ 5 \\
\hline
0
\end{array}
$$

The motorcycle cost $1700.

7. Ben's commission rate is 16%. He receives a commission of $268 from sales of clothing. How many dollars worth of clothing were sold?

$1675

Do Exercise 7.

c | Discount

Suppose that the regular price of a rug is $60, and the rug is on sale at 25% off. Since 25% of $60 is $15, the sale price is $60 − $15, or $45. We call $60 the **original**, or **marked price**, 25% the **rate of discount**, $15 the **discount**, and $45 the **sale price**. Note that discount problems are a type of percent of decrease problem.

> **Discount** = Rate of discount · Original price
>
> **Sale price** = Original price − Discount

Answers on page A-23

Example 7 *Rug Prices.* A rug marked $240 is on sale at 25% off. What is the discount? the sale price?

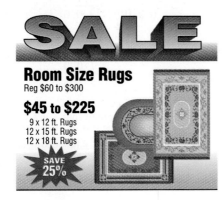

a) *Discount = Rate of discount · Original price*

$$D = 25\% \cdot 240$$

This tells us what to do. We convert 25% to decimal notation and multiply.

```
        2 4 0
   ×    0.2 5        25% = 0.25
        1 2 0 0
        4 8 0 0
       6 0.0 0
```

The discount is $60.

b) *Sale price = Marked price − Discount*

$$S = 240 - 60$$

This tells us what to do. We subtract.

```
      2 4 0
   −    6 0
      1 8 0
```

To check, note that the sale price is 75% of the marked price: $0.75 \times 240 = 180$.

The sale price is $180.

Do Exercise 8.

Example 8 *Antique Pricing.* An antique table is marked down from $620 to $527. What is the rate of discount?

We first find the discount by subtracting the sale price from the original price:

```
      6 2 0
   − 5 2 7
        9 3.
```

The discount is $93.

Next, we use the equation for discount:

Discount = Rate of discount · Original price

$$93 = r \cdot 620.$$

8. A suit marked $140 is on sale at 24% off. What is the discount? the sale price?

$33.60; $106.40

Answer on page A-23

9. A pair of running shoes is reduced from $75 to $60. Find the rate of discount.

20%

To solve, we divide by 620 on both sides:

$$\frac{93}{620} = \frac{r \cdot 620}{620}$$

$$0.15 = r$$

$$15\% = r.$$

```
        0.1 5
6 2 0 ) 9 3.0 0
        6 2 0
        3 1 0 0
        3 1 0 0
              0
```

The discount rate is 15%.

To check, note that a 15% discount rate means that 85% of the original price is paid:
$$0.85 \cdot 620 = 527.$$

Do Exercise 9.

Calculator Spotlight

% Key.   Many calculators have a percent key. This key can be useful in calculations like 20% · $25,560, as in Example 4, but you may need to change the order to 25,560 · 20%. To do the calculation, press

| 2 | 5 | 5 | 6 | 0 | × | 2 | 0 | SHIFT | % | .

The displayed result is

5112 .

Check your manual for other procedures for determining percents.

Exercises

Calculate.

1. 250 · 20%   50

2. 37% · 18,924   7001.88

3. 67.2% · 124,898   83,931.456

4. 56,788.22 · 64.2%   36,458.03724

On many calculators, there is a fast way to increase or decrease a number by any given percentage. In Example 1, the result of taking 6% of $41.85 and adding it to $41.85 can often be found by pressing

| 4 | 1 | . | 8 | 5 | × | 6 | SHIFT | % | + | .

The displayed result would be

44.361 .

If the price had been *reduced* by 6%, the computation would be

| 4 | 1 | . | 8 | 5 | × | 6 | SHIFT | % | − | .

The displayed result would be

39.339 .

Check your manual for other procedures for determining percents.

Exercise

Use a calculator with a % key to confirm your answers to Margin Exercises 5 and 8.

Answer on page A-23

Exercise Set 8.5

a Solve.

1. *Indiana Sales Tax.* The sales tax rate in Indiana is 5%. How much tax is charged on a generator costing $586? What is the total price? $29.30; $615.30

2. *New York City Sales Tax.* The sales tax rate in New York City is 8.25%. How much tax is charged on photo equipment costing $248? What is the total price? $20.46; $268.46

3. *Illinois Sales Tax.* The sales tax rate in Illinois is 6.25%. How much tax is charged on a purchase of 5 telephones at $53 apiece? What is the total price?

   $16.56; $281.56

4. *California Sales Tax.* The sales tax rate in California is 6%. How much tax is charged on a purchase of 5 teapots at $37.99 apiece? What is the total price?

   $11.40; $201.35

5. *Mountain Bike Sales.* The sales tax is $15.96 on the purchase of a mountain bike that sells for $399. What is the sales tax rate? 4%

6. *Jewelry Sales.* The sales tax is $15 on the purchase of a diamond ring that sells for $500. What is the sales tax rate? 3%

7. The sales tax is $44.75 on the purchase of a fiberglass canoe that sells for $895. What is the sales tax rate? 5%

8. The sales tax is $9.12 on the purchase of a patio set that sells for $456. What is the sales tax rate? 2%

9. *Truck Sales.* The sales tax on a used pickup truck is $250 and the sales tax rate is 5%. Find the purchase price (the price before taxes are added). $5000

10. *Motorboat Sales.* The sales tax on the purchase of a motorboat is $112 and the sales tax rate is 2%. Find the purchase price. $5600

11. The sales tax on a dining room set is $28 and the sales tax rate is 3.5%. Find the purchase price.

    $800

12. The sales tax on a home-theater speaker system is $66 and the sales tax rate is 5.5%. Find the purchase price. $1200

13. The sales tax rate in Dallas is 2% for the city and 6.25% for the state. Find the total amount paid for 2 shower units at $332.50 apiece.

$719.86

14. The sales tax rate in Omaha is 1% for the city and 5% for the state. Find the total amount paid for 3 air conditioners at $260 apiece.

$826.80

15. The sales tax is $1030.40 on the purchase of a used Chevrolet Camaro for $18,400. What is the sales tax rate?

5.6%

16. The sales tax is $979.60 on the purchase of a used Dodge Caravan for $15,800. What is the sales tax rate?

6.2%

b Solve.

17. Kelly is about to receive her commission of 35% for selling $2580 of Amstar products. How much commission will Kelly receive?

$903

18. Jose's commission rate is 32%. What is the commission from the sale of $12,500 worth of sailboards?

$4000

19. Bernie receives $87 as commission for selling $174 worth of cosmetics. What is the commission rate?

50%

20. Donna earns $408 selling $3400 worth of running shoes. What is the commission rate?

12%

21. An art gallery's commission rate is 40%. They receive a commission of $392. How many dollars worth of artwork were sold?

$980

22. A real estate agent's commission rate is 7%. She receives a commission of $5600 on the sale of a home. How much did the home sell for?

$80,000

23. A real estate commission is 6%. What is the commission on the sale of a $98,000 home?

$5880

24. A real estate commission is 8%. What is the commission on the sale of a piece of land for $68,000?

$5440

25. Bonnie earns $280.80 selling $2340 worth of tee shirts. What is the commission rate?

12%

26. Chuck earns $1147.50 selling $7650 worth of ski passes. What is the commission rate?

15%

27. Miguel's commission is increased according to how much he sells. He receives a commission of 5% for the first $2000 and 8% on the amount over $2000. What is the total commission on sales of $6000?

$420

28. Lucinda earns a salary of $500 a month, plus a 2% commission on software sales. One month, she sold $8700 worth of software. What were her wages that month?

$674

c Find what is missing.

29.

Marked Price	Rate of Discount	Discount	Sale Price
$300	10%	$30	$270

30.

Marked Price	Rate of Discount	Discount	Sale Price
$2000	40%	$800	$1200

31.

$17.00	15%	$2.55	$14.45

32.

$20.00	25%	$5	$15

33.

$125	10%	$12.50	$112.50

34.

$438	15%	$65.70	$372.30

35.

$600	40%	$240	$360

36.

$12,800	15%	$1920	$10,880

37. Find the discount and the rate of discount for the ring in this ad. $387; 30.4%

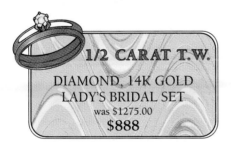

1/2 CARAT T.W.

DIAMOND, 14K GOLD
LADY'S BRIDAL SET
was $1275.00
$888

38. Find the discount and the rate of discount for the calculator in this ad. $45.02; 39.1%

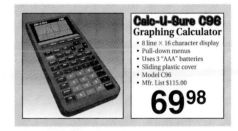

Calc-U-Sure C96
Graphing Calculator
• 8 line × 16 character display
• Pull-down menus
• Uses 3 "AAA" batteries
• Sliding plastic cover
• Model C96
• Mfr. List $115.00
69⁹⁸

39. Find the marked price and the rate of discount for the camcorder in this ad. $460; about 18%

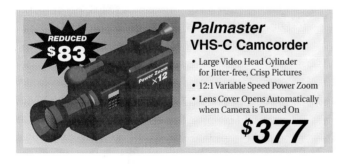

REDUCED
$83

Palmaster
VHS-C Camcorder
• Large Video Head Cylinder for Jitter-free, Crisp Pictures
• 12:1 Variable Speed Power Zoom
• Lens Cover Opens Automatically when Camera is Turned On
$377

40. Find the marked price and the rate of discount for the cedar chest in this ad. $299.99; about 16.7%

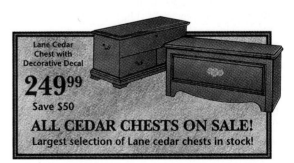

Lane Cedar
Chest with
Decorative Decal
249⁹⁹
Save $50
ALL CEDAR CHESTS ON SALE!
Largest selection of Lane cedar chests in stock!

Solve. [7.3b]

41. $\dfrac{x}{12} = \dfrac{24}{16}$ 18

42. $\dfrac{7}{2} = \dfrac{11}{x}$ $\frac{22}{7}$

Graph. [6.4b]

43. $y = \dfrac{4}{3}x$

Answer graph below.

44. $y = -\dfrac{4}{3}x + 1$

Answer graph below.

Write decimal notation. [5.1c]

45. $\dfrac{5}{9}$ $0.\overline{5}$

46. $\dfrac{23}{11}$ $2.\overline{09}$

47. $-\dfrac{11}{12}$ $-0.91\overline{6}$

48. $-\dfrac{13}{7}$ $-1.\overline{857142}$

Synthesis

49. ◆ Carl's Car Care mistakenly charged Dawn 5% tax for a cleaning job that was all labor. To correct the mistake, they subtracted 5% from what Dawn paid. Was this correct? Why or why not?

50. ◆Is the following ad mathematically correct? Why or why not?

43.

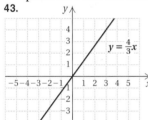

44.

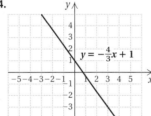

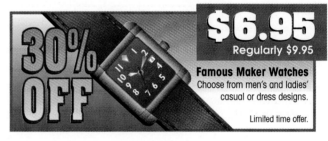

51. ◆ An item that is no longer on sale at "25% off" receives a price tag that is $33\frac{1}{3}\%$ more than the sale price. Has the item price been restored to its original price? Why or why not?

52. ◆ Which is better, a discount of 40% on a book's list price or a discount of 20% on list price followed by another discount of 20% on the reduced price? Explain.

53. ▦ A real estate commission rate is 7.5%. A house sells for $98,500. How much does the seller get for the house after paying the commission? $91,112.50

54. ▦ *People Magazine.* In a recent subscription drive, *People* offered a subscription of 52 weekly issues for a price of $1.89 per issue. They advertised that this was a savings of 29.7% off the newsstand price. What was the newsstand price? $2.69

55. ▦ Gordon receives a 10% commission on the first $5000 in sales and 15% on all sales beyond $5000. If Gordon receives a commission of $2405, how much did he sell? Use a calculator and trial and error if you wish. $17,700

56. Tee shirts are being sold at the mall for $5 each, or 3 for $10. If you buy three tee shirts, what is the rate of discount? $33\frac{1}{3}\%$

57. Herb collects baseball memorabilia. He bought two autographed plaques, but became short of funds and had to sell them quickly for $200 each. On one, he made a 20% profit and on the other, he lost 20%. Did he make or lose money on the sale?

He bought the plaques for $166\frac{2}{3}$ + $250, or $416\frac{2}{3}$, and sold them for $400, so he lost money.

Calculate the costs associated with the purchase of a car or truck.

Collaborative Learning Manual

8.6 Consumer Applications: Interest

a Simple Interest

Suppose you put $100 into an investment for 1 year. The $100 is called the **principal**. If the **interest rate** is 8%, in addition to the principal, you will get back 8% of the principal, which is

8% of $100, or 0.08 · 100, or $8.00.

The $8.00 is called the **interest**, or more precisely, the **simple interest**. It is, in effect, the price that a financial institution pays for the use of the money over time.

> The **simple interest** *I* on principal *P*, invested for *t* years at interest rate *r*, is given by
> $$I = P \cdot r \cdot t.$$

Example 1 What is the interest on $2500 invested at an interest rate of 6% for 1 year?

We use the formula $I = P \cdot r \cdot t$:

$$I = P \cdot r \cdot t = \$2500 \cdot 6\% \cdot 1$$
$$= \$2500 \cdot 0.06$$
$$= \$150.$$

```
   2 5 0 0
×    0.0 6
 1 5 0.0 0
```

The interest for 1 year is $150.

Do Exercise 1.

Example 2 What is the interest on a principal of $2500 invested at an interest rate of 6% for $\frac{1}{4}$ year?

We use the formula $I = P \cdot r \cdot t$:

$$I = P \cdot r \cdot t = \$2500 \cdot 6\% \cdot \frac{1}{4}$$
$$= \frac{\$2500 \cdot 0.06}{4}$$
$$= \$37.50.$$

```
        3 7.5
  4 ) 1 5 0.0
      1 2 0
        3 0
        2 8
          2 0
          2 0
            0
```

> We could have instead found $\frac{1}{4}$ of 6% and then multiplied by 2500.

The interest for $\frac{1}{4}$ year is $37.50.

Do Exercise 2.

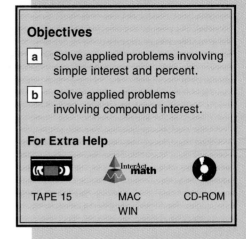

1. What is the interest on $4300 invested at an interest rate of 14% for 1 year?

$602

2. What is the interest on a principal of $4300 invested at an interest rate of 14% for $\frac{3}{4}$ year?

$451.50

Answers on page A-23

3. The Glass Nook borrows $4800 at 7% for 30 days. Find (a) the amount of simple interest due and (b) the total amount that must be paid after 30 days.

$27.62; $4827.62

Unless specified otherwise, it is understood that interest rates refer to the *yearly* rate at which interest is paid. This means that when a time period is given in days, we must divide it by 365 to express the time as a fractional part of a year.

Example 3 To pay for a shipment of tee shirts, New Wave Designs borrows $8000 at 9% for 60 days. Find (a) the amount of simple interest that is due and (b) the total amount that must be paid after 60 days.

a) We express 60 days as a fractional part of a year:

$$I = P \cdot r \cdot t = \$8000 \cdot 9\% \cdot \frac{60}{365} \quad \text{Note that 60 days} = \frac{60}{365} \text{ year.}$$

$$= \$8000 \cdot 0.09 \cdot \frac{60}{365}$$

$$\approx \$118.36. \quad \text{Using a calculator}$$

The interest due for 60 days is $118.36.

b) The total amount to be paid after 60 days is the principal plus the interest:

$$\$8000 + \$118.36 = \$8118.36.$$

The total amount due is $8118.36.

Do Exercise 3.

b Compound Interest

Simple interest is interest paid on principal only. When interest is paid on the accumulated interest as well as on the principal, we call it **compound interest.** This is the type of interest usually paid on investments. Suppose you have $5000 in a savings account at 6%. In 1 year, the account will contain the original $5000 plus 6% of $5000. Thus the total in the account after 1 year will be

106% of $5000, or 1.06 · $5000, or $5300.

Now suppose that the total of $5300 remains in the account for another year. At the end of this second year, the account will contain the $5300 plus 6% of $5300. The total in the account would thus be

106% of $5300, or 1.06 · $5300, or $5618.

Note that in the second year, interest is earned on the first year's interest. When this happens, we say that interest is **compounded annually.**

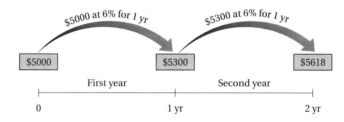

Answer on page A-23

Example 4 Find the amount in an account if $2000 is invested at 8%, compounded annually, for 2 years.

a) After 1 year, the account will contain 108% of $2000:

$1.08 \cdot \$2000 = \$2160.$

$$
\begin{array}{r}
2\ 0\ 0\ 0 \\
\times\ \ \ \ \ 1.0\ 8 \\
\hline
1\ 6\ 0\ 0\ 0 \\
0\ 0\ 0\ 0 \\
2\ 0\ 0\ 0 \\
\hline
2\ 1\ 6\ 0.0\ 0
\end{array}
$$

b) At the end of the second year, the account will contain 108% of $2160:

$1.08 \cdot \$2160 = \$2332.80.$

$$
\begin{array}{r}
2\ 1\ 6\ 0 \\
\times\ \ \ \ \ 1.0\ 8 \\
\hline
1\ 7\ 2\ 8\ 0 \\
0\ 0\ 0\ 0 \\
2\ 1\ 6\ 0 \\
\hline
2\ 3\ 3\ 2.8\ 0
\end{array}
$$

The amount in the account after 2 years is $2332.80.

Do Exercise 4.

Suppose that the interest in Example 4 were **compounded semi-annually**—that is, every half year. Interest would then be calculated twice a year at a rate of 8% ÷ 2, or 4%, each time. The approach used in Example 4 can then be adapted, as follows.

After the first $\frac{1}{2}$ year, the account will contain 104% of $2000:

$1.04(\$2000) = \$2080.$ **These calculations can be confirmed with a calculator.**

After a second $\frac{1}{2}$ year (1 full year), the account will contain 104% of $2080:

$1.04(\$2080) = \$2163.20.$

After a third $\frac{1}{2}$ year $\left(1\frac{1}{2}\text{ full years}\right)$, the account will contain 104% of $2163.20:

$1.04(\$2163.20) = \$2249.728$

$\approx \$2249.73.$ **Rounding to the nearest cent**

Finally, after a fourth $\frac{1}{2}$ year (2 full years), the account will contain 104% of $2249.73:

$1.04(\$2249.73) = \$2339.7192$

$\approx \$2339.72.$ **Rounding to the nearest cent**

Note that each multiplication was by 1.04 and that

$\$2000 \cdot 1.04^4 = \$2339.72.$ **Using a calculator and rounding to the nearest cent**

4. Find the amount in an account if $2000 is invested at 11%, compounded annually, for 2 years.

$2464.20

Answer on page A-23

5. A couple invests $7000 in an account paying 10%, compounded semiannually. Find the amount in the account after $1\frac{1}{2}$ years.

$8103.38

We have illustrated the following result.

> ▶ If a principal P has been invested at interest rate r, compounded n times a year, in t years it will grow to an amount A given by
> $$A = P \cdot \left(1 + \frac{r}{n}\right)^{n \cdot t}, \quad \text{where } r \text{ is written in decimal notation.}$$
> $\left(\text{Here } n \cdot t \text{ is the number of compounding periods and } \frac{r}{n} \text{ is the interest rate for each period.}\right)$

Example 5 The Ibsens invest $7000 in an account paying 8%, compounded quarterly. Find the amount in the account after $2\frac{1}{2}$ years.

We substitute $7000 for P, 0.08 for r, 4 for n, and $2\frac{1}{2}$ for t and solve for A:

$$A = P \cdot \left(1 + \frac{r}{n}\right)^{n \cdot t}$$

$$= 7000 \cdot \left(1 + \frac{0.08}{4}\right)^{4 \cdot (5/2)} \qquad \text{Writing } 2\frac{1}{2} \text{ as } \frac{5}{2}$$

$$= 7000 \cdot (1 + 0.02)^{10} \qquad 4 \cdot \frac{5}{2} = \frac{20}{2} = 10$$

$$= 7000 \cdot (1.02)^{10}$$

$$\approx 8532.96. \qquad \textbf{Using a calculator}$$

The amount in the account after $2\frac{1}{2}$ years is $8532.96.

Do Exercise 5.

Calculator Spotlight

When using a calculator for interest computations, it is important to remember the order in which operations are performed and to minimize "round-off error." For example, to find the amount due on a $20,000 loan made for 25 days at 11%, compounded daily, we press the following sequence of keys:

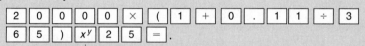

| 2 | 0 | 0 | 0 | 0 | × | (| 1 | + | 0 | . | 1 | 1 | ÷ | 3 |
| 6 | 5 |) | x^y | 2 | 5 | = |

This key may appear differently. See p. 75.

Without parentheses keys, we would press

| 1 | + | 0 | . | 1 | 1 | ÷ | 3 | 6 | 5 | = | x^y | 2 | 5 | = |
| × | 2 | 0 | 0 | 0 | 0 | = |

Note that in both sequences of keystrokes we raise $1 + \frac{0.11}{365}$, not just $\frac{0.11}{365}$, to the power. After 25 days, $20,151.23 is due.

Exercises

1. Find the amount due on a $16,000 loan made for 62 days at 13%, compounded daily. $16,357.18

2. An investment of $12,500 is made for 90 days at 8.5%, compounded daily. How much is the investment worth after 90 days? $12,764.72

Answer on page A-23

Exercise Set 8.6

a Find the *simple* interest.

	Principal	Rate of interest	Time
1.	$200	13%	1 year
	$26		
2.	$450	18%	1 year
	$81		
3.	$2000	12.4%	$\frac{1}{2}$ year
	$124		
4.	$200	7.7%	$\frac{1}{2}$ year
	$7.70		
5.	$4300	14%	$\frac{1}{4}$ year
	$150.50		
6.	$2000	15%	$\frac{1}{4}$ year
	$75		

Solve. Assume that simple interest is being calculated in each case.

7. CopiPix, Inc., borrows $10,000 at 9% for 60 days. Find (a) the amount of interest due and (b) the total amount that must be paid after 60 days.

(a) $147.95; **(b)** $10,147.95

8. Sal's Laundry borrows $8000 at 10% for 90 days. Find (a) the amount of interest due and (b) the total amount that must be paid after 90 days.

(a) $197.26; **(b)** $8197.26

9. Animal Instinct, a pet supply shop, borrows $6500 at 8% for 90 days. Find (a) the amount of interest due and (b) the total amount that must be paid after 90 days.

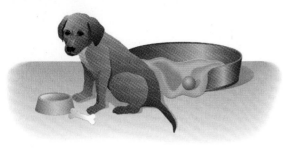

(a) $128.22; (b) $6628.22

10. Andante's Cafe borrows $4500 at 9% for 60 days. Find (a) the amount of interest due and (b) the total amount that must be paid after 60 days.

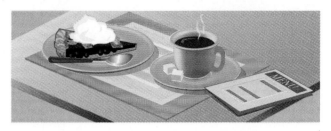

(a) $66.58; (b) $4566.58

11. Jean's Garage borrows $5600 at 10% for 30 days. Find (a) the amount of interest due and (b) the total amount that must be paid after 30 days.

(a) $46.03; (b) $5646.03

12. Shear Delights, a hair salon, borrows $3600 at 8% for 30 days. Find (a) the amount of interest due and (b) the total amount that must be paid after 30 days.

(a) $23.67;   (b) $3623.67

b Interest is compounded annually. Find the amount in the account after the given length of time. Round to the nearest cent.

	Principal	Rate of interest	Time
13.	$400	10%	2 years
	$484		
14.	$400	7.7%	2 years
	$463.97		
15.	$200	8.8%	2 years
	$236.75		
16.	$1000	15%	2 years
	$1322.50		

Interest is compounded semiannually. Find the amount in the account after the given length of time. Round to the nearest cent.

Principal	Rate of interest	Time
17. $4000	7%	1 year
$4284.90		
18. $1000	5%	1 year
$1050.63		
19. ▦ $2000	9%	3 years
$2604.52		
20. ▦ $5000	8%	30 months
$6083.26		

Solve.

21. ▦ A family invests $4000 in an account paying 6%, compounded monthly. How much is in the account after 5 months?

$4101.01

22. ▦ A couple invests $2500 in an account paying 9%, compounded monthly. How much is in the account after 6 months?

$2614.63

23. ▦ A couple invests $1200 in an account paying 10%, compounded quarterly. How much is in the account after 1 year?

$1324.58

24. ▦ The O'Hares invest $6000 in an account paying 8%, compounded quarterly. How much is in the account after 18 months?

$6756.97

Skill Maintenance

Solve. [7.3b]

25. $\dfrac{9}{10} = \dfrac{x}{5}$ 4.5

26. $\dfrac{7}{x} = \dfrac{4}{5}$ $8\dfrac{3}{4}$

27. $\dfrac{3}{4} = \dfrac{6}{x}$ 8

28. $\dfrac{7}{8} = \dfrac{x}{100}$ 87.5

Convert to a mixed numeral. [4.5b]

29. $-\dfrac{64}{17}$ $-3\dfrac{13}{17}$

30. $\dfrac{38}{11}$ $3\dfrac{5}{11}$

Convert from a mixed numeral to fractional notation. [4.5a]

31. $1\dfrac{1}{17}$ $\dfrac{18}{17}$

32. $20\dfrac{9}{10}$ $\dfrac{209}{10}$

Synthesis

33. ◆ Which is a better investment and why: $1000 invested at $14\frac{3}{4}\%$ simple interest for 1 year, or $1000 invested at 14% compounded monthly for 1 year?

34. ◆ A firm must choose between borrowing $5000 at 10% for 30 days and borrowing $10,000 at 8% for 60 days. Give arguments in favor of and against each option.

35. ◆ Without performing the multiplications, determine which gives the most interest: $1000 × 8% × $\frac{1}{12}$, or $1000 × 8% × $\frac{30}{365}$? How did you decide?

36. ▦ What is the simple interest on $24,680 at 7.75% for $\frac{3}{4}$ year? $1434.53

37. ▦ Interest is compounded semiannually. Find the value of the investment if $24,800 is invested at 6.4% for 5 years. $33,981.98

38. ▦ Interest is compounded quarterly. Find the value of the investment if $125,000 is invested at 9.2% for $2\frac{1}{2}$ years. $156,915.68

Effective Yield. The *effective yield* is the yearly rate of simple interest that corresponds to an interest rate that is compounded two or more times a year. For example, if P is invested at 12%, compounded quarterly, we would multiply P by $(1 + 0.12/4)^4$, or 1.03^4. Since $1.03^4 \approx 1.126$ or 112.6%, the 12% compounded quarterly corresponds to an effective yield of approximately 12.6%. In Exercises 39 and 40, find the effective yield for the indicated account.

39. ▦ The account pays 9% compounded monthly.
9.38%

40. ▦ The account pays 10% compounded daily.
10.5%

41. ▦ Rather than spend $20,000 on a new car that will lose 30% of its value in 1 year, the Coniglios invest the money at 9%, compounded daily. After 1 year, how much have the Coniglios saved by not buying the car?
$7883.24

Prepare an amortization table for a car loan.

Summary and Review Exercises: Chapter 8

Important Properties and Formulas

Commission = Commission rate × Sales
Sale price = Original price − Discount
Compound Interest: $A = P \cdot \left(1 + \dfrac{r}{n}\right)^{n \cdot t}$

Discount = Rate of discount × Original price
Simple Interest: $I = P \cdot r \cdot t$

Write percent notation. [8.1b]

1. 0.483

2. 0.36

Write percent notation. [8.1c]

3. $\dfrac{3}{8}$

4. $\dfrac{1}{3}$

Write decimal notation. [8.1b]

5. 73.5%

6. $6\dfrac{1}{2}\%$

Write fractional notation. [8.1c]

7. 24%

8. 6.3%

Translate to an equation. Then solve. [8.3a, b]

9. 30.6 is what percent of 90?

10. 63 is 84 percent of what?

11. What is $38\dfrac{1}{2}\%$ of 168?

Translate to a proportion. Then solve. [8.2a, b]

12. 24 percent of what is 16.8?

13. 42 is what percent of 30?

14. What is 10.5% of 84?

Solve. [8.4a, b]

15. Food expenses account for 26% of the average family's budget. A family makes $2300 one month. How much do they spend for food?

16. The price of a television set was reduced from $350 to $308. Find the percent of decrease in price.

17. Jerome County has a population that is increasing 3% each year. This year the population is 80,000. What will it be next year?

18. The price of a box of cookies increased from $1.70 to $2.04. What was the percent of increase in the price?

19. Carney College has a student body of 960 students. Of these, 17.5% are seniors. How many students are seniors?

Solve. [8.5a, b, c]

20. A city charges a meals tax of $4\dfrac{1}{2}\%$. What is the meals tax charged on a dinner party costing $320?

21. In Massachusetts, a sales tax of $378 is collected on the purchase of a used car for $7560. What is the sales tax rate?

22. Kim earns $753.50 selling $6850 worth of televisions. What is the commission rate?

23. An air conditioner has a marked price of $350. It is placed on sale at 12% off. What are the discount and the sale price?

24. A fax machine priced at $305 is discounted at the rate of 14%. What are the discount and the sale price?

25. An insurance salesperson receives a 7% commission. If $42,000 worth of life insurance is sold, what is the commission?

Solve. [8.6a, b]

26. What is the simple interest on $1800 at 6% for $\frac{1}{3}$ year?

27. The Dress Shack borrows $24,000 at 10% simple interest for 60 days. Find (a) the amount of interest due and (b) the total amount that must be paid after 60 days.

28. What is the simple interest on $2200 principal at the interest rate of 5.5% for 1 year?

29. The Kleins invest $7500 in an investment account paying 12%, compounded monthly. How much is in the account after 3 months?

30. Find the amount in an investment account if $8000 is invested at 9%, compounded annually, for 2 years.

31. Find the rate of discount. [8.5c]

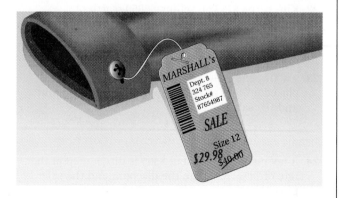

Solve. [7.3b]

32. $\frac{3}{8} = \frac{7}{x}$

33. $\frac{1}{6} = \frac{7}{x}$

Graph. [6.4b]

34. $y = 2x - 4$

35. $y = -\frac{1}{3}x - 4$

Convert to decimal notation. [5.5a]

36. $\frac{11}{3}$

37. $\frac{11}{7}$

Convert to a mixed numeral. [4.5b]

38. $\frac{11}{3}$

39. $\frac{121}{7}$

Synthesis

40. ◈ Ollie buys a microwave oven during a 10%-off sale. The sale price that Ollie paid was $162. To find the original price, Ollie calculates 10% of $162 and adds that to $162. Is this correct? Why or why not? [8.5c]

41. ◈ Which is a better deal for a consumer and why: a discount of 40% or a discount of 20% followed by another of 22%? [8.5c]

42. ▦ *Land Area of the United States.* When Hawaii and Alaska became states, the total land area of the United States increased from 2,963,681 mi² to 3,540,939 mi². What was the percent of increase? [8.4b]

43. Rhonda's Dress Shop reduces the price of a dress by 40% during a sale. By what percent must the store increase the sale price, after the sale, to get back to the original price? [8.5c]

44. A $200 coat is marked up 20%. After 30 days, it is marked down 30% and sold. What was the final selling price of the coat? [8.5c]

45. How many successive 10% discounts are necessary to lower the price of an item to below 50% of its original price? [8.5c]

Test: Chapter 8

1. Write decimal notation for 89%.

2. Write percent notation for 0.674.

3. Write percent notation for $\frac{11}{8}$.

4. Write fractional notation for 65%.

5. Translate to an equation. Then solve.

   What is 40% of 55?

6. Translate to a proportion. Then solve.

   What percent of 80 is 65?

Solve.

7. *Weight of Muscles.* The weight of muscles in an adult woman is about 23% of total body weight. A woman weighs 125 lb. What do the muscles weigh?

8. *Population Growth.* The population of Rippington increased from 1500 to 3600. Write the percent of increase in population.

9. *Arizona Tax Rate.* The sales tax rate in Arizona is 5%. How much tax is charged on a purchase of $324? What is the total price?

10. *Sales Commissions.* Gwen's commission rate is 15%. What is the commission from the sale of $4200 worth of merchandise?

11. The marked price of a CD player is $200 and the item is on sale at 20% off. What are the discount and the sale price?

12. What is the simple interest on a principal of $120 at the interest rate of 7.1% for 1 year?

13. The Burnham Parents–Teachers Association invests $5200 at 6% simple interest. How much is in the account after $\frac{1}{2}$ year?

14. Write the amount in an account if $1000 is invested at 5%, compounded annually, for 2 years.

Answers

1. [8.1b] 0.89

2. [8.1b] 67.4%

3. [8.1c] 137.5%

4. [8.1c] $\frac{13}{20}$

5. [8.3a, b] $a = 40\% \cdot 55$; 22

6. [8.2a, b] $\frac{N}{100} = \frac{65}{80}$; 81.25%

7. [8.4a] 28.75 lb

8. [8.4b] 140%

9. [8.5a] $16.20; $340.20

10. [8.5b] $630

11. [8.5c] $40; $160

12. [8.6a] $8.52

13. [8.6a] $5356

14. [8.6b] $1102.50

15. The Suarez family invests $10,000 at 9%, compounded monthly. How much is in the account after 3 months?

17.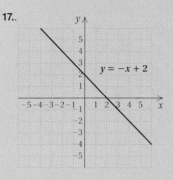

16. Find the discount and the discount rate of the bed in this ad.

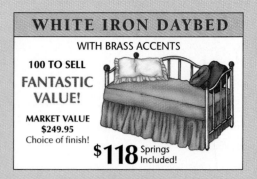

Skill Maintenance

17. Graph: $y = -x + 2$.

18. Solve: $\dfrac{5}{8} = \dfrac{10}{x}$.

19. Convert to decimal notation: $\dfrac{17}{12}$.

20. Convert to a mixed numeral: $\dfrac{153}{44}$.

Synthesis

21. By selling a home without using a realtor, Juan and Marie can avoid paying a 7.5% commission. They receive an offer of $109,000 from a potential buyer. In order to give a comparable offer, for what price would a realtor need to sell the house? Round to the nearest hundred.

22. Karen's commission rate is 16%. She invests her commission from the sale of $15,000 worth of merchandise at the interest rate of 12%, compounded quarterly. How much is Karen's investment worth after 6 months?

23. A housing development is constructed on a dead-end road along a river and ends in a cul-de-sac, as shown in the figure.

The property owners agree to share the cost of maintaining the road in the following manner. The first fifth of the road in front of lot 1 is to be shared equally among all five lot owners. The cost of the second fifth in front of lot 2 is to be shared equally among the owners of lots 2–5, and so on. Assume that all five sections of the road cost the same to maintain.

a) What fractional part of the cost is paid by each owner?
b) What percent of the cost is paid by each owner?
c) If lots 3, 4, and 5 were all owned by the same person, what percent of the cost of maintenance would this person pay?

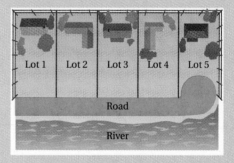

Cumulative Review: Chapters 1–8

1. Write fractional notation for 0.091.

2. Write decimal notation for $\frac{13}{6}$.

3. Write decimal notation for 3%.

4. Write percent notation for $\frac{9}{8}$.

5. Write fractional notation for the ratio 5 to 0.5.

6. Write the rate in kilometers per hour.

   350 km,   15 hr

Use <, >, or = for ▨ to write a true sentence.

7. $\frac{5}{7}$ ▨ $\frac{6}{8}$

8. -3.78 ▨ -37.8

Estimate the sum or difference by rounding to the nearest hundred.

9. $263{,}961 + 32{,}090 + 127.89$

10. $73{,}510 - 23{,}450$

11. Calculate: $46 - [4(6 + 4 \div 2) + 2 \times 3 - 5]$

12. Combine like terms: $5x - 9 - 7x - 5$.

Peform the indicated operation and simplify.

13. $\frac{6}{5} + 1\frac{5}{6}$

14. $-46.9 + 32.7$

15.
$$\begin{array}{r} 4\,8\,7{,}0\,9\,4 \\ 6{,}9\,3\,6 \\ +\quad 2\,1{,}1\,2\,0 \\ \hline \end{array}$$

16. $35 - 34.98$

17. $3\frac{1}{3} - 2\frac{2}{3}$

18. $-\frac{8}{9} - \frac{6}{7}$

19. $\frac{7}{9} \cdot \frac{3}{14}$

20. $(-32)(-4)(-3)$

21.
$$\begin{array}{r} 4\,6.0\,1\,2 \\ \times\quad 0.0\,3 \\ \hline \end{array}$$

22. $6\frac{3}{5} \div 4\frac{2}{5}$

23. $431.2 \div 35.2$

24. $15\,\overline{)\,1\,8\,5\,0}$

Solve.

25. $36 \cdot x = 3420$

26. $y + 142.87 = 151$

27. $\frac{2}{15} \cdot t = -\frac{6}{5}$

28. $\frac{3}{4} + x = \frac{5}{6}$

29. $3(x - 7) + 2 = 12x - 3$

30. $\frac{16}{n} = \frac{21}{11}$

31. In what quadrant does the point $(-3, -5)$ lie?

32. Graph on a plane: $y = -\frac{3}{5}x$.

33. Find the mean: 19, 29, 34, 39, 45.

34. Find the median: 7, 7, 12, 15, 19.

35. Find the perimeter of a 15-in. by 15-in. chessboard.

36. Find the area of a 40-yd by 80-yd soccer field.

Solve.

37. A 12-oz box of cereal costs $1.80. Find the unit price in cents per ounce.

38. A bus travels 456 km in 6 hr. At this rate, how far would the bus travel in 8 hr?

39. In a recent year, Americans recycled 37 million lb of paper. It is projected that this will increase to 53 million lb in 2005. Find the percent of increase.

40. The state of Utah has an area of 1,722,850 mi^2. Of this area, 60% is owned by the government. How many square miles are owned by the government?

41. How many pieces of ribbon $1\frac{4}{5}$ yd long can be cut from a length of ribbon 9 yd long?

42. Bobbie walked $\frac{7}{10}$ km to school and then $\frac{8}{10}$ km to the library. How far did she walk?

Synthesis

On a trip through the mountains, a Dodge hatchback traveled 240 mi on $7\frac{1}{2}$ gal of gasoline. Going across the plains, the same car averaged 36 miles per gallon.

43. What was the percent of increase or decrease in miles per gallon when the car left the mountains for the plains?

44. How many miles per gallon did the Dodge average over the entire trip if it used 5 gal of gas to cross the plains?

The bar graph below shows how the winning times in the Olympic marathon and the qualifying times for the Boston Marathon have changed over time.

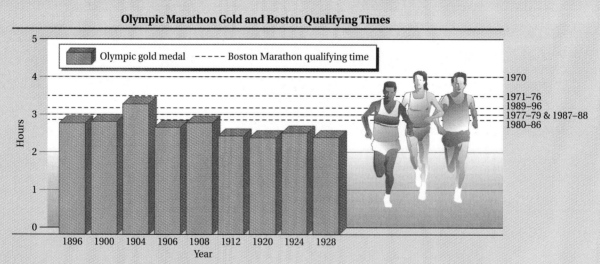

Olympic Marathon Gold and Boston Qualifying Times

Source: Boston Athletic Association; *Guinness Book of Olympics*

45. During which of the years listed would the winner of the Olympic marathon have qualified for the 1985 Boston Marathon?

46. What was the first year in which the Boston Marathon's qualifying time was lower than a time that had been good enough to win an Olympic gold medal?

9

Geometry and Measures

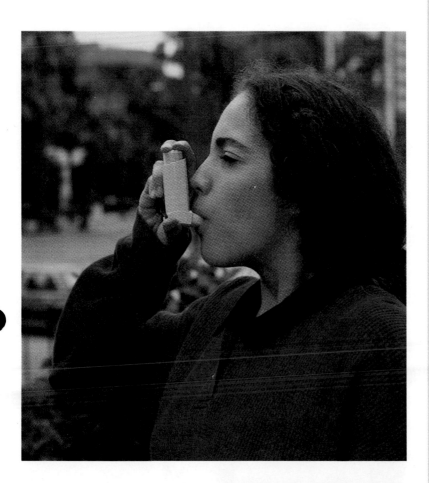

Introduction

This chapter introduces American and metric systems used to measure length, area, volume, weight, mass, and temperature. Parallelograms, trapezoids, circles, and angles are also studied.

An Application	The Mathematics

The medicine Albuterol is used for the treatment of asthma. It typically comes in an inhaler that contains 18 g. If one actuation, or spray, delivers 90 mg, how many actuations are in one inhaler?

This problem appears as Exercise 81 in Section 9.7.

Before dividing by 90, we convert 18 g to milligrams:

$$18 \text{ g} = 18 \text{ g} \cdot \frac{1000 \text{ mg}}{1 \text{ g}}.$$

These are units of measure.

World Wide Web   For more information, visit us at www.mathmax.com

Pretest: Chapter 9

Complete.

1. 9 ft = _____ in.

2. 8 in. = _____ ft

3. 7.32 km = _____ m

4. 7.5 mm = _____ cm

5. 3 ft^2 = _____ in^2

6. 108 ft^2 = _____ yd^2

7. 4.2 cm^2 = _____ mm^2

8. 7 gal = _____ oz

9. 7 T = _____ lb

10. 48 oz = _____ lb

11. 423 g = _____ kg

12. 0.4 kg = _____ mg

Find each area. Use 3.14 for π.

13.

11 ft

10 ft

15 ft

14.

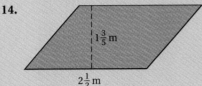

$1\frac{3}{5}$ m

$2\frac{1}{2}$ m

15.

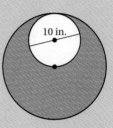

10 in.

16. Find the length of a diameter of a circle with a radius of 9.4 m.

17. Find the circumference of a 70-cm–diameter bicycle wheel. Use $\frac{22}{7}$ for π.

18. Find the area of a 20-cm–wide circular mat. Use 3.14 for π.

19. A nurse administers a 45-mL allergy shot. How many liters are injected?

In a right triangle, find the length of the side not given. Assume that c represents the length of the hypotenuse and a and b are lengths of legs. Find an exact answer and an approximation to three decimal places.

20. $a = 12$, $b = 16$

21. $a = 2$, $c = 7$

Find each volume. Use $\frac{22}{7}$ for π.

22.

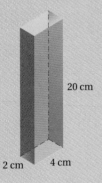

20 cm

2 cm   4 cm

23.

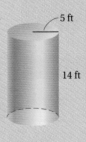

5 ft

14 ft

24.

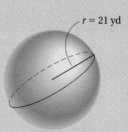

$r = 21$ yd

25. Find the measure of a complement of a 42° angle.

26. Find the measure of a supplement of a 25° angle.

27. Convert 77°F to Celsius.

28. Convert 37°C to Fahrenheit.

9.1 Systems of Linear Measurement

Length, or distance, is one kind of measure. To find lengths, we start with some **unit segment** and assign to it a measure of 1. Suppose $\overline{AB}$ below is a unit segment.

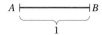

Let's measure segment $\overline{CD}$ below, using $\overline{AB}$ as our unit segment.

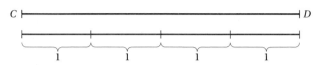

Since 4 unit segments fit end to end along $\overline{CD}$, the measure of $\overline{CD}$ is 4.

Sometimes we have to use parts of units. For example, the measure of the segment $\overline{MN}$ below is $1\frac{1}{2}$.

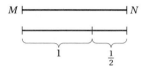

Do Exercises 1–4.

a | American Measures

American units of length are related as follows.

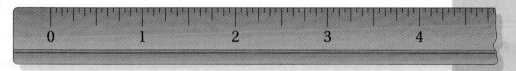

(Actual size, in inches)

> **AMERICAN UNITS OF LENGTH**
>
> 12 inches (in.) = 1 foot (ft)   3 feet = 1 yard (yd)
> 36 inches = 1 yard   5280 feet = 1 mile (mi)

The symbolism 13 in. = 13″ and 27 ft = 27′ is also used for inches and feet. American units have also been called "English," or "British–American," because at one time they were used by both countries. Today, both Canada and England have officially converted to the metric system. However, if you travel in England, you will still see units such as "miles" on road signs.

Example 1   Complete: 5 yd = _____ in.

$$5 \text{ yd} = 5 \cdot 1 \text{ yd}$$
$$= 5 \cdot 36 \text{ in.} \qquad \textbf{Substituting 36 in. for 1 yd}$$
$$= 180 \text{ in.} \qquad \textbf{Multiplying}$$

Objectives

a Convert from one American unit of length to another.

b Convert from one metric unit of length to another.

c Convert between American and metric units of length.

For Extra Help

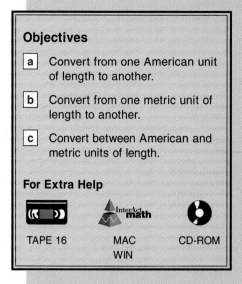

TAPE 16   MAC   CD-ROM
              WIN

Use the unit below to measure the length of each segment or object.

$$A \vdash\!\!-\!\!-\!\!\dashv B$$
$$1$$

1. $\vdash\!\!-\!\!-\!\!-\!\!-\!\!-\!\!-\!\!-\!\!\dashv$
2

2.

3

3.

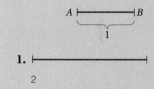

$1\frac{1}{2}$

4.

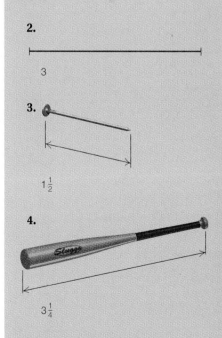

$3\frac{1}{4}$

Answers on page A-24

Complete.

5. 8 yd = ___288___ in.

6. 14.5 yd = ___43.5___ ft

7. 3.8 mi = ___240,768___ in.

Complete.

8. 72 in. = ___6___ ft

9. 24 ft = ___8___ yd

Complete.

10. 18 yd = ___54___ ft

11. 35 ft = $\underline{11\frac{2}{3}, \text{ or } 11.\overline{6}}$ yd

Answers on page A-24

Example 2   Complete: 2 mi = _____ in.

$$2 \text{ mi} = 2 \cdot 1 \text{ mi}$$
$$= 2 \cdot 5280 \text{ ft} \qquad \text{Substituting 5280 ft for 1 mi}$$
$$= 10{,}560 \cdot 1 \text{ ft}$$
$$= 10{,}560 \cdot 12 \text{ in.} \qquad \text{Substituting 12 in. for 1 ft}$$
$$= 126{,}720 \text{ in.} \qquad \text{The student should check the multiplication.}$$

Do Exercises 5–7.

Sometimes it helps to use multiplying by 1 when making conversions. For example, 12 in. = 1 ft, so we might choose to write 1 as

$$\frac{12 \text{ in.}}{1 \text{ ft}} \quad \text{or} \quad \frac{1 \text{ ft}}{12 \text{ in.}}.$$

Example 3   Complete: 48 in. = _____ ft.

To convert from "in." to "ft," we multiply by 1 using a symbol for 1 with "in." on the bottom and "ft" on the top. This process introduces feet and at the same time eliminates inches.

$$48 \text{ in.} = \frac{48 \text{ in.}}{1} \cdot \frac{1 \text{ ft}}{12 \text{ in.}} \qquad \text{Multiplying by 1 using } \frac{1 \text{ ft}}{12 \text{ in.}} \text{ to eliminate in.}$$
$$= \frac{48 \text{ in.}}{12 \text{ in.}} \cdot 1 \text{ ft} \qquad \text{Pay careful attention to the units.}$$
$$= \frac{48}{12} \cdot \frac{\text{in.}}{\text{in.}} \cdot 1 \text{ ft} \qquad \text{The } \frac{\text{in.}}{\text{in.}} \text{ acts like 1, so we can omit it.}$$
$$= 4 \cdot 1 \text{ ft} \qquad \text{Dividing by 12}$$
$$= 4 \text{ ft.}$$

The conversion can also be regarded as "canceling" units:

$$48 \text{ in.} = \frac{48 \text{ in.}}{1} \cdot \frac{1 \text{ ft}}{12 \text{ in.}} = \frac{48}{12} \cdot 1 \text{ ft} = 4 \text{ ft.}$$

Do Exercises 8 and 9.

In Examples 4 and 5, we will use only the "canceling" method.

Example 4   Complete: 75 yd = _____ ft.

Since we are converting from "yd" to "ft," we choose a symbol for 1 with "ft" on the top and "yd" on the bottom:

$$75 \text{ yd} = 75 \text{ yd} \cdot \frac{3 \text{ ft}}{1 \text{ yd}}$$
$$= 75 \cdot 3 \text{ ft}$$
$$= 225 \text{ ft.} \qquad \text{Multiplying by 3}$$

Do Exercises 10 and 11.

Example 5 Complete: 23,760 ft = _____ mi.

We choose a symbol for 1 with "mi" on the top and "ft" on the bottom:

$$23{,}760 \text{ ft} = 23{,}760 \text{ ft} \cdot \frac{1 \text{ mi}}{5280 \text{ ft}} \qquad 5280 \text{ ft} = 1 \text{ mi, so } \frac{1 \text{ mi}}{5280 \text{ ft}} = 1.$$

$$= \frac{23{,}760}{5280} \cdot 1 \text{ mi}$$

$$= 4.5 \cdot 1 \text{ mi} \qquad \text{Dividing by 5280}$$

$$= 4.5 \text{ mi.}$$

Do Exercises 12 and 13.

b | The Metric System

The **metric system** is used in most countries of the world, and the United States is now making greater use of it as well. The metric system does not use inches, feet, pounds, and so on, although units for time and electricity are the same as those you use now.

An advantage of the metric system is that it is easier to convert from one unit to another. That is because the metric system is based on the number 10.

The basic unit of length is the **meter**. It is just over a yard. In fact, 1 meter ≈ 1.1 yd.

(Comparative sizes are shown.)

1 Meter

1 Yard

The other units of length are multiples of the length of a meter:

10 times a meter,   100 times a meter,   1000 times a meter,

or fractions of a meter:

$\frac{1}{10}$ of a meter, $\frac{1}{100}$ of a meter, $\frac{1}{1000}$ of a meter.

> **METRIC UNITS OF LENGTH**
>   1 *kilo*meter (km) = 1000 meters (m)
>   1 *hecto*meter (hm) = 100 meters (m)
>   1 *deka*meter (dam) = 10 meters (m)
>   1 meter (m) | *hm, dam* and *dm* are not often used. |
>   1 *deci*meter (dm) = $\frac{1}{10}$ meter (m)
>   1 *centi*meter (cm) = $\frac{1}{100}$ meter (m)
>   1 *milli*meter (mm) = $\frac{1}{1000}$ meter (m)

It is important to remember these names and abbreviations. The prefixes *kilo-* for 1000, *deci-* for $\frac{1}{10}$, *centi-* for $\frac{1}{100}$, and *milli-* for $\frac{1}{1000}$ are used the most. These prefixes are also used when measuring capacity (volume) and mass (weight).

Complete.

12. 26,400 ft = __5__ mi

13. 6 mi = __31,680__ ft

Answers on page A-24

Complete.

14. 23 km = __23,000__ m

To familiarize yourself with metric units, consider the following.

1 kilometer (1000 meters)	is slightly more than $\frac{1}{2}$ mile ($\approx$0.6 mi).
1 meter	is just over a yard ($\approx$1.1 yd).
1 centimeter (0.01 meter)	is a little more than the width of a jumbo paperclip ($\approx$0.3937 inch).
1 millimeter	is about the diameter of a paperclip wire.

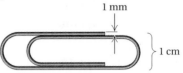

1 inch is about 2.54 centimeters.

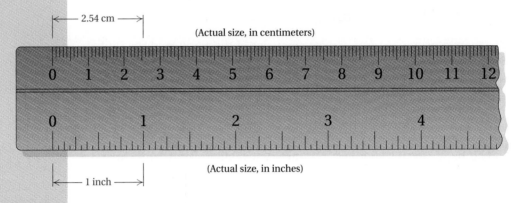

Example 6 Complete: 4 km = _____ m.

$$4 \text{ km} = 4 \cdot 1 \text{ km}$$
$$= 4 \cdot 1000 \text{ m} \qquad \text{Substituting 1000 m for 1 km}$$
$$= 4000 \text{ m} \qquad \text{Multiplying by 1000}$$

15. 4 hm = __400__ m

Do Exercises 14 and 15.

Since

$$\frac{1}{10} \text{ m} = 1 \text{ dm}, \qquad \frac{1}{100} \text{ m} = 1 \text{ cm}, \quad \text{and} \quad \frac{1}{1000} \text{ m} = 1 \text{ mm},$$

it follows that

> 1 m = 10 dm,   1 m = 100 cm,   and   1 m = 1000 mm.

Memorizing these equations will help you to write forms of 1 when canceling to make conversions. The procedure is the same as that used in Examples 4 and 5.

Example 7 Complete: 93.4 m = _____ cm.

To convert from "m" to "cm," we multiply by 1 using a symbol for 1 with "m" on the bottom and "cm" on the top. This process introduces centimeters and at the same time eliminates meters.

$$93.4 \text{ m} = 93.4 \text{ m} \cdot \frac{100 \text{ cm}}{1 \text{ m}} \qquad \text{Multiplying by 1 using } \frac{100 \text{ cm}}{1 \text{ m}}$$

$$= 93.4 \text{ m} \cdot \frac{100 \text{ cm}}{1 \text{ m}} = 93.4 \cdot 100 \text{ cm} = 9340 \text{ cm}$$

Answers on page A-24

Example 8 Complete: 0.248 m = _____ mm.

We are converting from "m" to "mm," so we choose a symbol for 1 with "mm" on the top and "m" on the bottom:

$$0.248 \text{ m} = 0.248 \text{ m} \cdot \frac{1000 \text{ mm}}{1 \text{ m}} = 0.248 \cdot 1000 \text{ mm} = 248 \text{ mm}.$$

Do Exercises 16 and 17.

Example 9 Complete: 2347 m = _____ km.

We multiply by 1 using $\frac{1 \text{ km}}{1000 \text{ m}}$:

$$2347 \text{ m} = 2347 \text{ m} \cdot \frac{1 \text{ km}}{1000 \text{ m}} = \frac{2347}{1000} \cdot 1 \text{ km} = 2.347 \text{ km}.$$

Do Exercises 18 and 19.

It is helpful to remember that 1000 mm = 100 cm and, more simply, 10 mm = 1 cm.

Example 10 Complete: 8.42 mm = _____ cm.

We can multiply by 1 using either $\frac{1 \text{ cm}}{10 \text{ mm}}$ or $\frac{100 \text{ cm}}{1000 \text{ mm}}$. Both expressions for 1 will eliminate mm and leave cm:

$$8.42 \text{ mm} = 8.42 \text{ mm} \cdot \frac{1 \text{ cm}}{10 \text{ mm}} = \frac{8.42}{10} \cdot 1 \text{ cm} = 0.842 \text{ cm}.$$

Do Exercises 20 and 21.

Mental Conversion

Note in Examples 6–10 that changing from one unit to another in the metric system involves moving a decimal point. This occurs because the metric system is based on 10. To find a faster way to convert, consider these equivalent ways of expressing the width of a standard sheet of paper.

> ▶ Width of a standard sheet of paper = 216 mm = 21.6 cm = 2.16 dm = 0.216 m = 0.0216 dam = 0.00216 hm = 0.000216 km

Each unit in the box above has a value that is ten times as large as the next smaller unit. Thus converting to the next larger unit means moving the decimal point one place to the left.

Example 11 Complete: 35.7 mm = _____ cm.

Think: Centimeters is the next larger unit after millimeters. Thus we move the decimal point one place to the left.

35.7   3.5.7   35.7 mm = 3.57 cm

Converting to the next *smaller* unit means moving the decimal point one place to the right.

Complete.

16. 1.78 m = ___178___ cm

17. 9.04 m = ___9040___ mm

Complete.

18. 7814 m = ___7.814___ km

19. 7814 m = ___781.4___ dam

Complete.

20. 87.2 mm = ___8.72___ cm

21. 89 km = _____ cm
      8,900,000

Answers on page A-24

Complete. Try to do this mentally using the table on page 515.

22. 6780 m = __6.78__ km

23. 9.74 cm = __97.4__ mm

24. 1 mm = __0.1__ cm

25. 845.1 mm = __8.451__ dm

Complete.

26. 100 yd = __90.909__ m
(The length of a football field)

27. 500 mi = __804.5__ km
(The Indianapolis 500-mile race)

28. 2383 km = __1479.843__ mi
(The distance from St. Louis to Phoenix)

Answers on page A-24

Example 12   Complete: 3 m = _____ cm.

Think: A meter is 100 times as large as a centimeter (100 cm = 1 m). Thus we move the decimal point two places to the right. To do so, we write two additional zeros.

$$3 \qquad 3.00. \qquad 3 \text{ m} = 300 \text{ cm}$$

Example 13   Complete: 4.37 km = _____ cm.

Think: Kilometers are 100,000 times as large as centimeters (100,000 cm = 1 km). Thus we move the decimal point five places to the right. This requires writting three additional zeros.

$$4.37 \qquad 4.37000. \qquad 4.37 \text{ km} = 437{,}000 \text{ cm}$$

> The most commonly used metric units of length are km, m, cm, and mm. We have purposely used these more often than the others in the exercises and examples.

Do Exercises 22–25.

c | Converting Between American and Metric Units

We can make conversions between American and metric units by using the following table. Again, we either make a substitution or multiply by 1 appropriately.

Metric	American
1 m	39.37 in.
1 m	3.3 ft
0.303 m	1 ft
2.54 cm	1 in.
1 km	0.621 mi
1.609 km	1 mi

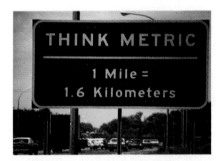

THINK METRIC
1 Mile = 1.6 Kilometers

Example 14   Complete: 26.2 mi = _____ km. (This is the approximate length of the Olympic marathon.)

$$26.2 \text{ mi} = 26.2 \cdot 1 \text{ mi}$$
$$\approx 26.2 \cdot 1.609 \text{ km}$$
$$\approx 42.1558 \text{ km}$$

Example 15   Complete: 100 m = _____ yd. (This is the length of a dash in track.)

$$100 \text{ m} = 100 \cdot 1 \text{ m} \approx 100 \cdot 3.3 \text{ ft} \approx 330 \text{ ft} \qquad \text{Converting to feet}$$
$$\approx 330 \text{ ft} \cdot \frac{1 \text{ yd}}{3 \text{ ft}} \approx \frac{330}{3} \text{ yd} \approx 110 \text{ yd} \qquad \text{Converting feet to yards}$$

Do Exercises 26–28.

Exercise Set 9.1

a Complete.

1. 1 ft = __12__ in.

2. 1 yd = __3__ ft

3. 1 in. = $\frac{1}{12}$ ft

4. 1 mi = __1760__ yd

5. 1 mi = __5280__ ft

6. 1 ft = $\frac{1}{3}$ yd

7. 4 yd = __144__ in.

8. 3 yd = __9__ ft

9. 84 in. = __7__ ft

10. 48 ft = __16__ yd

11. 18 in. = $1\frac{1}{2}$ ft

12. 29 ft = $9\frac{2}{3}$ yd

13. 5 mi = __26,400__ ft

14. 5 mi = __8800__ yd

15. 48 in. = __4__ ft

16. 11,616 ft = __2.2__ mi

17. 19 ft = $6\frac{1}{3}$ yd

18. 5.2 yd = __15.6__ ft

19. 10 mi = __52,800__ ft

20. 15,840 ft = __3__ mi

21. $7\frac{1}{2}$ ft = $2\frac{1}{2}$ yd

22. 36 in. = __3__ ft

23. 360 in. = __10__ yd

24. 7.2 ft = __86.4__ in.

25. 330 ft = __110__ yd

26. 1760 yd = __1__ mi

27. 3520 yd = __2__ mi

28. 25 mi = __132,000__ ft

29. 100 yd = __300__ ft

30. 240 in. = __20__ ft

31. 63,360 in. = __1__ mi

32. 2 mi = __126,720__ in.

b Complete. Do as much as possible mentally.

33. a) 1 km = <u>1000</u> m   **34. a)** 1 hm = <u>100</u> m   **35. a)** 1 dam = <u>10</u> m

b) 1 m = <u>0.001</u> km   **b)** 1 m = <u>0.01</u> hm   **b)** 1 m = <u>0.1</u> dam

36. a) 1 dm = <u>0.1</u> m   **37. a)** 1 cm = <u>0.01</u> m   **38. a)** 1 mm = <u>0.001</u> m

b) 1 m = <u>10</u> dm   **b)** 1 m = <u>100</u> cm   **b)** 1 m = <u>1000</u> mm

39. 6.7 km = <u>6700</u> m   **40.** 27 km = <u>27,000</u> m   **41.** 98 cm = <u>0.98</u> m

42. 53 cm = <u>0.53</u> m   **43.** 8921 m = <u>8.921</u> km   **44.** 8664 m = <u>8.664</u> km

45. 56.66 m = <u>0.05666</u> km   **46.** 4.733 m = <u>0.004733</u> km   **47.** 5666 m = <u>566,600</u> cm

48. 869 m = <u>86,900</u> cm   **49.** 477 cm = <u>4.77</u> m   **50.** 6.27 mm = <u>0.00627</u> m

51. 6.88 m = <u>688</u> cm   **52.** 6.88 m = <u>68.8</u> dm   **53.** 1 mm = <u>0.1</u> cm

54. 1 cm = <u>0.00001</u> km   **55.** 1 km = <u>100,000</u> cm   **56.** 2 km = <u>200,000</u> cm

57. 14.2 cm = __142__ mm   **58.** 25.3 cm = __253__ mm   **59.** 8.2 mm = __0.82__ cm

60. 9.7 mm = __0.97__ cm   **61.** 4500 mm = __450__ cm   **62.** 8,000,000 m = __8000__ km

63. 0.024 mm = __0.000024__ m   **64.** 60,000 mm = __6__ dam   **65.** 6.88 m = __0.688__ dam

66. 7.44 m = __0.0744__ hm   **67.** 2.3 dam = __230__ dm   **68.** 9 km = __90__ hm

[c] Complete. Answers mary vary slightly, depending on the conversion used.

69. 10 km = __6.21__ mi
(A common running distance)

70. 5 mi = __8.045__ km
(A common running distance)

71. 14 in. = __35.56__ cm
(A common paper length)

72. 400 m = __440__ yd
(A common race distance)

73. 65 mph = __104.585__ km/h
(A common speed limit in the
United States)

74. 100 km/h = __62.1__ mph
(A common speed limit in
Canada)

75. 330 ft = __100__ m
(The length of most baseball
foul lines)

76. 165 cm = __64.96__ in.
(A common height for a
woman)

77. 180 cm = __70.866__ in.
(A common snowboard length)

78. 450 ft = __136.36__ m
(The length of a long home run
in baseball)

79. 36 yd = __32.727__ m
(A common length for a roll
of tape)

80. 70 in. = __177.8__ cm
(A common height for a man)

Solve.

81. $-7x - 9x = 24$ [5.7b] $-\frac{3}{2}$

82. $-2a + 9 = 5a + 23$ [5.7b] -2

83. If 3 calculators cost $43.50, how much would 7 calculators cost?   [7.4a] $101.50

84. A principal of $500 is invested at a rate of 8.9% for 1 year. Find the simple interest.   [8.6a] $44.50

Convert to percent notation.

85. 0.47   [8.1b]   47%

86. $\frac{7}{20}$ [8.1c]   35%

Synthesis

87. ◆ A student writes the following conversion:
    23 in. = 23 · (12 ft) = 276 ft.
    What mistake has been made?

88. ◆ Explain in your own words why metric units are easier to work with than American units.

89. ◆ Would you expect the world record for the 100-m dash to be longer or shorter than the record for the 100-yd dash? Why?

Complete. Answers may vary, depending on the conversion used.

90. ▦ 2 mi = _____ cm   321,800

91. ▦ 10 km = _____ in.   393,700

92. ▦ Audio cassettes are generally played at a rate of $1\frac{7}{8}$ in. per second. How many meters of tape are used for a 60-min cassette? (*Note*: A 60-min cassette has 30 min of playing time on each side.)
    85.725 m

93. ▦ In a recent year, the world record for the 100-m dash was 9.86 sec. How fast is this in miles per hour? Round to the nearest tenth of a mile per hour.   22.7 mph

94. ▦ *National Debt.* Recently the national debt was $5.103 trillion. To get an idea of this amount, picture that if that many $1 bills were stacked on top of each other, they would reach 1.382 times the distance to the moon. The distance to the moon is 238,866 mi. How thick, in inches, is a $1 bill?   0.0041 in.

Use < or > to complete the following. Perform only approximate, mental calculations.

95. 59 in. ▨ 59 cm   >

96. 35 yd ▨ 35 m   <

97. 7 km ▨ 6 mi   <

98. 9 mi ▨ 18 km   <

99. 24 ft ▨ 6 m   >

100. 30 in. ▨ 90 cm   <

Collaborative Learning Manual

Practice conversions with old British monetary units.

9.2 More with Perimeter and Area

We have already studied how to find the perimeter of polygons and the area of squares, rectangles, and triangles. In this section, we learn how to find the area of *parallelograms, trapezoids,* and *circles.* We also learn how to calculate the perimeter, or *circumference,* of a circle.

Objectives

a Find the area of a parallelogram or trapezoid.

b Find the circumference, area, radius, or diameter of a circle, given the length of a radius or diameter.

For Extra Help

TAPE 16

MAC
WIN

CD-ROM

a Parallelograms and Trapezoids

A **parallelogram** is a four-sided figure with two pairs of parallel sides, as shown below.

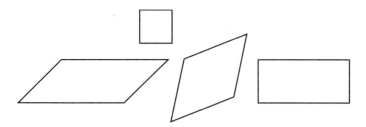

To find the area of a parallelogram, consider the one below.

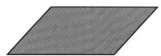

If we cut off a piece and move it to the other end, we get a rectangle.

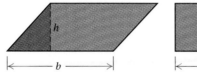

We can find the area by multiplying the length *b*, called a **base**, by *h*, called the **height**.

> The **area of a parallelogram** is the product of the length of a base *b* and the height *h*:
>
> $$A = b \cdot h.$$
>
>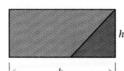

Example 1 Find the area of this parallelogram.

$$A = b \cdot h$$
$$= 7 \text{ km} \cdot 5 \text{ km}$$
$$= 35 \text{ km}^2$$

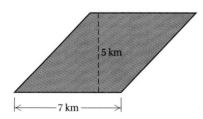

Find the area.

1.

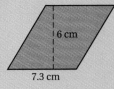

6 cm

7.3 cm

43.8 cm²

2.

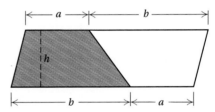

5.5 km

2.25 km

12.375 km²

Answers on page A-25

Example 2   Find the area of this parallelogram.

$$A = b \cdot h$$
$$= (1.2 \text{ m}) \cdot (6 \text{ m})$$
$$= 7.2 \text{ m}^2$$

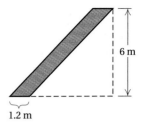

6 m

1.2 m

Do Exercises 1 and 2.

Trapezoids

A **trapezoid** is a polygon with four sides, two of which, the **bases**, are parallel to each other.*

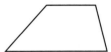

To find the area of a trapezoid, think of cutting out another just like it.

a

b

Then place the second one like this.

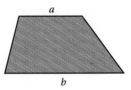

a   *b*

h

b   *a*

The resulting figure is a parallelogram with an area of

$$h \cdot (a + b).$$ The base is *a* + *b*.

The trapezoid we started with has half the area of the parallelogram, or

$$\frac{1}{2} \cdot h \cdot (a + b).$$

> The **area of a trapezoid** is half the product of the height and the sum of the lengths of the parallel sides, or the product of the height and the average length of the bases:
>
> $$A = \frac{1}{2} \cdot h \cdot (a + b) = h \cdot \frac{a + b}{2}.$$

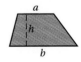

a

h

b

*Some definitions of trapezoid specify *exactly* two parallel sides. We refrain from doing so. Thus we consider a parallelogram a special type of trapezoid.

Example 3 Find the area of this trapezoid.

$$A = \frac{1}{2} \cdot h \cdot (a + b)$$

$$= \frac{1}{2} \cdot 7 \text{ cm} \cdot (12 + 18) \text{ cm}$$

$$= \frac{7 \cdot 30}{2} \cdot \text{cm}^2 = \frac{7 \cdot 15 \cdot \cancel{2}}{1 \cdot \cancel{2}} \text{ cm}^2$$

$$= 105 \text{ cm}^2 \qquad \textbf{Removing a factor equal to 1: } \tfrac{2}{2} = 1$$

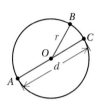

Do Exercises 3 and 4.

b | Circles

Radius and Diameter

At right is a circle with center O. Segment $\overline{AC}$ is a *diameter*. A **diameter** is a segment that passes through the center of the circle and has endpoints on the circle. Segment $\overline{OB}$ is called a *radius*. A **radius** is a segment with one endpoint on the center and the other endpoint on the circle. The words *radius* and *diameter* are also used to represent the lengths of a circle's radius and diameter, respectively.

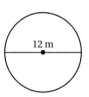

Suppose that d is the diameter of a circle and r is the radius. Then

$$d = 2 \cdot r \quad \text{or} \quad r = \frac{d}{2}.$$

Example 4 Find the length of a radius of this circle.

$$r = \frac{d}{2}$$

$$= \frac{12 \text{ m}}{2}$$

$$= 6 \text{ m}$$

12 m

The radius is 6 m.

Example 5 Find the length of a diameter of this circle.

$$d = 2 \cdot r$$

$$= 2 \cdot \frac{1}{4} \text{ ft}$$

$$= \frac{1}{2} \text{ ft}$$

$\frac{1}{4}$ ft

The diameter is $\frac{1}{2}$ ft.

Do Exercises 5 and 6.

Find the area.

3.

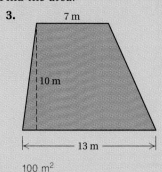

100 m²

4.

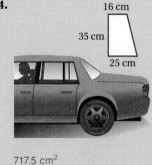

717.5 cm²

5. Find the length of a radius.

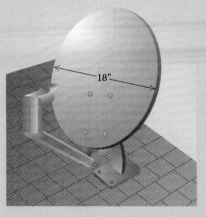

9 in.

6. Find the length of a diameter.

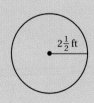

5 ft

Answers on page A-25

7. Find the circumference of this circle. Use 3.14 for π.

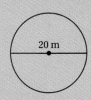

20 m

62.8 m

Circumference

The perimeter of a circle is called its **circumference**. Take a 12-oz soda can and measure its circumference C and diameter d. Next, consider the ratio C/d:

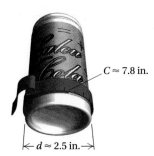

$C \approx 7.8$ in.

$\leftarrow d \approx 2.5$ in. $\rightarrow$

$$\frac{C}{d} = \frac{7.8 \text{ in.}}{2.5 \text{ in.}} \approx 3.1.$$

Suppose we found this ratio for cans and circles of several sizes. We would always get a number close to 3.1. Any time we divide the circumference C by the diameter d, we get the same number. We call this number π (pi).

> $\frac{C}{d} = \pi$ or $C = \pi \cdot d$.   The number π is about 3.14, or about $\frac{22}{7}$.

Example 6   Find the circumference of this circle. Use 3.14 for π.

$C = \pi \cdot d$

   $\approx 3.14 \cdot 6$ cm

   ≈ 18.84 cm

6 cm

The circumference is about 18.84 cm.

Do Exercise 7.

Since $d = 2 \cdot r$, where r is the length of a radius, it follows that

$C = \pi \cdot d = \pi \cdot (2 \cdot r)$.

> $C = 2 \cdot \pi \cdot r$

Example 7   Find the circumference of this circle. Use $\frac{22}{7}$ for π.

$C = 2 \cdot \pi \cdot r$

   $\approx 2 \cdot \dfrac{22}{7} \cdot 70$ in.

   $\approx 2 \cdot 22 \cdot \dfrac{70}{7}$ in.

   $\approx 44 \cdot 10$ in.

   ≈ 440 in.

70 in.

The circumference is about 440 in.

Answer on page A-25

Example 8 Find the perimeter of this figure. Use 3.14 for π.

We let P = the perimeter. We see that we have half a circle attached to three sides of a square. Thus we add half the circumference to the lengths of the three line segments.

$$P = 3 \cdot 9.4 \text{ km} + \frac{1}{2} \cdot 2 \cdot \pi \cdot 4.7 \text{ km}$$

$$\approx 28.2 \text{ km} + 3.14 \cdot 4.7 \text{ km}$$

$$\approx 28.2 \text{ km} + 14.758 \text{ km}$$

$$\approx 42.958 \text{ km}$$

The perimeter is about 42.958 km.

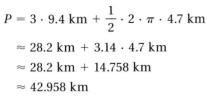

Do Exercises 8–10.

Area

To find the area of a circle, consider cutting half a circular region into small slices and arranging them as shown below.

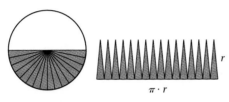

Then imagine slicing the other half of the circular region and arranging the pieces in between the others as shown below.

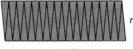

This is almost a parallelogram. The base has length $\frac{1}{2} \cdot 2 \cdot \pi \cdot r$, or $\pi \cdot r$ (half the circumference) and the height is r. Thus the area is

$$(\pi \cdot r) \cdot r.$$

This is the area of a circle.

> The **area of a circle** with radius of length r is given by
> $$A = \pi \cdot r \cdot r, \quad \text{or} \quad A = \pi \cdot r^2.$$

Example 9 Find the area of this circle. Use $\frac{22}{7}$ for π.

$$A = \pi \cdot r^2 = \pi \cdot r \cdot r$$

$$\approx \frac{22}{7} \cdot 14 \text{ cm} \cdot 14 \text{ cm}$$

$$\approx \frac{22}{\cancel{7}} \cdot \frac{\cancel{7} \cdot 2}{1} \text{ cm} \cdot 14 \text{ cm}$$

$$\approx 616 \text{ cm}^2 \quad \textbf{Note: } r^2 \neq 2r.$$

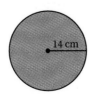

The area is about 616 cm².

Do Exercise 11.

---

8. Find the circumference of this circle. Use 3.14 for π.

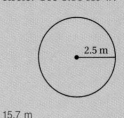

15.7 m

9. Find the circumference of this bicycle wheel. Use $\frac{22}{7}$ for π.

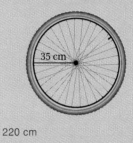

220 cm

10. Find the perimeter of this figure. Use 3.14 for π.

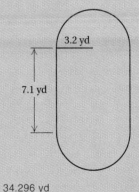

34.296 yd

11. Find the area of this circle. Use $\frac{22}{7}$ for π.

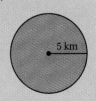

$78\frac{4}{7}$ km²

Answer on page A-25

12. Find the area of this circle. Use 3.14 for π.

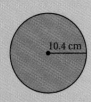

10.4 cm

339.6 cm²

13. Which is larger and by how much: a 10-ft square flower bed or a 12-ft diameter flower bed?

A 12-ft diameter flower bed is 13.04 ft² larger.

Calculator Spotlight

On certain calculators, there is a pi key, $\boxed{\pi}$. You can use a $\boxed{\pi}$ key for most computations instead of stopping to round the value of π. Rounding, if necessary, is done at the end.

Exercises

1. If you have a $\boxed{\pi}$ key on your calculator, to how many decimal places does this key give the value of π?

2. Find the circumference and the area of a circle with a radius of 225.68 in.

3. Find the area of a circle with a diameter of $46\frac{12}{13}$ in.

4. Find the area of a large irrigated farming circle with a diameter of 400 ft.

1. Answers will vary.
2. 1417.99 in.; 160,005.91 in²
3. 1729.27 in² 4. 125,663.71 ft²

Answers on page A-25

Example 10 Find the area of this circle. Use 3.14 for π. Round to the nearest hundredth.

$$A = \pi \cdot r \cdot r$$
$$\approx 3.14 \cdot 2.1 \text{ m} \cdot 2.1 \text{ m}$$
$$\approx 3.14 \cdot 4.41 \text{ m}^2$$
$$\approx 13.8474 \text{ m}^2 \approx 13.85 \text{ m}^2$$

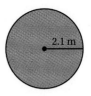

2.1 m

The area is about 13.85 m².

Do Exercise 12.

Example 11 *Area of a Pizza Pan.* Which makes a larger pizza and by how much: a 16-in. square pizza pan or a 16-in. diameter circular pizza pan?

1. Familiarize. From examining a picture of each, we see that the square pan has the larger area. We let D = the difference in area.

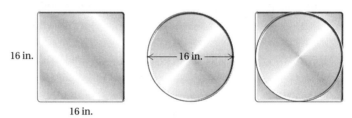

16 in.

16 in.

16 in.

2. Translate. The problem can be rephrased as follows.

Area of square pan	minus	Area of circular pan	is	Difference in area
$s \cdot s$	$-$	$\pi \cdot r \cdot r$	$=$	D

3. Solve. We use 3.14 for π and substitute:

$$16 \text{ in.} \cdot 16 \text{ in.} - 3.14 \cdot 8 \text{ in.} \cdot 8 \text{ in.} \approx D \qquad \textbf{Substituting}$$
$$256 \text{ in}^2 - 200.96 \text{ in}^2 \approx D$$
$$55.04 \text{ in}^2 \approx D.$$

4. Check. We can check by repeating our calculations. Note also that the area of the square pan is larger, as we expected.

5. State. The square pan is larger by about 55.04 in².

Do Exercise 13.

Area of a parallelogram: $A = b \cdot h$

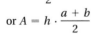
h

b

Area of a trapezoid: $A = \dfrac{1}{2} \cdot h \cdot (a + b)$

or $A = h \cdot \dfrac{a + b}{2}$

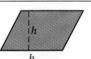
a

h

b

Circumference of a circle: $C = \pi \cdot d$
or $C = 2 \cdot \pi \cdot r$

Area of a circle: $A = \pi \cdot r^2$

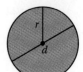
r

d

Note: $d = 2r$ and $\pi \approx 3.14 \approx \frac{22}{7}$.

Exercise Set 9.2

a Find the area of each parallelogram or trapezoid.

1.

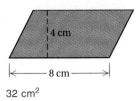

4 cm
8 cm

32 cm^2

2.

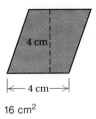

4 cm
4 cm

16 cm^2

3.

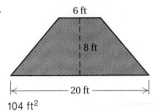

6 ft
8 ft
20 ft

104 ft^2

4.

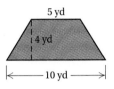

5 yd
4 yd
10 yd

30 yd^2

5.

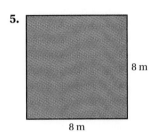

8 m
8 m

64 m^2

6.

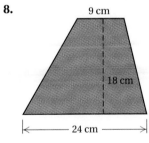

4.5 in.
7 in.
8.5 in.

45.5 in^2

7.

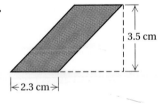

3.5 cm
2.3 cm

8.05 cm^2

8.

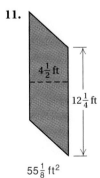

9 cm
18 cm
24 cm

297 cm^2

9.

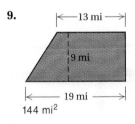

13 mi
9 mi
19 mi

144 mi^2

10.

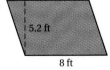

5.2 ft
8 ft

41.6 ft^2

11.

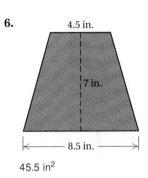

$4\frac{1}{2}$ ft
$12\frac{1}{4}$ ft

$55\frac{1}{8}$ ft^2

12.

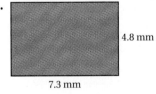

4.8 mm
7.3 mm

35.04 mm^2

13.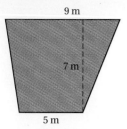

9 m

7 m

5 m

49 m²

14.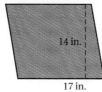

14 in.

17 in.

238 in²

15.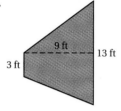

9 cm

12 cm

108 cm²

16.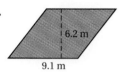

6.2 m

9.1 m

56.42 m²

17.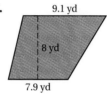

9.1 yd

8 yd

7.9 yd

68 yd²

18.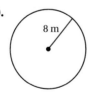

9 ft

13 ft

3 ft

72 ft²

b Find the length of a diameter of each circle.

19.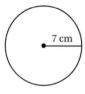

7 cm

14 cm

20.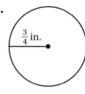

8 m

16 m

21.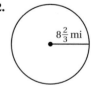

$\frac{3}{4}$ in.

$1\frac{1}{2}$ in.

22.

$8\frac{2}{3}$ mi

$17\frac{1}{3}$ mi

Find the length of a radius of each circle.

23.
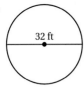
32 ft

16 ft

24.
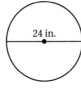
24 in.

12 in.

25.
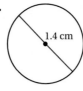
1.4 cm

0.7 cm

26.
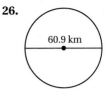
60.9 km

30.45 km

Find the circumference of each circle in Exercises 19–22. Use $\frac{22}{7}$ for π.

27. Exercise 19

44 cm

28. Exercise 20

$50\frac{2}{7}$ m

29. Exercise 21

$4\frac{5}{7}$ in.

30. Exercise 22

$54\frac{10}{21}$ mi

Find the circumference of each circle in Exercises 23–26. Use 3.14 for π.

31. Exercise 23

100.48 ft;

32. Exercise 24

75.36 in.

33. Exercise 25

4.396 cm

34. Exercise 26

191.226 km

Find the area of each circle in Exercises 19–22. Use $\frac{22}{7}$ for π.

35. Exercise 19

154 cm²

36. Exercise 20

$201\frac{1}{7}$ m²

37. Exercise 21

$1\frac{43}{56}$ in²

38. Exercise 22

$236\frac{4}{63}$ mi²

Find the area of each circle in Exercises 23–26. Use 3.14 for π.

39. Exercise 23

803.84 ft²

40. Exercise 24

452.16 in²

41. Exercise 25

1.5386 cm²

42. Exercise 26

2911.41585 km²

Solve. Use 3.14 for π.

43. A penny has a 1-cm radius. What is its diameter? circumference? area?

2 cm; 6.28 cm; 3.14 cm^2

44. The top of a soda can has a 6-cm diameter. What is its radius? circumference? area?

3 cm; 18.84 cm; 28.26 cm^2

45. A radio station is allowed by the FCC to broadcast over an area with a radius of 220 mi. How much area is this?   151,976 mi^2

46. Which is larger and by how much: a 12-in. circular pizza or a 12-in. square pizza?

A 12-in. square pizza is 30.96 in^2 larger.

47. The diameter of a quarter is 2.5 cm. What is the circumference? area?

7.85 cm; 4.90625 cm^2

48. The diameter of a dime is 1.8 cm. What is the circumference? area?

5.652 cm.; 2.5434 cm^2

49. *Botany.* To protect an elm tree, a 47.1-in. gypsy moth tape is wrapped once around the trunk. What is the diameter of the tree?   15 in.

50. *Farming.* The circumference of a silo is 62.8 ft. What is the diameter of the silo?   20 ft

51. *Track and Field.* Track meets take place on a track similar to the one shown below. Find the shortest distance around the track.   439.7784 yd

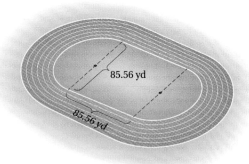

85.56 yd

85.56 yd

52. *Masonry.* Iris plans to install a 1-yd–wide walk around a circular swimming pool. The diameter of the pool is 8 yd. What will the area of the walk be?

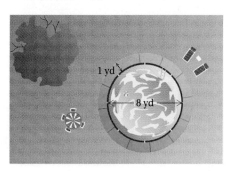

1 yd

8 yd

28.26 yd^2

Find the perimeter of each figure. Use 3.14 for π.

53.

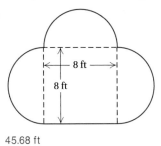

8 ft

8 ft

45.68 ft

54.

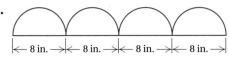

8 in.   8 in.   8 in.   8 in.

82.24 in.

55.

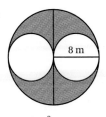

10 yd

10 yd

45.7 yd

56.

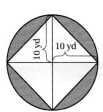

12.8 cm

10.2 cm

57.628 cm

Find the area of the shaded region in each figure. Use 3.14 for π.

57.

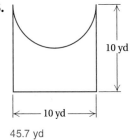

8 m

100.48 m²

58.

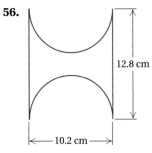

10 yd   10 yd

114 yd²

59.

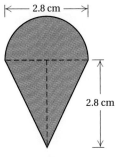

2.8 cm

2.8 cm

6.9972 cm²

60.

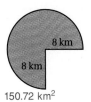

8 km

8 km

150.72 km²

Skill Maintenance

Convert to fractional notation.   [8.1c]

61. 9.25% $\dfrac{37}{400}$

62. $87\dfrac{1}{2}$% $\dfrac{7}{8}$

Convert to percent notation.   [8.1c]

63. $\dfrac{11}{8}$ 137.5%

64. $\dfrac{2}{3}$ $66.\overline{6}$% or $66\frac{2}{3}$%

65. $\dfrac{5}{4}$ 125%

66. $\dfrac{8}{5}$ 160%

Synthesis

67. ◆ Explain why a 16-in.–diameter pizza that costs $16.25 is a better buy than a 10-in.–diameter pizza that costs $7.85.

68. ◆ The radius of one circle is twice the length of another circle's radius. Is the area of the first circle twice the area of the other circle? Why or why not?

69. ◆ The radius of one circle is twice the size of another circle's radius. Is the circumference of the first circle twice the circumference of the other circle? Why or why not?

70. ▦ Calculate the surface area of an unopened steel can that has a height of 3.5 in. and a diameter of 2.5 in. (*Hint*: Make a sketch and "unroll" the sides of the can.) Use 3.14 for π.   37.2875 in²

71. ▦ The sides of a cake box are trapezoidal, as shown in the figure. Determine the surface area of the box.   1267 cm²

72. ▦ $\pi \approx \dfrac{3927}{1250}$ is another approximation for π. Find decimal notation using a calculator. Round to the nearest thousandth.   3.142

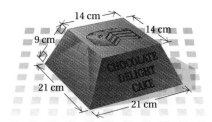

73. ▦ The distance from Kansas City to Indianapolis is 500 mi. A car was driven this distance using tires with a radius of 14 in. How many revolutions of each tire occurred on the trip? Use $\dfrac{22}{7}$ for π.   360,000

74. ◆ ▦ *Urban Planning.* Years ago, when a 12-in.–diameter tree was cut down in New York City, new trees with a combined diameter of 12 in. had to be planted. Now, instead of being able to use four 3-in.–diameter trees as replacement, a total of *sixteen* 3-in.–diameter trees must be planted. (*Source*: *The New York Times* 7/24/88, p. 6; article by David W. Dunlap). Consider area and explain why the new replacement calculation is more correct mathematically.

75. *Sports Marketing.* Tennis balls are generally packed vertically, three in a can, one on top of another. Without using a calculator, determine the larger measurement: the can's circumference or the can's height.   Circumference

76. ▦ *Landscaping.* Seed is needed for the field surrounded by the track in Exercise 51. If seed comes in 3-lb boxes, and each pound covers 120 ft², how many boxes must be purchased?   327

Collaborative Learning Manual

Verify the formulas for the area of a parallelogram, triangle, and trapezoid. Estimate the value of π.

9.3 Converting Units of Area

a | American Units

It is often necessary to convert units of area. First we will convert from one American unit of area to another.

Objectives

a Convert from one American unit of area to another.

b Convert from one metric unit of area to another.

For Extra Help

TAPE 16   MAC   CD-ROM
                 WIN

Example 1 Complete: $1 \text{ yd}^2 = $ _____ ft^2.

We recall that 1 yd = 3 ft and make a sketch. Note that $1 \text{ yd}^2 = 9 \text{ ft}^2$. The same result can be found as follows:

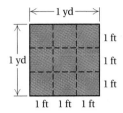

$$1 \text{ yd}^2 = 1 \cdot (3 \text{ ft})^2 \quad \textbf{Substituting 3 ft for 1 yd}$$
$$= 3 \text{ ft} \cdot 3 \text{ ft}$$
$$= 9 \text{ ft}^2. \quad \textbf{Note that ft} \cdot \textbf{ft} = \textbf{ft}^2.$$

Example 2 Complete: $2 \text{ ft}^2 = $ _____ in.^2.

$$2 \text{ ft}^2 = 2 \cdot (12 \text{ in.})^2 \quad \textbf{Substituting 12 in. for 1 ft}$$
$$= 2 \cdot 12 \text{ in.} \cdot 12 \text{ in.}$$
$$= 288 \text{ in.}^2 \quad \textbf{Note that in.} \cdot \textbf{in.} = \textbf{in.}^2.$$

Do Exercises 1–3.

American units of area are related as follows.

> 1 square yard (yd^2) = 9 square feet (ft^2)
> 1 square foot (ft^2) = 144 square inches (in^2)
> 1 square mile (mi^2) = 640 acres
> 1 acre = 43,560 ft^2

Example 3 Complete: $36 \text{ ft}^2 = $ _____ yd^2.

We are converting from "ft^2" to "yd^2". Thus we choose a symbol for 1 with yd^2 on top and ft^2 on the bottom.

$$36 \text{ ft}^2 = 36 \text{ ft}^2 \cdot \frac{1 \text{ yd}^2}{9 \text{ ft}^2} \quad \textbf{Multiplying by 1 using } \frac{\textbf{1 yd}^2}{\textbf{9 ft}^2}$$
$$= \frac{36}{9} \cdot \text{yd}^2 = 4 \text{ yd}^2$$

Example 4 Complete: $7 \text{ mi}^2 = $ _____ acres.

$$7 \text{ mi}^2 = 7 \cdot 640 \text{ acres} \quad \textbf{Substituting 640 acres for 1 mi}^2$$
$$= 4480 \text{ acres}$$

Had we used canceling, we could have multiplied 7 mi^2 by $\frac{640 \text{ acres}}{1 \text{ mi}^2}$:

$$7 \text{ mi}^2 = 7 \text{ mi}^2 \cdot \frac{640 \text{ acres}}{1 \text{ mi}^2} = 4480 \text{ acres}.$$

Do Exercises 4 and 5.

Complete.

1. $1 \text{ ft}^2 = $ __144__ in.^2

2. $10 \text{ ft}^2 = $ __1440__ in.^2

3. $7 \text{ yd}^2 = $ __63__ ft^2

Complete.

4. $360 \text{ in.}^2 = $ __2.5__ ft^2

5. $5 \text{ mi}^2 = $ __3200__ acres

Answers on page A-25

Complete.

6. $1 \text{ m}^2 =$ _____ mm^2

1,000,000

7. $1 \text{ cm}^2 =$ __100__ mm^2

Complete.

8. $2.88 \text{ m}^2 =$ __28,800__ cm^2

9. $4.3 \text{ mm}^2 =$ __0.043__ cm^2

10. $678,000 \text{ m}^2 =$ __0.678__ km^2

Answers on page A-25

---

b | **Metric Units**

We next convert from one metric unit of area to another.

Example 5   Complete: $1 \text{ km}^2 =$ _____ m^2.

$$1 \text{ km}^2 = 1 \cdot (1000 \text{ m})^2 \qquad \text{Substituting 1000 m for 1 km}$$
$$= 1000 \text{ m} \cdot 1000 \text{ m}$$
$$= 1,000,000 \text{ m}^2 \qquad \text{Note that m} \cdot \text{m} = \text{m}^2.$$

Example 6   Complete: $1 \text{ m}^2 =$ _____ cm^2.

$$1 \text{ m}^2 = 1 \cdot (100 \text{ cm})^2 \qquad \text{Substituting 100 cm for 1 m}$$
$$= 100 \text{ cm} \cdot 100 \text{ cm}$$
$$= 10,000 \text{ cm}^2 \qquad \text{Note that cm} \cdot \text{cm} = \text{cm}^2.$$

Do Exercises 6 and 7.

Mental Conversion

Note in Example 5 that whereas it takes 1000 m to make 1 km, it takes 1,000,000 m^2 to make 1 km^2. Similarly, in Example 6, we saw that although it takes 100 cm to make 1 m, it takes 10,000 cm^2 to make 1 m^2. In general, if a *length* conversion requires moving the decimal point n places, the corresponding *area* conversion requires moving the decimal point $2n$ places. For example, below we list four equivalent ways of expressing the area of a standard sheet of paper.

Area of a standard sheet of paper $= 60,264 \text{ mm}^2$
$= 602.64 \text{ cm}^2$
$= 0.060264 \text{ m}^2$
$\approx 0.00000006 \text{ km}^2$

Example 7   Complete: $3.48 \text{ km}^2 =$ _____ m^2.

Think: A kilometer is 1000 times as big as a meter, so 1 km^2 is 1,000,000 times as big as 1 m^2. We shift the decimal point *six* places to the right.

$$3.48 \qquad 3.480000. \qquad 3.48 \text{ km}^2 = 3,480,000 \text{ m}^2$$

Example 8   Complete: $586.78 \text{ cm}^2 =$ _____ m^2.

Think: To convert from cm to m, we shift the decimal point two places to the left. To convert from cm^2 to m^2, we shift the decimal point *four* places to the left.

$$586.78 \qquad 0.0586.78 \qquad 586.78 \text{ cm}^2 = 0.058678 \text{ m}^2$$

Do Exercises 8–10.

Exercise Set 9.3

a Complete.

1. 4 yd^2 = _____36_____ ft^2

2. 5 ft^2 = _____720_____ in^2

3. 7 ft^2 = _____1008_____ in^2

4. 2 acres = _____87,120_____ ft^2

5. 432 in^2 = _____3_____ ft^2

6. 54 ft^2 = _____6_____ yd^2

7. 22 yd^2 = _____198_____ ft^2

8. 40 ft^2 = _____5760_____ in^2

9. 44 yd^2 = _____396_____ ft^2

10. 144 ft^2 = _____16_____ yd^2

11. 20 mi^2 = _____12,800_____ acres

12. 576 in^2 = _____4_____ ft^2

13. 69 ft^2 = _____$7\frac{2}{3}$_____ yd^2

14. 1 mi^2 = _____ yd^2 3,097,600

15. 720 in.^{2} = _____5_____ ft^2

16. 27 ft^2 = _____3_____ yd^2

17. 1 in.^{2} = ___$\frac{1}{144}$___ ft^2

18. 72 in.^{2} = ___$\frac{1}{2}$___ ft^2

19. 1 acre = ___$\frac{1}{640}$___ mi^2

20. 4 acres = __174,240__ ft^2

b Complete.

21. 17 km^2 = _____ m^2 17,000,000

22. 65 km^2 = _____ m^2 65,000,000

23. 6.31 m^2 = __63,100__ cm^2

24. 2.7 m^2 = __2,700,000__ mm^2

25. 2345.6 mm^2 = __23.456__ cm^2

26. 8.38 cm^2 = __838__ mm^2

27. 349 cm^2 = __0.0349__ m^2

28. 125 mm^2 = _____ m^2 0.000125

29. 250,000 mm² = __2500__ cm²

30. 2400 mm² = __24__ cm²

31. 472,800 m² = __0.4728__ km²

32. 1.37 cm² = __137__ mm²

Find the area of the shaded region of each figure. Give the answer in square feet. (Figures are not drawn to scale.)

33.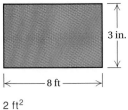

3 in.

8 ft

2 ft²

34.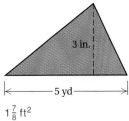

3 in.

5 yd

$1\frac{7}{8}$ ft²

35.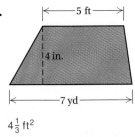

5 ft

4 in.

7 yd

$4\frac{1}{3}$ ft²

36.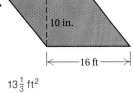

10 in.

16 ft

$13\frac{1}{3}$ ft²

Find the area of the shaded region of each figure.

37.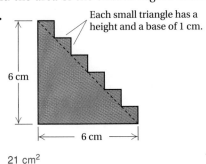

Each small triangle has a height and a base of 1 cm.

6 cm

6 cm

21 cm²

38.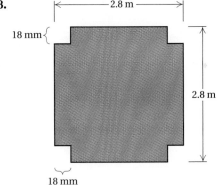

2.8 m

18 mm

2.8 m

18 mm

7.838704 m², or 7,838,704 mm²

Skill Maintenance

Find the simple interest.   [8.6a]

Principal	Rate of interest	Time
39. $700	5%	$\frac{1}{2}$ year $17.50
40. $450	6%	$\frac{1}{4}$ year $6.75
41. $1200	8.9%	30 days $8.78
42. $1800	12%	60 days $35.51

Synthesis

43. ◆ Which is larger and why: one square meter or nine square feet?

44. ◆ What advantage do metric units offer over American units when we are converting area measurements?

45. ◆ Why might a scientist choose to give area measurements in mm^2 rather than cm^2?

46. ▦ A 30-ft by 60-ft ballroom is to be turned into a nightclub by placing an 18-ft by 42-ft dance floor in the middle and carpeting the rest of the room. The new dance floor is laid in tiles that are 8 in. by 8 in. squares. How many such tiles are needed? What percent of the area is the dance floor?   1701; 42%

Complete. Answers may vary slightly, depending on the conversion used.

47. ▦ 1 m^2 = __10.89__ ft^2

48. ▦ 1 in^2 = __6.4516__ cm^2

49. ▦ 2 yd^2 = __1.65__ m^2

50. ▦ 1 acre = __4000__ m^2

51. ▦ The president's family has about 20,175 ft^2 of living area in the White House. Estimate the living area in square meters.   1852.6 m^2

52. A handwoven scarf is 2 m long and 10 in. wide. Find its area in square centimeters.   5080 cm^2

53. ▦ In order to remodel an office, a carpenter needs to purchase carpeting, at $8.45 a square yard, and molding for the base of the walls, at $0.87 a foot. If the room is 9 ft by 12 ft, with a 3-ft doorway, what will the materials cost? $135.33

Collaborative
Learning Manual

Verify the conversions between American units of area.

9.4 Angles

a | Measuring Angles

An **angle** is a set of points consisting of two **rays**, or half-lines, with a common endpoint. The endpoint is called the **vertex**.

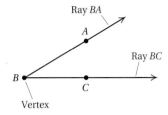

The rays are called the *sides*. The angle above can be named

angle *ABC*,   angle *CBA*,   angle *B*,   ∠*ABC*,   ∠*CBA*,   or   ∠*B*.

Note that the name of the vertex is either in the middle or, if no confusion results, listed by itself.

Do Exercises 1 and 2.

To measure angles, we start with some unit angle and assign to it a measure of 1. Suppose that ∠*U*, below, is a unit angle. To measure ∠*DEF*, we find that 3 copies of ∠*U* will "fill up" ∠*DEF*. Thus the measure of ∠*DEF* would be 3.

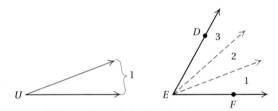

The unit most commonly used for angle measure is the degree. Below is such a unit. Its measure is 1 degree, or 1°.

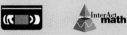

A device called a **protractor** is used to measure angles. Protractors have two scales. To measure an angle like ∠*Q* below, we place the protractor's ▲ at the vertex and line up one of the angle's sides at 0°. Then we check where the angle's other side crosses the scale. In the figure below, 0° is on the inside scale, so we check where the angle's other side crosses the inside scale. We see that *m*∠*Q* = 145°. The notation *m*∠*Q* is read "the measure of angle *Q*."

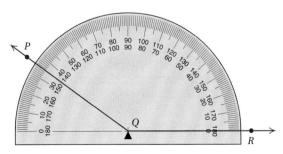

Do Exercise 3.

Objectives

a Name a given angle in four different ways and given an angle, measure it with a protractor.

b Classify an angle as right, straight, acute, or obtuse.

c Identify complementary and supplementary angles and find the measure of a complement or a supplement of a given angle.

For Extra Help

TAPE 16   MAC   CD-ROM
                 WIN

Name each angle in six different ways.

1.

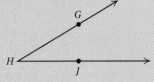

Angle *GHJ*, angle *JHG*, angle *H*, ∠*GHJ*, ∠*JHG*, or ∠*H*

2.

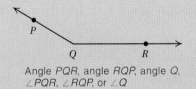

Angle *PQR*, angle *RQP*, angle *Q*, ∠*PQR*, ∠*RQP*, or ∠*Q*

3. Use a protractor to measure this angle.   126°

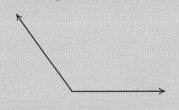

Answers on page A-25

9.4 Angles

541

4. Use a protractor to measure this angle.   33°

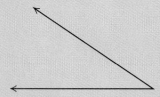

5. *Lengths of Engagement of Married Couples.* The data below relate the percent of married couples who were engaged for a certain time period before marriage (**Source:** Bruskin Goldring Research). Use this information to draw a circle graph.

Less than 1 yr:	24%
1–2 yr:	21%
More than 2 yr:	35%
Never engaged:	20%

Times of Engagement of Married Couples

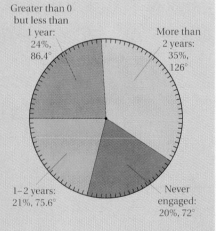

Greater than 0 but less than 1 year: 24%, 86.4°

More than 2 years: 35%, 126°

1–2 years: 21%, 75.6°

Never engaged: 20%, 72°

Answers on page A-25

Let's find the measure of ∠ABC. This time we will use the 0° on the outside scale. We see that $m \angle ABC = 42°$.

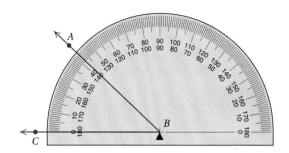

Do Exercise 4.

Protractors are needed when drawing circle graphs by hand.

Example 1   *Water Supplies.* Predictions indicate that by the year 2050, water supplies will be scarce in 18% of the world, stressed in 24% of the world, and sufficient in just 58% of the world (**Source:** Simon, Paul, *Tapped Out,* New York, 1998, Welcome Rain Publishers). Draw a circle graph to represent these figures.

Every circle graph contains a total of 360°. Thus,

24% of the circle is a 0.24(360°), or 86.4° angle;

18% of the circle is a 0.18(360°), or 64.8° angle; and

58% of the circle is a 0.58(360°), or 208.8° angle.

To draw an 86.4° angle, we first draw a horizontal segment and use a progractor to mark off an 86.4° angle. From that mark, we draw a segment to complete the angle. From that segment, we repeat the procedure to draw a 64.8° angle.

To confirm that the remainder of the circle is indeed 208.8°, we measure 180°, make a mark, and from there measure another 28.8°.

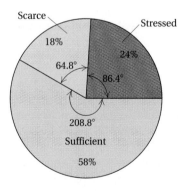

Scarce
18%

Stressed
24%

64.8°

86.4°

208.8°

Sufficient
58%

Do Exercise 5.

b | Classifying Angles

The following are ways in which we classify angles.

> **Right angle:** An angle that measures 90°.
> **Straight angle:** An angle that measures 180°.
> **Acute angle:** An angle that measures more than 0° and less than 90°.
> **Obtuse angle:** An angle that measures more than 90° and less than 180°.

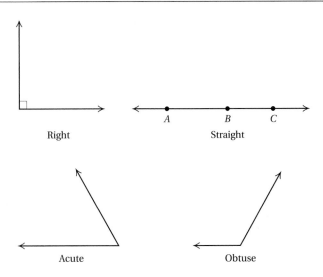

Right   Straight

Acute   Obtuse

Do Exercises 6–9.

c | Complementary and Supplementary Angles

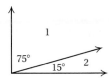

∠1 and ∠2 above are **complementary** angles.

$$m\angle 1 + m\angle 2 = 90°$$
$$75° \quad + \quad 15° \quad = 90°$$

> Two angles are **complementary** if the sum of their measures is 90°. Each angle is called a **complement** of the other.

If two angles are complementary, each is an acute angle. When complementary angles are adjacent to each other, they form a right angle.

Classify each angle as right, straight, acute, or obtuse. Use a protractor if necessary.

6.
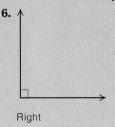
Right

7.
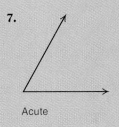
Acute

8.
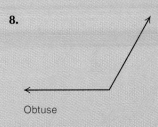
Obtuse

9.
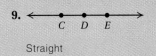
Straight

Answers on page A-25

10. Identify each pair of complementary angles.

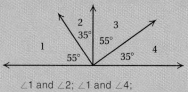

∠1 and ∠2; ∠1 and ∠4;
∠2 and ∠3; ∠3 and ∠4

Find the measure of a complement of the angle.

11.

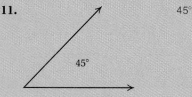

45°

12.

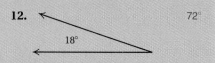

72°

13.

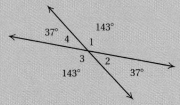

5°

14. Identify each pair of supplementary angles.

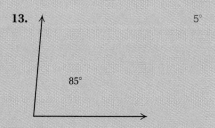

∠1 and ∠2; ∠1 and ∠4;
∠2 and ∠3; ∠3 and ∠4

Find the measure of a supplement of an angle with the given measure.

15. 38° 142°

16. 157° 23°

17. 90° 90°

Answers on page A-25

Example 2 Identify each pair of complementary angles.

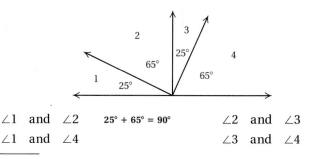

∠1 and ∠2   25° + 65° = 90°   ∠2 and ∠3
∠1 and ∠4   ∠3 and ∠4

Example 3 Find the measure of a complement of an angle of 39°.

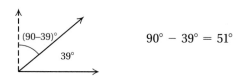

90° − 39° = 51°

The measure of a complement is 51°.

Do Exercises 10–13.

Next, consider ∠1 and ∠2 as shown below. Because the sum of their measures is 180°, ∠1 and ∠2 are said to be **supplementary**. Note that when supplementary angles are adjacent, they form a straight angle.

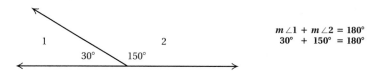

$m \angle 1 + m \angle 2 = 180°$
$30° + 150° = 180°$

> Two angles are **supplementary** if the sum of their measures is 180°. Each angle is called a **supplement** of the other.

Example 4 Identify each pair of supplementary angles.

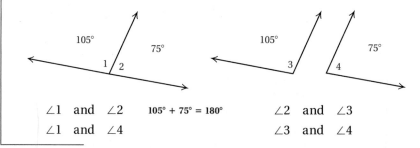

∠1 and ∠2   105° + 75° = 180°   ∠2 and ∠3
∠1 and ∠4   ∠3 and ∠4

Example 5 Find the measure of a supplement of an angle of 112°.

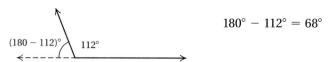

180° − 112° = 68°

The measure of a supplement is 68°.

Do Exercises 14–17.

Exercise Set 9.4

a Name each angle in six different ways.

1.

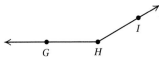

Angle *GHI*, angle *IHG*, angle *H*, ∠*GHI*, ∠*IHG*, or ∠*H*

2.

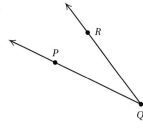

Angle *PQR*, angle *RQP*, angle *Q*, ∠*PQR*, ∠*RQP*, or ∠*Q*

Use a protractor to measure each angle.

3.

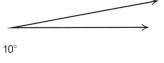

10°

4.

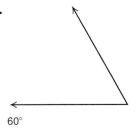

60°

5.

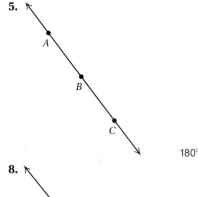

180°

6.

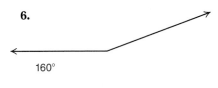

160°

7.

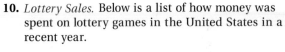

90°

8.

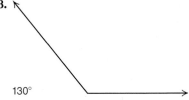

130°

Use the given information and a protractor to draw a circle graph.

9. *Sporting Goods Purchases.* Below is a list of educational backgrounds of people who purchase sporting goods.

Less than high school:	10%
High school:	26%
Some college:	35%
College graduate:	29%

Source: The Sporting Goods Market in 1997. Mt. Prospect, IL: National Sporting Goods Association (copyright).

Sporting Goods Purchases

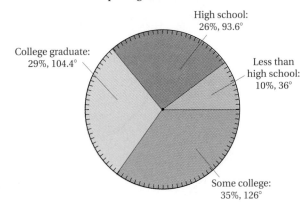

High school: 26%, 93.6°

College graduate: 29%, 104.4°

Less than high school: 10%, 36°

Some college: 35%, 126°

10. *Lottery Sales.* Below is a list of how money was spent on lottery games in the United States in a recent year.

Lotto:	28%	Instant:	40%
4-digit:	6%	Other:	10%
3-digit:	16%		

Source: 1998 *World Lottery Almanac* annual. Boyds, MD: TLF Publications, Inc.; *LaFleur's Fiscal 1997 Lottery Special Report*; and *LaFleur's Lottery World Government Profits Report* (copyright).

Money Spent on Lotteries

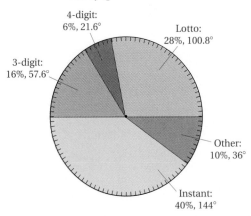

4-digit: 6%, 21.6°

Lotto: 28%, 100.8°

3-digit: 16%, 57.6°

Other: 10%, 36°

Instant: 40%, 144°

11.–18. Classify each of the angles in Exercises 1–8 as right, straight, acute, or obtuse.

11. Obtuse **12.** Acute **13.** Acute **14.** Acute
15. Straight **16.** Obtuse **17.** Right **18.** Obtuse

19.–22. Classify each of the angles in Margin Exercises 1–4 as right, straight, acute, or obtuse.

19. Acute **20.** Obtuse **21.** Obtuse **22.** Acute

c Find the measure of a complement of an angle with the given measure.

23. 11° 79°

24. 83° 7°

25. 67° 23°

26. 5° 85°

27. 58° 32°

28. 32° 58°

29. 29° 61°

30. 54° 36°

Find the measure of a supplement of an angle with the given measure.

31. 3° 177°

32. 54° 126°

33. 139° 41°

34. 13° 167°

35. 85° 95°

36. 129° 51°

37. 102° 78°

38. 45° 135°

Skill Maintenance

39. Convert to decimal notation: 56.1%. [8.1b] 0.561

40. Convert to percent notation: 0.6734. [8.1b] 67.34%

41. Solve: $3.1x + 4.3 = x + 9.55$. [5.7b] 2.5

42. Convert to percent notation: $\dfrac{9}{8}$. [8.1c] 112.5%

43. Add: $-9.7 + 3.8$. [5.2c] −5.9

44. Subtract: $-4.3 - (-9.8)$. [5.2c] 5.5

Synthesis

45. ◈ Do parallelograms always contain two acute and two obtuse angles? Why or why not?

46. ◈ Explain a procedure that could be used to determine the measure of an angle's supplement from the measure of the angle's complement.

47. ◈ Is it possible that both an angle and its supplement can be obtuse? Why or why not?

48. ▦ In the figure, $m\angle 1 = 79.8°$ and $m\angle 6 = 33.07°$. Find $m\angle 2$, $m\angle 3$, $m\angle 4$, and $m\angle 5$.

49. ▦ In the figure, $m\angle 2 = 42.17°$ and $m\angle 3 = 81.9°$. Find $m\angle 1$, $m\angle 4$, $m\angle 5$, and $m\angle 6$.

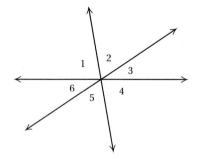

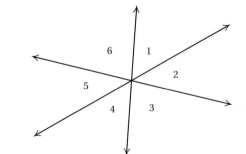

50. For any triangle, the sum of the measures of the angles is 180°. Use this fact to help find $m\angle ACB$, $m\angle CAB$, $m\angle EBC$, $m\angle EBA$, $m\angle AEB$, and $m\angle ADB$ in the rectangle shown at right.

$m\angle ACB = 50°$; $m\angle CAB = 40°$; $m\angle EBC = 50°$;
$m\angle EBA = 40°$; $m\angle AEB = 100°$; $m\angle ADB = 50°$

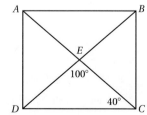

48. $m\angle 2 = 67.13°$; $m\angle 3 = 33.07°$; $m\angle 4 = 79.8°$; $m\angle 5 = 67.13°$
49. $m\angle 1 = 55.93°$; $m\angle 4 = 55.93°$; $m\angle 5 = 42.17°$; $m\angle 6 = 81.9°$

9.5 Square Roots and the Pythagorean Theorem

a Square Roots

> If a number is a product of a factor times itself, then that factor is a **square root** of the number. (If $c^2 = a$, then c is a square root of a.)

For example, 36 has two square roots, 6 and -6. To see this, note that $6 \cdot 6 = 36$ and $(-6) \cdot (-6) = 36$.

Example 1 Find the square roots of 25.

The square roots of 25 are 5 and -5, because $5^2 = 25$ and $(-5)^2 = 25$.

CAUTION! To find the *square* of a number, multiply the number by itself. To find a *square root* of a number, find a number that, when squared, gives the original number.

Do Exercises 1–12.

Since every positive number has two square roots, the symbol $\sqrt{}$ (called a *radical* sign) is used to denote the positive square root of the number underneath. Thus, $\sqrt{9}$ means 3, not -3. When we refer to *the* square root of some number n, we mean the positive square root, $\sqrt{n}$.

Examples Simplify.

2. $\sqrt{36} = 6$ The square root of 36 is 6 because $6^2 = 36$ and 6 is positive.

3. $\sqrt{25} = 5$ Note that $5^2 = 25$.

4. $\sqrt{144} = 12$ Note that $12^2 = 144$.

5. $\sqrt{256} = 16$ Note that $16^2 = 256$.

Do Exercises 13–22.

b Approximating Square Roots

Many square roots can't be written as whole numbers or fractions. For example,

$$\sqrt{2}, \quad \sqrt{3}, \quad \sqrt{39}, \quad \text{and} \quad \sqrt{70}$$

cannot be precisely represented in decimal notation. To see this, consider the following decimal approximations for $\sqrt{2}$. Each gives a closer approximation, but none is exactly $\sqrt{2}$:

$\sqrt{2} \approx 1.4$ because $(1.4)^2 = 1.96$;

$\sqrt{2} \approx 1.41$ because $(1.41)^2 = 1.9881$;

$\sqrt{2} \approx 1.414$ because $(1.414)^2 = 1.999396$;

$\sqrt{2} \approx 1.4142$ because $(1.4142)^2 = 1.99996164$.

Decimal approximations like these are commonly found by using a calculator.

Objectives

a Simplify square roots of squares such as $\sqrt{25}$.

b Approximate square roots.

c Given the lengths of any two sides of a right triangle, find the length of the third side.

For Extra Help

TAPE 17   MAC WIN   CD-ROM

Find each square.

1. 9^2 81   **2.** $(-10)^2$ 100

3. 11^2 121   **4.** 12^2 144

> It would be helpful to memorize the squares of numbers from 1 to 25.

5. 13^2 169   **6.** 14^2 196

7. 15^2 225   **8.** 16^2 256

Find all square roots. Use the results of Exercises 1–8 above, if necessary.

9. 100 $-10, 10$ **10.** 81 $-9, 9$

11. 49 $-7, 7$ **12.** 196 $-14, 14$

Simplify. Use the results of Exercises 1–8 above, if necessary.

13. $\sqrt{49}$ 7   **14.** $\sqrt{16}$ 4

15. $\sqrt{121}$ 11   **16.** $\sqrt{100}$ 10

17. $\sqrt{81}$ 9   **18.** $\sqrt{64}$ 8

19. $\sqrt{225}$ 15   **20.** $\sqrt{169}$ 13

21. $\sqrt{1}$ 1   **22.** $\sqrt{0}$ 0

Answers on page A-25

Approximate to three decimal places.

23. $\sqrt{5}$ 2.236

24. $\sqrt{78}$ 8.832

25. $\sqrt{168}$ 12.961

Answers on pages A-25 and A-26

Example 6 Approximate $\sqrt{3}$, $\sqrt{27}$, and $\sqrt{180}$ to three decimal places. Use a calculator.

We use a calculator to find each square root. Since more than three decimal places are given, we round back to three places.

$$\sqrt{3} \approx 1.732,$$
$$\sqrt{27} \approx 5.196,$$
$$\sqrt{180} \approx 13.416$$

As a check, note that because $1 \cdot 1 = 1$ and $2 \cdot 2 = 4$, we expect $\sqrt{3}$ to be between 1 and 2. Similarly, we expect $\sqrt{27}$ to be between 5 and 6 and $\sqrt{180}$ to be between 13 and 14.

Do Exercises 23–25.

c | The Pythagorean Theorem

A **right triangle** is a triangle with a 90° angle, as shown here.

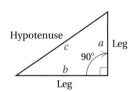

In a right triangle, the longest side is called the **hypotenuse**. It is also the side opposite the right angle. The other two sides are called **legs**. We generally use the letters a and b for the lengths of the legs and c for the length of the hypotenuse. They are related as follows.

> **THE PYTHAGOREAN THEOREM**
>
> In any right triangle, if a and b are the lengths of the legs and c is the length of the hypotenuse, then
> $$a^2 + b^2 = c^2, \quad \text{or}$$
> $$(\text{Leg})^2 + (\text{Other leg})^2 = (\text{Hypotenuse})^2.$$
>
>
>
> The equation $a^2 + b^2 = c^2$ is called the **Pythagorean equation.***

It is important to remember this theorem because it is extremely useful. By using the Pythagorean theorem, we can find the length of any side in a right triangle if the lengths of the other sides are known.

---

*The *converse* of the Pythagorean theorem is also true. That is, if $a^2 + b^2 = c^2$, then the triangle is a right triangle.

Example 7 Find the length of the hypotenuse of this right triangle. Give an exact answer and an approximation to three decimal places.

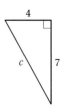

We substitute in the Pythagorean equation:

$$a^2 + b^2 = c^2$$
$$4^2 + 7^2 = c^2 \qquad \text{Substituting}$$
$$16 + 49 = c^2$$
$$65 = c^2.$$

The solutions of this equation are the square roots of 65. Thus, we would ordinarily say that the numbers $\sqrt{65}$ and $-\sqrt{65}$ are solutions. In this case, however, since we are solving for a length, only positive answers are acceptable.

> *Exact answer:* $\qquad c = \sqrt{65}$
>
> *Approximate answer:* $\quad c \approx 8.062 \qquad$ **Using a calculator**

Do Exercise 26.

Example 8 Find the length b for the right triangle shown. Give an exact answer and an approximation to three decimal places.

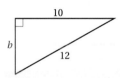

We substitute in the Pythagorean equation. Then we solve for b^2 and b, as follows:

$$a^2 + b^2 = c^2$$
$$10^2 + b^2 = 12^2 \qquad \text{Substituting}$$
$$100 + b^2 = 144$$
$$100 + b^2 - 100 = 144 - 100 \qquad \text{Subtracting 100 on both sides}$$
$$b^2 = 144 - 100$$
$$b^2 = 44$$

> *Exact answer:* $\qquad b = \sqrt{44}$
>
> *Approximation:* $\quad b \approx 6.633. \qquad$ **Using a calculator**

Do Exercises 27–29.

26. Find the length of the hypotenuse of this right triangle. Give an exact answer and an approximation to three decimal places.

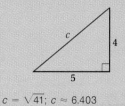

$c = \sqrt{41}; c \approx 6.403$

Find the length of the unknown leg of each right triangle. Give an exact answer and an approximation to three decimal places.

27.

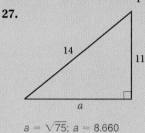

$a = \sqrt{75}; a \approx 8.660$

28.

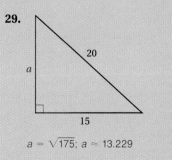

$b = \sqrt{120}; b \approx 10.954$

29.

$a = \sqrt{175}; a \approx 13.229$

Answers on page A-26

30. How long is a guy wire reaching from the top of an 18-ft pole to a point on the ground 10 ft from the pole? Give an exact answer and an approximation to the nearest tenth of a foot.

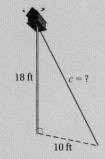

18 ft $c = ?$

10 ft

$\sqrt{424}$ ft ≈ 20.6 ft

Example 9 *Height of Ladder.* A 12-ft ladder leans against a building. The bottom of the ladder is 7 ft from the building. How high is the top of the ladder? Give an exact answer and an approximation to the nearest tenth of a foot.

1. Familiarize. We first make a drawing. In it we see a right triangle. We let h = the unknown height.

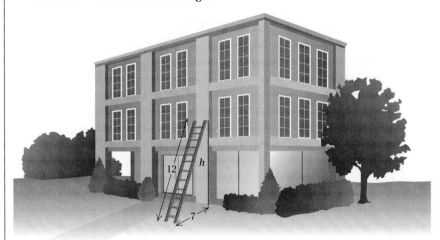

2. Translate. We substitute 7 for a, h for b, and 12 for c in the Pythagorean equation:

$$a^2 + b^2 = c^2 \quad \text{Pythagorean equation}$$
$$7^2 + h^2 = 12^2.$$

3. Solve. We solve for h^2 and then h:

$$49 + h^2 = 144$$
$$49 + h^2 - 49 = 144 - 49$$
$$h^2 = 95$$

Exact answer: $\quad h = \sqrt{95}$

Approximation: $\quad h \approx 9.7$ ft.

4. Check. $7^2 + (\sqrt{95})^2 = 49 + 95 = 144 = 12^2$.

5. State. The top of the ladder is $\sqrt{95}$, or about 9.7 ft from the ground.

Do Exercise 30.

The Pythagorean theorem is named for the Greek mathematician Pythagoras (569?–500? B.C.). In the diagram below, we show one way in which the theorem can be visualized.

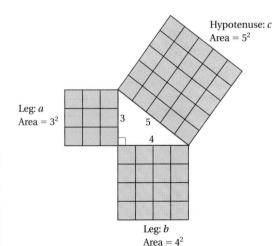

Hypotenuse: c
Area = 5^2

Leg: a
Area = 3^2

3
5
4

Leg: b
Area = 4^2

$a^2 + b^2 = c^2$
$3^2 + 4^2 = 5^2$
$9 + 16 = 25$

Answer on page A-26

Exercise Set 9.5

a Find all square roots.

1. 16 −4, 4   **2.** 9 −3, 3   **3.** 121 −11, 11   **4.** 49 −7, 7

5. 169 −13, 13   **6.** 144 −12, 12   **7.** 6400 −80, 80   **8.** 3600 −60, 60

Simplify.

9. $\sqrt{49}$

7

10. $\sqrt{4}$

2

11. $\sqrt{81}$

9

12. $\sqrt{64}$

8

13. $\sqrt{225}$

15

14. $\sqrt{121}$

11

15. $\sqrt{625}$

25

16. $\sqrt{900}$

30

17. $\sqrt{400}$

20

18. $\sqrt{169}$

13

19. $\sqrt{10,000}$

100

20. $\sqrt{1,000,000}$

1000

b Approximate each number to three decimal places.

21. $\sqrt{48}$
6.928

22. $\sqrt{17}$
4.123

23. $\sqrt{8}$
2.828

24. $\sqrt{7}$
2.646

25. $\sqrt{3}$
1.732

26. $\sqrt{6}$
2.449

27. $\sqrt{12}$
3.464

28. $\sqrt{18}$
4.243

29. $\sqrt{19}$
4.359

30. $\sqrt{75}$
8.660

31. $\sqrt{110}$
10.488

32. $\sqrt{10}$
3.162

c Find the length of each third side of each right triangle. Give an exact answer and, when appropriate, an approximation to three decimal places.

33.

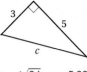

$c = \sqrt{34}$; $c \approx 5.831$

34.

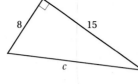

$c = 17$

35.

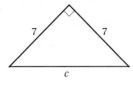

$c = \sqrt{98}$; $c \approx 9.899$

36.

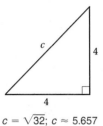

$c = \sqrt{32}$; $c \approx 5.657$

37.

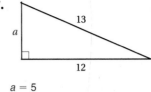

$a = 5$

38.

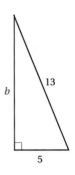

$b = 12$

39.

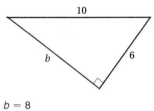

$b = 8$

40.

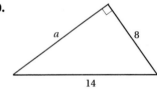

$a = \sqrt{132}$; $a \approx 11.489$

For each right triangle, find the length of the side not given. Assume that c represents the length of the hypotenuse. Give an exact answer and, when appropriate, an approximation to three decimal places.

41. $a = 10$, $b = 24$

$c = 26$

42. $a = 5$, $b = 12$

$c = 13$

43. $a = 9$, $c = 15$

$b = 12$

44. $a = 18$, $c = 30$

$b = 24$

45. $a = 1$, $c = 32$

$b = \sqrt{1023}$; $b = 31.984$

46. $b = 1$, $c = 20$

$a = \sqrt{399}$; $a \approx 19.975$

47. $a = 4$, $b = 3$

$c = 5$

48. $a = 1$, $c = 15$

$b = \sqrt{224}$; $b \approx 14.967$

In Exercises 49–56, give an exact answer and an approximation to the nearest tenth.

49. How long is a string of lights reaching from the top of a 12-ft pole to a point 8 ft from the base of the pole?

$\sqrt{208}$ ft ≈ 14.4 ft

50. How long must a wire be in order to reach from the top of a 13-m telephone pole to a point on the ground 9 m from the base of the pole?

$\sqrt{250}$ m ≈ 15.8 m

51. *Baseball Diamond.* A baseball diamond is actually a square 90 ft on a side. How far is it from home plate to second base?

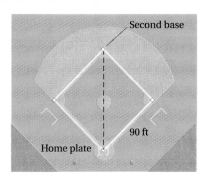

$\sqrt{16,200}$ ft ≈ 127.3 ft

52. *Softball Diamond.* A slow-pitch softball diamond is actually a square 65 ft on a side. How far is it from home plate to second base?

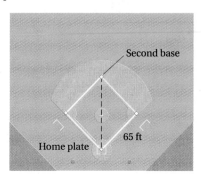

$\sqrt{8450}$ ft ≈ 91.9 ft

53. How tall is this tree?

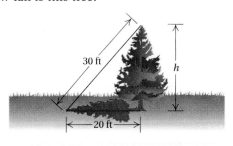

$\sqrt{500}$ ft ≈ 22.4 ft

54. How far is the base of the fence post from point *A*?

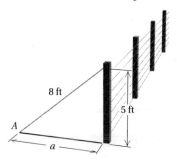

$\sqrt{39}$ ft ≈ 6.2 ft

55. An airplane is flying at an altitude of 4100 ft. The slanted distance directly to the airport is 15,100 ft. How far is the airplane horizontally from the airport? $\sqrt{211,200,000}$ ft ≈ 14,532.7 ft

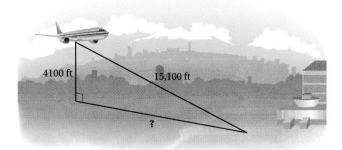

56. A surveyor had poles located at points *P*, *Q*, and *R* around a lake. The distances that the surveyor was able to measure are marked on the drawing. What is the distance from *P* to *R* across the lake?

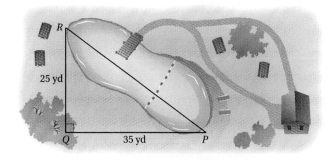

$\sqrt{1850}$ yd ≈ 43.0 yd

Solve.

57. Food expenses account for 26% of the average family's budget. A family makes $1800 one month. How much do they spend for food? [8.4a] $468

58. The price of a cellular phone was reduced from $350 to $308. Find the percent of decrease in price. [8.4b] 12%

59. A county has a population that is increasing by 4% each year. This year the population is 180,000. What will it be next year? [8.4b] 187,200

60. The price of a box of cookies increased from $2.85 to $3.99. What was the percent of increase in the price? [8.4b] 40%

61. A college has a student body of 1850 students. Of these, 17.5% are seniors. How many students are seniors? [8.4a] About 324

62. A state charges a meals tax of $4\frac{1}{2}$%. What is the meals tax charged on a dinner party costing $540? [8.5a] $24.30

Synthesis

63. ◈ Explain how the Pythagorean theorem can be used to prove that a triangle is a *right* triangle.

64. ◈ Write a problem similar to Exercises 49–52 for a classmate to solve. Design the problem so that its solution involves the length $\sqrt{58}$ m.

65. ◈ Give an argument that could be used to convince a classmate that $\sqrt{2501}$ is not a whole number. Do not use a calculator.

66. ▦ Find the area of the trapezoid shown. Round to the nearest hundredth. 47.80 cm²

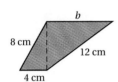

67. Which of the triangles below has the larger area?

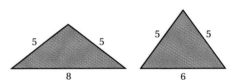

The areas are the same.

68. A 19-in. television set has a rectangular screen that measures 19 in. diagonally. The ratio of length to width in a conventional television set is 4 to 3. Find the length and the width of the screen.

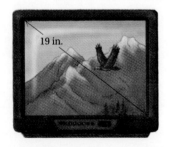

Length: 15.2 in.; width: 11.4 in.

69. A Philips 42-in. plasma television has a rectangular screen that measures 42 in. diagonally. The ratio of length to width is 16 to 9. Find the length and the width of the screen.

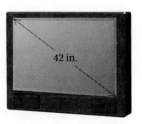

Length: 36.6 in.; width: 20.6 in.

9.6 Volume and Capacity

a | Volume

The **volume** of a **rectangular solid** is the number of unit cubes needed to fill it.

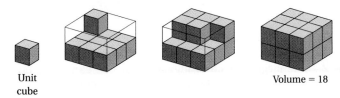

Two other units are shown below.

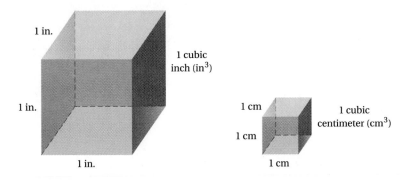

Example 1 Find the volume.

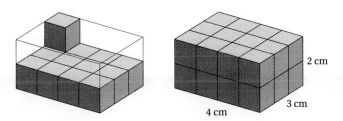

The figure is made up of 2 layers of 12 cubes each, so its volume is 24 cubic centimeters (cm³).

Do Exercise 1.

The volume of a rectangular solid can be thought of as the product of the area of the base times the height:

$$V = l \cdot w \cdot h$$
$$= (l \cdot w) \cdot h$$
$$= (\text{Area of the base}) \cdot h$$
$$= B \cdot h,$$

Area of base $= B = l \cdot w$

where B is the area of the base.

Objectives

a | Find the volume of a rectangular solid, a cylinder, and a sphere.

b | Convert from one unit of capacity to another.

c | Solve applied problems involving capacity.

For Extra Help

TAPE 17   MAC WIN   CD-ROM

1. Find the volume.   12 cm³

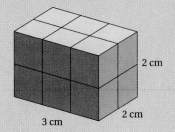

Answer on page A-26

2. In a recent year, people in the United States bought enough unpopped popcorn to provide every person in the country with a bag of popped corn measuring 2 ft by 2 ft by 5 ft. Find the volume of such a bag.

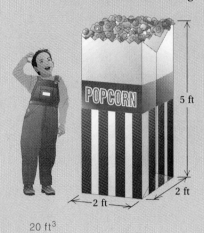

5 ft

2 ft

2 ft

20 ft³

3. *Cord of Wood.* A cord of firewood measures 4 ft by 4 ft by 8 ft. What is the volume of a cord of firewood?

128 ft³

Answers on page A-26

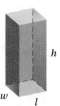 The **volume of a rectangular solid** is found by multiplying length by width by height:

$$V = \underbrace{l \cdot w}_{\substack{\text{Area} \\ \text{of} \\ \text{base}}} \cdot \underset{\text{Height}}{h}.$$

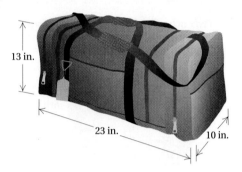

h

w l

Example 2   The largest piece of luggage that you can carry on an airplane measures 23 in. by 10 in. by 13 in. Find the volume of this solid.

$$V = l \cdot w \cdot h$$
$$= 23 \text{ in.} \cdot 10 \text{ in.} \cdot 13 \text{ in.}$$
$$= 230 \cdot 13 \text{ in}^3$$
$$= 2990 \text{ in}^3$$

13 in.

23 in.

10 in.

Do Exercises 2 and 3.

Cylinders

Like rectangular solids, **circular cylinders** have tops and bottoms of equal area that lie in parallel planes. The bases of circular cylinders are circular regions.

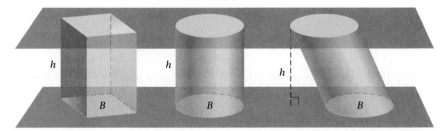

h h h

B B B

The volume of a circular cylinder is also the product of the area of the base times the height. The height is always measured perpendicular to—that is, at a 90° angle from—the base.

The volume of a circular cylinder of radius r is the product of the area of the base B and the height h:

$$V = B \cdot h, \quad \text{or} \quad V = \pi \cdot r^2 \cdot h.$$

Example 3 Find the volume of this circular cylinder. Use 3.14 to approximate π.

$$V = Bh = \pi \cdot r^2 \cdot h$$
$$\approx 3.14 \cdot 4 \text{ cm} \cdot 4 \text{ cm} \cdot 12 \text{ cm}$$
$$\approx 602.88 \text{ cm}^3$$

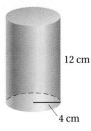

12 cm

4 cm

Do Exercises 4 and 5.

Spheres

A **sphere** is the three-dimensional counterpart of a circle. It is the set of all points in space that are a given distance (the radius) from a given point (the center). The volume of a sphere depends on its radius.

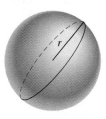

> The volume of a sphere of radius r is given by
>
> $$V = \frac{4}{3} \cdot \pi \cdot r^3.$$

Example 4 *Bowling.* The radius of a standard-sized bowling ball is about 11 cm. Find the volume of a standard-sized bowling ball. Round to the nearest cubic centimeter. Use 3.14 for π.

$$V = \frac{4}{3} \cdot \pi \cdot r^3 \approx \frac{4}{3} \cdot 3.14 \cdot (11 \text{ cm})^3$$
$$\approx \frac{4 \cdot 3.14 \cdot 1331 \text{ cm}^3}{3} \approx 5572 \text{ cm}^3$$

Do Exercises 6 and 7.

b Capacity

Since many substances come in containers that have irregular shape, to answer a question like "How much soda is in the bottle?" we need measures of **capacity**. American units of capacity are ounces, cups, pints, quarts, and gallons. These units are related as follows.

> **AMERICAN UNITS OF CAPACITY**
>
> 1 gallon (gal) = 4 quarts (qt)   1 pt = 2 cups = 16 ounces (oz)
>
> 1 qt = 2 pints (pt)   1 cup = 8 oz

---

4. Find the volume of the cylinder. Use 3.14 to approximate π.

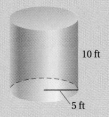

10 ft

5 ft

785 ft^3

5. Find the volume of the cylinder. Use $\frac{22}{7}$ to approximate π.

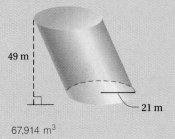

49 m

21 m

67,914 m^3

6. Find the volume of the sphere. Use 3.14 for π.

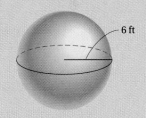

6 ft

904.32 ft^3

7. The radius of a standard-sized golf ball is about $\frac{4}{5}$ in. Find its volume. Use $\frac{22}{7}$ for π.

$\frac{5632}{2625}$ in^3

Answers on page A-26

Complete

8. 80 qt = _____20_____ gal.

Complete.

9. 4 gal = _____32_____ pt.

Answers on page A-26

Example 5   Complete: 24 qt = _____ gal.

In this case, we multiply by 1 using 1 gal in the numerator, since we are converting to gallons, and 4 qt in the denominator, since we are converting from quarts.

$$24 \text{ qt} = 24 \text{ qt} \cdot \frac{1 \text{ gal}}{4 \text{ qt}} = \frac{24}{4} \cdot 1 \text{ gal} = 6 \text{ gal}$$

To check that our answer is reasonable, note that since we are converting from smaller to larger units, our answer is a smaller number than the one with which we started.

Do Exercise 8.

Example 6   Complete: 9 gal = _____ oz.

First, we multiply by 1 using 4 qt on the top and 1 gal on the bottom:

$$9 \text{ gal} = 9 \text{ gal} \cdot \frac{4 \text{ qt}}{1 \text{ gal}} \quad \text{This converts from gallons to quarts.}$$
$$= 9 \cdot 4 \text{ qt} = 36 \text{ qt}.$$

Next, we convert 36 qt to ounces by multiplying by 32 oz/1 qt:

$$9 \text{ gal} = 36 \text{ qt} = 36 \text{ qt} \cdot \frac{32 \text{ oz}}{1 \text{ qt}}$$
$$= 36 \cdot 32 \text{ oz} = 1152 \text{ oz}.$$

This conversion could have been done in one step had we known that 1 gal = 128 oz. We then would have multiplied 9 gal by 128 oz/1 gal.

Do Exercise 9.

The basic unit of capacity for the metric system is the **liter**. A liter is just a bit more than a quart (1 liter = 1.06 quarts). It is defined as follows.

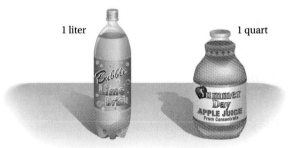

1 liter   1 quart

> **METRIC UNITS OF CAPACITY**
>
> 1 liter (L) = 1000 cubic centimeters (1000 cm^3)
>
> The script letter ℓ is also used for "liter."

Metric prefixes are also used with liters. The most common is **milli-**. The milliliter (mL) is, then, $\frac{1}{1000}$ liter. Thus,

> ▶ $1 \text{ L} = 1000 \text{ mL} = 1000 \text{ cm}^3$;
> $0.001 \text{ L} = 1 \text{ mL} = 1 \text{ cm}^3$.

A preferred unit for drug dosage is the milliliter (mL) or the cubic centimeter (cm³). The notation "cc" is also used for cubic centimeter, especially in medicine. A milliliter and a cubic centimeter are the same size. Each is about the size of a sugar cube.

> ▶ $1 \text{ mL} = 1 \text{ cm}^3 = 1 \text{ cc}$

Volumes for which quarts and gallons are used are expressed in liters. Large volumes may be expressed using cubic meters (m³).

Do Exercises 10–13.

Example 7 Complete: $4.5 \text{ L} =$ _____ mL.

$$4.5 \text{ L} = 4.5 \,\cancel{\text{L}} \cdot \frac{1000 \text{ mL}}{1 \,\cancel{\text{L}}}$$
$$= 4.5 \cdot 1000 \text{ mL}$$
$$= 4500 \text{ mL}$$

Example 8 Complete: $280 \text{ mL} =$ _____ L.

$$280 \text{ mL} = 280 \,\cancel{\text{mL}} \cdot \frac{1 \text{ L}}{1000 \,\cancel{\text{mL}}}$$
$$= \frac{280}{1000} \text{ L}$$
$$= 0.28 \text{ L}$$

Do Exercises 14 and 15.

c | Solving Problems

Example 9 At a self-service gasoline station, 89-octane gasoline sells for 28.3¢ a liter. Estimate the price of 1 gal in dollars.

Since 1 liter is about 1 quart and there are 4 quarts in a gallon, the price of a gallon is about 4 times the price of a liter:

$$4 \cdot 28.3\text{¢} = 113.2\text{¢} = \$1.132.$$

Thus 89-octane gasoline sells for about $1.13 a gallon.

Do Exercise 16.

Complete with mL or L.

10. To prevent infection, a patient received an injection of 2 __mL__ of penicillin.

11. There are 250__mL__ in a coffee cup.

12. The gas tank holds 80 __L__ .

13. Bring home 8 __L__ of milk.

Complete.

14. $0.97 \text{ L} = $ __970__ mL

15. $8990 \text{ mL} = $ __8.99__ L

16. At the same station, the price of 87-octane gasoline is 26.9 cents a liter. Estimate the price of 1 gallon in dollars.

$1.08

Answers on page A-26

17. *Medicine Capsule.* A cold capsule is 8 mm long and 4 mm in diameter. Find the volume of the capsule. Use 3.14 for π. (*Hint*: First find the length of the cylindrical section.) 83.73 mm³

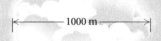
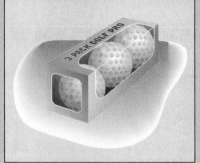
Answer on page A-26

Example 10   *Propane Gas Tank.* A propane gas tank is shaped like a circular cylinder with half of a sphere at each end. Find the volume of the tank if the cylindrical section is 5 ft long with a 4-ft diameter. Use 3.14 for π.

1. Familiarize.   We first make a drawing.

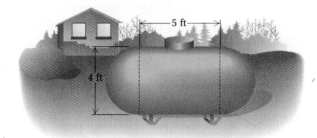

2. Translate.   This is a two-step problem. We first find the volume of the cylindrical portion. Then we find the volume of the two ends and add. Note that the radius is 2 ft and that together the two ends make a sphere. We let V = the total volume.

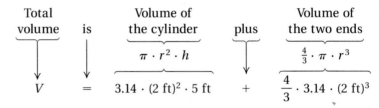

Total volume	is	Volume of the cylinder	plus	Volume of the two ends
		$\pi \cdot r^2 \cdot h$		$\frac{4}{3} \cdot \pi \cdot r^3$
V	$=$	$3.14 \cdot (2 \text{ ft})^2 \cdot 5 \text{ ft}$	$+$	$\frac{4}{3} \cdot 3.14 \cdot (2 \text{ ft})^3$

3. Solve.   The volume of the cylinder is approximately

$$3.14 \cdot (2 \text{ ft})^2 \cdot 5 \text{ ft} \approx 3.14 \cdot 2 \text{ ft} \cdot 2 \text{ ft} \cdot 5 \text{ ft}$$
$$\approx 62.8 \text{ ft}^3.$$

The volume of the two ends is approximately

$$\frac{4}{3} \cdot 3.14 \cdot (2 \text{ ft})^3 \approx 1.33 \cdot 3.14 \cdot 2 \text{ ft} \cdot 2 \text{ ft} \cdot 2 \text{ ft}$$
$$\approx 33.4 \text{ ft}^3.$$

The total volume is approximately

$$62.8 \text{ ft}^3 + 33.4 \text{ ft}^3 = 96.2 \text{ ft}^3.$$

4. Check.   The check is left to the student.

5. State.   The volume of the tank is about 96.2 ft³.

Do Exercise 17.

Exercise Set 9.6

a Find each volume. Use 3.14 for π in Exercises 9–12 and 15–18. Use $\frac{22}{7}$ for π in Exercises 13, 14, 19, and 20.

1.

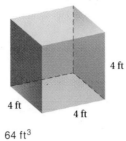

5 cm

10 cm   5 cm

250 cm³

2.

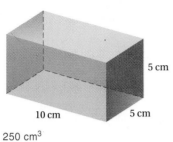

4 ft

4 ft   4 ft

64 ft³

3.

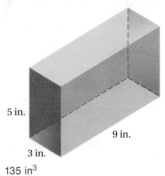

5 in.   9 in.

3 in.

135 in³

4.

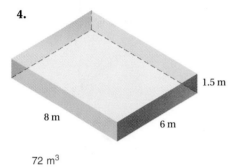

1.5 m

8 m   6 m

72 m³

5.

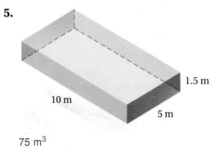

10 m   1.5 m

5 m

75 m³

6.

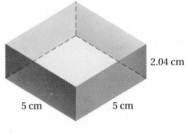

2.04 cm

5 cm   5 cm

51 cm³

7.

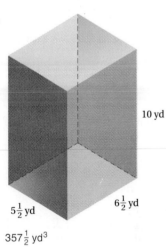

10 yd

$5\frac{1}{2}$ yd $6\frac{1}{2}$ yd

$357\frac{1}{2}$ yd³

8.

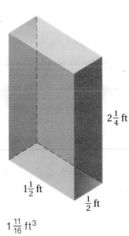

$2\frac{1}{4}$ ft

$1\frac{1}{2}$ ft $\frac{1}{2}$ ft

$1\frac{11}{16}$ ft³

9.

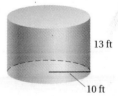

13 ft

10 ft

4082 ft³

10.

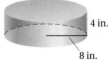

4 in.

8 in.

803.84 in³

11.

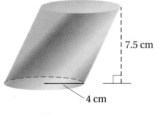

7.5 cm

4 cm

376.8 cm³

12.

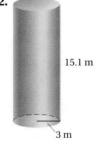

15.1 m

3 m

426.726 m³

13.

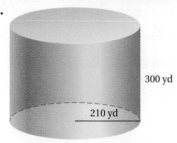

300 yd

210 yd

41,580,000 yd³

14.

28 km

4 km

1408 km³

15.

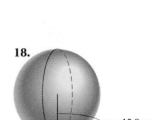

r = 100 in.

4,186,666.6̄ in³

16.

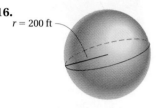

r = 200 ft

33,493,333.3̄ ft³

17.

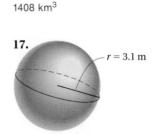

r = 3.1 m

Approximately 124.725 m³

18.

r = 15.2 cm

Approximately 14,702.769 cm³

19.

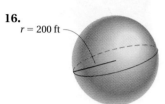

r = 7 km

$1437\frac{1}{3}$ km³

20.

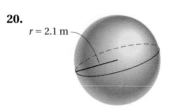

r = 2.1 m

38.808 m³

b Complete.

21. 1 L = __1000__ mL = __1000__ cm³

22. __0.001__ L = 1 mL = __1__ cm³

23. 87 L = __87,000__ mL

24. 806 L = __806,000__ mL

25. 49 mL = __0.049__ L

26. 19 mL = __0.019__ L

27. 27.3 L = __27,300__ cm³

28. 49.2 L = __49,200__ cm³

29. 5 gal = __40__ pt

30. 48 oz = __3__ pt

31. 10 qt = __320__ oz

32. 2 gal = __32__ cups

33. 24 oz = __3__ cups

34. 20 cups = __10__ pt

35. 8 gal = __32__ qt

36. 5 gal = __80__ cups

37. 3 gal = __48__ cups

38. 72 oz = __9__ cups

39. 15 pt = __$1\frac{7}{8}$__ gal

40. 9 qt = __$2\frac{1}{4}$__ gal

c Solve.

41. *Medicine.* Dr. Carey ordered 0.5 L of normal saline solution. How many milliliters were ordered?

500 mL

42. *Medicine.* Ingrid receives 84 mL per hour of normal saline solution. How many liters did Ingrid receive in a 24-hr period?   2.016 L

43. *Medicine.* Dr. Norris tells a patient to purchase 0.5 L of hydrogen peroxide. Commercially, hydrogen peroxide is found on the shelf in bottles that hold 4 oz, 8 oz, and 16 oz. Which bottle comes closest to filling the prescription?   16 oz

44. *Medicine.* Dr. Gomez wants a patient to receive 3 L of a normal glucose solution in a 24-hr period. How many milliliters per hour should the patient receive?

125 mL

45. A rung of a ladder is 2 in. in diameter and 18 in. long. Find the volume. Use 3.14 for π.

56.52 in³

46. The diameter of a cylindrical trashcan is 0.7 yd. The height is 1.1 yd. Find the volume. Use $\frac{22}{7}$ for π.

0.4235 yd³

47. An oak log has a diameter of 12 cm and a length of 42 cm. Find the volume. Use 3.14 for π.   4747.68 cm³

48. *Farming.* A barn silo, excluding the top, is a circular cylinder. The silo is 6 m in diameter and the height is 13 m. Find the volume. Use 3.14 for π.   367.38 m³

49. *Merchandising.* Tennis balls are generally packaged in circular cylinders that hold 3 balls each. The diameter of a tennis ball is 6.5 cm. Find the volume of a can of tennis balls. Use 3.14 for π.   646.74 cm³

50. *Oceanography.* A research submarine is capsule-shaped. Find the volume of the submarine if it has a length of 10 m and a diameter of 8 m. Use 3.14 for π. (*Hint:* First find the length of the cylindrical section.)   368.42$\overline{6}$ m³

51. *Metallurgy.* If all the gold in the world could be gathered together, it would form a cube 18 yd on a side. Find the volume of the world's gold.   5832 yd³

52. *Astronomy.* The radius of Pluto's moon is about 500 km. Find the volume of this satellite. Use $\frac{22}{7}$ for π.   523,809,523.8 km³

53. *Farming.* A water storage tank is a right circular cylinder with a radius of 14 cm and a height of 100 cm. What is the tank's volume? How many liters can it hold? Use $\frac{22}{7}$ for π.   61,600 cm³; 61.6 L

54. *Conservation.* Many people leave the water running while brushing their teeth. Suppose that one person wastes 32 oz of water in such a manner each day. How much water, in gallons, would that person waste in a week? in 30 days? in a year? If each of the 261 million people in this country wastes water this way, estimate how much water is wasted in a year.

$1\frac{3}{4}$ gal; 7.5 gal; $91\frac{1}{4}$ gal; about 24,000,000,000 gal

Skill Maintenance

55. Find the simple interest on \$600 at 8% for $\frac{1}{2}$ yr.
[8.6a]   \$24

56. Find the simple interest on \$5000 at 7% for $\frac{1}{2}$ yr.
[8.6a]   \$175

57. If 9 pens cost \$8.01, how much would 12 pens cost?
[7.4a]   \$10.68

58. Solve: $9(x - 1) = 3x + 5$.   [5.7b] $\frac{7}{3}$

59. Solve: $-5y + 3 = -12y - 4$.   [5.7b] -1

60. A barge travels 320 km in 15 days. At this rate, how far will it travel in 21 days?   [7.4a]   448 km

Synthesis

61. ◆ Which occupies more volume: two spheres, each with radius r, or one sphere with radius $2r$? Explain why.

62. ◆What advantages do metric units of capacity have over American units?

63. ◆ How could you use the volume formulas in this section to help estimate the volume of an egg?

64. ▦ Audio-cassette cases are typically 7 cm by 10.75 cm by 1.5 cm and contain 90 min of music. Compact-disc cases are typically 12.4 cm by 14.1 cm by 1 cm and contain 50 min of music. Which container holds the most music per cubic centimeter?   Audio-cassette cases

65. ▦ A 2-cm–wide stream of water passes through a 30-m long garden hose. At the instant that the water is turned off, how many liters of water are in the hose? Use 3.141593 for π.   9.424779 L

66. ▦ The volume of a basketball is 2304π cm^3. Find the volume of a cube-shaped box that is just large enough to hold the ball.   13,824 cm^3

67. ▦ The width of a dollar bill is 2.3125 in., the length is 6.0625 in., and the thickness is 0.0041 in. Find the volume occupied by one million one-dollar bills.
57,480 in^3

68. ▦ A sphere with diameter 1 m is circumscribed by a cube. How much more volume is in the cube?

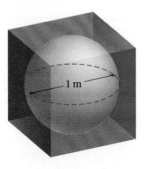

0.476 m^3

69. ▦ A cube is circumscribed by a sphere with a 1-m diameter. How much more volume is in the sphere?

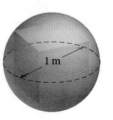

0.331 m^3

Copyright © 2000 Addison Wesley Longman

9.7 Weight, Mass, and Temperature

a | Weight: The American System

The American units of weight are as follows.

> **AMERICAN UNITS OF WEIGHT**
>
> 1 ton (T) = 2000 pounds (lb)
>
> 1 lb = 16 ounces (oz)

The term "ounce" used here for weight is different from the "ounce" we used for capacity in Section 9.6.

Example 1 A well-known hamburger is called a "quarter-pounder." Find its name in ounces: a "_____ ouncer."

$$\frac{1}{4} \text{ lb} = \frac{1}{4} \cdot 1 \text{ lb}$$

$$= \frac{1}{4} \cdot 16 \text{ oz} \qquad \text{Substituting 16 oz for 1 lb}$$

$$= 4 \text{ oz}$$

A "quarter-pounder" can also be called a "four-ouncer."

Example 2 Complete: 15,360 lb = _____ T.

$$15{,}360 \text{ lb} = 15{,}360 \text{ lb} \cdot \frac{1 \text{ T}}{2000 \text{ lb}} \qquad \textbf{Multiplying by 1}$$

$$= \frac{15{,}360}{2000} \text{ T} \qquad \textbf{Dividing by 2000}$$

$$= 7.68 \text{ T}$$

Do Exercises 1–3.

b | Mass: The Metric System

There is a difference between **mass** and **weight**, but the terms are often used interchangeably. People sometimes use the word "weight" instead of "mass." Weight is related to the force of gravity. The farther you are from the center of the earth, the less you weigh. Your mass stays the same no matter where you are.

The basic unit of mass is the **gram** (g), which is the mass of 1 cubic centimeter (1 cm³ or 1 mL) of water. Since a cubic centimeter is small, a gram is a small unit of mass.

$$1 \text{ g} = 1 \text{ gram} = \text{the mass of 1 cm}^3 \text{ (1 mL) of water}$$

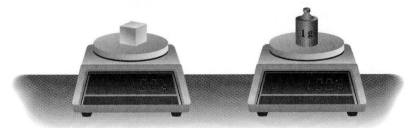

Complete.

1. 5 lb = ____80____ oz

2. 8640 lb = ____4.32____ T

3. 1 T = ____32,000____ oz

Answers on page A-26

Complete with mg, g, kg, or t.

4. A laptop computer has a mass of 2 ___kg___ .

5. Rosita has a body mass of 56 ___kg___ .

6. The athlete took a 200-___mg___ pain reliever.

7. A pen has a mass of 12 ___g___ .

8. A pickup truck has a mass of 1.5 ___t___ .

Answers on page A-26

The metric prefixes for mass are the same as those used for length.

> **METRIC UNITS OF MASS**
>
> 1 metric ton (t) = 1000 kilograms (kg)
>
> 1 *kilo*gram (kg) = 1000 grams (g)
>
> 1 *hecto*gram (hg) = 100 grams (g)
>
> 1 *deka*gram (dag) = 10 grams (g)
>
> 1 gram (g)
>
> 1 *deci*gram (dg) = $\frac{1}{10}$ gram (g)
>
> 1 *centi*gram (cg) = $\frac{1}{100}$ gram (g)
>
> 1 *milli*gram (mg) = $\frac{1}{1000}$ gram (g)

Thinking Metric

The mass of 1 raisin or 1 paperclip is approximately 1 gram (g). Since 1 metric ton is 1000 kg and 1 kg is about 2.2 lb, it follows that 1 metric ton (t) is about 2200 lb, or about 10% more than 1 American ton (T). The metric ton is used for very large masses, such as vehicles; the kilogram is used for masses of people or larger food packages; the gram is used for smaller food packages or objects like a coin or a ring; the milligram is used for even smaller masses like a dosage of medicine.

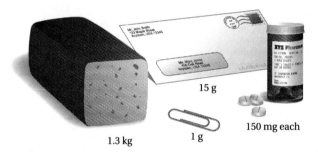

15 g

1.3 kg   1 g   150 mg each

Do Exercises 4–8.

Changing Units Mentally

As before, changing from one metric unit to another amounts to only the movement of a decimal point. Consider these equivalent masses.

> **MASS OF A STANDARD SHEET OF PAPER**
>
> 4260 mg = 426 cg = 4.26 g = 0.00426 kg

Example 3   Complete: 8 kg = _____ g.

Think: A kilogram is 1000 times the mass of a gram. Thus we move the decimal point three places to the right.

8.0   8.000.   8 kg = 8000 g

Example 4 Complete: 4235 g = _____ kg.

Think: There are 1000 grams in 1 kilogram. Thus we move the decimal point three places to the left.

$$4235.0 \qquad 4{.}235.0 \qquad 4235 \text{ g} = 4.235 \text{ kg}$$

Example 5 Complete: 6.98 cg = _____ mg.

Think: One centigram has the mass of 10 milligrams. Thus we move the decimal point one place to the right.

$$6.98 \qquad 6.9{.}8 \qquad 6.98 \text{ cg} = 69.8 \text{ mg}$$

The most commonly used metric units of mass are kg, g, cg, and mg. We have purposely used those more often than the others in the exercises.

Do Exercises 9–12.

c Temperature

Estimated Conversions

Below are two temperature scales: **Fahrenheit** for American measure and **Celsius** for metric measure.

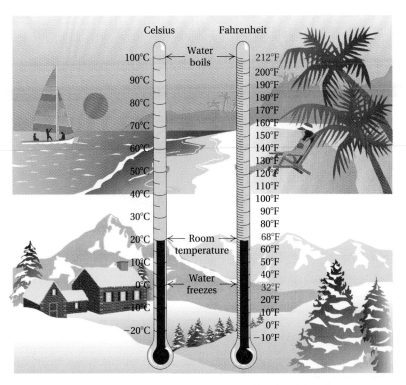

By laying a straightedge horizontally between the scales, we can approximate conversions between Celsius and Fahrenheit.

Complete.

9. 6.2 kg = ___6200___ g

10. 79.3 g = ___0.0793___ kg

11. 7.7 cg = ___77___ mg

12. 2344 mg = ___234.4___ cg

Answers on page A-26

Use a straightedge to convert the following temperatures to either Celsius or Fahrenheit. Answers may be approximate.

13. 25°F (Cold day)   −4°C

14. 30°C (Warm beach day)   85°F

15. −10°F (Extremely cold day)
  −25°C

16. 10°C (A cold bath)   50°F

Convert to Fahrenheit or Celsius.

17. 80°C   176°F

18. 35°C   95°F

19. 95°F   35°C

20. 113°F   45°C

Answers on page A-26

Examples   Use a straightedge to approximate each of the following conversions. Use the scales on p. 567.

6. 110°F (Hot bath) ≈ 43°C

7. 50°C (Warm food) = 122°F

8. 160°F (Temperature of a sauna) ≈ 72°C

9. 0°C (Freezing point of water) = 32°F   **This is exact.**

Do Exercises 13–16.

Exact Conversions

A formula allows us to make exact conversions from Celsius to Fahrenheit.

$$F = \frac{9}{5} \cdot C + 32, \quad \text{or} \quad F = 1.8 \cdot C + 32$$

$$\left(\text{Multiply the Celsius temperature by } \frac{9}{5}, \text{ or } 1.8, \text{ and add 32.}\right)$$

Examples   Convert to Fahrenheit.

10. 0°C $F = \frac{9}{5} \cdot 0 + 32 = 0 + 32 = 32°$ **Substituting 0 for C**

Thus, 0°C = 32°F.

11. 37°C $F = 1.8 \cdot 37 + 32 = 66.6 + 32 = 98.6°$ **Substituting 37 for C**

Thus, 37°C = 98.6°F. This is normal body temperature.

A second formula gives exact conversions from Fahrenheit to Celsius.

$$C = \frac{5}{9} \cdot (F - 32)$$

$$\left(\text{Subtract 32 from the Fahrenheit temperature and multiply by } \frac{5}{9}.\right)$$

Examples   Convert to Celsius.

12. 212°F $C = \frac{5}{9} \cdot (F - 32)$

$$= \frac{5}{9} \cdot (212 - 32) = \frac{5}{9} \cdot 180 = 100°$$

Thus, 212°F = 100°C.

13. 77°F $C = \frac{5}{9} \cdot (F - 32)$

$$= \frac{5}{9} \cdot (77 - 32) = \frac{5}{9} \cdot 45 = 25°$$

Thus, 77°F = 25°C.

Do Exercises 17–20.

Exercise Set 9.7

a Complete.

1. 1 lb = <u>16</u> oz

2. 1 T = <u>2000</u> lb

3. 6000 lb = <u>3</u> T

4. 5 T = <u>10,000</u> lb

5. 3 lb = <u>48</u> oz

6. 10 lb = <u>160</u> oz

7. 3.5 T = <u>7000</u> lb

8. 2.5 T = <u>5000</u> lb

9. 4800 lb = <u>2.4</u> T

10. 7500 lb = <u>3.75</u> T

11. 72 oz = <u>4.5</u> lb

12. 960 oz = <u>60</u> lb

b Complete.

13. 1 kg = <u>1000</u> g

14. 6 kg = <u>6000</u> g

15. 1 g = <u>0.001</u> kg

16. 1 dg = <u>0.1</u> g

17. 1 cg = <u>0.01</u> g

18. 1 mg = <u>0.001</u> g

19. 1 g = <u>1000</u> mg

20. 1 g = <u>100</u> cg

21. 1 g = <u>10</u> dg

22. 45 kg = <u>45,000</u> g

23. 725 kg = <u>725,000</u> g

24. 678 g = <u>0.678</u> kg

25. 6345 g = <u>6.345</u> kg

26. 42.75 kg = <u>42,750</u> g

27. 897 mg = <u>0.000897</u> kg

28. 45 cg = ___0.45___ g   **29.** 7.32 kg = ___7320___ g   **30.** 0.439 cg = ___4.39___ mg

31. 6780 g = ___6.78___ kg   **32.** 5677 g = ___5.677___ kg   **33.** 69 mg = ___6.9___ cg

34. 76.1 mg = ___7.61___ cg   **35.** 8 kg = ___800,000___ cg   **36.** 0.02 kg = ___20,000___ mg

37. 1 t = ___1000___ kg   **38.** 2 t = ___2000___ kg

39. 3.4 cg = ___0.0034___ dag   **40.** 9.34 g = ___9340___ mg

c Convert to Celsius. Round the answer to the nearest ten degrees. Use the scales on p. 567.

41. 178°F   80°C   **42.** 195°F   90°C   **43.** 140°F   60°C   **44.** 107°F   40°C

45. 68°F   20°C   **46.** 45°F   10°C   **47.** 10°F   −10°C   **48.** 120°F   50°C

Convert to Fahrenheit. Round the answer to the nearest ten degrees. Use the scales on p. 567.

49. 86°C   190°F   **50.** 93°C   200°F   **51.** 58°C   140°F   **52.** 33°C   90°F

53. −10°C   10°F   **54.** −5°C   20°F   **55.** 5°C   40°F   **56.** 15°C   60°F

Convert to Fahrenheit. Use the formula $F = \dfrac{9}{5} \cdot C + 32$.

57. 25°C 77°F

58. 85°C 185°F

59. 40°C 104°F

60. 90°C 194°F

61. 3000°C (melting point of iron) 5432°F

62. 1000°C (melting point of gold) 1832°F

Convert to Celsius. Use the formula $C = \dfrac{5}{9} \cdot (F - 32)$.

63. 86°F 30°C

64. 59°F 15°C

65. 131°F 55°C

66. 140°F 60°C

67. 98.6°F (normal body temperature) 37°C

68. 104°F (high-fevered body temperature) 40°C

Skill Maintenance

Convert to percent notation. [8.1b]

69. 0.0043 0.43%

70. 2.31 231%

71. If 2 cans of tomato paste cost $1.49, how many cans of tomato paste can you buy for $7.45? [7.4a] 10

72.

Sound Levels

Whisper	15
Tick of watch	30
Speaking aloud	60
Noisy factory	90
Moving car	80
Car horn	98
Subway	104

10 20 30 40 50 60 70 80 90 100 110
Loudness (in decibels)

72. *Sound Levels.* Make a horizontal bar graph to show the loudness of various sounds, as listed below. A decibel is a measure of the loudness of sounds. [6.2b]

Sound	Loudness (in decibels)
Whisper	15
Tick of watch	30
Speaking aloud	60
Noisy factory	90
Moving car	80
Car horn	98
Subway	104

73. Solve: $9(x - 3) = 4x - 5$. [5.7b] $\dfrac{22}{5}$

74. Solve: $34.1 - 17.4x = 2.1x - 14.65$. [5.7b] 2.5

75. ◆ Near the Canadian border, a radio forecast calls for an overnight low of 60. Was the temperature given in Celsius or Fahrenheit? Explain how you can tell.

76. ◆ Give at least two reasons why someone might prefer the use of grams to the use of ounces.

77. ◆ Describe a situation in which one object weighs 70 kg, another object weighs 3 g, and a third object weighs 125 mg.

Complete. Use 1 kg = 2.205 lb and 453.5 g = 1 lb. Round to four decimal places.

78. 🔢 1 lb = __0.4535__ kg

79. 🔢 1 g = __0.0022__ lb

80. Use the formula $F = \frac{9}{5} \cdot C + 32$ to find the temperature that is the same for both the Fahrenheit and Celsius scales. −40°

81. *Medicine.* The medicine Albuterol is used for the treatment of asthma. It typically comes in an inhaler that contains 18 g. One actuation, or spray, is 90 mg.

   a) How many actuations are in one inhaler? 200
   b) Myra is going away for 4 months of college and wants to take enough Albuterol to last for that time. Assuming that Myra will need 4 actuations per day, estimate the number of inhalers she will need for the 4-month period. 3

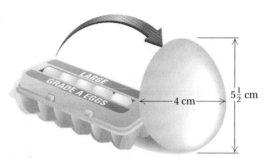

82. *Chemistry.* Another temperature scale often used is the **Kelvin** scale. Conversions from Celsius to Kelvin can be carried out using the formula

$$K = C + 273.$$

A chemistry textbook describes an experiment in which a reaction takes place at a temperature of 400° Kelvin. A student wishes to perform the experiment, but has only a Fahrenheit thermometer. At what Fahrenheit temperature will the reaction take place? 260.6°F

83. 🔢 A large egg is about $5\frac{1}{2}$ cm tall with a diameter of 4 cm. Estimate the mass of such an egg by averaging the volumes of two spheres. (*Hint*: 1 cc of water has a mass of 1 g.) 60 g

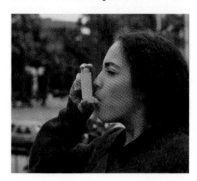

84. *Medicine.* Quinidine is a medicine that comes mixed with water. There are 80 mg of Quinidine in every milliliter of liquid. A standard dosage requires 200 mg of Quinidine. How much of the liquid mixture would be required in order to achieve this dosage? 2.5 mL

85. *Medicine.* A medicine called cephalexin is available in a liquid mixture, part medicine and part water. There are 250 mg of cephalexin in 5 mL of liquid. A standard dosage is 400 mg. How much of the liquid would be required in order to achieve this dosage?

   8 mL

86. 🔢 *Track and Field.* A man's shot put weighs 16 lb and has a 5-in. diameter. Find its mass per cubic centimeter. About 6.6 g/cm³

87. 🔢 *Track and Field.* A woman's shot put weighs 8.8 lb and has a 4.5-in. diameter. Find its mass per cubic centimeter. About 5.1 g/cm³

Summary and Review: Chapter 9

Important Properties and Formulas

Area of a Parallelogram:	$A = b \cdot h$
Area of a Trapezoid:	$A = \frac{1}{2} \cdot h \cdot (a + b)$
Radius and Diameter of a Circle:	$d = 2 \cdot r$, or $r = \frac{d}{2}$
Circumference of a Circle:	$C = \pi \cdot d$, or $C = 2 \cdot \pi \cdot r$
Area of a Circle:	$A = \pi \cdot r \cdot r$, or $A = \pi \cdot r^2$
Pythagorean Equation:	$a^2 + b^2 = c^2$
Volume of a Rectangular Solid:	$V = l \cdot w \cdot h$
Volume of a Circular Cylinder:	$V = \pi \cdot r^2 \cdot h$
Volume of a Sphere:	$V = \frac{4}{3} \cdot \pi \cdot r^3$
Temperature Conversion:	$F = \frac{9}{5} \cdot C + 32$; $C = \frac{5}{9} \cdot (F - 32)$

See tables inside chapter for units of length, weight, mass, and capacity.

Review Exercises

Complete.

1. 10 ft = _____ yd
[9.1a]

2. $\frac{5}{6}$ yd = _____ in.
[9.1a]

3. 0.7 mm = _____ cm
[9.1b]

4. 9 m = _____ km
[9.1b]

5. 4 km = _____ cm
[9.1b]

6. 14 in. = _____ ft
[9.1a]

7. 9 lb = _____ oz
[9.7a]

8. 4 g = _____ kg
[9.7b]

9. 54 qt = _____ gal
[9.6b]

10. 32 gal = _____ pt
[9.6b]

11. 60 mL = _____ L
[9.6b]

12. 0.4 L = _____ mL
[9.6b]

13. 0.8 T = _____ lb
[9.7a]

14. 0.2 g = _____ mg
[9.7b]

15. 4.7 kg = _____ g
[9.7b]

16. 4 cg = _____ g
[9.7b]

17. 5 yd^2 = _____ ft^2
[9.3a]

18. 0.7 km^2 = _____ m^2
[9.3b]

19. 1008 in^2 = _____ ft^2
[9.3a]

20. 570 cm^2 = _____ m^2
[9.3b]

21. Find the circumference of a circle of radius 5 m. Use 3.14 for π.   [9.2b]

22. Find the length of a radius of the circle.   [9.2b]

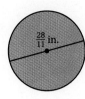

28⁄11 in.

23. Find the length of a diameter of the circle.   [9.2b]

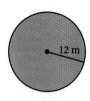

12 m

Find the area of each figure in Exercises 24–29.
[9.2a, b]

24.

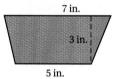

7 in.

3 in.

5 in.

25.

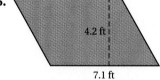

4.2 ft

7.1 ft

26.

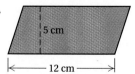

5 cm

12 cm

27.

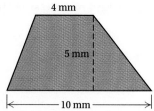

4 mm

5 mm

10 mm

28. Use $\frac{22}{7}$ for π.

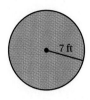

7 ft

29. Use 3.14 for π.

10 cm

30. A "Norman" window is designed with dimensions as shown. Find its area. Use 3.14 for π.   [9.2b]

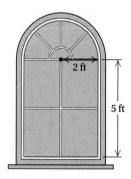

2 ft

5 ft

31. Find the measure of a complement of $\angle BAC$.
[9.4c]

C

41°   120°   D

B   A

32. Find the measure of a supplement of a 44° angle.
[9.4c]

For each right triangle, find the length of the side not given. Find an exact answer and an approximation to three decimal places. Assume that c represents the length of the hypotenuse. [9.5c]

33. $a = 15$, $b = 25$ **34.** $a = 4$, $c = 10$

35.

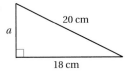

36.

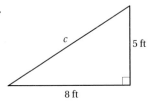

Find the volume of each figure. Use 3.14 for π. [9.6a]

37.

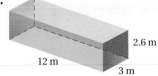

38.

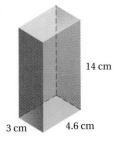

39.

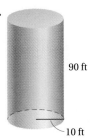

40.

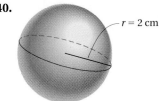

41.

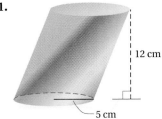

42. Convert 35°C to Fahrenheit. [9.7c]

43. Convert 68°F to Celsius. [9.7c]

44. A physician prescribed 650 mL per hour of a saline solution for a patient. How many liters of fluid did this patient receive in one day? [9.6c]

45. Find the simple interest on $5000 at 9.5% for 30 days. [8.6a]

46. Convert to percent notation: 0.47. [8.1b]

47. Convert to decimal notation: 56.7%. [8.1b]

48. Solve: $9x + 4 = 3x - 23$. [5.7b]

49. A hot air balloon travels 5 mi in $2\frac{1}{2}$ hr. At this rate, how far will the balloon travel in 12 hr? [7.4a]

50. Solve: $5(x - 1.5) = x + 2.5$. [5.7b]

Synthesis

51. ◈ Is a square a special type of parallelogram? Why or why not? [9.2a]

52. ◈ Which is a larger measure of volume: 1 m^3 or 27 ft^3? Explain how you can tell without using a calculator. [9.1c], [9.6a]

53. ◈ What weighs more: 32 oz or 1 kg? Explain how you can tell without using a calculator. [9.7a, b]

54. ▦ Find the area of the largest round pizza that can be baked in a 35-cm by 50-cm pan. [9.2b]

55. ▦ One lap around a standard running track is 440 yd. A marathon is 26 mi, 385 yd long. How many laps around a track does a marathon require? [9.1a]

56. Lumber that starts out at a certain measure must be trimmed to take out warps and get boards that are straight. Because of trimming, a "two-by-four" is trimmed to an actual size of $1\frac{1}{2}$ in. by $3\frac{1}{2}$ in. What percent of the wood in a 10-ft board is lost by trimming? [9.6c]

57. A community center has a rectangular swimming pool that is 50 ft wide, 100 ft long, and 10 ft deep. The center decides to fill the pool with water to a line that is 1 ft from the top. Water costs $2.25 per 1000 ft^3. How much does it cost to fill the pool? [9.6c]

Test: Chapter 9

Complete.

1. 9 ft = _____ in.

2. 280 cm = _____ m

3. 2 yd^2 = _____ ft^2

4. 5 km = _____ m

5. 8.7 mm = _____ cm

6. 4520 m^2 = _____ km^2

7. 3080 mL = _____ L

8. 3.8 kg = _____ g

9. 10 gal = _____ oz

10. 0.24 L = _____ mL

11. 4 lb = _____ oz

12. 4.11 T = _____ lb

13. Find the length of a radius of this circle.

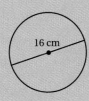

16 cm

14. Find the area of a circle of radius 4 m. Use 3.14 for π.

15. Find the circumference of a circle of radius 14 ft. Use $\frac{22}{7}$ for π.

Find the area.

16.

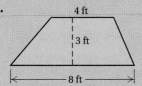

2.5 cm

10 cm

17.

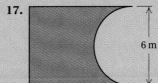

6 m

8 m

18.

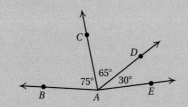

4 ft

3 ft

8 ft

19. A 5-in. by 7-in. photo is mounted on matting board that is 6 in. by 8 in. What is the area of the border?

20. Find the measure of a supplement of $\angle CAD$.

C

D

65°

75° 30°

B   A   E

1. [9.1a] 108

2. [9.1b] 2.8

3. [9.3a] 18

4. [9.1b] 5000

5. [9.1b] 0.87

6. [9.3b] 0.00452

7. [9.6b] 3.08

8. [9.7b] 3800

9. [9.6b] 1280

10. [9.6b] 240

11. [9.7a] 64

12. [9.7a] 8220

13. [9.2b] 8 cm

14. [9.2b] 50.24 m^2

15. [9.2b] 88 ft

16. [9.2a] 25 cm^2

17. [9.2b] 33.87 m^2

18. [9.2a] 18 ft^2

19. [9.2a] 13 in^2

20. [9.4c] 115°

For each right triangle, find the length of the side not given. Find an exact answer and an approximation to three decimal places.

21.

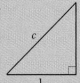

22.

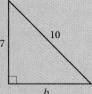

23. Find $\sqrt{121}$.

24. A ring box measures 6 cm by 8 cm by 4 cm. What is its volume?

In Exercises 25–27, find the volume in each figure. Use 3.14 for π.

25.

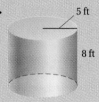

5 ft

8 ft

26.

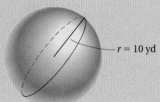

$r = 10$ yd

27.

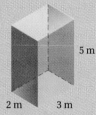

5 m

2 m   3 m

28. Dr. Pietrofiro wants a patient to receive 0.5 L of a dextrose solution every 8 hr. How many milliliters will the patient have received after one 48-hr period?

29. Convert 86°F to Celsius.

30. Convert 45°C to Fahrenheit.

Skill Maintenance

31. Find the simple interest on $5000 at 8.8% for 1 year.

32. Convert to percent notation: 0.93.

33. Convert to decimal notation: 93.2%.

34. Solve: $5 - 2x = 7(3 - x) + 4$.

35. If 5 gal of gas costs $7.45, how much will 9 gal cost?

36. Solve: $7x - 3.6 = 3x + 6.4$.

Synthesis

37. The measure of $\angle SMC$ is three times that of its complement. Find the measure of $\angle SMC$.

38. 🖩 A *board foot* is the amount of wood in a piece 12 in. by 12 in. by 1 in. A carpenter places the following order for a certain kind of lumber:

25 pieces: 2 in. by 4 in. by 8 ft;
32 pieces: 2 in. by 6 in. by 10 ft;
24 pieces: 2 in. by 8 in. by 12 ft.

The price of this type of lumber is $225 per thousand board feet. What is the total cost of the carpenter's order?

Cumulative Review: Chapters 1–9

Perform the indicated operations and simplify.

1. $4\dfrac{2}{3} + 5\dfrac{1}{2}$

2. $\left(\dfrac{1}{4}\right)^2 \div \left(\dfrac{1}{2}\right)^3 \times 2^4 + (10.3)(4)$

3. $120.5 - 32.98$

4. $-27{,}148 \div 22$

5. $14 \div [33 \div 11 + 8 \times 2 - (15 - 3)]$

6. $8^3 + 45 \cdot 24 - 9^2 \div 3$

Find fractional notation.

7. -6.23

8. 210%

Use $<$, $>$, or $=$ for ▩ to write a true sentence.

9. $\dfrac{5}{6}$ ▩ $\dfrac{7}{8}$

10. $\dfrac{5}{12}$ ▩ $\dfrac{3}{10}$

Complete.

11. $6 \text{ oz} = \underline{\hspace{1cm}} \text{ lb}$

12. $15°C = \underline{\hspace{1cm}} °F$

13. $0.087 \text{ L} = \underline{\hspace{1cm}} \text{ mL}$

14. $2.5 \text{ yd} = \underline{\hspace{1cm}} \text{ in.}$

15. $3 \text{ yd}^2 = \underline{\hspace{1cm}} \text{ ft}^2$

16. $17 \text{ cm} = \underline{\hspace{1cm}} \text{ m}$

17. Find the perimeter and the area.

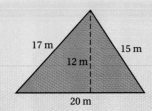

17 m 15 m 12 m 20 m

18. Combine like terms: $12a - 7 - 3a - 9$.

19. Graph: $y = -\dfrac{1}{3}x + 2$.

The line graph at right shows the average number of pounds of bananas eaten per person in the United States for the years 1991–1995 (**Source**: U.S. Department of Agriculture).

20. What was the average number of pounds of bananas that each person ate in 1995?

21. In what year did banana consumption peak?

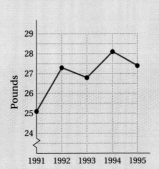

Solve.

22. $\dfrac{12}{15} = \dfrac{x}{18}$

23. $1 - 7x = 4 - (x + 9)$

24. $-15x = 265$

25. $x + \dfrac{3}{4} = \dfrac{7}{8}$

26. A case of returnable bottles contains 24 bottles. Several students find that together they have 168 bottles. How many cases can they fill?

27. Americans own 52 million dogs, 56 million cats, 45 million birds, 250 million fish, and 125 million other creatures as house pets. How many pets do Americans own?

28. Find the mean: 49, 53, 60, 62, 69.

29. What is the simple interest on $800 at 12% for $\frac{1}{4}$ year?

30. How long must a rope be in order to reach from the top of an 8-m tree to a point on the ground 15 m from the bottom of the tree?

31. The sales tax on a purchase of $5.50 is $0.33. What is the sales tax rate?

32. A bolt of fabric in a fabric store has $10\frac{3}{4}$ yd on it. A customer purchases $8\frac{5}{8}$ yd. How many yards remain on the bolt?

33. What is the cost, in dollars, of 15.6 gal of gasoline at 108.9¢ per gallon? Round to the nearest cent.

34. A box of powdered milk that makes 20 qt costs $4.99. A box that makes 8 qt costs $1.99. Which size has the lower unit price?

35. It is $\frac{7}{10}$ km from Ida's dormitory to the library. She starts to walk there, changes her mind after going $\frac{1}{4}$ of the distance, and returns home. How far did Ida walk?

Synthesis

36. A house sits on a lot measuring 75 ft by 200 ft. The lot is a corner lot, so there are sidewalks on two sides of the lot. If the sidewalks are 3 ft wide and 4 in. of snow falls, what volume of snow must be shoveled?

37. The U.S. Postal Service will not ship a box if the sum of the box's lengthwise perimeter and widthwise perimeter exceeds 108 in. Will a 1-ft by 2-ft by 3-ft box be accepted for shipping? Support your answer mathematically.

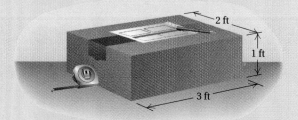

10

Polynomials

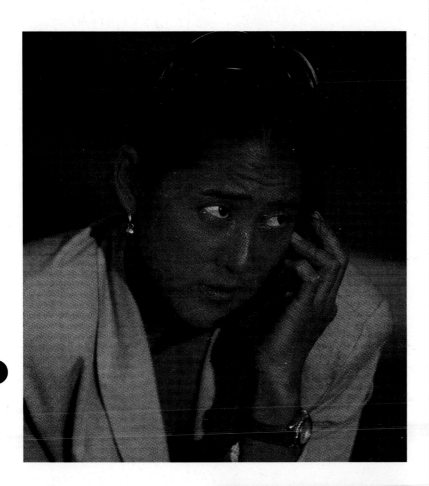

An Application

The *polynomial*

$$0.04x^3 - 0.23x^2 + 0.94x - 0.05$$

can be used to estimate the number of cellular phones in use, in millions, *x* years after 1985.

This problem appears as Exercise 79 in Section 10.1.

The Mathematics

We can evaluate this polynomial to estimate how many millions of cellular phones will be in use in 2004.

Pretest: Chapter 10

1. Add: $(5x^2 - 6x + 3) + (7x^2 + 4x - 13)$.

2. Find two equivalent expressions for the opposite of $6a^3b^2 - 7a^2b - 5$.

3. Subtract: $(3x^2 - 6x + 8) - (7x^2 + 11x - 13)$.

Evaluate.

4. 57^1

5. $(-23)^0$

6. $2x^3 - 5x^2$, for $x = 4$

Multiply.

7. $9a^3b(-2a^2b^2)$

8. $5x^2(7x^3 - 4x + 1)$

9. $(a + 4)(a - 7)$

10. $(a^2 - a)(2a^3 - a + 3)$

Factor.

11. $21a^3 + 30a^2 - 12a$

12. $15x^2y - 20xy^3$

Write an equivalent expression with positive exponents. Then simplify, if possible.

13. 7^{-2}

14. $5x^{-3}$

15. $\dfrac{a^{-8}}{b^{-5}c}$

16. $\left(\dfrac{5}{2}\right)^{-2}$

17. Write an expression equivalent to $\dfrac{1}{x^9}$ using a negative exponent.

Simplify. Use positive exponents in the answer.

18. $a^{-4} \cdot a^{-7}$

19. $(4x^7y^{-3})(-6x^2y^{-2})$

10.1 Addition and Subtraction of Polynomials

In Section 2.7, we defined a *term* as a number, a variable, a product of numbers and/or variables, or a quotient of numbers and/or variables. Thus expressions like

$$5x^2, \quad -34, \quad \frac{3}{4}ab^2, \quad xy^3z^5 \quad \text{and} \quad \frac{7n}{m}$$

are terms. A term is sometimes called a **monomial** if there is no division by a variable. Thus all of the expressions above, with the exception of $7n/m$, are monomials. Monomials are used to form **polynomials** like the following:

$$a^2b + c^3, \quad 5y + 3, \quad 3x^2 + 2x - 5, \quad -7a^3 + \tfrac{1}{2}a, \quad 37p^4, \quad x, \quad 0.$$

> A **polynomial** is a monomial or a combination of sums and/or differences of monomials.

The following algebraic expressions are *not* polynomials:

$$\textbf{(1)} \; \frac{x+3}{x-4}, \qquad \textbf{(2)} \; 5x^3 - 2x^2 + \frac{1}{x}, \qquad \textbf{(3)} \; \frac{1}{x^3-2}.$$

Expressions (1) and (3) are not polynomials because they represent quotients, not sums or differences. Expression (2) is not a polynomial because the term

$$\frac{1}{x}$$

is not a monomial.

a | Adding Polynomials

Recall that the commutative and associative laws are often used to make addition easier to perform. For example,

$$(9 + 17) + (1 + 13)$$

can be rewritten as the equivalent expression

$$(9 + 1) + (17 + 13), \quad \text{or} \quad 10 + 30.$$

A similar approach can be used for adding polynomials.

Example 1 Add: $(5x^3 + 4x^2 + 3x) + (2x^3 + 5x^2 - x)$.

$(5x^3 + 4x^2 + 3x) + (2x^3 + 5x^2 - x)$

$= (5x^3 + 2x^3) + (4x^2 + 5x^2) + (3x - x)$ Using the commutative and associative laws to pair up like terms

$= 7x^3 + 9x^2 + 2x$ Combining like terms. Remember that x means $1x$.

Objectives

a   Add polynomials.

b   Find the opposite of a polynomial.

c   Subtract polynomials.

d   Evaluate a polynomial.

For Extra Help

TAPE 18   MAC WIN   CD-ROM

Add.

1. $(7a^2 + 2a + 8) +$
$(2a^2 + a - 9)$ $9a^2 + 3a - 1$

Polynomials can be added even if their terms do not all form pairs of similar (like) terms.

Example 2   Add: $(3a^2 + 7a^2b) + (5a^2 - 6ab^2)$.

$$(3a^2 + 7a^2b) + (5a^2 - 6ab^2)$$
$$= (3a^2 + 5a^2) + 7a^2b - 6ab^2 \qquad \text{Note that } 7a^2b \text{ and } -6ab^2 \text{ are}$$
$$\qquad\qquad\qquad\qquad\qquad\qquad\quad \textit{not} \text{ similar terms.}$$
$$= 8a^2 + 7a^2b - 6ab^2 \qquad\quad \textbf{Combining like terms}$$

Example 3   Add: $(7x^2 + 5) + (5x^3 + 4x)$.

$$(7x^2 + 5) + (5x^3 + 4x) = 7x^2 + 5 + 5x^3 + 4x \qquad \text{There are no similar}$$
$$\qquad\qquad\qquad\qquad\qquad\qquad\qquad\qquad\qquad \text{terms here.}$$
$$= 5x^3 + 7x^2 + 4x + 5 \qquad \textbf{Rearranging the order}$$

2. $(5x^2y + 3x^2 + 4) +$
$(2x^2y + 4x)$

$7x^2y + 3x^2 + 4x + 4$

Note that in Example 3 we wrote the answer so that the powers of x decrease as we read from left to right. This **descending order** is the traditional way of expressing an answer, especially when the polynomials in the statement of the problem are given in descending order.

Do Exercises 1–3.

b | Opposites of Polynomials

To subtract a number, we can add its opposite. We can similarly subtract a polynomial by adding its opposite. To determine when two polynomials are opposites, recall that 5 and -5 are opposites, because $5 + (-5) = 0$.

> Two polynomials are **opposites,** or **additive inverses,** of each other if their sum is zero.

3. $(2a^3 + 17) + (2a^2 - 9a)$

$2a^3 + 2a^2 - 9a + 17$

To develop a method for finding the opposite of a polynomial, consider that

$$(5t^3 - 2) + (-5t^3 + 2) = 0 \quad \text{and} \quad (-9x^2 + x - 7) + (9x^2 - x + 7) = 0.$$

Since $(5t^3 - 2) + (-5t^3 + 2) = 0$, we see that the opposite of $(5t^3 - 2)$ is $(-5t^3 + 2)$. This can be said with purely algebraic symbolism:

The opposite of $(5t^3 - 2)$ is $-5t^3 + 2.$

$$- \qquad (5t^3 - 2) \qquad = \qquad -5t^3 + 2.$$

Similarly,

The opposite of $(-9x^2 + x - 7)$ is $9x^2 - x + 7.$

$$- \qquad (-9x^2 + x - 7) \qquad = \qquad 9x^2 - x + 7.$$

> We can find an equivalent polynomial for the opposite, or additive inverse, of a polynomial by replacing each term with its opposite—that is, *changing the sign of every term.*

Answers on page A-27

Example 4 Find two equivalent expressions for the opposite of

$$4x^5 - 7x^3 - 8x + \tfrac{5}{6}.$$

a) $-\left(4x^5 - 7x^3 - 8x + \tfrac{5}{6}\right)$ This is one expression for the opposite of $4x^5 - 7x^3 - 8x + \tfrac{5}{6}$.

b) $-4x^5 + 7x^3 + 8x - \tfrac{5}{6}$ Changing the sign of every term

Thus, $-\left(4x^5 - 7x^3 - 8x + \tfrac{5}{6}\right)$ is equivalent to $-4x^5 + 7x^3 + 8x - \tfrac{5}{6}$, and each is the opposite of the original polynomial $4x^5 - 7x^3 - 8x + \tfrac{5}{6}$.

Do Exercises 4–7.

Example 5 Simplify: $-\left(-7x^4 - \tfrac{5}{9}x^3 + 8x^2 - x + 67\right)$.

$$-\left(-7x^4 - \tfrac{5}{9}x^3 + 8x^2 - x + 67\right) = 7x^4 + \tfrac{5}{9}x^3 - 8x^2 + x - 67$$

Do Exercises 8–10.

c | Subtracting Polynomials

We can now subtract a polynomial by adding the opposite of that polynomial. That is, for any polynomials p and q, $p - q = p + (-q)$.

Example 6 Subtract:

$$(9x^5 + x^3 - 2x^2 + 4) - (2x^5 + x^4 - 4x^3 - 3x^2).$$

We have

$(9x^5 + x^3 - 2x^2 + 4) - (2x^5 + x^4 - 4x^3 - 3x^2)$

$= (9x^5 + x^3 - 2x^2 + 4) + [-(2x^5 + x^4 - 4x^3 - 3x^2)]$ Adding the opposite

$= (9x^5 + x^3 - 2x^2 + 4) + [-2x^5 - x^4 + 4x^3 + 3x^2]$ Finding the opposite by changing the sign of *each* term

$= 9x^5 + x^3 - 2x^2 + 4 - 2x^5 - x^4 + 4x^3 + 3x^2$

$= 7x^5 - x^4 + 5x^3 + x^2 + 4.$ Combining like terms

Do Exercises 11 and 12.

To shorten our work, we often begin by changing the sign of each term in the polynomial being subtracted.

Example 7 Subtract:

$$(5a^4 - 7a^3 + 5a^2b) - (-3a^4 + 4a^2b + 6).$$

We have

$(5a^4 - 7a^3 + 5a^2b) - (-3a^4 + 4a^2b + 6)$

$= 5a^4 - 7a^3 + 5a^2b + 3a^4 - 4a^2b - 6$

$= 8a^4 - 7a^3 + a^2b - 6.$ Combining like terms

Do Exercise 13.

Find two equivalent expressions for the opposite of each polynomial.

4. $12x^4 - 3x^2 + 4x$

$-(12x^4 - 3x^2 + 4x);$
$-12x^4 + 3x^2 - 4x$

5. $-4x^4 + 3x^2 - 4x$

$-(-4x^4 + 3x^2 - 4x);$
$4x^4 - 3x^2 + 4x)$

6. $-13x^6 + 2x^4 - 3x^2 + x - \tfrac{5}{13}$

$-\left(-13x^6 + 2x^4 - 3x^2 + x - \tfrac{5}{13}\right);$
$13x^6 - 2x^4 + 3x^2 - x + \tfrac{5}{13}$

7. $-8a^3b + 5ab^2 - 2ab$

$-(-8a^3b + 5ab^2 - 2ab);$
$8a^3b - 5ab^2 + 2ab$

Simplify.

8. $-(4x^3 - 6x + 3)$

$-4x^3 + 6x - 3$

9. $-(5x^3y + 3x^2y^2 - 7xy^3)$

$-5x^3y - 3x^2y^2 + 7xy^3$

10. $-\left(14x^{10} - \tfrac{1}{2}x^5 + 5x^3 - x^2 + 3x\right)$

$-14x^{10} + \tfrac{1}{2}x^5 - 5x^3 + x^2 - 3x$

Subtract.

11. $(7x^3 + 2x + 4) - (5x^3 - 4)$

$2x^3 + 2x + 8$

12. $(-3x^2 + 5x - 4) - (-4x^2 + 11x - 2)$

$x^2 - 6x - 2$

13. Subtract

$(7x^3 + 3x^2 - xy) - (5x^3 + 3xy + 2).$

$2x^3 + 3x^2 - 4xy - 2$

Answers on page A-27

14. Evaluate each expression for $a = 2$. (See Margin Exercise 1.)

a) $(7a^2 + 2a + 8) +$
$(2a^2 + a - 9)$ 41

b) $9a^2 + 3a - 1$ 41

15. In the situation of Example 9, what is the total number of games to be played in a league of 12 teams?   132

The perimeter of a square of side x is given by the polynomial $4x$.

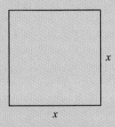

16. A baseball diamond is a square 90 ft on a side. Find the perimeter of a baseball diamond.   360 ft

17. Find the perimeter of a softball diamond that is 65 ft on a side.   260 ft

Answers on page A-27

---

d | **Evaluating Polynomials and Applications**

It is important to keep in mind that when we are finding the sum or difference of two polynomials, we are *not* solving an equation. Rather, we are finding an equivalent expression that is usually more concise. One reason we do this is to make it easier to evaluate the original expression.

Example 8 Evaluate both $(5x^3 + 4x^2 + 3x) + (2x^3 + 5x^2 - x)$ and $7x^3 + 9x^2 + 2x$ for $x = 2$ (see Example 1).

a) When x is replaced by 2 in $(5x^3 + 4x^2 + 3x) + (2x^3 + 5x^2 - x)$, we have

$$5 \cdot 2^3 + 4 \cdot 2^2 + 3 \cdot 2 + 2 \cdot 2^3 + 5 \cdot 2^2 - 2,$$

or $5 \cdot 8 + 4 \cdot 4 + 6 + 2 \cdot 8 + 5 \cdot 4 - 2,$

or $40 + 16 + 6 + 16 + 20 - 2,$ which is 96.

b) Similarly, when x is replaced by 2 in $7x^3 + 9x^2 + 2x$, we have

$$7 \cdot 2^3 + 9 \cdot 2^2 + 2 \cdot 2,$$

or $7 \cdot 8 + 9 \cdot 4 + 4,$

or $56 + 36 + 4.$ As expected, this is also 96.

Do Exercise 14.

Polynomials are frequently evaluated in real-world situations.

Example 9 *Athletics.* In a sports league of n teams in which all teams play each other twice, the total number of games to be played is given by the polynomial

$$n^2 - n.$$

A women's softball league has 10 teams. If each team plays every other team twice, what is the total number of games to be played?

We evaluate the polynomial for $n = 10$:

$$n^2 - n = 10^2 - 10 = 100 - 10 = 90.$$

The league plays 90 games.

Do Exercises 15–17.

Exercise Set 10.1

a Add.

1. $(2x + 7) + (-4x + 3)$ $-2x + 10$

2. $(6x + 1) + (-7x + 2)$ $-x + 3$

3. $(-9x + 5) + (x^2 + x - 3)$ $x^2 - 8x + 2$

4. $(x^2 - 5x + 4) + (8x - 9)$ $x^2 + 3x - 5$

5. $(x^2 - 7) + (x^2 + 7)$ $2x^2$

6. $(x^3 + x^2) + (2x^3 - 5x^2)$ $3x^3 - 4x^2$

7. $(6t^4 + 4t^3 - 1) + (5t^2 - t + 1)$ $6t^4 + 4t^3 + 5t^2 - t$

8. $(5t^2 - 3t + 12) + (2t^2 + 8t - 30)$ $7t^2 + 5t - 18$

9. $(3 + 4x + 6x^2 + 7x^3) + (6 - 4x + 6x^2 - 7x^3)$
$9 + 12x^2$

10. $(3x^4 - 6x - 5x^2 + 5) + (6x^2 - 4x^3 - 1 + 7x)$
$3x^4 - 4x^3 + x^2 + x + 4$

11. $(9x^8 - 7x^4 + 2x^2 + 5) + (8x^7 + 4x^4 - 2x)$
$9x^8 + 8x^7 - 3x^4 + 2x^2 - 2x + 5$

12. $(4x^5 - 6x^3 - 9x + 1) + (6x^3 + 9x^2 + 9x)$
$4x^5 + 9x^2 + 1$

13. $(9t^4 + 6t^3 - t^2 + 3t) + (5t^4 - 2t^3 + t - 7)$
$14t^4 + 4t^3 - t^2 + 4t - 7$

14. $(7t^5 - 3t^4 - 2t^2 + 5) + (3t^5 - 2t^4 + 4t^3 - t^2)$
$10t^5 - 5t^4 + 4t^3 - 3t^2 + 5$

15. $(-5x^4y^3 + 7x^3y^2 - 4xy^2) + (2x^3y^3 - 3x^3y^2 - 5xy)$
$-5x^4y^3 + 2x^3y^3 + 4x^3y^2 - 4xy^2 - 5xy$

16. $(-9a^5b^4 + 7a^3b^3 + 2a^2b^2) + (2a^4b^4 - 5a^3b^3 - a^2b^2)$
$-9a^5b^4 + 2a^4b^4 + 2a^3b^3 + a^2b^2$

17. $(8a^3b^2 + 5a^2b^2 + 6ab^2) + (5a^3b^2 - a^2b^2 - 4a^2b)$
$13a^3b^2 + 4a^2b^2 - 4a^2b + 6ab^2$

18. $(6x^3y^3 - 4x^2y^2 + 3xy^2) + (x^3y^3 + 7x^3y^2 - 2xy^2)$
$7x^3y^3 + 7x^3y^2 - 4x^2y^2 + xy^2$

19. $(17.5abc^3 + 4.3a^2bc) + (-4.9a^2bc - 5.2abc)$
$-0.6a^2bc + 17.5abc^3 - 5.2abc$

20. $(23.9x^3yz - 19.7x^2y^2z) + (-14.6x^3yz - 8x^2yz)$
$9.3x^3yz - 19.7x^2y^2z - 8x^2yz$

b Find two equivalent expressions for the opposite of each polynomial.

21. $-5x$ $-(-5x); 5x$

22. $x^2 - 3x$ $-(x^2 - 3x); -x^2 + 3x$

23. $-x^2 + 10x - 2$
$-(-x^2 + 10x - 2); x^2 - 10x + 2$

24. $-4x^3 - x^2 - x$
$-(-4x^3 - x^2 - x); 4x^3 + x^2 + x$

25. $12x^4 - 3x^3 + 3$
$-(12x^4 - 3x^3 + 3); -12x^4 + 3x^3 - 3$

26. $4x^3 - 6x^2 - 8x + 1$
$-(4x^3 - 6x^2 - 8x + 1);$
$-4x^3 + 6x^2 + 8x - 1$

Simplify.

27. $-(3x - 7)$ $-3x + 7$

28. $-(-2x + 4)$ $2x - 4$

29. $-(4x^2 - 3x + 2)$ $-4x^2 + 3x - 2$

30. $-(-6a^3 + 2a^2 - 9a + 1)$
$6a^3 - 2a^2 + 9a - 1$

31. $-\left(-4x^4 + 6x^2 + \frac{3}{4}x - 8\right)$
$4x^4 - 6x^2 - \frac{3}{4}x + 8$

32. $-(-5x^4 + 4x^3 - x^2 + 0.9)$
$5x^4 - 4x^3 + x^2 - 0.9$

c Subtract.

33. $(3x + 2) - (-4x + 3)$ $7x - 1$

34. $(6x + 1) - (-7x + 2)$ $13x - 1$

35. $(9t^2 + 7t + 5) - (5t^2 + t - 1)$ $4t^2 + 6t + 6$

36. $(8t^2 - 5t + 7) - (3t^2 - 2t + 1)$ $5t^2 - 3t + 6$

37. $(-6x + 2) - (x^2 + x - 3)$ $-x^2 - 7x + 5$

38. $(x^2 - 5x + 4) - (8x - 9)$ $x^2 - 13x + 13$

39. $(7a^2 + 5a - 9) - (2a^2 + 7)$ $5a^2 + 5a - 16$

40. $(8a^2 - 6a + 5) - (2a^2 - 19a)$ $6a^2 + 13a + 5$

41. $(6x^4 + 3x^3 - 1) - (4x^2 - 3x + 3)$
$6x^4 + 3x^3 - 4x^2 + 3x - 4$

42. $(-4x^2 + 2x) - (3x^3 - 5x^2 + 3)$
$-3x^3 + x^2 + 2x - 3$

43. $(1.2x^3 + 4.5x^2 - 3.8x) - (-3.4x^3 - 4.7x^2 + 23)$
$4.6x^3 + 9.2x^2 - 3.8x - 23$

44. $(0.5x^4 - 0.6x^2 + 0.7) - (2.3x^4 + 1.8x - 3.9)$
$-1.8x^4 - 0.6x^2 - 1.8x + 4.6$

45. $\left(\frac{5}{8}x^3 - \frac{1}{4}x - \frac{1}{3}\right) - \left(-\frac{1}{8}x^3 + \frac{1}{4}x - \frac{1}{3}\right)$ $\frac{3}{4}x^3 - \frac{1}{2}x$

46. $\left(\frac{1}{5}x^3 + 2x^2 - 0.1\right) - \left(-\frac{2}{5}x^3 + 2x^2 + 0.01\right)$ $\frac{3}{5}x^3 - 0.11$

47. $(5x^3y^3 + 8x^2y^2 + 7xy) - (3x^3y^3 - 2x^2y + 3xy)$
$2x^3y^3 + 8x^2y^2 + 2x^2y + 4xy$

48. $(3x^4y + 2x^3y - 7x^2y) - (5x^4y + 2x^2y^2 - 2x^2y)$
$-2x^4y + 2x^3y - 2x^2y^2 - 5x^2y$

|d| Evaluate each polynomial for $x = 4$.

49. $-5x + 2$ −18

50. $-3x + 1$ −11

51. $2x^2 - 5x + 7$ 19

52. $3x^2 + x + 7$ 59

53. $x^3 - 5x^2 + x$ −12

54. $7 - x + 3x^2$ 51

Evaluate each polynomial for $x = -1$.

55. $3x + 5$ 2

56. $6 - 2x$ 8

57. $x^2 - 2x + 1$ 4

58. $5x - 6 + x^2$ −10

59. $-3x^3 + 7x^2 - 3x - 2$ 11

60. $-2x^3 - 5x^2 + 4x + 3$ −4

Daily Accidents. The daily number of accidents N (average number of accidents per day) involving drivers of age a is approximated by the polynomial

$$N = 0.4a^2 - 40a + 1039.$$

61. Evaluate the polynomial for $a = 18$ to find the daily number of accidents involving 18-year-old drivers.

About 449

62. Evaluate the polynomial for $a = 20$ to find the daily number of accidents involving 20-year-old drivers.

399

Falling Distance. The distance s, in feet, traveled by a body falling freely from rest in t seconds is approximated by the polynomial

$$s = 16t^2.$$

$s = 16t^2$

63. A stone is dropped from a cliff and takes 8 sec to hit the ground. How high is the cliff?   1024 ft

64. A brick is dropped from a building and takes 3 sec to hit the ground. How high is the building?   144 ft

Total Revenue. Cutting Edge Electronics is marketing a new kind of stereo. *Total revenue* is the total amount of money taken in. The firm determines that when it sells x stereos, it will take in

$$280x - 0.4x^2 \text{ dollars.}$$

65. What is the total revenue from the sale of 75 stereos? $18,750

66. What is the total revenue from the sale of 100 stereos? $24,000

Total Cost. Cutting Edge Electronics determines that the total cost of producing x stereos is given by

$$5000 + 0.6x^2 \text{ dollars.}$$

67. What is the total cost of producing 500 stereos?

$155,000

68. What is the total cost of producing 650 stereos?

$258,500

69. A 10-lb fish serves 7 people. What is the ratio of servings to pounds?   [7.1a] $\frac{7}{10}$ serving per pound

70. A bicycle salesperson's commission rate is 22%. A commission of $783.20 is received. How many dollars worth of bicycles were sold?   [8.5b]

$3560

71. In 1998, the sales tax rate in Vermont was 5%. How much tax would be paid in Vermont for a computer that sold for $1350?   [8.5a] $67.50

72. Find the area of a rectangle that is 6.5 m by 4 m.   [5.8a]   26 m^2

73. Find the area of a circle with radius 20 cm. Use 3.14 for π.   [9.2b]   1256 cm^2

74. Melba earned $4740 for working 12 weeks. What was the rate of pay?   [7.2a] $395 per week

---

Synthesis

75. ◈ Is every term a monomial? Why or why not?

76. ◈ Suppose that two polynomials, each containing 3 terms, are added. Is it possible for the sum to contain more than 3 terms? fewer than 3 terms? exactly 3 terms? Explain.

77. ◈ Explain how the associative and commutative laws can be used when adding polynomials.

78. ▦ *Medicine.* When a person swallows 400 mg of ibuprofen, the number of milligrams in the bloodstream t hours later can be approximated by the polynomial

$$0.5t^4 + 3.45t^3 - 96.65t^2 + 347.7t$$
(where $0 \le t \le 6$).

Determine the amount of ibuprofen in the bloodstream **(a)** 1 hr after swallowing 400 mg; **(b)** 2 hr after swallowing 400 mg; **(c)** 6 hr after swallowing 400 mg.   **(a)** 255 mg; **(b)** 344.4 mg; **(c)** 0 mg

79. ▦ *Cellular Phone Sales.* The polynomial
$$0.04x^3 - 0.23x^2 + 0.94x - 0.05$$
can be used to estimate the number of cellular phones in use, in millions, x years after 1985. Predict the number of cellular phones in use in 2004.   209 million

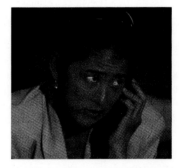

Perform the indicated operations and simplify.

80. $(7y^2 - 5y + 6) - (3y^2 + 8y - 12) + (8y^2 - 10y + 3)$

$12y^2 - 23y + 21$

81. $(3x^2 - 4x + 6) - (-2x^2 + 4) + (-5x - 3)$

$5x^2 - 9x - 1$

82. $(-y^4 - 7y^3 + y^2) + (-2y^4 + 5y - 2) - (-6y^3 + y^2)$

$-3y^4 - y^3 + 5y - 2$

83. $(-4 + x^2 + 2x^3) - (-6 - x + 3x^3) - (-x^2 - 5x^3)$

$2 + x + 2x^2 + 4x^3$

84. Complete: $9x^4 + \underline{\ 3x^4\ } + 5x^2 - 7x^3 + \underline{\ 2x^3\ } - 9 + \underline{\ (-7)\ } = 12x^4 - 5x^3 + 5x^2 - 16.$

85. Complete: $8t^4 + \underline{\ 9t^3\ } - 2t^3 + \underline{\ 2t^2\ } - 2t^2 + t - \underline{\ 4t\ } - 3 + \underline{\ 7\ } = 8t^4 + 7t^3 - 3t + 4.$

Collaborative Learning Manual

Determine the number of handshakes possible in a group.

10.2 Introduction to Multiplying and Factoring Polynomials

We now study how to multiply and factor certain polynomials.

a Multiplying Monomials

Recall that the area of a square with sides of length x is x^2.

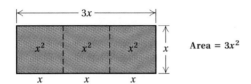

x Area $= x^2$

x

If a rectangle is 3 times as long as it is wide, we can represent its width by x and its length by $3x$.

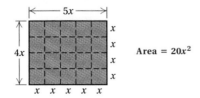

The area, $3x^2$, is the product of $3x$ and x. This product can be found using an associative law:

$$(3x)x = 3(xx) = 3x^2.$$

To find other products of monomials, we may need to use a commutative law as well.

Example 1   Multiply: $(4x)(5x)$.

$$
\begin{aligned}
(4x)(5x) &= 4 \cdot x \cdot 5 \cdot x && \text{Using an associative law}\\
&= 4 \cdot 5 \cdot x \cdot x && \text{Using a commutative law}\\
&= (4 \cdot 5)(xx) && \text{Using an associative law}\\
&= 20x^2
\end{aligned}
$$

Example 1 can be regarded as finding the area of a rectangle of width $4x$ and length $5x$. Note that the area consists of 20 squares, each of which has area x^2.

Area $= 20x^2$

Do Exercises 1 and 2.

Objectives

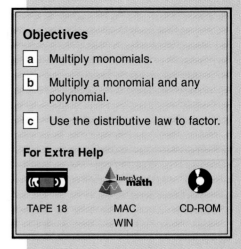

a   Multiply monomials.

b   Multiply a monomial and any polynomial.

c   Use the distributive law to factor.

For Extra Help

TAPE 18   InterAct math

MAC WIN   CD-ROM

Multiply.

1. $(6a)(3a)$ $18a^2$

2. $(-7x)(2x)$ $-14x^2$

Answers on page A-27

Multiply.

3. $(4a)(12a)$ $48a^2$

4. $(-m)(5m)$ $-5m^2$

5. $(-6a)(-7b)$ $42ab$

Multiply.

6. $a^5 \cdot a^4$ a^9

7. $(2x^8)(4x^5)$ $8x^{13}$

8. $(-7m^4)(-5m^7)$ $35m^{11}$

9. $(3a^5b^4)(5a^2b^8)$ $15a^7b^{12}$

Answers on page A-27

Usually the steps in Example 1 are combined: We multiply coefficients and we multiply variables.

Examples Multiply.

2. $(5x)(6x) = (5 \cdot 6)(x \cdot x)$ Multiplying the coefficients.
$= 30x^2$ Simplifying

3. $(3x)(-x) = (3x)(-1x)$ Rewriting $-x$ as $-1x$
$= (3)(-1)(x \cdot x)$
$= -3x^2$

4. $(7x)(4y) = (7 \cdot 4)(x \cdot y)$
$= 28xy$

Do Exercises 3–5.

Multiplying Powers with Like Bases

In later courses, you will likely learn several rules for manipulating exponents. The one rule that we develop now is useful when multiplying powers with like bases. Consider the following:

$$a^3 \cdot a^2 = \underbrace{(a \cdot a \cdot a)}_{3\ \text{factors}}\underbrace{(a \cdot a)}_{2\ \text{factors}} = \underbrace{a \cdot a \cdot a \cdot a \cdot a}_{5\ \text{factors}} = a^5.$$

Note that the exponent in a^5 is the sum of those in $a^3 \cdot a^2$. That is, $3 + 2 = 5$. Likewise,

$$b^4 \cdot b^3 = (b \cdot b \cdot b \cdot b)(b \cdot b \cdot b) = b^7, \quad \text{where} \quad 4 + 3 = 7.$$

Adding the exponents gives the correct result.

> ► **THE PRODUCT RULE**
>
> For any number a and any positive integers m and n,
> $$a^m \cdot a^n = a^{m+n}.$$
> (When multiplying with exponential notation, if the bases are the same, keep the base and add the exponents.)

Examples Multiply and simplify.

5. $x^2 \cdot x^5 = x^{2+5}$ Adding exponents
$= x^7$

6. $(3a^4)(5a^2) = (3 \cdot 5)(a^4 \cdot a^2)$ Multiplying coefficients; adding exponents
$= 15a^6$

7. $(-4x^2y^3)(3x^6y^7) = (-4 \cdot 3)(x^2 \cdot x^6)(y^3 \cdot y^7)$
$= -12x^8y^{10}$

Do Exercises 6–9.

We have not yet determined what the number 1 will mean when used as an exponent. Consider the following:

$$m \cdot m^2 = m \cdot m \cdot m = m^3;$$

$$x \cdot x^3 = x \cdot x \cdot x \cdot x = x^4;$$

and $a \cdot a^4 = a \cdot a \cdot a \cdot a \cdot a = a^5.$

Note that if $m = m^1$, $x = x^1$, and $a = a^1$, the same results can be found using the product rule:

$$m \cdot m^2 = m^1 \cdot m^2 = m^3;$$

$$x \cdot x^3 = x^1 \cdot x^3 = x^4;$$

and $a \cdot a^4 = a^1 \cdot a^4 = a^5.$

This suggests the following definition.

> ▶ $b^1 = b$ for any number b.

Example 8 Evaluate 5^1 and -23^1.

$5^1 = 5;$

$-23^1 = -23.$ We read -23^1 as "the opposite of 23^1."
To write -23 to the first, we would write $(-23)^1$.

Do Exercise 10.

b | Multiplying a Monomial and Any Polynomial

When a polynomial contains two terms, it is called a **binomial**. The product of the monomial x and the binomial $x + 2$ can be visualized as the area of a rectangle with width x and length $x + 2$.

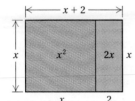

Area $= x(x + 2)$
$= x \cdot x + x \cdot 2$
$= x^2 + 2x$

Although many products of monomials and polynomials are difficult to visualize geometrically, the distributive law can always be used to find these products algebraically (pronounced al-je-bray´-ik-ally).

Example 9 Multiply: $2x$ and $5x + 3$.

$2x(5x + 3) = 2x \cdot 5x + 2x \cdot 3$ Using the distributive law

$= 10x^2 + 6x$ Multiplying the monomials

10. Evaluate 7^1 and -19^1. $7; -19$

Answer on page A-27

Multiply.

11. $4x$ and $3x + 5$ $12x^2 + 20x$

12. $3a(2a^2 - 5a + 7)$

$6a^3 - 15a^2 + 21a$

13. $4a^3b^2(2a^2 + 5b^4)$

$8a^5b^2 + 20a^3b^6$

Answers on page A-27

Example 10   Multiply: $5x(2x^2 - 3x + 4)$.

$$5x(2x^2 - 3x + 4) = 5x \cdot 2x^2 - 5x \cdot 3x + 5x \cdot 4$$
$$= 10x^3 - 15x^2 + 20x \qquad \text{Note that } x \cdot x^2 = x^1 \cdot x^2 = x^3.$$

Example 11   Multiply: $-3r^2s(2r^3s^2 - 5rs)$.

$$-3r^2s(2r^3s^2 - 5rs) = -3r^2s \cdot 2r^3s^2 - (-3r^2s)5rs$$
$$= -6r^5s^3 + 15r^3s^2$$

Do Exercises 11–13.

c Factoring

Factoring is the reverse of multiplying. To factor, we use the distributive law, beginning with a sum or a difference of two terms that contain a common factor:

$$ab + ac = a(b + c) \quad \text{and} \quad rs - rt = r(s - t).$$

> To **factor** an expression is to find an equivalent expression that is a product.

We have already factored polynomials in this text, although we did not call the process factoring at the time. For example, in Section 2.7, we factored when we first learned how to combine like terms (see p. 123).

$$5x + 3x = (5 + 3)x \qquad \text{Here we factored } 5x + 3x.$$
$$= 8x. \qquad \text{See also Sections 4.3 and 5.2.}$$

To *factor* an expression like $10y + 15$, we find an equivalent expression that is a product. To do this, we look to see if both of the terms have a factor in common. If there *is* a common factor, we can "factor it out" using the distributive law. Note the following:

$10y$ has the factors 10, 5, 2, 1, y, $2y$, $5y$, and $10y$;

15 has the factors 15, 5, 3, 1.

We generally factor out the largest common factor. In this case, that factor is 5 (which is the *only* common factor here). Thus,

$$10y + 15 = 5 \cdot 2y + 5 \cdot 3 \qquad \text{Try to do this step mentally.}$$
$$= 5(2y + 3). \qquad \text{Using the distributive law}$$

Examples Factor.

12. $5x - 10 = 5 \cdot x - 5 \cdot 2$ Try to do this step mentally.

$\qquad = 5(x - 2)$ You can check by multiplying.

13. $9x + 27y - 9 = 9 \cdot x + 9 \cdot 3y - 9 \cdot 1$

$\qquad\qquad\qquad = 9(x + 3y - 1)$

CAUTION! Note that although $3(3x + 9y - 3)$ is also equivalent to $9x + 27y - 9$, it is *not* factored "completely." However, we can complete the process by factoring out another factor of 3:

$$9x + 27y - 9 = 3(3x + 9y - 3) = 3 \cdot 3(x + 3y - 1) = 9(x + 3y - 1).$$

Remember to factor out the *largest common factor.*

Examples Factor. Try to write just the answer.

14. $-3x + 6y - 9z = -3(x - 2y + 3z)$

We generally factor out a negative when the first coefficient is negative. The way we factor can depend on the situation in which we are working. We might also factor as follows:

$$-3x + 6y - 9z = 3(-x + 2y - 3z).$$

15. $18z - 12x - 24 = 6(3z - 2x - 4)$ To check, multiply:

$$6(3z - 2x - 4) = 6 \cdot 3z - 6 \cdot 2x - 6 \cdot 4$$
$$= 18z - 12x - 24.$$

Remember: An expression is factored when it is written as a product.

Do Exercises 14–17.

When exponents appear, it is important to keep in mind the product rule.

Examples Factor.

16. $7x^2 + 7x = 7x(x + 1)$ The largest common factor is 7x.

17. $10a^5 + 5a^3 + 15a^2 = 5a^2(2a^3 + a + 3)$ The largest common factor of 10, 5, and 15 is 5. The largest common factor of a^5, a^3, and a^2 is a^2.

18. $8xy^3 - 6x^2y = 2xy(4y^2 - 3x)$ To check, multiply:

$$2xy(4y^2 - 3x) = 2xy \cdot 4y^2 - 2xy \cdot 3x$$
$$= 8xy^3 - 6x^2y.$$

Note in Example 17 that the *largest* common factor of a is the *smallest* of the three powers that appear in the original polynomial.

Do Exercises 18–20.

Factor.

14. $6z - 12$ $6(z - 2)$

15. $3x - 6y + 9$ $3(x - 2y + 3)$

16. $16a - 36b + 42$

$2(8a - 18b + 21)$

17. $-12x + 32y - 16z$

$-4(3x - 8y + 4z)$

Factor.

18. $5a^3 + 5a$ $5a(a^2 + 1)$

19. $14x^3 - 7x^2 + 21x$

$7x(2x^2 - x + 3)$

20. $9a^2b - 6ab^2$ $3ab(3a - 2b)$

Answers on page A-27

Improving Your Math Study Skills

Preparing for a Final Exam

Best Scenario: Two Weeks of Study Time

The best scenario for preparing for a final exam is to do so over a period of at least two weeks. Work in a diligent, disciplined manner, doing some final-exam preparation *each* day. Here is a detailed plan that many find useful.

1. **Begin by browsing through each chapter, reviewing the highlighted or boxed information regarding important formulas in both the text and the Summary and Review.** There may be some formulas that you will need to memorize.

2. **Retake all chapter tests that you took, assuming your instructor has returned them. Otherwise, use the chapter tests in the book.** Restudy the objectives in the text that correspond to each question you missed.

3. **Then work the Cumulative Review that covers all chapters up to that point.** Be careful to avoid any questions corresponding to objectives not covered. Again, restudy the objectives in the text that correspond to each question you missed.

4. **If you are still having difficulty, use the supplements for extra review.** For example, you might check out the videotapes, the *Student's Solutions Manual,* or the InterAct Math Tutorial Software.

5. **For remaining difficulties, see your instructor, go to a tutoring session, or participate in a study group.**

6. **Check for former final exams that may be on file in the math department or a study center, or with students who have already taken the course.** Use them for practice, being alert to trouble spots.

7. **Take the Final Examination in the text during the last couple of days before the final.** Set aside the same amount of time that you will have for the final. See how much of the final exam you can complete under test-like conditions.

Moderate Scenario: Three Days to Two Weeks of Study Time

1. **Begin by browsing through each chapter, reviewing the highlighted or boxed information regarding important formulas in both the text and the Summary and Review.** There may be some formulas that you will need to memorize.

2. **Retake all chapter tests that you took, assuming your instructor has returned them. Otherwise, use the chapter tests in the book.** Restudy the objectives in the text that correspond to each question you missed.

3. **Then work the last Cumulative Review in the portion of the text that you covered.** Avoid any questions corresponding to objectives not covered. Again, restudy the objectives in the text that correspond to each question you missed.

4. **For remaining difficulties, see your instructor, go to a tutoring session, or participate in a study group.**

5. **Take the Final Examination in the text during the last couple of days before the final.** Set aside the same amount of time that you will have for the final. See how much of the final exam you can complete under test-like conditions.

Worst Scenario: One or Two Days of Study Time

1. **Begin by browsing through each chapter, reviewing the highlighted or boxed information regarding important formulas in both the text and the Summary and Review.** There may be some formulas that you will need to memorize.

2. **Then work the last Cumulative Review in the portion of the text that you covered.** Avoid any questions corresponding to objectives not covered. Restudy the objectives in the text that correspond to each question you missed.

3. **Attend a final-exam review session if one is available.**

4. **Take the Final Examination in the text as preparation for the final.** Set aside the same amount of time that you will have for the final. See how much of the final exam you can complete under test-like conditions.

Promise yourself that next semester you will allow a more appropriate amount of time for final exam preparation.

Exercise Set 10.2

a Multiply.

1. $(5a)(9a)$ $45a^2$

2. $(7x)(6x)$ $42x^2$

3. $(-4x)(15x)$ $-60x^2$

4. $(-9a)(10a)$ $-90a^2$

5. $(7x^5)(4x^3)$ $28x^8$

6. $(10a^2)(3a^2)$ $30a^4$

7. $(-0.1x^6)(0.2x^4)$ $-0.02x^{10}$

8. $(0.3x^3)(-0.4x^6)$ $-0.12x^9$

9. $(5x^2y^3)(7x^4y^9)$ $35x^6y^{12}$

10. $(6a^3b^4)(2a^4b^7)$ $12a^7b^{11}$

11. $(4a^3b^4c^2)(3a^5b^4)$ $12a^8b^8c^2$

12. $(7x^3y^5z^2)(8x^3z^4)$ $56x^6y^5z^6$

13. $(3x^2)(-4x^3)(2x^6)$ $-24x^{11}$

14. $(-2y^5)(10y^4)(-3y^3)$ $60y^{12}$

b Multiply.

15. $3x(-x + 5)$ $-3x^2 + 15x$

16. $2x(4x - 6)$ $8x^2 - 12x$

17. $-3x(x - 1)$ $-3x^2 + 3x$

18. $-5x(-x - 1)$ $5x^2 + 5x$

19. $x^2(x^3 + 1)$ $x^5 + x^2$

20. $-2x^3(x^2 - 1)$ $-2x^5 + 2x^3$

21. $3x(2x^2 - 6x + 1)$
  $6x^3 - 18x^2 + 3x$

22. $-4x(2x^3 - 6x^2 - 5x + 1)$
  $-8x^4 + 24x^3 + 20x^2 - 4x$

23. $4xy(3x^2 + 2y)$
  $12x^3y + 8xy^2$

24. $5xy(3x^2 - 6y^2)$
  $15x^3y - 30xy^3$

25. $3a^2b(4a^5b^2 - 3a^2b^2)$
  $12a^7b^3 - 9a^4b^3$

26. $4a^2b^2(2a^3b - 5ab^2)$
  $8a^5b^3 - 20a^3b^4$

c Factor. Check by multiplying.

27. $2x + 6$ $2(x + 3)$

28. $3x + 12$ $3(x + 4)$

29. $7a - 21$ $7(a - 3)$

30. $9a - 18$ $9(a - 2)$

31. $14x + 21y$

$7(2x + 3y)$

32. $8x - 10y$

$2(4x - 5y)$

33. $9a - 27b + 81$

$9(a - 3b + 9)$

34. $5x + 10 + 15y$

$5(x + 2 + 3y)$

35. $24 - 6m$

$6(4 - m)$

36. $32 - 4y$

$4(8 - y)$

37. $-16 - 8x + 40y$

$-8(2 + x - 5y)$

38. $-35 + 14x - 21y$

$-7(5 - 2x + 3y)$

39. $3x^5 + 3x$

$3x(x^4 + 1)$

40. $5x^6 + 5x$

$5x(x^5 + 1)$

41. $a^3 - 8a^2$

$a^2(a - 8)$

42. $a^5 - 9a^2$

$a^2(a^3 - 9)$

43. $8x^3 - 6x^2 + 2x$

$2x(4x^2 - 3x + 1)$

44. $9x^4 - 12x^3 + 3x$

$3x(3x^3 - 4x^2 + 1)$

45. $12a^4b^3 + 18a^5b^2$

$6a^4b^2(2b + 3a)$

46. $15a^5b^2 + 20a^2b^3$

$5a^2b^2(3a^3 + 4b)$

Skill Maintenance

47. When used for a singles match, a regulation tennis court is 27 ft by 78 ft. Find its perimeter. [2.7c]

210 ft

48. The Floral Doctor's delivery van traveled 147 mi on 10.5 gal of gas. How many miles per gallon did the van get? [7.2a]   14 mpg

49. Ramon's new truck gets 21 miles per gallon. This is 20% more than the mileage his old truck got. What mileage did the old truck get? [8.4b]   17.5 mpg

50. A 5% sales tax is added to the price of a two-speed washing machine. If the machine is priced at $399, find the total amount paid. [8.5a] $418.95

51. Of the 8 fish Mac caught, 3 were trout. What percentage were not trout? [8.4a]   62.5%

52. The diameter of a compact disc is 12 cm. What is its circumference? (Use 3.14 for π.) [9.2b]   37.68 cm

Synthesis

53. ◈ Describe a method for creating a binomial that has $5x^2$ as its largest common factor.

54. ◈ If all of a polynomial's coefficients are prime, is it still possible to factor the polynomial? Why or why not?

55. ◈ Explain in your own words why the product rule "works."

Factor.

56. ▦ $391x^{391} + 299x^{299}$ $23x^{299}(17x^{92} + 13)$

57. ▦ $703a^{437} + 437a^{703}$ $19a^{437}(37 + 23a^{266})$

58. $84a^7b^9c^{11} - 42a^8b^6c^{10} + 49a^9b^7c^8$ $7a^7b^6c^8(12b^3c^3 - 6ac^2 + 7a^2b)$

59. Draw a figure similar to those preceding Examples 1 and 9 to show that $2x \cdot 3x = 6x^2$.   Answer to Exercise 59 can be found on p. A-28.

10.3 More Multiplication of Polynomials

a | Multiplying Two Binomials

To find an equivalent expression for the product of two binomials, we use the distributive law more than once. In the example that follows, the distributive law is used three times.

Example 1 Multiply: $x + 5$ and $x + 4$.

$$(\boxed{x + 5})(x + 4) = (\boxed{x + 5})x + (\boxed{x + 5})4 \qquad \text{Using the distributive law}$$

$$= x \cdot x + 5 \cdot x + x \cdot 4 + 5 \cdot 4 \qquad \text{Using the distributive law on each part}$$

$$= x^2 + 5x + 4x + 20 \qquad \text{Multiplying the monomials}$$

$$= x^2 + 9x + 20 \qquad \text{Combining like terms}$$

Do Exercises 1 and 2.

We can visualize the product $(x + 5)(x + 4)$ as the area of a rectangle with width $x + 4$ and length $x + 5$. Note that the total area is the sum of the four smaller areas.

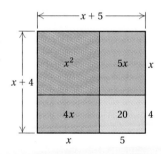

Area $= (x + 5)(x + 4)$
$= x \cdot x + 4x + 5x + 5 \cdot 4$
$= x^2 + 9x + 20$

More complicated products of binomials are not as easily visualized, but can be simplified using the steps of Example 1.

Example 2 Multiply: $4x + 3$ and $x - 2$.

$$(4x + 3)(x - 2) = (4x + 3)(x + (-2)) \qquad \text{Rewriting } x - 2 \text{ as } x + (-2)$$

$$= (\boxed{4x + 3})x + (\boxed{4x + 3})(-2) \qquad \text{Using the distributive law}$$

$$= 4x \cdot x + 3 \cdot x + 4x(-2) + 3(-2) \qquad \text{Using the distributive law on each part}$$

$$= 4x^2 + 3x + (-8x) + (-6) \qquad \text{Multiplying monomials}$$

$$= 4x^2 - 5x - 6 \qquad \text{Combining like terms}$$

Do Exercises 3 and 4.

Note in Example 1 that four products were found: $x \cdot x$, $x \cdot 4$, $5 \cdot x$, and $5 \cdot 4$. Similarly, in Example 2 we found $4x \cdot x$, $4x(-2)$, $3 \cdot x$, and $3(-2)$. These products are found by multiplying the First terms, the Outer terms, the Inner terms, and the Last terms in the binomials. We use the word FOIL to help remember these products.

Objectives

a Multiply two binomials.

b Multiply any two polynomials.

For Extra Help

TAPE 18   InterAct math   CD-ROM
           MAC
           WIN

Multiply.

1. $x + 8$ and $x + 5$

$x^2 + 13x + 40$

2. $(x + 5)(x - 4)$

$x^2 + x - 20$

Multiply.

3. $5x + 3$ and $x - 4$

$5x^2 - 17x - 12$

4. $(2x - 3)(3x - 5)$

$6x^2 - 19x + 15$

Answers on page A-28

Use FOIL to multiply.

5. $(x + 3)(x + 5)$ $x^2 + 8x + 15$

6. $(x - 3)(x - 8)$ $x^2 - 11x + 24$

Multiply.

7. $(x^2 + 3x - 4)(x^2 + 5)$

$x^4 + 3x^3 + x^2 + 15x - 20$

8. $(3y^2 - 7)(2y^3 - 2y + 5)$

$6y^5 - 20y^3 + 15y^2 + 14y - 35$

Multiply.

9. $3x^2 - 2x + 4$

$\underline{ x + 5}$

$3x^3 + 13x^2 - 6x + 20$

Answers on page A-28

Example 3   Use FOIL to multiply $(x + 3)(x + 7)$.

We have

First   Last

$(x + 3)(x + 7)$

Inner

Outer

$$\begin{array}{cccc} \text{F} & \text{O} & \text{I} & \text{L} \end{array}$$
$$(x + 3)(x + 7) = x \cdot x + 7 \cdot x + 3 \cdot x + 3 \cdot 7$$
$$= x^2 + 7x + 3x + 21$$
$$= x^2 + 10x + 21.$$

Do Exercises 5 and 6.

b | Multiplying Any Polynomials

A polynomial containing three terms is called a **trinomial**. To find the product of a binomial and a trinomial, we again use the distributive law.

Example 4   Multiply: $(x^2 + 2x - 3)(x^2 + 4)$.

$$(\boxed{x^2 + 2x - 3})(x^2 + 4) = (\boxed{x^2 + 2x - 3})x^2 + (\boxed{x^2 + 2x - 3})4$$
$$= x^2x^2 + 2xx^2 - 3x^2 + x^2 \cdot 4 + 2x \cdot 4 - 3 \cdot 4$$
$$= x^4 + 2x^3 - 3x^2 + 4x^2 + 8x - 12$$
$$= x^4 + 2x^3 + x^2 + 8x - 12 \qquad \text{Combining like terms}$$

Do Exercises 7 and 8.

> To multiply two polynomials P and Q, select one of the polynomials—say, P. Then multiply each term of P by every term of Q and combine like terms.

Columns can be used for long multiplication. To do so, we multiply each term at the top by every term below. We write like terms in columns and add the results. Such multiplication is like multiplying numbers:

$$\begin{array}{r} 2\ 3\ 1 \\ \times\ \ 3\ 2 \\ \hline 4\ 6\ 2 \\ 6\ 9\ 3\ 0 \\ \hline 7\ 3\ 9\ 2 \end{array}$$

$$\begin{array}{r} 2\ 3\ 1 \\ \times\ \ \ \ 3\ 2 \\ \hline 400 + 60 + 2 \\ 6000 +\ 900 + 30 \\ \hline 6000 + 1300 + 90 + 2 \end{array}$$

$= 200 + 30 + 1$
$= 30 + 2$
$= 2(231) = 2(200 + 30 + 1)$
$= 30(231) = 30(200 + 30 + 1)$
$= 7392$

Example 5   Multiply: $(4x^2 - 2x + 3)(x + 2)$.

$$\begin{array}{r} 4x^2 - 2x + 3 \\ x + 2 \\ \hline 8x^2 - 4x + 6 \\ 4x^3 - 2x^2 + 3x \\ \hline 4x^3 + 6x^2 - \ x + 6 \end{array}$$

It helps that both polynomials are in descending order.

Multiplying the top row by 2

Multiplying the top row by x

Combining like terms

Line up like terms in columns.

Do Exercise 9.

Exercise Set 10.3

a Multiply.

1. $(x + 7)(x + 2)$
$x^2 + 9x + 14$

2. $(x + 5)(x + 2)$
$x^2 + 7x + 10$

3. $(x + 5)(x - 2)$
$x^2 + 3x - 10$

4. $(x + 1)(x - 3)$
$x^2 - 2x - 3$

5. $(x + 6)(x - 2)$
$x^2 + 4x - 12$

6. $(x - 4)(x - 3)$
$x^2 - 7x + 12$

7. $(x - 7)(x - 3)$
$x^2 - 10x + 21$

8. $(x + 3)(x - 3)$
$x^2 - 9$

9. $(x + 6)(x - 6)$
$x^2 - 36$

10. $(5 - x)(5 - 2x)$
$25 - 15x + 2x^2$

11. $(3 + x)(6 + 2x)$
$18 + 12x + 2x^2$

12. $(2x + 5)(2x + 5)$
$4x^2 + 20x + 25$

13. $(3x - 4)(3x - 4)$
$9x^2 - 24x + 16$

14. $(5x - 1)(5x + 2)$
$25x^2 + 5x - 2$

15. $\left(x - \frac{5}{2}\right)\left(x + \frac{2}{5}\right)$
$x^2 - \frac{21}{10}x - 1$

16. $\left(x + \frac{4}{3}\right)\left(x + \frac{3}{2}\right)$
$x^2 + \frac{17}{6}x + 2$

b Multiply.

17. $(x^2 + x + 1)(x - 1)$ $x^3 - 1$

18. $(x^2 - x + 2)(x + 2)$ $x^3 + x^2 + 4$

19. $(2x + 1)(2x^2 + 6x + 1)$
$4x^3 + 14x^2 + 8x + 1$

20. $(3x - 1)(4x^2 - 2x - 1)$
$12x^3 - 10x^2 - x + 1$

21. $(y^2 - 3)(3y^2 - 6y + 2)$
$3y^4 - 6y^3 - 7y^2 + 18y - 6$

22. $(3y^2 - 3)(y^2 + 6y + 1)$
$3y^4 + 18y^3 - 18y - 3$

23. $(x^3 + x^2)(x^3 + x^2 - x)$
$x^6 + 2x^5 - x^3$

24. $(x^3 - x^2)(x^3 - x^2 + x)$
$x^6 - 2x^5 + 2x^4 - x^3$

25. $(2t^2 - t - 4)(3t^2 + 2t - 1)$
$6t^4 + t^3 - 16t^2 - 7t + 4$

26. $(3a^2 - 5a + 2)(2a^2 - 3a + 4)$
$6a^4 - 19a^3 + 31a^2 - 26a + 8$

27. $(x - x^3 + x^5)(x^2 - 1 + x^4)$
$x^9 - x^5 + 2x^3 - x$

28. $(x - x^3 + x^5)(3x^2 + 3x^6 + 3x^4)$
$3x^{11} + 3x^7 + 3x^3$

Skill Maintenance

29. A sidewalk of uniform width is built around three sides of a store, as shown in the figure. What is the area of the sidewalk? [1.8a] 912 m²

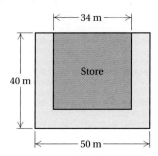

30. A real estate agent's commission rate is 6%. A commission of $7380 is received on the sale of a home. For how much did the home sell? [8.5b]

$123,000

31. What percent of 24 is 32? [8.3b] $133\frac{1}{3}$%, or 133.$\overline{3}$%

32. 39 is 150% of what number? [8.3b] 26

33. In 1998, the New York Yankees won 111 of their 162 games. What percentage of their games did the Yankees win? [7.4a] 68.5%

34. The Sanchez's flower garden covers a 14-ft–wide circular region of their yard. Find the garden's area. Use $\frac{22}{7}$ for π. [9.2b] 154 ft²

Synthesis

35. ◆ A student insists that since $x \cdot x$ is x^2 and $5 \cdot 4 = 20$, it follows that $(x + 5)(x + 4) = x^2 + 20$. How could you convince the student that this is not correct?

36. ◆ Is the product of two binomials always a trinomial? Why or why not?

37. ◆ Ron says that since $(xy)^2 = (xy) \cdot (xy) = x^2y^2$, it follows that $(x + y)^2 = x^2 + y^2$. Is he correct? Why or why not?

38. ▦ (See Example 4.) Check that the expressions $(x^2 + 2x - 3)(x^2 + 4)$ and $x^4 + 2x^3 + x^2 + 8x - 12$ are equivalent by evaluating both expressions for $x = 5$, $x = 3.5$, and $x = -1.2$.

928, 928: 264.0625, 264.0625; −21.5424, −21.5424

39. Simplify: $(x + 2)(x + 3) + (x - 4)^2$. $2x^2 - 3x + 22$

For each figure below, find a simplified expression for **(a)** the perimeter and **(b)** the area.

40.

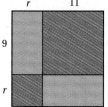

r   11

9

r

(a) $4r + 40$; **(b)** $r^2 + 20r + 99$

41.

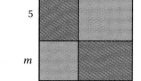

5

m

m   5

(a) $4m + 20$; **(b)** $m^2 + 10m + 25$

42. Find a polynomial for the shaded area. $78t^2 + 40t$

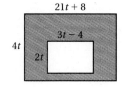

21*t* + 8

4*t*   3*t* − 4   2*t*

43. A box with a square bottom is to be made from a 12-in.–square piece of cardboard. Squares with side x are cut out of the corners and the sides are folded up. Find polynomials for the volume and the outside surface area of the box.

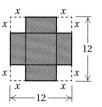

$V = 4x^3 - 48x^2 + 144x$; $S = -4x^2 + 144$

Multiply.

44. $(3x - 5)^2$ $9x^2 - 30x + 25$

45. $(9x + 4)^2$ $81x^2 + 72x + 16$

Visualize polynomials for factoring.

Collaborative Learning Manual

10.4 Integers as Exponents

We have already used the numbers 1, 2, 3, . . . , as exponents. Here we consider 0, as well as negative integers, as exponents.

a Zero as an Exponent

Look for a pattern in the following:

$$8 \cdot 8 \cdot 8 \cdot 8 = 8^4$$
$$8 \cdot 8 \cdot 8 = 8^3$$
$$8 \cdot 8 = 8^2$$
$$8 = 8^1$$
$$1 = 8^?.$$

We divide by 8 each time.

The exponents decrease by 1 each time. To continue the pattern, we would say that

$$1 = 8^0.$$

We make the following definition.

> $b^0 = 1$, for any nonzero number b.

We leave 0^0 undefined.

Example 1 Evaluate 3^0 and $(-7.3)^0$.

$$3^0 = 1;$$
$$(-7.3)^0 = 1 \qquad \text{Note that } -7.3^0 = -1 \cdot 7.3^0 = -1 \cdot 1 = -1 \neq (-7.3)^0.$$

Do Exercises 1–3.

Example 2 Evaluate $m^0 + 5$ for $m = 9$.

$$m^0 + 5 = 9^0 + 5 = 1 + 5 = 6$$

Example 3 Evaluate $(3x + 2)^0$ for $x = -5$.

We substitute -5 for x and follow the rules for order of operations:

$$(3x + 2)^0 = (3(-5) + 2)^0 \qquad \text{Substituting}$$
$$= (-15 + 2)^0 \qquad \text{Multiplying}$$
$$= (-13)^0$$
$$= 1.$$

CAUTION! Students often confuse the powers 1 and 0. Be careful: $8^0 = 1$, whereas $8^1 = 8$.

Do Exercises 4 and 5.

Objectives

a Evaluate algebraic expressions containing whole-number exponents.

b Express exponential expressions involving negative exponents as equivalent expressions containing positive exponents.

For Extra Help

TAPE 18   MAC   CD-ROM
            WIN

Evaluate.

1. 7^0 1

2. 6^1 6

3. $(-47)^0$ 1

4. Evaluate $t^0 - 4$ for $t = 7$.

   -3

5. Evaluate $(2x - 9)^0$ for $x = 3$.

   1

Answers on page A-28

Write an equivalent expression with positive exponents. Then simplify.

6. 4^{-3}

$\dfrac{1}{4^3}; \dfrac{1}{64}$

7. 5^{-2}

$\dfrac{1}{5^2}; \dfrac{1}{25}$

8. 2^{-4}

$\dfrac{1}{2^4}; \dfrac{1}{16}$

9. $(-2)^{-3}$

$\dfrac{1}{(-2)^3}; -\dfrac{1}{8}$

10. $\left(\dfrac{5}{3}\right)^{-2}$ $\left(\dfrac{3}{5}\right)^2; \dfrac{9}{25}$

Answers on page A-28

b | Negative Integers as Exponents

The pattern used to help define the exponent 0 can also be used to define negative-integer exponents:

$$8 \cdot 8 \cdot 8 = 8^3$$
$$8 \cdot 8 = 8^2$$
$$8 = 8^1$$
$$1 = 8^0$$
$$\dfrac{1}{8} = 8^?$$
$$\dfrac{1}{8 \cdot 8} = 8^?.$$

We divide by 8 each time.

The exponents decrease by 1 each time. To continue the pattern, we would say that

$$\dfrac{1}{8} = 8^{-1}$$

and $$\dfrac{1}{8 \cdot 8} = 8^{-2}.$$

Thus, if we are to preserve the above pattern, we must have

$$\dfrac{1}{8^1} = 8^{-1} \quad \text{and} \quad \dfrac{1}{8^2} = 8^{-2}.$$

This leads to our definition of negative exponents:

> For any nonzero numbers a and b, and any integer n,
> $$a^{-n} = \dfrac{1}{a^n}, \quad \text{and} \quad \left(\dfrac{a}{b}\right)^{-n} = \left(\dfrac{b}{a}\right)^n.$$
> (A base raised to a negative exponent is equal to the reciprocal of the base raised to a positive exponent.)

Examples   Write an equivalent expression using positive exponents. Then simplify.

4. $4^{-2} = \dfrac{1}{4^2} = \dfrac{1}{16}$ Note that 4^{-2} represents a *positive* number.

5. $(-3)^{-2} = \dfrac{1}{(-3)^2} = \dfrac{1}{(-3)(-3)} = \dfrac{1}{9}$

6. $m^{-3} = \dfrac{1}{m^3}$

7. $ab^{-1} = a\left(\dfrac{1}{b^1}\right) = a\left(\dfrac{1}{b}\right) = \dfrac{a}{b}$ Think of a as $\dfrac{a}{1}$ if you wish.

8. $\left(\dfrac{5}{6}\right)^{-2} = \left(\dfrac{6}{5}\right)^2$ $\left(\dfrac{a}{b}\right)^{-n} = \left(\dfrac{b}{a}\right)^n$

$= \dfrac{6}{5} \cdot \dfrac{6}{5} = \dfrac{36}{25}$

CAUTION! Note in Example 4 that

$$4^{-2} \neq 4(-2) \quad \text{and} \quad \frac{1}{4^2} \neq 4(-2).$$

Similarly, in Example 5,

$$(-3)^{-2} \neq (-3)(-2) \quad \text{and} \quad \frac{1}{(-3)^2} \neq (-3)(-2).$$

In general, $a^{-n} \neq a(-n)$. The negative exponent also does not mean to take the opposite of the denominator. That is,

$$4^{-2} = \frac{1}{16}, \quad not \quad \frac{1}{-16}.$$

Do Exercises 6–10 on the preceding page.

Examples Write an equivalent expression using negative exponents.

9. $\dfrac{1}{7^2} = 7^{-2}$ Reading $a^{-n} = \dfrac{1}{a^n}$ from right to left: $\dfrac{1}{a^n} = a^{-n}$

10. $\dfrac{5}{x^8} = 5 \cdot \dfrac{1}{x^8} = 5x^{-8}$

Do Exercises 11 and 12.

Consider an expression like

$$\frac{a^2}{b^{-3}},$$

in which the denominator is a negative power. We can simplify as follows:

$$\frac{a^2}{b^{-3}} = \frac{a^2}{\dfrac{1}{b^3}} \qquad \text{Rewriting } b^{-3} \text{ as } \dfrac{1}{b^3}$$

$$= a^2 \cdot \frac{b^3}{1} \qquad \begin{array}{l}\text{To divide by a fractional expression,}\\ \text{we multiply by its reciprocal.}\end{array}$$

$$= a^2 b^3.$$

Do Exercises 13 and 14.

Our work above indicates that to divide by a base raised to a negative power, we can instead multiply by the opposite power of the same base. This will shorten our work.

Examples Write an equivalent expression using positive exponents.

11. $\dfrac{x^3}{y^{-2}} = x^3 y^2$ $\begin{array}{l}\text{Instead of dividing by } y^{-2},\\ \text{multiply by } y^2.\end{array}$

12. $\dfrac{a^2 b^5}{c^{-6}} = a^2 b^5 c^6$ $\begin{array}{l}\text{Instead of dividing by } c^{-6},\\ \text{multiply by } c^6.\end{array}$

13. $\dfrac{x^{-2} y}{z^{-3}} = x^{-2} y z^3 = \dfrac{yz^3}{x^2}$

Do Exercises 15–17.

Write an equivalent expression with negative exponents.

11. $\dfrac{1}{9^2}$ 9^{-2}

12. $\dfrac{7}{x^4}$ $7x^{-4}$

Write an equivalent expression with positive exponents.

13. $\dfrac{m^3}{n^{-5}}$ $m^3 n^5$

14. $\dfrac{ab}{c^{-1}}$ abc

Write an equivalent expression with positive exponents.

15. $\dfrac{a^4}{b^{-6}}$ $a^4 b^6$

16. $\dfrac{x^7 y}{z^{-4}}$ $x^7 y z^4$

17. $\dfrac{a^4 b^{-7}}{c^{-3}}$ $\dfrac{a^4 c^3}{b^7}$

Answers on page A-28

Simplify. Use positive powers in the answer.

18. $5^{-2} \cdot 5^4$ 5^2, or 25

The product rule, developed in Section 10.2, still holds when exponents are zero or negative.

Examples Simplify. Use positive powers in the answer.

14. $7^{-3} \cdot 7^6 = 7^{-3+6}$ **Adding exponents**

$\qquad\qquad = 7^3$

15. $x^4 \cdot x^{-3} = x^{4+(-3)} = x^1 = x$

16. $(2a^3b^{-4})(3a^2b^7) = 2 \cdot 3 \cdot a^3 \cdot a^2 \cdot b^{-4} \cdot b^7$ **Using the commutative and associative laws**

$\qquad\qquad\qquad = 6a^{3+2}b^{-4+7}$ **Using the product rule**

$\qquad\qquad\qquad = 6a^5b^3$

19. $x^{-3} \cdot x^{-4}$

$\dfrac{1}{x^7}$

17. $(x^{-4}y^5)(x^7y^{-11}) = x^{-4+7}y^{5+(-11)}$

$\qquad\qquad\qquad = x^3y^{-6}$

$\qquad\qquad\qquad = \dfrac{x^3}{y^6}$

Do Exercises 18–21.

20. $(5x^{-3}y)(4x^{12}y^5)$ $20x^9y^6$

21. $(a^{-9}b^{-4})(a^2b^7)$

$\dfrac{b^3}{a^7}$

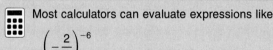
Answers on page A-28

4. −0.0484002582; −0.0484002582   **6.** 0.4932701843; 0.4932701843

Exercise Set 10.4

a Evaluate.

1. 9^0 1

2. 17^0 1

3. 3.14^0 1

4. 2.67^1 2.67

5. $(-19.57)^1$ −19.57

6. $(-34.6)^0$ 1

7. $(-5.43)^0$ 1

8. $(-98.6)^1$ −98.6

9. x^0, $x \neq 0$
1

10. a^0, $a \neq 0$
1

11. $(3x - 17)^0$, for $x = 10$
1

12. $(7x - 45)^0$, for $x = 8$
1

13. $(5x - 3)^1$, for $x = 4$
17

14. $(35 - 4x)^1$, for $x = 8$
3

15. $(4m - 19)^0$, for $m = 3$
1

16. $(9 - 2x)^0$, for $x = 5$
1

17. $3x^0 + 4$, for $x = -2$
7

18. $7x^0 + 6$, for $x = -3$
13

19. $(3x)^0 + 4$, for $x = -2$
5

20. $(7x)^0 + 6$, for $x = -3$
7

21. $(5 - 3x^0)^1$, for $x = 19$
2

22. $(5x^1 - 29)^0$, for $x = 4$
1

b Write an equivalent expression with positive exponents. Then simplify, if possible.

23. 3^{-2}

$\dfrac{1}{3^2}; \dfrac{1}{9}$

24. 2^{-3}

$\dfrac{1}{2^3}; \dfrac{1}{8}$

25. 10^{-4}

$\dfrac{1}{10^4}; \dfrac{1}{10,000}$

26. 5^{-6}

$\dfrac{1}{5^6}; \dfrac{1}{15,625}$

27. a^{-3}

$\dfrac{1}{a^3}$

28. x^{-2}

$\dfrac{1}{x^2}$

29. $(-5)^{-2}$

$\dfrac{1}{(-5)^2}; \dfrac{1}{25}$

30. $(-4)^{-3}$

$\dfrac{1}{(-4)^3}; \dfrac{1}{-64}$

31. $3x^{-7}$ $\dfrac{3}{x^7}$

32. $-6y^{-2}$ $-\dfrac{6}{y^2}$

33. $\dfrac{x}{y^{-4}}$ xy^4

34. $\dfrac{r}{t^{-7}}$ rt^7

35. $\dfrac{a^3}{b^{-4}}$ a^3b^4

36. $\dfrac{x^7}{y^{-5}}$ x^7y^5

37. $-7a^{-9}$ $\dfrac{-7}{a^9}$

38. $9p^{-4}$ $\dfrac{9}{p^4}$

39. $\left(\dfrac{2}{5}\right)^{-2}$ $\dfrac{25}{4}$

40. $\left(\dfrac{3}{7}\right)^{-2}$ $\dfrac{49}{9}$

41. $\left(\dfrac{5}{a}\right)^{-3}$ $\dfrac{a^3}{125}$

42. $\left(\dfrac{x}{3}\right)^{-4}$ $\dfrac{81}{x^4}$

Write an equivalent expression using negative exponents.

43. $\dfrac{1}{4^3}$ 4^{-3}

44. $\dfrac{1}{5^2}$ 5^{-2}

45. $\dfrac{9}{x^3}$ $9x^{-3}$

46. $\dfrac{4}{y^2}$ $4y^{-2}$

Simplify. Do not use negative exponents in the answer.

47. $x^{-2} \cdot x$ $\dfrac{1}{x}$

48. $x \cdot x^{-1}$ 1

49. $x^4 \cdot x^{-4}$ 1

50. $x^9 \cdot x^{-9}$ 1

51. $x^{-7} \cdot x^{-6}$ $\dfrac{1}{x^{13}}$

52. $y^{-5} \cdot y^{-8}$ $\dfrac{1}{y^{13}}$

53. $(3a^2b^{-7})(2ab^9)$ $6a^3b^2$

54. $(5xy^8)(3x^4y^{-5})$ $15x^5y^3$

55. $(-2x^{-3}y^8)(3xy^{-2})$ $-\dfrac{6y^6}{x^2}$

56. $(5a^{-1}b^{-7})(-2a^4b^2)$ $\dfrac{-10a^3}{b^5}$

57. $(3a^{-4}bc^2)(2a^{-2}b^{-5}c)$ $\dfrac{6c^3}{a^6b^4}$

58. $(5x^2y^{-7}z)(-4xy^{-3}z^{-4})$ $\dfrac{-20x^3}{y^{10}z^3}$

Skill Maintenance

59. George's Geo is driven 450 km in 9 hr. What is the rate in kilometers per hour? [7.2a] 50 km/h

60. A field hockey team won 18 of its 30 games. What percentage of its games did it win? [8.4a] 60%

61. The Jets once won 14 of their 16 games. What percentage of their games did they win? [8.4a]

87.5%

62. The sales tax is $27.60 on a purchase of $460. What is the sales tax rate? [8.5a] 6%

63. A circle has radius 5 cm. Find its circumference. Use 3.14 for π. [9.2b] 31.4 cm

64. Becky drove 326 mi on 14.5 gal of gas. What was her mileage? [7.2a] 22.5 mpg

---

Synthesis

65. ◆ Is there any choice of y for which $(5y)^0$ and $5y^0$ give the same result? Why or why not?

66. ◆ Consider the expression x^{-3}. When evaluated, will the expression always be negative? Will it *ever* be negative? Explain.

67. ◆ What number is larger and why: 5^{-8} or 6^{-8}? Do not use a calculator.

68. ▦ Evaluate $\dfrac{3^x}{3^{x-1}}$ for $x = -4$ and then for $x = -40$.

3; 3

69. ▦ Evaluate $\dfrac{5^x}{5^{x+1}}$ for $x = -3$ and then for $x = -30$.

$\frac{1}{5}$, or 0.2; $\frac{1}{5}$, or 0.2

70. ◆ How can negative exponents and the product rule be used to answer Exercises 68 and 69 without using a calculator?

Simplify.

71. $(y^{2x})(y^{3x})$ y^{5x}

72. $a^{5k} \div a^{3k}$ a^{2k}

73. $\dfrac{a^{6t}(a^{7t})}{a^{9t}}$ a^{4t}

Discover the pattern for negative integer exponents.

Collaborative
Learning Manual

Summary and Review: Chapter 10

Important Properties and Formulas

The Product Rule: $a^m \cdot a^n = a^{m+n}$

Negative exponents: $a^{-n} = \dfrac{1}{a^n}$ and $\left(\dfrac{a}{b}\right)^{-n} = \left(\dfrac{b}{a}\right)^n$

Review Exercises

Perform the indicated operation. [10.1a, c]

1. $(-5x + 9) + (7x - 13)$

2. $(5x^4 - 7x^3 + 3x - 5) + (3x^3 - 4x + 3)$

3. $(9a^5 + 8a^3 + 4a + 7) - (a^5 - 4a^3 + a^2 - 2)$

4. $(7a^3b^3 + 9a^2b^3) - (2a^3b^3 - 3a^2b^3 + 7)$

5. Find two equivalent expressions for the opposite of $12x^3 - 4x^2 + 9x - 3$. [10.1b]

Evaluate.

6. $(-72)^1$ [10.2a]

7. $(4x - 17)^0$, for $x = 5$ [10.4a]

8. $5t^3 + t$, for $t = -2$ [10.1d]

Multiply.

9. $(5x^3)(6x^4)$ [10.2a]

10. $3x(6x^3 - 4x - 1)$ [10.2b]

11. $2a^4b(7a^3b^3 + 5a^2b^3)$ [10.2b]

12. $(x - 7)(x + 9)$ [10.3a]

13. $(2x - 1)(5x - 3)$ [10.3a]

14. $(a^2 - 1)(a^2 + 2a - 1)$ [10.3b]

Factor. [10.2c]

15. $45x^3 - 10x$

16. $7a - 35b - 49ac$

17. $6x^3y - 9x^2y^5$

Write an equivalent expression using positive exponents. Then simplify, if possible. [10.4b]

18. 12^{-2}

19. $8a^{-7}$

20. $\dfrac{x^{-3}}{y^5z^{-6}}$

21. $\left(\dfrac{4}{5}\right)^{-2}$

22. Write an expression equivalent to $\dfrac{1}{x^7}$ using a negative exponent. [10.4b]

Simplify. Use positive exponents in the answer. [10.4b]

23. $x^{-5} \cdot x^{-12}$

24. $(-5x^4y^{-7})(-3x^5y^{-2})$

25. Willie eats 4 slices of pizza in 30 min. What is his rate in slices per minute? in minutes per slice? [7.2a]

26. In a sample of 40 tapes, 12 were defective. What percent were defective? What percent were not defective? [8.4a]

27. Phi purchases 4 tires at $45 apiece. If the sales tax rate is 5%, what will the total price be? [8.5a]

28. A round serving platter has a diameter of 21 in. Find its area. Use $\frac{22}{7}$ for π. [9.2b]

Synthesis

29. ◈ Can x^{-2} represent a negative number? Why or why not? [10.4b]

30. ◈ A student claims that
$$(3x^{-5})(-4x^{-2}) = -x^{10}.$$
What mistake(s) is the student probably making? [10.4b]

Simplify.

31. ▦ $(2349x^7 - 357x^2)(493x^{10} + 597x^5)$ [10.3a]

32. $-3x^5 \cdot 3x^3 - x^6(2x)^2 + (3x^4)^2 + (2x^4)^2 - 40x^2(x^3)^2$ [10.2a]

Factor. [10.2c]

33. $39a^3b^7c^6 - 130a^2b^5c^8 + 52a^4b^6c^5$

34. $w^5x^6y^4z^5 - w^7x^3y^7z^3 + w^6x^2y^5z^6 - w^6x^7y^3z^4$

Test: Chapter 10

1. Add: $(10a^3 - 9a^2 + 7) + (7a^3 + 4a^2 - a)$.

2. Find two equivalent expressions for the opposite of $-9a^4 + 7b^2 - ab + 3$.

[10.1b] $-(-9a^4 + 7b^2 - ab + 3)$; $9a^4 - 7b^2 + ab - 3$

2. _____

[10.1c]
3. $4x^4 - x^2 - 13$

3. Subtract: $(13x^4 + 7x^2 - 8) - (9x^4 + 8x^2 + 5)$.

4. [10.2a] 193

Evaluate.

4. 193^1

5. $(3x - 7)^0$, for $x = 2$

5. [10.4a] 1

6. The height h, in meters, of a ball t seconds after it has been thrown is approximated by the polynomial $h = -4.9t^2 + 15t + 2$. How high is the ball 2 sec after it has been thrown?

6. [10.1d] 12.4 m

7. [10.2a] $-10x^6y^8$

Multiply.

7. $(-5x^4y^3)(2x^2y^5)$

8. $5a(7a^2 - 4a + 3)$

[10.2b]
8. $35a^3 - 20a^2 + 15a$

9. $(x - 6)(x + 7)$

10. $(2a + 1)(a^2 - 3a + 2)$

9. [10.3a] $x^2 + x - 42$

[10.3b]
10. $2a^3 - 5a^2 + a + 2$

Factor.

11. $35x^6 - 25x^3 + 15x^2$

12. $6ab - 9bc + 12ac$

[10.2c]
11. $5x^2(7x^4 - 5x + 3)$

[10.2c]
12. $3(2ab - 3bc + 4ac)$

Write an equivalent expression with positive exponents. Then simplify, if possible.

13. 5^{-3}

14. $\dfrac{5a^{-3}}{b^{-2}}$

15. $\left(\dfrac{3}{5}\right)^{-3}$

---

13. [10.4b] $\dfrac{1}{5^3}$; $\dfrac{1}{125}$

14. [10.4b] $\dfrac{5b^2}{a^3}$

15. [10.4b] $\left(\dfrac{5}{3}\right)^3$; $\dfrac{125}{27}$

16. [10.4b] $\dfrac{1}{x^{16}}$

17. [10.4b] $\dfrac{-6a^3}{b^3}$

18. [7.2a] $\dfrac{5}{3}$ nails per minute; $\dfrac{3}{5}$ minute per nail

19. [8.4a] 40% satisfied; 60% not satisfied

20. [8.5a] $8500

21. [9.2b] 94.2 cm

22. [10.1d] 2.92 L

23. [10.2c], [10.3a], [10.4b] $\dfrac{3a^4}{a^4 - 6a^2 + 9}$

Simplify. Use positive exponents in the answer.

16. $x^{-7} \cdot x^{-9}$

17. $(3a^{-7}b^9)(-2a^{10}b^{-12})$

Skill Maintenance

18. Charlene hammers 25 nails in 15 min. What is her rate in nails per minute? in minutes per nail?

19. Of 55 people surveyed, 22 felt satisfied with their diets. What percent felt satisfied? What percent did not feel satisfied?

20. Gina pays $340 in tax on the purchase of a used car. If the sales tax rate is 4%, what was the price of the car before tax?

21. A juggler's hoop has a diameter of 30 cm. Find its circumference. Use 3.14 for π.

Synthesis

22. The polynomial

$$0.041h - 0.018A - 2.69$$

can be used to estimate the lung capacity, in liters, of a female of height h, in centimeters, and age A, in years. Find the lung capacity of a 30-yr-old woman who is 150 cm tall.

23. Write an equivalent expression with positive exponents and then simplify:

$$12a^6(2a^3 - 6a)^{-2}.$$

Final Examination

This exam reviews the entire textbook. A question may arise as to what notation to use for a particular problem or exercise. Although there is no hard-and-fast rule, especially as you use mathematics outside the classroom, here is the guideline that we follow: Use the notation given in the problem. That is, if the problem is given using mixed numerals, give the answer in mixed numerals. If the problem is given in decimal notation, give the answer in decimal notation.

1. In 46,301, what digit tells the number of thousands?

2. Write expanded notation for 8409.

Add and, if possible, simplify.

3.
$$
\begin{array}{r}
7\ 4\ 3 \\
+\ 2\ 7\ 5 \\
\hline
\end{array}
$$

4.
$$
\begin{array}{r}
4\ 9\ 0\ 3 \\
5\ 2\ 7\ 8 \\
6\ 3\ 9\ 1 \\
+\ 4\ 5\ 1\ 3 \\
\hline
\end{array}
$$

5. $\dfrac{4}{13} + \dfrac{1}{26}$

6.
$$
\begin{array}{r}
5\dfrac{4}{9} \\
+\ 3\dfrac{1}{3} \\
\hline
\end{array}
$$

7. $-29 + 53$

8. $-543 + (-219)$

9. $-34.56 + 2.783 + 0.433 + (-13.02)$

10. $(4x^5 + 7x^4 - 3x^2 + 9) + (6x^5 - 8x^4 + 2x^3 - 7)$

Subtract and, if possible, simplify.

11.
$$
\begin{array}{r}
6\ 7\ 4 \\
-\ 4\ 3\ 1 \\
\hline
\end{array}
$$

12. $-7x - 12x$

13. $\dfrac{2}{5} - \dfrac{7}{8}$

14.
$$
\begin{array}{r}
4\dfrac{1}{3} \\
-\ 1\dfrac{5}{8} \\
\hline
\end{array}
$$

15.
$$
\begin{array}{r}
2\ 0.0 \\
-\ \ \ \ 0.0\ 0\ 2\ 7 \\
\hline
\end{array}
$$

16. $(7x^3 + 2x^2 - x) - (5x^3 - 3x^2 - 8x)$

17. $(9a^2b + 3ab) - (13a^2b - 4ab)$

Multiply and, if possible, simplify.

18.
$$
\begin{array}{r}
2\ 9\ 7 \\
\times\ \ \ 1\ 6 \\
\hline
\end{array}
$$

19. $349 \cdot (-213)$

20. $2\dfrac{3}{4} \cdot 1\dfrac{2}{3}$

Answers

1. [1.1e] 6

2. [1.1a] 8 thousands + 4 hundreds + 9 ones

3. [1.2b] 1018

4. [1.2b] 21,085

5. [4.2b] $\dfrac{9}{26}$

6. [4.6a] $8\dfrac{7}{9}$

7. [2.2a] 24

8. [2.2a] -762

9. [5.2c] -44.364

10. [10.1a] $10x^5 - x^4 + 2x^3 - 3x^2 + 2$

11. [1.3d] 243

12. [2.7b] $-19x$

13. [4.3a] $-\dfrac{19}{40}$

14. [4.6b] $2\dfrac{17}{24}$

15. [5.2b] 19.9973

16. [10.1c] $2x^3 + 5x^2 + 7x$

17. [10.1c] $-4a^2b + 7ab$

18. [1.5b] 4752

19. [2.4a] $-74,337$

20. [4.7a] $4\dfrac{7}{12}$

21. [3.6a] $-\frac{6}{5}$

22. [3.6a] 10

23. [5.3a] 259.084

24. [2.7a] $24x - 15$

25. [10.2a] $27a^8b^3$

26. [10.2b] $21x^5 - 14x^3 + 56x^2$

27. [10.3a] $x^2 - 5x - 14$

28. [10.3b] $a^3 - 2a^2 - 11a + 12$

29. [1.6c] 573

30. [1.6c] 56 R 10

31. [3.7b] $-\frac{3}{2}$

32. [4.7b] $\frac{7}{90}$

33. [5.4a] 39

34. [4.5c] $56\frac{5}{17}$

35. [1.9c] 75

36. [1.9c], [2.1c] -2

37. [1.9a] 17^4

38. [1.4a] 68,000

39. [5.5b] 21.84

40. [3.1b] Yes

41. [3.2a] 1, 3, 5, 15

42. [4.1a] 105

43. [3.5b] $\frac{7}{10}$

44. [3.5b] $-\frac{58}{3}$

21. $-\dfrac{9}{7} \cdot \dfrac{14}{15}$

22. $12 \cdot \dfrac{5}{6}$

23.
$$\begin{array}{r} 3\,4.0\,9 \\ \times \quad\ \ 7.6 \\ \hline \end{array}$$

24. $3(8x - 5)$

25. $(9a^3b^2)(3a^5b)$

26. $7x^2(3x^3 - 2x + 8)$

27. $(x + 2)(x - 7)$

28. $(a + 3)(a^2 - 5a + 4)$

Divide and simplify. State the answer using a remainder when appropriate.

29. $6\,\overline{)\,3\ 4\ 3\ 8}$

30. $3\ 4\,\overline{)\,1\ 9\ 1\ 4}$

Divide and simplify.

31. $\dfrac{4}{5} \div \left(-\dfrac{8}{15}\right)$

32. $-2\dfrac{1}{3} \div (-30)$

33. $2.7\,\overline{)\,1\ 0\ 5.3}$

34. Write a mixed numeral for the quotient in Question 30.

Simplify.

35. $10 \div 2 \times 20 - 5^2$

36. $\dfrac{|3^2 - 5^2|}{2 - 2 \cdot 5}$

37. Write exponential notation: $17 \cdot 17 \cdot 17 \cdot 17$.

38. Round 68,489 to the nearest thousand.

39. Round $21.\overline{83}$ to the nearest hundredth.

40. Determine whether 1368 is divisible by 3.

41. Find all the factors of 15.

42. Find the LCM of 15 and 35.

Simplify.

43. $\dfrac{21}{30}$

44. $\dfrac{-290}{15}$

45. Convert to a mixed numeral: $-\dfrac{18}{5}$.

46. Use < or > for ▓ to write a true sentence:

$$-17 \ \blacksquare \ -29.$$

47. Use < or > for ▓ to write a true sentence:

$$\frac{4}{7} \ \blacksquare \ \frac{3}{5}.$$

48. Which number is greater, 1.001 or 0.9976?

49. Evaluate $\dfrac{a^2 - b}{3}$ for $a = -9$ and $b = -6$.

Factor.

50. $40 - 5t$

51. $18a^3 - 15a^2 + 6a$

52. What part is shaded?

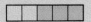

Convert to decimal notation.

53. $\dfrac{37}{1000}$

54. $-\dfrac{13}{25}$

55. $\dfrac{8}{9}$

56. 7%

Convert to fractional notation.

57. 6.71

58. $-7\dfrac{1}{4}$

59. 40%

Convert to percent notation.

60. $\dfrac{17}{20}$

61. 1.5

62. Estimate the sum $9.389 + 4.2105$ to the nearest tenth.

Solve.

63. $234 + y = 789$

64. $3.9a = 249.6$

65. $\dfrac{2}{3} \cdot t = \dfrac{5}{6}$

66. $\dfrac{8}{17} = \dfrac{36}{x}$

67. $7x - 9 = 26$

68. $-2(x - 5) = 3x + 12$

Answers

69. [6.5a] $23.75

70. [1.8a] 65 min

71. [4.6c] 25\frac{3}{4}$

72. [5.8a] 485.9 mi

73. [1.8a] $24,000

74. [1.8a] $595

75. [3.4c] $\frac{3}{10}$ km

76. [5.8a] $84.96

77. [7.4a] 13 gal

78. [7.2b] 17 $\frac{¢}{oz}$

79. [8.6a] $240

80. [8.5b] 7%

81. [8.4b] 30,160

82. [5.8a] 220 mi

83. [1.9b] 324

84. [10.4a] 1

85. [9.5a] 11

86. [10.4b] $\frac{1}{4^3}$; $\frac{1}{64}$

87. [10.4b] $\left(\frac{4}{5}\right)^2$; $\frac{16}{25}$

Final Examination

616

Solve.

69. Margie donated $20 to the Humane Society, $30 to the Red Cross, $25 to the Salvation Army, and $20 to Amnesty International. What was the average size of the donations?

70. A machine wraps 134 candy bars per minute. How long does it take this machine to wrap 8710 bars?

71. A share of IDX stock bought for 29\frac{5}{8}$ dropped 3\frac{7}{8}$ before it was resold. What was the price when it was resold?

72. At the start of a trip, the odometer on the Montgomery's Toyota read 27,428.6 mi and at the end of the trip the reading was 27,914.5 mi. How long was the trip?

73. From an income of $32,000, amounts of $6400 and $1600 are paid for federal and state taxes. How much remains after these taxes have been paid?

74. Shannon is paid $85 a day for 7 days work as a lifeguard. How much will she be paid?

75. A toddler walks $\frac{3}{5}$ km per hour. At this rate, how far would the child walk in $\frac{1}{2}$ hr?

76. Eight identical dresses cost a total of $679.68. What is the cost of each dress?

77. Eight gallons of paint covers 2000 ft^2. How much paint is needed to cover 3250 ft^2?

78. Eighteen ounces of a fruit "smoothie" costs $3.06. Find the unit price in cents per ounce.

79. What is the simple interest on $4000 principal at 8% for $\frac{3}{4}$ year?

80. Baldacci Real Estate received $5880 commission on the sale of an $84,000 home. What was the rate of commission?

81. The population of Bridgeton is 29,000 this year and is increasing at 4% per year. What will the population be next year?

82. Ace Car Rentals charges $35 a day plus 15 cents a mile for a van rental. If a couple's one-day van rental cost $68, how many miles did they drive?

Evaluate.

83. 18^2

84. 37^0

85. $\sqrt{121}$

Express with positive exponents. Then simplify, if possible.

86. 4^{-3}

87. $\left(\frac{5}{4}\right)^{-2}$

The following line graph show the driver fatality rate during a recent year. Use the line graph for Questions 88 and 89.

Driver Fatality Rate in 1996, By Age Per 100 Million Vehicle Miles Traveled

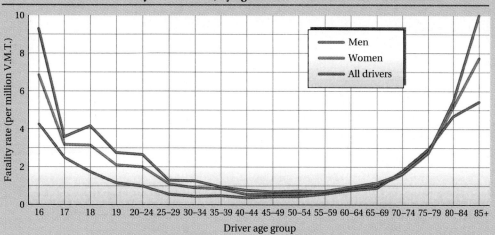

Source: National Highway Traffic Safety Administration; *The New York Times*, 10/21/98, p. 16

88. When all drivers are considered, what age group has the highest fatality rate? What is the rate?

89. Approximate the fatality rate for drivers aged 20–24.

90. The ages of students in a community college math lab are as follows:

18, 20, 27, 35, 20, 52, 26.

Find the mean, the median, and the mode of the ages.

91. In Sam's writing lab, 3 of the 20 students are left-handed. If a student is randomly selected, what is the probability that he or she is left-handed?

92. Plot the following points:
(−5, 2), (4, 0), (3, −4), (0, 2).

93. Graph: $y = -\frac{1}{3}x$.

94. These triangles are similar. Find the missing lengths.

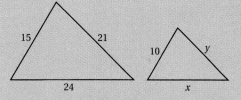

Complete.

95. $\frac{1}{3}$ yd = _____ in.

96. 4280 mm = _____ cm

97. 3.7 km = _____ m

98. 20,000 g = _____ kg

99. 10 lb = _____ oz

100. 0.008 cg = _____ mg

101. 8190 mL = _____ L

102. 20 qt = _____ gal

Answers

88. [6.2c] 85+; 8 fatalities per 100 million vehicle miles traveled

89. [6.2c] 1 fatality per 100 million vehicle miles traveled

90. [6.5a, b, c] Mean: $28\frac{2}{7}$; median: 26; mode: 20

91. [6.6b] $\frac{3}{20}$

92. [6.3a] See graph on p. A-29.

93. [6.4b] See graph on p. A-29.

94. [7.5a] $x = 16$, $y = 14$

95. [9.1a] 12

96. [9.1b] 428

97. [9.1b] 3700

98. [9.7b] 20

99. [9.7a] 160

100. [9.7b] 0.08

101. [9.6b] 8.19

102. [9.6b] 5

103. A rectangular picture frame measures 20 in. by 24 in. Find its perimeter.

Find the area of each figure.

104.

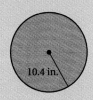

4 cm

15.4 cm

105.

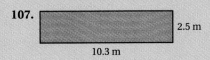

5 in.

10 in.

106.

10.8 yd

8.3 yd

20.2 yd

107.

2.5 m

10.3 m

108. Find the diameter, the circumference, and the area of this circle. Use 3.14 for π.

[9.2b] Diameter: 20.8 in.;
circumference: 65.312 in.; area: 339.6224 in²

10.4 in.

Find the volume of each shape. Use 3.14 for π.

109.

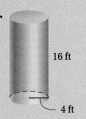

2.3 m

2.3 m

10 m

110.

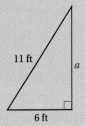

16 ft

4 ft

111.

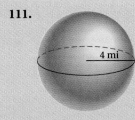

4 mi

112. Find the length of the third side of this right triangle. Give an exact answer and an approximation to three decimal places.

11 ft

a

6 ft

Developmental Units

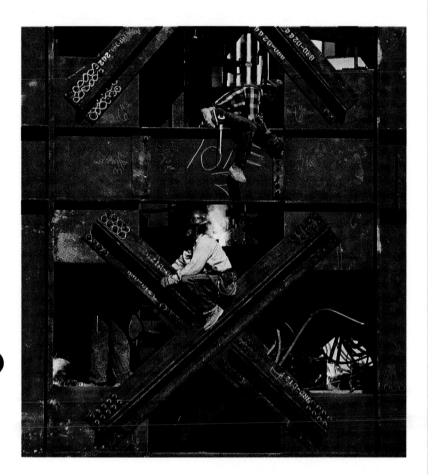

Introduction

These developmental units are meant to provide extra instruction for students who have difficulty with any of Sections 1.2, 1.3, 1.5, or 1.6. After reading one of these developmental units and doing the exercises in its exercise set, the student should restudy the appropriate section in Chapter 1.

A Addition
S Subtraction
M Multiplication
D Division

World Wide Web   For more information, visit us at www.mathmax.com

A Addition

a | Basic Addition

Basic addition can be explained by counting. The sum

$$3 + 4$$

can be found by counting out a set of 3 objects and a separate set of 4 objects, putting them together, and counting all the objects.

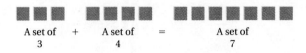

A set of 3   +   A set of 4   =   A set of 7

The numbers to be added are called **addends**. The result is the **sum**.

$$\underset{\text{Addend}}{3} \quad + \quad \underset{\text{Addend}}{4} \quad = \quad \underset{\text{Sum}}{7}$$

Examples   Add. Think of putting sets of objects together.

1. $5 + 6 = 11$

$$\begin{array}{r} 5 \\ + 6 \\ \hline 11 \end{array}$$

2. $8 + 5 = 13$

$$\begin{array}{r} 8 \\ + 5 \\ \hline 13 \end{array}$$

We can also do these problems by counting up from one of the numbers. For example, in Example 1, we start at 5 and count up 6 times: 6, 7, 8, 9, 10, 11.

Do Exercises 1–6.

What happens when we add 0? Think of a set of 5 objects. If we add 0 objects to it, we still have 5 objects. Similarly, if we have a set with 0 objects in it and add 5 objects to it, we have a set with 5 objects. Thus,

$$5 + 0 = 5 \quad \text{and} \quad 0 + 5 = 5.$$

> Adding 0 to a number does not change the number:
> $$a + 0 = 0 + a = a.$$
> We say that 0 is the **additive identity.**

Objectives

a   Add any two of the numbers 0, 1, 2, 3, 4, 5, 6, 7, 8, 9.

b   Find certain sums of three numbers such as $1 + 7 + 9$.

c   Add two whole numbers when carrying is not necessary.

d   Add two whole numbers when carrying is necessary.

Add; think of joining sets of objects.

1. $4 + 5$

9

2. $3 + 4$

7

3. $\begin{array}{r} 9 \\ + 5 \\ \hline \end{array}$

14

4. $\begin{array}{r} 8 \\ + 8 \\ \hline \end{array}$

16

5. $\begin{array}{r} 9 \\ + 7 \\ \hline \end{array}$

16

6. $\begin{array}{r} 7 \\ + 9 \\ \hline \end{array}$

16

The first printed use of the + symbol was in a book by a German, Johann Widmann, in 1498.

Answers on page A-29

Examples Add.

3. $0 + 9 = 9$

$$\begin{array}{r} 0 \\ +\ 9 \\ \hline 9 \end{array}$$

4. $0 + 0 = 0$

$$\begin{array}{r} 0 \\ +\ 0 \\ \hline 0 \end{array}$$

5. $97 + 0 = 97$

$$\begin{array}{r} 97 \\ +\ \ 0 \\ \hline 97 \end{array}$$

Do Exercises 7–12.

Your objective for this part of the section is to be able to add any of the numbers 0, 1, 2, 3, 4, 5, 6, 7, 8, 9. Adding 0 is easy. The rest of the sums are listed in this table. Memorize the table by saying it to yourself over and over or by using flash cards.

+	1	2	3	4	5	6	7	8	9
1	2	3	4	5	6	7	8	9	10
2	3	4	5	6	7	8	9	10	11
3	4	5	6	7	8	9	10	11	12
4	5	6	7	8	9	10	11	12	13
5	6	7	8	9	10	11	12	13	14
6	7	8	9	10	11	12	13	14	15
7	8	9	10	11	12	13	14	15	16
8	9	10	11	12	13	14	15	16	17
9	10	11	12	13	14	15	16	17	18

$6 + 7 = 13$
Find 6 at the left, and 7 at the top.

$7 + 6 = 13$
Find 7 at the left, and 6 at the top.

It is very important that you *memorize* the basic addition facts! If you do not, you will always have trouble with addition.

Note the following.

$3 + 4 = 7$	$7 + 6 = 13$	$7 + 2 = 9$
$4 + 3 = 7$	$6 + 7 = 13$	$2 + 7 = 9$

We can add whole numbers in any order. This is the *commutative law of addition*. Because of this law, you need to learn only about half the table above, as shown by the shading.

Do Exercises 13 and 14.

b Certain Sums of Three Numbers

To add $3 + 5 + 4$, we can add 3 and 5, then 4:

$$3 + 5 + 4$$
$$8 + 4$$
$$12.$$

We can also add 5 and 4, then 3:

$$3 + 5 + 4$$
$$3 + 9$$
$$12.$$

Either way we get 12.

Add.

7. $8 + 0$
8

8. $0 + 8$
8

9.
$$\begin{array}{r} 7 \\ +\ 0 \\ \hline 7 \end{array}$$

10.
$$\begin{array}{r} 46 \\ +\ \ 0 \\ \hline 46 \end{array}$$

11. $0 + 13$
13

12. $58 + 0$
58

Complete the table.

13.

+	1	2	3	4	5
1	2	3	4	5	6
2	3	4	5	6	7
3	4	5	6	7	8
4	5	6	7	8	9
5	6	7	8	9	10

14.

+	6	5	7	4	9
7	13	12	14	11	16
9	15	14	16	13	18
5	11	10	12	9	14
8	14	13	15	12	17
4	10	9	11	8	13

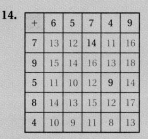

Answers on page A-29

Add from the top mentally.

15.
```
   1
   6
 + 9
  16
```

16.
```
   2
   3
 + 4
   9
```

17.
```
   6
   1
 + 4
  11
```

18.
```
   5
   2
 + 8
  15
```

Add.

19.
```
   2 4
 + 3 5
    59
```

20.
```
   3 4 6
 + 2 0 3
     549
```

21.
```
   8 3 2 7
 + 1 6 5 2
     9979
```

22.
```
   3 4 6 1
 + 2 0 3 5
     5496
```

Example 6 Add from the top mentally.

```
   1     We first add 1 and 7,
   7     getting 8. Then we add
 + 9     8 and 9, getting 17.
```

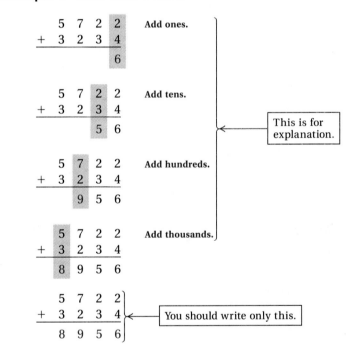

Example 7 Add from the top mentally.

```
   2
   4  →  6
 + 8     8  →  14
```

Do Exercises 15–18.

c | Addition (No Carrying)

We now move to a more gradual, conceptual development of the addition procedure you considered in Section 1.2. It is intended to provide you with a greater understanding so that your skill level will increase.

To add larger numbers, we can add the ones first, then the tens, then the hundreds, and so on.

Example 8 Add: 5722 + 3234.

```
   5 7 2 2     Add ones.
 + 3 2 3 4
         6


   5 7 2 2     Add tens.
 + 3 2 3 4
       5 6                    This is for
                             explanation.

   5 7 2 2     Add hundreds.
 + 3 2 3 4
     9 5 6


   5 7 2 2     Add thousands.
 + 3 2 3 4
   8 9 5 6


   5 7 2 2
 + 3 2 3 4                   You should write only this.
   8 9 5 6
```

Do Exercises 19–22.

d Addition (With Carrying)

Carrying Tens

Example 9 Add: 18 + 27.

```
  1  8      Add ones.      Think:        8
+ 2  7                                 + 7
     ?                                 1  5
```

15 ones = 10 ones + 5 ones
= 1 ten + 5 ones

```
   1
   1  8    Write 5 in the ones column.
 + 2  7    Write 1 for a reminder above the tens.
      5    This is called carrying.
```

```
   1
   1  8    Add tens.
 + 2  7
   4  5
```

We can use money to help explain Example 9.

```
   1  8¢ ──→ 1 dime and 8 pennies
 + 2  7¢ ──→ 2 dimes and 7 pennies
     15¢    We first add the pennies.
```

```
    1 dime
    1  8       We exchange ten pennies for a dime.
  + 2  7
  5 pennies
```

```
   1
   1  8       We now add the dimes. The result is
 + 2  7       4 dimes and 5 pennies.
   4  5
```

Do Exercises 23 and 24.

Carrying Hundreds

Example 10 Add: 256 + 391.

```
  2  5  6    Add ones.
+ 3  9  1
        7
```

```
   1
  2  5  6    Add tens. We get 14 tens. Now 14 tens = 10 tens + 4 tens =
+ 3  9  1    1 hundred + 4 tens. Write 4 in the tens column and a 1 above
     4  7    the hundreds.
```

> The carrying here is like exchanging 14 dimes
> for a 1 dollar bill and 4 dimes.

```
   1
  2  5  6    Add hundreds.
+ 3  9  1
  6  4  7
```

Add.

23.
```
   1 9
 + 3 7
   56
```

24.
```
   4 6
 + 3 9
   85
```

Add.

25.
```
   3 4 1
 + 4 8 8
   829
```

26.
```
   7 3 0
 + 2 9 6
   1026
```

Answers on page A-29

Do Exercises 25 and 26 on the preceding page.

Carrying Thousands

Example 11   Add: 4803 + 3792.

```
    4  8  0  3      Add ones.
 +  3  7  9  2
 ──────────────
             5
```

```
    4  8  0  3      Add tens.
 +  3  7  9  2
 ──────────────
          9  5
```

```
 1
    4  8  0  3      Add hundreds. We get 15 hundreds. Now 15 hundreds =
 +  3  7  9  2      10 hundreds + 5 hundreds = 1 thousand + 5 hundreds.
 ──────────────     Write 5 in the hundreds column and 1 above the thousands.
       5  9  5
```

```
 1
    4  8  0  3      Add thousands.
 +  3  7  9  2
 ──────────────
    8  5  9  5
```

Do Exercise 27.

Carrying More Than Once

Sometimes we must carry more than once.

Example 12   Add: 5767 + 4993.

```
          1
    5  7  6  7      Add ones. We get 10 ones. Now 10 ones = 1 ten +
 +  4  9  9  3      0 ones. Write 0 in the ones column and 1 above the tens.
 ──────────────
             0
```

```
       1  1
    5  7  6  7      Add tens. We get 16 tens. Now 16 tens = 1 hundred +
 +  4  9  9  3      6 tens. Write 6 in the tens column and 1 above
 ──────────────     the hundreds.
          6  0
```

```
    1  1  1
    5  7  6  7      Add hundreds. We get 17 hundreds. Now 17 hundreds =
 +  4  9  9  3      1 thousand + 7 hundreds. Write 7 in the hundreds column
 ──────────────     and 1 above the thousands.
       7  6  0
```

```
 1  1  1
    5  7  6  7      Add thousands. We get 10 thousands.
 +  4  9  9  3
 ──────────────
 1  0  7  6  0
```

Do Exercises 28 and 29.

---

27. Add.

```
    7 8 5 0
 +  4 8 4 8
 ───────────
   12,698
```

Add.

28.
```
    7 9 8 9
 +  5 6 7 2
 ───────────
   13,661
```

29.
```
    5 6,7 8 9
 +  1 4,5 3 9
 ────────────
   71,328
```

To the student: *If you had trouble with Section 1.2 and have studied Developmental Unit A, you should go back and work through Section 1.2 after completing Exercise Set A.*

Answers on page A-29

Exercise Set A

a Add. Try to do these mentally. If you have trouble, think of putting objects together.

1. 8 + 9 17	**2.** 8 + 7 15	**3.** 6 + 7 13	**4.** 9 + 5 14	**5.** 5 + 7 12	**6.** 5 + 6 11
7. 9 + 8 17	**8.** 9 + 7 16	**9.** 8 + 4 12	**10.** 9 + 1 10	**11.** 8 + 2 10	**12.** 3 + 8 11
13. 0 + 7 7	**14.** 4 + 3 7	**15.** 2 + 9 11	**16.** 0 + 0 0	**17.** 3 + 0 3	**18.** 9 + 9 18
19. 8 + 6 14	**20.** 3 + 7 10	**21.** 2 + 2 4	**22.** 7 + 7 14	**23.** 6 + 5 11	**24.** 7 + 8 15
25. 8 + 8 16	**26.** 8 + 1 9	**27.** 5 + 8 13	**28.** 5 + 9 14	**29.** 4 + 7 11	**30.** 6 + 1 7

31. 6 + 7
13

32. 7 + 7
14

33. 3 + 9
12

34. 6 + 0
6

35. 6 + 4
10

36. 9 + 3
12

37. 5 + 5
10

38. 5 + 3
8

39. 1 + 1
2

40. 4 + 5
9

41. 9 + 4
13

42. 0 + 8
8

43. 4 + 6
10

44. 2 + 7
9

45. 3 + 7
10

46. 3 + 3
6

47. 5 + 8
13

48. 3 + 6
9

49. 4 + 4
8

50. 4 + 7
11

b Add from the top mentally.

51. 1 8 + 3 12	**52.** 1 7 + 5 13	**53.** 3 2 + 5 10	**54.** 4 3 + 5 12	**55.** 1 7 + 9 17
56. 5 2 + 6 13	**57.** 4 5 + 1 10	**58.** 1 9 + 6 16	**59.** 1 8 + 7 16	**60.** 1 6 + 8 15

c Add.

61.
```
   2 3
 + 1 6
```
39

62.
```
   5 4
 + 3 5
```
89

63.
```
   6 7
 + 2 0
```
87

64.
```
   4 9 6
 + 5 0 3
```
999

65.
```
   7 0 0
 + 2 0 0
```
900

66.
```
   8 0 1
 +   6 7
```
868

67.
```
   6 6 6
 + 3 3 3
```
999

68.
```
   5 2 3
 + 3 2 5
```
848

69.
```
   7 4 7
 + 1 3 0
```
877

70.
```
   8 2 5 0
 + 9 4 3 0
```
17,680

71.
```
   6 5 5 2
 + 4 3 2 1
```
10,873

72.
```
   3 4 0 6
 + 1 2 9 3
```
4699

73.
```
   7 3 4 0
 + 3 5 2 7
```
10,867

74.
```
   4 8 2 5
 + 5 0 7 0
```
9895

75.
```
   2 0 7 3
 + 1 9 2 5
```
3998

76.
```
   9 1 1 1
 + 9 1 1 1
```
18,222

77.
```
   7 8 8 9
 + 9 0 0 0
```
16,889

78.
```
   5 2,4 3 3
 + 1 2,0 5 6
```
64,489

79.
```
   4 3,7 2 3
 + 5 6,2 7 6
```
99,999

80.
```
   5 1,6 7 0
 + 2 6,1 0 7
```
77,777

d Add.

81.
```
   3 8
 +   8
```
46

82.
```
   1 7
 +   9
```
26

83.
```
   1 7
 + 3 8
```
55

84.
```
   9 5
 +   6
```
101

85.
```
   8 6 2
 + 7 8 1
```
1643

86.
```
   6 1 3
 + 7 9 9
```
1412

87.
```
   3 5 5
 + 4 9 1
```
846

88.
```
   2 8 0
 + 3 4 8
```
628

89.
```
   8 1 4
 + 3 9 0
```
1204

90.
```
   2 7 4
 + 3 3 3
```
607

91.
```
   9 9 9 0
 +     1 0
```
10,000

92.
```
   9 9 9
 +   1 1
```
1010

93.
```
   9 9 9
 + 1 1 1
```
1110

94.
```
   8 3 9
 + 3 8 8
```
1227

95.
```
   9 0 9
 + 2 0 2
```
1111

96.
```
   8 0 8
 + 9 0 9
```
1717

97.
```
   8 7 1 8
 + 1 4 2 0
```
10,138

98.
```
   3 8 5 4
 + 2 7 0 0
```
6554

99.
```
   4 8 2 8
 + 1 2 8 3
```
6111

100.
```
   6 9 9 5
 + 1 4 3 2
```
8427

101.
```
   9 8 8 9
 +       1
```
9890

102.
```
   6 8 8 9
 + 4 7 2 3
```
11,612

103.
```
   9 1 2 8
 + 1 9 9 7
```
11,125

104.
```
   8 8 9 8
 + 6 6 4 5
```
15,543

105.
```
   9 9 8 9
 + 6 7 8 5
```
16,774

106.
```
   4 6,8 8 9
 + 2 1,7 8 6
```
68,675

107.
```
   2 3,4 4 8
 + 1 0,9 8 9
```
34,437

108.
```
   6 7,6 5 8
 + 9 8,7 8 6
```
166,444

109.
```
   7 7,5 4 8
 + 2 3,7 6 7
```
101,315

110.
```
   4 4,6 8 4
 +   4,7 6 5
```
49,449

S Subtraction

a | Basic Subtraction

Subtraction can be explained by taking away part of a set.

Example 1 Subtract: $7 - 3$.

We can do this by counting out 7 objects and then taking away 3 of them. Then we count the number that remain: $7 - 3 = 4$.

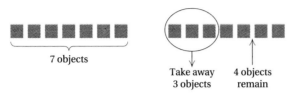

7 objects

Take away   4 objects
3 objects   remain

We could also do this mentally by starting at 7 and counting down 3 times: 6, 5, 4.

Examples Subtract. Think of "take away."

2. $11 - 6 = 5$ *Take away*: "11 take away 6 is 5."

$$\begin{array}{r} 11 \\ -\ 6 \\ \hline 5 \end{array}$$

3. $17 - 9 = 8$

$$\begin{array}{r} 17 \\ -\ 9 \\ \hline 8 \end{array}$$

Do Exercises 1–4.

In Developmental Unit A, you memorized an addition table. That table will enable you to subtract also. First, let's recall how addition and subtraction are related.

An addition:

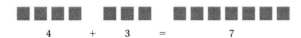

4   +   3   =   7

Two related subtractions.

A.

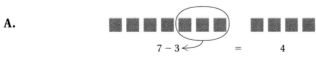

$7 - 3 \leftarrow$ =   4

B.

$7 - 4 \leftarrow$ =   3

Objectives

a Find basic differences such as $5 - 3$, $13 - 8$, and so on.

b Subtract one whole number from another when borrowing is not necessary.

c Subtract one whole number from another when borrowing is necessary.

Subtract.

1. $10 - 6$

4

2. $11 - 4$

7

3. $\begin{array}{r} 16 \\ -\ 8 \\ \hline 8 \end{array}$

4. $\begin{array}{r} 10 \\ -\ 7 \\ \hline 3 \end{array}$

Answers on page A-30

Since we know that

$$4 + 3 = 7, \qquad \text{A basic addition fact}$$

we also know the two subtraction facts

$$7 - 3 = 4 \quad \text{and} \quad 7 - 4 = 3.$$

Example 4 From $8 + 9 = 17$, write two subtraction facts.

a) The addend 8 is subtracted from the sum 17.

$8 + 9 = 17$ The related sentence is $17 - 8 = 9$.

b) The addend 9 is subtracted from the sum 17.

$8 + 9 = 17$ The related sentence is $17 - 9 = 8$.

Do Exercises 5 and 6.

We can use the idea that subtraction is defined in terms of addition to think of subtraction as "how much more."

Example 5 Find: $13 - 6$.

To find $13 - 6$, we ask, "6 plus what number is 13?"

$$6 + \boxed{} = 13$$

+	1	2	3	4	5	6	7	8	9
1	2	3	4	5	6	7	8	9	10
2	3	4	5	6	7	8	9	10	11
3	4	5	6	7	8	9	10	11	12
4	5	6	7	8	9	10	11	12	13
5	6	7	8	9	10	11	12	13	14
6	7	8	9	10	11	12	13	14	15
7	8	9	10	11	12	13	14	15	16
8	9	10	11	12	13	14	15	16	17
9	10	11	12	13	14	15	16	17	18

$13 - 6 = 7$

Using the addition table above, we find 13 inside the table and 6 at the left. Then we read the answer 7 from the top. Thus we have $13 - 6 = 7$. Strive to do this kind of thinking mentally as fast as you can, without having to use the table.

Do Exercises 7–10.

Answers on page A-30

b Subtraction (No Borrowing)

We now move to a more gradual, conceptual development of the subtraction procedure you considered in Section 1.3. It is intended to provide you with a greater understanding so that your skill level will increase.

To subtract larger numbers, we can subtract the ones first, then the tens, then the hundreds, and so on.

Example 6 Subtract: 5787 − 3214.

$$\begin{array}{r} 5\ 7\ 8\ \boxed{7} \\ -\ 3\ 2\ 1\ \boxed{4} \\ \hline \boxed{3} \end{array}$$ Subtract ones.

$$\begin{array}{r} 5\ 7\ \boxed{8}\ 7 \\ -\ 3\ 2\ \boxed{1}\ 4 \\ \hline \boxed{7}\ 3 \end{array}$$ Subtract tens.

This is the explanation.

$$\begin{array}{r} 5\ \boxed{7}\ 8\ 7 \\ -\ 3\ \boxed{2}\ 1\ 4 \\ \hline \boxed{5}\ 7\ 3 \end{array}$$ Subtract hundreds.

$$\begin{array}{r} \boxed{5}\ 7\ 8\ 7 \\ -\ \boxed{3}\ 2\ 1\ 4 \\ \hline \boxed{2}\ 5\ 7\ 3 \end{array}$$ Subtract thousands.

$$\begin{array}{r} 5\ 7\ 8\ 7 \\ -\ 3\ 2\ 1\ 4 \\ \hline 2\ 5\ 7\ 3 \end{array}$$ You should write only this.

Do Exercises 11–14.

c Subtraction (with Borrowing)

We now consider subtraction when borrowing is necessary.

Borrowing from the Tens Place

Example 7 Subtract: 37 − 18.

$$\begin{array}{r} 3\ \boxed{7} \\ -\ 1\ \boxed{8} \\ \hline \boxed{?} \end{array}$$ Try to subtract ones: 7 − 8 is not a whole number.

$$\begin{array}{r} {}^{2}\ {}^{17} \\ \not3\ \not7 \\ -\ 1\ \ 8 \end{array}$$ Borrow a ten. That is, 1 ten = 10 ones, and 10 ones + 7 ones = 17 ones. Write 2 above the tens column and 17 above the ones.

$$\begin{array}{r} {}^{2}\ \boxed{{}^{17}} \\ \not3\ \not7 \\ -\ 1\ \boxed{8} \\ \hline \boxed{9} \end{array}$$ Subtract ones.

The borrowing here is like exchanging 3 dimes and 7 pennies for 2 dimes and 17 pennies.

Subtract.

11.
$$\begin{array}{r} 7\ 8 \\ -\ 6\ 4 \\ \hline 14 \end{array}$$

12.
$$\begin{array}{r} 2\ 9 \\ -\ \ 9 \\ \hline 20 \end{array}$$

13.
$$\begin{array}{r} 5\ 4\ 2 \\ -\ 3\ 0\ 1 \\ \hline 241 \end{array}$$

14.
$$\begin{array}{r} 6\ 8\ 9\ 6 \\ -\ 4\ 8\ 7\ 1 \\ \hline 2025 \end{array}$$

Answers on page A-30

Subtract.

15.
```
   4 6
 − 2 9
```
17

16.
```
   7 4
 − 3 8
```
36

Subtract.

17.
```
   6 4 6
 − 1 9 2
```
454

18.
```
   7 3 3
 − 4 8 3
```
250

```
    2  17
    3̸  7̸      Subtract tens.
 − 1  8
 _____
    1  9
```

```
    2  17
    3̸  7̸      You should write only this.
 − 1  8
 _____
    1  9
```

Do Exercises 15 and 16.

Borrowing Hundreds

Example 8   Subtract: $538 − 275$.

```
   5  3  8     Subtract ones.
 − 2  7  5
 _____
          3
```

```
   5  3  8     Try to subtract tens: 3 tens − 7 tens is not a whole number.
 − 2  7  5
 _____
      ?  3
```

```
   4  13
   5̸  3̸  8     Borrow a hundred. That is, 1 hundred = 10 tens, and
 − 2  7  5     10 tens + 3 tens = 13 tens. Write 4 above the hundreds
 _____   column and 13 above the tens.
          3
```

> The borrowing is like exchanging 5 dollars, 3 dimes, and 8 pennies for 4 dollars, 13 dimes, and 8 pennies.

```
   4  13
   5̸  3̸  8     Subtract tens.
 − 2  7  5
 _____
      6  3
```

```
   4  13
   5̸  3̸  8     Subtract hundreds.
 − 2  7  5
 _____
   2  6  3
```

```
   4  13
   5̸  3̸  8     You should write only this.
 − 2  7  5
 _____
   2  6  3
```

Do Exercises 17 and 18.

Borrowing More Than Once

Sometimes we must borrow more than once.

Example 9 Subtract: 672 − 394.

$$\begin{array}{r} \overset{6\ \ 12}{6\ \not7\ \not2} \\ -\ 3\ 9\ 4 \\ \hline 8 \end{array}$$ Borrowing a ten to subtract ones

$$\begin{array}{r} \overset{\ \ 16}{\overset{5\ \not6\ 12}{\not6\ \not7\ \not2}} \\ -\ 3\ 9\ 4 \\ \hline 2\ 7\ 8 \end{array}$$ Borrowing a hundred to subtract tens

Do Exercises 19 and 20.

Example 10 Subtract: 6357 − 1769.

$$\begin{array}{r} \overset{\ \ \ 4\ 17}{6\ 3\ \not5\ \not7} \\ -\ 1\ 7\ 6\ 9 \\ \hline 8 \end{array}$$ We cannot subtract 9 from 7.
We borrow a ten.

$$\begin{array}{r} \overset{\ \ 14}{\overset{2\ \not4\ 17}{6\ \not3\ \not5\ \not7}} \\ -\ 1\ 7\ 6\ 9 \\ \hline 8\ 8 \end{array}$$ We cannot subtract 6 tens from 4 tens.
We borrow a hundred.

$$\begin{array}{r} \overset{12\ 14}{\overset{5\ \not2\ \not4\ 17}{\not6\ \not3\ \not5\ \not7}} \\ -\ 1\ 7\ 6\ 9 \\ \hline 4\ 5\ 8\ 8 \end{array}$$ We cannot subtract 7 hundreds from 2 hundreds.
We borrow a thousand.

We can always check by adding the answer to the number being subtracted.

Example 11 Subtract: 8341 − 2673. Check by adding.

We check by adding 5668 and 2673.

$$\begin{array}{r} \overset{12\ 13}{\overset{7\ \not2\ \not3\ 11}{\not8\ \not3\ \not4\ \not1}} \\ -\ 2\ 6\ 7\ 3 \\ \hline 5\ 6\ 6\ 8 \end{array}$$ *Check:* $\begin{array}{r} \overset{1\ \ 1\ \ 1}{5\ 6\ 6\ 8} \\ +\ 2\ 6\ 7\ 3 \\ \hline 8\ 3\ 4\ 1 \end{array}$

Do Exercises 21 and 22.

Zeros in Subtraction

Before subtracting, note the following:

50 is 5 tens;

70 is 7 tens.

Then

100 is 10 tens;

200 is 20 tens.

Do Exercises 23–26.

Subtract.

19.
$$\begin{array}{r} 5\ 6\ 3 \\ -\ 1\ 8\ 7 \\ \hline 376 \end{array}$$

20.
$$\begin{array}{r} 7\ 3\ 3 \\ -\ 4\ 8\ 8 \\ \hline 245 \end{array}$$

Subtract. Check by adding.

21.
$$\begin{array}{r} 4\ 2\ 3\ 6 \\ -\ 1\ 6\ 7\ 9 \\ \hline 2557 \end{array}$$

22.
$$\begin{array}{r} 7\ 5\ 4\ 1 \\ -\ 3\ 8\ 6\ 7 \\ \hline 3674 \end{array}$$

Complete.

23. 80 = _____8_____ tens

24. 60 = _____6_____ tens

25. 300 = _____30_____ tens

26. 900 = _____90_____ tens

Answers on page A-30

Complete.

27. $5000 = \underline{\quad 500 \quad}$ tens

28. $9000 = \underline{\quad 900 \quad}$ tens

29. $5380 = \underline{\quad 538 \quad}$ tens

30. $6770 = \underline{\quad 677 \quad}$ tens

Subtract.

31.
$$\begin{array}{r} 6\,0 \\ -\,1\,8 \\ \hline 42 \end{array}$$

32.
$$\begin{array}{r} 4\,8\,0 \\ -\,2\,5\,6 \\ \hline 224 \end{array}$$

Subtract.

33.
$$\begin{array}{r} 6\,0\,2 \\ -\,4\,6\,4 \\ \hline 138 \end{array}$$

34.
$$\begin{array}{r} 4\,0\,8 \\ -\,3\,6\,4 \\ \hline 44 \end{array}$$

Subtract.

35.
$$\begin{array}{r} 4\,0\,0\,6 \\ -\,1\,2\,3\,8 \\ \hline 2768 \end{array}$$

36.
$$\begin{array}{r} 9\,0\,0\,1 \\ -\,7\,8\,0\,4 \\ \hline 1197 \end{array}$$

Subtract.

37.
$$\begin{array}{r} 3\,0\,0\,0 \\ -\,1\,7\,5\,4 \\ \hline 1246 \end{array}$$

38.
$$\begin{array}{r} 8\,0\,1\,7 \\ -\,3\,2\,8\,9 \\ \hline 4728 \end{array}$$

To the student: *If you had trouble with Section 1.3 and have studied Developmental Unit S, you should go back and work through Section 1.3 after completing Exercise Set S.*

Answers on page A-30

Also,

> 230 is 2 hundreds + 3 tens
> or 20 tens + 3 tens
> or 23 tens.

Similarly,

> 1000 is 100 tens;
> 2000 is 200 tens;
> 4670 is 467 tens.

Do Exercises 27–30.

Example 12   Subtract: $50 - 37$.

$$\begin{array}{r} \overset{4\ \ 10}{\cancel{5}\ \cancel{0}} \\ -\,3\,7 \\ \hline 1\,3 \end{array}$$

We have 5 tens.
We keep 4 of them in the tens column.
We put 1 ten, or 10 ones, with the ones.

Do Exercises 31 and 32.

Example 13   Subtract: $803 - 547$.

$$\begin{array}{r} \overset{7\ \ 9\ \ 13}{8\,0\,\cancel{3}} \\ -\,5\,4\,7 \\ \hline 2\,5\,6 \end{array}$$

We have 8 hundreds, or 80 tens.
We keep 79 tens.
We put 1 ten, or 10 ones, with the ones.

Do Exercises 33 and 34.

Example 14   Subtract: $9003 - 2789$.

$$\begin{array}{r} \overset{8\ \ 9\ \ 9\ \ 13}{9\,0\,0\,\cancel{3}} \\ -\,2\,7\,8\,9 \\ \hline 6\,2\,1\,4 \end{array}$$

We have 9 thousands, or 900 tens.
We keep 899 tens.
We put 1 ten, or 10 ones, with the ones.

Do Exercises 35 and 36.

Examples   Subtract.

15.
$$\begin{array}{r} \overset{4\ \ 9\ \ 9\ \ 10}{5\,0\,0\,0} \\ -\,2\,8\,6\,1 \\ \hline 2\,1\,3\,9 \end{array}$$

16.
$$\begin{array}{r} \overset{4\ \ 9\ \ \overset{10}{0}\ \ 13}{5\,0\,1\,3} \\ -\,1\,8\,5\,7 \\ \hline 3\,1\,5\,6 \end{array}$$

We have 5 thousands, or 49 hundreds and 10 tens.

Do Exercises 37 and 38.

Exercise Set S

a Subtract. Try to do these mentally.

1.	**2.**	**3.**	**4.**	**5.**
7	8	7	8	5
− 0	− 8	− 7	− 3	− 2
7	0	0	5	3

6.	**7.**	**8.**	**9.**	**10.**
16	17	12	11	12
− 8	− 9	− 6	− 4	− 9
8	8	6	7	3

11.	**12.**	**13.**	**14.**	**15.**
14	18	13	15	9
− 7	− 9	− 7	− 9	− 7
7	9	6	6	2

16. 7 − 3
4

17. 4 − 1
3

18. 2 − 0
2

19. 3 − 3
0

20. 6 − 3
3

21. 7 − 6
1

22. 9 − 8
1

23. 10 − 3
7

24. 6 − 6
0

25. 11 − 7
4

26. 12 − 8
4

27. 5 − 0
5

28. 4 − 0
4

29. 13 − 9
4

30. 14 − 9
5

31. 11 − 2
9

32. 12 − 3
9

33. 16 − 9
7

34. 18 − 9
9

35. 11 − 5
6

36. 10 − 4
6

37. 10 − 8
2

38. 14 − 8
6

39. 15 − 8
7

40. 10 − 2
8

b Subtract.

41.	**42.**	**43.**	**44.**	**45.**
6 4	5 5	5 4 8	5 9 6	7 0 0
− 3 1	− 3 4	− 3 0 1	− 4 0 3	− 2 0 0
33	21	247	193	500

46. 765
       −111
654

47. 525
       −323
202

48. 747
       −130
617

49. 988
       −700
288

50. 9450
       −8230
1220

51. 6552
       −4321
2231

52. 7547
       −3421
4126

53. 5875
       −2111
3764

54. 38,695
       −37,004
1691

55. 67,899
       −66,673
1226

56. 99,999
       −   1
99,998

57. 56,780
       −56,770
10

58. 42,111
       −32,010
10,101

59. 77,654
       −66,611
11,043

60. 23,456
       −12,345
11,111

---

c Subtract.

61. 93
       −28
65

62. 42
       −13
29

63. 86
       −78
8

64. 98
       −89
9

65. 625
       −317
308

66. 735
       −609
126

67. 853
       −236
617

68. 961
       −747
214

69. 787
       −698
89

70. 6769
       −2367
4402

71. 6431
       −2876
3555

72. 7654
       −1765
5889

73. 5246
       −2859
2387

74. 6328
       −2679
3649

75. 7641
       −3809
3832

76. 8743
       − 599
8144

77. 12,647
       − 4,897
7750

78. 16,222
       − 5,777
10,445

79. 46,781
       −12,988
33,793

80. 470
       −189
281

81. 690
       −235
455

82. 703
       −132
571

83. 6406
       − 258
6148

84. 2309
       − 109
2200

85. 3406
       −1293
2113

86. 6807
       −3059
3748

87. 8000
       −2794
5206

88. 8002
       −6543
1459

89. 38,000
       −37,695
305

90. 16,043
       −11,588
4455

Developmental Units

634

M Multiplication

a | Basic Multiplication

To multiply, we begin with two numbers, called **factors**, and get a third number, called a **product**. Multiplication can be explained by counting. The product 3×5 can be found by counting out 3 sets of 5 objects each, joining them (in a rectangular array if desired), and counting all the objects.

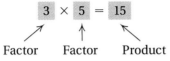

Factor   Factor   Product

We can also think of multiplication as repeated addition.

$$3 \times 5 = \underbrace{5 + 5 + 5}_{\text{3 addends of 5}} = 15$$

Examples Multiply. If you have trouble, think either of putting sets of objects together in a rectangular array or of repeated addition.

1. $5 \times 6 = 30$

$$\begin{array}{r} 6 \\ \times\ 5 \\ \hline 30 \end{array}$$

2. $8 \times 4 = 32$

$$\begin{array}{r} 4 \\ \times\ 8 \\ \hline 32 \end{array}$$

Do Exercises 1–4.

Multiplying by 0

How do we multiply by 0? Consider $4 \cdot 0$. Using repeated addition, we see that

$$4 \cdot 0 = \underbrace{0 + 0 + 0 + 0}_{\text{4 addends of 0}} = 0.$$

We can also think of this using sets. That is, $4 \cdot 0$ is 4 sets with 0 objects in each set, so the total is 0.

Consider $0 \cdot 4$. Using repeated addition, we say that this is 0 addends of 4, which is 0. Using sets, we say that this is 0 sets with 4 objects in each set, which is 0. Thus we have the following.

> Multiplying by 0 gives 0.

Examples Multiply.

3. $13 \times 0 = 0$

$$\begin{array}{r} 0 \\ \times 13 \\ \hline 0 \end{array}$$

4. $0 \cdot 11 = 0$

$$\begin{array}{r} 11 \\ \times\ 0 \\ \hline 0 \end{array}$$

5. $0 \cdot 0 = 0$

$$\begin{array}{r} 0 \\ \times 0 \\ \hline 0 \end{array}$$

Do Exercises 5 and 6.

Objectives

a Multiply any two of the numbers 0, 1, 2, 3, 4, 5, 6, 7, 8, 9.

b Multiply by multiples of 10, 100, and 1000.

c Multiply larger numbers by 0, 1, 2, 3, 4, 5, 6, 7, 8, 9.

d Multiply by multiples of 10, 100, and 1000.

Multiply. Think of joining sets in a rectangular array or of repeated addition.

1. $7 \cdot 8$ (The dot "$\cdot$" means the same as "$\times$".)

56

2. $\begin{array}{r} 9 \\ \times\ 4 \\ \hline \end{array}$

36

3. $4 \cdot 7$

28

4. $\begin{array}{r} 7 \\ \times\ 6 \\ \hline \end{array}$

42

Multiply.

5. $8 \cdot 0$

0

6. $\begin{array}{r} 17 \\ \times\ 0 \\ \hline \end{array}$

0

Answers on page A-30

Multiply.

7. 8 · 1

8

8.   2 3
    ×   1
   ___
    2 3

9. Complete the table.

×	2	3	4	5
2	4	6	8	10
3	6	9	12	15
4	8	12	16	20
5	10	15	20	25
6	12	18	24	30

10.

×	6	7	8	9
5	30	35	40	45
6	36	42	48	54
7	42	49	56	63
8	48	56	64	72
9	54	63	72	81

Answers on page A-30

Multiplying by 1

How do we multiply by 1? Consider 5 · 1. Using repeated addition, we see that

$$5 \cdot 1 = \underbrace{1 + 1 + 1 + 1 + 1}_{\text{5 addends of 1}} = 5.$$

We can also think of this using sets. That is, 5 · 1 is 5 sets with 1 object in each set, so the total is 5.

Consider 1 · 5. Using repeated addition, we say that this is 1 addend of 5, which is 5. Using sets, we say that this is 1 set of 5 objects, which is 5. Thus we have the following.

> Multiplying a number by 1 does not change the number:
> $$a \cdot 1 = 1 \cdot a = a.$$
> We say that 1 is the **multiplicative identity.**

This is a very important property.

Examples   Multiply.

6. $13 \cdot 1 = 13$

   1
  × 13
  ___
  13

7. $1 \cdot 7 = 7$

   7
  × 1
  ___
   7

8. $1 \cdot 1 = 1$

   1
  × 1
  ___
   1

Do Exercises 7 and 8.

You should be able to multiply any of the numbers 0, 1, 2, 3, 4, 5, 6, 7, 8, 9. Multiplying by 0 and 1 is easy. The rest of the products are listed in the following table.

×	2	3	4	5	6	7	8	9
2	4	6	8	10	12	14	16	18
3	6	9	12	15	18	21	24	27
4	8	12	16	20	24	28	32	36
5	10	15	20	25	30	35	40	45
6	12	18	24	30	36	42	48	54
7	14	21	28	35	42	49	56	63
8	16	24	32	40	48	56	64	72
9	18	27	36	45	54	63	72	81

$5 \times 7 = 35$
Find 5 at the left, and 7 at the top.

$8 \cdot 4 = 32$
Find 8 at the left, and 4 at the top.

It is *very* important that you have the basic multiplication facts *memorized.* If you do not, you will always have trouble with multiplication.

The *commutative law of multiplication* says that we can multiply numbers in any order. Thus you need to learn only about half the table, as shown by the shading.

Do Exercises 9 and 10.

b Multiplying Multiples of 10, 100, and 1000

We now move to a more gradual, conceptual development of the multiplication procedure you considered in Section 1.5. It is intended to provide you with a greater understanding so that your skill level will increase.

We begin by considering multiplication by multiples of 10, 100, and 1000. These are numbers such as 10, 20, 30, 100, 400, 1000, and 7000.

Multiplying by a Multiple of 10

We know that

$$50 = 5 \text{ tens} \qquad 340 = 34 \text{ tens} \quad \text{and} \quad 2340 = 234 \text{ tens}$$
$$= 5 \cdot 10, \qquad = 34 \cdot 10, \qquad = 234 \cdot 10.$$

Turning this around, we see that to multiply any number by 10, all we need do is write a 0 on the end of the number.

> To multiply a number by 10, write 0 on the end of the number.

Examples Multiply.

9. $10 \cdot 6 = 60$

10. $10 \cdot 47 = 470$

11. $10 \cdot 583 = 5830$

Do Exercises 11–15.

Let's find $4 \cdot 90$. This is $4 \cdot (9 \text{ tens})$, or 36 tens. The procedure is the same as multiplying 4 and 9 and writing a 0 on the end. Thus, $4 \cdot 90 = 360$.

Examples Multiply.

12. $5 \cdot 70 = 350$ — $5 \cdot 7$, then write a 0

13. $8 \cdot 80 = 640$

14. $5 \cdot 60 = 300$

Do Exercises 16 and 17.

Multiplying by a Multiple of 100

Note the following:

$$300 = 3 \text{ hundreds} \qquad 4700 = 47 \text{ hundreds} \quad \text{and} \quad 56{,}800 = 568 \text{ hundreds}$$
$$= 3 \cdot 100, \qquad = 47 \cdot 100, \qquad = 568 \cdot 100.$$

Turning this around, we see that to multiply any number by 100, all we need do is write two 0's on the end of the number.

> To multiply a number by 100, write two 0's on the end of the number.

Multiply.

11. $10 \cdot 7$

70

12. $10 \cdot 45$

450

13. $10 \cdot 273$

2730

14. $10 \cdot 10$

100

15. $10 \cdot 100$

1000

Multiply.

16. $\begin{array}{r} 7\,0 \\ \times \quad 8 \\ \hline 560 \end{array}$

17. $\begin{array}{r} 6\,0 \\ \times \quad 6 \\ \hline 360 \end{array}$

Answers on page A-30

Multiply.

18. 100 · 7

700

19. 100 · 23

2300

20. 100 · 723

72,300

21. 100 · 100

10,000

22. 100 · 1000

100,000

Multiply.

23.

```
   7 0 0
 ×     8
 ─────────
   5600
```

24.

```
   4 0 0
 ×     4
 ─────────
   1600
```

Multiply.

25. 1000 · 9

9000

26. 1000 · 852

852,000

27. 1000 · 10

10,000

28. 3 · 4000

12,000

29. 9 · 8000

72,000

Answers on page A-30

Examples Multiply.

15. 100 · 6 = 600

16. 100 · 39 = 3900

17. 100 · 448 = 44,800

Do Exercises 18–22.

Let's find 4 · 900. This is 4 · (9 hundreds), or 36 hundreds. The procedure is the same as multiplying 4 and 9 and writing two 0's on the end. Thus, 4 · 900 = 3600.

Examples Multiply.

18. 6 · 800 = 4800

        6 · 8, then write 00

19. 9 · 700 = 6300

20. 5 · 500 = 2500

Do Exercises 23 and 24.

Multiplying by a Multiple of 1000

Note the following:

$$6000 = 6 \text{ thousands} \quad \text{and} \quad 19,000 = 19 \text{ thousands}$$
$$= 6 \cdot 1000 \qquad\qquad = 19 \cdot 1000.$$

Turning this around, we see that to multiply any number by 1000, all we need do is write three 0's on the end of the number.

> To multiply a number by 1000, write three 0's on the end of the number.

Examples Multiply.

21. 1000 · 8 = 8000

22. 2000 · 13 = 26,000

23. 1000 · 567 = 567,000

Do Exercises 25–29.

Multiplying Multiples by Multiples

Let's multiply 50 and 30. This is 50 · (3 tens), or 150 tens, or 1500. The procedure is the same as multiplying 5 and 3 and writing two 0's on the end.

To multiply multiples of tens, hundreds, thousands, and so on:

a) Multiply the one-digit numbers.

b) Count the number of zeros.

c) Write that many 0's on the end.

Examples Multiply.

24.
```
      80      1 zero at end
 ×    60      1 zero at end
    4800
      ⤷——— 6 · 8, then write 00
```

25.
```
     800      2 zeros at end
 ×    60      1 zero at end
   48,000
      ⤷——— 6 · 8, then write 000
```

26.
```
     800      2 zeros at end
 ×   600      2 zeros at end
  480,000
      ⤷——— 6 · 8, then write
            0,000
```

27.
```
     800      2 zeros at end
 ×    50      1 zero at end
   40,000
      ⤷——— 5 · 8, then write
            000
```

Do Exercises 30–33.

c | Multiplying Larger Numbers

The product 3 × 24 can be represented as

$$3 \times (2 \text{ tens} + 4) = (2 \text{ tens} + 4) + (2 \text{ tens} + 4) + (2 \text{ tens} + 4)$$
$$= 6 \text{ tens} + 12$$
$$= 6 \text{ tens} + 1 \text{ ten} + 2$$
$$= 7 \text{ tens} + 2$$
$$= 72.$$

We multiply the 4 ones by 3, getting   12
We multiply the 2 tens by 3, getting   + 60
               Then we add: 72

Example 28 Multiply: 3 × 24.

```
     2 4
 ×     3
     1 2  ← Multiply the 4 ones by 3.
     6 0  ← Multiply the 2 tens by 3.
     7 2  ← Add.
```

Do Exercises 34–36.

Example 29 Multiply: 5 × 734.

```
       7 3 4
 ×         5
        2 0  ← Multiply the 4 ones by 5.
      1 5 0  ← Multiply the 3 tens by 5.
    3 5 0 0  ← Multiply the 7 hundreds by 5.
    3 6 7 0  ← Add.
```

Do Exercises 37 and 38.

Multiply.

30.
```
   9 0 0 0
 ×       6
  54,000
```

31.
```
      8 0
 ×  7 0
   5600
```

32.
```
    8 0 0
 ×   7 0
  56,000
```

33.
```
    6 0 0
 ×   3 0
  18,000
```

Multiply.

34.
```
   1 4
 ×   2
   28
```

35.
```
   5 8
 ×   2
  116
```

36.
```
   3 7
 ×   4
  148
```

Multiply.

37.
```
   8 2 3
 ×     6
  4938
```

38.
```
   1 3 4 8
 ×       5
    6740
```

Answers on page A-30

Multiply using the short form.

39.
$$\begin{array}{r} 5\,8 \\ \times\ \ 2 \\ \hline 116 \end{array}$$

40.
$$\begin{array}{r} 3\,7 \\ \times\ \ 4 \\ \hline 148 \end{array}$$

41.
$$\begin{array}{r} 8\,2\,3 \\ \times\ \ \ \ 6 \\ \hline 4938 \end{array}$$

42.
$$\begin{array}{r} 1\,3\,4\,8 \\ \times\ \ \ \ \ \ 5 \\ \hline 6740 \end{array}$$

Multiply.

43.
$$\begin{array}{r} 7\,4\,6 \\ \times\ \ \ \ 8 \\ \hline 5968 \end{array}$$

44.
$$\begin{array}{r} 7\,4\,6 \\ \times\ \ \ 8\,0 \\ \hline 59{,}680 \end{array}$$

45.
$$\begin{array}{r} 7\,4\,6 \\ \times\ 8\,0\,0 \\ \hline 596{,}800 \end{array}$$

To the student: *If you had trouble with Section 1.5 and have studied Developmental Unit M, you should go back and work through Section 1.5 after completing Exercise Set M.*

Answers on page A-30

Let's look at Example 29 again. Instead of writing each product on a separate line, we can use a shorter form.

Example 30 Multiply: 5×734.

Multiply the ones by 5: $5 \cdot (4\ \text{ones}) = 20\ \text{ones} = 2\ \text{tens} + 0\ \text{ones}$. Write 0 in the ones column and 2 above the tens.

Multiply the 3 tens by 5 and add 2 tens: $5 \cdot (3\ \text{tens}) = 15\ \text{tens}$, $15\ \text{tens} + 2\ \text{tens} = 17\ \text{tens} = 1\ \text{hundred} + 7\ \text{tens}$. Write 7 in the tens column and 1 above the hundreds.

Multiply the 7 hundreds by 5 and add 1 hundred: $5 \cdot (7\ \text{hundreds}) = 35\ \text{hundreds}$, $35\ \text{hundreds} + 1\ \text{hundred} = 36\ \text{hundreds}$.

$$\begin{array}{r} {}^{1}\,{}^{2}\ \ \ \\ 7\ 3\ 4 \\ \times\ \ \ \ \ 5 \\ \hline 3\ 6\ 7\ 0 \end{array}$$ You should write only this.

Try to avoid writing the reminders unless necessary.

Do Exercises 39–42.

---

d | Multiplying by Multiples of 10, 100, and 1000

To multiply 327 by 50, we multiply by 10 (write a 0), and then multiply 327 by 5.

$$\begin{array}{r} 3\ 2\ 7 \\ \times\ \ \ \ 5\,\boxed{0} \\ \hline 1\ 6{,}3\ 5\ 0 \end{array}$$ ← Write a 0.

Multiply $5 \cdot 327$.

Example 31 Multiply: 400×289.

$$\begin{array}{r} 2\ 8\ 9 \\ \times\ 4\,\boxed{0\ 0} \\ \hline 0\ 0 \end{array}$$ ← Write two 0's.

Multiply 4 and 289:

$$\begin{array}{r} 2\ 8\ 9 \\ \times\ \ \ \ 4\ 0\ 0 \\ \hline 1\ 1\ 5{,}6\ 0\ 0 \end{array}$$

$$\begin{array}{r} {}^{3}\,{}^{3}\ \ \\ 2\ 8\ 9 \\ \times\ \ \ \ 4 \\ \hline 1\ 1\ 5\ 6 \end{array}$$

$$\begin{array}{r} {}^{3}\,{}^{3}\ \ \ \ \\ 2\ 8\ 9 \\ \times\ \ \ \ 4\ 0\ 0 \\ \hline 1\ 1\ 5{,}6\ 0\ 0 \end{array}$$ You should write only this.

Do Exercises 43–45.

Exercise Set M

a Multiply. Try to do these mentally.

1. 3×4	2. 6×0	3. 7×1	4. 0×2	5. 10×1	6. 6×5
12	0	7	0	10	30

7. 5×2	8. 9×7	9. 9×6	10. 2×6	11. 7×0	12. 8×9
10	63	54	12	0	72

13. 1×8	14. 8×0	15. 4×7	16. 3×8	17. 5×9	18. 2×9
8	0	28	24	45	18

19. 0×7	20. 5×7	21. 9×5	22. 5×8	23. 0×0	24. 2×8
0	35	45	40	0	16

25. $5 \cdot 5$	26. $9 \cdot 9$	27. $1 \cdot 1$	28. $0 \cdot 0$	29. $2 \cdot 2$
25	81	1	0	4

30. $6 \cdot 6$	31. $1 \cdot 8$	32. $0 \cdot 1$	33. $3 \cdot 9$	34. $2 \cdot 9$
36	8	0	27	18

35. $6 \cdot 0$	36. $10 \cdot 1$	37. $6 \cdot 8$	38. $9 \cdot 6$	39. $8 \cdot 0$
0	10	48	54	0

40. $9 \cdot 8$	41. $3 \cdot 5$	42. $1 \cdot 8$	43. $1 \cdot 9$	44. $2 \cdot 1$
72	15	8	9	2

45. $8 \cdot 4$	46. $3 \cdot 2$	47. $5 \cdot 3$	48. $1 \cdot 6$	49. $4 \cdot 2$
32	6	15	6	8

50. $4 \cdot 5$	51. $5 \cdot 4$	52. $4 \cdot 4$	53. $5 \cdot 2$	54. $8 \cdot 0$
20	20	16	10	0

b Multiply.

55.	10 × 8 80	56.	7 ×10 70	57.	20 × 8 160	58.	30 × 7 210	59.	45 ×10 450

60. 78
   ×10
   780

61. 80
   × 7
   560

62. 90
   × 4
   360

63. 100
   × 8
   800

64. 100
   × 3
   300

65. 100
   × 9
   900

66. 100
   × 10
   1000

67. 3457
   × 100
   345,700

68. 400
   × 3
   1200

69. 700
   × 7
   4900

70. 500
   × 8
   4000

71. 100
   ×100
   10,000

72. 1000
   × 7
   7000

73. 1000
   × 9
   9000

74. 1000
   × 2
   2000

75. 457
   ×1000
   457,000

76. 6769
   ×1000
   6,769,000

77. 2000
   × 9
   18,000

78. 5000
   × 4
   20,000

79. 6000
   × 8
   48,000

80. 8000
   × 2
   16,000

81. 3000
   × 2
   6000

82. 1000
   ×1000
   1,000,000

83. 40
   ×30
   1200

84. 20
   ×10
   200

85. 80
   ×50
   4000

86. 50
   ×50
   2500

87. 400
   × 30
   12,000

88. 200
   × 30
   6000

89. 700
   × 90
   63,000

90. 400
   ×300
   120,000

91. 4000
   × 200
   800,000

92. 6000
   × 20
   120,000

93. 4000
   ×4000
   16,000,000

94. 8000
   × 10
   80,000

c Multiply.

95. 49
   × 3
   147

96. 74
   × 6
   444

97. 593
   × 5
   2965

98. 609
   × 8
   4872

99. 899
   × 7
   6293

100. 865
   × 4
   3460

101. 8118
   × 2
   16,236

102. 6754
   × 2
   13,508

103. 43,777
   × 2
   87,554

104. 32,564
   × 6
   195,384

d Multiply.

105. 58
   ×60
   3480

106. 93
   ×30
   2790

107. 42
   ×80
   3360

108. 78
   ×90
   7020

109. 346
   × 60
   20,760

110. 267
   × 40
   10,680

111. 897
   ×400
   358,800

112. 366
   ×300
   109,800

113. 834
   ×700
   583,800

114. 333
   ×900
   299,700

115. 5673
   ×2000
   11,346,000

116. 4678
   ×5000
   23,390,000

117. 6788
   ×9000
   61,092,000

118. 9129
   ×8000
   73,032,000

Developmental Units

D Division

a | Basic Division

Division can be explained by arranging a set of objects in a rectangular array. This can be done in two ways.

Example 1 Divide: $18 \div 6$.

METHOD 1 We can do this division by taking 18 objects and determining into how many rows, each with 6 objects, we can arrange the objects.

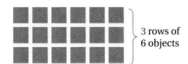

} 3 rows of 6 objects

Since there are 3 rows of 6 objects, we have

$$18 \div 6 = 3.$$

METHOD 2 We can also arrange the objects into 6 rows and determine how many objects are in each row.

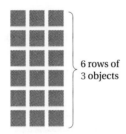

} 6 rows of 3 objects

Since there are 3 objects in each of the 6 rows, we have

$$18 \div 6 = 3.$$

We can also use fractional notation for division. That is,

$$18 \div 6 = 18/6 = \frac{18}{6}.$$

Examples Divide.

2. $9 \overline{)\ 3\ 6}^{\ 4}$ *Think*: 36 objects: How many rows, each with 9 objects? or 36 objects: How many objects in each of 9 rows?

3. $42 \div 7 = 6$

4. $\dfrac{24}{3} = 8$

Do Exercises 1–4.

Objectives

a Find basic quotients such as $20 \div 5$, $56 \div 7$, and so on.

b Divide using the "guess, multiply, and subtract" method.

c Divide by estimating multiples of thousands, hundreds, tens, and ones.

Divide.

1. $24 \div 6$ 4

2. $64 \div 8$ 8

3. $\dfrac{63}{7}$ 9

4. $\dfrac{27}{9}$ 3

Answers on page A-30

For each multiplication fact, write two division facts.

5. 6 · 2 = 12

  12 ÷ 2 = 6; 12 ÷ 6 = 2

6. 7 × 6 = 42

  42 ÷ 6 = 7; 42 ÷ 7 = 6

In Developmental Unit M, you memorized a multiplication table. That table will enable you to divide as well. First, let's recall how multiplication and division are related.

A multiplication: 5 · 4 = 20.

Two related divisions:

A.    20 ÷ 5 = 4.

4 rows of 5 objects

B.   20 ÷ 4 = 5.

5 rows of 4 objects

Since we know that

  5 · 4 = 20,   **A basic multiplication fact**

we also know the two division facts

  20 ÷ 5 = 4   and   20 ÷ 4 = 5.

Example 5   From 7 · 8 = 56, write two division facts.

a) We have

  7 · 8 = 56   **Division sentence**

  7 = 56 ÷ 8.   **Related multiplication sentence**

b) We also have

  7 · 8 = 56   **Division sentence**

  8 = 56 ÷ 7.   **Related multiplication sentence**

Do Exercises 5 and 6.

We can use the idea that division is defined in terms of multiplication to do basic divisions.

Example 6 Find: $35 \div 5$.

To find $35 \div 5$, we ask, "5 times what number is 35?"

$$5 \cdot \blacksquare = 35$$

×	2	3	4	5	6	7	8	9
2	4	6	8	10	12	14	16	18
3	6	9	12	15	18	21	24	27
4	8	12	16	20	24	28	32	36
5	10	15	20	25	30	35	40	45
6	12	18	24	30	36	42	48	54
7	14	21	28	35	42	49	56	63
8	16	24	32	40	48	56	64	72
9	18	27	36	45	54	63	72	81

$35 \div 5 = 7$

Using the multiplication table above, we find 35 inside the table and 5 at the left. Then we read the answer 7 from the top. Thus we have $35 \div 5 = 7$. Strive to do this kind of thinking mentally as fast as you can, without having to use the table.

Do Exercises 7–10.

Division by 1

Note that

$$3 \div 1 = 3 \quad \text{because} \quad 3 = 3 \cdot 1; \qquad \frac{14}{1} = 14 \quad \text{because} \quad 14 = 14 \cdot 1.$$

> Any number divided by 1 is that same number:
> $$a \div 1 = \frac{a}{1} = a.$$

Examples Divide.

7. $\dfrac{8}{1} = 8$

8. $6 \div 1 = 6$

9. $34 \div 1 = 34$

Do Exercises 11–13.

Division by 0

Why can't we divide by 0? Suppose the number 4 could be divided by 0. Then if $\square$ were the answer,

$$4 \div 0 = \square$$

and since 0 times any number is 0, we would have

$$4 = \square \cdot 0 = 0. \quad \text{False!}$$

Divide.

7. $28 \div 4$ 7

8. $81 \div 9$ 9

9. $\dfrac{16}{2}$ 8

10. $\dfrac{54}{6}$ 9

Divide.

11. $6 \div 1$ 6

12. $\dfrac{13}{1}$ 13

13. $1 \div 1$ 1

Answers on page A-30

D Division

645

Divide, if possible. If not possible, write "not defined."

14. $\dfrac{8}{4}$

2

15. $\dfrac{5}{0}$

Not defined

16. $\dfrac{0}{5}$

0

17. $\dfrac{0}{0}$

Not defined

18. $12 \div 0$

Not defined

19. $100 \div 10$

10

20. $\dfrac{5}{3-3}$

Not defined

21. $\dfrac{8-8}{4}$

0

Answers on page A-30

Suppose 12 could be divided by 0. If $\square$ were the answer,

$$12 \div 0 = \square$$

and since 0 times any number is 0, we would have

$$12 = \square \cdot 0 = 0. \qquad \text{False!}$$

Thus, $a \div 0$ would be some number $\square$ such that $a = \square \cdot 0 = 0$. So the only possible number that could be divided by 0 would be 0 itself.

But such a division would give us any number we wish, for

$$0 \div 0 = 8 \quad \text{because} \quad 0 = 8 \cdot 0;$$
$$0 \div 0 = 3 \quad \text{because} \quad 0 = 3 \cdot 0; \quad \Big\} \quad \text{All true!}$$
$$0 \div 0 = 7 \quad \text{because} \quad 0 = 7 \cdot 0.$$

We avoid the preceding difficulties by agreeing to exclude division by 0.

> ▶ Division by 0 is not defined. (We agree not to divide by 0.)

Dividing 0 by Other Numbers

Note that

$$0 \div 3 = 0 \quad \text{because} \quad 0 = 0 \cdot 3; \qquad \frac{0}{12} = 0 \quad \text{because } 0 = 0 \cdot 12.$$

> ▶ Zero divided by any number greater than 0 is 0:
>
> $$\frac{0}{a} = 0, \quad a > 0.$$

Examples Divide.

10. $0 \div 8 = 0$

11. $0 \div 22 = 0$

12. $\dfrac{0}{9} = 0$

Do Exercises 14–21.

Division of a Number by Itself

Note that

$$3 \div 3 = 1 \quad \text{because} \quad 3 = 1 \cdot 3; \qquad \frac{34}{34} = 1 \quad \text{because} \quad 34 = 1 \cdot 34.$$

> Any number greater than 0 divided by itself is 1:
>
> $$\frac{a}{a} = 1, \quad a > 0.$$

Examples Divide.

13. $8 \div 8 = 1$

14. $27 \div 27 = 1$

15. $\frac{32}{32} = 1$

Do Exercises 22–27.

b | Dividing by "Guess, Multiply, and Subtract"

To understand the process of division, we use a method known as "guess, multiply, and subtract." We do this to develop a shorter way that is understandable.

Example 16 Divide $275 \div 4$. Use "guess, multiply, and subtract."

We *guess* a partial quotient of 35. We could guess *any* number—say, 4, 16, or 30. We *multiply* and *subtract* as follows:

```
          3 5 ←— Partial quotient
    4 ) 2 7 5
        1 4 0 ←— 35 · 4
        1 3 5 ←— Remainder
```

Next, we look at 135 and *guess* another partial quotient—say, 20. Then we *multiply* and *subtract*:

```
          2 0 ←— Second partial quotient
          3 5
    4 ) 2 7 5
        1 4 0
        1 3 5
          8 0 ←— 20 · 4
          5 5 ←— Remainder
```

Next, we look at 55 and *guess* another partial quotient—say, 13. Then we *multiply* and *subtract*:

```
          1 3 ←— Third partial quotient
          2 0
          3 5
    4 ) 2 7 5
        1 4 0
        1 3 5
          8 0
          5 5
          5 2 ←— 13 · 4
            3 ←— Remainder is less than 4
```

Divide.

22. $23 \div 23$ 1

23. $\frac{67}{67}$ 1

24. $\frac{41}{41}$ 1

25. $17 \div 17$ 1

26. $17 \div 1$ 17

27. $\frac{54}{54}$ 1

Divide using the "guess, multiply, and subtract" method.

28. $6 \overline{) 4\ 5\ 4}$

75 R 4

29. $3\ 2 \overline{) 7\ 4\ 7}$

23 R 11

Answers on page A-30

Divide using the "guess, multiply, and subtract" method.

30. $7 \overline{\smash{)}\, 6789}$

969 R 6

31. $64 \overline{\smash{)}\, 3012}$

47 R 4

Since we cannot subtract any more 4's, the division is finished. We add our partial quotients.

```
          6 8 ←—— Quotient (sum of guesses)
          1 3
          2 0
          3 5
    4 ) 2 7 5         CHECK:    275 = (4 × 68) + 3
        1 4 0                   275 ? 272 + 3
        1 3 5                       | 275
          8 0
          5 5
          5 2
            3
```

The answer is 68 R 3. This tells us that with 275 objects, we could make 68 rows of 4 and have 3 left over.

The partial quotients (guesses) can be made in any manner so long as subtraction is possible.

Do Exercises 28 and 29 on the preceding page.

Example 17 Divide: $1506 \div 32$.

```
              4 7 ←—— Quotient (sum of guesses)
            2 0 ⎫
              2 ⎬
            2 0 ⎭ ←— Guesses
              5 ⎭
    3 2 ) 1 5 0 6
          1 6 0 ←— 5 · 32
          1 3 4 6
            6 4 0 ←— 20 · 32
            7 0 6
              6 4 ←— 2 · 32
            6 4 2
            6 4 0 ←— 20 · 32
                2 ←— Remainder: smaller than the divisor, 32
```

The answer is 47 R 2.

Remember, you can *guess any partial quotient* so long as subtraction is possible.

Do Exercises 30 and 31.

c Dividing by Estimating Multiples

Let's refine the guessing process. We guess multiples of 10, 100, and 1000, and so on.

Answers on page A-30

Example 18 Divide: 7643 ÷ 3.

a) Are there any thousands in the quotient? Yes, $3 \cdot 1000 = 3000$, which is less than 7643. To find how many thousands, we find products of 3 and multiples of 1000.

$$3 \cdot 1000 = 3000$$
$$3 \cdot 2000 = 6000$$
$$3 \cdot 3000 = 9000$$

← 7643 is here, so there are 2000 threes in the quotient.

$$
\begin{array}{r}
2\,0\,0\,0 \\
3\,)\,\overline{7\,6\,4\,3} \\
6\,0\,0\,0 \\
\hline
1\,6\,4\,3
\end{array}
$$

b) Now go to the hundreds place. Are there any hundreds in the quotient?

$$3 \cdot 100 = 300$$
$$3 \cdot 200 = 600$$
$$3 \cdot 300 = 900$$
$$3 \cdot 400 = 1200$$
$$3 \cdot 500 = 1500$$
$$3 \cdot 600 = 1800$$

← 1643

$$
\begin{array}{r}
5\,0\,0 \\
2\,0\,0\,0 \\
3\,)\,\overline{7\,6\,4\,3} \\
6\,0\,0\,0 \\
\hline
1\,6\,4\,3 \\
1\,5\,0\,0 \\
\hline
1\,4\,3
\end{array}
$$

c) Now go to the tens place. Are there any tens in the quotient?

$$3 \cdot 10 = 30$$
$$3 \cdot 20 = 60$$
$$3 \cdot 30 = 90$$
$$3 \cdot 40 = 120$$
$$3 \cdot 50 = 150$$

← 143

$$
\begin{array}{r}
4\,0 \\
5\,0\,0 \\
2\,0\,0\,0 \\
3\,)\,\overline{7\,6\,4\,3} \\
6\,0\,0\,0 \\
\hline
1\,6\,4\,3 \\
1\,5\,0\,0 \\
\hline
1\,4\,3 \\
1\,2\,0 \\
\hline
2\,3
\end{array}
$$

d) Now go to the ones place. Are there any ones in the quotient?

$$3 \cdot 1 = 3$$
$$3 \cdot 2 = 6$$
$$3 \cdot 3 = 9$$
$$3 \cdot 4 = 12$$
$$3 \cdot 5 = 15$$
$$3 \cdot 6 = 18$$
$$3 \cdot 7 = 21$$
$$3 \cdot 8 = 24$$

← 23

$$
\begin{array}{r}
2\,5\,4\,7 \\
7 \\
4\,0 \\
5\,0\,0 \\
2\,0\,0\,0 \\
3\,)\,\overline{7\,6\,4\,3} \\
6\,0\,0\,0 \\
\hline
1\,6\,4\,3 \\
1\,5\,0\,0 \\
\hline
1\,4\,3 \\
1\,2\,0 \\
\hline
2\,3 \\
2\,1 \\
\hline
2
\end{array}
$$

The answer is 2547 R 2.

Do Exercises 32 and 33.

Divide.

32. $4\,)\,\overline{3\,8\,5}$

96 R 1

33. $7\,)\,\overline{8\,8\,4\,6}$

1263 R 5

Answers on page A-30

Divide using the short form.

34. 2) 6 4 8

324

35. 9) 3 7 5 8

417 R 5

Divide.

36. 1 1) 4 1 5

37 R 8

37. 4 6) 1 0 7 5

23 R 17

To the student: *If you had trouble with Section 1.6 and have studied Developmental Unit D, you should go back and work through Section 1.6 after completing Exercise Set D.*

Answers on page A-30

A Short Form

Here is a shorter way to write Example 18.

Instead of this,

$$
\begin{array}{r}
2\ 5\ 4\ 7 \\
\hline
7 \\
4\ 0 \\
5\ 0\ 0 \\
2\ 0\ 0\ 0 \\
3\ )\ 7\ 6\ 4\ 3 \\
6\ 0\ 0\ 0 \\
\hline
1\ 6\ 4\ 3 \\
1\ 5\ 0\ 0 \\
\hline
1\ 4\ 3 \\
1\ 2\ 0 \\
\hline
2\ 3 \\
2\ 1 \\
\hline
2
\end{array}
$$

Short form

we write this.

$$
\begin{array}{r}
2\ 5\ 4\ 7 \\
3\ )\ 7\ 6\ 4\ 3 \\
6\ 0\ 0\ 0 \\
\hline
1\ 6\ 4\ 3 \\
1\ 5\ 0\ 0 \\
\hline
1\ 4\ 3 \\
1\ 2\ 0 \\
\hline
2\ 3 \\
2\ 1 \\
\hline
2
\end{array}
$$

We write a 2 above the thousands digit in the dividend to record 2000.
We write a 5 to record 500.
We write a 4 to record 40.
We write a 7 to record 7.

Do Exercises 34 and 35.

Example 19 Divide $2637 \div 41$. Use the short form.

$$
\begin{array}{r}
6 \\
4\ 1\ )\ 2\ 6\ 3\ 7 \\
2\ 4\ 6\ 0 \\
\hline
1\ 7\ 7
\end{array}
$$

$$
\begin{array}{r}
6\ 4 \\
4\ 1\ )\ 2\ 6\ 3\ 7 \\
2\ 4\ 6\ 0 \\
\hline
1\ 7\ 7 \\
1\ 6\ 4 \\
\hline
1\ 3
\end{array}
$$

The answer is 64 R 13.

Do Exercises 36 and 37.

In Section 1.6, the process of long division was refined with an estimation method. After doing Exercise Set D, you should restudy that procedure.

Exercise Set D

a Divide, if possible.

1. $24 \div 8$ 3

2. $72 \div 9$ 8

3. $28 \div 7$ 4

4. $22 \div 22$ 1

5. $32 \div 1$ 32

6. $45 \div 5$ 9

7. $14 \div 2$ 7

8. $40 \div 8$ 5

9. $37 \div 1$ 37

10. $10 \div 2$ 5

11. $36 \div 4$ 9

12. $12 \div 3$ 4

13. $54 \div 9$ 6

14. $18 \div 2$ 9

15. $20 \div 4$ 5

16. $16 \div 2$ 8

17. $72 \div 8$ 9

18. $42 \div 7$ 6

19. $12 \div 4$ 3

20. $8 \div 4$ 2

21. $54 \div 6$ 9

22. $18 \div 9$ 2

23. $9 \div 3$ 3

24. $28 \div 4$ 7

25. $56 \div 7$ 8

26. $24 \div 6$ 4

27. $14 \div 2$ 7

28. $14 \div 7$ 2

29. $21 \div 7$ 3

30. $36 \div 6$ 6

31. $8 \div 8$ 1

32. $32 \div 8$ 4

33. $30 \div 5$ 6

34. $18 \div 6$ 3

35. $49 \div 7$ 7

36. $81 \div 9$ 9

37. $0 \div 7$ 0

38. $9 \div 0$ Not defined

39. $16 \div 0$ Not defined

40. $42 \div 6$ 7

41. $\dfrac{48}{6}$ 8

42. $\dfrac{35}{5}$ 7

43. $\dfrac{9}{9}$ 1

44. $\dfrac{45}{9}$ 5

45. $\dfrac{0}{5}$ 0

46. $\dfrac{0}{8}$ 0

47. $\dfrac{6}{2}$ 3

48. $\dfrac{3}{3}$ 1

49. $\dfrac{8}{2}$ 4

50. $\dfrac{7}{1}$ 7

51. $\dfrac{5}{5}$ 1

52. $\dfrac{6}{1}$ 6

53. $\dfrac{2}{2}$ 1

54. $\dfrac{25}{5}$ 5

55. $\dfrac{4}{2}$ 2

56. $\dfrac{24}{3}$ 8

57. $\dfrac{0}{9}$ 0

58. $\dfrac{0}{4}$ 0

59. $\dfrac{40}{5}$ 8

60. $\dfrac{3}{1}$ 3

61. $\dfrac{16}{4}$ 4

62. $\dfrac{9}{0}$ Not defined

63. $\dfrac{32}{8}$ 4

64. $\dfrac{9}{9}$ 1

b Divide using the "guess, multiply, and subtract" method.

65. $4 \overline{)277}$
69 R 1

66. $2 \overline{)399}$
199 R 1

67. $8 \overline{)737}$
92 R 1

68. $6 \overline{)831}$
138 R 3

69. $5 \overline{)8619}$
1723 R 4

70. $3 \overline{)8775}$
2925

71. $9 \overline{)7777}$
864 R 1

72. $8 \overline{)4179}$
522 R 3

73. $7 \overline{)3691}$
527 R 2

74. $2 \overline{)5794}$
2897

75. $20 \overline{)875}$
43 R 15

76. $30 \overline{)987}$
32 R 27

77. $21 \overline{)999}$
47 R 12

78. $23 \overline{)975}$
42 R 9

79. $85 \overline{)7757}$
91 R 22

80. $54 \overline{)2821}$
52 R 13

81. $111 \overline{)3219}$
29

82. $102 \overline{)5612}$
55 R 2

83. $346 \overline{)78,910}$
228 R 22

84. $781 \overline{)15,999}$
20 R 379

c Divide.

85. $5 \overline{)105}$
21

86. $6 \overline{)708}$
118

87. $9 \overline{)820}$
91 R 1

88. $3 \overline{)965}$
321 R 2

89. $5 \overline{)4823}$
964 R 3

90. $8 \overline{)5437}$
679 R 5

91. $7 \overline{)9298}$
1328 R 2

92. $41 \overline{)1115}$
27 R 8

93. $46 \overline{)1058}$
23

94. $24 \overline{)7722}$
321 R 18

95. $38 \overline{)8522}$
224 R 10

96. $81 \overline{)2247}$
27 R 60

97. $94 \overline{)2153}$
22 R 85

98. $82 \overline{)4064}$
49 R 46

99. $117 \overline{)44,902}$
383 R 91

100. $740 \overline{)55,200}$
74 R 440

Answers

Diagnostic Pretest, p. xxiii

1. [1.2b] 4313   **2.** [1.7b] 28   **3.** [1.5b] 16,761
4. [1.8a] 23; 2   **5.** [2.6a] 150   **6.** [2.1d] 17
7. [2.2a] -13 **8.** [2.2a] -3 **9.** [2.3a] -17
10. [2.3a] 5   **11.** [2.4a] 54   **12.** [2.5b] 7
13. [2.7c] 70 ft   **14.** [2.7b] $7x + 13$ **15.** [2.8a] -17
16. [2.8b] 4   **17.** [3.6a] $-\frac{3}{2}$ **18.** [3.8a] -40
19. [3.5a] $\frac{35}{40}$ **20.** [3.7c] $\frac{3}{20}$ **21.** [4.3b] $\frac{1}{10}$
22. [4.7b] $4\frac{2}{3}$ **23.** [4.6a], [4.7b] $3\frac{1}{4}$ **24.** [4.4a] $\frac{12}{25}$
25. [5.2a] 8.976   **26.** [5.4a] -101.8
27. [5.2d] $2.5x - 7.3y$ **28.** [5.7a] 2.4
29. [6.4b]

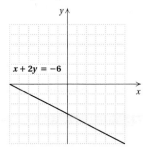

30. [6.5a, b, c] 14; 13; 12   **31.** [7.4a] 4   **32.** [7.5a] 7.5 ft
33. [8.1c] 62.5%   **34.** [8.1b] 0.024   **35.** [8.4b] 20%
36. [8.6a] $2090   **37.** [9.1a] 72   **38.** [9.1b] 0.00004
39. [9.7a] 4   **40.** [9.7b] 0.005   **41.** [9.3a] 18
42. [9.6b] 2.5   **43.** [9.2b] 36π cm^2; 12π cm
44. [9.6a] 125 m^3 **45.** [10.1a] $8x^3 - 3x^2 - 10$
46. [10.1c] $4x^4 - 8x^3 - x^2 - 2$
47. [10.3a] $2x^2 + 5x - 3$ **48.** [10.2c] $2x^3(5x^2 + 4x - 6)$
49. [10.4a] 1   **50.** [10.4b] $10a^4b^5$

Chapter 1

Pretest: Chapter 1, p. 2

1. [1.1c] Three million, seventy-eight thousand, fifty-nine   **2.** [1.1a] 6 thousands + 9 hundreds + 8 tens + 7 ones   **3.** [1.1d] 2,047,398,589
4. [1.1e] 6 ten thousands   **5.** [1.4a] 956,000
6. [1.5c] 60,000   **7.** [1.2b] 10,216   **8.** [1.3d] 4108
9. [1.5b] 22,976   **10.** [1.6c] 503 R 11   **11.** [1.4c] $<$
12. [1.4c] $>$ **13.** [1.7b] 5542   **14.** [1.7b] 22

15. [1.7b] 34   **16.** [1.7b] 25   **17.** [1.8a] 12 lb
18. [1.8a] 126   **19.** [1.8a] 22,981,000
20. [1.8a] 2292 sq ft   **21.** [1.9b] 25   **22.** [1.9b] 64
23. [1.9c] 0   **24.** [1.9d] 0

Margin Exercises, Section 1.1, pp. 3–6

1. 1 thousand + 8 hundreds + 0 tens + 5 ones, or 1 thousand + 8 hundreds + 5 ones   **2.** 3 ten thousands + 6 thousands + 2 hundreds + 2 tens + 3 ones   **3.** 3 thousands + 2 hundreds + 1 ten
4. 2 thousands + 9 ones   **5.** 5 thousands + 7 hundreds   **6.** 5689   **7.** 87,128   **8.** 9003
9. Fifty-seven   **10.** Twenty-nine   **11.** Eighty-eight
12. Two hundred four   **13.** Seventy-nine thousand, two hundred four   **14.** One million, eight hundred seventy-nine thousand, two hundred four
15. Twenty-two billion, three hundred one million, eight hundred seventy-nine thousand, two hundred four   **16.** 213,105,329   **17.** 2 ten thousands
18. 2 hundred thousands   **19.** 2 millions
20. 2 ten millions   **21.** 6   **22.** 8   **23.** 4   **24.** 5

Exercise Set 1.1, p. 7

1. 5 thousands + 7 hundreds + 4 tens + 2 ones
3. 2 ten thousands + 7 thousands + 3 hundreds + 4 tens + 2 ones   **5.** 5 thousands + 6 hundreds + 9 ones   **7.** 2 thousands + 3 hundreds   **9.** 2475
11. 68,939   **13.** 7304   **15.** 1009   **17.** Eighty-five
19. Eighty-eight thousand   **21.** One hundred twenty-three thousand, seven hundred sixty-five
23. Seven billion, seven hundred fifty-four million, two hundred eleven thousand, five hundred seventy-seven
25. One million, eight hundred sixty-seven thousand
27. One billion, five hundred eighty-three million, one hundred forty-one thousand   **29.** 2,233,812
31. 8,000,000,000   **33.** 9,460,000,000,000
35. 2,974,600   **37.** 5 thousands   **39.** 5 hundreds
41. 3   **43.** 0   **45.** ◈   **47.** All 9's as digits. Answers may vary. For an 8-digit readout, it would be 99,999,999. This number has three periods.

Margin Exercises, Section 1.2, pp. 9–13

1. $8 + 2 = 10$ **2.** $45 + $33 = 78 **3.** 100 mi + 93 mi = 193 mi   **4.** 5 ft + 7 ft = 12 ft   **5.** 4 in. + 5 in. + 9 in. + 6 in. + 5 in. = 29 in.   **6.** 5 ft + 6 ft + 5 ft + 6 ft = 22 ft   **7.** 30,000 sq ft + 40,000 sq ft = 70,000 sq ft   **8.** 8 sq yd + 9 sq yd = 17 sq yd
9. 6 cu yd + 8 cu yd = 14 cu yd   **10.** 80 gal + 56 gal = 136 gal   **11.** 9745   **12.** 13,465   **13.** 16,182
14. 27   **15.** 34   **16.** 27   **17.** 38   **18.** 47   **19.** 61
20. 27,474

Exercise Set 1.2, p. 15

1. 7 + 8 = 15 **3.** 500 acres + 300 acres = 800 acres
5. 114 mi **7.** 52 in. **9.** 1300 ft **11.** 387
13. 5188 **15.** 164 **17.** 100 **19.** 900 **21.** 1010
23. 8503 **25.** 5266 **27.** 4466 **29.** 8310 **31.** 6608
33. 16,784 **35.** 34,432 **37.** 101,310 **39.** 100,101
41. 28 **43.** 26 **45.** 67 **47.** 230 **49.** 130
51. 1349 **53.** 36,926 **55.** 18,424 **57.** 2320
59. 31,685 **61.** 11,679 **63.** 22,654 **65.** 12,765,097
67. 7992 **68.** Nine hundred twenty-four million, six
hundred thousand **69.** 8 ten thousands
70. 23,000,000 **71.** ◈ **73.** 56,055,667
75. 1 + 99 = 100, 2 + 98 = 100, . . . , 49 + 51 = 100.
Then 49 · 100 = 4900 and 4900 + 50 + 100 = 5050.

Margin Exercises, Section 1.3, pp. 19–22

1. 67 cu yd − 5 cu yd = 62 cu yd **2.** 20,000 sq ft −
12,000 sq ft = 8,000 sq ft **3.** 7 = 2 + 5, or 7 = 5 + 2
4. 17 = 9 + 8, or 17 = 8 + 9 **5.** 5 = 13 − 8;
8 = 13 − 5 **6.** 11 = 14 − 3; 3 = 14 − 11
7. 67 + ▧ = 348; ▧ = 348 − 67
8. 800 + ▧ = 1200; ▧ = 1200 − 800
9. 3801 **10.** 6328 **11.** 4747 **12.** 56 **13.** 205
14. 658 **15.** 2851 **16.** 1546

Exercise Set 1.3, p. 23

1. $1260 − $450 = ▧ **3.** 16 oz − 5 oz = ▧
5. 7 = 3 + 4, or 7 = 4 + 3 **7.** 13 = 5 + 8, or
13 = 8 + 5 **9.** 23 = 14 + 9, or 23 = 9 + 14
11. 43 = 27 + 16, or 43 = 16 + 27 **13.** 6 = 15 − 9;
9 = 15 − 6 **15.** 8 = 15 − 7; 7 = 15 − 8
17. 17 = 23 − 6; 6 = 23 − 17 **19.** 23 = 32 − 9;
9 = 32 − 23 **21.** 17 + ▧ = 32; ▧ = 32 − 17
23. 10 + ▧ = 23; ▧ = 23 − 10 **25.** 12 **27.** 44
29. 533 **31.** 1126 **33.** 39 **35.** 298 **37.** 226
39. 234 **41.** 5382 **43.** 1493 **45.** 2187 **47.** 3831
49. 7748 **51.** 33,794 **53.** 2168 **55.** 43,028
57. 56 **59.** 36 **61.** 84 **63.** 454 **65.** 771
67. 2191 **69.** 3749 **71.** 7019 **73.** 5745 **75.** 95,974
77. 9989 **79.** 83,818 **81.** 4206 **83.** 10,305
85. 7 ten thousands **86.** Six million, three hundred
seventy-five thousand, six hundred two **87.** 29,708
88. 22,692 **89.** ◈ **91.** 2,829,177 **93.** 3; 4

Margin Exercises, Section 1.4, pp. 27–30

1. 40 **2.** 50 **3.** 70 **4.** 100 **5.** 40 **6.** 80 **7.** 90
8. 140 **9.** 470 **10.** 240 **11.** 300 **12.** 600
13. 800 **14.** 800 **15.** 9300 **16.** 8000 **17.** 8000
18. 20,000 **19.** 69,000 **20.** 200 **21.** 1800
22. 2600 **23.** 11,000 **24.** < **25.** > **26.** >
27. < **28.** < **29.** >

Exercise Set 1.4, p. 31

1. 50 **3.** 70 **5.** 730 **7.** 900 **9.** 100 **11.** 1000
13. 9100 **15.** 32,900 **17.** 6000 **19.** 8000
21. 45,000 **23.** 373,000 **25.** 180 **27.** 5720
29. 220; incorrect **31.** 890; incorrect **33.** 16,500
35. 5200 **37.** 1600 **39.** 1500 **41.** 31,000
43. 69,000 **45.** < **47.** > **49.** < **51.** > **53.** >
55. > **57.** 86,754 **58.** 13,589 **59.** 48,824
60. 4415 **61.** ◈ **63.** 30,411 **65.** 69,594

Margin Exercises, Section 1.5, pp. 34–38

1. 8 · 7 = 56 **2.** 10 · 75 = 750 mL
3. 8 · 8 = 64 **4.** 4 · 6 = 24 sq ft **5.** 1035
6. 3024 **7.** 46,252 **8.** 205,065 **9.** 144,432
10. 287,232 **11.** 14,075,720 **12.** 391,760
13. 17,345,600 **14.** 56,200 **15.** 562,000
16. (a) 1081; **(b)** 1081; **(c)** same **17.** 40 **18.** 15
19. 210,000; 160,000

Exercise Set 1.5, p. 39

1. 21 · 21 = 441 **3.** 8 · 12 oz = 96 oz **5.** 18 sq ft
7. 121 sq yd **9.** 144 sq mm **11.** 870 **13.** 2,340,000
15. 520 **17.** 564 **19.** 65,200 **21.** 4,371,000
23. 1527 **25.** 64,603 **27.** 4770 **29.** 3995
31. 46,080 **33.** 14,652 **35.** 207,672 **37.** 798,408
39. 166,260 **41.** 11,794,332 **43.** 20,723,872
45. 362,128 **47.** 20,064,048 **49.** 25,236,000
51. 302,220 **53.** 49,101,136 **55.** 30,525
57. 298,738 **59.** 50 · 70 = 3500 **61.** 30 · 30 = 900
63. 900 · 300 = 270,000 **65.** 400 · 200 = 80,000
67. 6000 · 5000 = 30,000,000
69. 8000 · 6000 = 48,000,000 **71.** 4370 **72.** 3109
73. 2350; 2300; 2000 **75.** ◈

Margin Exercises, Section 1.6, pp. 44–49

1. 112 ÷ 14 = ▧ **2.** 112 ÷ 8 = ▧ **3.** 15 = 5 · 3, or
15 = 3 · 5 **4.** 72 = 9 · 8, or 72 = 8 · 9
5. 6 = 12 ÷ 2; 2 = 12 ÷ 6 **6.** 6 = 42 ÷ 7;
7 = 42 ÷ 6 **7.** 6; 6 · 9 = 54 **8.** 6 R 7; 6 · 9 = 54,
54 + 7 = 61 **9.** 4 R 5; 4 · 12 = 48, 48 + 5 = 53
10. 6 R 13; 6 · 24 = 144, 144 + 13 = 157 **11.** 59 R 3
12. 1475 R 5 **13.** 1015 **14.** 134 **15.** 63 R 12
16. 807 R 4 **17.** 1088 **18.** 360 R 4 **19.** 800 R 47

Calculator Spotlight, p. 48

1. 1475 R 5 **2.** 360 R 4 **3.** 800 R 47 **4.** 134

Exercise Set 1.6, p. 51

1. 760 ÷ 4 = ▧ **3.** 455 ÷ 5 = ▧ **5.** 18 = 3 · 6, or
18 = 6 · 3 **7.** 22 = 22 · 1, or 22 = 1 · 22
9. 54 = 6 · 9, or 54 = 9 · 6 **11.** 37 = 1 · 37, or
37 = 37 · 1 **13.** 9 = 45 ÷ 5; 5 = 45 ÷ 9

15. $37 = 37 \div 1;\ 1 = 37 \div 37$　**17.** $8 = 64 \div 8$
19. $11 = 66 \div 6;\ 6 = 66 \div 11$　**21.** 55 R 2　**23.** 108
25. 307　**27.** 753 R 3　**29.** 74 R 1　**31.** 92 R 2
33. 1703　**35.** 987 R 5　**37.** 12,700　**39.** 127
41. 52 R 52　**43.** 29 R 5　**45.** 40 R 12
47. 90 R 22　**49.** 29　**51.** 105 R 3　**53.** 1609 R 2
55. 1007 R 1　**57.** 23　**59.** 107 R 1　**61.** 370
63. 609 R 15　**65.** 304　**67.** 3508 R 219　**69.** 8070
71. 7 thousands + 8 hundreds + 8 tens + 2 ones
72. >　**73.** $21 = 16 + 5$, or $21 = 5 + 16$
74. $56 = 14 + 42$, or $56 = 42 + 14$　**75.** $47 = 56 - 9$;
$9 = 56 - 47$　**76.** $350 = 414 - 64;\ 64 = 414 - 350$
77. ◆　**79.** 30

Margin Exercises, Section 1.7, pp. 55–58

1. 7　**2.** 5　**3.** No　**4.** Yes　**5.** 5　**6.** 10　**7.** 5
8. 22　**9.** 22,490　**10.** 9022　**11.** 570　**12.** 3661
13. 8　**14.** 45　**15.** 77　**16.** 3311　**17.** 6114　**18.** 8
19. 16　**20.** 644　**21.** 96　**22.** 94

Exercise Set 1.7, p. 59

1. 14　**3.** 0　**5.** 29　**7.** 0　**9.** 8　**11.** 14　**13.** 1035
15. 25　**17.** 450　**19.** 90,900　**21.** 32　**23.** 143
25. 79　**27.** 45　**29.** 324　**31.** 743　**33.** 37　**35.** 66
37. 15　**39.** 48　**41.** 175　**43.** 335　**45.** 104
47. 45　**49.** 4056　**51.** 17,603　**53.** 18,252　**55.** 205
57. $7 = 15 - 8;\ 8 = 15 - 7$　**58.** $6 = 48 \div 8$;
$8 = 48 \div 6$　**59.** <　**60.** >　**61.** 142 R 5
62. 334 R 11　**63.** ◆　**65.** 347

Margin Exercises, Section 1.8, pp. 62–68

1. 1,424,000　**2.** $369　**3.** $18　**4.** $38,988
5. 9180 sq in.　**6.** 378 packages; 1 can left over
7. 37 gal　**8.** 70 min, or 1 hr, 10 min　**9.** 106

Exercise Set 1.8, p. 69

1. $12,276　**3.** $7,004,000,000　**5.** $64,000,000
7. 4007 mi　**9.** 384 in.　**11.** 4500　**13.** 7280
15. $247　**17.** 54 weeks; 1 episode left over
19. 168 hr　**21.** $400　**23.** (a) 4700 sq ft; (b) 288 ft
25. 44　**27.** 56 cartons; 11 books left over
29. 1600 mi; 27 in.　**31.** 18　**33.** 22　**35.** $704
37. 525 min, or 8 hr, 45 min　**39.** 3000 sq in.
41. 234,600　**42.** 235,000　**43.** 22,000　**44.** 16,000
45. 320,000　**46.** 720,000　**47.** ◆　**49.** 792,000 mi;
1,386,000 mi

Margin Exercises, Section 1.9, pp. 73–76

1. 5^4　**2.** 5^5　**3.** 10^2　**4.** 10^4　**5.** 10,000　**6.** 100
7. 512　**8.** 32　**9.** 51　**10.** 30　**11.** 584　**12.** 84
13. 4; 1　**14.** 52; 52　**15.** 29　**16.** 1880　**17.** 253
18. 93　**19.** 1880　**20.** 305　**21.** 93　**22.** 87 in.
23. 46　**24.** 4

Calculator Spotlight, p. 75

1. 1024　**2.** 40,353,607　**3.** 1,048,576　**4.** 49　**5.** 85
6. 135　**7.** 176

Exercise Set 1.9, p. 77

1. 3^4　**3.** 5^2　**5.** 7^5　**7.** 10^3　**9.** 49　**11.** 729
13. 20,736　**15.** 121　**17.** 22　**19.** 20　**21.** 100
23. 1　**25.** 49　**27.** 5　**29.** 434　**31.** 41　**33.** 88
35. 4　**37.** 303　**39.** 20　**41.** 70　**43.** 295　**45.** 32
47. 906　**49.** 62　**51.** 102　**53.** $94　**55.** 110　**57.** 7
59. 544　**61.** 708　**63.** 452　**64.** 13
65. 102,600 mi^2　**66.** 98 gal　**67.** ◆　**69.** 675
71. 24; $1 + 5 \cdot (4 + 3) = 36$
73. 7; $12 \div (4 + 2) \cdot 3 - 2 = 4$

Summary and Review: Chapter 1, p. 79

1. 2 thousands + 7 hundreds + 9 tens + 3 ones
2. 5 ten thousands + 6 thousands + 7 tens + 8 ones
3. 8669　**4.** 90,844　**5.** Sixty-seven thousand, eight
hundred nineteen　**6.** Two million, seven hundred
eighty-one thousand, four hundred twenty-seven
7. 476,588　**8.** 36,260,064　**9.** 8 thousands
10. 3　**11.** $406 + $78 = $484, or $78 + $406 = $484
12. 986 yd　**13.** 14,272　**14.** 66,024　**15.** 22,098
16. 98,921　**17.** 151 lb − 12 lb = 139 lb
18. $340 − $196 = $144　**19.** $10 = 6 + 4$, or
$10 = 4 + 6$　**20.** $8 = 11 - 3;\ 3 = 11 - 8$　**21.** 5148
22. 1153　**23.** 2274　**24.** 17,757　**25.** 345,800
26. 345,760　**27.** 346,000　**28.** $41,300 + 19,700 =$
$61,000$　**29.** $38,700 - 24,500 = 14,200$
30. $400 \cdot 700 = 280,000$　**31.** >　**32.** <
33. $32 \cdot 15 = 480$　**34.** $125 \cdot 368 = 46,000$ yd^2
35. 420,000　**36.** 6,276,800　**37.** 506,748　**38.** 27,589
39. 5,331,810　**40.** $176 \div 4 = $ ▇　**41.** $222 \div 6 = $ ▇
42. $56 = 8 \cdot 7$, or $56 = 7 \cdot 8$　**43.** $4 = 52 \div 13$;
$13 = 52 \div 4$　**44.** 12 R 3　**45.** 5　**46.** 913 R 3
47. 384 R 1　**48.** 4 R 46　**49.** 54　**50.** 452
51. 5008　**52.** 4389　**53.** 8　**54.** 45　**55.** 546
56. $2413　**57.** 1982　**58.** $19,748　**59.** 137 beakers
filled; 13 mL of alcohol left over　**60.** 4^3　**61.** 10,000
62. 36　**63.** 65　**64.** 233　**65.** 56　**66.** 32
67. 260　**68.** 165
69. ◆ A vat contains 1152 oz of hot sauce. If
144 bottles are to be filled equally, how much will each
bottle contain? Answers may vary.
70. ◆ No; if subtraction were associative, then
$a - (b - c) = (a - b) - c$ for any a, b, and c. But, for
example,
$$12 - (8 - 4) = 12 - 4 = 8,$$
whereas
$$(12 - 8) - 4 = 4 - 4 = 0.$$
Since $8 \neq 0$, this example shows that subtraction is not
associative.
71. $d = 8$　**72.** $a = 8,\ b = 4$　**73.** 7 days

Test: Chapter 1, p. 81

1. [1.1a] 8 thousands + 8 hundreds + 4 tens + 3 ones
2. [1.1c] Thirty-eight million, four hundred three thousand, two hundred seventy-seven   **3.** [1.1e] 5
4. [1.2b] 9989   **5.** [1.2b] 63,791   **6.** [1.2b] 34
7. [1.2b] 10,515   **8.** [1.3d] 3630   **9.** [1.3d] 1039
10. [1.3d] 6848   **11.** [1.3d] 5175   **12.** [1.5b] 41,112
13. [1.5b] 5,325,600   **14.** [1.5b] 2405
15. [1.5b] 534,264   **16.** [1.6c] 3 R 3   **17.** [1.6c] 70
18. [1.6c] 97   **19.** [1.6c] 805 R 8   **20.** [1.8a] 1955
21. [1.8a] 92 packages, 3 cans left over
22. [1.8a] 62,811 mi^2 **23.** [1.8a] 120,000 m^2; 1600 m
24. [1.8a] 1808 lb   **25.** [1.8a] 20   **26.** [1.7b] 46
27. [1.7b] 13   **28.** [1.7b] 14   **29.** [1.4a] 35,000
30. [1.4a] 34,580   **31.** [1.4a] 34,600
32. [1.4b] 23,600 + 54,700 = 78,300
33. [1.4b] 54,800 − 23,600 = 31,200
34. [1.5c] 800 · 500 = 400,000   **35.** [1.4c] >
36. [1.4c] <   **37.** [1.9a] 12^4 **38.** [1.9b] 343
39. [1.9b] 8   **40.** [1.9c] 64   **41.** [1.9c] 96
42. [1.9c] 2   **43.** [1.9d] 216   **44.** [1.9c] 18
45. [1.9c] 92   **46.** [1.5a], [1.8a] 336 in^2 **47.** [1.8a] 80
48. [1.9c] 83   **49.** [1.9c] 9

Chapter 2

Pretest: Chapter 2, p. 84

1. [2.1a] −35; 67   **2.** [2.1b] <   **3.** [2.1b] >
4. [2.1b] <   **5.** [2.1c] 73   **6.** [2.1c] 57   **7.** [2.1d] 32
8. [2.1d] 17   **9.** [2.2a] −18   **10.** [2.2a] 6
11. [2.2a] −9   **12.** [2.2a] 0   **13.** [2.3a] −16
14. [2.3a] 2   **15.** [2.3a] 18   **16.** [2.3a] −6
17. [2.4a] 0   **18.** [2.4a] 48   **19.** [2.4b] −64
20. [2.5a] −5   **21.** [2.5a] 11   **22.** [2.5a] −80
23. [2.5a] 0   **24.** [2.5b] 0   **25.** [2.6a] −13
26. [2.7a] 3x + 15   **27.** [2.7a] 14x − 21y − 7
28. [2.7b] 15a   **29.** [2.7b] −10x + 15   **30.** [2.7c] 64 ft
31. [2.8b] −18   **32.** [2.8a] 22   **33.** [2.8b] 6

Margin Exercises, Section 2.1, pp. 86–89

1. 8; −5   **2.** 134; −80   **3.** −10; 148   **4.** −137; 289
5. >   **6.** >   **7.** <   **8.** >   **9.** 18   **10.** 9   **11.** 29
12. 52   **13.** −1   **14.** 2   **15.** 0   **16.** 4   **17.** 13
18. −28   **19.** 0   **20.** 7   **21.** 1   **22.** −6   **23.** −2

Calculator Spotlight, p. 86

1.–3. Keystrokes will vary by calculator.

Exercise Set 2.1, p. 91

1. −2   **3.** −1286; 29,028   **5.** 850; −432   **7.** >
9. <   **11.** <   **13.** <   **15.** >   **17.** <   **19.** 23
21. 0   **23.** 24   **25.** 53   **27.** 8   **29.** 8   **31.** 7
33. 0   **35.** 19   **37.** −42   **39.** 8   **41.** −7
43. 29   **45.** 22   **47.** −1   **49.** 3   **51.** −8
53. 2   **55.** 0   **57.** −34   **59.** 825   **60.** 125

61. 7106   **62.** 4   **63.** 81   **64.** 1550   **65.** ◆
67. ◆   **69.** [3] [2] [7] [×] [8] [3] [=] [+/−].
Answers may vary.   **71.** −8   **73.** −7   **75.** −1, 0, 1
77. −100, −5, 0, |3|, 4, |−6|, 7^2, 10^2, 2^7, 2^{10}

Margin Exercises, Section 2.2, pp. 93–94

1. −1   **2.** −8   **3.** 4   **4.** 0   **5.** 4 + (−5) = −1
6. −2 + (−4) = −6   **7.** −3 + 8 = 5   **8.** −11
9. −12   **10.** −34   **11.** −22   **12.** 2   **13.** −4
14. −2   **15.** 3   **16.** 0   **17.** 0   **18.** 0   **19.** 0
20. −58   **21.** −56   **22.** −12

Exercise Set 2.2, p. 95

1. −5   **3.** −4   **5.** 6   **7.** 0   **9.** −4   **11.** −15
13. −11   **15.** 0   **17.** 0   **19.** 8   **21.** −8
23. −25   **25.** −27   **27.** 0   **29.** 0   **31.** 3
33. −9   **35.** −5   **37.** 9   **39.** −3   **41.** 0
43. −10   **45.** −24   **47.** −5   **49.** −21   **51.** 2
53. −26   **55.** −21   **57.** 25   **59.** −17   **61.** 6
63. 8   **65.** −160   **67.** −62   **69.** 3 ten thousands + 9 thousands + 4 hundreds + 1 ten + 7 ones   **70.** 700
71. 33,000   **72.** 2352   **73.** 32   **74.** 3500   **75.** ◆
77. ◆   **79.** 17   **81.** −2531   **83.** All numbers less than 7   **85.** Positive   **87.** Positive

Margin Exercises, Section 2.3, pp. 97–99

1. −10   **2.** 3   **3.** −5   **4.** −2   **5.** −11   **6.** 4
7. −2   **8.** 3 − 10 = 3 + (−10); three minus ten is three plus negative ten.   **9.** 13 − 5 = 13 + (−5); thirteen minus five is thirteen plus negative five.
10. −12 − (−9) = −12 + 9; negative twelve minus negative nine is negative twelve plus nine.
11. −12 − 10 = −12 + (−10); negative twelve minus ten is negative twelve plus negative ten.
12. −14 − (−14) = −14 + 14; negative fourteen minus negative fourteen is negative fourteen plus fourteen.
13. −6   **14.** −16   **15.** 5   **16.** 3   **17.** −6   **18.** 13
19. −9   **20.** 17
21.

National League			
	HRs hit	HRs allowed	Diff.
Atlanta	215	117	98
St. Louis	223	151	72
Chicago	212	180	32
San Diego	167	139	28
Los Angeles	159	135	24
Houston	166	147	19
Colorado	183	174	9
Montreal	147	156	−9
San Francisco	161	171	−10
New York	136	152	−16
Arizona	159	188	−29
Cincinnati	138	170	−32
Milwaukee	152	188	−36
Pittsburgh	107	147	−40
Philadelphia	126	188	−62
Florida	114	182	−68

22. 50°C

Exercise Set 2.3, p. 101

1. −3 **3.** −8 **5.** −4 **7.** 0 **9.** −5 **11.** −7
13. −4 **15.** 0 **17.** 0 **19.** 14 **21.** 11 **23.** −14
25. 5 **27.** −7 **29.** −1 **31.** 18 **33.** −10 **35.** −3
37. −21 **39.** 5 **41.** −8 **43.** 12 **45.** −23
47. −68 **49.** −73 **51.** 116 **53.** 0 **55.** 55
57. 19 **59.** −62 **61.** −139 **63.** 6 **65.** 107
67. 219 **69.** −7 min **71.** $470 **73.** −3220 ft
75. 64 **76.** 1 **77.** 8 **78.** 288 oz **79.** 35 **80.** 3
81. ◈ **83.** ◈ **85.** 83,443 **87.** False; $0 − 3 \neq 3$
89. True **91.** False; $3 − 3 = 0$, but $3 \neq −3$
93. (a) −2; (b) yes

Margin Exercises, Section 2.4, pp. 105–108

1. 20; 10; 0; −10; −20; −30 **2.** −18 **3.** −100
4. −9 **5.** −10; 0; 10; 20; 30 **6.** 12 **7.** 32 **8.** 7
9. 0 **10.** 0 **11.** 120 **12.** −120 **13.** 6 **14.** −8
15. 81 **16.** −1 **17.** −25 **18.** Negative eight
squared; the opposite of eight squared

Calculator Spotlight, p. 108

1. 148,035,889 **2.** −1,419,857 **3.** −1,124,864
4. 1,048,576 **5.** −531,441 **6.** −117,649
7. −7776 **8.** −19,683

Exercise Set 2.4, p. 109

1. −21 **3.** −18 **5.** −48 **7.** −30 **9.** 10 **11.** 18
13. 42 **15.** 30 **17.** −120 **19.** 300 **21.** 72
23. −340 **25.** 0 **27.** 0 **29.** −96 **31.** 420
33. −70 **35.** 30 **37.** 0 **39.** −294 **41.** 25
43. −125 **45.** 10,000 **47.** −16 **49.** −243 **51.** 1
53. −729 **55.** −125 **57.** The opposite of seven to
the fourth power **59.** Negative nine to the sixth
power **61.** 532,500 **62.** 60,000,000 **63.** 80
64. 2550 **65.** 40 sq ft **66.** 240 **67.** ◈
69. ◈ **71.** −8 **73.** 25 **75.** 294 **77.** −85,525,504
79. −32 m **81.** (a) m and n must have different signs.
(b) At least one of m and n must be zero. (c) m and n
must have the same sign.

Margin Exercises, Section 2.5, pp. 111–112

1. −2 **2.** 5 **3.** −3 **4.** 0 **5.** −6 **6.** −5
7. Undefined **8.** 0 **9.** Undefined **10.** 68 **11.** 3
12. −15

Calculator Spotlight, p. 112

1. −4 **2.** −2 **3.** 787

Exercise Set 2.5, p. 113

1. −7 **3.** −14 **5.** −9 **7.** 4 **9.** −9 **11.** 2
13. −43 **15.** −8 **17.** Undefined **19.** −8 **21.** −23
23. 0 **25.** −19 **27.** −41 **29.** −7 **31.** 20

33. −334 **35.** 23 **37.** 8 **39.** 12 **41.** −10
43. −86 **45.** −9 **47.** 0 **49.** 10 **51.** −25
53. −7988 **55.** −3000 **57.** 60 **59.** 1 **61.** 2
63. 7 **65.** 2 **67.** 0 **69.** 28 sq in. **70.** 42
71. 14 gal **72.** 17 gal **73.** 150 calories **74.** 96 g
75. ◈ **77.** ◈ **79.** 0 **81.** −159 **83.** Negative
85. Negative

Margin Exercises, Section 2.6, pp. 115–116

1. 64 **2.** 28 **3.** −60 **4.** $-\dfrac{7}{x}; \dfrac{7}{-x}$ **5.** $\dfrac{-m}{n}; \dfrac{m}{-n}$
6. $-\dfrac{r}{4}; \dfrac{-r}{4}$ **7.** −7; −7; −7 **8.** 50 **9.** 48; 48
10. 81; 81 **11.** 9; −9 **12.** 4; −4 **13.** 32; −32

Exercise Set 2.6, p. 117

1. 14¢ **3.** −3 **5.** 1 **7.** 2 **9.** 13 **11.** 14 ft
13. 14 ft **15.** 21 **17.** 21 **19.** 400 ft **21.** −52
23. 10 **25.** −26 **27.** 36 **29.** $\dfrac{-3}{a}; \dfrac{3}{-a}$
31. $\dfrac{n}{-b}; -\dfrac{n}{b}$ **33.** $\dfrac{-9}{p}; -\dfrac{9}{p}$ **35.** $\dfrac{14}{-w}; -\dfrac{14}{w}$
37. −5; −5; −5 **39.** −27; −27; −27 **41.** 441; −147
43. 20; 20 **45.** 216; −216 **47.** 1; 1 **49.** 128; −128
51. −20 **53.** 370 **55.** 21 **57.** 100
59. Twenty-three million, forty-three thousand, nine
hundred twenty-one **60.** 901
61. $5280 − 2480 = 2800$ **62.** 994 **63.** 17 in.
64. 5 in. **65.** ◈ **67.** ◈ **69.** −8454 **71.** 2
73. 20 **75.** False; $2^3 = 8$, but $−2^3 = −8$ **77.** True

Margin Exercises, Section 2.7, pp. 121–126

1.

	$1 \cdot x$	x
$x = 3$	3	3
$x = -6$	−6	−6
$x = 0$	0	0

2.

	$-1 \cdot x$	$-x$
$x = 2$	−2	−2
$x = -6$	6	6
$x = 0$	0	0

3. $4a + 4b$ **4.** $5x + 5y + 5z$ **5.** $3x − 3y$
6. $2a − 2b + 2c$ **7.** $3x − 15$ **8.** $5x − 5y + 20$
9. $−2x + 6$ **10.** $−5x + 10y − 20z$ **11.** $5x; −4y; 3$
12. $−4y; −2x; \dfrac{x}{y}$ **13.** $9a^3$ and a^3; $4ab$ and $3ab$
14. $3xy$ and $−4xy$ **15.** $11a$ **16.** $7x^2 − 6$
17. $5m − n^2 − 4$ **18.** 26 cm **19.** 45 mm
20. 12 cm **21.** 24 ft **22.** 40 km **23.** 24 ft

Exercise Set 2.7, p. 127

1. $5a + 5b$ **3.** $4x + 4$ **5.** $2b + 10$ **7.** $7 - 7t$
9. $30x + 12$ **11.** $8x + 56 + 48y$ **13.** $-7y + 14$
15. $45x + 54y - 72$ **17.** $-4x + 12y + 8z$
19. $8a - 24b + 8c$ **21.** $4x - 12y - 28z$
23. $20a - 25b + 5c - 10d$ **25.** $19a$ **27.** $9a$
29. $11x + 6z$ **31.** $-13a + 62$ **33.** $-4 + 4t + 6y$
35. $-7x$ **37.** $-16y$ **39.** $-1 + 17a - 12b$
41. $6x + 3y$ **43.** $7x + y$ **45.** $6a + 4b - 2$
47. $x^3 + 9x$ **49.** $2a^2 + 8a^3 + 5$ **51.** $7xy + 6y^2 - 1$
53. $4a^2b - 3ab^2 + 2ab$ **55.** $-4x^4 + 6y^4 + 8x^4y^4$
57. 17 mm **59.** 18 m **61.** 20 in. **63.** 300 yd
65. 124 yd **67.** 52 ft **69.** 56 in. **71.** 300 cm
73. 64 ft **75.** 17 **76.** 210 **77.** 3174 **78.** Three
million, five hundred thirty-four thousand, five
hundred twelve **79.** 709 R 4 **80.** 811 **81.** ◈
83. ◈ **85.** $59 \boxed{\times} 17 \boxed{+} 59 \boxed{\times} 8 = 1475$
87. $7x + 1$ **89.** $-29 - 3a$ **91.** $-10 - x - 27y$
93. $29.75

Margin Exercises, Section 2.8, pp. 132–134

1. 24 **2.** -3 **3.** 25 **4.** -14 **5.** 6 **6.** -8
7. -9 **8.** -12 **9.** 26 **10.** -50 **11.** -4

Exercise Set 2.8, p. 135

1. 12 **3.** -3 **5.** 8 **7.** -12 **9.** 23 **11.** -12
13. 17 **15.** -14 **17.** 8 **19.** -4 **21.** 13 **23.** 8
25. -27 **27.** -83 **29.** 7 **31.** 475 **33.** 5
35. -15 **37.** 35 **39.** 45 **41.** -7 **43.** -9
45. -190 **47.** -81 **49.** 29 **50.** 7 **51.** 8 **52.** 27
53. 16 **54.** 26 **55.** ◈ **57.** ◈ **59.** 19 **61.** 3
63. $-\frac{4913}{3375}$ **65.** 45 **67.** 7 **69.** -10

Summary and Review: Chapter 2, p. 137

1. $527; -53$ **2.** $>$ **3.** $<$ **4.** $>$ **5.** 39 **6.** 12
7. 0 **8.** 53 **9.** 29 **10.** -9 **11.** -11 **12.** 6
13. -24 **14.** -9 **15.** 23 **16.** -1 **17.** 7
18. -4 **19.** 12 **20.** 92 **21.** -84 **22.** -40
23. -3 **24.** -5 **25.** 0 **26.** -25 **27.** -20
28. 7 **29.** $-4; -4; -4$ **30.** $20x + 36$
31. $6a - 12b + 15$ **32.** $18a$ **33.** $6x$
34. $-3m + 6$ **35.** 36 in. **36.** 100 cm **37.** -8
38. -9 **39.** -6 **40.** Three hundred eighty-six
thousand, four hundred fifty-one
41. $7300 - 2740 = 4560$ **42.** $2500 - 1700 = 800$
43. 136 **44.** 25,485 **45.** 21,286
46. ◈ The notation "$-x$" means "the opposite of x." If
x is a negative number, then $-x$ is a positive number.
For example, if $x = -2$, then $-x = 2$.
47. ◈ The expressions $(a - b)^2$ and $(b - a)^2$ are
equivalent for all choices of a and b because $a - b$ and
$b - a$ are opposites. When opposites are raised to an
even power, the results are the same.
48. 662,582 **49.** $-88,174$ **50.** -240

51. For all negative values of x **52.** For all values of
x less than -2

Test: Chapter 2, p. 139

1. [2.1a] $-542; 307$ **2.** [2.1b] $>$ **3.** [2.1c] 429
4. [2.1d] -19 **5.** [2.2a] -11 **6.** [2.2a] -21
7. [2.2a] 9 **8.** [2.3a] -12 **9.** [2.3a] -15
10. [2.3a] -24 **11.** [2.3a] 19 **12.** [2.3a] 24
13. [2.4b] -64 **14.** [2.4a] -130 **15.** [2.4a] 0
16. [2.5a] 8 **17.** [2.5a] -8 **18.** [2.5b] -1
19. [2.5b] 25 **20.** [2.3b] 13°F **21.** [2.6a] -3
22. [2.7a] $14x + 21y - 7$ **23.** [2.7b] $4x - 17$
24. [2.8b] 5 **25.** [2.8a] -12 **26.** [1.1c] Two million,
three hundred eight thousand, four hundred
fifty-one **27.** [1.4b] $3200 - 1920 = 1280$
28. [1.4b] $9200 - 2900 = 6300$ **29.** [1.8a] 21
30. [1.5b] 5648 **31.** [1.5b] 20,536 **32.** [2.7c] 66 ft
33. [2.7a, b] $35x - 7$ **34.** [2.7a, b] $-24x - 57$

Cumulative Review: Chapters 1–2, p. 141

1. [1.1d] 584,017,800 **2.** [1.1c] Five million, three
hundred eighty thousand, six hundred twenty-one
3. [1.2b] 17,797 **4.** [1.2b] 8857 **5.** [1.3d] 4946
6. [1.3d] 1425 **7.** [1.5b] 16,767 **8.** [1.5b] 8,266,500
9. [2.4a] -248 **10.** [2.4a] 72 **11.** [1.6c] 241 R 1
12. [1.6c] 62 **13.** [2.5a] 0 **14.** [2.5a] -5
15. [1.4a] 428,000 **16.** [1.4a] 5300
17. [1.4b] $749,600 + 301,400 = 1,051,000$
18. [1.5c] $700 \times 500 = 350,000$ **19.** [2.1b] $<$
20. [2.1c] 279 **21.** [1.9c] 36 **22.** [1.9d] 2
23. [2.5b] -86 **24.** [2.4b] 125 **25.** [2.6a] 3
26. [2.6a] 28 **27.** [2.7a] $-2x - 10$
28. [2.7a] $18x - 12y + 24$ **29.** [2.2a] -26
30. [2.3a] -31 **31.** [2.3a] -15 **32.** [2.3a] 13
33. [1.7b] 27 **34.** [2.8b] -3 **35.** [2.8a] -3
36. [1.7b] 24 **37.** [1.8a] 78,425 sq ft **38.** [1.8a] 13,931
39. [1.8a] $75 **40.** [1.8a] Westside Appliance
41. [2.7b] $23x - 14$ **42.** [1.8a] 5 cases, 3 six-packs,
4 loose cans **43.** [1.9d], [2.7b] $4a$

Chapter 3

Pretest: Chapter 3, p. 144

1. [3.1b] Yes **2.** [3.1b] Yes **3.** [3.2b] Prime
4. [3.2c] $2 \cdot 2 \cdot 2 \cdot 5 \cdot 7$ **5.** [3.3c] 1 **6.** [3.3c] $7x$
7. [3.3c] 0 **8.** [3.5b] $-\dfrac{1}{4}$ **9.** [3.5b] $\dfrac{2}{7}$ **10.** [3.5a] $\dfrac{12}{28}$
11. [3.6a] $\dfrac{6}{5}$ **12.** [3.6a] -20 **13.** [3.6a] $\dfrac{5a}{4}$
14. [3.7a] $\dfrac{8}{7}$ **15.** [3.7a] $\dfrac{1}{11}$ **16.** [3.7b] 24
17. [3.7b] $-\dfrac{3}{4}$ **18.** [3.7b] $\dfrac{2}{9x}$ **19.** [3.8a] $-\dfrac{2}{7}$
20. [3.8a] 30 **21.** [3.8a] $\dfrac{5}{8}$ **22.** [3.6b] $54

23. [3.7c] $\frac{1}{24}$ m   **24.** [3.6b] 26 ft^2

Margin Exercises, Section 3.1, pp. 145–149

1. $5 = 1 \cdot 5$; $45 = 9 \cdot 5$; $100 = 20 \cdot 5$ **2.** $10 = 1 \cdot 10$; $60 = 6 \cdot 10$; $110 = 11 \cdot 10$ **3.** 5, 10, 15, 20, 25, 30, 35, 40, 45, 50   **4.** Yes   **5.** Yes   **6.** No   **7.** Yes   **8.** No   **9.** Yes   **10.** No   **11.** Yes   **12.** No   **13.** Yes   **14.** No   **15.** Yes   **16.** No   **17.** No   **18.** Yes   **19.** No   **20.** Yes   **21.** No   **22.** Yes   **23.** No   **24.** Yes   **25.** No   **26.** Yes   **27.** Yes   **28.** No   **29.** No   **30.** Yes

Calculator Spotlight, p. 146

1. Yes   **2.** No   **3.** No   **4.** Yes

Exercise Set 3.1, p. 151

1. 6, 12, 18, 24, 30, 36, 42, 48, 54, 60   **3.** 20, 40, 60, 80, 100, 120, 140, 160, 180, 200   **5.** 3, 6, 9, 12, 15, 18, 21, 24, 27, 30   **7.** 13, 26, 39, 52, 65, 78, 91, 104, 117, 130   **9.** 10, 20, 30, 40, 50, 60, 70, 80, 90, 100   **11.** 9, 18, 27, 36, 45, 54, 63, 72, 81, 90   **13.** No   **15.** Yes   **17.** No   **19.** No   **21.** No   **23.** 46, 224, 300, 36, 45,270, 4444, 256, 8064, 21,568   **25.** 300, 45,270   **27.** 300, 36, 45,270, 8064   **29.** 324, 42, 501, 3009, 75, 2001, 402, 111,111, 1005   **31.** 55,555, 200, 75, 2345, 35, 1005   **33.** 324   **35.** 53   **36.** 5   **37.** −8   **38.** −24   **39.** $680   **40.** 42   **41.** ◈   **43.** ◈   **45.** 99,969   **47.** 30   **49.** 60   **51.** 121

Margin Exercises, Section 3.2, pp. 153–156

1. 1, 2, 3, 6   **2.** 1, 2, 4, 8   **3.** 1, 2, 5, 10   **4.** 1, 2, 4, 8, 16, 32   **5.** 13, 19, 41 are prime; 4, 6, 8 are composite; 1 is neither   **6.** $2 \cdot 3$ **7.** $2 \cdot 2 \cdot 3$ **8.** $3 \cdot 3 \cdot 5$ **9.** $2 \cdot 7 \cdot 7$ **10.** $2 \cdot 3 \cdot 3 \cdot 7$ **11.** $2 \cdot 2 \cdot 2 \cdot 2 \cdot 3 \cdot 3$

Exercise Set 3.2, p. 157

1. 1, 2, 3, 6, 9, 18   **3.** 1, 2, 3, 6, 9, 18, 27, 54   **5.** 1, 2, 4   **7.** 1, 7   **9.** 1   **11.** 1, 2, 7, 14, 49, 98   **13.** 1, 2, 3, 6, 7, 14, 21, 42   **15.** 1, 5, 7, 11, 35, 55, 77, 385   **17.** 1, 2, 3, 4, 6, 9, 12, 18, 36   **19.** 1, 3, 5, 9, 15, 25, 45, 75, 225   **21.** Prime   **23.** Composite   **25.** Composite   **27.** Prime   **29.** Neither   **31.** Composite   **33.** Prime   **35.** Prime   **37.** $2 \cdot 2 \cdot 2 \cdot 2$ **39.** $2 \cdot 7$ **41.** $2 \cdot 11$ **43.** $5 \cdot 5$ **45.** $2 \cdot 31$ **47.** $2 \cdot 2 \cdot 5 \cdot 7$ **49.** $2 \cdot 2 \cdot 5 \cdot 5$ **51.** $5 \cdot 7$ **53.** $2 \cdot 3 \cdot 13$ **55.** $7 \cdot 11$ **57.** $2 \cdot 2 \cdot 2 \cdot 2 \cdot 7$ **59.** $2 \cdot 2 \cdot 3 \cdot 5 \cdot 5$ **61.** −26   **62.** 256   **63.** 8   **64.** −23   **65.** 0   **66.** 1   **67.** ◈   **69.** ◈   **71.** $53 \cdot 53 \cdot 73 \cdot 139$ **73.** $2 \cdot 2 \cdot 2 \cdot 3 \cdot 3 \cdot 5 \cdot 7$ **75.** $2 \cdot 3 \cdot 3 \cdot 3 \cdot 37$ **77.** Answers may vary. One arrangement is a three-dimensional rectangular array consisting of 2 tiers of 12 objects each, where each tier consists of a rectangular array of 4 rows with 3 objects each.

Margin Exercises, Section 3.3, pp. 159–162

1. 5, numerator; 7, denominator   **2.** $5a$, numerator; $7b$, denominator   **3.** −22, numerator; 3, denominator   **4.** $\frac{1}{2}$ **5.** $\frac{1}{3}$ mi   **6.** $\frac{1}{3}$ gal   **7.** $\frac{1}{6}$ hr   **8.** $\frac{5}{8}$ **9.** $\frac{2}{3}$ mi   **10.** $\frac{3}{4}$ gal   **11.** $\frac{4}{6}$ yr   **12.** $\frac{4}{3}$ mi   **13.** $\frac{5}{5}$ **14.** $\frac{5}{4}$ mi   **15.** $\frac{7}{4}$ gal   **16.** $\frac{4}{7}$ **17.** $\frac{2}{3}$ **18.** $\frac{2}{6}$; $\frac{4}{6}$ **19.** 1   **20.** 1   **21.** 1   **22.** 1   **23.** 1   **24.** 1   **25.** 0   **26.** 0   **27.** 0   **28.** 0   **29.** Undefined   **30.** Undefined   **31.** 8   **32.** −10   **33.** −346   **34.** 1

Exercise Set 3.3, p. 163

1. 3, numerator; 4, denominator   **3.** 7, numerator; −9, denominator   **5.** $2x$, numerator; $3z$, denominator   **7.** $\frac{3}{4}$ **9.** $\frac{2}{8}$ mi   **11.** $\frac{4}{3}$ L   **13.** $\frac{3}{4}$ acre   **15.** $\frac{8}{16}$ lb   **17.** $\frac{5}{12}$ **19.** $\frac{1}{4}$ **21.** 0   **23.** 15   **25.** 1   **27.** 1   **29.** 0   **31.** 1   **33.** 1   **35.** −63   **37.** 0   **39.** Undefined   **41.** $7n$ **43.** Undefined   **45.** −210   **46.** −322   **47.** 0   **48.** 0   **49.** $13,772   **50.** 201 min   **51.** ◈   **53.** ◈   **55.** $\frac{52}{365}$ **57.** $\frac{9}{39}$

Margin Exercises, Section 3.4, pp. 165–168

1. $\frac{2}{3}$ **2.** $\frac{5}{8}$ **3.** $\frac{10}{3}$ **4.** $-\frac{33}{8}$ or $\frac{-33}{8}$ **5.** $\frac{46}{5}$ **6.** $\frac{4x}{9}$ **7.** $\frac{15}{56}$ **8.** $\frac{32}{15}$ **9.** $\frac{3}{100}$ **10.** $-\frac{7a}{b}$ or $\frac{-7a}{b}$ **11.**

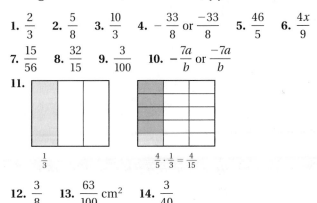

$\frac{1}{3}$ $\frac{4}{5} \cdot \frac{1}{3} = \frac{4}{15}$

12. $\frac{3}{8}$ **13.** $\frac{63}{100}$ cm^2 **14.** $\frac{3}{40}$

Exercise Set 3.4, p. 169

1. $\frac{3}{7}$ **3.** $\frac{-5}{6}$ or $-\frac{5}{6}$ **5.** $\frac{14}{3}$ **7.** $-\frac{7}{9}$ or $\frac{-7}{9}$ **9.** $\frac{2x}{5}$ **11.** $-\frac{6}{5}$ or $\frac{-6}{5}$ **13.** $\frac{3a}{4}$ **15.** $\frac{17m}{6}$ **17.** $\frac{6}{5}$ **19.** $\frac{2x}{7}$ **21.** $\frac{1}{10}$ **23.** $-\frac{1}{40}$ or $\frac{-1}{40}$ **25.** $\frac{2}{15}$ **27.** $\frac{2x}{5y}$ **29.** $\frac{9}{16}$ **31.** $\frac{14}{39}$ **33.** $-\frac{3}{50}$ or $\frac{-3}{50}$ **35.** $\frac{7a}{64}$ **37.** $\frac{1}{100y}$ **39.** $\frac{-182}{285}$ or $-\frac{182}{285}$ **41.** $\frac{12}{25}$ m^2 **43.** $\frac{1}{80}$ gal   **45.** $\frac{6}{12}$ cup   **47.** $\frac{2}{30}$ **49.** −4   **50.** 4   **51.** 76   **52.** 102   **53.** 6 hundred thousands   **54.** 4 millions   **55.** ◈   **57.** ◈   **59.** $-\frac{185,193}{226,981}$ or $\frac{-185,193}{226,981}$ **61.** $-\frac{3}{160}$ or $\frac{-3}{160}$ **63.** $\frac{4}{105}$

Margin Exercises, Section 3.5, pp. 171–173

1. $\dfrac{8}{16}$ 2. $\dfrac{3x}{5x}$ 3. $-\dfrac{52}{100}$ 4. $\dfrac{-16}{-6}$ 5. $\dfrac{12}{9}$ 6. $\dfrac{-18}{-24}$

7. $\dfrac{9x}{10x}$ 8. $\dfrac{9}{45}$ 9. $\dfrac{-56}{49}$ 10. $\dfrac{3}{7}$ 11. $\dfrac{-5}{6}$ 12. 5

13. $\dfrac{4}{3}$ 14. $-\dfrac{5}{3}$ 15. $\dfrac{7}{8}$ 16. $\dfrac{89}{78}$ 17. $\dfrac{-8}{7}$

18. $\dfrac{2}{100}=\dfrac{1}{50}$; $\dfrac{4}{100}=\dfrac{1}{25}$; $\dfrac{32}{100}=\dfrac{8}{25}$; $\dfrac{44}{100}=\dfrac{11}{25}$; $\dfrac{18}{100}=\dfrac{9}{50}$

Calculator Spotlight, p. 174

1. $\dfrac{14}{15}$ 2. $\dfrac{7}{8}$ 3. $\dfrac{138}{167}$ 4. $\dfrac{7}{25}$

Exercise Set 3.5, p. 175

1. $\dfrac{5}{10}$ 3. $\dfrac{-36}{-48}$ 5. $\dfrac{27}{30}$ 7. $\dfrac{11t}{5t}$ 9. $\dfrac{20}{48}$ 11. $-\dfrac{51}{54}$

13. $\dfrac{10}{-25}$ 15. $\dfrac{-42}{132}$ 17. $\dfrac{5x}{8x}$ 19. $\dfrac{7m}{11m}$ 21. $\dfrac{4ab}{9ab}$

23. $\dfrac{12b}{27b}$ 25. $\dfrac{1}{2}$ 27. $-\dfrac{2}{3}$ 29. $\dfrac{2}{5}$ 31. -3 33. $\dfrac{3}{4}$

35. $-\dfrac{12}{7}$ 37. $\dfrac{1}{3}$ 39. $\dfrac{-1}{3}$ 41. $\dfrac{7}{8}$ 43. $\dfrac{8}{9}$ 45. $\dfrac{3}{8}$

47. $\dfrac{3y}{2}$ 49. 3600 yd^2 50. $928 51. -5 52. -18

53. 186 54. 2737 55. -5 56. 3520 57. ◆

59. ◆ 61. $\dfrac{11b}{13c}$ 63. $-\dfrac{11a}{17b}$ 65. $\dfrac{151}{139}$ 67. 69

69. (a) $1200; (b) $\dfrac{1}{12}$

Margin Exercises, Section 3.6, pp. 178–180

1. $\dfrac{7}{12}$ 2. $-\dfrac{1}{3}$ 3. 6 4. $\dfrac{15}{x}$ 5. 10 lb 6. 96 m^2

7. $\dfrac{66}{5}$ cm^2 8. 100 in^2

Exercise Set 3.6, p. 181

1. $\dfrac{5}{8}$ 3. $-\dfrac{1}{8}$ 5. $\dfrac{3}{20}$ 7. $\dfrac{2}{9}$ 9. $-\dfrac{27}{10}$ 11. $\dfrac{7x}{9}$

13. 2 15. 5 17. -9 19. $3a$ 21. 1 23. 1

25. $\dfrac{40a}{3}$ 27. $-\dfrac{88}{3}$ 29. 1 31. 3 33. $\dfrac{119}{750}$

35. $-\dfrac{20}{187}$ 37. $-\dfrac{42}{275}$ 39. $-\dfrac{16}{5}$ 41. $-\dfrac{11}{40}$ 43. $\dfrac{5}{14}$

45. $42 47. 12 lb 49. 260 51. $\dfrac{1}{3}$ cup

53. $93,000 55. 160 mi 57. $6750 for food; $5400 for housing; $2700 for clothing; $3000 for savings; $6750 for taxes; $2400 for other expenses 59. 60 in^2

61. $\dfrac{35}{4}$ mm^2 63. $\dfrac{63}{8}$ m^2 65. 92 mi^2 67. 6800 ft^2

69. 35 70. 8546 71. 477 72. 70 73. -111

74. -22 75. ◆ 77. ◆ 79. $\dfrac{219}{355}$ 81. 432 ft^2

83. $\dfrac{1}{12}$ 85. $\dfrac{1}{168}$

Margin Exercises, Section 3.7, pp. 187–190

1. $\dfrac{5}{2}$ 2. $\dfrac{x}{-6}$ 3. $\dfrac{1}{9}$ 4. 5 5. $-\dfrac{10}{3}$ 6. $\dfrac{8}{7}$ 7. $-\dfrac{8}{3}$

8. $\dfrac{1}{10}$ 9. $\dfrac{100}{a}$ 10. -1 11. $\dfrac{14}{15}$ 12. 320 13. 12

Exercise Set 3.7, p. 191

1. $\dfrac{3}{7}$ 3. $\dfrac{1}{4}$ 5. 6 7. $-\dfrac{3}{10}$ 9. $\dfrac{21}{2}$ 11. $\dfrac{m}{-3n}$

13. $\dfrac{-15}{7}$ 15. $\dfrac{1}{7m}$ 17. $\dfrac{4}{5}$ 19. $-\dfrac{7}{10}$ 21. 4 23. -2

25. $\dfrac{1}{64}$ 27. $\dfrac{3}{7x}$ 29. -8 31. $35a$ 33. 1 35. $-\dfrac{2}{3}$

37. $\dfrac{99}{224}$ 39. $\dfrac{112a}{3}$ 41. 88 43. 9 days 45. 20

47. $\dfrac{3}{64}$ acre 49. $\dfrac{1}{10}$ m 51. 32 53. 32 55. 510

56. -292 57. 27; -27 58. 80; 80 59. 147, 147

60. 343; -343 61. ◆ 63. ◆ 65. $-\dfrac{15}{196}$ 67. $\dfrac{35}{33}$

69. $\dfrac{7}{5}$

Margin Exercises, Section 3.8, pp. 195–196

1. 15 2. -28 3. $-\dfrac{9}{32}$ 4. $-\dfrac{3}{4}$

Exercise Set 3.8, p. 197

1. 10 3. 9 5. -42 7. $\dfrac{2}{17}$ 9. $\dfrac{10}{21}$ 11. $-\dfrac{16}{21}$

13. $-\dfrac{2}{25}$ 15. $\dfrac{1}{6}$ 17. $-\dfrac{80}{3}$ 19. $-\dfrac{1}{6}$ 21. $-\dfrac{9}{13}$

23. $\dfrac{27}{31}$ 25. $\dfrac{5}{7}$ 27. $\dfrac{12}{5}$ 29. $-\dfrac{10}{7}$ 31. $\dfrac{24}{7}$ 33. 14

35. $\dfrac{10}{7}$ 37. 20 38. 6 39. $17x$ 40. $4a$

41. $7a+3$ 42. $4x-7$ 43. ◆ 45. ◆

47. $-\dfrac{432}{49}$ 49. 400 km; 160 km 51. $\dfrac{8}{21}$ mi

Summary and Review: Chapter 3, p. 199

1. No 2. No 3. Yes 4. $2\cdot5\cdot7$

5. $2\cdot2\cdot2\cdot3\cdot3$ 6. $2\cdot3\cdot5\cdot5$ 7. Prime

8. 9, numerator; 7, denominator 9. $\dfrac{3}{5}$ 10. $\dfrac{3}{8}$

11. 0 12. 1 13. 48 14. 1 15. $-\dfrac{2}{3}$ 16. $\dfrac{1}{4}$

17. -1 18. $\dfrac{3}{4}$ 19. $\dfrac{2}{5}$ 20. Undefined 21. $9n$

22. $\dfrac{1}{3}$ 23. $\dfrac{15}{21}$ 24. $\dfrac{-30}{55}$ 25. $\dfrac{9}{5}$ 26. $-\dfrac{1}{7}$ 27. 8

28. $\dfrac{5y}{3x}$ 29. $\dfrac{6}{35}$ 30. $\dfrac{4y}{9x}$ 31. $\dfrac{2}{3}$ 32. $-\dfrac{1}{14}$ 33. $\dfrac{1}{25}$

34. 1   **35.** $\frac{18}{5}$ **36.** $\frac{1}{4}$ **37.** 300   **38.** $\frac{1}{15}$ **39.** $4a$

40. -1 **41.** 220 mi   **42.** $\frac{3}{8}$ cup   **43.** $\frac{1}{6}$ mi   **44.** 18

45. 42 m^2 **46.** $\frac{35}{2}$ ft^2 **47.** 240   **48.** $-\frac{3}{10}$ **49.** 24

50. 11   **51.** 14   **52.** 27   **53.** ◈ To simplify fractional notation, first factor the numerator and the denominator into prime numbers. Examine the factorizations for factors common to both the numerator and the denominator. Change the order of the factorizations, if necessary, so that the pairs of like factors are above and below each other. Factor the fraction, with each pair of like factors forming a factor equal to 1. Remove the factors equal to 1, and multiply the remaining factors in the numerator and in the denominator, if necessary.   **54.** ◈ The fraction is equivalent to $\frac{2}{8}$, but it is not in simplest form. Fractional notation is not simplified until the numerator and the denominator contain no common factors. The notation $\frac{20}{80}$ simplifies to $\frac{1}{4}$.

55. $\frac{3}{17}$ **56.** $\frac{17}{6}$ **57.** 2, 8

Test: Chapter 3, p. 201

1. [3.1b] Yes   **2.** [3.1b] No   **3.** [3.2c] $2 \cdot 2 \cdot 3 \cdot 3$
4. [3.2c] $2 \cdot 2 \cdot 3 \cdot 5$ **5.** [3.2b] Composite

6. [3.3a] 4, numerator; 9, denominator   **7.** [3.3b] $\frac{3}{4}$

8. [3.3c] 26   **9.** [3.3c] 1   **10.** [3.3c] 0   **11.** [3.5b] $\frac{-1}{3}$

12. [3.5b] $\frac{1}{9}$ **13.** [3.5b] $\frac{1}{14}$ **14.** [3.5a] $\frac{15}{40}$

15. [3.7a] $\frac{27}{x}$ **16.** [3.7a] $-\frac{1}{9}$ **17.** [3.4b] $\frac{35}{18}$

18. [3.7a] $\frac{28}{33}$ **19.** [3.4a] $\frac{3x}{8}$ **20.** [3.7b] $-\frac{98}{3}$

21. [3.6a] $\frac{6}{65}$ **22.** [3.7c] $\frac{3}{20}$ lb   **23.** [3.6b] 125 lb

24. [3.8a] 64   **25.** [3.8a] $-\frac{7}{4}$ **26.** [3.6b] $\frac{91}{2}$ m^2

27. [1.9c] 41   **28.** [1.7b], [2.8b] 101   **29.** [2.2a] -167

30. [2.4a] 63   **31.** [3.6b] $\frac{15}{8}$ tsp   **32.** [3.6b] $\frac{7}{48}$ acre

33. [3.6a], [3.7b] $-\frac{7}{960}$ **34.** [3.8a] $\frac{7}{5}$

Cumulative Review: Chapters 1–3, p. 203

1. [1.1c] Two million, fifty-six thousand, seven hundred eighty-three   **2.** [1.2b] 10,982   **3.** [2.2a] -43
4. [2.2a] -33 **5.** [1.3d] 2129   **6.** [2.3a] -23
7. [2.3a] -8 **8.** [1.5b] 16,905   **9.** [2.4a] -312
10. [3.6a] $-30x$ **11.** [3.6a] $\frac{7}{15}$ **12.** [1.6c] 235 R 3
13. [2.5a] -17 **14.** [3.7b] -28 **15.** [3.7b] $\frac{2}{3}$
16. [1.4a] 4510   **17.** [1.5c] $900 \times 500 = 450,000$

18. [2.1c] 879   **19.** [2.5b] 8   **20.** [3.2b] Composite
21. [2.6a] -21 **22.** [1.7b], [2.8a] 25
23. [1.7b], [2.8b] 9   **24.** [3.8a] -45 **25.** [1.8a] 8 mpg
26. [1.8a] 8 oz   **27.** [2.7b] $2x - 4$ **28.** [2.7b] $3x + 7y$
29. [3.3c] 1   **30.** [3.3c] 59   **31.** [3.3c] 0
32. [3.5b] $-\frac{5}{27}$ **33.** [3.7a] $\frac{5}{2}$ **34.** [3.7a] $\frac{1}{17}$
35. [3.5a] $\frac{21}{70}$ **36.** [3.6b] \$36   **37.** [3.7c] 12
38. [3.6b] $\frac{3}{5}$ mi   **39.** [2.6a], [3.6a], [3.7b] $-\frac{54}{169}$
40. [2.1c], [2.6a], [3.6a] $-\frac{9}{100}$ **41.** [3.6b] \$468

Chapter 4

Pretest: Chapter 4, p. 206

1. [4.1a] 75   **2.** [4.2c] $<$ **3.** [4.2a] $-\frac{1}{4}$ **4.** [4.2b] $\frac{11}{90}$
5. [4.3a] $\frac{9}{35}$ **6.** [4.5a] $\frac{43}{8}$ **7.** [4.5b] $3\frac{1}{4}$ **8.** [4.5c] $399\frac{1}{12}$
9. [4.6b] $6\frac{11}{30}$ **10.** [4.3b] $\frac{2}{9}$ **11.** [4.4a] -9
12. [4.7a] $18\frac{7}{11}$ **13.** [4.7a] $36\frac{5}{12}$ **14.** [4.7b] $-7\frac{5}{7}$
15. [4.7b] $1\frac{14}{39}$ **16.** [4.7c] $8\frac{26}{35}$ **17.** [4.6c] $38\frac{1}{4}$ lb
18. [4.7d] $4\frac{1}{4}$ cu ft   **19.** [4.7d] $1577\frac{1}{2}$ mi
20. [4.6c] $6\frac{1}{4}$ cups

Margin Exercises, Section 4.1, pp. 207–210

1. 45   **2.** 40   **3.** 18   **4.** 24   **5.** 10   **6.** 200   **7.** 40
8. 360   **9.** 18   **10.** 24   **11.** 2520   **12.** xyz
13. $5a^3b$

Exercise Set 4.1, p. 211

1. 4   **3.** 50   **5.** 40   **7.** 54   **9.** 150   **11.** 120
13. 72   **15.** 420   **17.** 144   **19.** 288   **21.** 30
23. 105   **25.** 72   **27.** 60   **29.** 36   **31.** 900
33. 300   **35.** abc **37.** $9x^2$ **39.** $4x^3y$ **41.** Once every 60 yr   **43.** 14   **44.** -27 **45.** 7935   **46.** $\frac{2}{3}$
47. $-\frac{8}{7}$ **48.** -167 **49.** ◈   **51.** ◈   **53.** 70,200
55. 2520   **57. (a)** Not the LCM because 8 is not a factor of $2 \cdot 2 \cdot 3 \cdot 3$; **(b)** not the LCM because 8 is not a factor of $2 \cdot 2 \cdot 3$; **(c)** not the LCM because neither 8 nor 12 is a factor of $2 \cdot 3 \cdot 3$; **(d)** the LCM because both 8 and 12 are factors of $2 \cdot 2 \cdot 2 \cdot 3$ and it is the smallest such number   **59.** 27 and 2; 27 and 6; 27 and 18

Margin Exercises, Section 4.2, pp. 213–218

1. $\frac{4}{5}$ **2.** 1   **3.** $\frac{1}{2}$ **4.** $-\frac{3}{8}$ **5.** $-\frac{4}{x}$ **6.** $\frac{2}{5}a$
7. $\frac{7}{19} + \frac{10}{19}x$ **8.** $\frac{5}{6}$ **9.** $\frac{29}{24}$ **10.** $\frac{2}{9}$ **11.** $\frac{38}{5}$
12. $\frac{413}{1000}$ **13.** $\frac{157}{210}$ **14.** $<$ **15.** $>$ **16.** $>$ **17.** $<$
18. $<$ **19.** $<$ **20.** $\frac{11}{10}$ lb

Calculator Spotlight, p. 218

1. $\frac{5}{8}$ **2.** $\frac{67}{60}$ **3.** $\frac{52}{21}$ **4.** $\frac{201}{140}$ **5.** $\frac{253}{150}$ **6.** $\frac{792}{667}$

Exercise Set 4.2, p. 219

1. 1 **3.** $\frac{3}{4}$ **5.** $\frac{2}{5}$ **7.** $\frac{13}{a}$ **9.** $-\frac{2}{11}$ **11.** $\frac{7}{9}x$

13. $\frac{3}{8} + \frac{1}{2}t$ **15.** $-\frac{10}{x}$ **17.** $\frac{7}{24}$ **19.** $-\frac{1}{10}$ **21.** $\frac{19}{24}$

23. $\frac{83}{20}$ **25.** $\frac{5}{24}$ **27.** $\frac{37}{100}x$ **29.** $\frac{41}{60}$ **31.** $-\frac{9}{100}$ **33.** $\frac{67}{12}$

35. $-\frac{33}{7}t$ **37.** $-\frac{17}{24}$ **39.** $\frac{437}{1000}$ **41.** $\frac{5}{4}$ **43.** $\frac{239}{78}$

45. $\frac{59}{90}$ **47.** < **49.** < **51.** > **53.** > **55.** >

57. > **59.** $\frac{4}{15}, \frac{3}{10}, \frac{5}{12}$ **61.** $\frac{5}{6}$ lb **63.** $\frac{9}{8}$ mi **65.** $\frac{43}{48}$ qt

67. 690 kg; $\frac{14}{23}$; $\frac{5}{23}$; $\frac{4}{23}$; 1 **69.** $\frac{33}{20}$ mi **71.** $\frac{51}{32}$ in.

73. -13 **74.** 4 **75.** -8 **76.** -31 **77.** $\frac{10}{3}$

78. 42; 42 **79.** ◆ **81.** ◆ **83.** $\frac{22}{45} + \frac{17}{42}x$ **85.** <

87. $\frac{4}{15}$; $320

Margin Exercises, Section 4.3, pp. 223–226

1. $\frac{1}{2}$ **2.** $\frac{3}{5a}$ **3.** $-\frac{1}{2}$ **4.** $\frac{1}{12}$ **5.** $\frac{1}{6}$ **6.** $-\frac{3}{10}$ **7.** $-\frac{1}{6}$

8. $\frac{9}{112}$ **9.** $\frac{3}{10}x$ **10.** $\frac{3}{5}$ **11.** $\frac{1}{6}$ **12.** $-\frac{59}{40}$ **13.** $\frac{2}{15}$ cup

Exercise Set 4.3, p. 227

1. $\frac{2}{3}$ **3.** $-\frac{1}{4}$ **5.** $\frac{4}{a}$ **7.** $\frac{2}{t}$ **9.** $-\frac{4}{5a}$ **11.** $\frac{13}{16}$

13. $-\frac{1}{3}$ **15.** $\frac{7}{10}$ **17.** $-\frac{17}{60}$ **19.** $\frac{53}{100}$ **21.** $\frac{26}{75}$ **23.** $-\frac{21}{100}$

25. $\frac{13}{24}$ **27.** $\frac{1}{10}$ **29.** $\frac{23}{72}$ **31.** $\frac{1}{360}$ **33.** $\frac{2}{9}x$ **35.** $-\frac{3}{20}a$

37. $\frac{7}{9}$ **39.** $\frac{6}{11}$ **41.** $\frac{1}{9}$ **43.** $\frac{9}{8}$ **45.** $\frac{2}{15}$ **47.** $-\frac{7}{24}$

49. $\frac{1}{15}$ **51.** $-\frac{5}{4}$ **53.** $\frac{5}{12}$ hr **55.** $\frac{13}{24}$ mi **57.** $\frac{1}{32}$ in.

59. $\frac{3}{2}$ **60.** $\frac{4}{21}$ **61.** -21 **62.** -32 **63.** 6 lb

64. 9 cups **65.** ◆ **67.** ◆ **69.** $\frac{41}{3289}$ **71.** $-\frac{11}{10}$

73. $-\frac{64}{35}$ **75.** $\frac{31}{32}$ in. **77.** $\frac{3}{16}$

Margin Exercises, Section 4.4, pp. 231–234

1. Yes **2.** No **3.** 26 **4.** -15 **5.** -16 **6.** $-\frac{18}{7}$

Exercise Set 4.4, p. 235

1. 3 **3.** 5 **5.** 7 **7.** 12 **9.** -7 **11.** -5 **13.** 25

15. 10 **17.** 20 **19.** $\frac{5}{6}$ **21.** $\frac{21}{5}$ **23.** 6 **25.** $\frac{17}{4}$

27. $\frac{3}{4}$ **29.** The balance has decreased $150.

30. $1180 profit **31.** $\frac{5}{7m}$ **32.** $20n$ **33.** $3a + 3b$

34. $7m - 21$ **35.** ◆ **37.** ◆ **39.** 4 **41.** $\frac{436}{35}$

43. 2 cm

Margin Exercises, Section 4.5, pp. 237–240

1. $1\frac{2}{3}$ **2.** $8\frac{3}{4}$ **3.** $12\frac{2}{3}$ **4.** $\frac{22}{5}$ **5.** $\frac{61}{10}$ **6.** $\frac{29}{6}$ **7.** $\frac{37}{4}$

8. $\frac{62}{3}$ **9.** $-\frac{32}{5}$ **10.** $-\frac{59}{7}$ **11.** $2\frac{1}{3}$ **12.** $1\frac{1}{10}$ **13.** $18\frac{1}{3}$

14. $-2\frac{2}{5}$ **15.** $-11\frac{1}{6}$ **16.** $807\frac{2}{3}$ **17.** $55\frac{3}{4}$ qt

Calculator Spotlight, p. 240

1. $1476\frac{1}{6}$ **2.** $676\frac{4}{9}$ **3.** $800\frac{51}{56}$ **4.** $13,031\frac{1}{2}$

5. $51,626\frac{9}{11}$ **6.** $7330\frac{7}{32}$ **7.** $134\frac{1}{15}$ **8.** $2666\frac{130}{213}$

9. $3571\frac{51}{112}$ **10.** $12\frac{169}{454}$

Exercise Set 4.5, p. 241

1. $\frac{17}{5}$ **3.** $\frac{25}{4}$ **5.** $-\frac{161}{8}$ **7.** $\frac{51}{10}$ **9.** $\frac{103}{5}$ **11.** $-\frac{59}{6}$

13. $\frac{69}{10}$ **15.** $-\frac{51}{4}$ **17.** $\frac{57}{10}$ **19.** $-\frac{507}{100}$ **21.** $4\frac{2}{3}$

23. $-4\frac{1}{2}$ **25.** $5\frac{7}{10}$ **27.** $7\frac{4}{7}$ **29.** $7\frac{1}{2}$ **31.** $11\frac{1}{2}$

33. $-1\frac{1}{2}$ **35.** $4\frac{2}{3}$ **37.** $-55\frac{3}{4}$ **39.** $108\frac{5}{8}$

41. $906\frac{3}{7}$ **43.** $40\frac{4}{7}$ **45.** $-20\frac{2}{15}$ **47.** $-22\frac{3}{7}$ **49.** $2\frac{1}{5}$ g

51. $2\frac{3}{10}$ **53.** $\frac{8}{9}$ **54.** 18 **55.** $-\frac{5}{2}$ **56.** $\frac{1}{4}$

57. ◆ **59.** ◆ **61.** $297\frac{23}{349}$ **63.** $6\frac{5}{6}$ **65.** $52\frac{2}{7}$

67. Wire length: 3 ft, 11 in. Diameter: $4\frac{3}{4}$ in.

Margin Exercises, Section 4.6, pp. 243–248

1. $7\frac{2}{5}$ **2.** $12\frac{1}{10}$ **3.** $13\frac{7}{12}$ **4.** $1\frac{1}{2}$ **5.** $3\frac{1}{6}$ **6.** $3\frac{1}{3}$

7. $3\frac{2}{3}$ **8.** $12\frac{5}{6}t$ **9.** $2\frac{1}{4}x$ **10.** $14\frac{1}{30}x$ **11.** $7\frac{1}{12}$ yd

12. $\frac{3}{8}$ in. **13.** $-\frac{3}{4}$ **14.** $-3\frac{3}{4}$ **15.** $-1\frac{5}{6}$ **16.** $-13\frac{7}{30}$

Exercise Set 4.6, p. 249

1. $9\frac{1}{2}$ **3.** $2\frac{11}{12}$ **5.** $13\frac{7}{12}$ **7.** $12\frac{1}{10}$ **9.** $17\frac{5}{24}$ **11.** $21\frac{1}{2}$

13. $27\frac{7}{8}$ **15.** $1\frac{3}{5}$ **17.** $4\frac{1}{10}$ **19.** $21\frac{17}{24}$ **21.** $12\frac{1}{4}$

23. $15\frac{3}{8}$ **25.** $7\frac{5}{12}$ **27.** $11\frac{5}{18}$ **29.** $8\frac{13}{42}t$ **31.** $2\frac{1}{8}x$

33. $8\frac{31}{40}t$ **35.** $11\frac{34}{45}t$ **37.** $6\frac{1}{6}x$ **39.** $9\frac{31}{33}x$ **41.** $4\frac{1}{4}$ lb

43. $6\frac{7}{20}$ cm **45.** $19\frac{1}{16}$ ft **47.** 39 in. **49.** $17\frac{1}{8}$

51. $20\frac{1}{8}$ in. **53.** $3\frac{4}{5}$ hr **55.** $28\frac{3}{4}$ yd **57.** $7\frac{3}{8}$ ft

59. $1\frac{9}{16}$ in. **61.** $-\frac{4}{5}$ **63.** $-3\frac{1}{4}$ **65.** $-3\frac{13}{15}$ **67.** $-7\frac{3}{5}$

69. $-10\frac{29}{35}$ **71.** $-1\frac{8}{9}$ **73.** $\frac{1}{10}$ **74.** $-\frac{10}{13}$ **75.** $\frac{8}{11}$

76. $-\frac{7}{9}$ **77.** ◆ **79.** ◆ **81.** $1888\frac{1053}{2279}$

83. $5\frac{3}{4}$ ft **85.** $56\frac{8}{45}$

Margin Exercises, Section 4.7, pp. 253–258

1. 20 **2.** $1\frac{7}{8}$ **3.** $-12\frac{4}{5}$ **4.** $8\frac{1}{3}$ **5.** 16 **6.** $1\frac{7}{8}$

7. $-\frac{7}{10}$ **8.** $175\frac{1}{2}$ **9.** $159\frac{4}{5}$ **10.** $5\frac{3}{4}$ **11.** $227\frac{1}{2}$ mi

12. 20 mpg **13.** $240\frac{3}{4}$ ft^2 **14.** $9\frac{7}{8}$ in.

Calculator Spotlight, p. 258

1. $\frac{5}{8}$ **2.** $\frac{7}{10}$ **3.** $\frac{5}{7}$ **4.** $\frac{133}{68}$ **5.** $\frac{73}{150}$ **6.** $\frac{97}{116}$ **7.** $24\frac{3}{7}$

8. $\frac{115}{147}$ **9.** $13\frac{41}{63}$ **10.** $5\frac{59}{72}$ **11.** $3\frac{5}{8}$ **12.** $19\frac{5}{8}$

Exercise Set 4.7, p. 259

1. $28\frac{1}{3}$ **3.** $1\frac{2}{3}$ **5.** $-73\frac{1}{3}$ **7.** $16\frac{1}{3}$ **9.** $-10\frac{3}{25}$

11. $35\frac{91}{100}$ **13.** $7\frac{9}{13}$ **15.** $1\frac{1}{5}$ **17.** $3\frac{9}{16}$ **19.** $-1\frac{1}{8}$

21. $1\frac{8}{43}$ **23.** $-\frac{9}{40}$ **25.** $23\frac{2}{5}$ **27.** $15\frac{5}{7}$ **29.** $-28\frac{28}{45}$

31. $-1\frac{1}{3}$ **33.** $12\frac{1}{4}$ **35.** $8\frac{3}{20}$ **37.** 24 **39.** $13\frac{1}{3}$ tsp

41. $16\frac{1}{2}$ **43.** $343\frac{3}{4}$ lb **45.** $82\frac{1}{2}$ in. **47.** 68°

49. 69 kg **51.** $2\frac{41}{128}$ lb **53.** $18\frac{3}{5}$ days **55.** $76\frac{1}{4}$ ft^2

57. Yes; $\frac{7}{8}$ in. **59.** $-8x + 24$ **60.** 19°F **61.** -21

62. 198 **63.** 33 **64.** 0 **65.** ◆ **67.** ◆

69. $352\frac{44}{93}$ **71.** $18\frac{43}{48}$ **73.** $1\frac{5}{8}$ **75.** $-30\frac{5}{8}$; $-30\frac{5}{8}$

77. 6 ft, $6\frac{4}{5}$ in.　**79.** 5 chicken bouillon cubes; $3\frac{3}{4}$ cups hot water; $7\frac{1}{2}$ tbsp margarine; $7\frac{1}{2}$ tbsp flour; $6\frac{1}{4}$ cups diced cooked chicken; $2\frac{1}{2}$ cups cooked peas; $2\frac{1}{2}$ 4-oz cans sliced mushrooms, drained; $\frac{5}{6}$ cups sliced cooked carrots; $\frac{5}{8}$ cups chopped onions; 5 tbsp chopped pimiento; $2\frac{1}{2}$ tsp salt.

Summary and Review: Chapter 4, p. 265

1. 36　**2.** 90　**3.** 30　**4.** $\frac{7}{9}$　**5.** $\frac{7}{a}$　**6.** $-\frac{7}{15}$
7. $\frac{7}{16}$　**8.** $\frac{1}{3}$　**9.** $-\frac{1}{8}$　**10.** $\frac{5}{27}$　**11.** $\frac{11}{18}$　**12.** $>$
13. $<$　**14.** $\frac{19}{40}$　**15.** 4　**16.** $-\frac{5}{6}$　**17.** $\frac{12}{25}$　**18.** $\frac{15}{2}$
19. $\frac{67}{8}$　**20.** $-\frac{13}{3}$　**21.** $\frac{75}{7}$　**22.** $2\frac{1}{3}$　**23.** $-6\frac{3}{4}$
24. $12\frac{3}{5}$　**25.** $3\frac{1}{2}$　**26.** $-877\frac{1}{3}$　**27.** $81\frac{1}{3}$　**28.** $10\frac{2}{5}$
29. $11\frac{11}{15}$　**30.** -9　**31.** $1\frac{3}{4}$　**32.** $7\frac{7}{9}$　**33.** $4\frac{11}{15}$
34. $-5\frac{1}{8}$　**35.** $-14\frac{1}{4}$　**36.** $\frac{7}{9}x$　**37.** $3\frac{7}{40}a$　**38.** 16
39. $-3\frac{1}{2}$　**40.** $2\frac{21}{50}$　**41.** 6　**42.** 12　**43.** $-1\frac{7}{17}$
44. $\frac{1}{8}$　**45.** $\frac{9}{10}$　**46.** $13\frac{5}{7}$　**47.** $2\frac{8}{11}$　**48.** 15　**49.** $\$70\frac{3}{8}$
50. $\frac{3}{5}$ mi　**51.** $8\frac{3}{8}$ cups　**52.** $177\frac{3}{4}$ in²　**53.** $50\frac{1}{4}$ in²
54. $-\frac{6}{5}$　**55.** $-\frac{3}{2}$　**56.** $\$30$ loss　**57.** $5a-45$
58. ◈ The student multiplied the whole numbers and multiplied the fractions. The mixed numerals should be converted to fractional notation before multiplying.
59. ◈ Yes. We may need to find a common denominator before adding or subtracting. To find the least common denominator, we use the least common multiple of the denominators.
60. $3 \cdot 23 \cdot 41 \cdot 47 \cdot 59$, or 7,844,817　**61.** $\frac{600}{13}$
62. (a) 6; **(b)** 5; **(c)** 12; **(d)** 18; **(e)** -101; **(f)** -155; **(g)** -3; **(h)** -1　**63. (a)** 6; **(b)** 10; **(c)** 46; **(d)** 1; **(e)** -14; **(f)** -28; **(g)** -2; **(h)** -1

Test: Chapter 4, p. 269

1. [4.1a] 48　**2.** [4.2a] 3　**3.** [4.2b] $-\frac{5}{24}$　**4.** [4.3a] $\frac{2}{t}$
5. [4.3a] $\frac{1}{12}$　**6.** [4.3a] $-\frac{1}{12}$　**7.** [4.2c] $>$　**8.** [4.3b] $\frac{1}{4}$
9. [4.4a] $-\frac{12}{5}$　**10.** [4.4a] 18　**11.** [4.5a] $\frac{7}{2}$
12. [4.5a] $-\frac{79}{8}$　**13.** [4.5b] $-8\frac{2}{9}$　**14.** [4.5c] $162\frac{7}{11}$
15. [4.6a] $14\frac{1}{5}$　**16.** [4.6a] $14\frac{5}{12}$　**17.** [4.6b] $4\frac{7}{24}$
18. [4.6d] $8\frac{4}{7}$　**19.** [4.6d] $-5\frac{7}{10}$　**20.** [4.3a] $-\frac{1}{8}x$
21. [4.6b] $1\frac{54}{55}a$　**22.** [4.7a] 39　**23.** [4.7a] -18
24. [4.7b] 6　**25.** [4.7b] 2　**26.** [4.7c] $19\frac{3}{5}$
27. [4.7c] $28\frac{1}{20}$　**28.** [4.7d] $7\frac{1}{2}$ lb　**29.** [4.7d] 80
30. [4.5c] $148\frac{1}{2}$ lb　**31.** [4.3c] $\frac{13}{200}$ m　**32.** [2.7a] $9x-54$
33. [3.7b] $\frac{8}{5}$　**34.** [3.6a] $\frac{10}{9}$　**35.** [2.3b] 1190 ft
36. [4.1a] $\frac{24}{25}$ min　**37.** [4.3c] Dolores; $\frac{17}{56}$ mi
38. [4.1a] **(a)** 24, 48, 72; **(b)** 24　**39.** [4.2b] **(a)** $\frac{1}{2}$; **(b)** $\frac{2}{3}$; **(c)** $\frac{3}{4}$; **(d)** $\frac{4}{5}$; **(e)** $\frac{9}{10}$

Cumulative Review: Chapters 1–4, p. 271

1. [1.1e] 5　**2.** [1.1a] 6 thousands + 7 tens + 5 ones
3. [1.1c] Twenty-nine thousand, five hundred
4. [1.2b] 623　**5.** [2.2a] -8　**6.** [4.2b] $\frac{5}{12}$　**7.** [4.6a] $8\frac{1}{4}$
8. [1.3d] 5124　**9.** [2.3a] 16　**10.** [4.3a] $-\frac{5}{12}$
11. [4.6b] $1\frac{1}{6}$　**12.** [1.5b] 5004　**13.** [2.4a] -145
14. [3.6a] $\frac{3}{2}$　**15.** [3.6a] -15　**16.** [4.7a] $7\frac{1}{3}$
17. [1.6c] 48 R 11　**18.** [1.6c] 56 R 11　**19.** [4.5c] $56\frac{11}{45}$
20. [3.7b] $-\frac{4}{7}$　**21.** [4.7b] $7\frac{1}{3}$　**22.** [1.4a] 38,500
23. [4.1a] 72　**24.** [3.1b] Yes　**25.** [3.2a] 1, 2, 4, 8, 16
26. [3.3b] $\frac{1}{6}$　**27.** [4.2c] $>$　**28.** [4.2c] $<$　**29.** [3.5b] $\frac{4}{5}$
30. [3.5b] -14　**31.** [4.5a] $\frac{37}{8}$　**32.** [4.5b] $-5\frac{2}{3}$
33. [1.7b], [2.8a] 93　**34.** [4.3b] $\frac{5}{9}$　**35.** [3.8a] $-\frac{12}{7}$
36. [4.4a] $\frac{2}{21}$　**37.** [2.6a] 4　**38.** [2.7a] $7b-35$
39. [2.7a] $-3x+6-3z$　**40.** [2.7b] $-6x-9$
41. [1.8a] $\$235$　**42.** [1.8a] $\$663$　**43.** [1.8a] 297 ft²
44. [1.8a] 31　**45.** [3.6b] $\frac{2}{5}$ tsp　**46.** [4.7d] 39 lb
47. [4.7d] 16　**48.** [4.2d] $\frac{19}{16}$ in.　**49.** [4.4a], [4.6a] $\frac{3}{7}$
50. [4.6c], [4.7d] 3780 m²

Chapter 5

Pretest: Chapter 5, p. 274

1. [5.1a] Seventeen and three hundred sixty-nine thousandths　**2.** [5.1a] Six hundred twenty-five and $\frac{27}{100}$ dollars　**3.** [5.1b] $\frac{21}{100}$　**4.** [5.1b] $\frac{5408}{1000}$
5. [5.1c] 3.79　**6.** [5.1c] -0.0079　**7.** [5.1e] 21.0
8. [5.2a] 607.219　**9.** [5.2b] 91.732　**10.** [5.3a] 4.688
11. [5.2c] -252.9937　**12.** [5.4a] -30.4
13. [5.2d] $12.9a$　**14.** [5.2d] $-6.9x+6.8$
15. [5.4b] -12.62　**16.** [5.6a] 7.6　**17.** [5.5c] 1.4
18. [5.5a] $4.\overline{142857}$　**19.** [5.5d] 1.7835
20. [5.5d] 4.34 m²　**21.** [5.7a] 3.35　**22.** [5.7a] -84.26
23. [5.7a] 5.4　**24.** [5.7b] 6　**25.** [5.7b] 4.55
26. [5.8a] $\$285.95$　**27.** [5.8a] 1081.6 mi
28. [5.8a] $\$89.70$　**29.** [5.8a] $\$3397.71$
30. [5.8a] 15.4 mpg

Margin Exercises, Section 5.1, pp. 276–280

1. Twenty and five tenths　**2.** Two and four thousand five hundred thirty-three ten-thousandths
3. Negative four hundred fifty-three and twenty-seven hundredths　**4.** Fifty-one thousand, seven hundred thirty-nine and eighty-two thousandths　**5.** Four thousand, two hundred seventeen and $\frac{56}{100}$ dollars
6. Thirteen and $\frac{98}{100}$ dollars　**7.** $\frac{896}{1000}$　**8.** $-\frac{3908}{100}$
9. $\frac{56,789}{10,000}$　**10.** $-\frac{37}{10}$　**11.** 7.43　**12.** 0.048
13. 6.7089　**14.** -0.9　**15.** -7.03　**16.** 23.047
17. 2.04　**18.** 0.06　**19.** 0.58　**20.** 1　**21.** 0.8989
22. 21.05　**23.** -34.008　**24.** -8.98　**25.** 2.8
26. 13.9　**27.** -234.4　**28.** 7.0　**29.** 0.64
30. -7.83　**31.** 34.70　**32.** -0.03　**33.** 0.943

34. −8.004   **35.** −43.112   **36.** 37.401   **37.** 7459.360
38. 7459.36   **39.** 7459.4   **40.** 7459   **41.** 7460
42. 7500   **43.** 7000

Exercise Set 5.1, p. 281

1. Four hundred eighty-one and twenty-seven
hundredths   **3.** One and five thousand five hundred
ninety-nine ten-thousandths   **5.** Thirty-four and
eight hundred ninety-one thousandths   **7.** Three
hundred twenty-six and $\frac{48}{100}$ dollars   **9.** Thirty-six and
$\frac{72}{100}$ dollars   **11.** $\frac{83}{10}$ **13.** $\frac{2036}{10}$ **15.** $-\frac{2703}{1000}$ **17.** $\frac{109}{10,000}$
19. $-\frac{6004}{1000}$ **21.** 0.8   **23.** −0.59   **25.** 3.798
27. 0.0078   **29.** −0.00018   **31.** 0.376193   **33.** 99.44
35. −8.431   **37.** 2.1739   **39.** 8.953073   **41.** 0.58
43. 0.91   **45.** −5.043   **47.** 235.07   **49.** $\frac{4}{100}$
51. −0.872   **53.** 0.1   **55.** −0.4   **57.** 3.0
59. −327.2   **61.** 0.89   **63.** −0.67   **65.** 1.00
67. −0.03   **69.** 0.325   **71.** 17.002   **73.** −20.202
75. 9.985   **77.** 809.5   **79.** 809.47   **81.** 0   **82.** $\frac{31}{45}$
83. $-\frac{2}{9}$ **84.** $-\frac{2}{7}$ **85.** $\frac{29}{3}$ **86.** $-\frac{1}{14}$ **87.** ◈   **89.** ◈
91. 1979   **93.** 1998   **95.** 0.07070

Margin Exercises, Section 5.2, pp. 283–286

1. 10.917   **2.** 34.2079   **3.** 4.969   **4.** 3.5617
5. 9.40544   **6.** 912.67   **7.** 2514.773   **8.** 10.754
9. 0.339   **10.** 1.47   **11.** 0.24238   **12.** 7.36992
13. 1194.22   **14.** 4.9911   **15.** −1.96   **16.** 3.159
17. −8.55   **18.** −4.16   **19.** −7.44   **20.** 12.4
21. −2.7   **22.** 4.7x **23.** 1.7a **24.** −2.7y + 5.4

Exercise Set 5.2, p. 287

1. 334.37   **3.** 1576.215   **5.** 132.56   **7.** 64.413
9. 50.0248   **11.** 0.835   **13.** 771.967   **15.** 20.8649
17. 227.468   **19.** 2.1   **21.** 49.02   **23.** 2.4975
25. 85.921   **27.** 1.6666   **29.** 4.0622   **31.** 8.85
33. 3.37   **35.** 1.045   **37.** 3.703   **39.** 0.9092
41. 605.21   **43.** 0.994   **45.** 161.62   **47.** 44.001
49. 1.71   **51.** −2.5   **53.** −7.2   **55.** 3.379   **57.** −22.6
59. 2.5   **61.** −3.519   **63.** 9.601   **65.** 14.5   **67.** 3.8
69. −10.292   **71.** −8.8   **73.** 8.7x **75.** 4.86a
77. 21.1t + 7.9   **79.** −5.311t **81.** 8.106y − 7.1
83. −0.9x + 3.1y **85.** 7.2 − 8.4t **87.** 0   **88.** $-\frac{1}{21}$
89. $-\frac{1}{10}$ **90.** $\frac{7}{3}$ **91.** 3   **92.** $-\frac{4}{9}$ **93.** ◈   **95.** ◈
97. −18.183x − 0.02058y − 91.127z **99.** 345.8
101. $8744.16 should be $8744.17; $8764.65 should be
$8723.68; $8848.65 should be $8808.68; $8801.05 should
be $8760.08; $8533.09 should be $8492.13

Margin Exercises, Section 5.3, pp. 292–296

1. 625.66   **2.** 21.4863   **3.** 0.00943   **4.** −12.535374
5. 35.9   **6.** 0.7324   **7.** −0.058   **8.** 0.07236
9. 539.17   **10.** −6241.7   **11.** 64,700   **12.** 430,100
13. 4,300,000   **14.** $44,100,000,000   **15.** 1569¢
16. 17¢   **17.** $0.35   **18.** $5.77   **19.** 6.656
20. 8.125 sq cm   **21.** 55.107

Calculator Spotlight, p. 296

2. (a) 8245.258176; (b) 1036.192585; (c) 11,814.1659

Exercise Set 5.3, p. 297

1. 47.6   **3.** 6.72   **5.** 0.252   **7.** 0.1032   **9.** 426.3
11. −783,686.852   **13.** −780   **15.** 7.918   **17.** 0.09768
19. −0.287   **21.** 43.68   **23.** 3.2472   **25.** 89.76
27. −322.07   **29.** 55.68   **31.** 3487.5   **33.** 0.1155
35. −9420   **37.** 0.00953   **39.** 2888¢   **41.** 66¢
43. $0.34   **45.** $34.45   **47.** $32,279,000,000
49. 1,030,000   **51.** 11,000   **53.** 26.025   **55.** (a) 44 ft;
(b) 118.75 sq ft   **57.** 1   **58.** $\frac{1}{15}$ **59.** $-\frac{1}{18}$ **60.** $\frac{2}{7}$
61. $\frac{3}{5}$ **62.** 0   **63.** ◈   **65.** ◈   **67.** 431.061084
69. 10^{15} **71.** $53.02

Margin Exercises, Section 5.4, pp. 299–304

1. 0.6   **2.** 1.5   **3.** 0.47   **4.** 0.32   **5.** −5.75   **6.** 0.25
7. (a) 375; (b) 15   **8.** 4.9   **9.** 12.8   **10.** 15.625
11. 12.78   **12.** 0.001278   **13.** 0.09847   **14.** −67.832
15. 0.2426   **16.** −7.4   **17.** 1.2825 billion

Calculator Spotlight, p. 300

1. 28 R 2   **2.** 116 R 3   **3.** 74 R 10   **4.** 415 R 3

Exercise Set 5.4, p. 305

1. 16.4   **3.** 23.78   **5.** 7.48   **7.** 7.2   **9.** −1.143
11. −0.9   **13.** 70   **15.** 40   **17.** −0.15   **19.** 48
21. 3.2   **23.** 0.625   **25.** 0.26   **27.** 2.34
29. −0.3045   **31.** −2.134567   **33.** 1023.7
35. −56,780   **37.** 9.7   **39.** −75,300   **41.** 230.01
43. 2107   **45.** −302.997   **47.** −178.1   **49.** 119.0176
51. −400.0108   **53.** 0.6725   **55.** 5.383   **57.** 10.5
59. 4.229 billion   **61.** 59.49°   **63.** $3\frac{1}{2}$ **64.** $-1\frac{1}{3}$
65. −8   **66.** $-\frac{29}{2}$, or $-14\frac{1}{2}$ **67.** 11   **68.** 15   **69.** ◈
71. ◈   **73.** 5.469156952   **75.** 10,000   **77.** 18.9
79. 590

Margin Exercises, Section 5.5, pp. 309–314

1. 0.4   **2.** 0.375   **3.** 0.1$\overline{6}$ **4.** 0.$\overline{6}$ **5.** 0.$\overline{45}$
6. −1.$\overline{09}$ **7.** 0.$\overline{714285}$ **8.** 0.7; 0.67; 0.667
9. 0.6; 0.61; 0.608   **10.** −7.3; −7.35; −7.349
11. 2.7; 2.69; 2.689   **12.** 0.8   **13.** −0.45   **14.** 0.035
15. 1.32   **16.** 0.72   **17.** 0.552   **18.** 4.225 ft^2

Calculator Spotlight, p. 314

1. 123.150432   **2.** 52.59026102

Exercise Set 5.5, p. 315

1. 0.3125   **3.** 0.475   **5.** −0.2   **7.** 0.65   **9.** 0.425
11. 1.225   **13.** −0.52   **15.** 20.016   **17.** −0.25
19. 0.575   **21.** −0.625   **23.** 1.48   **25.** 0.5$\overline{3}$
27. 0.$\overline{3}$ **29.** −1.$\overline{3}$ **31.** 1.1$\overline{6}$ **33.** 0.$\overline{571428}$
35. −0.91$\overline{6}$ **37.** 0.5; 0.53; 0.533   **39.** 0.3; 0.33; 0.333

41. −1.3; −1.33; −1.333   **43.** 1.2; 1.17; 1.167
45. 0.6; 0.57; 0.571   **47.** −0.9; −0.92; −0.917
49. 0.7; 0.75; 0.747   **51.** −8.0; −7.97; −7.967
53. 9.485   **55.** −417.51$\overline{6}$ **57.** 0.09705   **59.** −1.5275
61. 24.375   **63.** 1.08 m^2 **65.** 5.78 cm^2 **67.** $3\frac{2}{5}$
68. $30\frac{7}{10}$ **69.** −95   **70.** −10   **71.** −7   **72.** 1
73. ◆   **75.** ◆   **77.** 0.$\overline{285714}$ **79.** 0.$\overline{571428}$
81. 0.$\overline{857142}$ **83.** 0.$\overline{01}$ **85.** 0.$\overline{0001}$ **87.** 6.16 cm^2
89. 63.585 yd^2 or 63.61725124 yd^2

Margin Exercises, Section 5.6, pp. 319–321

1. $540   **2.** $160   **3.** $1320   **4.** 4   **5.** 16   **6.** 18
7. 470   **8.** 0.07   **9.** 18   **10.** 125   **11.** (c)   **12.** (a)
13. (c)   **14.** (c)

Exercise Set 5.6, p. 323

1. $360   **3.** $50   **5.** $2700   **7.** 5   **9.** 1.6   **11.** 6
13. 60   **15.** 2.3   **17.** 180   **19.** (a)   **21.** (c)   **23.** (b)
25. (b)   **27.** 8000   **29.** $2 \cdot 2 \cdot 3 \cdot 3 \cdot 3$
30. $2 \cdot 2 \cdot 2 \cdot 2 \cdot 5 \cdot 5$ **31.** $5 \cdot 5 \cdot 13$ **32.** $2 \cdot 3 \cdot 3 \cdot 37$
33. $\frac{5}{16}$ **34.** $\frac{129}{251}$ **35.** $\frac{8}{9}$ **36.** $\frac{13}{25}$ **37.** ◆   **39.** ◆
41. No   **43.** Yes

Margin Exercises, Section 5.7, pp. 325–328

1. 4.2   **2.** 5.7   **3.** 2.6   **4.** −10.8   **5.** 3.6   **6.** −1.9
7. 3.5   **8.** 2.2   **9.** −4.5   **10.** 1.25

Exercise Set 5.7, p. 329

1. 5.4   **3.** 0.5239   **5.** −4.5   **7.** 10.3   **9.** 43.78
11. 7.7   **13.** −9.7   **15.** 5   **17.** 2.5   **19.** −2.8
21. −4.7   **23.** 1.7   **25.** 9   **27.** 1.25   **29.** −3.25
31. 30   **33.** 3.2   **35.** 4   **37.** 8.5   **39.** 2.9
41. 3.8575   **43.** −4.6   **45.** 7   **47.** −2.5   **49.** 1
50. $\frac{23}{18}$ **51.** $-\frac{29}{50}$ **52.** 0   **53.** −2   **54.** 8
55. ◆   **57.** ◆   **59.** −2.7   **61.** 1

Margin Exercises, Section 5.8, pp. 333–338

1. 8.4°   **2.** $37.28   **3.** $189.50   **4.** 28.6 mpg
5. 13.76 in^2 **6.** 1.25 hr

Exercise Set 5.8, p. 339

1. $230.86   **3.** $26.50   **5.** $5.32   **7.** 8.17 mg
9. $368.75   **11.** 1.65 mg   **13.** $21,219.17
15. 4523.76 cm^2 **17.** 93.9 km   **19.** $956.16
21. 78.1 cm   **23.** 28.5 cm   **25.** 2.31 cm
27. 20.2 mpg   **29.** $11.03   **31.** 331.74 ft^2
33. 39.585 ft^2 **35.** $505.75   **37.** 450.5 mi
39. 8.125 hr   **41.** 2.5 hr   **43.** 2152.56 yd^2 **45.** 17
47. 0   **48.** $-\frac{1}{10}$ **49.** $-\frac{20}{33}$ **50.** −4   **51.** $6\frac{5}{6}$
52. 1   **53.** ◆   **55.** ◆   **57.** 3
59. 25 cm^2. We assume that the figures are nested squares formed by connecting the midpoints of consecutive sides of the next larger square.
61. $1.32

1. Three and forty-seven hundredths
2. Five hundred ninety-seven and $\frac{25}{100}$ dollars
3. $\frac{9}{100}$ **4.** $-\frac{30,227}{10,000}$ **5.** −0.034   **6.** 27.91   **7.** 0.034
8. −0.19   **9.** 39.4   **10.** 39.43   **11.** 499.829
12. 29.148   **13.** 229.1   **14.** 685.0519   **15.** −57.3
16. 2.37   **17.** 12.96   **18.** −1.073   **19.** 24,680
20. 3.2   **21.** −1.6   **22.** 0.2763   **23.** $2.2x − 9.1y$
24. $−2.84a + 12.57$ **25.** 925   **26.** 40.84   **27.** 11.3
28. 20   **29.** (c)   **30.** $15.49   **31.** 248.27   **32.** 2.6
33. 1.28   **34.** 3.25   **35.** $-1.1\overline{6}$ **36.** 21.08   **37.** −3.2
38. −3   **39.** −7.5   **40.** 6.5   **41.** 11.16   **42.** 89.4 sec
43. 6365.1 bushels   **44.** $32.59   **45.** 24.36; 104.4
46. 8.4 mi   **47.** 1   **48.** $\frac{1}{18}$ **49.** $\frac{3}{10}$ **50.** $-\frac{1}{4}x - \frac{1}{4}y$
51. ◆ Each decimal place in the decimal notation corresponds to one zero in the denominator of the fractional notation. When the fractions are multiplied, the number of zeros in the denominator of the product is the sum of the number of zeros in each factor. So the number of decimal places in the product will be the sum of the number of decimal places in each factor.
52. ◆ The decimal points must be lined up before adding.   **53.** $\frac{-13}{15}, \frac{-17}{20}, -\frac{11}{13}, -\frac{15}{19}, \frac{-5}{7}, -\frac{2}{3}$ **54.** $35

Test: Chapter 5, p. 347

1. [5.1a] Six and four hundred one ten-thousandths
2. [5.1a] One thousand two hundred thirty-four and $\frac{78}{100}$ dollars   **3.** [5.1b] $-\frac{2}{10}$ **4.** [5.1b] $\frac{7308}{1000}$
5. [5.1c] 0.0049   **6.** [5.1c] −5.28   **7.** [5.1d] 0.162
8. [5.1d] −0.173   **9.** [5.1e] 9.5   **10.** [5.1e] 9.452
11. [5.2a] 405.219   **12.** [5.3a] 0.03   **13.** [5.3a] 0.21345
14. [5.2b] 44.746   **15.** [5.2a] 356.37   **16.** [5.2c] −2.2
17. [5.2b] 1.9946   **18.** [5.4a] 0.44   **19.** [5.4a] 30.4
20. [5.4a] −0.34682   **21.** [5.3b] 17,982¢
22. [5.2d] $9.8x − 3.9y − 4.6$ **23.** [5.3c] 11.6
24. [5.4b] 7.6   **25.** [5.6a] 8 gal   **26.** [5.5b] 48.7
27. [5.5c] 1.6   **28.** [5.5c] 5.25   **29.** [5.5a] −0.4375
30. [5.5a] $1.\overline{2}$ **31.** [5.5d] 9.72   **32.** [5.7a] −3.24
33. [5.7b] 10   **34.** [5.7b] 1.4   **35.** [5.8a] $1209.22
36. [5.8a] 33.46 sec   **37.** [5.8a] $119.70
38. [5.8a] 8.2 mi   **39.** [5.8a] 1.5 hr   **40.** [3.3c] 0
41. [4.2b] $\frac{3}{7}$ **42.** [4.3a] $-\frac{1}{30}$ **43.** [4.3a] $\frac{7}{10}x + \frac{1}{15}y$
44. [5.3a] (a) Always; (b) never; (c) sometimes; (d) sometimes

Cumulative Review: Chapters 1–5, p. 349

1. [1.1a] 1 ten thousand + 2 thousands + 7 hundreds + 5 tens + 8 ones   **2.** [5.1a] Eight hundred two and $\frac{53}{100}$ dollars   **3.** [5.1b] $\frac{1009}{100}$ **4.** [4.5a] $\frac{27}{8}$
5. [5.1c] −0.035   **6.** [3.2a] 1, 2, 3, 6, 11, 22, 33, 66
7. [3.2c] $2 \cdot 3 \cdot 11$ **8.** [4.1a] 140   **9.** [1.4a] 7000
10. [5.1e] 6962.47   **11.** [4.6a] $6\frac{2}{9}$ **12.** [5.2a] 235.397
13. [1.2b] 5495   **14.** [4.2b] $-\frac{1}{30}$ **15.** [2.3a] 46
16. [5.2b] 8446.53   **17.** [4.3a] $\frac{1}{72}$ **18.** [4.6b] $3\frac{2}{5}$

19. [5.3a] 4.78 **20.** [3.6a] $-\frac{2}{7}$ **21.** [4.7a] $13\frac{7}{11}$
22. [3.6a] $\frac{3}{2}$ **23.** [4.7b] $1\frac{1}{2}$ **24.** [3.7b] $\frac{48}{35}$
25. [5.4a] $-43{,}795$ **26.** [5.4a] 20.6 **27.** [4.2c] $>$
28. [2.1b] $>$ **29.** [2.6a] -2 **30.** [2.7a] $4x - 4y + 12$
31. [2.7b] $7p - 5$ **32.** [2.7b] $14x - 11$ **33.** [5.7a] 0.78
34. [2.8b], [3.8b] -28 **35.** [5.7a] 8.62
36. [2.8a] 369,375 **37.** [4.3b] $\frac{1}{18}$ **38.** [3.8b] $\frac{1}{2}$
39. [5.7a] 3.8125 **40.** [4.4a] -15 **41.** [1.8a] 19,299
42. [3.7c] $500 **43.** [1.8a] 86,400 **44.** [3.6b] $2800
45. [5.8a] $258.77 **46.** [4.6c] $6\frac{1}{2}$ lb **47.** [3.6b] 88 ft^2
48. [5.8a] 467.28 ft^2 **49.** [4.7d] 144 **50.** [5.8a] $1.58

Chapter 6

Pretest: Chapter 6, p. 352

1. [6.1a] **(a)** $298; **(b)** $172; **(c)** $134
2. [6.2b]

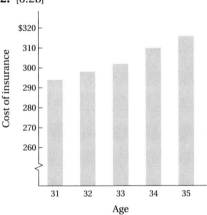

3. [6.2d]

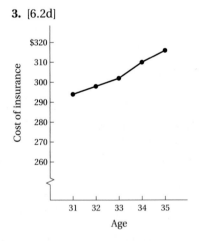

4. [6.2c] 260
5. [6.2c] 160 occurrences per 1000 people

6. [6.3a]

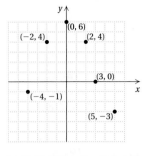

7. [6.3b] II **8.** [6.3c] No
9. [6.4b] **10.** [6.4b]

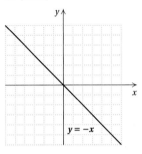
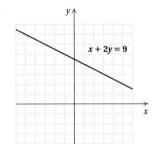

11. [6.4b]

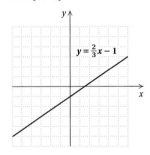

12. [6.5a, b, c] **(a)** 51; **(b)** 51.5; **(c)** None exists.
13. [6.5a, b, c] **(a)** 3; **(b)** 3; **(c)** 5, 1
14. [6.5a, b, c] **(a)** 12.75; **(b)** 17; **(c)** 4 **15.** [6.5a] 55 mph
16. [6.5a] 86 **17.** [6.6a] 50 per 1000 people
18. [6.6b] $\frac{1}{6}$

Margin Exercises, Section 6.1, pp. 353–356

1. Kellogg's Complete Bran Flakes **2.** Kellogg's
Special K **3.** Kellogg's Special K, Wheaties
4. Ralston Rice Chex, Kellogg's Complete Bran Flakes,
Honey Nut Cheerios **5.** 510.66 mg **6.** AT&T, LCI
7. GTE **8.** 11.7¢/min **9.** 14.7¢/min
10. 795 cups; answers may vary **11.** 750 cups;
answers may vary **12.** 1650 cups; answers may vary
13.

Total Gross Revenue

Boyz II Men				
REM				
Kiss				

= $10,000,000

Exercise Set 6.1, p. 357

1. 483,612,200 mi **3.** Neptune **5.** All **7.** 11
9. 27,884.$\overline{1}$ mi **11.** 1992 **13.** 59.29°, 59.58°
15. 59.50°, 59.56125°, 0.06125° **17.** 1989 and 1990
19. 1.0 billion **21.** 1999 **23.** 1650 and 1850
25. 2.0 billion **27.** 1995 **29.** 8 hr **31.** 4 hr/wk
33. 1991 and 1992, or 1992 and 1993, or 1995 and 1996
35.

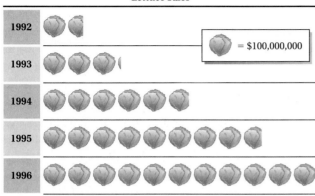

Lettuce Sales

36. −2 **37.** −3 **38.** 1 **39.** 0.375 **40.** 0.06
41. 1.16 **42.** 0.8$\overline{3}$ **43.** ◈ **45.** ◈ **47.** 0.5$\overline{3}$ hr

Margin Exercises, Section 6.2, pp. 363–367

1. 16 g **2.** Big Bacon Classic **3.** Chicken Club, Big
Bacon Classic, Single with Everything **4.** 60
5. 85+ **6.** 60–64 **7.** Yes
8.

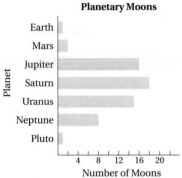

Planetary Moons

9. Month 7 **10.** Months 1 and 2, 4 and 5, 6 and 7, 11
and 12 **11.** Months 2, 5, 6, 7, 8, 9, 12
12.

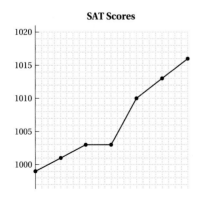

SAT Scores

Exercise Set 6.2, p. 369

1. 190 **3.** 1 slice of chocolate cake with fudge frosting
5. 1 cup of premium chocolate ice cream
7. 120 calories **9.** 920 calories **11.** 28 lb
13. 920,000 hectares **15.** Latin America
17. Africa **19.** 880,000 hectares
21.

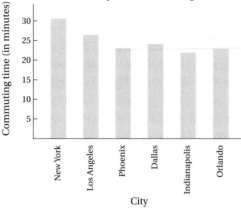

Metropolitan Commuting

23. Indianapolis **25.** 28.5 min
27. 580 calories **29.** 1930 calories **31.** 1998
33. About $0.55 million **35.** 1994 and 1995
37.

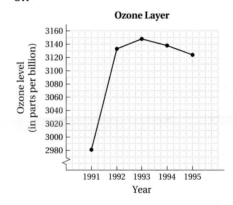

Ozone Layer

39. 1994 and 1995
41. 3135.75 parts per billion **43.** 1995 and 1996
45. $48.35 million **47.** 34 **48.** $\frac{9}{50}$ **49.** 72 fl oz
50. 32 **51.** 50 **52.** 18 **53.** ◈ **55.** ◈
57. 268 per 100,000

Margin Exercises, Section 6.3, pp. 375–378

1., 2.

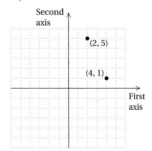

3.–8.

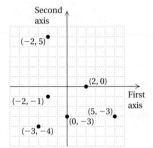

9. *A*: (−5, 1); *B*: (−3, 2); *C*: (0, 4); *D*: (3, 3); *E*: (1, 0); *F*: (0, −3); *G*: (−5, −4) **10.** Both are negative numbers. **11.** The first, or horizontal, coordinate is positive; the second, or vertical, coordinate is negative. **12.** I **13.** III **14.** IV **15.** II **16.** No **17.** Yes

Calculator Spotlight, p. 378

1. Yes **2.** No **3.** No **4.** Yes **5.** No **6.** Yes **7.** Yes **8.** No

Exercise Set 6.3, p. 379

1.

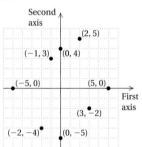

3.

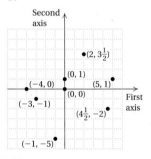

5. *A*: (3, 3); *B*: (0, −4); *C*: (−5, 0); *D*: (−1, −1); *E*: (2, 0); *F*: (−3, 5) **7.** *A*: (5, 0); *B*: (0, 5); *C*: (−3, 4); *D*: (2, −4); *E*: (2, 3); *F*: (−4, −2) **9.** II **11.** IV **13.** III **15.** I **17.** Positive; negative **19.** III **21.** IV; positive **23.** Yes **25.** No **27.** Yes **29.** No **31.** Yes **33.** No **35.** 7 **36.** 9 **37.** 3 **38.** $\frac{30}{17}$ **39.** $\frac{61}{33}a$ **40.** $7x - 24$ **41.** ◈ **43.** ◈ **45.** No **47.** III, IV **49.** II, IV **51.** (5, 2); (−7, 2); (3, −8)

53.

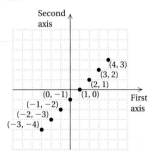

Answers may vary.
55. 65

Margin Exercises, Section 6.4, pp. 383–387

1. (8, 5) **2.** (1, 5); (3, −5) **3.** (1, 3), (7, 0), (5, 1) **4.** (0, 7), (2, 3), (−2, 11)

5.

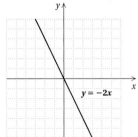

6.

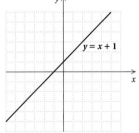

7.

8.

9.

10.

11.

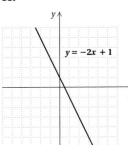

$y = -2x + 1$

12.

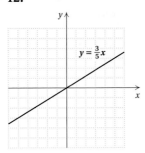

$y = \frac{3}{5}x$

45.

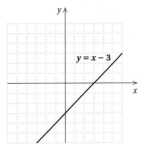

$y = x - 3$

47.

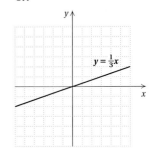

$y = \frac{1}{3}x$

Calculator Spotlight, p. 388

1.

$y = \frac{2}{3}x$

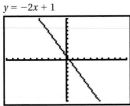

2.

$y = x + 1$

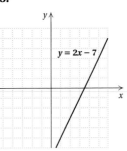

49.

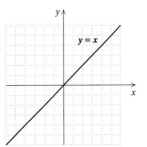

$y = x$

51.

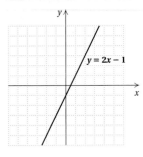

$y = 2x - 1$

3.

$y = -2x + 1$

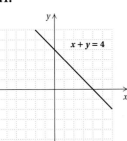

4.

$y = \frac{3}{5}x$

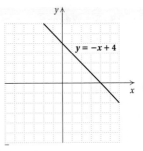

53.

$y = 2x - 7$

55.

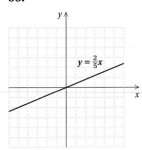

$y = \frac{2}{5}x$

57.

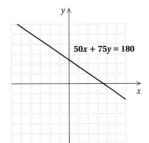

$y = -x + 4$

Exercise Set 6.4, p. 389

1. (8, 5)   **3.** (3, 1)   **5.** (5, 14)   **7.** (7, −2)   **9.** (1, 3)
11. (2, −1)   **13.** (−1, 8); (4, 3)   **15.** (7, 3); (10, 6)
17. (3, 3); (6, 1)   **19.** (3, −2); (1, 3)
21. (1, 4); (−2, −8)   **23.** $\left(0, \frac{3}{5}\right)$; $\left(\frac{3}{2}, 0\right)$
25. (0, 12), (5, 7), (14, −2)   **27.** (0, 0), (1, 4), (2, 8)
29. (0, 13), (1, 10), (2, 7)   **31.** (0, −1), (2, 5), (−1, −4)
33. (0, 0), (1, −5), (−1, 5)   **35.** (0, −4), (4, 0), (1, −3)
37. (0, 6), (4, 0), $\left(1, \frac{9}{2}\right)$ **39.** (0, 2), (3, 3), (−3, 1)
41.

$x + y = 4$

43.

$x - 1 = y$

59. $1\frac{7}{8}$ cup   **60.** $-\frac{7}{11}$ **61.** 42   **62.** $-\frac{5}{8}$ **63.** 2.6
64. 2   **65.** ◈   **67.** ◈
69. (−3, 4.4), (−3.9, 5), (3, 0.4)

$50x + 75y = 180$

71. (2, 4), (−3, −1), (−5, −3); answers may vary.
73. Answers may vary, but all should appear on this graph:

Margin Exercises, Section 6.5, pp. 393–396

1. 75   **2.** 54.9   **3.** 81   **4.** 19.4   **5.** 0.4 lb
6. 2.5   **7.** 94   **8.** 17   **9.** 17   **10.** 91   **11.** $1700
12. 67.5   **13.** 45   **14.** 34, 67   **15.** No mode exists
16. (a) 17 g; **(b)** 18 g; **(c)** 19 g2

Calculator Spotlight, p. 395

1. $203.\overline{3}$ **2.** The answers are the same.

Exercise Set 6.5, p. 397

1. Mean: 20; median: 18; mode: 29   **3.** Mean: 20;
median: 20; modes: 5, 20   **5.** Mean: 5.2; median: 5.7;
mode: 7.4   **7.** Mean: 137.5; median: 128.5; mode: 128
9. Mean: 21.2; median: 21; mode: 23   **11.** 33 mpg
13. 2.9   **15.** Mean: $9.19; median: $9.49; mode: $7.99
17. 90   **19.** 263 days   **21.** 196   **22.** 16   **23.** 1.96
24. $-\frac{10}{30}$ **25.** 2.5 hr   **26.** 6 hr   **27.** ◆   **29.** ◆
31. 171   **33.** 10   **35.** $3475

Margin Exercises, Section 6.6, pp. 399–402

1. 111 million   **2.** 94%   **3. (a)** $\frac{4}{25}$, or 0.16; **(b)** $\frac{6}{25}$, or
0.24; **(c)** $\frac{3}{5}$, or 0.6   **4. (a)** $\frac{1}{4}$, or 0.25; **(b)** $\frac{2}{13}$

Exercise Set 6.6, p. 403

1. 83   **3.** 3112 parts per billion   **5.** $148.8 billion
7. $27.30   **9.** $\frac{1}{6}$, or $0.1\overline{6}$ **11.** $\frac{1}{2}$, or 0.5   **13.** $\frac{1}{52}$
15. $\frac{2}{13}$ **17.** $\frac{3}{26}$ **19.** $\frac{4}{39}$ **21.** $\frac{34}{39}$ **23.** 3   **24.** $-\frac{5}{2}$
25. $-\frac{11}{5}$ **26.** 0.4   **27.** $1.1\overline{3}$ **28.** −0.625   **29.** ◆
31. ◆   **33.** $\frac{1}{2}$, or 0.5   **35.** $\frac{31}{366}$

Summary and Review: Chapter 6, p. 407

1. 179 lb   **2.** 118 lb   **3.** 5 ft, 3 in., medium frame
4. 5 ft, 11 in., medium frame
5.

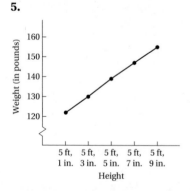

6. 14,000   **7.** Los Angeles   **8.** Houston
9. 12,500   **10.** 2.5 million   **11.** Birds   **12.** Reptiles

13. 6 million   **14.** True   **15.** False   **16.** Under 20
17. Approximately 12
18. Approximately 13 per 100 drivers
19. Between 45 and 74   **20.** Approximately 11
21. Under 20   **22.** (−5, −1)   **23.** (−2, 5)   **24.** (3, 0)
25. (4, −2)
26.–28.

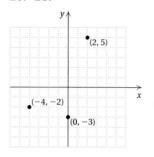

29. IV   **30.** III   **31.** I   **32.** No   **33.** Yes
34.   **35.**

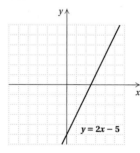   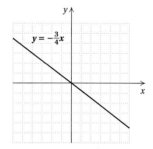

36.   **37.**

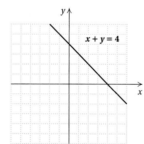   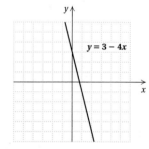

38. (a) 36; **(b)** 34; **(c)** 26   **39. (a)** 14; **(b)** 14; **(c)** 11, 17
40. (a) 322.5; **(b)** 375; **(c)** 470   **41. (a)** 1800; **(b)** 1900;
(c) 700   **42. (a)** $17.50; **(b)** $17; **(c)** $17
43. (a) $37,500; **(b)** $27,500; **(c)** None exists.
44. $310.50, $307   **45.** $66\frac{1}{6}°$ **46.** 96
47. 28   **48.** $\frac{1}{52}$ **49.** $\frac{1}{2}$ **50.** −135   **51.** $\frac{1}{3}$ m²
52. −8   **53.** −1.45
54. ◆ It is not possible for the graph of a linear
equation to pass through all four quadrants. Lines can
be drawn through two quadrants, or three, but not four.
Since the graph of a linear equation is a straight line,
one will not pass through all four quadrants.
55. ◆ The attendance at four college football games
was 21,500, 23,800, 24,400, and 27,000. What was the
average attendance?

56. $(1, 1.404255319), (0, 2.127659574), (2.941176471, 0)$;

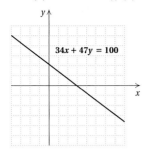

$34x + 47y = 100$

57. $11.52   **58.** 40.8 million   **59.** 35.75 million
60. Yes   **61.** Yes

62.

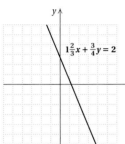

$1\frac{2}{3}x + \frac{3}{4}y = 2$

63.

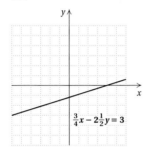

$\frac{3}{4}x - 2\frac{1}{2}y = 3$

Test: Chapter 6, p. 411

1. [6.1a] Hiking with a 20-lb load   **2.** [6.1a] Hiking with a 10-lb load
3. [6.2b]

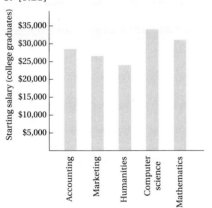

4. [6.1b] 175   **5.** [6.1b] Alex Rodriguez
6. [6.1b] Aaron Boone   **7.** [6.1b] Tony Gwynn and Tony Fernandez   **8.** [6.2c] About $6.5 billion
9. [6.2c], [6.5a] About $5.3 billion
10. [6.2c] About $5.8 billion   **11.** [6.2c] 1997
12. [6.2c], [6.5b] About $4.5 billion   **13.** [6.6a] About $11.9 billion   **14.** [6.3b] II   **15.** [6.3b] III
16. [6.3a] $(3, 4)$ **17.** [6.3a] $(0, -4)$ **18.** [6.3a] $(-4, 2)$
19. [6.3c] Yes

20. [6.4b]

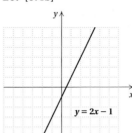

$y = 2x - 1$

21. [6.4b]

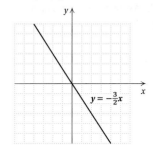

$y = -\frac{3}{2}x$

22. [6.4b]

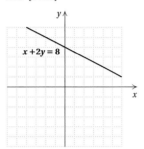

$x + 2y = 8$

23. [6.5a] 50   **24.** [6.5a] 3   **25.** [6.5a] 15.5
26. [6.5b, c] Median: 50.5; mode: 54
27. [6.5b, c] Median: 3; no mode exists
28. [6.5b, c] Median: 17.5; modes: 17, 18
29. [6.5a] 58 km/h   **30.** [6.5a] 76   **31.** [6.6b] $\frac{1}{4}$
32. [2.5a] -20 **33.** [3.5b] $\frac{5}{3}$ **34.** [3.4c] $\frac{1}{4}$ lb
35. [5.7a] -1.62
36. [6.4b]

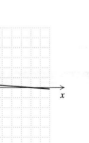

$\frac{1}{4}x + 3\frac{1}{2}y = 1$

37. [6.4b]

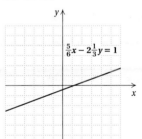

$\frac{5}{6}x - 2\frac{1}{3}y = 1$

38. [6.3a] 56

Cumulative Review: Chapters 1–6, p. 415

1. [1.1a] 3 thousands + 6 hundreds + 7 tens + 1 one
2. [1.8a] 115 mi   **3.** [1.1d] 8,000,000,000
4. [1.8a], [2.7c] Perimeter: 22 cm; area: 28 cm^2
5. [1.8a] 216 g   **6.** [1.9a] 7^4 **7.** [2.1a] $-9, 4$
8. [2.1b] $>$ **9.** [4.2c] $>$ **10.** [5.1d] $<$ **11.** [2.1d] 5
12. [2.1d] 17   **13.** [2.6a] -2 **14.** [2.7b] $-2x + y$
15. [3.2a] 1, 2, 3, 4, 6, 9, 12, 18, 36   **16.** [3.1b] Yes
17. [2.6a] $\dfrac{7}{\frac{3}{7}x}$; $-\dfrac{7}{x}$ **18.** [2.7a] $10a - 15b + 5$
19. [3.3b] $\frac{3}{7}$ **20.** [3.5a] $\frac{10}{35}$ **21.** [1.3d] 29
22. [1.5b] 476   **23.** [2.5a] -9 **24.** [2.2a] -115
25. [4.2a] $\frac{5}{7}$ **26.** [3.7b] $\frac{5}{21}$ **27.** [4.3a] $\frac{13}{18}$ **28.** [4.2b] $\frac{1}{6}$
29. [3.6a] 1   **30.** [4.6a] $9\frac{1}{8}$ **31.** [4.6b] $2\frac{5}{12}x$

32. [4.7a] $13\frac{1}{5}$ **33.** [5.2a] 83.28   **34.** [5.4a] 62.345
35. [5.3a] -42.282 **36.** [3.3c] 1   **37.** [3.3c] $4x$
38. [3.3c] 0   **39.** [4.3b] $-\frac{16}{15}$ **40.** [4.4a] 32
41. [5.7b] $-\frac{17}{4}$ **42.** [6.3b] II
43. [6.4b]

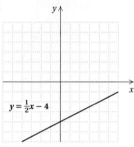

$y = \frac{1}{2}x - 4$

44. [6.5a] 36   **45.** [6.5b] 10.5   **46.** [6.5c] 49
47. [6.5a] $19\frac{2}{3}$ km/h   **48.** [1.9c], [3.6a], [4.6b], [4.7a] $\frac{9}{32}$
49. [4.5b], [4.6a] $7\frac{47}{1000}$ **50.** [6.3a] $(-2, -1)$, $(-2, 7)$,
$(6, 7)$, $(6, -1)$

Chapter 7

Pretest: Chapter 7, p. 418

1. [7.1a] $\frac{31}{54}$ **2.** [7.1b] $\frac{3}{7}$ **3.** [7.2a] 24 $\dfrac{\text{mi}}{\text{gal}}$

4. [7.2b] 0.0656 $\dfrac{\text{dollars}}{\text{oz}}$ **5.** [7.2b] Cleary's

6. [7.3a] Yes   **7.** [7.3b] 22.5   **8.** [7.3b] 0.75
9. [7.4a] 12 min   **10.** [7.4a] Approximately 394 mi
11. [7.5b] $x = 3\frac{3}{4}$, $y = 2\frac{1}{2}$, $z = 3\frac{3}{4}$ **12.** [7.5a] 60 ft

Margin Exercises, Section 7.1, pp. 419–420

1. $\frac{5}{11}$ **2.** $\frac{57.3}{86.1}$ **3.** $\dfrac{6\frac{3}{4}}{7\frac{2}{5}}$ **4.** $\frac{7410}{28,500}$ **5.** $\frac{21.1}{182.5}$ **6.** $\frac{5}{9}$ **7.** $\frac{9}{5}$
8. $\frac{73}{27}$ **9.** $\frac{3}{4}$ **10.** 18 is to 27 as 2 is to 3.
11. 3.6 is to 12 as 3 is to 10.
12. 1.2 is to 1.5 as 4 is to 5.

Exercise Set 7.1, p. 421

1. $\frac{4}{5}$ **3.** $\frac{178}{572}$ **5.** $\frac{0.4}{12}$ **7.** $\frac{3.8}{7.4}$ **9.** $\frac{56.78}{98.35}$ **11.** $\dfrac{8\frac{3}{4}}{9\frac{5}{6}}$
13. $\frac{1}{4}$; $\frac{3}{1}$ **15.** $\frac{4}{1}$ **17.** $\frac{478}{213}$; $\frac{213}{478}$ **19.** $\frac{2}{3}$ **21.** $\frac{3}{4}$ **23.** $\frac{12}{25}$
25. $\frac{7}{9}$ **27.** $\frac{2}{3}$ **29.** $\frac{14}{25}$ **31.** $\frac{1}{2}$ **33.** $\frac{3}{4}$ **35.** $\frac{51}{49}$ **37.** $\frac{32}{101}$
39. $<$ **40.** $<$ **41.** $>$ **42.** $<$ **43.** $6\frac{7}{20}$ cm
44. $17\frac{11}{20}$ cm   **45.** ◈   **47.** ◈   **49.** 1.011399197 to 1
51. $\frac{1}{3}$; $\frac{3}{2}$

Margin Exercises, Section 7.2, pp. 423–424

1. 5 mi/hr   **2.** 12 mi/hr   **3.** 0.3 mi/hr
4. 1100 ft/sec   **5.** 4 ft/sec   **6.** 14.5 ft/sec
7. 250 ft/sec   **8.** 2 gal/day   **9.** 20.64¢/oz
10. Container B

Exercise Set 7.2, p. 425

1. 40 km/h   **3.** 11 m/sec   **5.** 152 yd/day

7. 25 mi/hr; 0.04 hr/mi   **9.** 57.5¢/min
11. 0.623 gal/ft^2 **13.** 1100 ft/sec   **15.** 124 km/h
17. 560 mi/hr   **19.** \$19.50/yd   **21.** 20.59¢/oz
23. \$4.34/lb   **25.** Tico's   **27.** Dell's   **29.** Shine
31. Big Net   **33.** Four 12-oz bottles   **35.** B
37. Bert's   **39.** 1.7 million   **40.** $25\frac{1}{2}$ **41.** 109.608
42. 67,819   **43.** IV   **44.** II   **45.** ◈   **47.** ◈
49. For about a month, the unit price decreased by
0.8¢/oz. Then it changed to the same unit cost as the
16-oz bottle.   **51.** 16-in. pizza
53. About 7.27 at-bats per home run.

Margin Exercises, Section 7.3, pp. 430–432

1. Yes   **2.** No   **3.** No   **4.** Yes   **5.** No   **6.** 14
7. $11\frac{1}{4}$ **8.** 10.5   **9.** 9   **10.** 10.8

Exercise Set 7.3, p. 433

1. No   **3.** Yes   **5.** Yes   **7.** No   **9.** 45   **11.** 12
13. 10   **15.** 20   **17.** 5   **19.** 18   **21.** 22   **23.** 28
25. $9\frac{1}{3}$ or $\frac{28}{3}$ **27.** $2\frac{8}{9}$ or $\frac{26}{9}$ **29.** 0.06   **31.** 5
33. 1   **35.** 1   **37.** 0   **39.** $\frac{51}{16}$, or $3\frac{3}{16}$ **41.** 12.5725
43. $\frac{1748}{249}$, or $7\frac{5}{249}$ **45.** III   **46.** II   **47.** IV   **48.** I
49. -52 **50.** -19.75 **51.** 290.5   **52.** $1523.\overline{1}$
53. ◈   **55.** ◈   **57.** Approximately 66.85   **59.** -10.5

Margin Exercises, Section 7.4, pp. 435–436

1. 1120 mi   **2.** 16 gal   **3.** 8   **4.** $42\frac{3}{4}$ in. or less

Exercise Set 7.4, p. 437

1. 9.75 gal   **3.** 175   **5.** 2975 ft^2 **7.** 450   **9.** 60
11. 13,500 mi   **13.** 120 lb   **15.** 64 cans   **17.** 650 mi
19. 7
21.

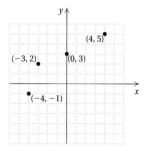

22. -79.13 **23.** -2.3 **24.** -7.3 **25.** -7.2
26. -1.8 **27.** ◈   **29.** ◈   **31.** \$2990   **33.** \$140,000

Margin Exercises, Section 7.5, pp. 439–441

1. 15   **2.** 24.75 ft   **3.** 34.9 ft   **4.** 21 cm   **5.** 29 ft

Calculator Spotlight 7.5, p. 442

1. 27.5625   **2.** 25.6   **3.** 15.140625   **4.** 41.6875
5. 40.03952941   **6.** 39.74857143   **7.** 2.615217391
8. 119

Exercise Set 7.5, p. 443

1. 25 **3.** $\frac{4}{3}$, or $1\frac{1}{3}$ **5.** $x = \frac{27}{4}$, or $6\frac{3}{4}$; $y = 9$
7. $x = 7.5$; $y = 7.2$ **9.** 1.25 m **11.** 36 ft
13. 7 ft **15.** 100 ft **17.** 4 **19.** $10\frac{1}{2}$
21. $x = 6$; $y = 5.25$; $z = 3$ **23.** $x = 5\frac{1}{3}$, or $5.\overline{3}$; $y = 4\frac{2}{3}$,
or $4.\overline{6}$; $z = 5\frac{1}{3}$, or $5.\overline{3}$ **25.** 20 ft **27.** $59.81
28. 9.63 **29.** -679.4928 **30.** 2.74568 **31.** 27,456.8
32. 0.549136 **33.** ◈ **35.** ◈ **37.** 19.25 ft
39. $x \approx 0.35$, $y = 0.4$ **41.** 86.68 cm^2

Summary and Review: Chapter 7, p. 447

1. $\frac{37}{85}$ **2.** $\frac{9}{10}$ **3.** $\frac{9}{11}$ **4.** $\frac{20}{57}$ km/min; 2.85 min/km
5. 3 min/mi **6.** $0.27/oz **7.** BiteFine **8.** No
9. 32 **10.** $\frac{1}{40}$ **11.** 7 **12.** 24 **13.** $6.65 **14.** 351
15. 6 **16.** 832 km **17.** 2,433,600 kg **18.** 9906
19. $\frac{14}{3}$ **20.** $x = \frac{56}{5}$, $y = \frac{63}{5}$ **21.** 40 ft
22. $x = 3$, $y = 9$, $z = 7\frac{1}{2}$ **23.** $1630.40
24. III, II, I, IV **25.** $-10,672.74$ **26.** 45.5
27. ◈ It took Leslie 4 gal of gasoline to drive 92 mi.
How many gallons would she need to go 368 mi?
28. ◈ In terms of cost, a low faculty-to-student ratio is
less expensive. In terms of quality education and
student satisfaction, a high faculty-to-student ratio is
better. To ensure a good education, the
student-to-faculty ratio should be low.
29. $\frac{1827}{12,704} \approx 0.14$ **30.** $\frac{3121}{12,754} \approx 0.24$ **31.** $35.53/person
32. $100.75/person **33.** 28 gal **34.** 105 min

Test: Chapter 7, p. 449

1. [7.1a] $\frac{83}{94}$ **2.** [7.1a] $\frac{0.34}{124}$ **3.** [7.1b] $\frac{32}{15}$
4. [7.2a] $\frac{5}{8}$ ft/sec **5.** [7.2a] $1\frac{2}{3}$ min/km
6. [7.2b] $0.35/oz **7.** [7.3a] No **8.** [7.3b] 12
9. [7.3b] 360 **10.** [7.4a] 1512 km **11.** [7.4a] 4.8 min
12. [7.4a] 525 mi **13.** [7.5a] 66 m **14.** [7.5a] $x = 8$,
$y = 8.8$ **15.** [7.5b] $x = 8$, $y = 8$, $z = 12$
16. [5.8a] 25.8 million lb **17.** [6.3b] II, IV, I, III
18. [5.3a] 173.736 **19.** [5.4a] -0.9944
20. [7.3b] $\frac{24}{13}$ **21.** [7.3b] $\frac{41}{10}$ **22.** [7.4a] 5888
23. [7.4a] $47.91 **24.** [7.5a] 10.5 ft

Cumulative Review: Chapters 1–7, p. 451

1. [5.2a] 643.502 **2.** [4.6a] $6\frac{3}{4}$ **3.** [4.2b] $\frac{7}{20}$
4. [5.2b] 50.501 **5.** [2.3a] -17 **6.** [4.3a] $\frac{7}{60}$
7. [5.3a] 222.076 **8.** [2.4a] -645 **9.** [4.7a] 3
10. [5.4a] 43 **11.** [2.5a] -51 **12.** [3.7b] $\frac{3}{2}$
13. [1.1a] 3 ten thousands + 7 tens + 4 ones
14. [5.1a] One hundred twenty and seven
hundredths **15.** [5.1d] 0.7 **16.** [5.1d] -0.799
17. [3.2c] $2 \cdot 2 \cdot 2 \cdot 2 \cdot 3 \cdot 3$ **18.** [4.1a] 220
19. [3.3b] $\frac{5}{8}$ **20.** [3.5b] $\frac{5}{8}$ **21.** [5.5d] 5.718
22. [5.4b] -25.56 **23.** [6.5a] 48.75 **24.** [7.3a] Yes

25. [6.4b]

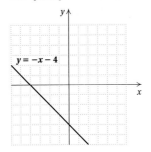

26. [2.6a] 5 **27.** [7.3b] $30\frac{6}{25}$ **28.** [2.8b], [3.8a] $-\frac{423}{16}$,
or $-26\frac{7}{16}$ **29.** [4.4a] -4 **30.** [5.7b] 3
31. [5.7a] 33.34 **32.** [3.8a] $\frac{8}{9}$ **33.** [7.4a] 42.2025 mi
34. [7.4a] 7 min **35.** [5.8a] 976.9 mi
36. [1.8a] 414,000 **37.** [3.6b] 10 ft^2 **38.** [3.7c] 12
39. [4.6c] $2\frac{1}{4}$ cups **40.** [5.8a] 132 **41.** [7.2a] 60 mph
42. [7.2b] The 12-oz bag **43.** [7.4a] No; the money
will be gone after 24 weeks. Hans will need $400
more. **44.** [7.4a] **(a)** CD player: $200; receiver–
amplifier: $600; speakers: $400; **(b)** CD player: $500;
receiver–amplifier: $1500; speakers: $1000

Chapter 8

Pretest: Chapter 8, p. 454

1. [8.1b] 0.87 **2.** [8.1b] 53.7% **3.** [8.1c] 75%
4. [8.1c] $\frac{37}{100}$ **5.** [8.3a, b] $a = 60\% \cdot 75$; 45
6. [8.2a, b] $\frac{n}{100} = \frac{35}{50}$; 70% **7.** [8.4a] 90 lb
8. [8.4b] 20% **9.** [8.5a] $17.16; $303.16
10. [8.5b] $5152
11. [8.5c] $112.50 discount; $337.50 sale price
12. [8.6a] $99.60 **13.** [8.6a] $20 **14.** [8.6b] $6242.40

Margin Exercises, Section 8.1, pp. 455–460

1.

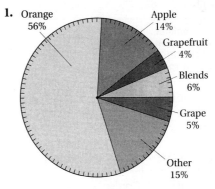

2. $\frac{70}{100}$; $70 \times \frac{1}{100}$; 70×0.01 **3.** $\frac{23.4}{100}$; $23.4 \times \frac{1}{100}$;
23.4×0.01 **4.** $\frac{100}{100}$; $100 \times \frac{1}{100}$; 100×0.01 **5.** 0.34
6. 0.789 **7.** 1.045 **8.** 0.042 **9.** 24% **10.** 347%
11. 100% **12.** 40% **13.** 25% **14.** 25% **15.** 87.5%
16. $66\frac{2}{3}$% **17.** 187.5% **18.** 57% **19.** 76% **20.** $\frac{9}{5}$
21. $\frac{13}{400}$ **22.** $\frac{2}{3}$

23.

$\frac{1}{5}$	$\frac{5}{6}$	$\frac{3}{8}$
0.2	$0.83\overline{3}$	0.375
20%	$83\frac{1}{3}\%$	$37\frac{1}{2}\%$

Calculator Spotlight, p. 459

1. 52% **2.** 38.46% **3.** 107.69% **4.** 171.43%
5. 59.62% **6.** 28.31%

Exercise Set 8.1, p. 461

1.

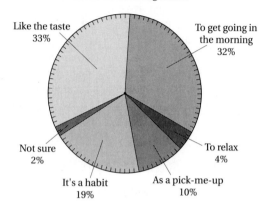

Reasons for Drinking Coffee

Like the taste 33%
To get going in the morning 32%
Not sure 2%
To relax 4%
It's a habit 19%
As a pick-me-up 10%

3. $\frac{90}{100}$; $90 \times \frac{1}{100}$; 90×0.01 **5.** $\frac{12.5}{100}$; $12.5 \times \frac{1}{100}$; 12.5×0.01 **7.** 0.12 **9.** 0.347 **11.** 0.5901
13. 0.1 **15.** 0.01 **17.** 3 **19.** 0.006 **21.** 0.0023
23. 1.0524 **25.** 0.4 **27.** 0.025 **29.** 0.622 **31.** 47%
33. 3% **35.** 870% **37.** 33.4% **39.** 75% **41.** 40%
43. 89.25% **45.** 0.0104% **47.** 24% **49.** 32.6%
51. 41% **53.** 5% **55.** 20% **57.** 28% **59.** 15%
61. 62.5%, or $62\frac{1}{2}\%$ **63.** 80% **65.** $66.\overline{6}\%$, or $66\frac{2}{3}\%$
67. 58% **69.** 36% **71.** $\frac{17}{20}$ **73.** $\frac{5}{8}$ **75.** $\frac{1}{3}$ **77.** $\frac{1}{6}$
79. $\frac{29}{400}$ **81.** $\frac{1}{125}$ **83.** 21% **85.** 24% **87.** $\frac{11}{20}$
89. $\frac{19}{50}$ **91.** $\frac{11}{100}$ **93.** $\frac{33}{125}$ **95.** $\frac{457}{1000}$
97.

Fractional Notation	Decimal Notation	Percent Notation
$\frac{1}{8}$	0.125	$12\frac{1}{2}\%$, or 12.5%
$\frac{1}{6}$	$0.1\overline{6}$	$16\frac{2}{3}\%$, or $16.\overline{6}\%$
$\frac{1}{5}$	0.2	20%
$\frac{1}{4}$	0.25	25%
$\frac{1}{3}$	$0.\overline{3}$	$33\frac{1}{3}\%$, or $33.\overline{3}\%$
$\frac{3}{8}$	0.375	$37\frac{1}{2}\%$, or 37.5%
$\frac{2}{5}$	0.4	40%
$\frac{1}{2}$	0.5	50%

99.

Fractional Notation	Decimal Notation	Percent Notation
$\frac{1}{2}$	0.5	50%
$\frac{1}{3}$	$0.\overline{3}$	$33\frac{1}{3}\%$, or $33.\overline{3}\%$
$\frac{1}{4}$	0.25	25%
$\frac{1}{6}$	$0.1\overline{6}$	$16\frac{2}{3}\%$, or $16.\overline{6}\%$
$\frac{1}{8}$	0.125	$12\frac{1}{2}\%$, or 12.5%
$\frac{3}{4}$	0.75	75%
$\frac{5}{6}$	$0.8\overline{3}$	$83\frac{1}{3}\%$, or $83.\overline{3}\%$
$\frac{3}{8}$	0.375	$37\frac{1}{2}\%$, or 37.5%

101. $33\frac{1}{3}$ **102.** $-37\frac{1}{2}$ **103.** 400 **104.** 18.75
105. 23.125 **106.** 25.5 **107.** ◈ **109.** ◈
111. $5.\overline{405}\%$ **113.** $329.\overline{38479}\%$ **115.** $0.0158\overline{3}$
117. $1.061\overline{6}$

Margin Exercises, Section 8.2, pp. 468–470

1. $\frac{12}{100} = \frac{a}{50}$ **2.** $\frac{40}{100} = \frac{a}{60}$ **3.** $\frac{130}{100} = \frac{a}{72}$ **4.** $\frac{20}{100} = \frac{45}{b}$
5. $\frac{120}{100} = \frac{60}{b}$ **6.** $\frac{N}{100} = \frac{16}{40}$ **7.** $\frac{N}{100} = \frac{10.5}{84}$
8. $225 **9.** 35.2 **10.** 6 **11.** 50 **12.** 30%
13. 12.5%

Exercise Set 8.2, p. 471

1. $\frac{37}{100} = \frac{a}{74}$ **3.** $\frac{N}{100} = \frac{4.3}{5.9}$ **5.** $\frac{25}{100} = \frac{14}{b}$
7. $\frac{9}{10} = \frac{37}{b}$ **9.** $\frac{70}{100} = \frac{a}{660}$ **11.** 40 **13.** 2.88
15. 25% **17.** 102% **19.** 25% **21.** 93.75% **23.** $72
25. 90 **27.** 88 **29.** 20 **31.** 25 **33.** $780.20
35. 7.9
37.

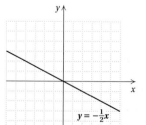

$y = -\frac{1}{2}x$

38.

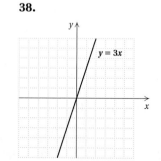

$y = 3x$

Answers

39.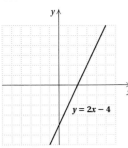

40.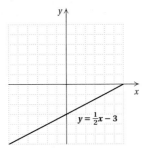

41. $\frac{43}{48}$ qt **42.** $\frac{1}{8}$ T **43.** ◈ **45.** ◈
47. 12,500 (can vary); 12,448

Margin Exercises, Section 8.3, pp. 473–476

1. $12\% \cdot 50 = a$ **2.** $a = 40\% \cdot 60$ **3.** $45 = 20\% \cdot t$
4. $120\% \cdot y = 60$ **5.** $16 = n \cdot 40$ **6.** $n \cdot 84 = 10.5$
7. 6 **8.** $35.20 **9.** 225 **10.** $50 **11.** 40%
12. 12.5%

Exercise Set 8.3, p. 477

1. $y = 32\% \cdot 78$ **3.** $89 = a \cdot 99$ **5.** $13 = 25\% \cdot y$
7. 234.6 **9.** 45 **11.** $18 **13.** 1.9 **15.** 78%
17. 200% **19.** 50% **21.** 125% **23.** 40 **25.** $40
27. 88 **29.** 20 **31.** 6.25 **33.** $846.60 **35.** 41.1
37. $\frac{623}{1000}$ **38.** $\frac{19}{10}$ **39.** $\frac{237}{100}$ **40.** 0.009 **41.** 0.39
42. 5.7 **43.** ◈ **45.** ◈
47. 62.5% (can vary); 64.5% **49.** $1875

Margin Exercises, Section 8.4, pp. 479–482

1. 16% **2.** 5 lb **3.** 4% **4.** $19,075 **5.** 9%

Exercise Set 8.4, p. 483

1. 20; 100 **3.** 402 **5.** 32.5%; 67.5%
7. 20.4 mL; 659.6 mL **9.** 25%
11. 166; 156; 146; 140; 122 **13.** 8% **15.** 20%
17. $30,030 **19.** $12,600
21. 6.096 billion; 6.194 billion; 6.293 billion
23. $36,400 **25.** $17.25; $39.10; $56.35
27. (a) 4.1%; **(b)** 31.0% **29.** 35.9% **31.** $2.\overline{27}$
32. 0.44 **33.** 3.375 **34.** $4.\overline{7}$ **35.** 0.92 **36.** $0.8\overline{3}$
37. 0.4375 **38.** 2.317 **39.** 3.4809 **40.** 0.675
41. ◈ **43.** ◈ **45.** About 5 ft, 6 in. **47.** $83\frac{1}{3}\%$
49. 19%

Margin Exercises, Section 8.5, pp. 487–492

1. $40.14; $709.09 **2.** $1.03; $15.78 **3.** 6% **4.** $420
5. $5628 **6.** 25% **7.** $1675 **8.** $33.60; $106.40
9. 20%

Calculator Spotlight, p. 492

1. 50 **2.** 7001.88 **3.** 83,931.456 **4.** 36,458.03724

Exercise Set 8.5, p. 493

1. $29.30; $615.30 **3.** $16.56; $281.56 **5.** 4% **7.** 5%
9. $5000 **11.** $800 **13.** $719.86 **15.** 5.6%
17. $903 **19.** 50% **21.** $980 **23.** $5880 **25.** 12%
27. $420 **29.** $30; $270 **31.** $2.55; $14.45
33. $125; $112.50 **35.** 40%; $360 **37.** $387; 30.4%
39. $460; about 18% **41.** 18 **42.** $\frac{22}{7}$
43. 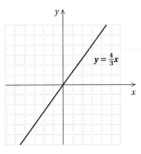 **44.**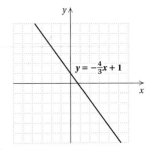

45. $0.\overline{5}$ **46.** $2.\overline{09}$ **47.** $-0.91\overline{6}$ **48.** $-1.\overline{857142}$
49. ◈ **51.** ◈ **53.** $91,112.50 **55.** $17,700
57. He bought the plaques for $166\frac{2}{3} + $250, or $416\frac{2}{3}$, and sold them for $400, so he lost money.

Margin Exercises, Section 8.6, pp. 497–500

1. $602 **2.** $451.50 **3.** $27.62; $4827.62
4. $2464.20 **5.** $8103.38

Calculator Spotlight, p. 500

1. $16,357.18 **2.** $12,764.72

Exercise Set 8.6, p. 501

1. $26 **3.** $124 **5.** $150.50 **7. (a)** $147.95;
(b) $10,147.95 **9. (a)** $128.22; **(b)** $6628.22
11. (a) $46.03; **(b)** $5646.03 **13.** $484 **15.** $236.75
17. $4284.90 **19.** $2604.52 **21.** $4101.01
23. $1324.58 **25.** 4.5 **26.** $8\frac{3}{4}$ **27.** 8 **28.** 87.5
29. $-3\frac{13}{17}$ **30.** $3\frac{5}{11}$ **31.** $\frac{18}{17}$ **32.** $\frac{209}{10}$ **33.** ◈
35. ◈ **37.** $33,981.98 **39.** 9.38%
41. $7883.24

Summary and Review: Chapter 8, p. 505

1. 48.3% **2.** 36% **3.** 37.5%, or $37\frac{1}{2}\%$ **4.** $33.\overline{3}\%$,
or $33\frac{1}{3}\%$ **5.** 0.735 **6.** 0.065 **7.** $\frac{6}{25}$ **8.** $\frac{63}{1000}$
9. $30.6 = x \times 90$; 34% **10.** $63 = 84\% \times n$; 75
11. $y = 38\frac{1}{2}\% \times 168$; 64.68 **12.** $\frac{24}{100} = \frac{16.8}{b}$; 70
13. $\frac{42}{30} = \frac{N}{100}$; 140% **14.** $\frac{10.5}{100} = \frac{a}{84}$; 8.82 **15.** $598
16. 12% **17.** 82,400 **18.** 20% **19.** 168 **20.** $14.40
21. 5% **22.** 11% **23.** $42; $308 **24.** $42.70;
$262.30 **25.** $2940 **26.** $36 **27. (a)** $394.52;
(b) $24,394.52 **28.** $121 **29.** $7727.26

30. $9504.80   **31.** Approximately 25%   **32.** $\frac{56}{3}$
33. 42
34.   **35.**

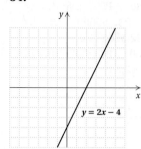

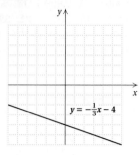

36. $3.\overline{6}$ **37.** $1.\overline{571428}$ **38.** $3\frac{2}{3}$ **39.** $17\frac{2}{7}$
40. ◈ No; the 10% discount was based on the original price rather than on the sale price.
41. ◈ A 40% discount is better. When successive discounts are taken, each is based on the previous discounted price, not the original price. A 20% discount followed by a 22% discount is the same as a 37.6% discount off the original price.
42. 19.5%   **43.** $66\frac{2}{3}$%   **44.** $168   **45.** 7

Test: Chapter 8, p. 507

1. [8.1b] 0.89   **2.** [8.1b] 67.4%   **3.** [8.1c] 137.5%
4. [8.1c] $\frac{13}{20}$ **5.** [8.3a, b] $a = 40\% \cdot 55$; 22
6. [8.2a, b] $\frac{N}{100} = \frac{65}{80}$; 81.25%   **7.** [8.4a] 28.75 lb
8. [8.4b] 140%   **9.** [8.5a] $16.20; $340.20
10. [8.5b] $630   **11.** [8.5c] $40; $160   **12.** [8.6a] $8.52
13. [8.6a] $5356   **14.** [8.6b] $1102.50
15. [8.6b] $10,226.69   **16.** [8.5c] $131.95; 52.8%
17. [6.4b]

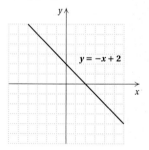

18. [7.3b] 16   **19.** [5.1c] $1.41\overline{6}$ **20.** [4.5b] $3\frac{21}{44}$
21. [8.5b] $117,800   **22.** [8.5b], [8.6b] $2546.16
23. (a) [3.6a], [4.2d] #1 pays $\frac{1}{25}$, #2 pays $\frac{9}{100}$, #3 pays $\frac{47}{300}$, #4 pays $\frac{77}{300}$, #5 pays $\frac{137}{300}$; (b) [8.1c], [8.4a] 4%, 9%, $15\frac{2}{3}$%, $25\frac{2}{3}$%, $45\frac{2}{3}$%; (c) [8.1c], [8.4a] 87%

Cumulative Review: Chapters 1–8, p. 507

1. [5.1b] $\frac{91}{1000}$ **2.** [5.5a] $2.1\overline{6}$ **3.** [8.1b] 0.03
4. [8.1c] 112.5%   **5.** [7.1a] $\frac{5}{0.5}$ **6.** [7.2a] $23\frac{1}{3}$ km/h

7. [4.2c] <   **8.** [5.1d] >   **9.** [5.6a] 296,200
10. [1.4b] 50,000   **11.** [1.9c] 13
12. [2.7b] $-2x - 14$ **13.** [4.6a] $3\frac{1}{30}$
14. [5.2c] -14.2 **15.** [1.2b] 515,150
16. [5.2b] 0.02   **17.** [4.6b] $\frac{2}{3}$ **18.** [4.3a] $-\frac{110}{63}$
19. [3.6a] $\frac{1}{6}$ **20.** [2.4a] -384
21. [5.3a] 1.38036   **22.** [4.7b] $1\frac{1}{2}$ **23.** [5.4a] 12.25
24. [1.6c] 123 R 5   **25.** [2.8b], [3.8a] 95
26. [5.7a] 8.13   **27.** [3.8a] -9 **28.** [4.3b] $\frac{1}{12}$
29. [5.7b] $-\frac{16}{9}$ **30.** [7.3b] $8\frac{8}{21}$ **31.** [6.3b] III
32. [6.4b]

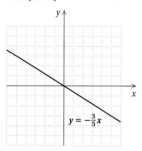

33. [6.5a] 33.2   **34.** [6.5b] 12   **35.** [2.7c] 60 in.
36. [1.5a] 3200 yd^2 **37.** [7.2b] $15\frac{\text{¢}}{\text{oz}}$ **38.** [7.4a] 608 km
39. [8.4b] 43.2%   **40.** [8.4a] 1,033,710 mi^2
41. [4.7d] 5   **42.** [4.2d] $\frac{3}{2}$ km
43. [8.4b] 12.5% increase   **44.** [4.7d], [6.5a] 33.6 mpg
45. [6.2a] 1906, 1912, 1920, 1924, 1928   **46.** [6.2a] 1977

Chapter 9

Pretest: Chapter 9, p. 512

1. [9.1a] 108   **2.** [9.1a] $\frac{2}{3}$ **3.** [9.1b] 7320
4. [9.1b] 0.75   **5.** [9.3a] 432   **6.** [9.3a] 12
7. [9.3b] 420   **8.** [9.6b] 896   **9.** [9.7a] 14,000
10. [9.7a] 3   **11.** [9.7b] 0.423   **12.** [9.7b] 400,000
13. [9.2a] 130 ft^2 **14.** [9.2a] 4 m^2
15. [9.2b] 235.5 in^2 **16.** [9.2b] 18.8 m
17. [9.2b] 220 cm   **18.** [9.2b] 314 cm^2
19. [9.6b] 0.045 L   **20.** [9.5c] $c = 20$
21. [9.5c] $b = \sqrt{45}$; $b \approx 6.708$ **22.** [9.6a] 160 cm^3
23. [9.6a] 1100 ft^3 **24.** [9.6a] 38,808 yd^3
25. [9.4c] 48°   **26.** [9.4c] 155°   **27.** [9.7c] 25°C
28. [9.7c] 98.6°F

Margin Exercises, Section 9.1, pp. 513–518

1. 2   **2.** 3   **3.** $1\frac{1}{2}$ **4.** $3\frac{1}{4}$ **5.** 288
6. 43.5   **7.** 240,768   **8.** 6   **9.** 8   **10.** 54
11. $11\frac{2}{3}$, or $11.\overline{6}$ **12.** 5   **13.** 31,680   **14.** 23,000
15. 400   **16.** 178   **17.** 9040   **18.** 7.814   **19.** 781.4
20. 8.72   **21.** 8,900,000   **22.** 6.78   **23.** 97.4
24. 0.1   **25.** 8.451   **26.** 90.909   **27.** 804.5
28. 1479.843

Exercise Set 9.1, p. 519

1. 12 **3.** $\frac{1}{12}$ **5.** 5280 **7.** 144 **9.** 7 **11.** $1\frac{1}{2}$
13. 26,400 **15.** 4 **17.** $6\frac{1}{3}$ **19.** 52,800 **21.** $2\frac{1}{2}$
23. 10 **25.** 110 **27.** 2 **29.** 300 **31.** 1
33. (a) 1000; (b) 0.001 **35.** (a) 10; (b) 0.1
37. (a) 0.01; (b) 100 **39.** 6700 **41.** 0.98
43. 8.921 **45.** 0.05666 **47.** 566,600 **49.** 4.77
51. 688 **53.** 0.1 **55.** 100,000 **57.** 142 **59.** 0.82
61. 450 **63.** 0.000024 **65.** 0.688 **67.** 230
69. 6.21 **71.** 35.56 **73.** 104.585 **75.** 100
77. 70.866 **79.** 32.727 **81.** $-\frac{3}{2}$ **82.** -2
83. $101.50 **84.** $44.50 **85.** 47% **86.** 35%
87. ◈ **89.** ◈ **91.** 393,700 **93.** 22.7 mph
95. > **97.** < **99.** >

Margin Exercises, Section 9.2, pp. 524–528

1. 43.8 cm^2 **2.** 12.375 km^2 **3.** 100 m^2
4. 717.5 cm^2 **5.** 9″ **6.** 5 ft **7.** 62.8 m **8.** 15.7 m
9. 220 cm **10.** 34.296 yd **11.** $78\frac{4}{7}$ km^2
12. 339.6 cm^2 **13.** A 12-ft–diameter flower bed is 13.04 ft^2 larger.

Calculator Spotlight, p. 528

1. Answers will vary. **2.** 1417.99 in.; 160,005.91 in^2
3. 1729.27 in^2 **4.** 125,663.71 ft^2

Exercise Set 9.2, p. 529

1. 32 cm^2 **3.** 104 ft^2 **5.** 64 m^2 **7.** 8.05 cm^2
9. 144 mi^2 **11.** $55\frac{1}{8}$ ft^2 **13.** 49 m^2 **15.** 108 cm^2
17. 68 yd^2 **19.** 14 cm **21.** $1\frac{1}{2}$ in. **23.** 16 ft
25. 0.7 cm **27.** 44 cm **29.** $4\frac{5}{7}$ in. **31.** 100.48 ft
33. 4.396 cm **35.** 154 cm^2 **37.** $1\frac{43}{56}$ in^2
39. 803.84 ft^2 **41.** 1.5386 cm^2
43. 2 cm; 6.28 cm; 3.14 cm^2 **45.** 151,976 mi^2
47. 7.85 cm; 4.90625 cm^2 **49.** 15 in.
51. 439.7784 yd **53.** 45.68 ft **55.** 45.7 yd
57. 100.48 m^2 **59.** 6.9972 cm^2 **61.** $\frac{37}{400}$
62. $\frac{7}{8}$ **63.** 137.5% **64.** 66.$\overline{6}$%, or $66\frac{2}{3}$%
65. 125% **66.** 160% **67.** ◈ **69.** ◈
71. 1267 cm^2 **73.** 360,000 **75.** Circumference

Margin Exercises, Section 9.3, pp. 535–536

1. 144 **2.** 1440 **3.** 63 **4.** 2.5 **5.** 3200
6. 1,000,000 **7.** 100 **8.** 28,800 **9.** 0.043
10. 0.678

Exercise Set 9.3, p. 537

1. 36 **3.** 1008 **5.** 3 **7.** 198 **9.** 396 **11.** 12,800
13. $7\frac{2}{3}$ **15.** 5 **17.** $\frac{1}{144}$ **19.** $\frac{1}{640}$ **21.** 17,000,000
23. 63,100 **25.** 23.456 **27.** 0.0349 **29.** 2500
31. 0.4728 **33.** 2 ft^2 **35.** $4\frac{1}{3}$ ft^2 **37.** 21 cm^2
39. $17.50 **40.** $6.75 **41.** $8.78 **42.** $35.51
43. ◈ **45.** ◈ **47.** 10.89 **49.** 1.65 **51.** 1852.6 m^2
53. $135.33

Margin Exercises, Section 9.4, pp. 541–544

1. Angle GHI, Angle IHG, Angle H, $\angle GHI$, $\angle IHG$, $\angle H$
2. Angle PQR, Angle RQP, Angle Q, $\angle PQR$, $\angle RQP$, $\angle Q$
3. 126° **4.** 33°
5. Times of Engagement of Married Couples

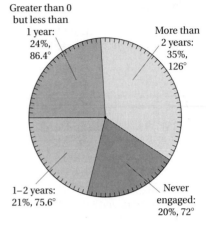

6. Right **7.** Acute **8.** Obtuse **9.** Straight
10. $\angle 1$ and $\angle 2$; $\angle 1$ and $\angle 4$; $\angle 2$ and $\angle 3$; $\angle 3$ and $\angle 4$
11. 45° **12.** 72° **13.** 5°
14. $\angle 1$ and $\angle 2$; $\angle 1$ and $\angle 4$; $\angle 2$ and $\angle 3$; $\angle 3$ and $\angle 4$
15. 142° **16.** 23° **17.** 90°

Exercise Set 9.4, p. 545

1. Angle GHJ, Angle JHG, Angle H, $\angle GHJ$, $\angle JHG$, $\angle H$
3. 10° **5.** 180° **7.** 90°
9. Sporting Goods Purchases

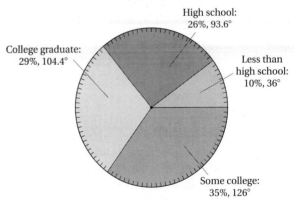

11. Obtuse **13.** Acute **15.** Straight **17.** Right
19. Acute **21.** Obtuse **23.** 79° **25.** 23° **27.** 32°
29. 61° **31.** 177° **33.** 41° **35.** 95° **37.** 78°
39. 0.561 **40.** 67.34% **41.** 2.5 **42.** 112.5%
43. -5.9 **44.** 5.5 **45.** ◈ **47.** ◈
49. $m\angle 1 = 55.93°$; $m\angle 4 = 55.93°$; $m\angle 5 = 42.17°$;
$m\angle 6 = 81.9°$

Margin Exercises, Section 9.5, pp. 547–550

1. 81 **2.** 100 **3.** 121 **4.** 144 **5.** 169 **6.** 196
7. 225 **8.** 256 **9.** $-10, 10$ **10.** $-9, 9$ **11.** $-7, 7$
12. $-14, 14$ **13.** 7 **14.** 4 **15.** 11 **16.** 10 **17.** 9

18. 8 **19.** 15 **20.** 13 **21.** 1 **22.** 0 **23.** 2.236
24. 8.832 **25.** 12.961 **26.** $c = \sqrt{41}$; $c \approx 6.403$
27. $a = \sqrt{75}$; $a \approx 8.660$ **28.** $b = \sqrt{120}$; $b \approx 10.954$
29. $a = \sqrt{175}$; $a \approx 13.229$ **30.** $\sqrt{424}$ ft ≈ 20.6 ft

Calculator Spotlight, p. 548

1. 6.6 **2.** 9.7 **3.** 19.8 **4.** 17.3 **5.** 24.9
6. 24.5 **7.** 121.2 **8.** 115.6 **9.** 16.2 **10.** 85.4

Exercise Set 9.5, p. 551

1. −4, 4 **3.** −11, 11 **5.** −13, 13 **7.** −80, 80 **9.** 7
11. 9 **13.** 15 **15.** 25 **17.** 20 **19.** 100 **21.** 6.928
23. 2.828 **25.** 1.732 **27.** 3.464 **29.** 4.359
31. 10.488 **33.** $c = \sqrt{34}$; $c \approx 5.831$ **35.** $c = \sqrt{98}$;
$c \approx 9.899$ **37.** $a = 5$ **39.** $b = 8$ **41.** $c = 26$
43. $b = 12$ **45.** $b = \sqrt{1023}$; $b \approx 31.984$ **47.** $c = 5$
49. $\sqrt{208}$ ft ≈ 14.4 ft **51.** $\sqrt{16,200}$ ft ≈ 127.3 ft
53. $\sqrt{500}$ ft ≈ 22.4 ft
55. $\sqrt{211,200,000}$ ft $\approx 14,532.7$ ft **57.** $468
58. 12% **59.** 187,200 **60.** 40% **61.** About 324
62. $24.30 **63.** ◈ **65.** ◈
67. The areas are the same.
69. Length: 36.6 in.; width: 20.6 in.

Margin Exercises, Section 9.6, pp. 555–560

1. 12 cm³ **2.** 20 ft³ **3.** 128 ft³ **4.** 785 ft³
5. 67,914 m³ **6.** 904.32 ft³ **7.** $\frac{5632}{2625}$ in³ **8.** 20
9. 32 **10.** mL **11.** mL **12.** L **13.** L **14.** 970
15. 8.99 **16.** $1.08 **17.** $83.7\overline{3}$ mm³

Calculator Spotlight, p. 560

1. 523,598,775.6 m³ **2.** 105.89 cm³

Exercise Set 9.6, p. 561

1. 250 cm³ **3.** 135 in³ **5.** 75 m³ **7.** $357\frac{1}{2}$ yd³
9. 4082 ft³ **11.** 376.8 cm³ **13.** 41,580,000 yd³
15. 4,186,666.$\overline{6}$ in³ **17.** Approximately 124.725 m³
19. $1437\frac{1}{3}$ km³ **21.** 1000; 1000 **23.** 87,000
25. 0.049 **27.** 27,300 **29.** 40 **31.** 320
33. 3 **35.** 32 **37.** 48 **39.** $1\frac{7}{8}$ **41.** 500 mL
43. 16 oz **45.** 56.52 in³ **47.** 4747.68 cm³
49. 646.74 cm³ **51.** 5832 yd³ **53.** 61,600 cm³; 61.6 L
55. $24 **56.** $175 **57.** $10.68 **58.** $\frac{7}{3}$ **59.** −1
60. 448 km **61.** ◈ **63.** ◈ **65.** 9.424779 L
67. 57,480 in³ **69.** 0.331 m³

Margin Exercises, Section 9.7, pp. 565–568

1. 80 **2.** 4.32 **3.** 32,000 **4.** kg **5.** kg **6.** mg
7. g **8.** t **9.** 6200 **10.** 0.0793 **11.** 77 **12.** 234.4
13. −4°C **14.** 85°F **15.** −25°C **16.** 50°F
17. 176°F **18.** 95°F **19.** 35°C **20.** 45°C

Exercise Set 9.7, p. 569

1. 16 **3.** 3 **5.** 48 **7.** 7000 **9.** 2.4 **11.** 4.5
13. 1000 **15.** 0.001 **17.** 0.01 **19.** 1000 **21.** 10
23. 725,000 **25.** 6.345 **27.** 0.000897 **29.** 7320
31. 6.78 **33.** 6.9 **35.** 800,000 **37.** 1000
39. 0.0034 **41.** 80°C **43.** 60°C **45.** 20°C
47. −10°C **49.** 190°F **51.** 140°F **53.** 10°F
55. 40°F **57.** 77°F **59.** 104°F **61.** 5432°F
63. 30°C **65.** 55°C **67.** 37°C **69.** 0.43%
70. 231% **71.** 10
72.

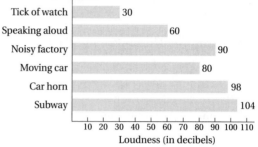

Sound Levels

Whisper	15
Tick of watch	30
Speaking aloud	60
Noisy factory	90
Moving car	80
Car horn	98
Subway	104

Loudness (in decibels)

73. $\frac{22}{5}$ **74.** 2.5 **75.** ◈ **77.** ◈ **79.** 0.0022
81. (a) 200; (b) 3 **83.** 60 g **85.** 8 mL
87. About 5.1 g/cm³

Summary and Review: Chapter 9, p. 573

1. $3\frac{1}{3}$ **2.** 30 **3.** 0.07 **4.** 0.009 **5.** 400,000 **6.** $1\frac{1}{6}$
7. 144 **8.** 0.004 **9.** $13\frac{1}{2}$ **10.** 256 **11.** 0.06
12. 400 **13.** 1600 **14.** 200 **15.** 4700 **16.** 0.04
17. 45 **18.** 700,000 **19.** 7 **20.** 0.057 **21.** 31.4 m
22. $\frac{14}{11}$ in. **23.** 24 m **24.** 18 in² **25.** 29.82 ft²
26. 60 cm² **27.** 35 mm² **28.** 154 ft² **29.** 314 cm²
30. 26.28 ft² **31.** 49° **32.** 136° **33.** $c = \sqrt{850}$;
$c \approx 29.155$ **34.** $b = \sqrt{84}$; $b \approx 9.165$ **35.** $c = \sqrt{89}$ ft;
$c \approx 9.434$ ft **36.** $a = \sqrt{76}$ cm; $a \approx 8.718$ cm
37. 93.6 m³ **38.** 193.2 cm³ **39.** 28,260 ft³
40. 33.49$\overline{3}$ cm³ **41.** 942 cm³ **42.** 95°F
43. 20°C **44.** 15.6 L **45.** $39.04 **46.** 47%
47. 0.567 **48.** −4.5 **49.** 24 mi **50.** 2.5
51. ◈ A square is a parallelogram because it is a
four-sided figure with two pairs of parallel sides.
52. ◈ Since 1 m is slightly more than 1 yd, it follows
that 1 m³ is larger than 1 yd³. Since 1 yd³ = 27 ft³, we
see that 1 m³ is larger than 27 ft³.
53. ◈ Since 1 kg is about 2.2 lb and 32 oz is 32/16, or
2 lb, 1 kg weighs more than 32 oz. **54.** 961.625 cm²
55. 104.875 **56.** 34.375% **57.** $101.25

Test: Chapter 9, p. 577

1. [9.1a] 108 **2.** [9.1b] 2.8 **3.** [9.3a] 18
4. [9.1b] 5000 **5.** [9.1b] 0.87 **6.** [9.3b] 0.00452
7. [9.6b] 3.08 **8.** [9.7b] 3800 **9.** [9.6b] 1280
10. [9.6b] 240 **11.** [9.7a] 64 **12.** [9.7a] 8220

13. [9.2b] 8 cm **14.** [9.2b] 50.24 m² **15.** [9.2b] 88 ft
16. [9.2a] 25 cm² **17.** [9.2b] 33.87 m²
18. [9.2a] 18 ft² **19.** [9.2a] 13 in²
20. [9.4c] 115° **21.** [9.5c] $c = \sqrt{2}$; $c \approx 1.414$
22. [9.5c] $b = \sqrt{51}$; $b \approx 7.141$ **23.** [9.5a] 11
24. [9.6a] 192 cm³ **25.** [9.6a] 628 ft³
26. [9.6a] $4186.\overline{6}$ yd³ **27.** [9.6a] 30 m³
28. [9.6c] 3000 mL **29.** [9.7c] 30°C **30.** [9.7c] 113°F
31. [8.6a] $440 **32.** [8.1b] 93% **33.** [8.1b] 0.932
34. [5.7b] 4 **35.** [7.4a] $13.41
36. [5.7b] 2.5 **37.** [9.4c] 67.5° **38.** [9.6c] $188.40

Cumulative Review: Chapters 1–9, p. 579

1. [4.6a] $10\frac{1}{6}$ **2.** [5.5d] 49.2 **3.** [5.2b] 87.52
4. [2.5a] −1234 **5.** [1.9d] 2 **6.** [1.9c] 1565
7. [5.1b] $-\frac{623}{100}$ **8.** [8.1c] $\frac{21}{10}$ **9.** [4.2c] <
10. [4.2c] > **11.** [9.7a] $\frac{3}{8}$ **12.** [9.7c] 59°F
13. [9.6b] 87 **14.** [9.1a] 90 **15.** [9.3a] 27
16. [9.1b] 0.17 **17.** [2.7c], [3.6b] 52 m; 120 m²
18. [2.7b] $9a - 16$
19. [6.4b]

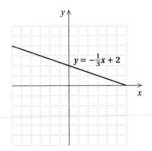

$y = -\frac{1}{3}x + 2$

20. [6.2c] 27.5 lb **21.** [6.2c] 1994 **22.** [7.3b] 14.4
23. [5.7b] 1 **24.** [2.8b], [3.8a] $-\frac{53}{3}$ **25.** [4.3b] $\frac{1}{8}$
26. [1.8a] 7 **27.** [1.8a] 528 million **28.** [6.5a] 58.6
29. [8.6a] $24 **30.** [9.5c] 17 m **31.** [8.5a] 6%
32. [4.6c] $2\frac{1}{8}$ yd **33.** [5.8a] $16.99
34. [7.2b] The 8-qt box **35.** [3.6b] $\frac{7}{20}$ km
36. [9.6c] 272 ft³ **37.** [2.7c] No; the sum of the
perimeters can be measured as 14 ft or 16 ft, or both of
which exceed 108 in.

Chapter 10

Pretest: Chapter 10, p. 582

1. [10.1a] $12x^2 - 2x - 10$
2. [10.1b] $-(6a^3b^2 - 7a^2b - 5)$, $-6a^3b^2 + 7a^2b + 5$
3. [10.1c] $-4x^2 - 17x + 21$ **4.** [10.2a] 57 **5.** [10.4a] 1
6. [10.1d] 48 **7.** [10.2a] $-18a^5b^3$
8. [10.2b] $35x^5 - 20x^3 + 5x^2$ **9.** [10.3a] $a^2 - 3a - 28$
10. [10.3b] $2a^5 - 2a^4 - a^3 + 4a^2 - 3a$
11. [10.2c] $3a(7a^2 + 10a - 4)$ **12.** [10.2c] $5xy(3x - 4y^2)$
13. [10.4b] $\frac{1}{7^2}$; $\frac{1}{49}$ **14.** [10.4b] $\frac{5}{x^3}$ **15.** [10.4b] $\frac{b^5}{a^8c}$
16. [10.4b] $\left(\frac{2}{5}\right)^2$; $\frac{4}{25}$ **17.** [10.4b] x^{-9} **18.** [10.4b] $\frac{1}{a^{11}}$
19. [10.4b] $\frac{-24x^9}{y^5}$

1. $9a^2 + 3a - 1$ **2.** $7x^2y + 3x^2 + 4x + 4$
3. $2a^3 + 2a^2 - 9a + 17$ **4.** $-(12x^4 - 3x^2 + 4x)$;
$-12x^4 + 3x^2 - 4x$ **5.** $-(-4x^4 + 3x^2 - 4x)$;
$4x^4 - 3x^2 + 4x$ **6.** $-\left(-13x^6 + 2x^4 - 3x^2 + x - \frac{5}{13}\right)$;
$13x^6 - 2x^4 + 3x^2 - x + \frac{5}{13}$
7. $-(-8a^3b + 5ab^2 - 2ab)$; $8a^3b - 5ab^2 + 2ab$
8. $-4x^3 + 6x - 3$ **9.** $-5x^3y - 3x^2y^2 + 7xy^3$
10. $-14x^{10} + \frac{1}{2}x^5 - 5x^3 + x^2 - 3x$ **11.** $2x^3 + 2x + 8$
12. $x^2 - 6x - 2$ **13.** $2x^3 + 3x^2 - 4xy - 2$
14. 41; 41 **15.** 132 **16.** 360 ft **17.** 260 ft

Exercise Set 10.1, p. 587

1. $-2x + 10$ **3.** $x^2 - 8x + 2$ **5.** $2x^2$
7. $6t^4 + 4t^3 + 5t^2 - t$ **9.** $9 + 12x^2$
11. $9x^8 + 8x^7 - 3x^4 + 2x^2 - 2x + 5$
13. $14t^4 + 4t^3 - t^2 + 4t - 7$
15. $-5x^4y^3 + 2x^3y^3 + 4x^3y^2 - 4xy^2 - 5xy$
17. $13a^3b^2 + 4a^2b^2 - 4a^2b + 6ab^2$
19. $-0.6a^2bc + 17.5abc^3 - 5.2abc$ **21.** $-(-5x)$; $5x$
23. $-(-x^2 + 10x - 2)$; $x^2 - 10x + 2$
25. $-(12x^4 - 3x^3 + 3)$; $-12x^4 + 3x^3 - 3$ **27.** $-3x + 7$
29. $-4x^2 + 3x - 2$ **31.** $4x^4 - 6x^2 - \frac{3}{4}x + 8$
33. $7x - 1$ **35.** $4t^2 + 6t + 6$ **37.** $-x^2 - 7x + 5$
39. $5a^2 + 5a - 16$ **41.** $6x^4 + 3x^3 - 4x^2 + 3x - 4$
43. $4.6x^3 + 9.2x^2 - 3.8x - 23$ **45.** $\frac{3}{4}x^3 - \frac{1}{2}x$
47. $2x^3y^3 + 8x^2y^2 + 2x^2y + 4xy$ **49.** −18 **51.** 19
53. −12 **55.** 2 **57.** 4 **59.** 11 **61.** About 449
63. 1024 ft **65.** $18,750 **67.** $155,000
69. $\frac{7}{10}$ serving per pound **70.** $3560 **71.** $67.50
72. 26 m² **73.** 1256 cm² **74.** $395 per week
75. ◆ **77.** ◆ **79.** 209 million **81.** $5x^2 - 9x - 1$
83. $2 + x + 2x^2 + 4x^3$ **85.** $8t^4 + 9t^3 - 2t^3 + 2t^2 - 2t^2 + t - 4t - 3 + 7 = 8t^4 + 7t^3 - 3t + 4$

Margin Exercises, Section 10.2,
pp. 591–595

1. $18a^2$ **2.** $-14x^2$ **3.** $48a^2$ **4.** $-5m^2$ **5.** $42ab$
6. a^9 **7.** $8x^{13}$ **8.** $35m^{11}$ **9.** $15a^7b^{12}$ **10.** 7; −19
11. $12x^2 + 20x$ **12.** $6a^3 - 15a^2 + 21a$
13. $8a^5b^2 + 20a^3b^6$ **14.** $6(z - 2)$ **15.** $3(x - 2y + 3)$
16. $2(8a - 18b + 21)$ **17.** $-4(3x - 8y + 4z)$
18. $5a(a^2 + 1)$ **19.** $7x(2x^2 - x + 3)$
20. $3ab(3a - 2b)$

Exercise Set 10.2, p. 597

1. $45a^2$ **3.** $-60x^2$ **5.** $28x^8$ **7.** $-0.02x^{10}$
9. $35x^6y^{12}$ **11.** $12a^8b^8c^2$ **13.** $-24x^{11}$
15. $-3x^2 + 15x$ **17.** $-3x^2 + 3x$ **19.** $x^5 + x^2$
21. $6x^3 - 18x^2 + 3x$ **23.** $12x^3y + 8xy^2$
25. $12a^7b^3 - 9a^4b^3$ **27.** $2(x + 3)$ **29.** $7(a - 3)$
31. $7(2x + 3y)$ **33.** $9(a - 3b + 9)$ **35.** $6(4 - m)$
37. $-8(2 + x - 5y)$ **39.** $3x(x^4 + 1)$ **41.** $a^2(a - 8)$

43. $2x(4x^2 - 3x + 1)$ **45.** $6a^4b^2(2b + 3a)$ **47.** 210 ft
48. 14 mpg   **49.** 17.5 mpg   **50.** $418.95   **51.** 62.5%
52. 37.68 cm   **53.** ◈   **55.** ◈
57. $19a^{437}(37 + 23a^{266})$
59.

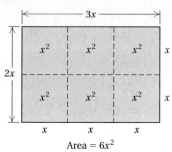

Area = $6x^2$

Margin Exercises, Section 10.3, pp. 599–600

1. $x^2 + 13x + 40$ **2.** $x^2 + x - 20$ **3.** $5x^2 - 17x - 12$
4. $6x^2 - 19x + 15$ **5.** $x^2 + 8x + 15$
6. $x^2 - 11x + 24$ **7.** $x^4 + 3x^3 + x^2 + 15x - 20$
8. $6y^5 - 20y^3 + 15y^2 + 14y - 35$
9. $3x^3 + 13x^2 - 6x + 20$

Exercise Set 10.3, p. 601

1. $x^2 + 9x + 14$ **3.** $x^2 + 3x - 10$ **5.** $x^2 + 8x + 15$
7. $x^2 - 10x + 21$ **9.** $x^2 - 36$ **11.** $18 + 12x + 2x^2$
13. $9x^2 - 24x + 16$ **15.** $x^2 - \frac{21}{10}x - 1$ **17.** $x^3 - 1$
19. $4x^3 + 14x^2 + 8x + 1$
21. $3y^4 - 6y^3 - 7y^2 + 18y - 6$ **23.** $x^6 + 2x^5 - x^3$
25. $6t^4 + t^3 - 16t^2 - 7t + 4$ **27.** $x^9 - x^5 + 2x^3 - x$
29. 912 m^2 **30.** $123,000   **31.** $133\frac{1}{3}$%, or 133.$\overline{3}$%
32. 26   **33.** 68.5%   **34.** 154 ft^2 **35.** ◈   **37.** ◈
39. $2x^2 - 3x + 22$
41. (a) $4m + 20$; (b) $m^2 + 10m + 25$
43. $V = 4x^3 - 48x^2 + 144x$; $S = -4x^2 + 144$
45. $81x^2 + 72x + 16$

Margin Exercises, Section 10.4, pp. 603–606

1. 1   **2.** 6   **3.** 1   **4.** -3 **5.** 1   **6.** $\frac{1}{4^3}$; $\frac{1}{64}$
7. $\frac{1}{5^2}$; $\frac{1}{25}$ **8.** $\frac{1}{2^4}$; $\frac{1}{16}$ **9.** $\frac{1}{(-2)^3}$; $\frac{1}{-8}$ **10.** $\left(\frac{3}{5}\right)^2$; $\frac{9}{25}$
11. 9^{-2} **12.** $7x^{-4}$ **13.** m^3n^5 **14.** abc **15.** a^4b^6
16. x^7yz^4 **17.** $\frac{a^4c^3}{b^7}$ **18.** 5^2, or 25   **19.** $\frac{1}{x^7}$
20. $20x^9y^6$ **21.** $\frac{b^3}{a^7}$

Calculator Spotlight, p. 606

1. 4.21399177; 4.21399177   **2.** 4.768371582; 4.768371582
3. -0.2097152; -0.2097152
4. -0.0484002582; -0.0484002582 **5.** 2.0736; 2.0736
6. 0.4932701843; 0.4932701843

Exercise Set 10.4, p. 607

1. 1   **3.** 1   **5.** -19.57 **7.** 1   **9.** 1   **11.** 1
13. 17   **15.** 1   **17.** 7   **19.** 5   **21.** 2   **23.** $\frac{1}{3^2}$; $\frac{1}{9}$
25. $\frac{1}{10^4}$; $\frac{1}{10,000}$ **27.** $\frac{1}{a^3}$ **29.** $\frac{1}{(-5)^2}$; $\frac{1}{25}$ **31.** $\frac{3}{x^7}$
33. xy^4 **35.** a^3b^4 **37.** $\frac{-7}{a^9}$ **39.** $\frac{25}{4}$
41. $\frac{a^3}{125}$ **43.** 4^{-3} **45.** $9x^{-3}$ **47.** $\frac{1}{x}$ **49.** 1
51. $\frac{1}{x^{13}}$ **53.** $6a^3b^2$ **55.** $-\frac{6y^6}{x^2}$ **57.** $\frac{6c^3}{a^6b^4}$
59. 50 km/h   **60.** 60%   **61.** 87.5%   **62.** 6%
63. 31.4 cm   **64.** 22.5 mpg   **65.** ◈   **67.** ◈
69. $\frac{1}{5}$, or 0.2; $\frac{1}{5}$, or 0.2   **71.** y^{5x} **73.** a^{4t}

Summary and Review: Chapter 10, p. 609

1. $2x - 4$ **2.** $5x^4 - 4x^3 - x - 2$
3. $8a^5 + 12a^3 - a^2 + 4a + 9$
4. $5a^3b^3 + 12a^2b^3 - 7$ **5.** $-(12x^3 - 4x^2 + 9x - 3)$;
$-12x^3 + 4x^2 - 9x + 3$ **6.** -72 **7.** 1   **8.** -42
9. $30x^7$ **10.** $18x^4 - 12x^2 - 3x$ **11.** $14a^7b^4 + 10a^6b^4$
12. $x^2 + 2x - 63$ **13.** $10x^2 - 11x + 3$
14. $a^4 + 2a^3 - 2a^2 - 2a + 1$ **15.** $5x(9x^2 - 2)$
16. $7(a - 5b - 7ac)$ **17.** $3x^2y(2x - 3y^4)$ **18.** $\frac{1}{12^2}$; $\frac{1}{144}$
19. $\frac{8}{a^7}$ **20.** $\frac{z^6}{x^3y^5}$ **21.** $\left(\frac{5}{4}\right)^2$; $\frac{25}{16}$ **22.** x^{-7} **23.** $\frac{1}{x^{17}}$
24. $\frac{15x^9}{y^9}$ **25.** $\frac{2}{15}$ slice per minute; $\frac{15}{2}$ minutes per slice
26. 30% defective; 70% not defective   **27.** $189
28. 346.5 in^2 **29.** ◈ The expression x^{-2} is equivalent
to $1/x^2$. Since x^2 means $x \cdot x$ and a number times itself
is never negative, x^2 can never be negative. Thus, $1/x^2$
and x^{-2} can never represent a negative number.
30. ◈ The student is probably adding the coefficients
and multiplying the exponents, instead of multiplying
the coefficients and adding the exponents.
31. $1,158,057x^{17} + 1,226,352x^{12} - 213,129x^7$
32. $-40x^8$ **33.** $13a^2b^5c^5(3ab^2c - 10c^3 + 4a^2b)$
34. $w^5x^2y^3z^3(x^4yz^2 - w^2xy^4 + wy^2z^3 - wx^5z)$

Test: Chapter 10, p. 611

1. [10.1a] $17a^3 - 5a^2 - a + 7$
2. [10.1b] $-(-9a^4 + 7b^2 - ab + 3)$;
$9a^4 - 7b^2 + ab - 3$ **3.** [10.1c] $4x^4 - x^2 - 13$
4. [10.2a] 193   **5.** [10.4a] 1   **6.** [10.1d] 12.4 m
7. [10.2a] $-10x^6y^8$ **8.** [10.2b] $35a^3 - 20a^2 + 15a$
9. [10.3a] $x^2 + x - 42$ **10.** [10.3b] $2a^3 - 5a^2 + a + 2$
11. [10.2c] $5x^2(7x^4 - 5x + 3)$
12. [10.2c] $3(2ab - 3bc + 4ac)$ **13.** [10.4b] $\frac{1}{5^3}$; $\frac{1}{125}$
14. [10.4b] $\frac{5b^2}{a^3}$ **15.** [10.4b] $\left(\frac{5}{3}\right)^3$; $\frac{125}{27}$

16. [10.4b] $\frac{1}{x^{16}}$　**17.** [10.4b] $\frac{-6a^3}{b^3}$

18. [7.2a] $\frac{5}{3}$ nails per minute; $\frac{3}{5}$ minute per nail

19. [8.4a] 40% satisfied; 60% not satisfied

20. [8.5a] $8500　**21.** [9.2b] 94.2 cm

22. [10.1d] 2.92 L

23. [10.2c], [10.3a], [10.4b] $\dfrac{3a^4}{a^4 - 6a^2 + 9}$

Final Examination, p. 613

1. [1.1e] 6　**2.** [1.1a] 8 thousands + 4 hundreds + 9 ones　**3.** [1.2b] 1018　**4.** [1.2b] 21,085
5. [4.2b] $\frac{9}{26}$　**6.** [4.6a] $8\frac{7}{9}$　**7.** [2.2a] 24
8. [2.2a] -762　**9.** [5.2c] -44.364
10. [10.1a] $10x^5 - x^4 + 2x^3 - 3x^2 + 2$
11. [1.3d] 243　**12.** [2.7b] $-19x$　**13.** [4.3a] $-\frac{19}{40}$
14. [4.6b] $2\frac{17}{24}$　**15.** [5.2b] 19.9973
16. [10.1c] $2x^3 + 5x^2 + 7x$　**17.** [10.1c] $-4a^2b + 7ab$
18. [1.5b] 4752　**19.** [2.4a] $-74,337$　**20.** [4.7a] $4\frac{7}{12}$
21. [3.6a] $-\frac{6}{5}$　**22.** [3.6a] 10　**23.** [5.3a] 259.084
24. [2.7a] $24x - 15$　**25.** [10.2a] $27a^8b^3$
26. [10.2b] $21x^5 - 14x^3 + 56x^2$
27. [10.3a] $x^2 - 5x - 14$
28. [10.3b] $a^3 - 2a^2 - 11a + 12$　**29.** [1.6c] 573
30. [1.6c] 56 R 10　**31.** [3.7b] $-\frac{3}{2}$　**32.** [4.7b] $\frac{7}{90}$
33. [5.4a] 39　**34.** [4.5c] $56\frac{5}{17}$　**35.** [1.9c] 75
36. [1.9c], [2.1c] -2　**37.** [1.9a] 17^4　**38.** [1.4a] 68,000
39. [5.5b] 21.84　**40.** [3.1b] Yes　**41.** [3.2a] 1, 3, 5, 15
42. [4.1a] 105　**43.** [3.5b] $\frac{7}{10}$　**44.** [3.5b] $-\frac{58}{3}$
45. [4.5b] $-3\frac{3}{5}$　**46.** [2.1b] $>$　**47.** [4.2c] $<$
48. [5.1d] 1.001　**49.** [2.6a] 29　**50.** [10.2c] $5(8 - t)$
51. [10.2c] $3a(6a^2 - 5a + 2)$　**52.** [3.3b] $\frac{3}{5}$
53. [5.1c] 0.037　**54.** [5.5a] -0.52　**55.** [5.5a] $0.\overline{8}$
56. [8.1b] 0.07　**57.** [5.1b] $\frac{671}{100}$　**58.** [4.5a] $-\frac{29}{4}$
59. [8.1c] $\frac{2}{5}$　**60.** [8.1c] 85%　**61.** [8.1b] 150%
62. [5.6a] 13.6　**63.** [2.8a] 555　**64.** [5.7a] 64
65. [3.8a] $\frac{5}{4}$　**66.** [7.3b] $\frac{153}{2}$　**67.** [4.4a] 5
68. [5.7b] $-\frac{2}{5}$　**69.** [6.5a] $23.75　**70.** [1.8a] 65 min
71. [4.6c] $25\frac{3}{4}$　**72.** [5.8a] 485.9 mi
73. [1.8a] $24,000　**74.** [1.8a] $595　**75.** [3.4c] $\frac{3}{10}$ km
76. [5.8a] $84.96　**77.** [7.4a] 13 gal　**78.** [7.2b] $17\frac{\cancel{c}}{oz}$
79. [8.6a] $240　**80.** [8.5b] 7%　**81.** [8.4b] 30,160
82. [5.8a] 220 mi　**83.** [1.9b] 324　**84.** [10.4a] 1
85. [9.5a] 11　**86.** [10.4b] $\frac{1}{4^3}$; $\frac{1}{64}$　**87.** [10.4b] $\left(\frac{4}{5}\right)^2$; $\frac{16}{25}$
88. [6.2c] 85+; 8 fatalities per 100 million vehicle miles traveled　**89.** [6.2c] 1 fatality per 100 million vehicle miles traveled　**90.** [6.5a, b, c] Mean: $28\frac{2}{7}$; median: 26; mode: 20　**91.** [6.6b] $\frac{3}{20}$
92. [6.3a]

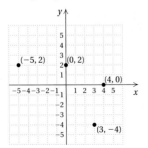

93. [6.4b]

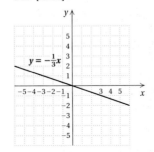

94. [7.5a] $x = 16$, $y = 14$　**95.** [9.1a] 12　**96.** [9.1b] 428
97. [9.1b] 3700　**98.** [9.7b] 20　**99.** [9.7a] 160
100. [9.7b] 0.08　**101.** [9.6b] 8.19　**102.** [9.6b] 5
103. [2.7c] 88 in.　**104.** [9.2a] 61.6 cm^2
105. [3.6b] 25 in^2　**106.** [9.2a] 128.65 yd^2
107. [5.8a] 25.75 m^2　**108.** [9.2b] Diameter: 20.8 in.; circumference: 65.312 in.; area: 339.6224 in^2
109. [9.6a] 52.9 m^3　**110.** [9.6a] 803.84 ft^3
111. [9.6a] $267.94\overline{6}$ mi^3　**112.** [9.5c] $\sqrt{85}$ ft; 9.220 ft

Developmental Units

Margin Exercises, Section A, pp. 620–624

1. 9　**2.** 7　**3.** 14　**4.** 16　**5.** 16　**6.** 16　**7.** 8
8. 8　**9.** 7　**10.** 46　**11.** 13　**12.** 58
13.

+	1	2	3	4	5
1	2	3	4	5	6
2	3	4	5	6	7
3	4	5	6	7	8
4	5	6	7	8	9
5	6	7	8	9	10

14.

+	6	5	7	4	9
7	13	12	14	11	16
9	15	14	16	13	18
5	11	10	12	9	14
8	14	13	15	12	17
4	10	9	11	8	13

15. 16　**16.** 9　**17.** 11　**18.** 15　**19.** 59　**20.** 549
21. 9979　**22.** 5496　**23.** 56　**24.** 85　**25.** 829
26. 1026　**27.** 12,698　**28.** 13,661　**29.** 71,328

Exercise Set A, p. 625

1. 17　**2.** 15　**3.** 13　**4.** 14　**5.** 12　**6.** 11　**7.** 17
8. 16　**9.** 12　**10.** 10　**11.** 10　**12.** 11　**13.** 7
14. 7　**15.** 11　**16.** 0　**17.** 3　**18.** 18　**19.** 14
20. 10　**21.** 4　**22.** 14　**23.** 11　**24.** 15　**25.** 16
26. 9　**27.** 13　**28.** 14　**29.** 11　**30.** 7　**31.** 13
32. 14　**33.** 12　**34.** 6　**35.** 10　**36.** 12　**37.** 10
38. 8　**39.** 2　**40.** 9　**41.** 13　**42.** 8　**43.** 10
44. 9　**45.** 10　**46.** 6　**47.** 13　**48.** 9　**49.** 8
50. 11　**51.** 12　**52.** 13　**53.** 10　**54.** 12　**55.** 17
56. 13　**57.** 10　**58.** 16　**59.** 16　**60.** 15　**61.** 39
62. 89　**63.** 87　**64.** 999　**65.** 900　**66.** 868
67. 999　**68.** 848　**69.** 877　**70.** 17,680　**71.** 10,873
72. 4699　**73.** 10,867　**74.** 9895　**75.** 3998
76. 18,222　**77.** 16,889　**78.** 64,489　**79.** 99,999
80. 77,777　**81.** 46　**82.** 26　**83.** 55　**84.** 101
85. 1643　**86.** 1412　**87.** 846　**88.** 628　**89.** 1204

90. 607   91. 10,000   92. 1010   93. 1110   94. 1227
95. 1111   96. 1717   97. 10,138   98. 6554   99. 6111
100. 8427   101. 9890   102. 11,612   103. 11,125
104. 15,543   105. 16,774   106. 68,675   107. 34,437
108. 166,444   109. 101,315   110. 49,449

Margin Exercises, Section S, pp. 627–632

1. 4   2. 7   3. 8   4. 3   5. $12 - 8 = 4$; $12 - 4 = 8$
6. $13 - 6 = 7$; $13 - 7 = 6$ 7. 8   8. 7   9. 9   10. 4
11. 14   12. 20   13. 241   14. 2025   15. 17   16. 36
17. 454   18. 250   19. 376   20. 245   21. 2557
22. 3674   23. 8   24. 6   25. 30   26. 90   27. 500
28. 900   29. 538   30. 677   31. 42   32. 224
33. 138   34. 44   35. 2768   36. 1197   37. 1246
38. 4728

Exercise Set S, p. 633

1. 7   2. 0   3. 0   4. 5   5. 3   6. 8   7. 8   8. 6
9. 7   10. 3   11. 7   12. 9   13. 6   14. 6   15. 2
16. 4   17. 3   18. 2   19. 0   20. 3   21. 1   22. 1
23. 7   24. 0   25. 4   26. 4   27. 5   28. 4   29. 4
30. 5   31. 9   32. 9   33. 7   34. 9   35. 6   36. 6
37. 2   38. 6   39. 7   40. 8   41. 33   42. 21
43. 247   44. 193   45. 500   46. 654   47. 202
48. 617   49. 288   50. 1220   51. 2231   52. 4126
53. 3764   54. 1691   55. 1226   56. 99,998   57. 10
58. 10,101   59. 11,043   60. 11,111   61. 65   62. 29
63. 8   64. 9   65. 308   66. 126   67. 617   68. 214
69. 89   70. 4402   71. 3555   72. 5889   73. 2387
74. 3649   75. 3832   76. 8144   77. 7750
78. 10,445   79. 33,793   80. 281   81. 455   82. 571
83. 6148   84. 2200   85. 2113   86. 3748   87. 5206
88. 1459   89. 305   90. 4455

Margin Exercises, Section M, pp. 635–640

1. 56   2. 36   3. 28   4. 42   5. 0   6. 0   7. 8
8. 23

9.

×	2	3	4	5
2	4	6	8	10
3	6	9	12	15
4	8	12	16	20
5	10	15	20	25
6	12	18	24	30

10.

×	6	7	8	9
5	30	35	40	45
6	36	42	48	54
7	42	49	56	63
8	48	56	64	72
9	54	63	72	81

11. 70   12. 450   13. 2730   14. 100   15. 1000
16. 560   17. 360   18. 700   19. 2300   20. 72,300
21. 10,000   22. 100,000   23. 5600   24. 1600
25. 9000   26. 852,000   27. 10,000   28. 12,000
29. 72,000   30. 54,000   31. 5600   32. 56,000
33. 18,000   34. 28   35. 116   36. 148   37. 4938
38. 6740   39. 116   40. 148   41. 4938   42. 6740
43. 5968   44. 59,680   45. 596,800

Exercise Set M, p. 641

1. 12   2. 0   3. 7   4. 0   5. 10   6. 30   7. 10
8. 63   9. 54   10. 12   11. 0   12. 72   13. 8   14. 0
15. 28   16. 24   17. 45   18. 18   19. 0   20. 35
21. 45   22. 40   23. 0   24. 16   25. 25   26. 81
27. 1   28. 0   29. 4   30. 36   31. 8   32. 0
33. 27   34. 18   35. 0   36. 10   37. 48   38. 54
39. 0   40. 72   41. 15   42. 8   43. 9   44. 2
45. 32   46. 6   47. 15   48. 6   49. 8   50. 20
51. 20   52. 16   53. 10   54. 0   55. 80   56. 70
57. 160   58. 210   59. 450   60. 780   61. 560
62. 360   63. 800   64. 300   65. 900   66. 1000
67. 345,700   68. 1200   69. 4900   70. 4000
71. 10,000   72. 7000   73. 9000   74. 2000
75. 457,000   76. 6,769,000   77. 18,000   78. 20,000
79. 48,000   80. 16,000   81. 6000   82. 1,000,000
83. 1200   84. 200   85. 4000   86. 2500   87. 12,000
88. 6000   89. 63,000   90. 120,000   91. 800,000
92. 120,000   93. 16,000,000   94. 80,000   95. 147
96. 444   97. 2965   98. 4872   99. 6293   100. 3460
101. 16,236   102. 13,508   103. 87,554   104. 195,384
105. 3480   106. 2790   107. 3360   108. 7020
109. 20,760   110. 10,680   111. 358,800   112. 109,800
113. 583,800   114. 299,700   115. 11,346,000
116. 23,390,000   117. 61,092,000   118. 73,032,000

Margin Exercises, Section D, pp. 643–650

1. 4   2. 8   3. 9   4. 3   5. $12 \div 2 = 6$; $12 \div 6 = 2$
6. $42 \div 6 = 7$; $42 \div 7 = 6$ 7. 7   8. 9   9. 8   10. 9
11. 6   12. 13   13. 1   14. 2   15. Not defined
16. 0   17. Not defined   18. Not defined   19. 10
20. Not defined   21. 0   22. 1   23. 1   24. 1
25. 1   26. 17   27. 1   28. 75 R 4   29. 23 R 11
30. 969 R 6   31. 47 R 4   32. 96 R 1   33. 1263 R 5
34. 324   35. 417 R 5   36. 37 R 8   37. 23 R 17

Exercise Set D, p. 651

1. 3   2. 8   3. 4   4. 1   5. 32   6. 9   7. 7   8. 5
9. 37   10. 5   11. 9   12. 4   13. 6   14. 9   15. 5
16. 8   17. 9   18. 6   19. 3   20. 2   21. 9   22. 2
23. 3   24. 7   25. 8   26. 4   27. 7   28. 2   29. 3
30. 6   31. 1   32. 4   33. 6   34. 3   35. 7   36. 9
37. 0   38. Not defined   39. Not defined   40. 7
41. 8   42. 7   43. 1   44. 5   45. 0   46. 0   47. 3
48. 1   49. 4   50. 7   51. 1   52. 6   53. 1   54. 5
55. 2   56. 8   57. 0   58. 0   59. 8   60. 3   61. 4
62. Not defined   63. 4   64. 1   65. 69 R 1
66. 199 R 1   67. 92 R 1   68. 138 R 3   69. 1723 R 4
70. 2925   71. 864 R 1   72. 522 R 3   73. 527 R 2
74. 2897   75. 43 R 15   76. 32 R 27   77. 47 R 12
78. 42 R 9   79. 91 R 22   80. 52 R 13   81. 29
82. 55 R 2   83. 228 R 22   84. 20 R 379   85. 21
86. 118   87. 91 R 1   88. 321 R 2   89. 964 R 3
90. 679 R 5   91. 1328 R 2   92. 27 R 8   93. 23
94. 321 R 18   95. 224 R 10   96. 27 R 60   97. 22 R 85
98. 49 R 46   99. 383 R 91   100. 74 R 440

Index

Negative integers, 85
  as exponents, 604, 609
Negative mixed numerals, 247
Negative numbers on a calculator, 86
Nine, divisibility by, 148
Notation
  decimal, 275
  expanded, 3
  exponential, 73
  fractional, 159
  percent, 455
  ratio, 419
  standard, for numbers, 3
Number line, 27
  addition on, 93
  order on, 87
Numbers
  composite, 154
  digits, 5
  equivalent, 171
  even, 147
  expanded notation, 3
  factoring, 153
  integers, 85
  natural, 3
  negative, on a calculator, 86
  periods, 4
  place-value, 4, 5, 275
  prime, 154
  rational, 275
  standard notation, 3
  whole, 3
  word names for, 4, 275
Numerals, mixed, 237. *See also*
    Mixed numerals.
Numerator, 159

O

Obtuse angle, 543
One
  division by, 162, 199, 645
  as an exponent, 593
  fractional notation for, 161, 199
  multiplying by, 171, 214, 224, 514,
    516, 518, 535, 558, 559, 565,
    636
Ones period, 5
Operations, order of, 74, 112
Opposite, 85, 88
  of a polynomial, 584
  and subtracting, 97, 585
Order
  of addition, *see* Commutative law
    of addition
  in decimal notation, 279
  descending, 584
  in fractional notation, 216
  of multiplication, *see* Commutative
    law of multiplication

on the number line, 87
of operations, 74, 112, 303
    and calculators, 75
of whole numbers, 30
Ordered pair, 375
  as the solution of an equation, 377
Origin, 375
Original price, 490, 505
Ounce, 557, 565

P

Parallelogram, 382, 523
  area, 523, 528, 573
Parentheses
  in multiplication, 33
  within parentheses, 76
Partial quotient, 647
Percent, *see* Percent notation
Percent key on a calculator, 492
Percent of decrease, 480–482
Percent of increase, 480–482
Percent notation, 455
  converting
      from/to decimal notation,
        456, 457
      from/to fractional notation,
        458–460
  solving problems involving,
    467–470, 473–476
Percent symbol, 456
Perimeter, 10, 125
  of a rectangle, 125, 137
  of a square, 126, 137
Periods in word names, 4
Pi (π), 337, 526, 534
  on a calculator, 314, 528
Picture graphs, 355
Pictographs, 355
Pie chart, 160, 455, 542
Pint, 557
Pixels, 39
Place-value, 4, 5, 275
Plane, 375
Plotting points, 375
Points, 375
Polygon, 125
Polynomials, 583
  addition of, 583
  additive inverse, 584
  applications, 581, 586, 590, 611, 612
  binomial, 593
  descending order, 584
  evaluating, 586
  factoring, 594
  monomials, 583
  multiplication of, 591–594, 599, 600
  opposite of, 584
  subtraction, 585

terms, 583
trinomial, 600
Positive integers, 85
Pound, 565
Power, 73
  of an integer, 107
Predictions, 399
Price
  marked, 490
  original, 490, 505
  purchase, 487
  sale, 490, 505
  total, 487
  unit, 424
Primary principle of probability, 402
Prime factorization, 155
  in finding LCMs, 208
Prime number, 154
Prime, relatively, 158
Principal, 497
Principles
  addition, 131, 231, 265
  multiplication, 195, 199, 231, 265
Probability, 401
  primary principle of, 402
Problem solving, 61. *See also* Applied
    problems, Index of
    Applications.
Product rule, 592, 609
Products, 33, 635
  cross, 429
  estimating, 38, 319
Proportional, 429
Proportions, 429
  and geometric figures, 441
  and similar triangles, 439
  solving, 430–432, 442
  used in solving percent problems,
    467–470
Protractor, 541
Purchase price, 487
Pythagoras, 550
Pythagorean equation, 548, 573
Pythagorean theorem, 548

Q

Quadrants, 377
Quart, 557
Quotient, 43
  estimating, 319
  as a mixed numeral, 240
  partial, 647
  zeros in, 49

R

Radical sign ($\sqrt{}$), 547
Radius, 337, 525, 573

Index of Applications